Surgery
of the Knee

Section Editors

W. Norman Scott, MD, FACS
Clinical Professor
Department of Orthopaedic Surgery
Albert Einstein College of Medicine
Associate Orthopaedic Attending
Lenox Hill Hospital
Director
Insall Scott Kelly Institute for Orthopaedics and Sports
  Medicine
New York, New York

Henry D. Clarke, MD
Assistant Professor of Orthopaedics
Mayo Clinic College of Medicine
Rochester, Minnesota
Senior Associate Consultant
Department of Orthopaedics
Mayo Clinic
Scottsdale, Arizona

Fred D. Cushner, MD
Assistant Clinical Professor
Department of Surgery
Division of Orthopaedic Surgery
Albert Einstein College of Medicine
Attending Orthopaedic Surgeon
Lenox Hill Hospital
Beth Israel Medical Center
Director
Insall Scott Kelly Institute for Orthopaedics and Sports
  Medicine
New York, New York

A. Seth Greenwald, DPhil (Oxon)
Director
Orthopaedic Research and Education
Orthopaedic Research Laboratories
Lutheran Hospital
Cleveland Clinic Health System
Cleveland, Ohio

George J. Haidukewych, MD
Orthopaedic Trauma and Adult Reconstruction
Florida Orthopaedic Institute
Temple Terrace, Florida

Mary I. O'Connor, MD
Chair
Department of Orthopaedic Surgery
Associate Professor
Mayo Clinic College of Medicine
Jacksonville, Florida

Susan Craig Scott, MD
Surgeon
Hand Surgery Service
Hospital for Joint Diseases
New York, New York

Giles R. Scuderi, MD
Assistant Clinical Professor of Orthopaedic Surgery
Albert Einstein College of Medicine
Orthopaedic Surgeon
Lenox Hill Hospital
Director
Insall Scott Kelly Institute for Orthopaedics and Sports
  Medicine
New York, New York

Carl L. Stanitski, MD
Professor of Orthopaedic Surgery and Pediatrics
Medical University of South Carolina
Charleston, South Carolina

INSALL & SCOTT

Surgery *of the* Knee

Fourth Edition

VOLUME 2

W. Norman Scott, MD, FACS
Clinical Professor
Department of Orthopaedic Surgery
Albert Einstein College of Medicine
Associate Orthopaedic Attending
Lenox Hill Hospital
Director
Insall Scott Kelly Institute for Orthopaedics and Sports Medicine
New York, New York

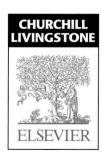

CHURCHILL
LIVINGSTONE

ELSEVIER

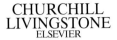

CHURCHILL
LIVINGSTONE
ELSEVIER

1600 John F. Kennedy Blvd.
Ste 1800
Philadelphia, PA 19103-2899

INSALL & SCOTT SURGERY OF THE KNEE

E-dition ISBN-13: 978-0443-06961-1
E-dition ISBN-10: 0443-06961-1
ISBN-13: 978-0-443-6671-1
ISBN-10: 0-443-6671-X
Volume 1: PN 9996000389
Volume 2: PN 9996001342

Copyright © 2006, 2001, 1993, 1984 by Elsevier Inc.

NOTICE

Knowledge and best practice in orthopaedic surgery are constantly changing. As new research and experience broaden our knowledge, changes in practice, treatment, and drug therapy may become necessary or appropriate. Readers are advised to check the most current information provided (i) on procedures featured or (ii) by the manufacturer of each product to be administered, to verify the recommended dose or formula, the method and duration of administration, and contraindications. It is the responsibility of the practitioner, relying on his or her own experience and knowledge of the patient, to make diagnoses, to determine dosages and the best treatment for each individual patient, and to take all appropriate safety precautions. To the fullest extent of the law, neither the publisher nor the editors assume any liability for any injury and/or damage to persons or property arising out of or related to any use of the material contained in this book.

The Publisher

Library of Congress Control Number 2005054901

ISBN-13: 978-0-443-06671-1
ISBN-10: 0-443-06671-X

Publishing Director: Kim Murphy
Developmental Editor: Janice Gaillard
Publishing Services Manager: Tina Rebane
Project Manager: Norm Stellander
Interior Design: Steven Stave
Cover Design: Louis Forgione

Printed in the United States of America

Last digit is the print number: 9 8 7 6 5 4 3 2 1

Dedication

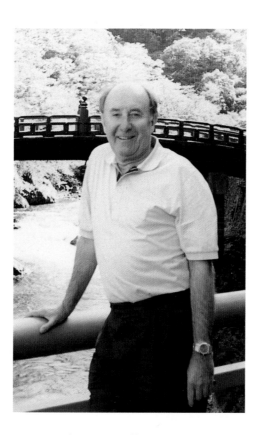

To John N. Insall (1930–2000)

He is greatly missed by all his students and friends,
whose lives have been enriched by his many contributions.

Contributors

Paolo Aglietti, MD
Professor of Orthopaedics and Traumatology, and Director, First Orthopaedic Clinic, University of Florence, Florence, Italy

J. Winslow Alford, MD
Staff Orthopaedic Surgeon, West Bay Orthopaedics, Shoulder and Sports Medicine Division, Warwick, Rhode Island

Annunziato Amendola, MD
Professor, Department of Orthopaedics and Rehabilitation, University of Iowa; Director, University of Iowa Sports Medicine Center, Department of Orthopaedic Surgery, University of Iowa Hospitals and Clinics, Iowa City, Iowa

Jean-Noël A. Argenson, MD
Professor and Chairman of Orthopaedic Surgery, Aix-Marseille University; Service de Chirurgie Orthopedique et de Traumatologie, Hôpitaux de Marseille, Marseille, France

Steven P. Arnoczky, DVM
Professor of Orthopaedic Surgery, College of Human Medicine and College of Orthopaedic Medicine, Michigan State University; Director, Laboratory for Comparative Orthopaedic Research, College of Veterinary Medicine, Michigan State University, East Lansing, Michigan

Bernard R. Bach, Jr., MD
The Claude N. Lambert, MD—Helen S. Thomson Professor, and Director, Division of Sports Medicine, Department of Orthopedic Surgery, Rush University Medical Center, Chicago, Illinois

David Backstein, MD, MEd, FRSC(C)
Assistant Professor of Surgery, and Director of Undergraduate Education, Department of Surgery, University of Toronto, Toronto, Ontario, Canada

Scott A. Banks, PhD
Assistant Professor, Mechanical and Aerospace Engineering, University of Florida, Gainesville; Technical Director, The BioMotion Foundation, West Palm Beach, Florida

Sanjiv Bansal, MD
Attending Orthopedic Surgeon, New York Westchester Square Medical Center and Our Lady of Mercy Medical Center, Bronx, and North Shore University Hospital, Queens, New York

Scott A. Barbour, MD
Founder, Comprehensive Orthopaedic Group, Northside Forsyth Hospital, Cumming, Georgia

Michael Battaglia, MD
Associate Clinical Professor, University of Washington, Seattle, Washington; Associate Clinical Professor, University of California, San Diego, La Jolla, California; Bethesda National Naval Medical Center, Bethesda, Maryland

Todd C. Battaglia, MD, MS
Fellow in Sports Medicine, Department of Orthopaedic Surgery, University of Virginia, Charlottesville, Virginia

Joshua Baumfeld, MD
Orthopaedic Surgery Resident, Mayo Clinic, Rochester, Minnesota; Sports Medicine/Orthopaedic Fellowship, University of Virginia, Charlottesville, Virginia

Christopher P. Beauchamp, MD
Associate Professor, Mayo Clinic Graduate School of Medicine; Chair, Department of Orthopaedics, Mayo Clinic Scottsdale, Scottsdale, Arizona

John A. Bergfeld, MD
Director of Medical Affairs, Cleveland Clinic Sports Health, Department of Orthopaedics, The Cleveland Clinic Foundation, Cleveland, Ohio

Thomas Bernasek, MD
Adult Reconstruction, Florida Orthopaedic Institute, Temple Terrace, Florida

J. David Blaha, MD
Professor, Department of Orthopaedic Surgery, University of Michigan, Ann Arbor, Michigan

Robert B. Bourne, MD, FRCSC
Professor and Chairman, Division of Orthopaedic Surgery, University of Western Ontario; Chief of Orthopaedics, London Health Sciences Centre, London, Ontario, Canada

Marc F. Brassard, MD, MS
Anne Arundel Medical Center, Annapolis, Maryland

K. K. Briggs, MPH
Director of Clinical Research, Steadman Hawkins Research Foundation, Vail, Colorado

Thomas E. Brown, MD
Assistant Professor, Department of Orthopaedic Surgery, and Co-Director, Orthopaedic Surgery Residency Program, University of Virginia, Charlottesville, Virginia

Richard Brull, MD, FRCPC
Lecturer, Department of Anesthesia, University of Toronto; Staff Anesthesiologist, Toronto Western Hospital, University Health Network, Toronto, Ontario, Canada

Joseph A. Buckwalter, MD
Professor and Head, Orthopaedic Surgery and Rehabilitation, Department of Orthopaedics, University of Iowa Hospitals, Iowa City, Iowa

William D. Bugbee, MD
Associate Professor, Department of Orthopaedic Surgery, University of California, San Diego, La Jolla, California

Michael T. Busch, MD
Orthopaedic Surgeon, Department of Pediatric Orthopaedics, Children's Healthcare of Atlanta at Scottish Rite; Surgical Director, Sports Medicine Program, Children's Healthcare of Atlanta, Atlanta, Georgia

David N. M. Caborn, MB, ChB
Professor, Orthopaedic Surgery, University of Louisville; Chief of Sports Medicine, Jewish Hospital, Louisville, Kentucky

John J. Callaghan, MD
The Lawrence and Marilyn Dorr Chair and Professor, University of Iowa Health Care, Iowa City, Iowa

Anikar Chhabra, MD, MS
Canyon Orthopaedic Surgeons, Ltd., Scottsdale, Arizona

Chang Haw Chong, MBBS, FRCS (Ed), FAMS
Consultant, Department of Orthopedic Surgery, Changi General Hospital, Singapore

Charles R. Clark, MD
Dr. Michael Bonfiglio Professor of Orthopaedics and Rehabilitation, and Professor of BioMedical Engineering, University of Iowa; Staff Physician, Department of Orthopaedics, University of Iowa Hospital and Clinics, Iowa City, Iowa

Henry D. Clarke, MD
Assistant Professor of Orthopaedics, Mayo Clinic College of Medicine, Rochester, Minnesota; Senior Associate Consultant, Department of Orthopaedics, Mayo Clinic, Scottsdale, Arizona

Brian J. Cole, MD, MBA
Associate Professor, Departments of Orthopedics and Anatomy and Cell Biology, Rush University; Director, Rush Cartilage Restoration Center, Rush University Medical Center, Chicago, Illinois

John P. Collier, DE
Myron Tribus Professor of Engineering, Senior Lecturer, and Director, Dartmouth Biomedical Engineering Center, Thayer School of Engineering, Dartmouth College, Hanover, New Hampshire

Matthew J. Crawford, DO, PhD
Clinical Instructor, Michigan State University, East Lansing, Michigan

R. Alexander Creighton, MD
Assistant Professor, Department of Orthopaedic Surgery, University of North Carolina at Chapel Hill, Chapel Hill, North Carolina

Pierluigi Cuomo, MD
First Orthopaedic Clinic, and PhD Candidate, University of Florence, Florence, Italy

Fred D. Cushner, MD
Assistant Clinical Professor, Department of Surgery, Division of Orthopaedic Surgery, Albert Einstein College of Medicine, Bronx; Attending Orthopaedic Surgeon, Lenox Hill Hospital and Beth Israel Medical Center; Director, Insall Scott Kelly Institute for Orthopaedics and Sports Medicine, New York, New York

Diane L. Dahm, MD
Assistant Professor of Orthopaedic Surgery, Mayo Clinic College of Medicine; Orthopaedic Surgeon, Mayo Clinic, Rochester, Minnesota

Timothy A. Damron, MD
David G. Murray Professor of Orthopedics, State University of New York Upstate Medical University; Adjunct Professor, Department of Bioengineering and Neuroscience, Syracuse University, and Department of Neuroscience and Physiology, State University of New York Upstate Medical University, Syracuse, New York

A. Lee Dellon, MD, FACS
Professor, Department of Plastic Surgery—Neurosurgery, Johns Hopkins University, Baltimore, Maryland; Professor of Plastic Surgery, Neurosurgery, and Anatomy, University of Arizona; and Director, Dellon Institute for Peripheral Nerve Surgery, Baltimore, Maryland

Douglas A. Dennis, MD
Adjunct Professor, Department of Biomedical
Engineering, University of Tennessee, Knoxville;
Medical Director, Center for Musculoskeletal
Research, Oak Ridge National Laboratory, Oak Ridge,
Tennessee

Ian D. Dickey, MD
Adjunct Professor of Orthopaedics, University of Maine;
Eastern Maine Medical Center, Cancer Care of Maine,
and Eastern Orthopaedic Oncologist, Bangor, Maine

Todd B. Dietrick, MD
Orthopaedic Surgeon, Congress Medical Associates, Inc.,
Pasadena, California

Anthony M. DiGioia III, MD
Senior Research Scientist and Co-Director, Center for
Medical Robotics and Computer Assisted Surgery,
Carnegie Mellon University; Director, Institute for
Computer Assisted Orthopaedic Surgery, The Western
Pennsylvania Hospital; Orthopaedic Surgeon,
Renaissance Orthopaedics, PC, Pittsburgh,
Pennsylvania

Thomas DiPasquale, DO
Affiliate Assistant Professor, University of South Florida,
Tampa; Associate Director of Orthopaedic Trauma
Service, Tampa General Hospital, Tampa, and Florida
Orthopaedic Institute, Temple Terrace, Florida

Julie A. Dodds, MD
Associate Professor, Michigan State University, East
Lansing, Michigan

Jeffrey B. Driban, MEd, ATC, CSCS
Kinesiology, Temple University, Philadelphia,
Pennsylvania

Zsófia Duska
Physiotherapist, Department of Orthopaedics, Uzsoki
Hospital, Budapest, Hungary

Mark E. Easley, MD
Assistant Professor, Duke University Medical Center;
Consultant, Veterans Administration Medical Center
and Durham Regional Medical Center, Durham, North
Carolina

Thomas H. Eickmann, MD
Orthopedic Surgeon, Centura Avista Adventist Hospital,
Louisville, Colorado

Gregory C. Fanelli, MD
Chief, Arthroscopic Surgery and Sports Medicine,
Geisinger Medical Center, Danville, Pennsylvania

Philip M. Faris, MD
Orthopaedic Surgeon, St. Frances Hospital, Mooresville,
Mooresville, Indiana

Christopher M. Farrell, MD
Fellow, Insall Scott Kelly Institute for Orthopaedics and
Sports Medicine, New York, New York

Thomas K. Fehring, MD
Attending Surgeon, OrthoCarolina Hip and Knee Center,
Charlotte, North Carolina

John M. Flynn, MD
Associate Chief of Orthopaedic Surgery and Associate
Professor of Orthopaedic Surgery, University of
Pennsylvania School of Medicine; Associate Chief of
Orthopaedic Surgery and Associate Orthopaedic
Surgeon, Children's Hospital of Philadelphia,
Philadelphia, Pennsylvania

Lynanne J. Foster, MD
Assistant Professor, Department of Orthopaedics,
University of Texas Health Sciences Center at Houston
Medical School, Houston, Texas

Andrew G. Franks, Jr., MD, FACP
Clinical Professor, New York University School of
Medicine; Attending Physician, Tisch Hospital, The
University Hospital of New York University, New
York, New York

Marc J. Friedman, MD
Assistant Clinical Professor, University of California, Los
Angeles, School of Medicine, Los Angeles; Attending
Surgeon, Southern California Orthopedic Institute,
Van Nuys, California

Richard J. Friedman, MD, FRCSC
Clinical Professor of Orthopaedic Surgery, Medical
University of South Carolina; Medical Director,
Charleston Orthopaedic Associates, Charleston, South
Carolina

Wolfgang Fitz, MD
Clinical Instructor, Orthopaedic Surgery, Harvard
Medical School; Associate Surgeon, Department of
Orthopaedic Surgery, Brigham and Women's Hospital,
Falkner Hospital, and New England Baptist Hospital,
Boston, Massachusetts

Freddie H. Fu, MD
David Silver Professor and Chairman of Orthopaedic
Surgery, University of Pittsburgh School of Medicine
and University of Pittsburgh Medical Center,
Pittsburgh, Pennsylvania

John P. Fulkerson, MD
Clinical Professor of Orthopedic Surgery, and Sports
Medicine Fellowship Director, University of
Connecticut, Farmington, Connecticut

John A. Gallagher, MBBS, FAACS
Fellow, University of Western Ontario, and London
Health Sciences Centre, London, Ontario, Canada

Theodore J. Ganley, MD
Assistant Professor of Orthopaedic Surgery, University of Pennsylvania; Attending Surgeon, and Orthopaedic Director of Sports Medicine, Department of Orthopaedic Surgery, Children's Hospital of Philadelphia, Philadelphia, Pennsylvania

Francesco Giron, MD, PhD
Lecturer, University of Florence, and Attending, First Orthopaedic Clinic, University of Florence, Florence, Italy

Vipool K. Goradia, MD
President, Goradia Orthopedics and Sports Medicine, Chester, Virginia

Robert S. Gotlin, DO
Assistant Professor, Rehabilitation Medicine, Albert Einstein College of Medicine, Bronx; Director, Orthopaedic and Sports Rehabilitation, Beth Israel Medical Center, New York, New York

A. Seth Greenwald, DPhil (Oxon)
Director, Orthopaedic Research and Education, Orthopaedic Research Laboratories, Lutheran Hospital, Cleveland Clinic Health System, Cleveland, Ohio

Allan Gross, MD, FRCSC
Bernard I. Ghert Foundation Chair, Lower Extremity Reconstruction Surgery, and Professor of Surgery, Faculty of Medicine, University of Toronto, Toronto, Ontario, Canada

Mahmoud A. Hafez, MD, FRCS Ed
Clinical Research Fellow, Institute for Computer Assisted Orthopaedic Surgery, The Western Pennsylvania Hospital, Pittsburgh, Pennsylvania

George J. Haidukewych, MD
Orthopaedic Trauma and Adult Reconstruction, Florida Orthopaedic Institute, Temple Terrace, Florida

Lázsló Hangody, MD, PhD, DSc
Head, Department of Orthopaedics, Uzsoki Hospital, Budapest, Hungary

Arlen D. Hanssen, MD
Professor of Orthopaedic Surgery, Mayo Clinic College of Medicine; Consultant in Orthopaedic Surgery, Mayo Clinic, Rochester, Minnesota

Melinda K. Harman, DPhil, MSc
Director of Research, The BioMotion Foundation, Palm Beach, Florida

Christopher D. Harner, MD
Professor, Department of Orthopedic Surgery, University of Pittsburgh School of Medicine; UPMC Center for Sports Medicine, Pittsburgh, Pennsylvania

David E. Haynes, MD
Orthopaedic Surgeon, Southwest Sports Medicine and Orthopaedics, Waco, Texas

William L. Healy, MD
Professor of Orthopaedic Surgery, Boston University School of Medicine, Boston; Chairman and Orthopaedic Surgeon, Lahey Clinic, Burlington, Massachusetts

Joseph E. Herrera, DO
Fellow, Orthopaedic Sports and Spine Rehabilitation, Beth Israel Medical Center, New York, New York

Richard Y. Hinton, MD, MPH
Attending, Union Memorial Hospital, Baltimore, Maryland

Aaron A. Hofmann, MD
Professor, Department of Orthopedic Surgery, University of Utah School of Medicine, Salt Lake City, Utah

Ginger E. Holt, MD
Assistant Professor, Division of Musculoskeletal Oncology, Department of Orthopaedic Surgery, Vanderbilt Medical Center, Nashville, Tennessee

Johnny Huard, PhD
Henry J. Mankin Associate Professor, Department of Orthopaedic Surgery, and Associate Professor, Molecular Genetics and Biochemistry and Bioengineering, University of Pittsburgh, School of Medicine; Director, Growth and Development Laboratory, Children's Hospital of Pittsburgh, Pittsburgh, Pennsylvania

David S. Hungerford, MD
Professor of Orthopaedic Surgery, Johns Hopkins University School of Medicine; Attending, Good Samaritan Hospital, Baltimore, Maryland

Marc W. Hungerford, MD
Johns Hopkins University School of Medicine, and Chief, Johns Hopkins Orthopedics at Good Samaritan Hospital, Baltimore, Maryland

Anthony Infante, DO
Clinical Faculty, Michigan State University, East Lansing, Michigan; Orthopaedic Traumatologist, General Orthopaedic Surgery, Tampa General Hospital, Brandon Regional Hospital, Tampa, Florida

John N. Insall, MD*
Formerly Clinical Professor of Orthopaedic Surgery,
Albert Einstein College of Medicine, Bronx; Director,
Insall Scott Kelly Institute for Orthopaedics and
Sports Medicine, Beth Israel Medical Center, New
York, New York

Richard Iorio, MD
Assistant Professor of Orthopaedic Surgery, Boston
University School of Medicine, Boston; Active Staff,
Department of Orthopaedic Surgery, Lahey Clinic,
Burlington, Massachusetts

David J. Jacofsky, MD
Chairman, The CORE Institute, The Center for
Orthopedic Research and Education, Sun City West,
Arizona

Branislav Jaramaz, PhD
Associate Professor, Robotics Institute, Carnegie Mellon
University; Scientific Director, Institute for Computer
Assisted Orthopaedic Surgery, The Western
Pennsylvania Hospital, Pittsburgh, Pennsylvania

James G. Jarvis, MD, FRCS(C)
Associate Professor of Surgery, University of Ottawa;
Chief, Division of Pediatric Orthopaedics, Children's
Hospital of Eastern Ontario, Ottawa, Ontario, Canada

Charles E. Johnston II, MD
Professor, Department of Orthopaedic Surgery,
University of Texas Southwestern Medical School;
Assistant Chief of Staff, Texas Scottish Rite Hospital
for Children, Dallas, Texas

Novák Pál Kaposi, MD
National Institute of Rheumatology and Physiotherapy,
Musculoskeletal Diagnostic Center, Budapest,
Hungary

Anastassios Karistinos, MD
Sports Medicine Fellow, Advanced Orthopaedics and
Sports Medicine, Salt Lake City, Utah; Attending
Physician, Department of Orthopaedic Surgery, Athens
Naval Hospital, Athens, Greece

Craig M. Kessler, MD
Professor of Medicine, Georgetown University Medical
Center, Washington, DC

Harpal S. Khanuja, MD
Assistant Professor, Department of Orthopaedic Surgery,
The Johns Hopkins University School of Medicine;
Attending, Good Samaritan Hospital, Baltimore,
Maryland

Warren King, MD
Team Physician, Oakland Raiders; USA Rugby Partner;
Fellowship Director, Sports Medicine, Palo Alto
Medical Clinic, Palo Alto, California

*Deceased.

John J. Klimkiewicz, MD
Assistant Professor, Department of Orthopaedic Surgery,
Georgetown University Hospital, Washington, DC

Kevin Klingele, MD
Attending Orthopaedic Surgeon, Columbus Children's
Hospital, Columbus, Ohio

Donald M. Knapke, MD
Attending Orthopedic Surgeon, Adult Reconstruction,
William Beaumont Hospital, Royal Oak, Michigan

Mininder S. Kocher, MD, MPH
Assistant Professor of Orthopaedic Surgery, Harvard
Medical School; Associate Director, Division of Sports
Medicine, Children's Hospital, Boston, Massachusetts

Richard D. Komistek, PhD
Professor, Biomedical Engineering, University of
Tennessee, Knoxville; Director, Center for
Musculoskeletal Research, Oak Ridge National
Laboratory, Oak Ridge, Tennessee

Kenneth A. Krackow, MD
Professor and Vice Chairman, Department of
Orthopaedic Surgery, State University of New York at
Buffalo; Clinical Director, Department of Orthopaedic
Surgery, Kaleida Health—Buffalo General Hospital,
Buffalo, New York

John E. Kuhn, MD
Associate Professor, Division of Sports Medicine,
Department of Orthopaedics and Rehabilitation,
Vanderbilt University Medical Center, Nashville,
Tennessee

Amit Lahav, MD
Fellow, Department of Orthopedic Surgery, University of
Utah School of Medicine, Salt Lake City, Utah

Jason E. Lang, MD
Chief Resident, Division of Orthopaedic Surgery, Duke
University Medical Center, Durham, North Carolina

James M. Leone, MD, FRCSC
Instructor of Orthopaedic Surgery, Mayo College of
Medicine, Rochester, Minnesota

Scott M. Lephart, PhD, ATC
Acting Chair, and Associate Professor, Department of
Sports Medicine and Nutrition, University of
Pittsburgh, Pittsburgh, Pennsylvania

Randall J. Lewis, MD
Clinical Professor, Department of Orthopaedic Surgery,
George Washington University Medical Center;
Director, Washington Center for Hip and Knee
Surgery, Washington, DC

Eric M. Lindvall, DO, MS
Orthopaedic Traumatologist, Tampa General Hospital, Tampa, Florida

David R. Lionberger, MD
Clinical Assistant Professor, Department of Orthopedic Surgery, Baylor College of Medicine, Houston; Active Staff, The Methodist Hospital and Twelve Oaks Hospital, Houston; and Active Staff, Bellville General Hospital, Bellville, Texas

Frank Liporace, MD
Attending Physician, Department of Orthopaedics, University of Medicine and Dentistry of New Jersey, Newark, New Jersey

Steve S. Liu, MD
Research Assistant, University of Iowa Health Care, Iowa City, Iowa

T. Thomas Liu, MD, PhD
Orthopaedic Surgery Resident, University of Pittsburgh Medical Center, Pittsburgh, Pennsylvania

Jess H. Lonner, MD
Director, Joint Arthroplasty Fellowship, and Director, Knee Replacement Surgery, Booth Bartolozzi Balderston Orthopaedics, Pennsylvania Hospital, Philadelphia, Pennsylvania

Paul A. Lotke, MD
Professor of Orthopaedic Surgery, University of Pennsylvania School of Medicine; Chief of Implant Service, Hospital of the University of Pennsylvania, Philadelphia, Pennsylvania

Steven Lyons, MD
Adult Reconstruction, Florida Orthopaedic Institute, Temple Terrace, Florida

Mohamed R. Mahfouz, PhD
Co-Director, Center for Musculoskeletal Research, University of Tennessee, Knoxville; Oak Ridge National Laboratory, Oak Ridge, Tennessee

Stephen G. Manifold, MD
Orthopaedic Surgeon, Bayhealth Medical Center, Dover, Delaware

J. Bohannon Mason, MD
Adjunct Professor, Department of Mechanical Engineering, University of North Carolina at Charlotte; Attending Surgeon, OrthoCarolina Hip and Knee Center, Charlotte, North Carolina

Henry Masur, MD
Clinical Professor of Medicine, George Washington University School of Medicine, Washington, DC; Chief, Critical Care Medicine, National Institutes of Health, Bethesda, Maryland

Kevin R. Math, MD
Associate Professor of Clinical Radiology, Albert Einstein College of Medicine, Bronx; Chief of Musculoskeletal Radiology, Beth Israel Medical Center, New York, New York

Leslie S. Matthews, MD, MBA
Assistant Clinical Professor, Johns Hopkins Hospital, and Chief of Orthopaedic Surgery, Union Memorial Hospital, Baltimore, Maryland

James P. McAuley, MD, FRCSC
Associate Clinical Professor, University of Maryland, Baltimore, Maryland; Consultant; Anderson Orthopaedic Clinic and Research Institute, Alexandria, Virginia

David A. McGuire, MD
Clinical Instructor, University of Washington, Seattle, Washington; Affiliate Professor, University of Alaska, Anchorage, Alaska

Nathan M. Melton, DO
Resident, Grandview Hospital, Dayton, Ohio

R. Michael Meneghini, MD
St. Vincent Center for Joint Replacement, Joint Replacement Surgeons of Indiana, Indianapolis, Indiana

Theodore T. Miller, MD
Associate Professor of Radiology, New York University School of Medicine, New York; Chief, Division of Musculoskeletal Imaging, Department of Radiology, North Shore University Hospital–Long Island Jewish Medical Center, Great Neck, New York

Tom Minas, MD, MS
Associate Professor, Harvard Medical School, Boston; Director, Cartilage Repair Center, Brigham and Women's Hospital, Chestnut Hill, Massachusetts

Timothy S. Mologne, MD
Sports Medicine Center, Appleton, Wisconsin

Michael A. Mont, MD
Director, Center for Joint Preservation and Reconstruction, Sinai Hospital of Baltimore, Rubin Institute for Advanced Orthopedics, Baltimore, Maryland

Adam Mor, MD
Research Fellow in Rheumatology, New York University School of Medicine, New York, New York

Edward A. Morra, MSME
Manager, Computational Testing Services, Orthopaedic Research Laboratories, Lutheran Hospital, Cleveland Clinic Health System, Cleveland, Ohio

Kevin J. Mulhall, MD, MCh, FRCSI(TR and Orth)
Fellow, Adult Reconstructive Surgery, Department of Orthopaedic Surgery, University of Virginia, Charlottesville, Virginia

Sandeep Munjal, MCh (Orth), MD
Orthopaedic Attending, Department of Orthopaedics, Physicians' Clinic of Iowa, Cedar Rapids, Iowa

Cass Nakasone, MD
Fellow, University of Southern California, Los Angeles, California

Michael D. Neel, MD
Clinical Assistant Professor in Orthopaedics, University of Tennessee; Adjunct Faculty, Department of Orthopaedics, St. Jude Children's Research Hospital, Memphis, Tennessee

Mary I. O'Connor, MD
Chair, Department of Orthopaedic Surgery, and Associate Professor, Mayo Clinic College of Medicine, Jacksonville, Florida

Mark W. Pagnano, MD
Associate Professor of Orthopaedic Surgery, Mayo College of Medicine; Consultant, Division of Adult Reconstruction, Department of Orthopaedic Surgery, Mayo Clinic, Rochester, Minnesota

Richard D. Parker, MD
Education and Fellowship Director, Cleveland Clinic Sports Health, Department of Orthopaedics, The Cleveland Clinic Foundation, Cleveland, Ohio

Todd A. Parker, MD
Senior Medical Officer, USS Gunston Hall

Lonnie E. Paulos, MD
Partner, Advanced Orthopedics and Sports Medicine, Salt Lake City, Utah

Henrik B. Pedersen, MD
Director of Medical Multimedia, Insall Scott Kelly Institute for Orthopaedics and Sports Medicine, New York, New York

Catherine Petchprapa, MD
Assistant Professor, Department of Radiology, Beth Israel Hospital, New York, New York

Lars Peterson, MD, PhD
Professor, Department of Orthopaedics, University of Goteborg; Clinical Director, Gothenburg Medical Center, Frolunda, Sweden

Russell S. Petrie, MD
Clinical Instructor, Western University Physician Assistant Program, Pomona; Chairman, Department of Orthopedic Surgery, Hoag Memorial Hospital Presbyterian, Newport Beach, California

Pascal Poilvache, MD
Associate Professor, Catholic University of Louvain; Chief, Hip and Knee Reconstruction, Saint-Luc University Hospital, Brussels, Belgium

W.R. Post, MD
Associate Professor, Vice-Chairman, Chief, Section of Sports Medicine and Shoulder Surgery, Department of Orthopedics, West Virginia University School of Medicine, Morgantown, West Virginia

Anthony H. Presutti, MD
Active Staff, Department of Surgery (Privileges in Orthopaedics), Cheshire Medical Center, Dartmouth-Hitchcock Keene, Keene, New Hampshire

Lisa A. Pruitt, PhD
Professor, Department of Mechanical Engineering, University of California, Berkeley, Berkeley, California

Craig S. Radnay, MD, MPH
Orthopaedic Fellow, Insall Scott Kelly Institute for Orthopaedics and Sports Medicine, New York, New York; Fellow, Florida Orthopaedic Institute, Tampa, Florida

Phillip S. Ragland, MD
Center for Joint Preservation and Reconstruction, Rubin Institute for Advanced Orthopedics, Sinai Hospital of Baltimore, Baltimore, Maryland

Robert Lor Randall, MD, FACS
Associate Professor, Department of Orthopaedics, and Director, Sarcoma Services, Huntsman Cancer Institute at the University of Utah and Primary Children's Medical Center, Salt Lake City, Utah

Robert Siskind Reiffel, MD
Attending and Chief Emeritus of Plastic Surgery, and Secretary/Treasurer, Medical Staff, White Plains Hospital, White Plains, New York

Michael D. Ries, MD
Professor of Orthopedic Surgery, Department of Orthopaedic Surgery, and Chief of Arthroplasty, University of California, San Francisco, San Francisco; Professor of Mechanical Engineering, Department of Mechanical Engineering, University of California, Berkeley, Berkeley, California

William G. Rodkey, DVM, Dip ACVS
Director, Basic Science Research and Assistant
 Fellowship Director, Steadman–Hawkins Research
 Foundation; Vice President, Scientific Affairs, ReGen
 Biologics, Inc., Vail, Colorado

Juan J. Rodrigo, MD
Adjunct Professor of Biomedical Engineering, Clemson
 University; Emeritus Professor of Orthopaedics,
 Department of Orthopaedics, University of California,
 Davis, Sacramento, California; Steadman-Hawkins
 Clinic of the Carolinas, Spartanburg, South Carolina

Cecil H. Rorabeck, MD, FRCSC
Professor, University of Western Ontario; Attending
 Orthopaedic Surgeon, Department of Orthopaedic
 Surgery, London Health Sciences Center, London,
 Ontario, Canada

Aaron G. Rosenberg, MD
Professor of Surgery and Director of Adult
 Reconstructive Orthopaedics, Rush University Medical
 Center, Chicago, Illinois

Oleg Safir, MD
Clinical Fellow, University of Toronto and Mount Sinai
 Hospital, Toronto, Ontario, Canada

**Khaled J. Saleh, MD, MSc (Epid),
FRCS(C), FACS**
Division Head and Fellowship Director, Adult
 Reconstruction; Associate Professor, Department of
 Orthopaedic Surgery; and Associate Professor, Health
 Evaluation Sciences, University of Virginia,
 Charlottesville, Virginia

Roy Sanders, MD
Clinical Professor of Orthopaedics, Department of
 Orthopaedic Surgery, University of South Florida;
 Chief, Department of Orthopaedics, Tampa General
 Hospital, Tampa, Florida

Richard D. Scott, MD
Professor of Orthopaedic Surgery, Harvard Medical
 School; Senior Surgeon, Brigham and Women's
 Hospital and New England Baptist Hospital, Boston,
 Massachusetts

Susan Craig Scott, MD
Surgeon, Hand Surgery Service, Hospital for Joint
 Diseases, New York, New York

W. Norman Scott, MD, FACS
Clinical Professor, Department of Orthopaedic
 Surgery, Albert Einstein College of Medicine;
 Associate Orthopaedic Attending, Lenox Hill
 Hospital; Director, Insall Scott Kelly Institute for
 Orthopaedics and Sports Medicine, New York, New
 York

Giles R. Scuderi, MD
Assistant Clinical Professor of Orthopaedic Surgery,
 Albert Einstein College of Medicine, Bronx;
 Orthopaedic Surgeon, Lenox Hill Hospital, and
 Director, Insall Scott Kelly Institute for Orthopaedics
 and Sports Medicine, New York, New York

Jon K. Sekiya, MD
Assistant Professor, Center for Sports Medicine,
 University of Pittsburgh Medical Center, Pittsburgh,
 Pennsylvania

Alison Selleck, MD
Clinic Physician, National Institute of Allergy and
 Infectious Disease, Warren G. Magnuson Clinical
 Center, National Institutes of Health Critical Care
 Medicine Department, Bethesda, Maryland

Krishn M. Sharma, MD
Resident, Orthopaedics, Union Memorial Hospital,
 Baltimore, Maryland

Nigel E. Sharrock, MB, ChB
Clinical Professor, Weill Medical College of Cornell
 University; Senior Scientist and Attending
 Anesthesiologist, Department of Anesthesiology, The
 Hospital for Special Surgery, New York, New York

Stephen G. Silver, MD
Attending, Lenox Hill Hospital, New York, New York;
 Attending, Hackensack Medical Center, Hackensack,
 New Jersey

Carl L. Stanitski, MD
Professor of Orthopaedic Surgery and Pediatrics, Medical
 University of South Carolina, Charleston, South
 Carolina

J. Richard Steadman, MD
Clinical Professor, University of Texas Southwestern
 Medical School, Dallas, Texas; Orthopaedic Surgeon
 and Chairman of the Board, Steadman-Hawkins Clinic
 and Research Foundation, Vail, Colorado

James B. Stiehl, MD
Clinical Associate Professor, Department of Orthopaedic
 Surgery, Medical College of Wisconsin; Staff
 Physician, Columbia St. Mary's Hospital, Milwaukee,
 Wisconsin

Michael J. Stuart, MD
Professor of Orthopaedics, Mayo Clinic College of
 Medicine; Co-Director, Sports Medicine Center, and
 Vice-Chairman, Department of Orthopaedics, Mayo
 Clinic, Rochester, Minnesota

S. David Stulberg, MD
Professor, Clinical Orthopaedic Surgery, Northwestern
University Feinberg School of Medicine; Director,
Section of Joint Reconstruction and Implant Surgery,
Northwestern Memorial Hospital, Northwestern
Orthopaedic Institute, Chicago, Illinois

Charles Buz Swanik, PhD, ATC
University of Delaware, Department of Health,
Nutrition, and Exercise Sciences, Human Performance
Laboratory, Newark, Delaware

Imre Szerb, MD
Assistant Leader of the Department of Orthopaedics,
Uzsoki Hospital, Budapest, Hungary

Kimberly Templeton, MD
Associate Professor of Orthopaedic Surgery and McCann
Professor of Women in Medicine and Science,
University of Kansas School of Medicine, Kansas City,
Kansas

Alfred J. Tria, Jr., MD
Clinical Professor of Orthopaedic Surgery, and Director
of Orthopaedic Fellowship Training, Robert Wood
Johnson Medical School, New Brunswick, New Jersey

Hans K. Uhthoff
Professor Emeritus, Research Associate, Ottawa Hospital,
Ottawa, Ontario, Canada

Anthony S. Unger, MD
Associate Professor, Department of Orthopaedic Surgery,
George Washington University Medical Center;
Director, Washington Center for Hip and Knee
Surgery, Washington, DC

Thomas Parker Vail, MD
Professor of Orthopaedic Surgery and Director of Adult
Reconstructive Surgery, Duke University Medical
Center, Durham, North Carolina

Douglas W. Van Citters, MS
PhD Candidate, Thayer School of Engineering,
Dartmouth College, Hanover, New Hampshire

Nikhil Verma, MD
Assistant Professor, Rush University Medical Center,
Chicago, Illinois

Vincent J. Vigorita, MD
Professor of Pathology and Orthopaedic Surgery,
Department of Pathology and Orthopaedic Surgery,
State University of New York Health Sciences Center
at Brooklyn/Downstate Medical Center, Brooklyn;
Director of Orthopaedic Research, St. Vincent's
Medical Center, New York, New York

Kelly G. Vince, MD
Associate Professor, University of Southern California
Center for Arthritis, Los Angeles, California

James A. Walker, PhD
Sports Science Director, The Orthopaedic Specialty
Hospital, Salt Lake City, Utah

Kurt R. Weiss, MD
Orthopaedic Surgery Resident, University of Pittsburgh
Medical Center, Pittsburgh, Pennsylvania

David R. Whiddon, MD
Bone and Joint/Sports Medicine Institute, Department of
Orthopaedic Surgery, Naval Medical Center,
Portsmouth, Virginia

Leo A. Whiteside, MD
Clinical Professor of Orthopaedic Surgery, St. Louis
University; Orthopaedic Surgeon, St. Joseph Hospital
of Kirkwood, and Director, Biomechanical Research
Foundation, Missouri Bone and Joint Center, St.
Louis, Missouri

Thomas L. Wickiewicz, MD
Professor, Weill Medical College of Cornell University,
and Chief, Sports Medicine and Shoulder Service,
Hospital for Special Surgery, New York, New York

William M. Wind, MD
University Sports Medicine, Buffalo Sports Medicine,
Buffalo, New York

Edward M. Wojtys, MD
Professor, Department of Orthopaedic Surgery, and
Director of Sports Medicine, University of Michigan
Health System, Ann Arbor, Michigan

Syed Furqan Zaidi, MD
Chief Resident of Diagnostic Radiology, Beth Israel
Medical Center, New York, New York

Foreword

In the past two decades knee surgery has progressed from a small specialty in its infancy, with a limited basic science foundation, crude imaging and diagnostic modalities, and rudimentary treatment methods, to a huge field that encompasses many subspecialties, each with its own core of knowledge and literature. The field has been dynamic, and much has been learned over a relatively short time period.

A field that has come into its own deserves a textbook that reflects this arrival: *Insall & Scott Surgery of the Knee* is a comprehensive textbook that fulfills this important role. The scope of this text is broad. The book covers basic science of knee disorders, ligament and tendon disorders and reconstruction, fractures about the knee, pediatric knee disorders, and the practice and biomechanics of knee replacement and its alternatives.

The quality of an undertaking of this magnitude is dependent on the individual contributions of each author. A review of chapter authorship reveals this text is written by masters—and in many cases the fathers—of each topic. Authors provide their best work when the subject is their passion and when the book in which their work is to appear is the standard-bearer for a profession. *Insall & Scott Surgery of the Knee* fulfills both criteria, which helps to explain the exceptional quality of the material.

Textbook editors are challenged to produce a text that stays current in the face of a rapidly evolving specialty.

The editors of this book address this dilemma with an innovative idea: a companion electronic version, to include cutting-edge monthly content updates to complement the book. Illustrating surgical technique in a manner that is useful to the surgeon also is a challenge for textbook editors. The editors of this text surmount the challenge with modern technology: an accompanying digital video disk augments the text and illustrates key operative techniques.

A textbook derives its content, organization, and style from its editors and section editors. This text already has a rich heritage. The late John Insall is widely acknowledged as the father of modern reconstructive knee surgery. Norman Scott has been one of the foremost practitioners and educators in the combined fields of sports medicine of the knee and reconstructive knee surgery for the past two decades. This book, their brainchild, now in its fourth edition, provides a comprehensive, authoritative, dynamic, and innovative text that will be the standard on the subject for today's knee surgeons.

Daniel J. Berry, MD
Professor and Chairman
Department of Orthopaedic Surgery
Mayo Clinic
Rochester, Minnesota

Preface

In 1984, John Insall almost single-handedly wrote the first edition of *Surgery of the Knee*. There were only 24 contributors to that single volume. In 1993, the second edition had 40 contributors and four associate editors and consisted of two volumes. In 2001, we combined efforts (*The Knee*, Mosby, 1994) to enhance the third edition (159 contributors) of *Surgery of the Knee*. Thus in 17 years three editions were published, and now the fourth edition has published less than five years later. This shortened publication time reflects our interest in being current and in using the latest technology and leading experts to inform our readers. In this fourth edition of *Surgery of the Knee*, we have updated basic chapters and introduced new information utilizing text and visual aids (DVDs), and we are inaugurating a new feature, a companion online e-dition: www.scottkneesurgery.com. The e-dition website will include full text search, hyperlinks to PubMed, an image library, and monthly content updates, to minimize the customary complaint of the "perpetual lag" inherent with textbooks in general. Our goal is to create an interactive current environment for all of us students of the diagnosis and treatment of knee disorders.

The fourth edition of *Surgery of the Knee* has 12 sections, 112 chapters, and 191 international contributors. The DVD sections include (1) a classic video recorded in 1994 (Drs. Insall and Scott) detailing "Exposures, Approaches and Soft Tissue Balancing in Knee Arthroplasty"; (2) interactive anatomical and physical examination recordings, which enhance the material presented in Chapters 1, 2, 3, 5, 6, and 7; and (3) three commonly used minimally invasive surgical techniques for knee arthroplasty.

In Section I, Basic Science, Chapters 1 to 5, the core information presented in the third edition is updated. The DVD of the Anatomy Section is interactive with the imaging in Section II, so the reader can see the normal and abnormal findings side by side. Chapter 3, Clinical Examination of the Knee, now, as mentioned, has the added feature of an actual examination on the DVD to enhance the text.

Section III, Biomechanics, has been expanded under the guidance of A. Seth Greenwald, DPhil (Oxon), to include soft issue and implant considerations that are essential to executing surgical decisions.

With the plethora of Internet information available to patients today, it behooves the knee physician to be absolutely familiar with the various nonoperative and operative alternatives for the treatment of articular cartilage and meniscal disorders (Section IV). Dr. Henry Clarke has done a magnificent job in assembling the innovators in the field. The 18 chapters in this section truly capture the basic science, including the potential of gene therapy, biomechanics, and various treatment options, presented in great detail with the most current results. The section is further highlighted by Dr. Clarke's algorithm for clinical management of articular cartilage injuries.

The advances in the treatment of knee ligament injuries since 1984 are, needless to say, overwhelming. The success achieved today in the treatment of ligament injuries would have been unimaginable 25 years ago. As Section Editor of Section V, Ligament Injuries, Dr. Fred Cushner has assembled most of the people associated with these improvements. The foundations for treatments, controversies, and specific techniques are well chronicled throughout this section. Similarly, Section VI, Patellar and Extensor Mechanism Disorders, represents an updated comprehensive review by Dr. Aglietti and surgical chapters by Drs. Fulkerson and Scuderi.

Sections VII and VIII are "must reads" for all knee clinicians. In addition to discussing the normal and abnormal synovium, we have recruited distinguished authors to discuss the application of current topics of concern to both the patient and clinician, e.g., HIV and hepatitis (Chapter 59), anesthesia for knee surgery (Chapter 60), and an understanding of reflex sympathetic dystrophy (Chapter 61). The orthopaedic knee surgeon must have an absolute awareness of the potential problems inherent in the skin about the knee. In Chapter 63, Soft-Tissue Healing, Drs. Susan Scott and Robert Reiffel give us a foundation for avoiding and treating these potential problems.

Section IX focuses on fractures about the knee and has been organized by Dr. George Haidukewych. These fracture experts have covered all the fractures that occur, including the difficult periprosthetic fractures. Treatment modalities are detailed and reflect the current options with the latest equipment.

Section X, Pediatric Knee, has been reinvigorated with the help of Carl Stanitski. We decided to present the orthopaedic pediatric approach, rather than the sole viewpoint of the knee physician who treats pediatric injuries. The section is well organized, comprehensive, and, I believe, an improvement over the third edition of *Surgery of the Knee*.

The largest section in this two-volume edition is Section XI, Joint Replacement and Its Alternatives. Dr. Gil Scuderi has organized this section of the surgical treatment of the arthritic knee, including osteotomy, unicompartment replacement, patellofemoral arthroplasty, total knee replacement, and the more challenging revision surgery. While establishing the indications and contraindications for techniques, he has been careful to include the identification and management of difficult complications, such as infection, bone defects, extensor mechanism disruption, blood management, and thrombophlebitis. The tremendous success achieved in knee arthroplasty has paralleled the improvements in surgical instrumentation. In this section several authors have detailed the current concepts of computer and navigation surgery, a truly exciting recent development. In the aforementioned e-dition version of *Surgery of the Knee*, the first several streaming videos will focus on specific techniques. Thus, these chapters provide an excellent foundation for interpreting the subsequent e-version techniques.

Dr. Mary O'Connor has developed Section XII, Tumors about the Knee, in a concise, clinically rational framework for those physicians who do not necessarily treat many of these difficult problems. Chapters 106 to 112 are well written and are truly outstanding contributions to this text.

Surgery of the Knee is a text that includes audiovisual teaching aids and now a monthly means of communicating current information in a timely audiovisual manner. To me, it's very exciting, and I look forward to integrating the contributions of these authors into a rapidly current technology for the benefit of all our patients.

W. Norman Scott, MD

Acknowledgments

I would like to express my appreciation to Dr. Henrik Pedersen, without whom the DVDs and e-version addition would not have been possible; to Kathleen Lenhardt for doing everything imaginable during the transition; and to Ruth O'Sullivan for being a reservoir of dependability.

Contents

Contents

Surgery
of the Knee

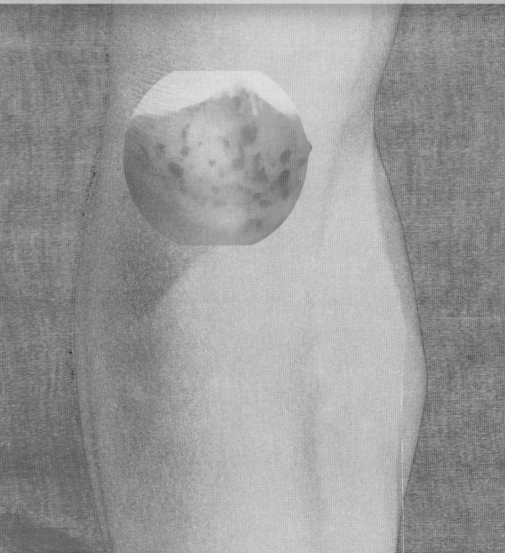

SECTION VII

Miscellaneous Conditions and Treatment

CHAPTER 56

Inflammatory Arthritis of the Knee

Andrew G. Franks, Jr. • *Adam Mor*

In inflammatory arthritis affecting the knee, classic signs of inflammation, such as heat, erythema, swelling, pain, and loss of function, may be variably present and thus suggest an array of diagnostic possibilities. Involvement of the knee may frequently be only part of a more generalized rheumatic disease or systemic illness. The key to successful diagnosis and treatment is a systematic approach to the patient that combines a thoughtful, detailed history, careful physical examination, and proper use and interpretation of all ancillary studies by the orthopedist and rheumatologist. The history should be structured to answer specific questions: Is the problem localized or generalized, symmetric or asymmetric, peripheral or central, and acute or chronic? Do the symptoms suggest inflammation or mechanical damage? Is there evidence of a systemic process? Are associated extra-articular features present? Does the patient have a family history of related problems? After a physical examination and x-ray films, the initial laboratory evaluation should include a complete blood count (CBC); serum chemistries, including liver function, calcium, phosphorus, and uric acid; and urinalysis. Other tests commonly used are the erythrocyte sedimentation rate, C-reactive protein, rheumatoid factor, antinuclear antibodies, and other autoantibodies, some of which correlate with specific diseases (Table 56–1). If the diagnosis continues to remain unclear, additional blood tests, radiographic studies, synovianalysis, and rarely, synovial biopsy or arthroscopy may be required. Synovianalysis is more clinically useful than synovial biopsy, with the exception of the granulomatous diseases and amyloidosis.[34]

DIFFERENTIAL DIAGNOSIS

In the last decade, the evolving etiology and prevalence of various inflammatory disorders affecting the knee include Lyme disease, human immunodeficiency virus (HIV)-associated arthritis, and hepatitis C; thus the physician must maintain a high index of suspicion and not concentrate prematurely on limited diagnostic possibilities (Box 56–1). The popularization of fitness and sports has dramatically increased acute injuries to the knee, and preexisting or concomitant inflammatory disorders of the knee may be pitfalls in accurate diagnosis and treatment. Moreover, as a result of advances in health care, an increasing proportion of the population is older, and not surprisingly, the prevalence of nontraumatic arthritis of the knee has also grown.

Major advances in our understanding of the pathogenesis of the two most common forms of arthritis, rheumatoid arthritis (RA) and osteoarthritis (OA), have occurred over the past decade.[3] The classic distinction between inflammatory and degenerative arthritis is rapidly waning. Current concepts regard OA as a mechanically driven disease mediated by inflammatory factors, unlike RA, which is defined as a primary autoimmune disease. In advanced stages, inflammatory OA can be confused with RA. Depending on the underlying pathophysiology, the inflammation of RA differs from that of OA and has different therapeutic implications. Knowledge of the pathogenesis of articular damage promises to bring highly specific and effective forms of therapy to decrease the inflammation and articular destruction occurring in these diseases. As more detailed information about the causes of the various forms of arthritis is formulated, more precise treatments directed against the specific causes are being developed and the use of nonspecific anti-inflammatory agents is lessening.

RA is the most prevalent chronic, symmetric polyarthritis affecting the younger adult population in the United States. The diagnosis of RA is supported by the presence of rheumatoid nodules over extensor surfaces, detection of rheumatoid factor in serum, x-ray changes consisting of marginal erosion and osteopenia, and inflammatory synovial fluid. OA is the most likely cause of progressive pain in the knees aggravated by weightbearing in the older adult population. It is a heterogeneous group of disorders, each of which leads to varying degrees of articular cartilage loss, destruction of bone, and formation of marginal osteophytes. However, a variety of other conditions can give rise to similar manifestations, and the specific diagnosis requires further laboratory data and radiographic imaging.

Spondyloarthropathies are a group of inflammatory diseases that are common and share several characteristic manifestations, such as sacroiliitis and the presence of HLA-B27. Several of the diseases in this group, including psoriatic arthritis, reactive arthritis, colitis-associated arthritis, and undifferentiated arthritis, have been shown to involve the knee. Lyme disease may cause a monoarticular or polyarticular inflammatory arthritis and may occur without a history of a tick bite, rash, or constitutional symptoms.[43] Although the diagnosis of Lyme disease is often made clinically, serological blood testing should be performed for confirmation of the arthritis, current practice being confirmation of all positive or equivocal enzyme-linked immunosorbent assay results with Western blot analysis.[42] HIV infection may lead to a

Table 56–1. Autoantibodies in Rheumatic Diseases

TYPE OF ANTIBODY	CLINICAL ASSOCIATIONS
Anti-dsDNA	SLE
Anti-histone	Drug-induced lupus
Anti-ENA (Sm and RNP)	SLE and MCTD
Anti-Ro and Anti-La	SLE, neonatal lupus, Sjögren's syndrome
Anti-centromere	Limited systemic sclerosis
Anti-Scl-70 (topoisomerase)	Diffuse systemic sclerosis
Anti-Jo-1	Polymyositis
Anti-CCP	Rheumatoid arthritis

CCP, citrulinated peptide; dsDNA, double-stranded DNA; ENA, extractable nuclear antibody; MCTD, mixed connective tissue disease; RNP, ribonucleoprotein; SLE, systemic lupus erythematosus.

Box 56–1. Inflammatory Causes of Knee Arthritis.

Crystal-Associated Arthritis
Gout
Calcium pyrophosphate disease
Calcium oxalate disease

Infectious Arthritis
Bacterial
Lyme
Mycobacterial
HIV
Viral hepatitis
Other viral diseases

Systemic Diseases Causing Knee Inflammation
Rheumatoid arthritis
Psoriatic arthritis
Reactive arthritis
Colitis-associated arthritis
Undifferentiated spondyloarthropathy
Lupus arthritis
Sarcoidosis
Behçet's disease
Other vasculitis syndromes

wide variety of arthritic syndromes, and appropriate testing should be performed in individuals at risk. In hepatitis C virus–infected patients, polyarthritis with rheumatoid factors may also develop and cause diagnostic confusion with classic RA.[28]

SYNOVIANALYSIS

When acute arthritis occurs without a history of trauma and bacterial infection or crystal-induced arthritis is suspected, arthrocentesis with a 19-gauge needle and synovianalysis performed immediately may guide initial therapy. Alternatively, in patients with more indolent disease in which ancillary studies, including radiographs, blood cultures, and chemical and serological investigations, are

Table 56–2. Normal Synovial Fluid

Volume (knee)	4 mL
Viscosity (string or mucin clot)	High
Color	Colorless/pale yellow
Clarity	Transparent
Total WBC/mm^3	200
Differential WBC count	
PMNs	25%
Lymphocytes	25%
Monocytes	50%
Crystals	None
Protein	2.5 g/dL
Glucose	90% of blood
Culture	Negative

PMN, polymorphonuclear cell; WBC, white blood cell.

unrevealing, synovianalysis may be performed later. Small effusions are analyzed before arthroscopy to avoid bleeding caused by introduction of the arthroscope or dilution with instilled saline and anesthetic. Two circumstances require careful exclusion before synovianalysis, whether by arthrocentesis or arthroscopy, to prevent septic contamination of a sterile joint. Patients with septicemia or with cutaneous or soft-tissue infection mimicking acute arthritis should not be subjected to arthrocentesis to avoid direct introduction of the offending organisms into the joint space.

Normal Synovial Fluid

The normal knee joint contains up to 4 mL of synovial fluid with fewer than 200 white cells per cubic millimeter. In general, small lymphocytes and monocytes predominate, with few, if any, polymorphonuclear cells. This fluid is not simply an ultrafiltrate of plasma as occurs in serous cavities because the synovial lining cells (synoviocytes) produce hyaluronate (mucin), a heavy, asymmetrically branched glycosaminoglycan that significantly alters viscosity as well as composition by diminishing water content and interfering with the permeability of large molecules such as fibrinogen, other clotting factors, and globulins. Therefore, normal synovial fluid has scant volume with few white cells, is highly viscous, does not clot, is transparent, and is colorless or pale yellow. These features are the basis for correct interpretation of synovianalysis of an abnormal knee joint (Table 56–2).

Abnormal Synovial Fluid

Diseases that affect the knee may change the normal characteristics of synovial fluid in a number of ways, thereby allowing distinctions to be made. Grossly increased volume, decreased viscosity, ability to clot, diminished clarity, and change in color all contribute to the interpretation of synovianalysis. Microscopic analysis for the number and type of cells, as well as the presence or absence of crystals, is equally important. The addition of bacteriological, chemical, and immunological tests further enhances the ability to discriminate between the vast number of disorders that may affect the knee. However, the total white blood cell count and identification of bacteria or crystals are considered the most important factors in the majority of diagnostic and therapeutic decisions.[36]

Initial descriptions of abnormal joint fluid were simply divided into those that were noninflammatory and those that were inflammatory. The usefulness of this division was eventually increased by the separation of fluids that were septic and those that were hemorrhagic. Therefore, at the present time, four clinically useful groups of abnormal synovial fluid (Table 56–3) have been defined. Distinction among these groups is based on synovial fluid volume, viscosity (hyaluronate), clarity, color, cellularity (amount and type), and culture. Further subdivision, particularly within inflammatory noninfectious (group II) synovial fluid, has recently been suggested.

Technique of Synovianalysis

Inadequate or improper technique in performing synovianalysis has been responsible for misinterpretation, sometimes diminishing its importance in assessing joint disease. It is often more informative than performing just a synovial biopsy.[36] Unfortunately, there are more pitfalls in its collection and preparation than with other body fluids, and many clinical and hospital laboratories are not thoroughly familiar with the preferred techniques.[12] Therefore, it becomes the responsibility of the physician who performs synovianalysis to become adept in this area, whether performing the tests personally or documenting the correct handling of specimens sent to the laboratory. Although a complete review of specific techniques is beyond the scope of this chapter, some general guidelines are suggested. The reader is referred to detailed descriptions of this subject in the references.

When profuse amounts of extraneous blood are caused by introduction of the needle or arthroscope, the validity of synovianalysis is questionable. However, in situations in which smaller numbers of red blood cells may interfere with white blood cell counts, lysing the red blood cells may be helpful (see later). Once synovial fluid is obtained, approximately 10 to 15 mL is sufficient for complete synovianalysis, although basic studies such as cell count and culture can be performed with smaller amounts.

The fluid is obtained in a sterile syringe and should be gently shaken. Any needle should be removed from the syringe, and then the fluid should be immediately separated as follows:

1. Sterile tube with sodium heparin (green-topped tubes in many laboratories, if sterile): 3 to 5 mL for stains and cultures, including aerobic, anaerobic, tubercular, and fungal vials and direct inoculation onto chocolate agar for gonococci. Use the same media as for blood cultures. Do not use transport media. Gram and special stains are best performed on a centrifuged aliquot.
2. Sterile tube with sodium heparin or ethylenediaminetetraacetic acid (EDTA) (green- or purple-topped tubes in many laboratories): 2 to 3 mL for cell counts, differential, cytology, and crystals.
3. Two clean tubes without anticoagulant (plain red-topped tubes in many laboratories): 1 to 2 mL for color, viscosity (string or mucin clot), inclusions, crystals (alternative to anticoagulated); 1 to 2 mL for total protein, rheumatoid factor, complement, and other such tests.
4. Clean tube with preservative (e.g., oxalate; gray-topped tube in many laboratories): 1 mL for glucose.

VOLUME

The total volume aspirated may help determine the severity of the disease process, although it is not generally helpful in distinguishing between the various groups of abnormal fluid. Low volume does not rule out significant disease; rather, the volume of synovial fluid removed on several subsequent synovianalyses is sometimes helpful in determining the response to treatment, such as in septic arthritis. Generally, more than 4 mL obtained from the knee is considered abnormal.

VISCOSITY

Reduced viscosity results from either degradation of hyaluronate secondary to inflammation or rapid accumulation of fluid after trauma, which dilutes the hyaluronate concentration. Direct measurement of viscosity or hyaluronate is not usually performed; instead, indirect assessment is based on two relatively simple procedures: the string and mucin clot tests.

When a drop of normal synovial fluid is held between the gloved thumb and index finger, a "string" effect will be noted as the fingers are slowly separated. If viscosity is reduced, separation of the fingers occurs without any bridge of synovial fluid between them. An alternative method is to express fluid one drop at a time from a syringe with the needle removed. Normal synovial fluid droplets form a long string, suggestive of honey, whereas low-viscosity fluid appears like water droplets with short tails.

The mucin clot test also correlates with the amount of hyaluronate present and therefore reflects viscosity. When one part normal synovial fluid is added to four parts 2% acetic acid and shaken, a firm button of clotted hyaluronate protein complex forms at the bottom of the tube after standing for 5 minutes. With degraded hyaluronate from inflammation, no button forms, and the synovial fluid may contain friable shreds of clotted material.

The string and mucin clot tests are generally interchangeable in the interpretation of synovial fluid

Table 56-3. Characteristics of Abnormal Synovial Fluid

GROUP I: NONINFLAMMATORY

Volume (knee)	Often >4 mL
Viscosity (string or mucin clot)	High
Color	Straw colored to yellow
Clarity	Transparent
Total WBC/mm^3	200-3000
Differential WBC count	
PMNs	≤25%
Lymphocytes	<25%
Monocytes	>50%
Crystals	None
Protein	Usually normal
Glucose	90% of blood
Culture	Negative

Partial List of Associated Conditions

Trauma

Internal derangement

Osteoarthritis

Aseptic necrosis

Osteochondritis dissecans

Osteochondromatosis

Polymyalgia rheumatica

Amyloidosis

Early or resolving inflammation

Acquired immunodeficiency syndrome

GROUP II: INFLAMMATORY

Volume (knee)	Often >4 mL
Viscosity (string or mucin clot)	Low
Color	Yellow to white
Clarity	Translucent
Total WBC/mm^3	2000-75,000
Differential WBC count	
PMNs	>50%
Lymphocytes	<25%
Monocytes	25%
Crystals	May be present
Protein	>32.0 g/dL
Glucose	75% of blood or lower
Culture	Negative for bacteria

Partial List of Associated Conditions

Often highly inflammatory
  Rheumatoid arthritis
  Crystal arthritis
  Reiter's syndrome
  Acute rheumatic fever
  Lyme disease

Often mildly inflammatory
  Psoriatic arthritis
  Bowel-related arthritis
  Juvenile arthritis
  Ankylosing spondylitis
  Connective tissue disease
  Viral arthritis (including parvovirus)[22]
  Tubercular or fungal arthritis

GROUP III: SEPTIC

Volume (knee)	Usually >4 mL
Viscosity (string or mucin clot)	Low
Color	Variable
Clarity	Opaque
Total WBC/mm^3	Usually >100,000
Differential WBC count	
PMNs	>75%
Lymphocytes	<10%
Monocytes	≤10%
Crystals	None
Protein	>3.0 g/dL
Glucose	50% of blood or lower
Culture	Positive for bacteria

Partial List of Associated Conditions

Bacterial infections

Tubercular or fungal arthritis (rare)

GROUP IV: HEMORRHAGIC

Volume (knee)	Usually >4 mL
Viscosity (string or mucin clot)	Variable
Color	Pink to bloody
Clarity	Variable
Total WBC/mm^3	Variable
Differential WBC count	
PMNs	Variable
Lymphocytes	Variable
Monocytes	Variable
Crystals	None
Protein	Variable
Glucose	Variable
Culture	Negative

Partial List of Associated Conditions

Trauma (exclude fracture)

Hemorrhagic diatheses
  Thrombocytopenia
  Anticoagulant therapy
  Hemophilia
  Sickle cell disease
  Malignancy

Neuroarthropathy (Charcot's joint)

Joint prostheses

Tumor
  Pigmented villonodular synovitis
  Synovial hemangioma

PMN, polymorphonuclear cell; WBC, white blood cell.

viscosity, with most clinicians preferring the former because of its simplicity.

CLARITY

The clarity of normal synovial fluid can be reduced by any particulate matter, most commonly increased cellularity, but also by crystals, inclusion bodies, and lipids. The method for detecting loss of clarity generally involves placing black text on a white background, such as newsprint, behind a test tube containing synovial fluid. If the text can be read through the fluid with a bright light, its clarity is normal (transparent).

COLOR

Normal synovial fluid is colorless or pale yellow (straw colored). When blood not caused by the procedure itself is found, it generally does not form clots and is evenly distributed throughout the fluid. Inflammatory fluid may appear deep yellow. Pus may be found, but large numbers of crystals or inflammatory debris may mimic its appearance.

CELL COUNTS

Grossly bloody fluid may result from introduction of the needle or arthroscope and is usually evident during the procedure; the blood may be unevenly distributed, often clots, and may decrease as the procedure continues. A hematocrit level from an anticoagulated tube should be obtained on all bloody effusions to determine whether it is blood per se because just moderate amounts of red cells may simulate the appearance of whole blood. If red cells are actually present in synovial fluid as a result of the disease process, they are usually evenly distributed, do not clot, and remain consistent throughout the procedure. Because the intra-articular breakdown of these disease-related red cells releases heme, a centrifuged specimen produces xanthochromia. Considered one of the most important aspects of synovianalysis, the total and differential white cell count may be inaccurate if precautions are not observed. It is important that synovial fluid be placed promptly in appropriate anticoagulant and that no clumps of cells be found after gently shaking the tube. Any remaining clots should alert one that the total white cell count may be falsely low. Even if the cell counts are performed correctly, differences may occur, depending on whether manual or automated methods are used. Manual counts are considered most accurate but have one pitfall: if acetic acid is inadvertently used as the diluent, synovial protein clots will entrap white cells and falsely lower the total count. Therefore, it is imperative that normal saline be used as the diluent. If the effusion is bloody, hypotonic (0.3%) saline should be used to lyse the red cells after a hematocrit is performed. Automated counters are not recommended because of the large number of technical artifacts that may occur.

CRYSTALS

The presence or absence of crystals in synovial fluid is as essential in the evaluation of disorders of the knee as the total cell count and differential, particularly since crystal-induced arthritis may produce inflammation with very high white cell counts overlapping those of septic arthritis. As with the cell count, precautions must be observed to obtain an accurate result. Considerable variation in correctly identifying crystals has been documented in clinical and hospital laboratories, and it is strongly recommended that the clinician perform the analysis personally to ensure accuracy, just as the hematologist does with the bone marrow examination.

Collection of the specimen into appropriate tubes is essential for success. As noted earlier, anticoagulated tubes may be used, but only with sodium heparin or EDTA. If lithium heparin or calcium oxalate is inadvertently used, crystalline artifacts will be produced and cause totally inaccurate results. Although nonanticoagulated specimens may also be used, inaccuracies may be caused by white cells clumps obscuring identification of crystals. An additional pitfall is the presence of corticosteroid crystals for weeks after instillation into the joint cavity.

Once the specimen is collected into a tube containing sodium heparin or EDTA, a wet mount should be prepared as soon as possible. This requires placing a drop of synovial fluid on a slide free of dust or scratches, placing a clean cover slip over the drop, and sealing it on all four sides with clear nail polish. Sealing the cover slip avoids streaming of cells, as well as de novo precipitation of crystals caused by dehydration of the specimen. Assuming correct collection of the specimen and preparation of the wet mount, identification of crystals requires the use of a compensated, polarized light microscope with a rotating stage. All clinicians who perform synovianalysis should have access to this equipment and be familiar with its use. Without it, significant joint disease will surely be missed. At the present time, four types of pathological crystals may be identified: monosodium urate monohydrate in gout, calcium pyrophosphate dihydrate in pseudogout, calcium oxalate in chronic dialysis arthropathy, and hydroxyapatite in rotator cuff (Milwaukee shoulder) syndrome and erosive osteoarthritis.

The purpose of the compensated, polarized light is twofold. It provides a black background that causes the crystalline material, which is most frequently found intracellularly, to stand out from the cells and other particulate material, thus allowing an estimation of size and shape. In addition, it provides two optical characteristics of crystals, extinction and elongation (birefringence), which further aids in differentiating the specific type of crystal seen. The reader is referred to the references for detailed discussions on identification of crystals.

Microbiology

Swift identification of septic arthritis of the knee depends on analysis of the synovial fluid. As noted earlier, in patients in whom septicemia or soft-tissue infection is suspected, synovianalysis should be deferred until ancillary data are obtained to avoid contaminating a sterile joint.

Once fluid is collected in a sterile tube, aliquots should be placed into both aerobic and anaerobic blood agar vials, including tubercular and fungal media, and an additional aliquot should be immediately inoculated onto chocolate agar if gonococcal disease is suspected. Gram stain for bacteria and special stains for mycobacteria and fungi are best performed on a concentrated (centrifuged) aliquot.

Chemistry and Serology

The total protein of normal synovial fluid is usually about 2 g/dL, or approximately 25% that of blood. If greater than 2.5 g/dL, it is abnormal, with higher levels reflecting the degree of inflammation present. Although fasting specimens are the most accurate, normal synovial fluid glucose is about 90% that of simultaneous blood. With inflammation, levels of synovial fluid glucose diminish, the lowest levels generally occurring in septic arthritis.

Rheumatoid factor may be found in synovial fluid, even in patients with negative serum levels. Presumably, this is due to production by the synovial cells themselves; the factor may be found as a nonspecific reaction to many kinds of inflammation and should not be used as an indicator of RA.

Many other components, such as antinuclear antibodies, DNA, complement, globulins, cryoprecipitates, and enzymes, may be found in synovial fluid, but they are of little clinical value at present and are mainly of research interest.

MEDICAL TREATMENT

A significant percentage of all drugs sold in the United States are intended to alleviate musculoskeletal pain and/or inflammation. Drugs for the treatment of inflammatory arthritis of the knee can be divided into four major categories: nonsteroidal anti-inflammatory drugs (NSAIDs); corticosteroids; disease-modifying antirheumatic drugs (DMARDs); and the new biological response modifiers (BRMs)—tumor necrosis factor-α (TNF-α) and interleukin-1 (IL-1) antagonists. Rapid advances in the biology of inflammation and the recent introduction of novel pharmacological agents have revolutionized the classic treatment algorithms for knee arthritis.

Nonsteroidal Anti-inflammatory Drugs

NSAIDs have been adequate as first-line agents for most patients with knee synovitis, including OA (primary and secondary) and RA. NSAIDs provide immediate pain relief and reduce mild inflammation. They owe their pharmacological actions principally to inhibition of the enzyme cyclooxygenase (COX), which is responsible for the conversion of arachidonic acid to prostaglandin and other inflammatory mediators. Side effects include dyspepsia, peptic ulceration, and gastrointestinal bleeding—a major iatrogenic concern. Risk factors for the development of gastrointestinal complications, such as advanced age, concomitant use of corticosteroids, and the presence of systemic inflammatory disease, are particularly relevant for patients with arthritis.[13] The discovery of at least two different COX enzymes, COX-1 and COX-2, has had significant clinical implications. The association of COX-1 inhibition with gastrointestinal side effects has led to the rapid development of COX-2 selective compounds, such as rofecoxib (Vioxx), celecoxib (Celebrex), and valdecoxib (Bextra).

The expectation was that a COX-1–sparing effect would result in fewer gastrointestinal complications. Although rofecoxib decreased the risk for gastrointestinal toxicity by 50% to 60% relative to naproxen in the VIGOR trial[4] (prospective study comparing rofecoxib with naproxen in patients with RA), the results with celecoxib from the CLASS trial (a study comparing gastrointestinal toxicity with celecoxib versus ibuprofen) are less clear.[41] From the same study concomitant use of aspirin for cardiovascular prophylaxis appeared to mitigate the protective effect of celecoxib. Furthermore, the VIGOR trial indicated an increased risk for cardiovascular events with rofecoxib versus naproxen. The APPROVe trial (a prospective, randomized, placebo-controlled clinical trial) was designed to evaluate the efficacy of rofecoxib in preventing recurrence of colorectal polyps in patients with a history of colorectal adenomas. In this study, patients taking rofecoxib had an increased relative risk, versus those taking placebo, for confirmed cardiovascular events, such as heart attack and stroke, beginning after 18 months of treatment. Rofecoxib was voluntarily withdrawn from the market in September 2004 by its manufacturer for this reason. Valdecoxib (Bextran) was removed from the market in April, 2005, for the same cardiovascular risk factors, as well as because of an increased incidence of serious skin reactions. Although the results of clinical studies with one drug in a given class are not necessarily applicable to others in the class, COX-2 selective inhibitors should be used with caution in patients with cardiovascular risk factors.

It is important to remember that as a class, COX-2 selective inhibitors are not more effective than NSAIDs in reducing symptoms. In the VACT study, celecoxib was not significantly better than acetaminophen, and rofecoxib produced a better outcome only in a dose double that recommended for OA.

NSAIDs, including the COX-2 selective inhibitors, may significantly reduce the production of renal vasodilatory prostaglandins. Although this effect may be inconsequential on normal kidneys, the presence of preexisting renal disease or conditions associated with a contracted plasma volume, such as hemorrhage, diuretic therapy, congestive heart failure, and cirrhosis with ascites, may lead to further renal compromise. Specifically, such problems include renal failure as a result of decreased glomerular filtration, papillary necrosis probably caused by medullary ischemia, sodium retention with edema, nephrotic syndrome (which may occur after discontinuing NSAIDs), and hyperkalemia and hyponatremia secondary to suppression of renin production.

Individual agents within the NSAID class, as well as the COX-2 selective inhibitors, are similarly efficacious, and preferences are usually based on tolerability, adverse effects, dosing schedule, and cost. Because the therapeutic goal with first-line drugs is relief of symptoms, guides to efficacy include patient preference, pain relief, relief of stiffness, and functional ability. Frequently, a sequence of these drugs, in varying doses, must be used on a trial-and-error basis. Generally, a 2- or 3-week trial is sufficient, along with suitable adjustments in dose frequency and strength. In patients with a high risk for gastrointestinal complications, adding a proton pump inhibitor should be considered first. Adding a COX-2 selective inhibitor should be considered after weighing the cardiovascular risk.[16]

Corticosteroids

Although corticosteroids are some of the most potent anti-inflammatory agents, the incidence of toxicity associated with systemic administration limits their use in patients with chronic forms of arthritis. Long-term use is associated with osteoporosis, osteonecrosis, hypertension, hyperglycemia, obesity, accelerated atherosclerotic disease, cataracts, skin fragility, and mood disturbance. In acute synovitis of the knee, their use should be restricted until the diagnosis is established, and then they should serve as therapeutic adjuncts while awaiting the delayed effect of DMARDs. Suggested guidelines for the prevention of osteoporosis secondary to the long-term use of corticosteroids include keeping the dose at a minimum as dictated by symptoms, performing bone densitometry (because even a daily dose of 5 mg of prednisone carries increased risk), and adding a bisphosphonate with 1500 mg of calcium and 400 to 800 IU of vitamin D daily. Lifestyle modifications that help prevent bone loss are smoking cessation, limitation of alcohol use, and weight-bearing exercises.

When major levels of disability are attributable to the knee, intra-articular administration of steroid preparations, as interim adjunctive treatment, may induce periods of improvement that last for several weeks or more. Injections in individual joints should not be repeated frequently because of the risk of accelerated cartilage destruction.

Disease-Modifying Antirheumatic Drugs

The ultimate goal of treatment is to prevent the progression of joint destruction from unremitting synovitis as may occur in RA and other inflammatory disorders. DMARDs, by definition as a class, should have the following disease-modifying effect: reduction or prevention of radiographic joint damage and preservation of joint function. Commonly used DMARDs are hydroxychloroquine (Plaquenil), sulfasalazine (Azulfidine), methotrexate (Rheumatrex), and leflunomide (Arava). Etanercept (Enbrel), infliximab (Remicade), anakinra (Kineret), and adalimumab (Humira) are novel additions to this group

and will be discussed separately (see later). Other agents used less frequently, which will not be discussed here, are azathioprine (Imuran), mycophenolate mofetil (CellCept), cyclosporine (Neoral), minocycline (Minocin), D-penicillamine (Depen), and gold salts (Solganal).

TREATMENT OF SPECIFIC FORMS OF CHRONIC KNEE SYNOVITIS

Rheumatoid Arthritis

Treatment of RA has changed dramatically over the course of the last decade. Cure still remains elusive; however, complete remission is an approachable goal. Traditional treatment of RA has been based on symptomatic management with NSAIDs and corticosteroids, followed by DMARDs, each with its own substantial drawbacks in terms of effectiveness or adverse effects. The traditional "pyramid" treatment algorithm, prescribing NSAIDs and steroids until joint deformity or radiographic erosion is evident and then stepping up to DMARDs, has undergone complete remodeling such that treatment is now started earlier and is more aggressive.[37] The use of early combinations of DMARDs and BRMs has gained acceptance because of greater efficacy and better outcome.[10]

ANTIMALARIALS

Hydroxychloroquine is used more often than chloroquine (Aralen) in the United States for the treatment of RA because of its lower toxicity. Hydroxychloroquine is a weak anti-inflammatory agent. By increasing the pH of intracellular lysosomes it may interfere with the processing and presentation of antigenic peptides by antigen-presenting cells (APCs) and thereby lead to decreased T-cell activation. Hydroxychloroquine has a slow onset of action, and patients usually require concomitant administration of NSAIDs to control symptoms. It improves the signs and symptoms of RA, especially in early, mild disease.[44] There is no clear evidence that it prevents radiographic progression when used alone. Hydroxychloroquine is usually limited to 400 to 600 mg/day because of its dose-dependent risk for retinal toxicity. Two to six months is required before maximal efficacy is seen. The most dreaded potential toxicity is retinopathy. Fortunately, when the recommended daily dosage is not exceeded and appropriate ophthalmological examinations are performed every 12 months, progression to loss of visual acuity is rare.[40] A number of other side effects may occur, including headache, rash, alopecia, leukopenia, nausea, and weight loss. It may also provoke hemolysis in individuals deficient in glucose-6-phosphate dehydrogenase.

SULFASALAZINE

Sulfasalazine has been in widespread use for chronic inflammatory bowel disease for many years. After oral intake, most of the drug is metabolized to 5-aminosalicylic acid and sulfapyridine by colonic bacteria. The remainder inhibits 5-aminoimidazole-4-carboxamide ribonucleotide transformylase, thereby leading to an increased level of adenosine.[14] Sulfasalazine also prevents activation of the nuclear factor NF-κB. Several trials have demonstrated that sulfasalazine produces a statistically significant improvement in signs and symptoms in patients with RA. Sulfasalazine was also demonstrated to slow radiographic progression.[27] It should be started at low doses and titrated up to 2 to 3 g daily to prevent gastrointestinal toxicity. Maximal benefit usually requires 1 to 2 months of treatment. Common adverse effects include nausea, vomiting, anorexia, diarrhea, headache, and oligospermia. Less frequent effects are hemolysis and rash. Idiosyncratic reactions include hepatitis, agranulocytosis, and aplastic anemia, so the CBC and liver function tests (LFTs) should be monitored regularly.

METHOTREXATE

Methotrexate has been used to treat psoriasis, psoriatic arthritis, RA, and other inflammatory conditions.[19] No drug used as monotherapy has yet been shown to be better than methotrexate in controlling the signs and symptoms of RA.[1] It inhibits the conversion of dihydrofolate to folinic acid by dihydrofolate reductase, a critical step in de novo purine synthesis. Its anti-inflammatory effect is also related to an increased extracellular level of adenosine. Adenosine has potent inhibitory effects on a variety of inflammatory cells, including neutrophils, monocytes, and lymphocytes. The drug was shown to delay progression of radiographic erosion and joint space narrowing and to improve functional status.[2] Recently, there has been new information about the beneficial effects of methotrexate on mortality associated with RA. It was shown to improve overall mortality, including cardiovascular events.[6] An acceptable regimen includes a starting dose of 7.5 mg/wk, with dose escalation to 15 mg/wk at week 4 and 20 mg/wk at week 8. Maximal benefit requires 4 to 8 weeks. Although it does suppress disease activity quickly in a high percentage of patients, rebound of activity often occurs within a few weeks of stopping therapy. Side effects are not uncommon and include vomiting, diarrhea, stomatitis, headache, hair loss, leukopenia, thrombocytopenia, interstitial lung disease, and hepatic toxicity. Liver biopsy after 2 years of continuous use or a cumulative dose of 1500 mg is no longer routinely performed; however, periodic evaluation of LFTs is mandatory. Many of the adverse reactions are prevented by daily folic acid supplementation. Leucovorin given after methotrexate may also help treat the side effects. Abstinence from alcohol is required. The CBC and creatinine should also be checked every 8 weeks.

LEFLUNOMIDE

Leflunomide is an immunosuppressive agent that inhibits de novo synthesis of pyrimidine. Its active metabolite does so by inhibiting dihydroorotate dehydrogenase. A decreased level of pyrimidine inhibits T-cell proliferation, which plays an important role in inflammation. A randomized double-blind, placebo-controlled trial of RA patients showed that leflunomide was equally effective as methotrexate in improving symptoms and slowing radiographic progression.[39] Another study that compared leflunomide and methotrexate found both to have similar efficacy for signs and symptoms. Because of its long half-life, an oral loading dose of 100 mg/day for 3 days is recommended, followed by a daily dose of either 10 or 20 mg. Leflunomide has a more rapid onset of action than methotrexate does, with benefit seen in as early as 3 weeks. Hepatotoxicity is the most important side effect. Cases of hepatic failure were described in patients receiving concomitant methotrexate. Patients taking leflunomide should have LFTs, CBC, and creatinine evaluated every 1 to 2 months.[39] Onset and exacerbation of hypertension have also been noted. Before planning pregnancy or in case of adverse effect, rapid elimination of the drug is necessary. This is done by applying a washout protocol based on cholestyramine followed by monitoring of serum metabolite levels.

BIOLOGICAL RESPONSE MODIFIERS

There is strong evidence that TNF-α and IL-1 play a critical role in the pathogenesis of RA. TNF-α leads to the activation of NF-κB inducible genes that encode adhesion molecules, proinflammatory cytokines (IL-1, IL-6, IL-8), and enzymes involved in the synthesis of COX-2, inducible nitric oxide synthase, and matrix metalloproteinases.[3] It is therefore not a surprise that agents capable of neutralizing these cytokines are able to halt the inflammatory process in many patients. At present, three agents that inhibit TNF-α and one that inhibits IL-1 are commercially available: etanercept, infliximab, adalimumab, and anakinra.

Individual patients differ in the aggressiveness of their disease and its concomitant structural damage. These factors must be examined when considering biological treatment because these agents are not free of toxicity. The current indication for treatment with BRMs is active RA after an adequate trial of another effective DMARD, of which methotrexate is the common example. BRMs can also be added to preexisting treatments or may replace previous DMARDs. Patients in whom other DMARDs are contraindicated may be considered for treatment with BRMs as the first-line drug. Use of these drugs requires physicians experienced in the diagnosis, treatment, and assessment of RA.

ETANERCEPT

Etanercept is a fusion protein made of two recombinant human TNF-α receptor p75 components fused with one Fc portion of the human IgG molecule. This fusion protein binds and inactivates circulating TNF-α by reducing the amount available for receptor binding. Addition of the Fc portion increases the protein's half-life. Either as monotherapy or as combination therapy with methotrexate it improves the signs and symptoms of RA. In early RA, etanercept and methotrexate were similarly useful in improving the signs and symptoms and in slowing radiographic progression. A 52-week open-label study demonstrated etanercept to be superior to methotrexate in reducing disease activity and improving functional outcome.[18] Patients need to be instructed on how to perform two self-administered subcutaneous injections of 25 mg/wk. Recently, a once per week 50-mg schedule has been introduced. Clinical response may occur within 2 weeks. Adverse events include serious infections, particularly the activation of latent tuberculosis, which may be atypical in manifestation. Etanercept has also been associated with central nervous system demyelinating disorders and the development of autoantibodies and lupus-like syndromes. Concern regarding increased risk for lymphoma has also emerged, although it is unclear whether it exceeds the risk in other RA patients. Local site irritation is the most frequently reported side effect and occurs in up to a third of all patients. Treatment should be withheld from patients with active infection. All patients should be screened with a chest radiograph and tuberculin skin test before treatment.

INFLIXIMAB

Another approach to blocking the effects of TNF-α is using specific monoclonal antibodies. Infliximab is a chimeric anti–TNF-α monoclonal antibody consisting of 75% human and 25% mouse protein sequences that binds circulating and membrane-bound TNF-α. The mouse portion consists of the Fab region, whereas the human portion is used to reduce antigenicity. The benefits of infliximab in controlling the signs and symptoms of RA were confirmed in the ATTRACT study. At 54 weeks significant improvement was observed in both radiographic progression and functional outcomes. Adverse effects were opportunistic infections, including extrapulmonary and disseminated tuberculosis.[17] It is recommended that all patients being considered for treatment be screened with a chest radiograph and tuberculin skin test. Prophylaxis should be given to carriers. Lupus-like syndrome and the induction of antinuclear antibodies and double-stranded DNA were reported. Infliximab is administered as a parenteral infusion given at doses of 3 mg/kg and repeated every 8 weeks. Infusion reactions are common and include chills, fever, headache, dyspnea, and pruritus. It has been approved for use only in combination with methotrexate.[23]

ADALIMUMAB

Adalimumab is a recombinant, fully human, anti–TNF-α monoclonal IgG antibody that binds to both circulating and cell-bound TNF-α. It has been shown to improve the signs and symptoms of RA, to slow radiographic progression, and to improve functional outcomes. Forty milligrams is given every 2 weeks by subcutaneous self-injection. Clinical response may occur within 2 weeks. Adverse effects are similar to those observed with infliximab and etanercept. Treatment should be withheld from patients with infection, including latent tuberculosis. Again, all patients should be screened with a chest radiograph and tuberculin skin test before treatment, and treatment of latent tuberculosis should be initiated before beginning therapy with any of these three agents.

ANAKINRA

Elevated levels of IL-1 are found systemically and in the joints of patients with RA. After IL-1 stimulation, fibroblasts release matrix metalloproteinases that degrade collagen and proteoglycans and finally lead to cartilage destruction. IL-1 also stimulates osteoclast-mediated bone resorption. IL-1 receptor antagonist is produced in healthy subjects and helps protect against the adverse effects associated with IL-1 overexpression. Anakinra is a recombinant form of IL-1 receptor antagonist approved for the treatment of RA. It is produced by cloning human IL-1 receptor antagonist complementary DNA and inserting it into an *Escherichia coli* expression vector. It was found to be superior to placebo in improving signs and symptoms, slowing radiographic progression, and improving functional outcomes. Combination therapy with anakinra and methotrexate was superior to either alone. A dose of 100 mg is administered once a day by subcutaneous injection. Effect may be seen in 4 weeks. The development of opportunistic infections has not yet been reported. Injection site reactions develop in many patients. Long-term safety profiles are not clear. Cases of reversible neutropenia have been reported, so checking the CBC every 3 months is recommended.

COSTIMULATORY BLOCKERS AND B-CELL INHIBITORS

The T cell has a pivotal role in the pathogenesis of RA. For antigen-presenting cells to activate specific T cells, it is not satisfactory to express the antigenic peptide adjacent to the major histocompatibility complex. Costimulation is required. One of the costimulatory pathways known to be critical for the activation of T cells is the CTLA4 pathway. In this pathway CD80/86 on the APC interacts with CD28 on the T cell. This interaction leads to expression of CTLA4 (CD152) on the T cell. The role of CD152 is to serve as negative feedback and turn "off" the activated cell. CTLA4-Ig (Abatacept) is a fusion protein consisting of the extracellular domain of cytotoxic T-lymphocyte antigen-4 and human IgG1 receptor immunoglobulin that can inhibit full T-cell activation. It blocks the interaction of CD28 with CD80/86(B7) by binding to the latter. This blockade leads to decreased CD40L expression on the T cell, thereby diminishing its ability to activate CD40-positive B cells farther downstream.[26] CTLA4-Ig was found to be effective in psoriasis. A recent study in patients with RA has shown promising results, both as monotherapy and in combination with methotrexate.[20]

B cells also have a potential role in RA. They interact directly with T cells and with APCs and are responsible for antibody production and secretion of cytokines. B cells specifically overexpress CD20, and therefore one of the anti–B-cell approaches is the use of anti-CD20 antibodies.[7] Rituximab, a chimeric monoclonal antibody directed at CD20 that is approved for use in B-cell lymphomas, is now being evaluated for treatment of RA. Rituximab decreases levels of B cells and consequently lowers immunoglobulin levels. Early studies show clinical improvement after a few doses. In a phase II trial all American College of Rheumatology responses were superior to those of methotrexate.

Psoriatic Arthritis

Psoriatic arthritis is a chronic inflammatory arthropathy that encompasses a heterogeneous group of joint diseases ranging from mild synovitis to severe erosive arthritis. Thirty percent to 50% of patients evaluated initially have monoarthritis or oligoarthritis, and the overall prevalence of knee involvement is between 40% and 60%. For most patients, psoriasis is present before the onset of arthritis. Inflammation at the site of attachment of tendons and ligaments to bones, or enthesitis, is common. The general principles of RA treatment also apply to psoriatic arthritis, but with some different aspects because additional factors may influence treatment, such as axial versus peripheral joint involvement and the extent of skin affected.

NSAIDs are effective in many patients and should be the initial drug therapy attempted for mild disease. They are commonly used to control symptoms related to mild synovitis. However, some of the most exciting advances in the treatment of psoriatic arthritis pertain to the emerging evidence for the benefit of TNF blockade in this disease, before the onset of early cartilage destruction.

DISEASE-MODIFYING ANTIRHEUMATIC DRUGS

DMARDs should be initiated as early as possible in any patient not responding to NSAIDs and in those who already have erosive articular disease, as well as those with the potential for progressive disease. Whether DMARDs can prevent structural damage, as in RA, is not completely clear.

Methotrexate is effective for both skin and joint disease. It is generally accepted as the DMARD of choice for psoriatic arthritis, but other issues, including age, sex, and comorbidity, may play an important role in the choice for an individual patient.[8] Both open-label and randomized controlled trials have demonstrated its efficacy for both peripheral arthritis and skin disease.[9]

Sulfasalazine is useful for peripheral arthritis, including the knee; however, it has no substantial effect on skin. It has been evaluated for psoriatic arthritis in several randomized controlled trials, and benefit in patients with peripheral joint activity has been observed.[31] The Cochrane Database confirmed that methotrexate and sulfasalazine are the only two agents outside TNF blockers with well-demonstrated published efficacy for peripheral synovitis in psoriatic arthritis.

Little evidence has emerged to recommend the use of other DMARDs in psoriatic arthritis. Cyclosporine may represent a second-choice treatment in patients with severe refractory psoriatic arthritis, but further controlled trials are necessary to better define its place. Leflunomide was evaluated in two small short-term open-label trials, and a reduction in measures of disease activity was observed. The TOPAS study, the first large randomized controlled trial, compared leflunomide with placebo in 190 patient over a period of 24 weeks. Fifty-eight percent of the leflunomide-treated patients with psoriatic arthritis met the response criteria as compared with 32% of the placebo group. Larger controlled trials are necessary to further substantiate the safety and efficacy of leflunomide.

Corticosteroids can be used in low doses, in combination with DMARDs, or as bridge therapy. Psoriasis flare on tapering high-dose corticosteroids is a concern.

BIOLOGICAL RESPONSE MODIFIERS

Several open-label studies and, more recently, two randomized controlled trials suggest that TNF inhibitors lead to improvement in skin and joint manifestations in psoriatic arthritis. For patients with aggressive and destructive disease and for those who respond poorly to a single agent, TNF inhibitors are recommended.

Mease demonstrated the safety and efficacy of etanercept at a dose of 25 mg subcutaneously twice weekly.[25] In this 12-week study of 60 patients with active psoriatic arthritis, 73% to 87% of patients treated with etanercept met the response criteria as compared with 13% to 23% of patients taking placebo. Subgroup analysis of patients receiving concomitant methotrexate therapy demonstrated that etanercept was still more effective than placebo. The most common adverse events were upper respiratory tract infections and injection site reactions.

Salvarani et al published the results of an open-label study in which 16 patients with psoriatic arthritis who were receiving a stable dosage of methotrexate were treated with infliximab (3 mg/kg) over a 30-week follow-up. At the end of study, significant improvement in the number of tender and swollen joints versus baseline was achieved. Severe allergic reactions developed in two patients and necessitated discontinuation of treatment.[35]

Recently, preliminary results from the Infliximab Multinational Psoriatic Arthritis Controlled Trial (IMPACT) were presented. In this study, Antoni et al randomized 102 patients with psoriatic arthritis to receive infliximab (5 mg/kg) or placebo in a 16-week double-blind phase followed by open-label extension. Response was achieved in 71% of the treatment group versus 10% of the placebo group.

Other potential therapeutic agents that are currently being tested for psoriatic arthritis include anti-CD3 therapy using the non–Fc receptor–binding humanized derivative of murine anti-CD3 antibody and alefacept, a leukocyte function-associated-3 (LFA-3)-IgG1 fusion protein.

Osteoarthritis

Despite an enormous increase in our understanding of the molecular biology of articular cartilage and the recognition that OA is not merely a disease of cartilage,[29] more efficacious treatment of OA is still somewhat discouraging and symptomatic.[5] In contrast to RA, no biological agents are available. Since the early 1960s, when Sir John Charnley succeeded in developing total arthroplasty, no pharmacological treatments approximate the effectiveness of arthroplasty.[21]

ACETAMINOPHEN (TYLENOL)

Acetaminophen, as recommended by the American College of Rheumatology, is considered the first-line therapy for mild to moderate OA.[15] It is more efficacious than placebo and is considered to be safe and well tolerated. Data from recent trials and the results of meta-analysis, however, show that acetaminophen is not as effective as NSAIDs for pain associated with OA.[32] Moreover, data suggest that use of acetaminophen at a dose greater than 2 g/day may increase the risk for gastrointestinal bleeding. The mechanism may be related to its ability to inhibit isoforms of COX-1. It should be avoided in patients with excessive alcohol consumption and abnormal LFT results.

NSAIDs AND COX-2 SELECTIVE INHIBITORS

The use of NSAIDs should be considered for patients with severe pain or failure to respond to acetaminophen.[33] NSAIDs combine analgesia with anti-inflammation and form the basis for current medical therapy. However, the magnitude of pain relief afforded by them is modest. No consistent evidence has suggested that one NSAIDs is better than another in relieving the pain associated with OA. The majority of clinical trials comparing NSAIDs with acetaminophen have shown a small benefit in favor of NSAIDs.[12] The small statistical difference between treatments does not necessarily translate into clinical differences because patients often prefer acetaminophen to NSAIDs.[38] COX-2 selective inhibitors have no greater efficacy than nonselective NSAIDs do for the treatment of OA. They may offer some gastrointestinal safety advantage, mainly for patients who are at increased risk. However, the adverse cardiovascular, renal, and thrombotic effects should be considered. An alternative for patients at risk is to use nonselective NSAIDs with gastroprotective agents, as discussed earlier. Topical NSAIDs for knee OA also demonstrated efficacy; however, no published trials have compared the same NSAIDs administered orally and topically.

TRAMADOL

Tramadol is a centrally acting analgesic that has an opioid agonist effect. It may be useful, continuously or intermittently, for moderate to severe OA, both as monotherapy and along with NSAIDs. Tolerance and dependence are uncommon, and its main side effect is constipation. In one study, the analgesia that was achieved with tramadol was not greater than that achieved with an acetaminophen-codeine formulation.

CORTICOSTEROIDS

Systemic corticosteroid treatment should generally not be used for OA because of limited, short-lived benefits and high toxicity. Aspiration as well as joint irrigation of acute or recurrent knee effusion may offer significant relief and may be combined with the instillation of corticosteroids. Intra-articular instillation of corticosteroids, though often helpful with recalcitrant flares, should be used judiciously because masking of the pain may accelerate joint deterioration. Cartilage and subchondral bone may also deteriorate more rapidly with frequent instillation.

INTRA-ARTICULAR HYALURONAN DERIVATIVE

The beneficial effect of intra-articular hyaluronan derivative on knee pain in selected patients with OA has been documented, and the derivative is currently available for this purpose. It is best combined with continuous NSAID treatment. However, its effects on the course of the disease, if any, remain to be elucidated. It was suggested that viscosupplementation is the basis for clinical improvement. For some patients the beneficial effects may last several months. In an analysis of 11 clinical trials of intra-articular hyaluronan treatment, it had only mild to moderate benefit. It is expensive and its cost-effectiveness is under debate. There is no evidence that reduction of the NSAID dose occurs in patients treated with intra-articular hyaluronan.

STRUCTURE-MODIFYING OSTEOARTHRITIS DRUGS

New concepts of etiopathogenesis-based treatment direct attention toward modifying the basic disease processes rather than serving as pure analgesics or NSAIDs. Despite the fact that our understanding of the pathogenesis of OA has increased in the past decade, this knowledge has not yet translated into better outcomes for patients. However, it has led to major interest in searching for new drugs whose main effect is not relief of symptoms, but rather slowing the progression of radiographic changes.

Glucosamine and Chondroitin Sulfate

Glucosamine and chondroitin sulfate have recently enjoyed popularity for the treatment of OA. These agents have been suggested to modulate cartilage constituents. Glucosamine sulfate is thought to slow cartilage breakdown, possibly by stimulating cartilage to synthesize glycosaminoglycans and proteoglycans and by inhibiting proteolytic enzymes that damage articular cartilage. Chondroitin sulfate is the predominant glycosaminoglycan found in articular cartilage. Studies have shown that the efficacy of glucosamine is greater than that of placebo and comparable to that of NSAIDs in patients with knee OA. However, these studies were not large and were not well designed. In a meta-analysis of six studies of glucosamine and nine of chondroitin sulfate, it was concluded that only moderate symptomatic benefit was demonstrated for both of these agents relative to placebo.[41]

A National Institutes of Health–supported multicenter study (GAIT) currently in progress is comparing glucosamine, chondroitin sulfate, a combination of the two, and celecoxib with placebo in patients with knee OA. Data from this study will be useful in defining the role of these agents in the treatment of OA.

Diacerein (ART-50)

Diacerein has been available for several years in some European countries. Rhein, the active metabolite of diacerein, inhibits IL-1, and consequently, collagenase activity in cartilage is reduced. Rhein also inhibits chemotaxis and the phagocytic activity of neutrophils and macrophages. In clinical trials, 50 mg of diacerein twice daily was associated with improvement in 57% to 85% of patients with OA.[11] Diacerein has efficacy similar to that of some NSAIDs, but with slower onset of action. Except for a moderate and transient adverse effect of diarrhea, the drug is well tolerated. Recent trials have demonstrated structure-modifying properties of diacerein.[30]

CONCLUSION

A review of the medical evaluation and treatment of inflammatory arthritis of the knee has been presented. Rapid advancement in therapeutics, especially with BRMs, is changing the currently accepted "standard" therapeutic algorithms in favor of early intervention with disease-modifying agents that have the potential to minimize cartilage destruction with lower morbidity, thereby optimizing the quality of life for our patients.

References

1. Alarcon GS: Methotrexate use in rheumatoid arthritis. A clinician's perspective. Immunopharmacology 47:259-271, 2000.
2. American College of Rheumatology Subcommittee on Rheumatoid Arthritis Guidelines: Guidelines for the management of rheumatoid arthritis: 2002 update. Arthritis Rheum 46:328-346, 2002.
3. Bingham CO 3rd: The pathogenesis of rheumatoid arthritis: Pivotal cytokines involved in bone degradation and inflammation. J Rheumatol Suppl 65:3-9, 2002.
4. Bombardier C, Laine L, Reicin A, et al: Comparison of upper gastrointestinal toxicity of rofecoxib and naproxen in patients with rheumatoid arthritis. VIGOR Study Group. N Engl J Med 343:1520-1528, 2 p following 1528, 2000.
5. Chard J, Dieppe P: Update: Treatment of osteoarthritis. Arthritis Rheum 47:686-690, 2002.
6. Choi H, Hernan MA, Seeger JD, et al: Methotrexate and mortality in patients with rheumatoid arthritis: A prospective study. Lancet 359:1173-1177, 2002.
7. Choy EH, Panayi GS: Cytokine pathways and joint inflammation in rheumatoid arthritis. N Engl J Med 344:907-916, 2001.
8. Cuellar ML, Espinoza LR: Methotrexate use in psoriasis and psoriatic arthritis. Rheum Dis Clin North Am 23:797-809, 1997.
9. Cutolo M, Seriolo B, Pizzorni C, et al: Methotrexate in psoriatic arthritis. Clin Exp Rheumatol 20(6 Suppl 28):S76-S80, 2002.
10. Durez P, Nzeusseu Toukap A, Lauwerys BR, et al: A randomised comparative study of the short term clinical and biological effects of intravenous pulse methylprednisolone and infliximab in patients with active rheumatoid arthritis despite methotrexate treatment. Ann Rheum Dis 63:1069-1074, 2004.
11. Falgarone G, Dougados M: Diacerein as a disease-modulating agent in osteoarthritis. Curr Rheumatol Rep 3:479-483, 2001.
12. Fraenkel L, Bogardus ST Jr, Concato J, Wittink DR: Treatment options in knee osteoarthritis: The patient's perspective. Arch Intern Med 164:1299-1304, 2004.
13. Fraenkel L, Wittink DR, Concato J, Fried T: Informed choice and the widespread use of antiinflammatory drugs. Arthritis Rheum 51:210-214, 2004.
14. Gadangi P, Longaker M, Naime D, et al: The anti-inflammatory mechanism of sulfasalazine is related to adenosine release at inflamed sites. J Immunol 156:1937-1941, 1996.
15. Golden HE, Moskowitz RW, Minic M: Analgesic efficacy and safety of nonprescription doses of naproxen sodium compared with acetaminophen in the treatment of osteoarthritis of the knee. Am J Therapeutics 11(2):85-94, 2004.
16. Hawkey CJ, Langman MJ: Non-steroidal anti-inflammatory drugs: Overall risks and management. Complementary roles for COX-2 inhibitors and proton pump inhibitors. Gut 52:600-608, 2003.
17. Keane J, Gershon S, Wise RP, et al: Tuberculosis associated with infliximab, a tumor necrosis factor alpha–neutralizing agent. N Engl J Med 345:1098-1104, 2001.
18. Keystone EC, Schiff MH, Kremer JM, et al: Once-weekly administration of 50 mg etanercept in patients with active rheumatoid arthritis: Results of a multicenter, randomized, double-blind, placebo-controlled trial. Arthritis Rheum 50:353-363, 2004.
19. Kremer JM: Toward a better understanding of methotrexate. Arthritis Rheum 50:1370-1382, 2004.
20. Kremer JM, Westhovens R, Leon M, et al: Treatment of rheumatoid arthritis by selective inhibition of T-cell activation with fusion protein CTLA4Ig. N Engl J Med 349:1907-1915, 2003.
21. Laufer S: Osteoarthritis therapy—are there still unmet needs? Rheumatology 43(Suppl 1):i9-i15, 2004.
22. Lehmann H, von Landenberg P, Modrow S: Parvovirus B19 infection and autoimmune disease. Autoimmun Rev 2:218-223, 2003.
23. Maini RN, Breedveld FC, Kalden JR et al: Sustained improvement over two years in physical function, structural damage, and signs and symptoms among patients with rheumatoid arthritis treated with infliximab and methotrexate. Arthritis Rheum 50:1051-1065, 2004.
24. McAlindon TE, LaValley MP, Gulin JP, Felson DT: Glucosamine and chondroitin for treatment of osteoarthritis: A systematic quality assessment and meta-analysis. JAMA 283:1469-1475, 2000.
25. Mease PJ: Recent advances in the management of psoriatic arthritis. Curr Opin Rheumatol 16:366-370, 2004.
26. Moreland LW, Alten R, Van den Bosch F, et al: Costimulatory blockade in patients with rheumatoid arthritis: A pilot, dose-finding, double-blind, placebo-controlled clinical trial evaluating CTLA-4Ig and LEA29Y eighty-five days after the first infusion. Arthritis Rheum 46:1470-1479, 2002.
27. O'Dell JR: Therapeutic strategies for rheumatoid arthritis. N Engl J Med 350:2591-2602, 2004.

28. Pearlman BL: Hepatitis C infection: A clinical review. South Med J 97:364-373, quiz 374, 2004.

29. Pelletier JP, Martel-Pelletier J, Abramson SB: Osteoarthritis, an inflammatory disease: Potential implication for the selection of new therapeutic targets. Arthritis Rheum 44:1237-1247, 2001.

30. Pelletier JP, Yaron M, Haraoui B, et al: Efficacy and safety of diacerein in osteoarthritis of the knee: A double-blind, placebo-controlled trial. The Diacerein Study Group. Arthritis Rheum 43:2339-2348, 2000.

31. Rahman P, Gladman DD, Cook RJ, et al: The use of sulfasalazine in psoriatic arthritis: A clinic experience. J Rheumatol 25:1957-1961, 1998.

32. Recommendations for the medical management of osteoarthritis of the hip and knee: 2000 update. American College of Rheumatology Subcommittee on Osteoarthritis Guidelines. Arthritis Rheum 43:1905-1915, 2000.

33. Saag KG, Olivieri JJ, Patino F, et al: Measuring quality in arthritis care: The Arthritis Foundation's quality indicator set for analgesics. Arthritis Rheum 51:337-349, 2004.

34. Saito T, Takeuchi R, Mitsuhashi S, et al: Use of joint fluid analysis for determining cartilage damage in osteonecrosis of the knee. Arthritis Rheum 46:1813-1819, 2002.

35. Salvarani C, Cantini F, Olivieri I, et al: Efficacy of infliximab in resistant psoriatic arthritis. Arthritis Rheum 49:541-545, 2003.

36. Schumacher HR Jr: Aspiration and injection therapies for joints. Arthritis Rheum 49:413-420, 2003.

37. Schumacher HR, Pessler F, Chen LX: Diagnosing early rheumatoid arthritis (RA). What are the problems and opportunities? Clin Exp Rheumatol 21(5 Suppl 31):S15-S19, 2003.

38. Shamoon MC: Treatment of osteoarthritis with acetaminophen: Efficacy, safety, and comparison with nonsteroidal anti-inflammatory drugs. Curr Rheumatol Rep 2:454-458, 2000.

39. Sharp JT, Strand V, Leung H, et al: Treatment with leflunomide slows radiographic progression of rheumatoid arthritis: Results from three randomized controlled trials of leflunomide in patients with active rheumatoid arthritis. Leflunomide Rheumatoid Arthritis Investigators Group (erratum appears in Arthritis Rheum Jun;43(6):1345). Arthritis Rheum 43:495-505, 2000.

40. Silman A, Shipley M: Ophthalmological monitoring for hydroxychloroquine toxicity: A scientific review of available data. Br J Rheumatol 36:599-601, 1997.

41. Silverstein FE, Faich G, Goldstein JL, et al: Gastrointestinal toxicity with celecoxib vs nonsteroidal anti-inflammatory drugs for osteoarthritis and rheumatoid arthritis: The CLASS study: A randomized controlled trial. Celecoxib Long-term Arthritis Safety Study. JAMA 284:1247-1255, 2000.

42. Stanek G, Strle F: Lyme borreliosis. Lancet 362:1639-1647, 2003.

43. Steere AC, Coburn J, Glickstein L: The emergence of Lyme disease. J Clin Invest 113:1093-1101, 2004.

44. Tsakonas E, Fitzgerald KAA, Fitzcharles MA, et al: Consequences of delayed therapy with second-line agents in rheumatoid arthritis: A 3 year followup on the hydroxychloroquine in early rheumatoid arthritis (HERA) study. J Rheumatol 27:623-629, 2000.

CHAPTER 57

The Synovium: Normal and Pathological Conditions*

Vincent J. Vigorita

NORMAL SYNOVIUM: MICROANATOMY AND FUNCTION

The major function of the synovium is to provide joint tissue with lubrication and nutrient oxygen and proteins. Its complex structure leads to central roles in mediating the inflammatory response to injury and disease.

The synovium forms when a primitive mesenchymal tissue cavitates, forming a recognizable joint space at approximately 8 weeks of embryonic life (Fig. 57–1). Mature synovium appears pale pink in color and architecturally covers all the surfaces of the joint space, excluding the articular cartilage and most fibrocartilaginous structures. Only in abnormal conditions does the synovium encroach on the surface of articular cartilage, a change classically seen in the reddish "pannus" or inflammatory synovial invasion of the articular cartilage in rheumatoid arthritis.

The synovial membrane, the most superficial layer of the synovium, lines the joint and forms the linings of tendon sheaths. Parietal and visceral synovium mimic their mesothelial-like counterparts in the thoracic and pericardial cavities. The extensive synovial-like lining cells of tendon sheaths and ligaments explain a host of reactive synovitis and painful clinical tenosynovitis, bursitis, and enthesopathy syndromes. Joint capsule fibrous connective tissue is thought to add to the joint's mechanical strength. The term *joint capsule* refers to the fibrofatty neurovascular tissue that envelops the nonarticular cartilaginous tissue of the joint space.[39]

In pathological states, synovial-like anatomic structures, not related to a joint space ("synovial metaplasia"), are known to form in a variety of circumstances, including (1) postsurgical states; (2) failed prostheses, including breast implants[28]; (3) mechanical damage to connective tissue; and (4) experimental settings (injected air or oil in subcutaneous soft tissue).[20] These structures histologically resemble normal synovium and often have demonstrably similar secretory and phagocytic function.

Normally the synovium appears smooth and transparent, but it turns thick, dull, and opaque with pathological change. With hemorrhage, it becomes obviously bloody, but in chronic hemarthrosis it turns a reddish or rusty brown (Fig. 57–2) owing to hemosiderin deposition and the release of iron from red blood cells. In cases of severe bleeding, a dark purple or rusty color may be noted. The appearance of reddish purple or rusty synovium indicates a hemangioma or bleeding and may be seen in trauma, bleeding disorders such as hemophilia, von Willebrand's disease, and pigmented villonodular synovitis. In ochronosis (alkaptonuria), the synovium may appear a dull gray, whereas fibrocartilage and articular cartilage are discolored black. Darkening or blackening also may be seen when there is extensive release of metallic debris. White foci in the synovium usually indicate gout (urate deposition), pseudogout (calcium pyrophosphate deposition [CPPD]), or soft-tissue calcifications (deposits caused by trauma or calcinosis syndromes). Cement debris also may lead to pallor. A yellow color ensues with xanthoma cell accumulaton, which may be a predominant feature of pigmented villonodular synovitis (PVNS) or xanthomatous disease.

Microanatomic Structure

The synovium consists of a thin layer of synovial cells or synoviocytes, the intimal layer, above a richly fibrovascular zone, the subintimal layer, which contains arterioles, fat, and other connective tissue cells, such as fibroblasts, histiocytes, and occasionally mast cells (Fig. 57–3). The intimal layer of lining cells is usually one to two cells thick with no discernible differences on light microscopy. The loose connective tissue subintimal zone layer becomes gradually more fibrous at capsular insertions.

The villous appearance of synovium is not abnormal, but rather nonspecific and may be seen in a broad range of conditions (Fig. 57–4). In general, traumatic synovitis and degenerative joint disease (DJD) (osteoarthritis) are attended by edematous change and mild villous hypertrophy. Inflammatory arthritis (classically rheumatoid arthritis) shows a dramatically reddish hyperplastic synovium with fibrinous exudation characterized by abundant tan fibrinous loose bodies, called *rice bodies,* and marked lymphoplasmacytic synovitis. In septic arthritis, leukocytes are seen in tissue. Neuropathic joints and rapidly destructive joint processes are characterized by bone and cartilage debris.

---

*Chapter adapted from Vigorita VJ: The synovium. In Vigorita VJ: Orthopaedic Pathology. Philadelphia, Lippincott/Williams & Wilkins, 1999.

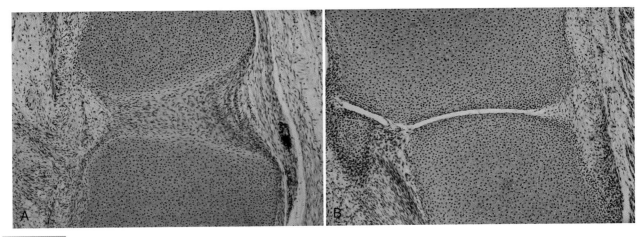

Figure 57–1. Embryonic joint showing evolution of primitive mesenchyme **(A)** into a joint space **(B)** at about 8 weeks of intrauterine life. (From Vigorita VJ: The synovium. In Vigorita VJ: Orthopedic Pathology. Philadelphia, Lippincott/Williams & Wilkins, 1999, pp 516-576.)

Ultrastructure

The intimal zone consists of an admixture of cell types often conveniently classified as cells exhibiting macrophage function (synovial A cells) and cells more synthesizing in function (synovial B cells) (Fig. 57–5).

Electron microscopy studies and immunophenotyping studies further characterized these cells. Ultrastructural studies show abundant mitochondria, Golgi apparatus, vacuoles, lysosomes, phagosomes, vesicles, and surface undulations (characteristics suited to macrophage activity) in type A cells, and rough endoplasmic reticulum, free ribosomes, and smoother cytoplasmic profiles (character-

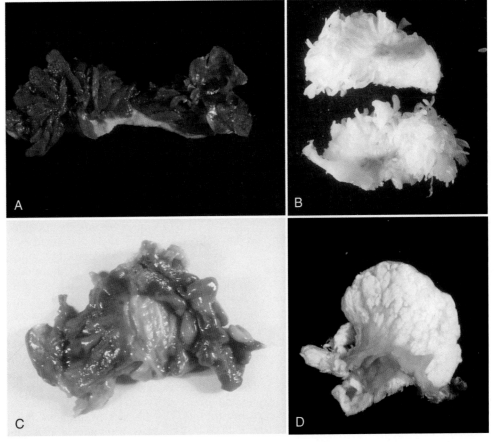

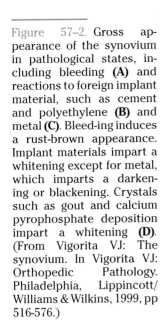

Figure 57–2. Gross appearance of the synovium in pathological states, including bleeding **(A)** and reactions to foreign implant material, such as cement and polyethylene **(B)** and metal **(C)**. Bleed-ing induces a rust-brown appearance. Implant materials impart a whitening except for metal, which imparts a darken-ing or blackening. Crystals such as gout and calcium pyrophosphate deposition impart a whitening **(D)**. (From Vigorita VJ: The synovium. In Vigorita VJ: Orthopedic Pathology. Philadelphia, Lippincott/ Williams & Wilkins, 1999, pp 516-576.)

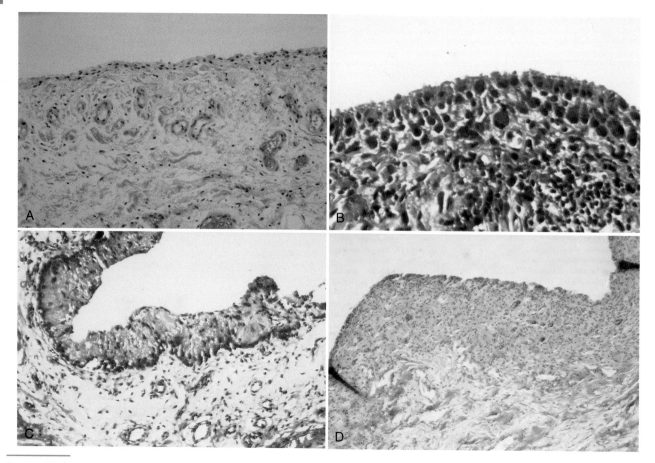

Figure 57–3. **A,** Normal synovium consists of a fine single or double layer of lining intimal cells on top of a subintimal zone of vascular and fatty tissue, fibroblasts, and rare histiocytes and mast cells. There is increasing collagen in the vicinity of dense connective tissue structures. **B,** Hyperplastic synovium showing moderate hypertrophy of cells confined to the surface with increasing hyperplasia and hyperplastic cells migrating into the subintimal zone with marked hypertrophy. **C,** Mucinous hyperplasia illustrating secretory potential of synovium. **D,** Superficial zone foreign-body giant cell reaction to failed prosthesis. (From Vigorita VJ: The synovium. In Vigorita VJ: Orthopedic Pathology. Philadelphia, Lippincott/Williams & Wilkins, 1999, pp 516-576.)

istics suited to synthetic activity) in type B. As might be expected, synoviocytes may be "intermediate" in nature, featuring organelle functions of types A and B. Some evidence supports the existence of other cells, such as antigen-type cells (HLA-DR, IA-like).

The use of special immunological techniques, including monoclonal antibodies, against a range of antigens can confirm that synovial cells consist of many different cell types. Three distinct populations can be defined immunologically.

Arbitrarily designated type 1 (synovial "A" cells) is a group of cells that seem to be related to mononuclear phagocytes based on their expression of antigen and derivation from cells of the monocyte macrophage cell lineage.[21] These cells exhibit phagocytosis and contain macrophage markers, abundant HLA-DR IA antigen, and Fc receptors. These cells constitute approximately one-third of the synovial cell population.

A second cell population, type 2, is characterized by nonphagocytic activity and a strong expression of IA antigen with the absence of IgG Fc receptors and antigens associated with the monocyte lineage, D and T lymphocytes, and fibroblasts. Type 2 cells include the IA antigen–positive dendritic cells. In rheumatoid arthritis, a considerable portion of the cells are type 2 cells.

A third cell population, type 3, is characterized by a nonlymphocytic population with characteristics typical of fibroblasts. These are the cells that usually predominate in tissue culture. They lack phagocytic activity and do not express monocyte antigens or IA antigens.

Cell types as defined by immunological studies are consistent with previous morphological observations. Type 1 cells expressing the monocyte macrophage antigens are similar to the cells historically described as characterized by phagocytosis type A and type C cells. Type 1 cells are most likely mononuclear phagocytes of bone marrow origin as ascertained by their antigenic marking with monocyte and IA antigen. Modifications in antigen expression suggest that they act more like tissue macrophages in the joint. The historically designated "type B" synovial cell that produces glycosaminoglycans is most likely of the type 3 cell variety, probably mesenchymal in origin. These cells lack IA antigens and most of the differentiated antigens of monocyte macrophage lineage.[10]

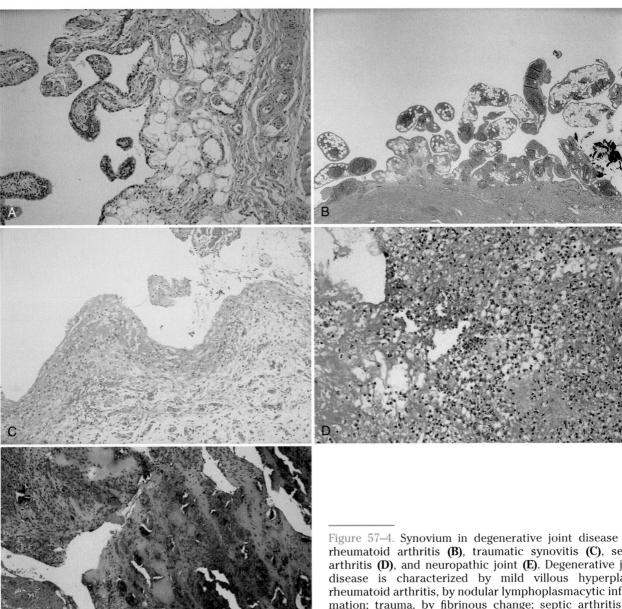

Figure 57–4. Synovium in degenerative joint disease **(A)**, rheumatoid arthritis **(B)**, traumatic synovitis **(C)**, septic arthritis **(D)**, and neuropathic joint **(E)**. Degenerative joint disease is characterized by mild villous hyperplasia; rheumatoid arthritis, by nodular lymphoplasmacytic inflammation; trauma, by fibrinous change; septic arthritis, by leukocytosis; and neuropathic joints, by abundant bone and cartilage detritus. (From Vigorita VJ: The synovium. In Vigorita VJ: Orthopedic Pathology. Philadelphia, Lippincott/ Williams & Wilkins, 1999, pp 516-576.)

The origin of normal synovial lining cells is controversial, but a dual-cell origin remains plausible with bone marrow derivation for the histiocytoid or type A cells and local mesenchymal tissue for fibroblast or type B cells. Many clinicians believe, however, the heterogeneity of synovial cells is more an expression of functional activity resulting from various factors, and the cell types are possibly interconvertible.

Although the synovial cells lack desmosomes or tight junctions, characteristic of epithelial tissue, the complexity of this cell structure is evident in the changes seen in various pathological states. Hyperplasia may be limited to a mild increase in intimal cell number, or there may be dramatic change, including large, bizarre cells, such as Grimley-Sokoloff giant cells or even striking mucin-producing cells. In this latter condition (mucinous hypertrophy of the synovium), the copious amount of material secreted testifies to the potential capacity of this membrane (see Fig. 57–3C). More recently, multipotential mesenchymal stem cells have been developed from the adult human synovial membrane and were inducible into chrondrogenesis, myogenesis, osteogenesis and adipogenesis.[15]

Functions of the Synovium

The functions of the synovium are best appreciated by understanding the characteristics of its cellular components and microarchitectural structure. The synovial A

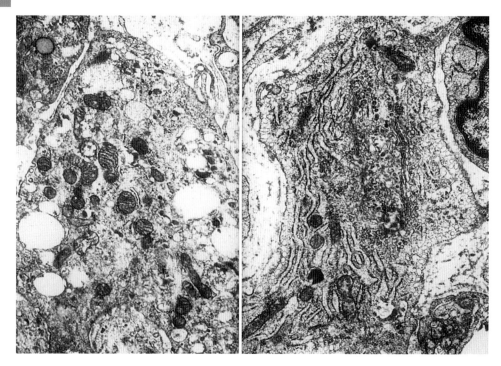

Figure 57–5. Ultrastructure of synovial intimal cells. Type A cells show prominent Golgi cells, vesicles, vacuoles, lysosomes, and mitochondria. Type B cells show abundant rough endoplasmic reticulum. There are no basal laminae separating lining cells from subintimal connective tissue and, unless inflamed, rarely cell junctions. (From Vigorita VJ: The synovium. In Vigorita VJ: Orthopedic Pathology. Philadelphia, Lippincott/Williams & Wilkins, 1999, pp 516-576.)

cells are suited to phagocytic (or macrophage) activity and ingest native or foreign material, such as hemosiderin in chronic bleeding conditions (hemophilia) or iatrogenically introduced substances (gold in the treatment of rheumatoid arthritis). Most recently, synovial giant cell reactions to viscosupplementation products have been identified (see later). The phagocytic potential of the synovium is probably best illustrated by the marked foreign-body giant cell and histiocytic reaction in some cases of loosened prostheses or in the resorption of bone and cartilage debris in rapidly destructive joint disease or neuropathic joints. Absorption of fluid material by synovial intimal cells is shown ultrastructurally by pinocytotic vesicles and vacuoles. Alternatively the synovial B cell is suited to synthetic function and most characteristically secretes the hyaluronate protein of synovial fluid, hyaluronate contributing to the lubrication of joint structures. Type A and type B cells seem to have secretory and phagocytic potential, however. Other functions in conjunction with the vascular and lymphatic systems of the synovium include the regulation of movement of physiologically important proteins and electrolytes. The lack of a basal lamina, the presence of gaps between synovial cells, and the lack of a basement membrane in synovial blood vessels facilitate interchange between synovial fluid and blood vessels.

Synovial Fluid

Synovial fluid, a dialysate of plasma, contains small amounts of hyaluronic acid, a copolymer of glucuronic acid, and an acetic glycocyamine, a protein complex hyaluronate synthesized by the cells of the synovial membrane. This material gives synovial fluid its high viscosity.

In addition, synovial fluid contains cells, mostly mononuclear phagocytes, and neutrophils. Synovial fluid content of glucose, uric acid, and lactate is similar to that in plasma, but there is less total protein. Albumin constitutes most of the total protein, whereas proteins of higher molecular weight, such as fibrinogen and other globulins, are relatively decreased compared with their plasma concentrations.

Arthrocentesis is the procedure whereby the synovial fluid is removed, a procedure that infrequently is complicated by infection. Arthrocentesis may be helpful in detecting crystal-induced synovitis, such as gout, CPPD disease, and hydroxyapatite crystal deposition disease. Blood is a nonspecific finding, which may be seen in a broad range of conditions, including trauma-induced hemarthrosis and PVNS, rheumatoid arthritis, and infection. Collection of synovial fluid in either heparin or liquid ethylenediamine-tetraacetic acid facilitates the identification of crystal deposition disorders. Heparinized tubes should be used for microbial cultures and Gram stain. For chemical analyses, observation of fresh synovial fluid in a clean test tube may be beneficial because normal synovial fluid does not clot (low fibrinogen concentration). Subsequent centrifugation can remove cells, fibrin, and other debris for further analysis for lactate, protein, uric acid, glucose, and other substances.

Synovial fluid analysis may be grouped for general classification of types of conditions producing synovial fluid (Fig. 57–6 and Table 57–1).[65] Noninflammatory conditions, such as DJD, trauma-induced arthritis, osteochondritis dissecans, and neuropathic arthropathies, or primary synovial metaplastic conditions, such as synovial chondromatosis, are characterized by a yellowish synovial fluid with high viscosity, low leukocyte counts, less than 10 mg/dL of glucose (i.e., below serum level), and low protein. Cultures are negative. This noninflammatory or class I type of synovial fluid group is distinct from the inflammatory or crystal-induced arthropathies, which are characterized by a synovial fluid with low viscosity, a yellow or whitish color, and a variable leukocyte count with a greater than 50% neutrophil population. Glucose

usually is elevated greater than 25 mg/dL with protein elevation greater than 3 g/dL.

Septic arthritis usually is characterized by a yellowish green fluid of low viscosity with an elevated leukocyte count with greater than 75% neutrophils. Glucose is usually greater than 25 mg/dL with increased protein levels. A wide range of conditions can induce a hemorrhagic arthropathy, including idiopathic hemosideric synovitis, trauma-induced arthritis, hemophilic arthropathy, and PVNS as a secondary change. These synovial disorders are characterized by a reddish brown color with decreased viscosity and a moderate elevation in white blood cell count with greater than 25% neutrophils. Glucose is in the normal range, usually 0 to 10 mg below serum level. Protein may be greater than 3 g/dL.

Normal synovial fluid is usually less than 3.5 mL and clear or faintly yellow in color with clear transparency. It has high viscosity as a result of hyaluronic acid and does not clot because of low concentrations of fibrinogen and other clotting factors. In normal synovial fluid, there are fewer than 200 cells/µL with a predominance of mononuclear phagocytes. There is a variable amount of lymphocytes, although lymphocytes and neutrophils increase dramatically in inflammatory arthropathies.

Eosinophilic synovitis has been described and may be associated with a mild to marked peripheral eosinophilia. Normal synovial fluid chemistries are typical. The differential diagnosis includes suppurative arthritis, tuberculosis and parasitic infections, allergies, and both degenerative and rheumatoid arthritis. The condition has been noted after arthrography and is usually accompanied by synovial fluid eosinophilia.

Crystal-induced arthropathy can be diagnosed with examination of synovial fluid using polarized light microscopy. Crystals other than gout (urate) and pseudogout (calcium pyrophosphate) may be seen. In chronic

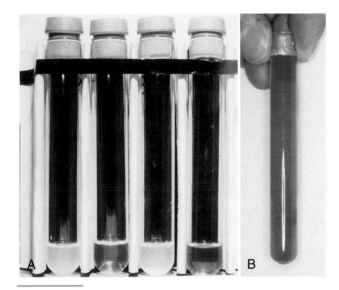

Figure 57–6. Synovial fluid composite. **A,** Synovial fluid from a patient with calcium pyrophosphate crystal deposition (cloudy), normal subject (clear amber), patient with rheumatoid arthritis (cloudy yellow), and trauma patient (blood stained). **B,** Pigmented villonodular synovitis, especially of the diffuse type, can give a bloody or rusty appearance. Septic arthritis yields a turbid yellowish green. (From Vigorita VJ: The synovium. In Vigorita VJ: Orthopedic Pathology. Philadelphia, Lippincott/Williams & Wilkins, 1999, pp 516-576.)

Table 57–1. Classification of Synovial Effusions

	NORMAL	NONINFLAMMATORY	INFLAMMATORY	SEPTIC
GROSS EXAMINATION OF SYNOVIAL FLUID				
Volume (mL) (knee)	<3.5	Often >3.5	Often >3.5	Often >3.5
Viscosity	High	High	Low	Variable
Color	Colorless to straw	Straw to yellow	Yellow	Variable
Clarity	Transparent	Transparent	Translucent	Opaque
Routine laboratory examination				
WBC (mm³)	<200	200-2000	2000-75,000	Often >100,000
PMN leukocytes (%)	<25%	<25%	Often >50%	>75%
Culture	Negative	Negative	Negative	Often positive
Mucin clot	Firm	Firm	Friable	Friable
Glucose (morning fasting)	Nearly equal to blood	Nearly equal to blood	<50 mg/dL lower than blood	>50 mg/dL lower than blood
PATHOLOGY				
		Osteoarthritis, osteochondromatosis, osteochondritis dissecans, neuroarthropathy	Rheumatoid arthritis, systemic lupus erythematosus, ankylosing spondylitis, gout, chondrocalcinosis (pseudogout)	Bacterial, fungal, and tuberculous infections

PMN, polymorphonuclear; WBC, white blood count.
Modified from Schumacher HR: Pathologic findings in rheumatoid arthritis. In Schumacher RH, Gall EP (eds): Rheumatoid Arthritis: An Illustrated Guide to Pathology, Diagnosis, and Management. Philadelphia, JB Lippincott, 1988, pp 4.1-4.36.

noninflammatory disorders, cholesterol crystals may be seen, which are square or rectangular with notched corners. Steroid injections may persist and be detectable as faintly birefringent.

IRON-RELATED CHANGES

Iron in tissue removed during orthopedic or related conditions usually is seen in the form of hemosiderin, typically identified as granular brown pigments in an intracytoplasmic localization. The presence of hemosiderin can be seen in a broad variety of conditions (Table 57–2).[65] Traumatic hemarthrosis is seen in association with soft-tissue injuries and fractures, including secondary fractures associated with other pathological states. Iron can be a contributing factor to the pathophysiology of disorders such as hemophilic arthropathy and transfusional hemosiderosis of thalassemia. Deposition at the mineralization front, causing osteoporosis or even osteomalacia, can be seen in primary or secondary hemochromatosis. The term *pigmented* in PVNS refers to the brown pigmentation caused by coincidental iron deposition in the synovial tissue surrounding the proliferating nodules of an essentially fibrous tumor. Yellow color may be seen as a result of the abundant presence of foamy histiocytes.

Incidental hemosiderin deposition seen in association with microscopic or macroscopic hemorrhage is usually of little pathophysiological consequence. Iron has been linked directly, however, to several important hemosiderin-driven osteoarticular pathologies, such as trauma-related hemosideric synovitis, hemophilic arthropathy, and osteoarticular iron osteopathy in hemochromatosis.

The most commonly encountered iron-related injury in orthopedics is that related to hemorrhage into the joint. Considering the rich vascularity of the subintimal layer of the synovium, microscopic bleeds from normal daily use of the joint may be expected. A few red blood cells are considered normal in joint fluid analysis. Trauma to the knee often is accompanied by significant hemarthrosis, however, an important association because bleeding—or perhaps more specifically the release of iron from ruptured red blood cells—stimulates clinically significant synovial changes, characterized clinically by pain and swelling.

Acute hemarthrosis of the knee in athletes may result from a wide range of injuries to the meniscus and the cruciate ligaments, fracture of the bone, and tear of synovial tissue.[48,63] In chronic hemarthrosis, iron accumulates in the synovium. Histopathological localization includes the synovial intimal cells and the histiocytic cells of the subintimal zone. Grossly the synovium may attain a "rusty" appearance (see Fig. 57–3).

Experimental evidence suggests that iron adversely affects synovial function. Chronic hemarthrosis may increase the synthetic function of the otherwise macrophagic synovial type A cell. Hemosideric synovitis without hemophilia is well described clinically.[22] Hemophilia represents this situation in a clinical extreme.

Findings on MRI in iron or hemosiderin accumulation are complex. In general, hemosiderin has a so-called paramagnetic or ferromagnetic property, causing a signal dropout[34] in most cases.

Hemosideric Synovitis

In hemorrhages that occur within the synovium, a highly vascularized tissue, red blood cells eventually disintegrate with phagocytosis occurring by histiocytes. Eventually the hemoglobin is broken down and processed into hemosiderin. Hemosiderin characteristically is seen as a brown-pigmented granular substance in cells of the synovium. Hemosiderin may occur as minute granules or accumulate into globules 25 μm in diameter. The intracellular deposition of hemosiderin is observed mostly in macrophages or histiocytes, but also may be seen engulfed in various trauma-associated conditions by the hypertrophied synovial lining cells. In joints subjected to hemorrhage, hemosiderin may be noted intracellularly or extracellularly. Cells within different compartments or layers of the synovium may be affected, ranging from the synovial lining cells to the subsynovial proliferating connective tissue cells. The gross appearance of the joint with chronic hemarthrosis is that of a rusty pigmentation, although more acute bleeding may be demonstrable as a blackish green discoloration.

The response of the human joint to bleeding is denoted clinically by the formation of a hyperplastic vascular synovium within a few days. Examination of the tissue reveals a proliferation of the synovial cells and other subsynovial lining cell connective tissue elements, including often inflammatory cells. Under electron microscope, iron-containing, electron-dense particles that are membrane bound, called *siderosomes,* are noted within the synovial cells and subsynovial macrophages.

Clinically, hemosideric synovitis may be due to a wide range of conditions, most notably trauma, particularly chronic trauma leading to chronic hemarthrosis. It also may be caused by the use of oral anticoagulant therapies, as a result of breakdown of synovial hemangiomas, or as a secondary phenomenon in conditions such as rheumatoid arthritis, PVNS, scurvy, and sickle cell anemia. The

Table 57–2. Causes of Hemarthrosis

Trauma (with or without fractures)	Von Willebrand's disease
	Anticoagulant therapy
Pigmented villonodular synovitis	Myeloproliferative disease with thrombocytosis
Synovioma and other tumors	Thrombocytopenia
Hemangioma	Scurvy
Charcot's joint or other severe joint destruction	Ruptured aneurysm
	Arteriovenous fistula
Hemophilia or other bleeding disorders	Idiopathic

Modified from Schumacher HR: Pathologic findings in rheumatoid arthritis. In Schumacher RH, Gall EP (eds): Rheumatoid Arthritis: An Illustrated Guide to Pathology, Diagnosis, and Management. Philadelphia, JB Lippincott, 1988, pp 4.1-4.36.

radiographic appearances may lead to joint space narrowing and may be confused with other ailments destructive to joints. Although most patients with chronic hemarthrosis or with an episode of hemarthrosis recover without any significant sequelae, the potential for joint destruction is present in any patient with bleeding into the joint.

With bleeding into the joint, two pathways may lead to damage. In one mechanism, the red blood cells may break down, causing macrophage activation. The ensuing inflammation may lead to destructive changes in and of itself, as seen in rheumatoid arthritis. Intracellular hemosiderin precipitates the release of leukocyte-derived and synovium-derived chondrolytic enzymes.[5] In excessive cases, the iron deposition in organs such as the meniscus may be severe enough to cause mechanical dysfunction and degenerative changes. In a second pathway, bleeding may lead directly to synovial proliferation, the release of an uncontrollable cascade of destructive substances such as proteases.

Hemophilia

The adverse effect on synovium in patients with chronic hemorrhage has been studied most extensively in the joint changes of hemophilic arthropathy of the knee. In tissue removed from hemophiliacs, the synovium shows marked villous hypertrophy with extensive hypertrophy and hyperplasia of the synovial lining cells and the subsynovial connective tissue components with abundant intracytoplasmic hemosiderin granule accumulation (Fig. 57–7). In tissue cultures of synovium in hemophilia, pigment-laden fibroblast cells have been shown to proliferate, and explants of the synovial cells have been shown to secrete large amounts of latent collagenase and neutral proteinases, establishing the destructive potential of the synovitis in hemophilia. Synovium incited by hemophilia produces enzymes and may do so without coincident inflammation, the latter a significant component to the destructive arthropathy seen in rheumatoid arthritis.

Iron accumulation may lead directly to chondrocyte destruction. In experiments aimed at developing a model for PVNS, a condition secondary to expanding nodules of proliferative fibroblasts and histiocytes, blood was experimentally injected into various animal models. The resultant proliferative synovitis was characterized by hyperplasia of fibroblasts, lipid-laden macrophages and giant cells, and extensive hemosiderin accumulation similar to that seen in reactive hemosideric synovitis or hemophilic arthropathy.

Although less visible, iron is known to accumulate in cartilage as well. Extensive hemosiderin deposition leading to grossly visible brown menisci has been observed clinically.[5] In studying hemophilic joints, iron has been localized to superficial chondrocytes, suggesting chondrocytic phagocytic uptake triggering a degradative enzyme release similar to that described in synovial cells. Iron has

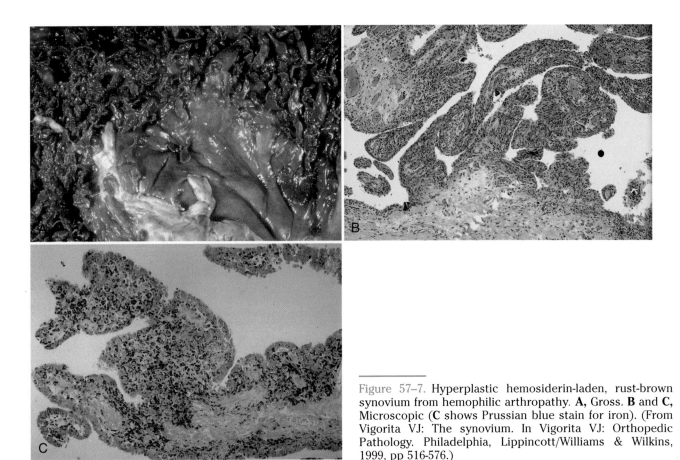

Figure 57–7. Hyperplastic hemosiderin-laden, rust-brown synovium from hemophilic arthropathy. **A,** Gross. **B** and **C,** Microscopic (**C** shows Prussian blue stain for iron). (From Vigorita VJ: The synovium. In Vigorita VJ: Orthopedic Pathology. Philadelphia, Lippincott/Williams & Wilkins, 1999, pp 516-576.)

been localized histochemically to the tidemark in lupus and in hemochromatosis. Hemophilia A and hemophilia B are inherited X-linked deficiencies of factor VIII and factor X.

Hemophilia A is the most common hereditary coagulation disorder, affecting 1 per 5000 live male births because of the deficiency, absence, or malfunction of coagulation factor VIII.[58] Roughly one-third of patients have no history of this disease. In normal patients, a very low concentration of factor VIII (0.2 mg/mL plasma) is sufficient for adequate coagulation. Bleeding leading to clinically perceptible illness requires a reduction of at least 75%.

Hemophilia A is a clinically heterogeneous disorder ranging from mild disease (1% to 4% deficiency) to severe disease. Patients with mild or moderate disease may not be recognized unless a significant traumatic event precipitates abnormal bleeding. Excessive bleeding during surgery may be the first clue. Therapy centers around replacement of factor VIII.[24] Replacement traditionally was done with shotgun frozen plasma, and cryoprecipitate became available in the 1960s. More recently, purified concentrates have been used. Current treatment consists of regularly scheduled replacement of deficient factor with recombinant proteins synthesized in tissue culture. In general, 1 U of factor VIII increases plasma activity by 0.024/mL. Because 0.3 U/mL usually is needed to treat a mild bleeding episode, clinical goals should strive for more than this amount. Therapy has improved morbidity significantly.

Clinically, bleeding is the key, especially into joints. Most commonly involved, in order of frequency, are the knees and elbows, followed by the ankles, shoulders, and hips. Not usually evident in infancy, childhood signs include mild discomfort and joint limitation. Pain and swelling ensue. Numerous damaging microhemarthroses have transpired before the initial arousal of clinical suspicion, delaying diagnosis. Hemosiderin deposition and synovial hypertrophy with joint destruction occur.

Radiographically, joint space narrowing, loss of articular cartilage, cystic remodeling of bone, and hemophilic pseudotumors characterize the illness. Strict adherence to maintenance of factor VIII levels to prevent spontaneous hemorrhage has been associated with significantly decreased morbidity and has halted radiographic progression of disease.

Surgical joint reconstruction in hemophiliacs has been attempted to preserve function, but radioactive synoviorthesis and arthroscopic synovectomy have been used.[5] Total knee arthroplasty performed for hemophilic arthropathy has a high risk of failure as a result of infection, which develops late and often is caused by *Staphylococcus epidermidis*.[54]

Intra-articular, intrabursal, and soft-tissue bleeding in hemophilia may result in painless masses clinically and radiographically mimicking a tumor, called *pseudotumors of hemophilia* (Fig. 57–8). These masses consist of spongy coagula of partially clotted blood encapsulated by thick fibrous membranes. Complications of these so-called hemophilic pseudotumors include muscle and bone damage, infection, and neuropathies. Surgical removal is not without danger. Pseudotumors occur in 1% to 2% of hemophiliacs[5] mostly in the lower extremity and pelvis.

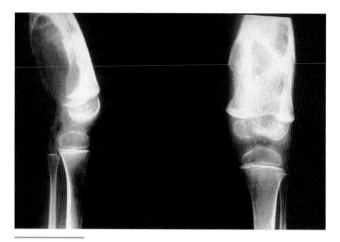

Figure 57–8. Radiograph of hemophilic pseudotumor. (From Vigorita VJ: The synovium. In Vigorita VJ: Orthopedic Pathology. Philadelphia, Lippincott/Williams & Wilkins, 1999, pp 516-576.)

Bleeding in the vicinity of the periosteum has been implicated in the peculiar juxtaosseous changes, among them cystlike bone changes and large soft-tissue masses eroding bone. MRI studies indicate low signal on T1-weighted imaging and high signal on T2-weighted imaging.

Before 1970, hemophilia A was still associated with significant severe disability and death at a young age. Median life expectancy grew significantly throughout the 20th century, however, from 11.4 years to 68 years in carefully monitored populations.[44] The transfusion of blood products, including factor VIII concentrates, has led to a well-recognized modern complication of hemophilia—transfusion-related acquired immunodeficiency syndrome (AIDS). Life expectancy now has reversed after considerable gains. Large numbers of hemophiliacs developed serologically detectable antibodies to human immunodeficiency virus (HIV) beginning around 1979. Approximately two-thirds of HIV-positive hemophiliacs have eventually died of AIDS. The risk to the surgeon is minimal if the proper precautions are taken.[29]

More recent therapy has used factor VIII concentrates exposed to vigorous virus-killing heat treatment or solvent cleaning. Genetically engineered products are now available and are being tested for complications. Expense is a significant consideration.

Another condition leading to a congenital deficiency is von Willebrand's disease. von Willebrand's factor is a protein that promotes the secretion of factor VIII and protects it from proteolytic inactivation. Mutations can lead to cases similar to mild to moderate hemophilia. Pedigree analysis, specific assays identifying factor VIII bonding to von Willebrand's factor, and specific molecular defect analysis are clinical and laboratory approaches to the diagnosis.

Hemochromatosis

Much current knowledge about the effect of iron on tissue comes from studies of hemochromatosis, the systemic disorder in which iron deposition is associated with tissue dysfunction. In general, iron overload has been studied in clinical situations in which there has been hyperplastic refractory anemia, excessive blood transfusions for underlying hematopoietic abnormalities (thalassemia), and hereditary forms of hemochromatosis. In the United States and northern Europe, hereditary hemochromatosis is a common cause of iron overload; 15% of the population exhibits the gene in its heterozygous state. The abnormal gene, located on the short arm of chromosome 6, is closely linked to the HLAA locus. In hereditary hemochromatosis, there is an increased absorption of dietary iron resulting in excess iron deposition in parenchymal tissues of endocrine organs, liver, and heart; death often results from heart failure or chronic liver disease.

In secondary hemochromatosis, the cause is ineffective erythropoiesis as seen in β-thalassemia and sideroblastic or aplastic anemia, for which the treatment may include repeated transfusions. Secondary hemochromatosis also may be caused by chronic liver disease, and in certain populations, such as within sub-Saharan Africa, hemochromatosis has been attributed to increased amounts of dietary iron intake, such as from large amounts of iron in beer brewed in steel drums. Inidividuals at greatest risk probably have a genetic predisposition.[26]

The deposition of iron in bone, particularly at the osteoblast-osteoid interface or at the mineralization front or as hemosiderosis within the hematopoietic cells of the marrow, is a relatively common sequela to primary and transfusional hemosiderosis. Although the primary organs involved are the heart and the liver with eventual development of cirrhosis and hepatocellular carcinoma and heart failure, endocrine organs are particularly involved. Joint pain in the clinical presentation of arthritis has been noted in 11% of patients carefully analyzed clinically; bone pain is a less frequent cause for presentation.[3]

First recognized in 1964 as a feature of hemochromatosis, arthropathy now generally is believed to be a common clinical symptom. In hemochromatosis, the joint changes may mimic DJD. Less than 50% of patients seem to have clinically osteoarticular problems. The metacarpophalangeal joints and interphalangeal joints are most frequently reported. Wrists, elbows, shoulders, hips, and knees are less frequently affected. Iron may inhibit the pyrophosphatase activity in cartilage tissue, leading to the precipitation of calcium pyrophosphate crystals, an association between the two that is well recognized.

LEAD SYNOVITIS

The signs and symptoms of lead poisoning are subtle, and recognition of this entity may be difficult. Plumbism is caused most commonly by ingestion of lead-based paint by children; by occupational exposure, such as painting, lead mining, and working in battery factories; and by the consumption of contaminated beverages, such as moonshine.[7]

A prototype of lead injury to the joint is the effect of retained bullet fragments.[8] Lead poisoning secondary to retained projectiles is rare (Fig. 57–9), but has been reported since the ancient Roman wars. Lead toxicity may cause convulsions, somnolence, mania, delirium tremens, coma, neuritis, nausea, vomiting, abdominal cramps, anorexia, weight loss, renal insufficiency, general malaise, and death. Orthopedic complications include bone cysts, localized arthropathy, pseudarthrosis, and gouty arthritis. Serum levels of lead of 920 μg/dL (44.40 mm/L) have been reported after retention of lead projectiles. The time between injury and onset of symptoms has ranged from 2 days to 40 years, although patients may be asymptomatic for long periods.

The location of the projectile in the body is a major factor in the likelihood of the development of lead intoxication. Exposure of lead to acidic synovial fluid results in greater dissolution than does exposure to human serum, water, or soft tissues. A second variable that may affect the duration of the symptomatic period is the surface area of the lead that is exposed to body tissue. Multiple small pellets have a greater surface area than one larger pellet, facilitating solubilization. Embedded lead particles usually are not absorbed systemically because they are encapsulated by dense, avascular fibrous tissue, inhibiting their dissolution in body fluids.

The diagnosis of lead intoxication routinely has included analysis of the levels of lead in serum and urine and clinical findings. Studies in which electron microscopy was used suggested that lead is incorporated into cells to a level that causes death of cells, resulting in extracellular deposition of lead. This finding suggests a need for removing lead fragments from the intra-articular space as soon as possible to avoid localized arthropathy.

The treatment of lead intoxication has consisted primarily of chelation therapy and open techniques for removal of the fragments. Symptomatic lead poisoning can be treated with arthroscopic removal of lead. This technique allows for removal of the fragments, extensive synovectomy, and débridement without the need for an open arthrotomy. Frequently, chelation therapy is given preoperatively to avoid sudden exacerbation of lead intoxication caused by the stress of the operation. Theoretically, lead, which is stored mostly in bone, can be released during stresses, such as an operation, fever, immobilization, acidosis, and other conditions, and this would increase symptoms dramatically. The level of lead might not increase, however, with intervention such as arthroscopy.

Chelation therapy has been given intravenously and orally. Multiple courses of chelation therapy may be needed to deplete the body stores of lead. It should be combined with operative removal of lead from the intra-articular space, and arthroscopic excision may be an effective way to achieve this goal.

Reported clinical effects of lead on articular structures include extracellular subsynovial lead deposition, synovial hypertrophy and inflammation, and intracellular lead uptake. Radiographic effects reported in animals include synovial lead uptake and arthropathies. The presence of lead near the joint space can induce microscopic degenerative changes in the joint structures. Lead-implanted knees yield significantly greater degeneration compared with knees with steel, knees undergoing simple arthrotomy, and control knees.

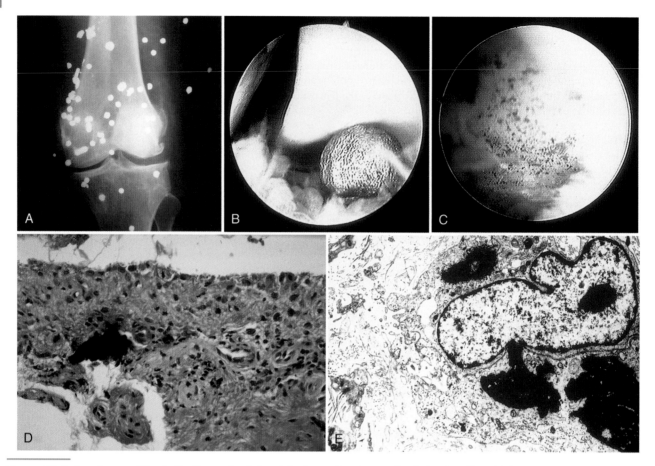

Figure 57–9. Lead synovitis. **A,** Radiograph of the right knee showing multiple lead pellets. **B,** Intraoperative view of the shotgun pellet in the intra-articular space (×10). **C,** Intraoperative view of minute particulate matter engulfing the articular surface of the tibial plateau (×10). **D,** Photomicrograph of hyperplastic and hypertrophied synovial tissue with irregular fragments of foreign material *(black)*. A sparse and patchy chronic inflammation is present (hematoxylin-eosin, ×255). **E,** Transmission electron micrograph of synovial tissue with cytoplasmic electron-dense particulate matter surrounding the nucleus *(right)* and at the left. The scale marker represents 1 μm (×9800). (From Vigorita VJ: The synovium. In Vigorita VJ: Orthopedic Pathology. Philadelphia, Lippincott/Williams & Wilkins, 1999, pp 516-576.)

ARTHRITIS

Degenerative Joint Disease and Rheumatoid Arthritis

Although a broad range of disorders may give rise to arthritis, de novo arthritis may be readily classified into two groups: (1) DJD or osteoarthritis and (2) rheumatoid arthritis.[30] They are distinct etiologically, clinically, radiographically, and pathologically (macroscopically and microscopically).

There are significant differences in the primary component of the joint involved. Notwithstanding experimental interest in synovial tissue modulation of cartilage destruction by cytokines, such as catabolin (interleukin-1), the synovium in DJD seems, at least initially, to be an innocent bystander, with the brunt of damage initially involving the articular cartilage (fibrillation and eventual denudement) and bone (subchondral cyst formation and sclerosis with marginal new bone formation or osteophy-

tosis). Biologically, osteoarthritis is associated with cartilage change, including reduction in the major proteoglycan, reduction in aggrecan, change in collagen fibril size and structure, and increased synthesis and degradation of matrix molecules.[47] Although the synovium may show hyperplasia, this is usually minimal and nonspecific. Synovitis is limited if present at all (Fig. 57–10). More active roles of the synovium in the pathogenesis of DJD have been proposed, including the reduction of the diffusion of synovial fluid and subchondral vascularization that accompanies high joint pressure, further deteriorating chondrocyte metabolism. Arthroscopic studies reveal that gross signs of inflammation in early DJD, in contrast to signs of rheumatoid arthritis, are limited anatomically to the points of the synovium in close proximity to articular cartilage. The overwhelming remaining synovium is essentially normal.

In rheumatoid arthritis, the synovium is the central inflammatory mediator. In acute rheumatoid arthritis, the synovium shows the most significant pathology (Fig. 57–11). Infiltrated by lymphocytes and plasma cells, the synovium becomes hyperplastic, and the surface exudes a

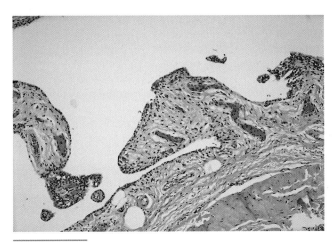

Figure 57–10. Synovium in degenerative joint disease. Villous change with mild hypertrophy and hyperplasia of synovial lining cells. (From Vigorita VJ: The synovium. In Vigorita VJ: Orthopedic Pathology. Philadelphia, Lippincott/Williams & Wilkins, 1999, pp 516-576.)

fibrinous exudate. Changes in the articular cartilage are truly secondary as the pannus, or inflammatory synovium, invades the surface of the joint, causing chondrolysis, eventual cartilage denudement, and, in chronic cases, the appearance of a secondary degenerative phenomenon.

Chondrolysis and osteoporosis characterize rheumatoid arthritis, however, distinguishing it clearly from DJD. This distinction is evident in laboratory diagnosis and monitoring. The inflammatory changes in rheumatoid arthritis are discernible in elevated sedimentation rates and positive rheumatoid factors (an elevated immunoglobulin protein, usually IgM, circulating in the serum). There is no equivalent useful laboratory monitor for DJD.

Radiographic changes initially show joint space narrowing and subchondral sclerosis. Eventually, new bone forms at the margins of articular cartilage (osteophytosis), which may give rise to villous synovial hypertrophy and metaplasia leading to chondro-osseous loose bodies.

Variants of DJD include an inflammatory type, characterized by more lymphocytic infiltration and hyperplasia of the synovium, and a rapidly destructive joint process that shows accelerated clinical and radiographic joint damage correlated pathologically by extensive cartilage and bone debris throughout the joint.[40]

Rheumatoid arthritis is classically a chronic, symmetric, persistent arthritis that may be associated with systemic symptoms and rheumatoid nodules (classically subcutaneous). Its cause is obscure, but laboratory studies and familial history suggest immunological and genetic factors in its expression. The rheumatoid synovium contains activated T cells, B cells, dendritic cells, and monocytes and macrophages. T cells are activated by

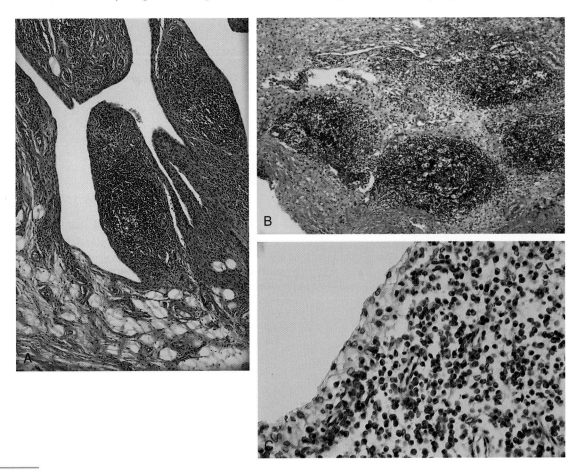

Figure 57–11. Synovium in rheumatoid arthritis. Synovial villi **(A)** with nodular lymphocytosis **(B)** and marked increase in plasma cells with synovial cell hyperplasia and hypertrophy **(C)**. (From Vigorita VJ: The synovium. In Vigorita VJ: Orthopedic Pathology. Philadelphia, Lippincott/Williams & Wilkins, 1999, pp 516-576.)

antigen-specific (signal 1) and costimulatory receptors (signal 2); the former are modulated through major histocompatibility peptide complexes.[42] Patients with class II major histocompatibility phenotypes, such as HLA-DR1 and HLA-DR4 (present in 80% of rheumatoid patients), are at risk because these molecules present antigens to CD4 and T cells. Proliferating T cells produce cytokines that can activate other inflammatory cells, such as macrophages, and cytokines such as tumor necrosis factor-α and interleukin-1 have become therapeutic targets. Molecular mimicry involving these steps has long implicated synovial proteins and infectious agents in the etiology of rheumatoid arthritis. Most patients with rheumatoid arthritis have a circulating protein in their blood, usually IgM, which is the basis for the rheumatoid factor test, a nonspecific but often useful serological test in corroborating the clinicopathological diagnosis. Atypical infections may trigger an as yet undetermined genetic predisposition. The presence of rheumatoid factor and elevated sedimentation rates correlates well with the characteristic synovial changes of a hyperemic synovial tissue infiltrated by a pronounced lymphocyte and plasma cell infiltration, often producing a fibrinous exudate. The latter proteinaceous exudation may override the articular bone surfaces of the joint, often creating tan, friable bodies (rice bodies).

Variants

Other disorders have been associated with rheumatoid-like inflammatory joint disease, but these "rheumatoid variants," such as psoriatic arthritis, Reiter's syndrome, and the arthritides associated with colitis, show fewer inflammatory synovial changes, vary in clinical progression of disease, and usually are not associated with a positive rheumatoid factor.

CRYSTAL-INDUCED SYNOVITIS

Although numerous crystals may deposit in the joint and in the bone proper, two crystals are particularly synoviotropic and associated with clinical articular and osseous pathology and should be specifically contrasted. Gout, resulting from the deposition of sodium urate, and CPPD (pseudogout, chondrocalcinosis) are frequently encountered crystal deposition disorders presenting with rheumatological or orthopedic complications.[32] In addition, hydroxyapatite crystals may be detected in synovial fluid in association with arthritis and degenerative joint changes. Other crystals, such as oxalosis and cystinosis, are rare and usually associated with renal disease.

Gout

Gout refers to the painful clinical syndrome associated with the precipitation of sodium urate crystals in and around joint surfaces characterized by synovitis and juxta-articular destruction of articular bone. Although gout often presents as a rheumatological or orthopedic syndrome, it is a systemic disorder preferentially depositing sodium urate crystals in and near joints. The ensuing inflammatory reaction or "tophus" may occur in virtually any organ in the body with the exception of the brain. Nonetheless, a severe form of hyperuricemia (Lesch-Nyhan syndrome) manifests with severe central nervous system clinical disease.

Gout is far more frequent in men and increases in incidence with age. Although there probably are asymptomatic deposits of crystals, gout usually is characterized by painful clinical attacks that are usually abrupt in onset involving the small peripheral joints, especially the metatarsophalangeal joints. The predilection for sodium urate gout crystals to deposit in the peripheral joints of the body suggests that multiple factors may be at work, including factors related to pH and temperature. A gouty attack may last a half day to several weeks. Although urate levels in the serum are usually elevated (approximately >8 mg/dL in men and >6.5 mg/dL in women), this may not be the case. Well-documented examples of gouty arthritis with large tophus deposits have been associated with normal uric acid levels, at least sporadically. The analysis of synovial fluid in gout cases reflects an inflammatory type of change with leukocytosis and the identification in sediment particularly of inflamed synovial fluid and of intracellular and extracellular needle-shaped crystals that have a characteristic negative birefringence on polarized light microscopy (Fig. 57–12). These morphological changes are useful in differentiating gouty crystals from synovial fluid, contrasting them with other crystals, such as those seen in CPPD disorders. A specific and sensitive technique is to use light microscopy and polarized light microscopy. The addition of a red filter clearly distinguishes the strongly "negative" birefringent crystals. The strongly birefringent crystals parallel to the orientation of the red filter are yellow, and perpendicular crystals are blue (U PAY PEB) (see Fig. 57–12). "Positive" birefringent crystals of CPPD oriented parallel are blue, and crystals oriented perpendicularly are yellow.

Although there may be a genetic component in a large percentage of gout cases, associated diseases are clearly demonstrable. They include, but are not limited to, diabetes, hypertension, hyperparathyroidism, and hypothyroidism. Gout may be precipitated by surgery, including localization around implanted prostheses. Additional associations or risk factors for gout include lymphoproliferative disorders, particularly polycythemia and diuretic therapy.

Perhaps the most important risk factor in gout is the intake of a purine-rich diet in patients genetically or otherwise susceptible to the disorder. Here the biochemical understanding of gout is particularly important. Purines and pyrimidines are nitrogen-containing compounds that may coalesce and, with sugars and phosphates, create nucleotides, which form the elements of RNA and DNA. The ability to synthesize purines is universal among living organisms; the final product of purine metabolism is uric acid.

Most gout is seen in men. A small group of younger patients, with Lesch-Nyhan syndrome, is of biochemical

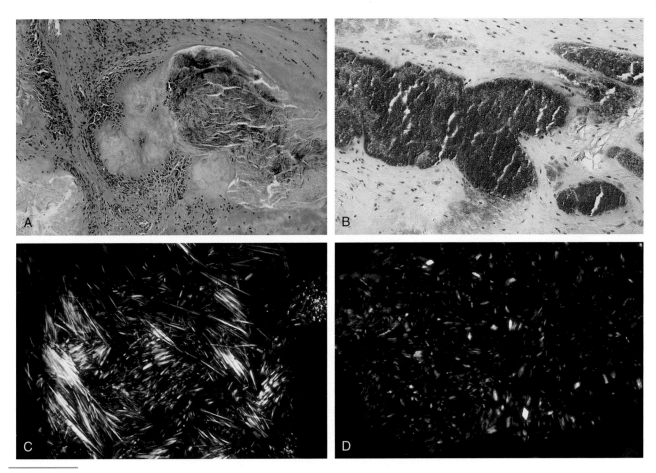

Figure 57–12. Gout versus calcium pyrophosphate crystals. In tissue section, gout **(A)** appears as brown accumulations if not dissolved in routine fixatives *(right)*; otherwise, amorphous whitish spaces remain *(left)*. There is always associated mononuclear and giant cell inflammation. Calcium pyrophosphate deposition (CPPD) **(B)** appears as purple deposits usually without associated inflammation. On polarized light microscopy, gout crystals appear needle-shaped and brilliantly refractive **(C)**. CPPD is less refractile, and crystals are rhomboid in shape **(D)**.

interest because it pinpoints the deficiency of the enzyme hypoxanthine-guanine phosphoribosine transferase, pointing to a primary metabolic defect in at least this rare age group with gout. In other patients, overproduction of uric acid can be linked to high activities of the enzyme phosphoribosyl pyrophosphate synthetase, leading to an increase in the endogenous production of uric acids. These conditions may be associated with genetically transmitted X-linked disorders.

The clinical manifestations of gout have been well described since antiquity. It is characterized clinically by extreme pain around the joints with evident red discoloration of the overlying skin in acute episodes.

Initially, radiographs are unremarkable, with only soft-tissue swelling. With progressive attacks and more urate crystal deposition, tophi, which are granulomatous aggregates of crystals, accumulate in the joint tissue, causing discrete radiolucent marginal erosions of the articular bone. Despite significant bone destruction, joint preservation may be well maintained until late in the disease. Gout may be associated with other crystal deposition disorders, particularly CPPD or hydroxyapatite deposition. Its characteristic radiolucent appearance at times may be admixed with radiodensities.

The gross appearance of gout is that of a chalk-white deposit of pastelike consistency (Fig. 57–13). Histologically, it is characterized in synovial fluid by needle-shaped crystals usually within polymorphonuclear leukocytes and, in tissue specimens, by a characteristic granulomatous inflammatory response. On routine hematoxylin-eosin stain, when crystals have not been dissolved, the crystals have a brown appearance, but sodium urate is particularly soluble in the water component of formalin preparations. More often than not, the deposition is noted by the characteristic amorphous-looking gray deposits surrounded by a mononuclear and giant cell reaction of varying degrees of severity (see Fig. 57–12). As with rheumatoid arthritis, the findings in synovial fluid are characterized by a leukocytosis and in tissue samples by a mononuclear cell population. Crystals from synovial fluid under polarized light often are phagocytosed by inflammatory cells.

Gout has been associated with major surgery, including joint replacements, and osteonecrosis, the mechanism of which is not understood.[4] The clinical differential diagnosis includes septic arthritis.[59] Finally, the relationship between lead toxicity and gout, first noted by Girrard in 1859 and involving renal dysfunction and hypertension,

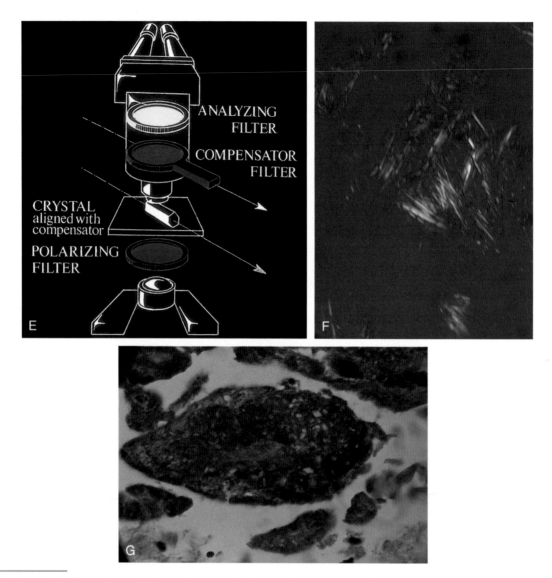

Figure 57–12, cont'd. On polarized light microscopy with a red compensator filter **(E)**, gout (*U*rate) crystals **(F)** are oriented to the red analyzer filter: *Pa*rallel, *y*ellow; *Pe*rpendicular, *blue (U Pay Peb)*. CPPD crystals **(G)** are less oriented, but often in the reverse orientation. By convention, the urate orientation of parallel yellow and perpendicular blue is considered negatively birefringent. Conversely, CPPD orientation is positively birefringent. (From Vigorita VJ: The synovium. In Vigorita VJ: Orthopedic Pathology. Philadelphia, Lippincott/Williams & Wilkins, 1999, pp 516-576.)

also is associated with attacks of acute gouty arthritis or saturnine gout.

Calcium Pyrophosphate Dihydrate Crystal Deposition*

CPPD crystals were first discovered in the early 1960s in the synovial fluid of patients with pseudogout syndrome. CPPD deposition now is well recognized by its radiographic appearance: radiodense linear calcifications seen

*CPPD refers to the crystal (calcium pyrophosphate) deposition in this disorder. *Pseudogout* refers to the occasional painful occurrence of CPPD-induced arthritis mimicking gout. *Chondrocalcinosis* refers to the fine linear radiopaque densities seen in the joint spaces of involved cases.

in articular cartilage, fibrocartilage, and soft tissues of the joints. Although CPPD crystal deposition is commonly seen with such diverse conditions as chronic degenerative arthropathy and acute arthritis, it is more common in older people and is seemingly an age-related phenomenon. It can be distinguished clinically, radiographically, and pathologically from gout (Table 57–3). CPPD crystal formation is seen in at least 25% of Americans by age 80. The variation in the reported incidence of CPPD depends on the site and method of detection. In tissue removed at knee replacement for DJD, CPPD crystals are grossly or microscopically seen in nearly 25% of patients. Although preferentially distributed in the meniscus and the layers of the articular cartilage, all tissue including synovial tissue, ligaments, and tendons may be involved (Fig. 57–14).[2] CPPD is characterized in routine hematoxylin-eosin stain by acellular purplish gray, granular deposits

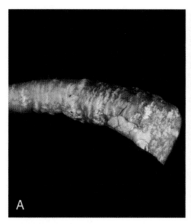
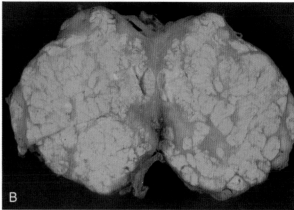

Figure 57–13. Urate crystals seen grossly involving the Achilles tendon **(A)** and synovium **(B)**. The chalk-white deposits have a paste-like consistency. (From Vigorita VJ: The synovium. In Vigorita VJ: Orthopedic Pathology. Philadelphia, Lippincott/Williams & Wilkins, 1999, pp 516-576.)

(see Fig. 57–12). Approximately 50% of the cases reveal positive birefringence on polarized light microscopy with a red analyzer filter. In other cases, crystals may have been cleared by formalin fixation. Inflammation confined to the sites of CPPD may be noted. This localized reaction is seen to a mild degree and usually consists of mononuclear cells. Inflammatory CPPD, or pseudogout, is associated with considerable inflammation, however. Occasionally, giant cells may be seen; the production of loose bodies associated with DJD also may be the site of CPPD deposition. These crystals also have been noted within the confines of other tissue, including cruciate ligaments.

Although the cause of CPPD remains obscure, it seems to be related temporally and microscopically to the degenerative process. Although some clinicians believe crystals are precipitated in the lacuna margin of dying chondrocytes, CPPD deposition has been linked to the deposition to abnormal hypertrophied chondrocytes.[67] Using special stains, Japanese investigators suggested that the proteoglycans normally inhibiting the mineralization are degraded and lost from the extracellular matrix around the chondrocytes, promoting crystal growth.[49] The presence of CPPD in noncartilaginous tissue, such as the synovium, may be explained by initial chondrometaplasia.[67]

Probably the most frequent observation of CPPD deposition is that seen in association with DJD, the cause of which is obscure. That DJD may be associated with changes in the inherent structures of the articular cartilage, such as collagen and proteoglycan, is of interest. Because the cause of CPPD is unknown, it seems that in some cases tissue differentiation toward cartilage may be a precipitating event or substrate for crystal deposition, a concept supported by noting that calcium pyrophosphate crystals deposit preferentially in fibrocartilage tissue throughout the body. It is possible that modification of the proteoglycan structure, such as that seen in chondrometaplasia and often noted in the vicinity of CPPD deposition, may permit calcification to proceed or perhaps that local activation of certain enzymes such as alkaline phosphatase or inorganic pyrophosphatase leads to inactivation of the calcification inhibitors. A subpopulation of patients with CPPD deposition are those in whom CPPD deposits take the form of bulky tumor-like masses in articular and para-articular tissues.[18]

Hydroxyapatite Deposition

Hydroxyapatite crystals are the major crystal component of bone, but extraosseous deposition in the soft tissues of the joint space, rotator cuff tendons, and even bursa suggests that precipitation of these crystals may induce an arthropathy in some clinical situations not dissimilar from

Table 57–3. Synoviotropic Crystal-Associated Disorders

VARIABLE	GOUT	PSEUDOGOUT
Crystal	Sodium urate	Calcium pyrophosphates
Radiograph	Early—soft tissue swelling; later—radiolucent erosions around edge of articular cartilage	Fine, radiopaque, linear deposits in the meniscus and articular cartilage
Frequency of occurrence in knee	Common	Very common; increases with age in DJD
Laboratory studies	Elevated serum uric acid	None
Crystal character with polarized light	Needle-shaped	Rhomboid
Crystal character with compensated polarized light	Parallel, yellow; perpendicular, blue	Parallel, blue; perpendicular, yellow
Birefringence	Negative	Positive

DJD, degenerative joint disease.
From Vigorita VJ: The synovium. In Vigorita VJ, Ghelman B (eds): Orthopaedic Pathology. Philadelphia, Lippincott/Williams & Wilkins, 1999.

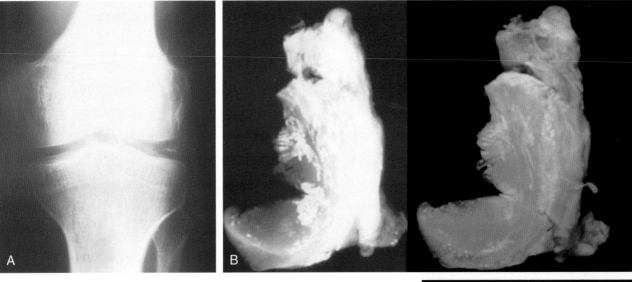

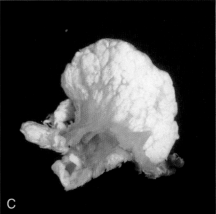

Figure 57–14. Radiograph of the knee in calcium pyrophosphate deposition **(A)**, meniscus gross and specimen x-ray film **(B)**, and synovium **(C)**. (From Vigorita VJ: The synovium. In Vigorita VJ: Orthopedic Pathology. Philadelphia, Lippincott/Williams & Wilkins, 1999, pp 516-576.)

gout or calcium pyrophosphate crystals. The process may be secondary to traumatic injury to the joint or joint structures, DJD, or a primary crystal-induced arthropathy.

Calcium hydroxyapatite is a basic calcium phosphate, and the calcium hydroxyapatite crystals are characteristically nonbirefringent, in contrast to the crystals of gout and pseudogout. Histologically, they are seen as dark-staining clumps usually bluish purple before decalcification and eosinophilic after decalcification. They are similar to bone in their staining characteristics, but can be contrasted with bone in that they lack osteocytes within the mineralized matrix. They may be discernible in synovial fluid and have a variable morphological appearance. The crystals in tissue removed for clinical symptoms may be seen in association with a usually sparse mononuclear and giant cell reaction, but significant erosive changes of adjacent bone may be noted. Radiographically, one observes radiodense calcifications in a wide spectrum of clinical appearances. There may be local deposition in a tumor mass–like fashion or more subtle depositions in periarticular soft tissue. In association with arthropathies, such as DJD, the release of apatite crystals from bone may be a secondary phenomenon in conditions in which crystals are uncovered in synovial fluid analysis. Calcium hydroxyapatite deposition has been described as monarthric and polyarthric, usually occurring in the later

adult years with equal distribution among men and women.

TRANSIENT SYNOVITIS

A common but poorly understood condition that must be differentiated from septic arthritis is transient synovitis. Pain and limitation of movement is common as in effusion (75%). It is seen most commonly in boys.

Effusion, although nonspecific, is the most common radiographic correlate by plain film, MRI, or ultrasound. In general, a temperature greater than 37°C, an erythrocyte sedimentation rate greater than 20 mm/hr, a C-reactive protein level greater than 1 mg/dL, a serum white blood cell count greater than 11,000/mm^3, and a joint space difference greater than 2 mm on radiographs favor septic arthritis.

HYLAN VISCOSUPPLEMENTATION

Hyaluronate, crucial for the normal viscoelasticity of synovial fluid and softening of load transmission, has been

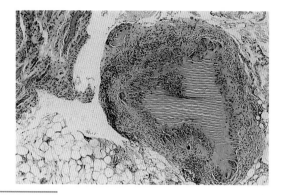

Figure 57–15. Granulomatous reaction to the viscosupplementation agent hylan G-F 20 (Synvisc). (Courtesy of Dr. Panna Desai.)

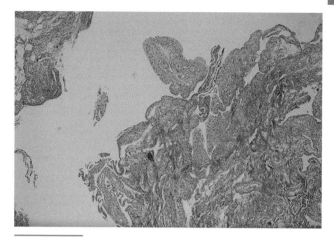

Figure 57–16. Synovial plica histology. Bland fibrous membrane lined with indistinct synovial-like lining cells. (From Vigorita VJ: The synovium. In Vigorita VJ: Orthopedic Pathology. Philadelphia, Lippincott/Williams & Wilkins, 1999, pp 516-576.)

exploited for its therapeutic potential. Commercial hyaluronan preparations, such as sodium hyaluronate (Hyalgan, Supartz) and hylan G-F 20 (Synvisc), are derived naturally and have been modified chemically and used extensively in efforts to relieve pain associated with DJD. Intra-articular injections of these viscous solutions, derived from rooster combs and composed of polymers of N-acetylglucosamine and N-acetylgalactosamine, have been associated with adverse reactions, the most common of which is an inflammatory reaction at the site of injection characterized by pain and swelling.[25] A pseudoseptic process also has been described characterized by inflammation within 24 to 72 hours after injection and by mononuclear cells including macrophages, neutrophils (often in high counts), and eosinophils.[25] Granulomatous inflammation also has been described with chronically inflamed synovium consisting of lymphocytes, monocytes, histiocytes, and foreign-body giant cell reactions surrounding cellular, amorphous material, the latter staining with alcian blue and hyaluronidase digestible, supporting hyaluronate as the culprit (Fig. 57–15).[11] Explanations for the reaction have ranged from immune-mediated reactions to components of the injectable products, direct stimulation of inflammatory and neutrophil mediators, vascular interruption through viscosity effects of hyaluronan, and direct tissue irritation from accompanying elements in the injection.[46]

PLICA

Symptomatic synovial plicae are a recognized but rare cause of anterior knee pain.[36] There are at least three generally recognized plicae: suprapatellar, infrapatellar, and mediopatellar. The mediopatellar plica is the synovial fold most often implicated in pathology of the anterior knee. The infrapatellar plica also is known as the ligamentum mucosum.

Synovial plicae are a common incidental finding at arthroscopy. They are the remnants of incompletely resorbed embryonic septum. Occasionally a medial plica can become inflamed by impinging on the anterior medial femoral condyle as the knee is flexed. When the condition is chronic, the plica becomes thickened and fibrotic. This

is the "medial shelf syndrome." Conservative therapy consisting of nonsteroidal anti-inflammatory drugs and quadriceps exercises is effective in most cases. Arthroscopic resection is indicated if the plica does not respond to conservative therapy. Histologically the resected plica is a nondescript fibrotic band covered with either normal or slightly inflamed synovium (Fig. 57–16).

TUMORS

The various components of the subintimal synovium explain the source of tumors reported in and around the joint:
- Hemangiomas (arterioles)
- Hemangiopericytoma (pericyte of the arteriole)
- Fibromas (fibroblast)
- Leiomyomas (smooth muscle of arteriole wall)
- Lipomas, Hoffa's disease (fat), and lipoma arborescens
- Synovial cysts/ganglion cysts
- Myxomas
- Synovial chondromatosis
- PVNS (fibrohistiocyte)

Malignant tumors arising near joints, such as synovial sarcomas, epithelioid sarcomas, clear cell sarcomas, alveolar soft part sarcomas, extraskeletal myxoid liposarcoma, and metastases, are rare.

Synovial Hemangioma

Synovium, the subintimal layer of which is rich in vasculature, may give rise to hemangiomas. They may be described as localized proliferative vascular tissue, which does not preclude their interpretation as a neoplasm, hamartomatous development, or arteriovenous malformation. All three interpretations have their proponents. Hemangiomas may arise from any structure lined by

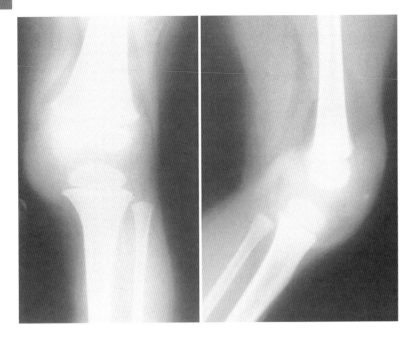

Figure 57–17. Radiograph of synovial hemangioma with increased articular space density. (From Vigorita VJ: The synovium. In Vigorita VJ: Orthopedic Pathology. Philadelphia, Lippincott/Williams & Wilkins, 1999, pp 516-576.)

synovium and have been described as intra-articular and arising from bursal spaces and tendon sheaths.[18]

Synovial hemangioma usually presents as a solitary benign vascular proliferation, most commonly seen in the knee joints of children and adolescents. In one large study, patient age ranged from 9 to 49 years (mean 25 years).[18] Although the patient may be asymptomatic, there may be swelling, mild pain, or limitation of motion, with the pain and swelling in some instances being of several years' duration. The knee is the most common location (60%) followed by the elbow (30%), a distribution similar to that of hemophilic hemarthrosis.

Radiological examination reveals a soft-tissue density suggesting a mass or synovial effusion (Fig. 57–17).[27] In severe cases, it may cause adjacent bone changes, such as periosteal reaction or lucent zones or phleboliths. On MRI, synovial hemangiomas have a high signal intensity on T2-weighted images and intermediate signal intensity on T1-weighted images often with contrast enhancement and fluid-fluid levels (Fig. 57–18).[27]

Gross examination of the knee joint reveals a soft, doughy, brown mass with proliferating villous synovium, frequently mahogany stained by hemosiderin deposition. Histologically, there is proliferation of vascular channels of various sizes and shapes with surrounding hyperplastic synovium (Fig. 57–19). Patterns described have been cavernous (dilated thin-walled vessels), capillary-size proliferation, and large thick-walled vessels predominating.

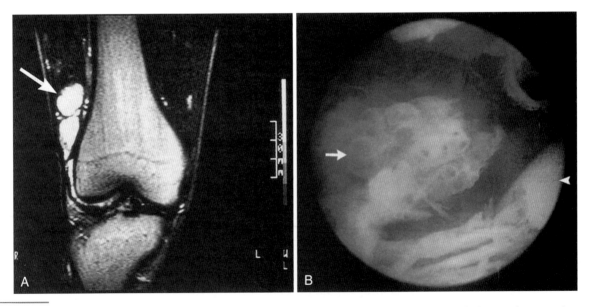

Figure 57–18. Synovial hemangioma. **A,** MRI showing hyperintense signal intensity with bulging of internal capsule. **B,** Arthroscopy showing pedunculated grapelike lesions. (From Macdonald O, Gollish J: Images in clinical medicine. N Engl J Med 341:336, 1999.)

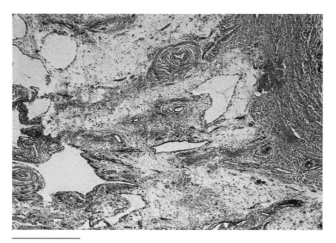

Figure 57–19. Synovial hemangioma. As with hemangiomas in soft tissue, pathology ranges from thick-walled to thin-walled vessels and may show considerable variation as in arteriovenous malformations. (From Vigorita VJ: The synovium. In Vigorita VJ: Orthopedic Pathology. Philadelphia, Lippincott/Williams & Wilkins, 1999, pp 516-576.)

No mitotic activity is seen. Copious hemosiderin may be seen in patients who have had repeated hemarthrosis. Giant cells, aggregates of inflammatory cells, are not seen. Treatment is surgical excision, after which there are no recurrences. The differential diagnosis includes chronic hemarthrosis, which is not characterized by nodular tumorous masses of proliferating blood vessels, and PVNS, a benign neoplasm of collagen-producing fibroblasts and histiocytes.

Hoffa's Disease and Lipoma Arborescens

Fatty proliferation beneath the synovial membrane associated with clinical and radiographic findings can be cat-egorized broadly into Hoffa's disease (infrapatellar fat pad impingement) and lipoma arborescens primarily affecting the suprapatellar region. First noted by Hoffa in 1904, accentuation of the infrapatellar fat pad characterized by hemorrhage, inflammation, fibrin deposition, macrophage infiltration, and degenerative lipocytes was believed to be due to repetitive trauma.[62] In the chronic state, fibrosis and cartilage and osseous metaplasia may ensue. Clinically characterized by anterior knee pain and loss of motion, radiographic features reflect the fat pad hypertrophy characterized on MRI by high signal on T2-weighted images exaggerated with fat saturation (Fig. 57–20). In the chronic state, fibrosis may ensue characterized by regions of decreased signal on T1-weighted images and T2-weighted images.

Lipoma arborescens is located most often in the supra-patella pouch and is characterized by slow-growing, painless swelling with intermittent effusions.[69] The macro-scopic hypertrophied fatty synovium is most frequently villous, but can be diffused or even nodular. MRI shows a high signal intensity similar to subcutaneous fat on T1-weighted images and T2-weighted images and low signal when fat suppressed or on short tau inversion recovery sequences. An intriguing hypothesis taking into consideration the inverse relationship between adipose differentiation and the osteogenic activity of bone marrow stromal cells is that lipoma arborescens and synovial chrondromatosis share a common etiology from reactive synovial change with different endpoints (fatty versus chrondro-osseous).[35]

Juxta-articular Myoma

The juxta-articular myoma or parameniscal cyst is a type of myxoma or ganglion. Typically a poorly circumscribed mass that may enlarge rapidly, it often is associated with pain or tenderness and may be symptomatic for weeks to

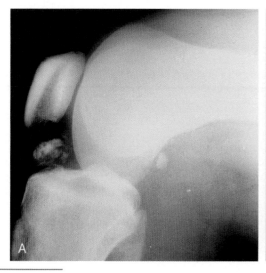
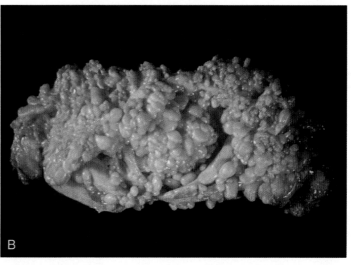

Figure 57–20. **A,** Hoffa's disease: infrapatellar soft-tissue (fatty) mass with circumscribed (secondary) calcification. **B,** Hoffa's disease: abundant excess of grossly identifiable fat. (From Vigorita VJ: The synovium. In Vigorita VJ: Orthopedic Pathology. Philadelphia, Lippincott/Williams & Wilkins, 1999, pp 516-576.)

years.[52] Juxta-articular myomas occur more frequently in men and are seen most typically in the knee followed by the shoulder and elbow. Many cases have been seen in association with DJD or meniscal tears. Histologically, they are composed of spindle and stellate fibroblasts in an abundant myxoid matrix. A secondary fibroblastic reaction may mimic sarcoma. Most myomas occur in the subcutaneous fat with extension to anatomic components of the joint, including the meniscus, tendons, capsule, and synovium.

Synovial (and Ganglion) Cysts

Cysts of the knee joint and related structures primarily may involve a synovial membrane, a bursa, or a poorly lined membranous structure, such as a ganglion. These cysts may be asymptomatic and noted by coincidental MRI or represent primary pathology presenting with pain or a palpable mass.

Popliteal (or Baker's) cysts are the most frequent and best defined anatomicly, the result of joint fluid accumulation between the medial head of the gastrocnemius and the semimembranosus tendon. Pathologically, this membrane-lined cyst often has a synovial-like lining from which it may originate.

A bursa may be defined as a space or potential space between anatomic planes. As such, they may or may not be in communication with the synovium; may or may not have a synovial-like lining; and may mimic all the inflammatory, infectious, hypertrophied, hyperplastic, traumatic, hemorrhagic, and even neoplastic changes of the synovium, including fluid-filled, synovial-like cyst formation.

Ganglion cysts most likely represent the accumulation of fluid within a mucoid cystic degenerative connective tissue matrix. They are characteristically gelatinous and lined by a relatively acellular membrane and located in areas of continuous stress. Popliteal artery aneurysms, popliteal vein varices, tumors such as synovial sarcoma, hematomas, and abscesses all are lesions that can mimic soft-tissue cysts of the knee.[50]

With regard to imaging of synovial cysts, sonography reliably shows a fluid collection and, when present, a rupture. CT shows a homogeneous mass with water density. MRI is characterized by a low signal on T1-weighted images and a high signal of T2-weighted images. Contrast material may enhance the cyst wall and show septations.

Loose Bodies ("Joint Mice")

Loose bodies may occur in any joint, may vary in size and number, and, depending on the cause, may present with a range of pathological tissue (Fig. 57–21).[41] They may be asymptomatic or cause pain and interfere mechanically with joint function, causing limited motion, locking, clicking, limping, and, in extreme cases, subluxation.

Typically consisting of metaplastic cartilage and bone, loose bodies may be formed of fibrin as a result of fibrinous exudation onto the synovial surface in the inflammatory arthritides. In rheumatoid arthritis, they are called rice bodies because of their soft, mushy texture and gross appearance. Synovial loose bodies may result from torsion and infarction of nodular PVNS.

Secondary Chondromatosis

Cartilaginous and osseous loose bodies are the result of DJD, neuropathic joint disease (Charcot's joints), osteochondritis dissecans, meniscal tears, or other trauma. These cartilage segments (with or without underlying bone) may dislodge, fall free into the joint, and continue to grow over prolonged periods. The synovial fluid acts as a virtual culture medium for their growth (Fig. 57–22). Grossly, they may be large or small, cartilaginous or osseous or both, and may or may not show obvious derivation from joint structures such as synovium and fibrocartilage.

Primary Synovial Chondromatosis (Synovial Osteochondromatosis)

The synovium, capable of undergoing metaplasia to cartilage in a broad range of conditions, including trauma and DJD, may produce de novo multiple cartilaginous and chondro-osseous loose bodies throughout the joint unrelated to underlying disease. This latter condition, primary synovial chondromatosis (synovial osteochondromatosis), is best characterized as a benign tumorous proliferation. Initially embedded in the synovium, the nodules may dislodge from the synovium and become free loose bodies ranging in number from a few to hundreds.

Synovial chondromatosis is a monoarthritic condition occurring in the 30s, 40s, and 50s, with predilection for the knee, which is involved in more than two-thirds of cases, followed by the elbow, ankle, hip, and shoulder. It is rare in childhood. It usually is associated with swelling and may be associated with pain, limitation of motion, and occasionally clicking or locking. Radiographically the condition is easily recognized if the cartilaginous bodies have undergone calcification or ossification, which they often do (Fig. 57–23). The numerous radiopaque densities range in size from 1 mm to several centimeters, varying considerably in the extent of calcification and size.[19] Arthrography is useful in diagnosing the noncalcified bodies. Grossly the synovium shows flakelike bodies, or it may possess an irregular nodular contour. Whitish or translucent bluish gray nodules, ranging greatly in size and shape, may be more obviously attached on the membrane or floating in the joint space.

Histopathological differences of these bodies supported a distinction between a secondary synovial chondromatosis associated with DJD and a primary synovial chondromatosis not associated with any underlying disorder. The loose bodies in the secondary synovial chondromatosis show more organized cellular growth, often in concentric

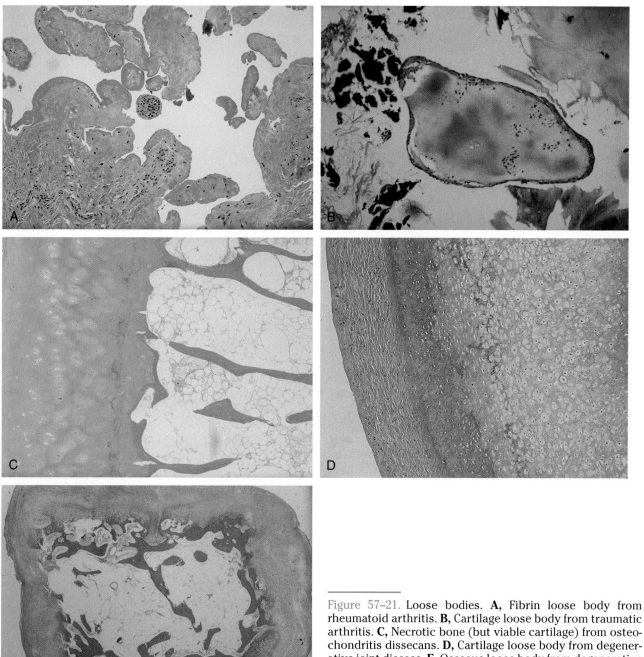

Figure 57–21. Loose bodies. **A,** Fibrin loose body from rheumatoid arthritis. **B,** Cartilage loose body from traumatic arthritis. **C,** Necrotic bone (but viable cartilage) from osteochondritis dissecans. **D,** Cartilage loose body from degenerative joint disease. **E,** Osseous loose body from degenerative joint disease. (From Vigorita VJ: The synovium. In Vigorita VJ: Orthopedic Pathology. Philadelphia, Lippincott/Williams & Wilkins, 1999, pp 516-576.)

rings. Progression is orderly with columns of cells usually identifiable. Zones of endochondral ossification are noted. Transformation between cartilage and bone may be abrupt, however. In the typical case, orderly zones of transformation from fibrocartilage to hyaline-type cartilage through endochondral ossification to bone may be noted.

In primary synovial chondromatosis, a more disorganized lobular proliferation of cartilage is apparent, resembling the lobular chondroid growth patterns of cartilage neoplasms (Fig. 57–24). There are increased chondrocytes, often crowded and irregular in spatial distribution.

Nuclei vary, and binucleate cells may be seen. Calcification may be patchy or diffuse. Endochondral ossification, causing confusion with secondary loose bodies, may be noted. Immunohistochemical studies, including studies showing proliferative cell nuclear antigen–positive chondrocytes, support the neoplastic nature of cartilage in primary synovial chrondromatosis.[64] Surgical removal of all the nodules is important in preventing recurrence.

If the chondro-osseous bodies are entirely free, loose within the joint, a thorough cleaning of the joint may suffice. The disorder may involve chondro-osseous change within the synovial subintimal connective tissue,

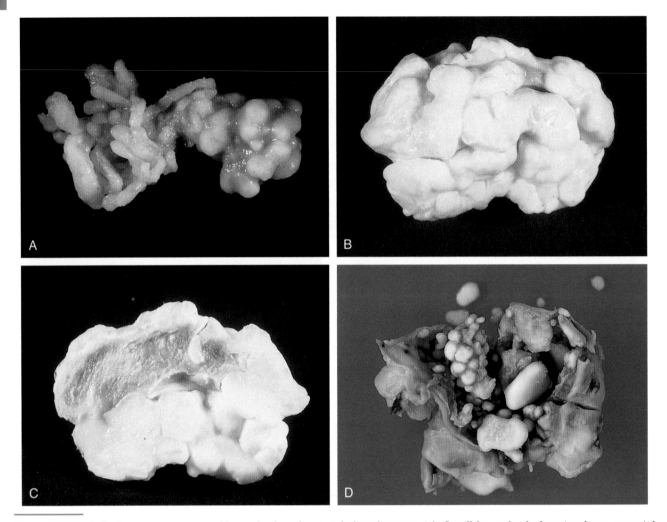

Figure 57–22. A-C, Gross appearance of loose bodies (synovial chondromatosis). Small loose body forming from synovial metaplasia **(A)**, in contrast to large, free-floating loose body with smooth bosselated cartilaginous surface and bony center (**B** and **C**, cross-section). **D,** Gross appearance of synovial chondromatosis. Numerous loose bodies of various sizes and shapes fill the joint space. (From Vigorita VJ: The synovium. In Vigorita VJ: Orthopedic Pathology. Philadelphia, Lippincott/Williams & Wilkins, 1999, pp 516-576.)

however, which may require total synovectomy to prevent recurrence.

Milgram and coworkers[53] suggested a temporal sequence for synovial chondromatosis beginning with active intrasynovial disease with no loose bodies, followed by transition lesions (intrasynovial and loose) and purely loose, floating intra-articular bodies. In this scheme, if the last phase could be identified, synovectomy would not be required.

The MRI appearance of synovial chondromatosis depends on the presence of calcium. Areas of calcification have low signal intensity. Without calcification, it is a low signal intensity equivalent to muscle on T1-weighted sequences with short repetition times and short echo times. With T2-weighted sequences (long repetition times and long echo times), the signal intensity is high, hyaline cartilage being high in water content. Fibrous tissue between the cartilage nodules gives rise to areas of lower signal intensity. A phenomenon similar to synovial chondromatosis may occur within bursae.

Synovial Chondrosarcoma

A malignant tumor arising within the joint is extremely rare. Chondrosarcomas may arise in the setting of synovial chondromatosis, however.[14] This condition is suspected when there is evidence of aggressive growth, such as invasion into adjacent extra-articular tissues. Focal areas of atypical and increased cellularity in an otherwise unremarkable case of synovial chondromatosis should not be overdiagnosed. Synovial chondrosarcoma also may arise as a de novo synovial malignancy. The clinical behavior of these neoplasms varies from that of low-grade neoplasms, with a propensity to recur locally, to neoplasms that may metastasize (primarily to the lungs).

Synovial chondrosarcomas have been reported throughout adult life and have been associated clinically with pain or swelling of usually long-standing duration. The tumor usually involves one joint, the knee more commonly than the hip, elbow, or ankle. Radiographically, there is little to

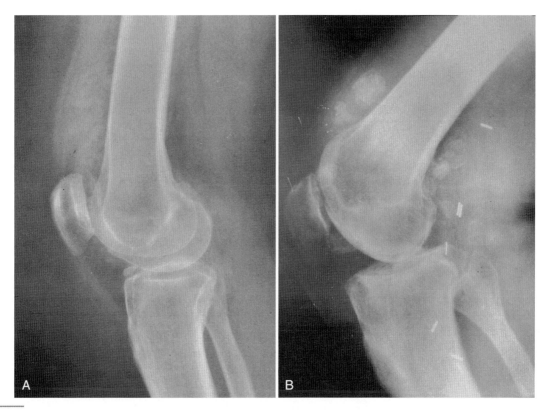

Figure 57–23. **A** and **B,** Synovial chondromatosis of the knee. Lateral radiographs of two different patients show large areas of calcification projecting inside the joint space, with most of the calcified bodies located in the suprapatellar bursa. The density, size, and definition of these bodies vary between the patients. (From Vigorita VJ: The synovium. In Vigorita VJ: Orthopedic Pathology. Philadelphia, Lippincott/Williams & Wilkins, 1999, pp 516-576.)

distinguish it from synovial chondromatosis except, when present, soft-tissue involvement and extensive bone erosion. At operation, cartilaginous lobules extend into the surrounding soft tissue beyond the confines of the joint capsule. Features of chondrosarcoma are seen histologically, including marked cellularity, increased cellularity and spindle cells at the periphery of lobules, scattered sheets of cells, and myxoid change. Treatment is aggressive surgical removal, resection with reconstruction when possible, and amputation if necessary.

The diagnosis of synovial chrondrosarcoma on imaging can be difficult or impossible. A classic case on MRI shows a large soft-tissue mass destroying the cortex infiltrating the bone marrow and often para-articular extension.

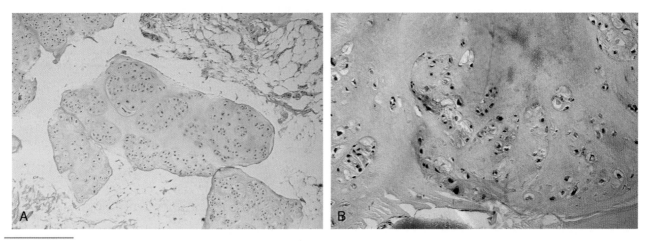

Figure 57–24. **A** and **B,** Primary synovial chondromatosis. Proliferating nodules of cartilage clones are evident, similar to other benign cartilaginous tumors. Atypia and cellularity vary. Calcification and endochondral ossification, when they occur, usually appear less orderly in secondary types. (From Vigorita VJ: The synovium. In Vigorita VJ: Orthopedic Pathology. Philadelphia, Lippincott/Williams & Wilkins, 1999, pp 516-576.)

Pigmented Villonodular Synovitis

PVNS is usually a localized monoarthritic, proliferative process that is found in synovial joints and tendon sheaths, most commonly the knee and the tendon sheaths of the digits of the hand (giant cell tumor of tendon sheath).[1,57] This lesion also is found in the hip, foot, wrist, shoulder, and rarely at other sites. The lesion is rarely polyarticular and does not metastasize, but it may invade bone locally. The localized tenosynovial and diffuse pigmented synovial lesions do not seem to be separate entities, judging from their similar histological characteristics and biological behavior. Tenosynovial nodules in the digits of the hand have been reported to recur in 7% to 45% of patients, and diffuse processes (PVNS) of the knee have been reported to recur in 45% of patients.

Clinical presentations depend on the site. In joint lesions, an insidious onset with swelling, stiffness, or discomfort is common. Swelling without trauma and out of proportion to the degree of discomfort is considered typical. The peak incidence of knee lesions is in the 30s.

The joint fluid color varies, ranging from normal to rusty or brownish red. The synovium may appear diffusely pigmented or, more commonly, focally pigmented. The pigment is due to hemosiderin accumulation from microscopic synovial hemorrhage (brown) and aggregations of lipid-laden macrophages (yellow) in the periphery of expanding nodules. Hyperplastic and pigmented changes mimicking changes of chronic hemarthrosis in the adjacent synovium are secondary in nature and do not represent the lesion proper.

At least five clinical types of PVNS are identified in the knee:[57] loose body, a localized nodule (pedunculated or embedded in the synovium), aggregates of nodules confined to one compartment, a truly diffuse involvement of the synovium, and synovial PVNS extending into bursa (Fig. 57–25). Localized nodular and nodular aggregate types of PVNS are most common.

Typically, PVNS is monoarthritic and usually is observed in early and middle adulthood and rarely at the extreme end of life. Symptoms may be gradual in onset. Clinically, patients may present with discomfort or pain.

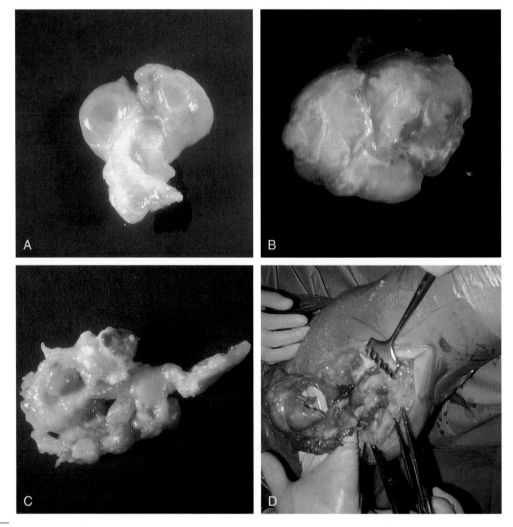

Figure 57–25. Pigmented villonodular synovitis/giant cell tumor of tendon sheath. **A,** Loose body. **B,** Localized nodule (gross appearance, cross-section). **C,** Localized aggregate of multiple nodules. **D,** Diffuse type throughout the joint. (From Vigorita VJ: The synovium. In Vigorita VJ: Orthopedic Pathology. Philadelphia, Lippincott/Williams & Wilkins, 1999, pp 516-576.)

Swelling, stiffness, locking, and instability of the knee may occur. Torsion of a pedunculated nodular form of PVNS has been associated with the unusual clinical presentation of acute pain.[14]

The radiological findings depend on the anatomy of the involved joint (Figs. 57–26 and 57–27). Articulations with close apposition of the capsule of the joint to the underlying bone, such as the hip, soon develop bone erosions secondary to the abnormal synovial masses. In other joints with greater separation between the capsule and bones, such as the knee, where the suprapatellar bursa is placed at a significant distance from the anterior surface of the femur, PVNS usually fails to cause significant bone erosions. The bone erosions are usually well defined, surrounded by minimal or no sclerosis. The erosions most often are located in the bare areas of bone but, at times, can be located in subchondral surfaces. PVNS does not calcify. Often the erosions are located in both sides of a joint, but at times the condition can be unifocal, causing erosions in only one side of the articular space.

The joint space is usually preserved because articular cartilage generally is not eroded. The hip represents an unusual situation because often these patients first present with narrowing of the joint space.

The differential diagnosis for PVNS includes any soft-tissue mass that causes erosions of adjacent bones, such as gout, rheumatoid nodules, tuberculosis arthritis, or juxtacortical chondromas. The absence of osteoporosis, joint space narrowing, or calcifications is helpful in making the correct diagnosis of PVNS.

The most common radiographic findings in the knee are soft-tissue swelling (see Fig. 57–26). Arthrograms may best show the nodules as discrete pitting defects. Bone changes are less frequent but may include erosions and degenerative changes. MRI has revealed an isointense or low signal intensity compared with that muscle on T1-weighted and T2-weighted images.[34] Findings vary, however, depending on the amount of hemosiderin, lipid, cellularity, and fibrosis. Edema leads to increased T2-weighted images. Significant enhancement after intravenous injection of gadolinium may be observed.

The treatment of PVNS is surgical. If an isolated loose body or nodule is confirmed, arthroscopic surgical excision may be attempted. The propensity of the lesions to

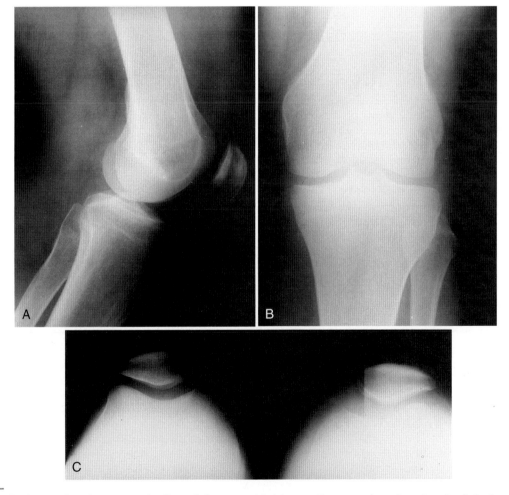

Figure 57–26. Radiographs of pigmented villonodular synovitis/giant cell tumor of tendon sheath of the knee. Soft-tissue masses as evidenced by fullness in posterior compartment **(A)**, fullness of lateral shadows on anteroposterior view **(B)**, and asymmetric shadowing on tunnel view **(C)**. (From Vigorita VJ: The synovium. In Vigorita VJ: Orthopedic Pathology. Philadelphia, Lippincott/Williams & Wilkins, 1999, pp 516-576.)

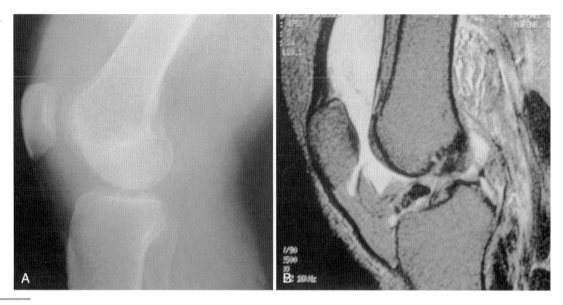

Figure 57–27. Pigmented villonodular synovitis. **A,** Lateral radiograph shows fullness of the suprapatellar region resulting from intra-articular effusion. **B,** T2-weighted sagittal MRI shows areas of signal void anterior to the anterior cruciate ligament and adjacent to the anterior border of the tibial plateau caused by hemosiderin deposition. Notice the large effusion in the suprapatellar bursa. (From Vigorita VJ: The synovium. In Vigorita VJ: Orthopedic Pathology. Philadelphia, Lippincott/Williams & Wilkins, 1999, pp 516-576.)

recur (in one third of cases) requires careful examination, however, of the remainder of the joint to exclude multiple foci. Smaller nodules may be missed, embedded as they are in the subintimal synovial layers. Recurrences may occur many years after initial treatment.

The diffuse form of PVNS is more problematic and requires total synovectomy. External-beam radiation and intra-articular radiation synovectomy have been used for problematic recurrent disease, the latter with dysprosium 165.[12] Maximum penetration of dysprosium has been estimated at 5.7 mm, roughly equivalent to inflamed synovium, and this probably is ineffective in very invasive disease.[12]

In one series, despite synovectomy for diffuse PVNS, complications included stiffness requiring manipulation, reflex sympathetic dystrophy, advanced osteoarthritis leading to joint replacement, and a recurrence rate of 18% despite operative and radiation treatment.[13] MRI may help in detecting recurrences elusive on clinical examination and recurrences with extrasynovial spread.[12]

If not removed, PVNS continues to grow and erodes into the articular bone. Bursal PVNS also requires adequate surgical excision and may extend deeply into surrounding soft tissue. On the basis of ultrastructural and immunohistochemical findings, PVNS/giant cell tumor of tendon sheath can be considered a tumorous proliferation of fibroblasts and histiocytes (i.e., a benign fibrous histiocytoma) (Fig. 57–28).[68]

Grossly the lesions usually are categorized as nodular or villonodular. Solitary nodules or aggregates of confluent nodules are designated nodular. Poorly delineated lesions, characterized by plump synovial villi and by small unencapsulated nodules, not contiguous to one another and often blending into the surrounding tissue, are designated villonodular.

No relationship between duration of symptoms and extent of the fibrosis is evident, indicating that these lesions do not become progressively fibrotic with time. Distinct hyperplasia of the synovial tissue adjacent to the lesion is often present. The giant cells usually are arranged in groups, and there are two types of these cells: One is a truly phagocytic, often densely staining multinucleated cell, and the other is a more inconspicuous cell whose characteristics suggest that it had been formed by fusion of the predominant vesicular, mononuclear, polyhedral stromal cells. Giant cells of the second type are seen commonly in rheumatoid synovitis and may represent multinucleated lining cells of the synovial membrane that are reacting to the proliferating lesions.

Although complete excision of a single nodule or multiple nodules is thought to be essential, total synovectomy may not be necessary. If total synovectomy is not performed, stiffness, a common postoperative complication of this procedure, may be prevented. Untreated, PVNS may erode and infiltrate surrounding structures, including bone.

Although it has been suggested that PVNS is an inflammatory process, its polyclonal proliferation, insignificant degree of inflammation, nodular growth pattern, propensity for recurrence after inadequate removal, and distinct lack of the changes characteristic of the lesion in the adjacent synovial tissue suggest that this is not the case. Inflammatory synovitis generally is a diffuse process without nodular changes. The evidence for an inflammatory cause was based partially on the observation that lesions tend to undergo progressive fibrosis. There does not seem to be any relationship between the degree of fibrosis and either the duration of symptoms or the size of the lesion, however. In patients for whom serial biopsy specimens were available or a recurrent lesion was

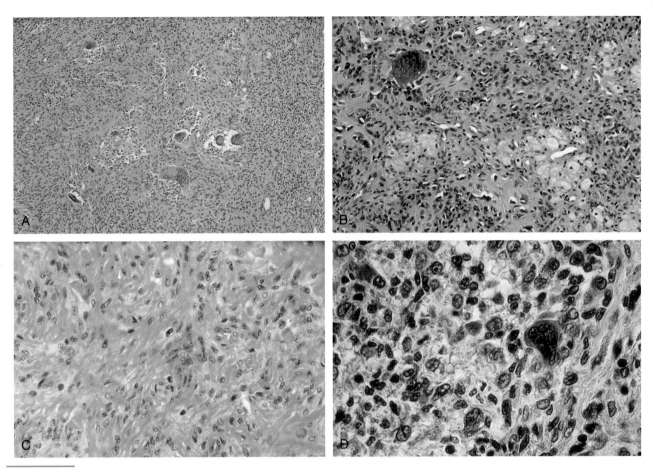

Figure 57–28. Pigmented villonodular synovitis/giant cell tumor of tendon sheath. **A,** Low power reveals sheets of mononuclear cells (fibroblasts and histiocytes) with interspersed giant cells awash in a collagen stroma. **B,** Higher power shows that xanthomatous cells are usually focal in distribution, notably in the periphery of lesions; little or no inflammation is evident. **C,** Collagen may predominate in a sea of spindly fibroblasts. **D,** Large multinucleated giant cell whose clear nucleus with prominent dense-staining nucleoli is similar to the proliferating surrounding mononuclear cells. (From Vigorita VJ: The synovium. In Vigorita VJ: Orthopedic Pathology. Philadelphia, Lippincott/Williams & Wilkins, 1999, pp 516-576.)

studied, no histological evidence of progressive fibrotic changes was seen. In most cases, PVNS seems to be a benign synovial neoplasm with the potential for local recurrence. Because pigmentation of the lesion is secondary to iron deposition, and the lesion is usually nodular and rarely shows inflammatory changes, its name is inappropriate.

The differential diagnosis includes benign and neoplastic conditions. Hemosideric synovitis, as is seen in hemophilia, and chronic synovitis, caused by either rheumatoid arthritis or trauma, do not have a distinct submembranous nodule or nodules composed of proliferating mononuclear and giant cells. Monophasic synovial sarcoma is differentiated by its characteristic increased cellularity, cellular pleomorphism, lack of fibrosis, and high mitotic counts. Other rare lesions, such as angioma, hemangiopericytoma, histiocytoma, and fibroma, are morphologically homogeneous and histologically distinct.

Atypical and malignant variants of PVNS have been described,[70] further substantiating the neoplastic nature of this lesion. Malignant PVNS has been described in the knee, ankle, cheek, foot, and thigh.[6] Cases of primary malignant and transformed benign PVNS are postulated.

Bertoni and associates[6] suggested the following features of malignancy:
1. Infiltrative pattern
2. Large, plump cells with eosinophilic cytoplasm
3. Large nuclei and prominent nucleoli
4. Necrotic areas

Four patients in Bertoni's series[6] died with metastases (four pulmonary nodes, two inguinal nodes). Patients with malignant PVNS tend to be older with a significant history of local recurrence. The presence of consistent chromosome trisomies in some patients with malignant disease has been suggested to support a neoplastic nature for PVNS.[45]

Synovium (Miscellaneous)

Synovial thickening manifest as a low signal on T2-weighted MRI includes fibrous lesions (e.g., synovial fibroma and PVNS) and amyloid deposition. Amyloid, most commonly deposited first in the walls of vessels, should be suspected in cases of renal failure, which is associated with β_2-microglobulin amyloidosis. All amyloids are characterized by apple-green birefringence on polarized light microscopy after staining the tissue with Congo red.

Malignant Tumors

EPITHELIOID SARCOMA

Epithelioid sarcoma is a malignant soft-tissue sarcoma of unknown histogenesis that primarily affects the subcutaneous tissue, fascia, and tendon sheaths of the extremities.[9] It is most commonly seen in the upper extremities as a small, painless, subcutaneous nodule. Because of associated inflammation and necrotizing granulomatous-like reactions, it may be confused with a benign process. It most often occurs in young men (mean age 23 years) and tends to recur locally after excision. Progression along tendon sheath and lymphatic pathways has been shown. A poor prognosis is associated with tumors larger than 3 cm; tumors that are deeply situated in the soft tissue; and tumors with high mitotic activity, nuclear pleomorphism, and vascular or nerve invasion.[61] Focal necrosis may indicate a worse prognosis.

Although it appears benign, epithelioid sarcoma must be removed at the initial approach. Poor results have been obtained with marginal resection. Wide or radical resection usually is required. Workup should include radiographs of the involved extremity and chest, MRI to assess local tumor spread, and CT scans of the chest for pulmonary metastases.

Microscopically, cells range from plump spindle cells to rounded or polygonal cells with deep eosinophilic cytoplasm. Resemblance to squamous cells or other epithelial cells has given rise to the name "epithelioid." Characteristic of epithelioid sarcoma is the macroscopic clustering of cells around areas of necrosis in a granulomatous-like fashion.

Varying degrees of fibrosis, cellularity, infiltration, necrosis, and mitotic activity have been described. Immunohistochemically the lesions are vimentin and keratin positive, a coexpression deemed typical. Metastases occur in approximately 40% of cases, unusually following multiple recurrences, which occur in about 70% of cases depending on the adequacy of initial excision.[61] The lungs are primarily involved in metastases.

CLEAR CELL SARCOMA

Clear cell sarcomas are rare neoplasms attached to tendons or aponeuroses. On MRI, the lesion has a slightly increased intensity on T1-weighted images compared with muscle in most cases. The lesions are slow growing and usually painless.

A clear cell sarcoma is composed of a compact mass of polygonal cells, some having a spindle appearance, often with multinucleation. Mitotic activity is scarce. The prognosis for patients with clear cell sarcoma is poor. The lesion has a high recurrence rate, and distant metastases occur within 10 years, often to the lung and bones. As with most soft-tissue sarcomas, size greater than 5 cm, necrosis and local recurrence are unfavorable prognostic factors.[16]

Clear cell sarcoma now is generally believed to originate from the neural crest based on the histochemical demonstration of melanin and the ultrastructural demonstration of premelanosomes. The immunophenotype is positive for S100 protein, HMB45, and other melanoma antigens in almost all cases. Its cytogenic hallmark is the presence of a reciprocal translocation, t(12;22) q13:q12), resulting in a fusion of the *EWS* (22q 12) and *ATF₁* (12q 13) genes.

ALVEOLAR SOFT PART SARCOMA

Alveolar soft part sarcoma constitutes less than 1% of soft tissue sarcomas and is characterized histologically by large granular cells dispersed in "alveolus"-like patterns separated by vascular channels. Seen most commonly in women in their 20s to 40s, it is slow growing but pulsatile, and bruits may be heard. Metastases to the lungs, bones, and brain occur. MRI patterns are high signal intensity relative to muscle on T1-weighted imaging with flow voids. Ten-year disease-free survival is about 50%.

Although there are no consistent immunohistochemical findings, a cytogenetic specific alteration, der (17) t(x;17) (p11; q25), has been shown to result in the fusion of the TFE_3 transcription factor. The lesion is highly metastatic. Poor prognostic factors include tumor size and the presence of matastases at diagnosis.[58]

SYNOVIAL SARCOMA

Synovial sarcoma is a malignant mesenchymal tumor that shows epithelial differentiation (often glandular) and has a specific chromosomal translocation: t(x;18) (p11;q11). It usually arises in structures adjacent to the joint, most often in a bursa or tenosynovium lining anatomic joint structures. It derives its name from the microscopic appearance, which mimics the histological appearance of the embryonic synovium. The anatomic location outside the joint and the occurrence of synovial sarcoma in tissue such as the pleura suggest that the tumor arises from mesenchymal tissue, not synovium. It occurs in close association with tendon sheaths, bursa, and joint capsules and has a propensity to differentiate toward a spindle cell–like or fibroblast-like mesoderm cell population and an epithelial population, giving it, in its classic presentation, a biphasic microscopic appearance. Intra-articular synovial sarcoma accounts for 10% of cases.[51] It is the fourth most common soft-tissue sarcoma, accounting for approximately 10% of all malignant mesenchymal neoplasms. It is most prevalent in patients between the ages of 15 and 35 years, and it characteristically presents as a painful, palpable soft-tissue mass.

The radiographic presentation of this malignant tumor is most often that of a soft-tissue mass, which in nearly 50% of cases is calcified. The calcifications can be dense, faint, or punctuated. The soft-tissue mass usually is located close to but outside a joint space. The growth of the tumor eventually results in extension into the adjacent joint and invasion and destruction of the adjacent bones.

CT and MRI are sensitive technologies in the demonstration of the soft-tissue tumor mass that forms synovial sarcoma. The adjacent anatomic structures (muscles, tendons, blood vessels, and nerves) are usually displaced, but at times may be invaded by the tumor. The calcifications of synovial sarcoma, if present, are best shown by CT. Areas of necrosis may develop, especially in the large synovial sarcomas, resulting in areas of lucency on CT hypointense compared with muscle on T1-weighted images and heterogeneous or high on T2-weighted images depending on the presence and degree of hemorrhage and necrosis. As with many soft-tissue sarcomas, a peripheral halo may suggest reactive edema. The dimensions of the tumor are a significant factor. In one multivariate analysis of 135 cases, size greater than 10 cm and size 5 to 10 cm were associated with an 18-fold increased risk of death compared with tumors smaller than 5 cm.[17] The more peripheral synovial sarcomas tend to have a better prognosis compared with tumors located more centrally.

Approximately 70% of synovial sarcomas occur in the lower extremity.

Histologically the tumor may be biphasic (approximately 15%), monophasic fibrous (approximately 63%), and poorly differentiated (22%). The biphasic tumor is diagnosed by the identification of a biphasic cell population (Fig. 57–29). Immunocytochemical and immunohistological staining showed a mesenchymal tissue in one component and epithelial differentiation in the other. Descriptions in the literature of monophasic variants of synovial sarcoma with a predominance of one of these two cell types raises questions about classification.

Monophasic variants tend to occur in distal extremity locations and may carry a poorer prognosis. Prognosis may be related to gross anatomic and histological findings, with a better prognosis in younger patients with tumors smaller than 5 cm, tumors located in the lower extremity with an epithelial gland cellularity greater than 50%, and a mitotic activity of less than 15 mitoses/10 high-power field.[55] Mast cells fewer than 20 mitoses/high-power field, tumor necrosis, presence of rhomboid cells, percent glandularity less than 50%, and later stage are possible additional poor prognostic factors.[55] An additional poor

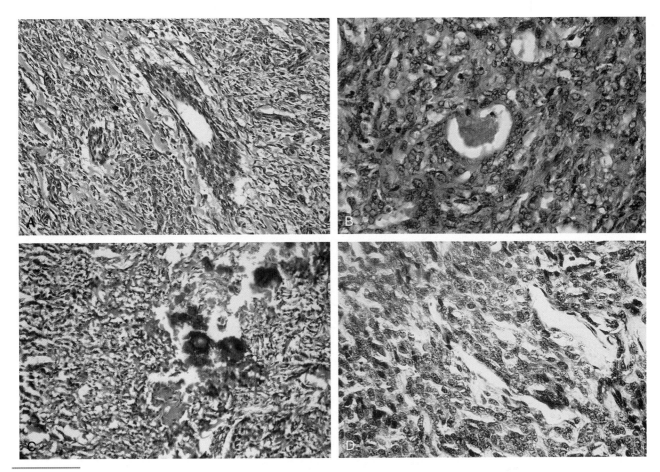

Figure 57–29. Synovial sarcoma. **A,** In biphasic synovial sarcoma, glandlike structures are seen in distinction with a spindle-shaped sarcomatous component. **B,** The epithelial (gland) structures may stand out or blend in with the stroma component. **C,** Calcification is irregular and may aggregate sufficiently to be seen radiographically. **D,** Monophasic synovial sarcoma is characterized by the typical cleftlike avascular spaces. (From Vigorita VJ: The synovium. In Vigorita VJ: Orthopedic Pathology. Philadelphia, Lippincott/Williams & Wilkins, 1999, pp 516-576.)

prognostic factor is increased staining with antibody to proliferating cell nuclear antigen.

These malignant lesions recur locally and spread by regional lymph node and pulmonary metastatic routes. Metastases to the lung occur in 75% of patients; to regional lymph nodes, in 15%; and to bone, in 10%.[37] It is the most common soft-tissue sarcoma to metastasize to lymph nodes. Five-year survival rates have been reported to be 21%.

Wide resection or amputation is the traditional approach to treatment. Patients with lesions greater than 5 cm or presenting with locally recurrent disease should be considered high risk and should receive adjuvant therapies (radiation or chemotherapy or both). A multimodality approach involving surgery, radiotherapy, and combined chemotherapy may improve survival in this highly malignant tumor. In one study of 14 patients with nonmetastasizing synovial sarcoma, encouraging results were achieved with intensive chemotherapy (high-dose cisplatin and doxorubicin or high-dose ifosfamide and cisplatin with doxorubicin) and local radiation followed by surgical resection and, in some patients, postoperative chemotherapy.[37] In a similar protocol, event-free survival at 5 years was 75%.[43] Chemotherapy (high-dose ifosfamide) may play a role in metastatic synovial sarcoma.[37]

Characteristic genetic findings include abnormal *bcl-2* proto-oncogene activity.[31] A characteristic *SYT-SSX* fusion gene resulting from the chromosome translocation t(X; 18) (p11; q11) is detectable in almost all synovial sarcomas and has been reported to be of prognostic significance. Kawai and coworkers[38] found a significant difference between monophasic and biphasic tumors. All biphasic tumors had a *SYT-SSX1* fusion transcript. All monophasic tumors that had a *SYT-SSX2* fusion had a significantly better metastasis-free survival.

References

1. Abdul-Karim FW, El-Naggar AK, Joyce MJ, et al: Diffuse and localized tenosynovial giant cell tumor and pigmented villonodular synovitis: A clinicopathologic and flow cytometric DNA analysis. Hum Pathol 23:729, 1992.
2. Abreu M, Johnson K, Chung CB, et al: Calcification in calcium pyrophosphate dehydrate (CPPD) crystalline deposits in the knee: Anatomic, radiographic, MR imaging, and histologic study in cadavers. Skeletal Radiol 33:392, 2004.
3. Adams PC, Kertesz AE, Valberg LS: Clinical presentation of hemochromatosis: A changing scene. Am J Med 90:445, 1991.
4. Archibeck MJ, Rosenberg AG, Sheinkop MB, et al: Gout induced arthropathy after total knee arthroplasty: A report of two cases. Clin Orthop 392:377, 2001.
5. Bennett GL, Leeson MC, Michael A: Extensive hemosiderin deposition in the medial meniscus of a knee: Its possible relationship to degenerative joint disease. Clin Orthop 230:182, 1988.
6. Bertoni F, Unni KK, Beabout JW, et al: Malignant giant cell tumor of the tendon sheaths and joints (malignant pigmented villonodular synovitis). Am J Pathol 21:153, 1997.
7. Bolanos AA, Demizio JP, Vigorita VJ, et al: Lead poisoning from an intra-articular shotgun pellet in the knee treated with arthroscopic extraction and chelation therapy: A case report. J Bone Joint Surg Am 78:422, 1996.
8. Bolanos AA, Vigorita VJ, Meyerson RI, et al: Intra-articular histopathologic changes secondary to local lead intoxication in rabbit knee joints. J Trauma 38:668, 1995.
9. Bos GD, Pritchard DJ, Reiman HM, et al: Epitheloid sarcoma: An analysis of 51cases. J Bone Joint Surg Am 70:862, 1988.
10. Burmester GR, Dimitriu-Bona A, Waters SJ, et al: Identification of three major living cell populations by monoclonal antibodies directed to Ia antigens and antigens associated with monocytes/macrophages and fibroblasts. Scand J Immunol 17:69, 1983.
11. Chen AL, Desai P, Adler EM, et al: Granulomatous inflammation after Hylan G-F 20 viscosupplementation of the knee: A report of six cases. J Bone Joint Surg Am 84:1142, 2002.
12. Chin KR, Barr SJ, Winalski C, et al: Treatment of advanced primary and recurrent diffuse pigmented villonodular synovium. J Bone Joint Surg Am 84:2192, 2002.
13. Chin KR, Brick GW: Extra-articular pigmented villonodular synovitis: A cause for failed knee arthropathy. Clin Orthop 404:330, 2002.
14. Davis RI, Hamilton A, Biggart JD: Primary synovial chrondromatosis: A clinicopathologic review and assessment of malignant potential. Hum Pathol 29:683, 1998.
15. DeBari C, Dell'Accio F, Tylzanowski P: Multipotential mesenchymal stem cells from adult human synovial membrane. Arthritis Rheum 44:1928, 2001.
16. Deenik W, Hooi WJ, Rutgers EJ, et al: Clear cell sarcoma (malignant melanoma) of soft parts: A clinicopathologic study of 30 cases. Cancer 86:969, 1999.
17. Deshmukh R, Mankin HJ, Singer S: Synovial sarcoma: The importance of size and location for survival. Clin Orthop 419:155, 2004.
18. Devaney K, Vinh TN, Sweet DE: Synovial hemangioma: A report of 20 cases with differential diagnostic considerations. Hum Pathol 24:737, 1993.
19. Edeiken J, Edeiken BS, Ayala AG, et al: Giant solitary synovial chondromatosis. Skeletal Radiol 23:23, 1994.
20. Edwards JCW, Sedgwick AD, Willoughby DA: The formation of a structure with the features of synovial lining by subcutaneous injection of air: An in vivo tissue culture system. J Pathol 134:147, 1981.
21. Firestein GS: Etiology and pathogenesis of rheumatoid arthritis. In Ruddy S, Harris E, Sledge C (eds): Kelly's Textbook of Rheumatology, 6th ed. Philadelphia, Saunders, 2001, pp 921-966.
22. France MP, Gupta SK: Nonhemophilic hemosiderotic synovitis of the shoulder: A case report. Clin Orthop 262:132, 1991.
23. Gaary E, Gorlin JB, Jaramillo D: Pseudotumor and arthropathy in the knees of a hemophiliac Skeletal Radiol 25:85, 1996.
24. Gilbert MS, Radomisli TE: Therapeutic options in the management of hemophilic synovitis. Clin Orthop 343:88, 1997.
25. Goldberg VM, Coutts RD: Pseudoseptic reactions to Hylan viscosupplementation: Diagnosis and treatment. Clin Orthop 419:130, 2004.
26. Gordeux V, Mukiibi J, Hasstedt SJ, et al: Iron overload in Africa: Interaction between a gene and dietary iron content. N Engl J Med 326:95, 1992.
27. Greenspan A, Azouz M, Matthews J, et al: Synovial hemangioma: Imaging features in eight histologically proven cases, review of the literature, and differential diagnosis. Skeletal Radiol 24:583, 1995.
28. Hameed MR, Erlandson R, Rosen PP: Capsular synovial-like hyperplasia around mammary implants similar to detritic synovitis: A morphologic and immunohistochemical study of 15 cases. Am J Surg Pathol 19:433, 1995.
29. Hamilton JB: Human immunodeficiency virus and the orthopaedic surgeon. Clin Orthop 328:31, 1996.
30. Hammerman D: The biology of osteoarthritis. N Engl J Med 320:1322, 1989.
31. Hirakawa N, Naka T, Yamamoto I, et al: Overexpression of bcl-2 protein in synovial sarcoma: A comparative study of other soft tissue spindle cell sarcomas and an additional analysis by fluorescence in situ hybridization. Hum Pathol 27:1060, 1996.
32. Ho G Jr, DeNuccio M: Gout and pseudogout in hospitalized patients. Arch Intern Med 153:2787, 1993.
33. Howie CR, Smith GD, Christie J, et al: Torsion of localized pigmented villonodular synovitis of the knee. J Bone Joint Surg Br 67:654, 1985.
34. Hughes TH, Sartoris DJ, Schweitzer ME, et al: Pigmented villonodular synovitis: MRI characteristics. Skeletal Radiol 24:7, 1995.
35. Ikushima K, Ueda T, Kudawara I, et al: Lipoma arborescens of the knee as a possible cause of osteoarthrosis. Orthopedica 24:603, 2001.

36. Johnson DP, Eastwood DM, Witherow PJ: Symptomatic synovial plicae of the knee. J Bone Joint Surg Am 75:1485, 1993.

37. Kampe CE, Rosen G, Eilber F, et al: Synovial sarcoma: A study of intensive chemotherapy in 14 patients with localized disease. Cancer 72:2161, 1993.

38. Kawai A, Woodruff J, Healey JH, et al: SYT-SSX gene fusion as a determinant of morphology and prognosis in synovial sarcoma. N Engl J Med 338:153, 1998.

39. Kleftogiannis F, Handley CJ, Campbell MA: Characterization of extracellular matrix macromolecules from bovine synovial capsule. J Orthop Res 12:365, 1994.

40. Komuya AS, Inoue A, Sasaguri Y, et al: Rapidly destructive arthropathy of the hip: Studies on bone resorption factors in joint with a theory of pathogenesis. Clin Orthop 284:273, 1992.

41. Krebs VE: The role of hip arthroscopy in the treatment of synovial disorders and loose bodies. Clin Orthop 406:48, 2003.

42. Kremer JM, Westhovens R, Leon M, et al: Treatment of rheumatoid arthritis by selective inhibition of T-cell activation with fusion protein CTLA 4 Ig. N Engl J Med 349:1907, 2003.

43. Ladenstein R, Treuner J, Koscielniak E, et al: Synovial sarcoma of childhood and adolescence: Report of the German CWS-81 study. Cancer 71:3647, 1993.

44. Larsson SA: Hemophilia in Sweden. Acta Med Scand 5(Suppl):1, 1984.

45. Layfield LJ, Meloni-Ehrig A, Liu K, et al: Malignant giant cell tumor of synovium (malignant pigmented villonodular synovitis). Arch Pathol Lab Med 124:1636, 2000.

46. Leopold SS, Warme WJ, Pettis PD, et al: Increased frequency of acute local reaction to intra-articular hylan G-F 20 (Synvisc) in patients receiving more than one course of treatment. J Bone Joint Surg Am 84:1619, 2002.

47. Liu W, Barton-Wurster N, Glant TT, et al: Spontaneous and experimental osteoarthritis in dog: Similarities and differences in proteoglycan levels. J Orthop Res 21:730, 2003.

48. Maffulli N, Binfield PM, King JB, et al: Acute haemarthrosis of the knee in athletes: A prospective study of 106 cases. J Bone Joint Surg Br 75:945, 1993.

49. Masuda I, Ishikawa K, Usuku G: A histologic and immunohistochemical study of calcium pyrophosphate dihydrate crystal deposition disease. Clin Orthop 263:272, 1991.

50. McCarthy CL, McNally EG: The MRI appearance of cystic lesions around the knee. Skeletal Radiol 33:187, 2004.

51. McKinney CD, Mills SE, Fechner RE: Intraarticular synovial sarcoma. Am J Surg Pathol 16:1017, 1992.

52. Meis JM, Enzinger FM: Juxta-articular myxoma: A clinical and pathologic study of 65 cases. Hum Pathol 23:639, 1992.

53. Milgram JW, Gilden JJ, Gilula LA: Multiple loose bodies: Formation revascularization and resorption: A 29-year follow-up study. Clin Orthop 322:152, 1996.

54. Norian JM, Ries MD, Karp S, et al: Total knee arthroplasty in hemophilic arthropathy. J Bone Joint Surg Am 84:1138, 2002.

55. Oda Y, Hashimoto H, Tsuneyoshi M, et al: Survival in synovial sarcoma: A multivariate study of prognostic factors with special emphasis on the comparison between early death and long-term survival. Am J Surg Pathol 17:35, 1993.

56. Portera CA Jr, Ho V, Pastel SR, et al: Alveolar soft part sarcoma: Clinical course and patterns of metastasis in 70 patients treated at a single institution. Cancer 91:585, 2001.

57. Rao S, Vigorita VJ: Pigmented villonodular synovitis (giant-cell tumor of the tendon sheath and synovial membrane): A review of eighty-one cases. J Bone Joint Surg Am 66:76, 1984.

58. Rodriguez-Merchan EC: Effects of hemophilia on articulations of children and adults. Clin Orthop 338:7, 1996.

59. Rogachefsky RA, Carneiro R, Altman RD, et al: Gout presenting as infectious arthritis. J Bone Joint Surg Am 76:269, 1994.

60. Rosen G, Forscher C, Lowenbraun S, et al: Synovial sarcoma: Uniform response of metastases to high dose ifosfamide. Cancer 73:2506, 1994.

61. Ross HM, Lewis JJ, Woodruff JM, et al: Epitheloid sarcoma: Clinical behavior and prognostic factors of survival. Ann Surg Oncol 4:491, 1997.

62. Saddik O, McNally EG, Richardson M: MRI for Hoffa's fat pad. Skeletal Radiol 33:433, 2004.

63. Safran MR, Johnston-Jones K, Kabo JM, et al: The effect of experimental hemarthrosis on joint stiffness and synovial histology in a rabbit model. Clin Orthop 303:280, 1994.

64. Salome K, Tamai K, Koguchi Y, et al: Growth potential of loose bodies: An immunohistochemical examination of primary and secondary synovial osteochandromatos. J Orthop Res 17:73, 1999.

65. Schumacher HR: Pathologic findings in rheumatoid arthritis. In Schumacher RH, Gall EP (eds): Rheumatoid Arthritis: An Illustrated Guide to Pathology, Diagnosis, and Management. Philadelphia, JB Lippincott, 1988, pp 4.1-4.36.

66. Sone M, Ehara S, Kashiwagi K, et al: Case report 859. Skeletal Radiol 23:475, 1994.

67. Vigorita VJ: Arthropathy in calcium pyrophosphate dihydrate crystal deposition disease. Arch Pathol Lab Med 107:275, 1993.

68. Vigorita VJ, Nakata K: Ultrastructural findings in nine cases of pigmented villonodular synovitis. Proceedings of the 29th Annual Meeting of the Orthopedic Research Society, Anaheim, CA, 1983, p 190.

69. Vilanova JC, Barcelo J, Villalon M, et al: MRI imaging of lipoma arborescens and the associated lesions. Skeletal Radiol 32:504, 2003.

70. Vogrincic GS, O'Connell JX, Gilks CB: Giant cell tumor of tendon sheath is a polyclonal cellular proliferation. Hum Pathol 28:815, 1997.

CHAPTER 58

Hemophilia and Pigmented Villonodular Synovitis

Anthony S. Unger • Craig Kessler • Randall J. Lewis

HEMOPHILIA

Hemophilia A (factor VIII:C deficiency) and hemophilia B (factor IX deficiency) are the two most commonly inherited deficiencies of coagulation proteins, occurring with an annual incidence of approximately 1 per 5000 male births and 1 per 30,000 female births. Hemophilia A must be differentiated from von Willebrand's disease (vWD), which occurs in 2% of the population and which is characterized by variable degrees of factor VIII:C deficiency. Hemophilia A and hemophilia B are clinically indistinguishable from each other and may be similar to the other, less common congenital bleeding disorders. The mild hemophilias (clotting factor activities >5% of normal) are not associated with spontaneous bleeding and often remain undiagnosed until adulthood when patients undergo a major surgical procedure.

One of the most important features of hemophilia A and hemophilia B is their sex-linked recessive familial bleeding pattern. This pattern is in contrast to the autosomal dominant inheritance pattern of vWD and the autosomal recessive patterns of the other inherited deficiencies of coagulation factor proteins. Hemophilia A and hemophilia B overwhelmingly affect males, although their mothers or sisters may manifest excessive bruising and bleeding tendencies as carriers if their factor activity levels exceed 50% of normal. If a female presents with clinical features consistent with hemophilia, she should be tested for vWD, the autosomal recessive coagulation factor deficiencies, and a hemophilia A or B carrier state.

The clinical severity of the hemophiliac is inversely proportional to the level of plasma coagulant factor activity. When factor VIII:C or factor IX activity levels are less than 1% of normal (severe hemophilia), frequent spontaneous bleeding (no overt trauma) into joints and soft tissues is expected, and prolonged, profuse bleeding typically accompanies trauma or surgery. If factor VIII:C or factor IX activities range from 1% to 5% of normal levels, there is a more moderate clinical course, characterized by occasional spontaneous bleeding and excessive bleeding with surgery or trauma. Factor VIII:C and factor IX levels greater than 5% of normal do not predispose patients to spontaneous bleeding events, although excessive bleeding with surgery or trauma can occur. Severe (<1% factor VIII:C activity) disease has been noted to occur in about 60% of patients with hemophilia A, whereas severe disease has been noted in about 20% to 45% of patients with hemophilia B (Table 58–1).

There is no single gene mutation responsible for hemophilia, in contrast to cystic fibrosis, sickle cell anemia, and Duchenne's muscular dystrophy, which are caused by one mutation or a limited number of mutations. Hundreds of point mutations, deletions, and inversions that cause hemophilia have been described throughout the factor VIII and factor IX genes.

Laboratory Evaluation

Normal factor VIII:C and factor IX activities range from 50% to 150%. A significantly prolonged activated partial thromboplastin time is the most common abnormal coagulation laboratory assay in hemophilia A and hemophilia B because factor VIII:C and factor IX lie within the intrinsic pathway of coagulation (Fig. 58–1). In North America, the one-stage clotting assay is performed on patient plasma to determine the exact level of clotting factor VIII:C and factor IX activity. This assay is based on the activated partial thromboplastin time and is reproducible, technically simple and automated, and inexpensive.

Hemophilia A and vWD are associated with deficiencies of factor VIII:C. Factor VIII:C synthesis is deficient in hemophilia A, but not in vWD, where factor VIII:C deficiency is due to defective stabilization of factor VIII:C by von Willebrand factor protein. von Willebrand factor protein complexes with factor VIII:C and chaperones it through the circulation and protects factor VIII:C from naturally occurring proteolytic degradation. Factor VIII:C decreases in vWD represent shortened circulating survival, but not decreased synthesis. Hemophilia A usually can be differentiated from vWD in the laboratory by the presence of normal or increased von Willebrand factor antigen and ristocetin cofactor activity.

Prolonged bleeding times are present in individuals with vWD, but individuals with hemophilia A or hemophilia B have normal bleeding times unless the patients have ingested aspirin or nonsteroidal anti-inflammatory drugs (NSAIDs). Platelet aggregation assays typically distinguish vWD from hemophilia A when ristocetin is used as the agonist or platelet activator. Ristocetin mediates platelet-platelet interactions by interacting with von Willebrand factor protein.

An inhibitor is an immunoglobulin, usually IgG, that interacts with and neutralizes the coagulation potential of factor VIII:C or factor IX. If it occurs in an individual with severe or moderately severe hemophilia, it is termed an *allogeneic antibody* and develops after the patient has been

Table 58–1. Hemophilia Clinical Severity

CLASS	FACTORS VII AND IX LEVEL (% NORMAL)	BLEEDING
Mild	>5	Bleeding only with significant trauma or surgery
Moderate	1-5	Occasional spontaneous bleeding; usually bleeding only with mild trauma
Severe	<1	Frequent spontaneous bleeding

exposed to sources of the missing clotting factor in replacement therapies employed to treat or prevent bleeding events. The potency of the inhibitors against factor VIII:C and factor IX activities is quantitated in Bethesda units (BU).

From the clinical perspective, an inhibitor targeting factor VIII:C or factor IX is clinically suspected when a bleeding episode fails to respond to an adequate dose of clotting factor concentrate replacement therapy. Surgical bleeding commonly is observed in individuals with allo-antibody inhibitors even at extremely low titers (e.g., >0.6 BU). Laboratory confirmation of the potency of the inhibitor is crucial to the diagnosis and subsequent treatment strategy.

Clinical Manifestations

Severe hemophilia A and hemophilia B (<1% normal clotting factor activity) are characterized by the occurrence of spontaneous bleeds into joints (hemarthrosis). These

joints are very painful (bleeding into a closed space) and swollen, and repetitive bleeds ultimately result in chronic inflammation of the synovium and deterioration of the cartilaginous and bony surfaces. Bleeding originates from the subsynovial venous plexus underlying the joint capsule.

Infants with severe hemophilia usually experience their first bleeding event between 12 and 18 months of age as they enter the toddler stage. Easy bruising also may be apparent. Patients with moderately severe or mild hemophilia have less bleeding and bruising, unless surgical or physical trauma is involved. Although patients with severe hemophilia can bleed from any anatomic site after negligible or unnoticed trauma, intra-articular and intramuscular bleeds are the most prevalent sites. Soft-tissue hemorrhages may be life-threatening if they occur in open spaces (e.g., retroperitoneum). Intracranial bleeds are the most common hemorrhagic cause of death. Hematuria and bleeding in the gastrointestinal tract are the most common sites of visceral problems, although usually not life-threatening. Isolated hemorrhage into closed spaces, such as into the extremities, may result in compartment syndromes with compromised nerve function and blood flow. If these conditions are not treated immediately by clotting factor replacement or surgical decompression, permanent neuropathy or limb-threatening tissue necrosis may develop. Compartment syndromes of the forearm can occur after faulty venipuncture, and retropharyngeal bleeds may compromise the airway after central venous access devices are placed.

Spontaneous intra-articular bleeds occur most commonly in the knees, followed by the elbows and ankles and less commonly in the shoulders, hips, and wrists. Acute bleeds produce a tingling or burning sensation in the joint area and progress to intense pain and swelling and reduced joint mobility. The acutely affected joint typically is fixed in a flexed position until the acute swelling subsides, and the intra-articular blood resorbs in response to replacement therapy with the deficient clotting factor. With repeat bleeds, arthritic changes and muscle atrophy occur, and pain may be constant.

Factor Replacement Therapy

The cessation of intra-articular bleeding in the hemophilias depends on adequate replacement of the deficient clotting factor protein to achieve hemostasis. The dose and choice of replacement product are influenced by the severity of the coagulopathy, the site and severity of the bleeding event, and the presence or absence of an alloantibody. The premise of replacement dosing relies on the fact that administration of 1 U/kg body weight of factor VIII:C–containing products ideally produces an incremental increase of 2% factor VIII:C activity in the one-stage coagulation assay. In comparison, 1 U/kg body weight replacement of factor IX ideally produces a 1% incremental rise in factor IX plasma activity in coagulation assays.

The commercially available clotting factor concentrates licensed in the United States are listed in Table 58–2.

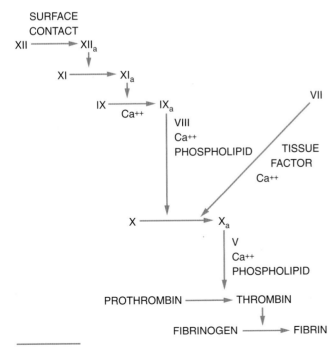

Figure 58–1. The coagulation cascade.

Table 58–2. Factor VIII and Factor IX Concentrates Available in the United States

VIRUCIDAL METHOD	TYPE/NAME OF PRODUCT	MANUFACTURER
Factor VIII		
Immunoaffinity chromatography	Advate	Baxter-Immuno
	Refacto	Wyeth-Ayerst
	Kogenate-FS	Bayer
	Helixate-FS	Bayer*
Immunoaffinity chromatography and pasteurization (60°C, 10 hr)	Monoclate P	ZLB-Behring
Immunoaffinity chromatography/solvent detergent, heat treatment (25°C, >10 hr)	Hemophil M	Baxter-Immuno
	Monarc M	Baxter-Immuno†
Affinity chromatography, solvent detergent, and terminal heating (80°C, 72 hr)	Alphanate SD	Griffols
Solvent detergent (TNBP/polysorbate 80)	Koate-HP	Bayer
Factor IX		
Affinity chromatography and ultrafiltration	BeneFIX	Wyeth-Ayerst
Dual-affinity chromatography, solvent detergent (TNBP/Polysorbate 80), and nanofiltration	AlphaNine SD	Griffols
Immunoaffinity chromatography, solvent detergent (sodium thiocyanate), and ultrafiltration	Mononine	ZLB-Behring
Dry heat (80°C, 72 hr)	Konyne 80	Bayer
Dry heat (68°C, 144 hr)	Proplex T	Baxter-Immuno

*Distributed by ZLB-Behring.
†Prepared from volunteer donor plasma provided by the American Red Cross.

There is no difference in the efficacies among these concentrates, but there may be perceived and real potential safety advantages of the recombinant products over the plasma-derived products, so greater than 90% of the replacement therapy for hemophilia A and hemophilia B in the United States is accomplished with recombinant products. With the advent of virtually safe viral attenuated clotting factor replacement therapies, fresh frozen plasma and cryoprecipitate rarely are used in the treatment of hemophilia A and hemophilia B. Rather, fresh frozen plasma is the preferred replacement therapy for the rare clotting factor deficiencies for which no specific replacement product exists (e.g., factor XI deficiency). Cryoprecipitate is hardly used in the United States as a replacement product except for patients with afibrinogenemia.

Potential Risks of Clotting Factor Concentrates: Blood-Borne Pathogens

Recombinant factor VIII:C and factor IX products introduced in the late 1980s and late 1990s are blood-borne viral safe. No transmission of human immunodeficiency virus (HIV); hepatitis A, B, or C; parvovirus; or new variant Creutzfeldt-Jakob disease has ever been reported with recombinant replacement concentrates. Virtually all patients with hemophilia A (and hemophilia B) who were exposed to plasma-derived concentrates manufactured before 1985 were likely to have been infected by hepatitis C, and greater than 80% of severe hemophilia A patients became HIV seropositive. Hepatitis B infections were almost eliminated by aggressive vaccination programs for hemophiliacs. Similar more recent vaccine initiatives have reduced the risks of hepatitis A transmission to

hemophiliacs. Currently available plasma-derived factor concentrates for hemophilia A or hemophilia B are virtually viral safe because the plasma donations are nucleic acid tested for the most common and lethal blood-borne viruses. New variant Creutzfeldt-Jakob prions may escape in vitro detection in plasma donations and are not amenable to the currently employed viral elimination techniques. The United Kingdom health authorities have informed individuals with hemophilia and other bleeding disorders that they are considered "at risk" for variant Creutzfeldt-Jakob disease if they used United Kingdom plasma products manufactured between 1980 and 1998. These products were made from plasma collected from donors in the United Kingdom who were later identified to have variant Creutzfeldt-Jakob disease or possibly from donors who still remain asymptomatic for variant Creutzfeldt-Jakob disease. To date, no cases of variant Creutzfeldt-Jakob disease are known to have been transmitted by any plasma replacement product, although transfusions of packed red blood cells has been associated with two cases of variant Creutzfeldt-Jakob disease.

Treatment of Inhibitors

The treatment of alloantibody inhibitors is determined by whether they are high-titer (>10 BU) or low-titer (<5 BU) antibodies. Low-titer inhibitors can be overwhelmed by administering large enough doses of human factor VIII or IX concentrates to saturate the inhibitor and to provide adequate clotting factor activity levels. High-titer factor VIII inhibitors cannot be overwhelmed with the specific clotting factor replacement therapy. Rather, coagulation must be achieved by using agents that "bypass" the effects of the inhibitor. Multiple treatment options are available and seem to be successful in about 80% of alloantibody-related bleeding episodes; however, no one agent is universally successful in treating bleeding complications in all patients. Factor IX complex concentrates (formerly prothrombin complex concentrates) of the standard (Konyne 80) or activated varieties (FEIBA) and recombinant activated factor VIIa concentrate (NovoSeven, Novo Nordisk) have become the first-line therapies for bleeding events.

Pathophysiology of Hemophilic Arthropathy

Hemophilia results in spontaneous bleeding into the knee. Repeated bleeds first cause a synovitis, which leads to articular cartilage destruction. The mechanism of joint damage is thought to be multifactorial. Chemical and inflammatory factors arise from the occurrence of bleeds in the joint. These two factors are followed by physical and biomechanical degradation of the articular cartilage.[28]

The reaction of the synovium to intra-articular bleeds results in vascular hyperplasia and friability of the synovial lining, which increases the potential for more bleeds. The synovial lining of the joint becomes fibrotic, leading to joint fibrosis and contracture. As this occurs, physiochemical alterations of the synovium cause articular cartilage damage.

When bleeding has occurred in the knee, hemosiderin-stained deposits appear in the synovium (Fig. 58–2). There is evidence that iron deposits in the synovium stimulate the production of cytokines. These proteins damage the articular cartilage. It seems likely that phagocytosis by the synovial cells leads to stimulation of cytokine production. Roosendal and coworkers[56] showed significantly higher production of interleukin-1, interleukin-6, and tumor necrosis factor in cultures of hemophilic synovial tissue compared with normal tissue. In addition, supernatant fluid from these cultures showed greater catabolic activity. Proteoglycan synthesis has been shown to be inhibited by these supernatants. Arnold and Hilgartner[1] have shown high levels of acid phosphatase and cathepsin D in hemophilic synovial tissue samples. Stein and Duthie[61] studied the histochemistry of synovium retrieved from hemophiliacs undergoing reconstructive surgery. They showed hemosiderin deposits in the synovium and articular cartilage. They postulated that the hypertrophic synovial membrane led to the release of lysosomal enzymes, such as cathepsin D, resulting in articular cartilage breakdown.

The direct effect of iron deposits on articular cartilage is not completely understood. Iron deposit within the articular cartilage is shown on histological examination. Electron microscopy has shown deposits within the cytoplasm of the chondrocytes. These deposits have been termed *siderosomes*. These cells all show signs of degeneration. The exact mechanism is not completely understood.

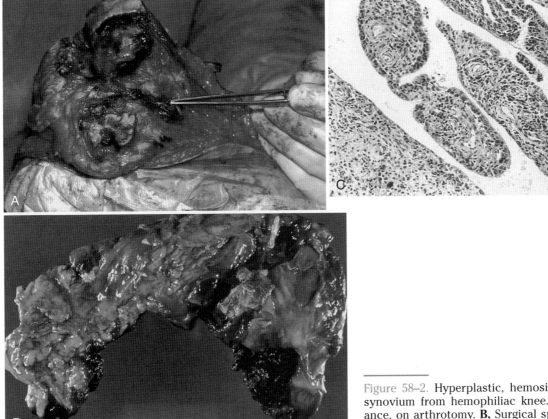

Figure 58–2. Hyperplastic, hemosiderin-laden brown synovium from hemophiliac knee. **A,** Gross appearance, on arthrotomy. **B,** Surgical specimen. **C,** Microscopic specimen.

One explanation is that the deposits inhibit the hydrolysis of calcium pyrophosphate, causing the precipitation of insoluble calcium pyrophosphatase crystals in the matrix, which leads to deterioration of the matrix and chondrocyte damage. Experimental evidence indicates that hemarthrosis has an inhibitory effect on proteoglycan synthesis. It is also thought that the deposits themselves may change the biomechanical properties of the matrix, leading to degeneration.

The cause of degeneration of the joint is probably multifactorial. Repeated bleeds into the joint result in synovial hypertrophy. This abnormal synovial tissue releases catabolic enzymes, which degrade the articular cartilage. In addition, there is evidence that the presence of blood itself within the joint leads to articular cartilage degeneration.

Radiology of Hemophilic Arthropathy of the Knee

Radiographic evaluation is the primary diagnostic tool to evaluate the knee in patients with hemophilia. Standing anteroposterior and lateral views should be taken. In addition, skyline or merchant views add valuable information about the presence of patellofemoral disease. MRI has been shown to be valuable in the evaluation of knees with minimal x-ray changes.[4,75] Often MRI shows evidence of synovial hypertrophy and other pathology before the standard x-ray. They may have particular value in the treatment of children with early disease who are candidates for synovectomy.[43] Wilson and colleagues[74] proposed the use of diagnostic ultrasound as an adjunct in the decision-making process for soft-tissue swelling around the hemophilic joint. Ultrasound may aid in the diagnosis of pseudotumors.

Two radiographic classification systems are in use today. Arnold and Hilgartner[1] described a five-stage system in 1977. This logical, simple system easily divides the presentation of joint changes into stages that have surgical significance. In 1979, Pettersson and associates[46] described an eight-stage system for grading arthropathy. Although this system is more detailed, it is not as commonly used today as the five-stage system of Arnold and Hilgartner (Table 58–3):

- *Stage 0:* A normal joint is seen.
- *Stage I:* No abnormalities are seen on the skeletal portion of the x-ray. There is soft-tissue swelling and x-ray evidence of a hemarthrosis.
- *Stage II:* The x-ray shows evidence of periarticular osteopenia with overgrowth of the epiphysis. There is no narrowing of the joint space and no bone cysts.
- *Stage III:* There is narrowing of the joint space, and subchondral cysts are present. The patella and femoral condyles may become square. The intercondylar notch is widened.
- *Stage IV:* Significant joint space narrowing is present. Cysts are larger and more common.
- *Stage V:* The joint is very arthritic by x-ray. The joint space is completely gone. Significant erosions and deformity are present. The joint is

Table 58–3. Arnold and Hilgartner's Radiographic Classification of Hemophilic Arthropathy

STAGE	RADIOGRAPHIC FINDING
0	Normal knee
I	Soft-tissue swelling
II	Soft-tissue swelling, osteopenia, epiphyseal overgrowth, no narrowing of joint space
III	No significant narrowing of joint space, subchondral cysts, osteopenia
IV	Destruction of cartilage and narrowing of joint space
V	End stage, with destruction of joint and gross bony changes

Data from Arnold WD, Hilgartner MW: Hemophilic arthropathy. J Bone Joint Surg Am 59:287, 1977.

contracted. There is loss of bone resulting in either valgus or varus deformity.

The classification system of Pettersson and associates[46] has eight different radiographic signs: osteoporosis, epiphyseal enlargement, joint margin erosion, irregular subchondral surface, joint incongruity, subchondral cysts, joint space narrowing, and angular deformity. Each sign is graded 0 points (no change), 1 point (slight change), or 2 points (severe changes). The total score yields a particular stage. Greene and colleagues[24] compared both of these systems and found that the Pettersson system was more accurate. A new system of four signs and seven points was proposed. This system was shown to be more accurate; however, the Arnold and Hilgartner system[1] remains the most commonly used system in the United States today.

Pseudotumors

Fernandez de Valderrama and Matthews first described a hemophilic pseudotumor as a progressive cystic swelling in the muscle; they believed this was due to recurrent hemorrhage into the muscle and was accompanied by bone involvement.[5] A pseudotumor presents in a hemophiliac as a slowly enlarging mass in a limb. It is often found in the muscles about the knee, such as the quadriceps (Fig. 58–3). These masses occur next to the femur, become encapsulated, and eventually erode into the bone, occasionally causing fracture.

Radiographic features show a large, sometimes calcified mass in the soft tissues. CT shows a fibrous walled mass with loculation. CT is good at delineating the bone destruction. MRI shows the soft-tissue detail to a better extent. The ability to produce multiplane cuts increases the visualization of the mass. Angiography often is used as a presurgical step to reduce the vascularity of the mass before surgical resection.

The treatment of pseudotumors is primarily surgical. Wide surgical excision should be undertaken as if the mass were a soft-tissue sarcoma. Before surgical intervention, radiation or embolization or both may be used to reduce the size and vascularity of the lesion.[57] Bone erosion that

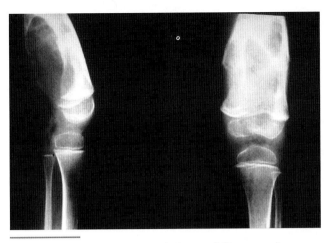

Figure 58–3. Radiograph of hemophilic pseudotumor. (From Vigorita VJ: The synovium. In Vigorita VJ, Ghelman B [eds]: Orthopaedic Pathology. Philadelphia, Lippincott Williams & Wilkins, 1999.)

may result in impending fractures must be stabilized at the time of resection. For large lesions that are considered unresectable or in a patient with other significant medical problems that may preclude surgical intervention, percutaneous embolization may be recommended. Caviglia and coworkers[7] presented their experience with percutaneous curettage of lesions followed by filling with fibrin seal and lyophilized bone graft. The best approach in the treatment of pseudotumors is prevention because the outcome of all of these treatments may have undesirable outcomes.

Treatment

NONSURGICAL

A hemophiliac who presents with an acutely painful and swollen joint should be treated for acute hemarthrosis. Most patients are treated with factor administration and immobilization. Usually, factor levels must be brought to the 100% level. There is little role for aspiration. Most acute cases of hemarthrosis resolve with this treatment. Occasionally, patients have recurrent hemarthrosis. The presumption is that they have a recalcitrant synovitis. These patients are best treated with prophylactic administration of factor or synovectomy or both.

Many hemophiliacs are immunocompromised. In 1984, the medical community noted the association of HIV disease and hemophilia. Consequently, any patient with hemophilia who does not respond to factor administration should be evaluated for infection. Wilkins and Weidel[73] reported a case of spontaneous pyarthrosis in a patient with hemophilia. The organism was *Staphylococcus aureus*. The patient required an open synovectomy to resolve the infection.

Prophylaxis

Prophylaxis is recommended most often to patients who have recurrent bleeding into their knee.[23,52] It is thought

that these patients have recalcitrant synovitis that creates hypervascular, friable synovium. This tissue is easily traumatized, and as a consequence there are repeated bleeds into the knee.

Prophylaxis usually requires the factor level to be maintained at the 100% level for at least 1 month. Often the next month the factor level is reduced to 75%. Oral steroids often are administered at the same time. We routinely administer 5 to 10 mg of prednisone per day to these patients.

Greene and associates[23] showed a significant reduction in the incidence of bleeding by the administration of factor to children for 9 months. Swedish authors have the most extensive data on prophylaxis. Nilsson and colleagues[41] reviewed their 25-year experience with prophylaxis in 65 children. The Pettersson score was almost 0 in this group when factor was started at an early age or the first sign of bleeding. Finally, Brettler and coworkers[6] showed that demand therapy prevents the progression of hemophilic arthropathy.

Medical Therapy

Patients with hemophilia who have recurrent bleeding in their knee ultimately develop arthropathy. Medical therapy should be instituted as a first step in the control of the symptoms of pain and stiffness. Available options include NSAIDs, intra-articular hyaluronic acid, steroid injection, brace therapy, and physical therapy.

Patients with hemophilia can receive NSAIDs if they are monitored carefully. We usually administer cyclooxygenase type 2 inhibitors, such as rofecoxib (Vioxx) or celecoxib (Celebrex). Occasionally, we administer a cyclooxygenase type 1 NSAID, such as ibuprofen or naproxen. The major concern with the administration of these drugs is the occurrence of a gastrointestinal bleed. Careful monitoring of the patient is required. Also, many of these patients have hepatic disease, and this may preclude the use of these drugs.

Intra-articular hyaluronic acid has been used with some success in patients with hemophilic arthropathy of the knee. Wallny and colleagues[69] noted significant improvement in the knee function of patients injected with five 20-mg injections of hyaluronic acid. Fernandez-Palazzi and coworkers[16] also noted satisfactory results when hylan G-F 20 (Synvisc) was injected into hemophilic knees. We have no personal experience with this type of therapy, but view it as a possible conservative option that might be offered to a patient who cannot undergo surgery.

Intra-articular steroids occasionally are offered to patients with hemophilic arthropathy of the knee. Sterile injection of 1 to 2 mL of triamcinolone (Kenalog) or betamethasone (Celestone) may be undertaken. We view this therapy as a temporary measure and offer it only to patients who are not candidates for surgery.

Physical therapy and brace therapy have a historic role in the treatment of hemophiliacs.[34] Today they are used infrequently. Reverse slings, traction, and other corrective systems previously were the only way that contractures could be corrected (Fig. 58–4). These modalities have few long-lasting effects and have been largely abandoned. Greene and associates[22] studied the effect of home-

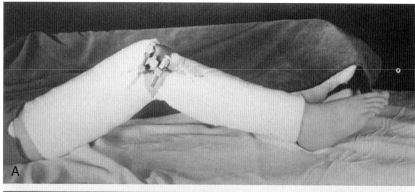

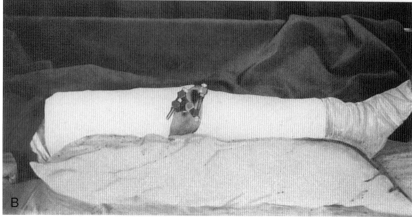

Figure 58–4. **A,** Extension-desubluxation cast on a patient with a 40-degree contracture. **B,** Flexion contracture reduced to 5 degrees after 12 days.

modified isokinetic strengthening on knee strength and contractures. The best results were in patients with stage III disease or less. Finally, physical therapy combined with factor administration does have some value in the maintenance of musculoskeletal function after repeated bleeds. Djourdjev and Pavlova[6] showed significant improvement of the function of patients treated with factor administration and physical therapy.

SURGICAL THERAPY

Open Synovectomy

Open synovectomy reduces the incidence of bleeding into the knee joint and delays the onset of end-stage arthropathy. Patients who have persistent bleeds with physical examination evidence of synovitis are candidates for open synovectomy. Medical management should be tried first for at least 3 to 6 months. If this fails, open synovectomy should be considered.

Patients with Arnold and Hilgartner stage III or less are candidates for synovectomy. Most patients have a full range of motion. Synovectomy rarely improves motion. Its primary indication is pain relief and reduced incidence of bleeding.

Patients who undergo synovectomy must be brought up to 100% factor levels before surgical intervention. We usually maintain this 100% level for at least 7 days, then reduce it to 50% for 2 weeks. Factor is then given to patients before physical therapy for at least 1 month, but

sometimes longer. Patients with inhibitors can be operated on if recombinant factor is available.

Open synovectomy is performed under tourniquet with prophylactic antibiotics. A midline "total knee" incision is used. A complete synovectomy is performed, including the medial and lateral gutters of the knee. There is almost never a good reason to perform surgery on the posterior aspect of the knee, and we do not recommend this be attempted because it may cause excessive bleeding and neurovascular compromise. The knee is immobilized in a postoperative "Jones-type" dressing with a drain for 24 to 48 hours before physical therapy is begun. We advise the surgeon to let the tourniquet down before closure to ensure adequate hemostasis is maintained.

Most reports of open synovectomy have shown positive results. Montane and associates[40] showed that the recurrent bleeding can be "effectively eliminated" for 12 years after synovectomy. Post and colleagues[40] also showed significant benefit from open synovectomy in 12 knees at 5 years' follow-up. Long-term studies show, however, that arthropathy eventually affects the knee even if synovectomy is performed.[19,26,37,44,63] Long-term studies from Norway and Spain showed joint function deterioration at follow-up of 12 to 17 years.[65]

Joint Débridement

Joint débridement is an alternative to total knee replacement. It is offered to patients who ordinarily are considered for total knee replacement, but are either too young or too ill to undergo this procedure. Joint débridement is done in the same fashion as an open synovectomy, but in addition osteophytes are removed, and the remaining articular cartilage is smoothed.

Joint débridement has been offered to patients in Europe, and the results have been fair. Rodriguez-Merchan and colleagues[54] reported the results in 11 knees at 5.4 years' follow-up. Eight of 11 patients had a good to excellent Hospital for Special Surgery rating. We have little experience with joint débridement and generally do not recommend it.

Arthroscopic Synovectomy

Arthroscopic synovectomy was introduced in the 1980s as an alternative to open synovectomy. This procedure has a lower morbidity because it is performed without an open arthrotomy. Consequently, there is less bleeding, and recovery is faster. All of the surgical indications for open synovectomy apply to arthroscopic synovectomy. These patients all have recalcitrant synovitis with an Arnold and Hilgartner stage of III or less.

Patients are prepared for surgery in the same manner as open synovectomy. Factor levels of 100% are required before surgical intervention and should be maintained for at least 1 week. Thereafter, the factor level is reduced to 50% for 2 weeks. Physical therapy is begun after 3 days of immobilization and is often required for 3 months. Arthroscopic synovectomy is tedious and requires the use of multiple portals. We do not recommend attempting to remove the synovium from the back of the knee by the use of a posterior portal. An arthroscopic shaver and an electrical cautery device must be employed to perform the synovectomy adequately and to reduce the amount of postoperative bleeding.

Eichhoff and coworkers[15] performed arthroscopic synovectomy on 32 knees, and 90% of the knees improved with this technique. Weidel[71] also showed significant benefit in nine knees with long-term follow-up of 10 to 15 years. Several other studies confirm these good results, but all the patients continue to show progression of arthropathy radiographically over time.[32,35,64] Whether the synovectomy is performed arthroscopically or by open methods, the disease progresses.

Radiation Synovectomy

Radiation synovectomy has been proposed as an alternative to surgical intervention.[11,25,38,47,55] This procedure has a role in the treatment of patients who cannot undergo surgery. Occasionally a hemophiliac is too ill to have either an open or an arthroscopic synovectomy. We would consider a radiation synovectomy under these circumstances.

Isotopes of gold, yttrium, dysprosium, rhenium, erbium, and phosphorus have been used. P-32 chromic phosphorus is favored in the United States. It is a beta particle emitter in colloidal form. The half-life is 14 days. Zuckerman and colleagues[76] treated six knees with P-32 phosphorus. The isotope has a penetration of 3 to 5 mm into the tissue. Four of the knees had significant improvement. Silva and associates[60] reported the results of

130 phosphorus (P-32) synovectomies with an average follow-up of 36.5 months. The results were excellent to good in 80%. Molho and coworkers[39] showed an 81% success rate in 90 radiation synovectomies performed with yttrium, rhenium, and erbium.

There is a concern that the phosphorus and other isotopes may accumulate in the bone marrow and other tissues. The possibility of malignant changes in the soft tissues surrounding the synovectomy was entertained. To date, however, no deleterious effects have been found. Fernandez-Palazzi and colleagues[16] showed that chromosomal damage did not occur in tissue adjacent to the radiation synovectomy. They studied tissue specimens from knees injected with gold, rhenium, and phosphorus. There is little information, however, about the long-term effects on articular cartilage. Although several investigators have shown few effects in animal models on the articular cartilage, we are concerned about the effect of radiation on already diseased human articular cartilage.

Radiation synovectomy is an option that can be used in a patient who is too ill to undergo surgery. We prefer an open or arthroscopic synovectomy. The long-term effects on human articular cartilage need to be studied.

Osteotomy

Repeated bleeds into the knee result in contracture of the knee (Fig. 58-5). The recurrent hemorrhages lead to progressive quadriceps atrophy and a fixed flexion contracture. In the early stages, extension splints, such as a

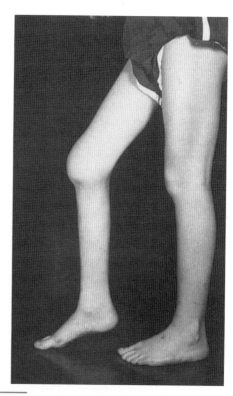

Figure 58-5. Significant knee flexion contracture in an 11-year-old with classic hemophilia.

Dynasplint, may have some value. The reverse dynamic slings reported by Stein and Dickson[62] and others are of historical interest but have little use today in clinical practice.

Soft-tissue hamstring release can be performed in early-stage disease. Generally, patients with Arnold and Hilgartner stage II or less are candidates. Rodriquez-Merchan[53] reported the results of 16 hamstring and posterior capsule releases. Indications were a flexion contracture of at least 30 degrees with minimal arthropathy. An average of 25 degrees of extension was obtained. The results were good in 11 of 16 knees at 9.5 years.

A more reproducible method of reducing the contracture is an extension osteotomy. Supracondylar extension osteotomy with internal fixation can eliminate or reduce contractures of 50 degrees. Caviglia and associates[7] showed significant correction in 19 patients over a 30-year period. Trieb and colleagues[67] noted that there were significant long-term benefits in patients with hemophilia, and the osteotomy may postpone the need for a knee replacement in young patients. Wallny and colleagues[70] showed that in 42 patients with 45 osteotomies there was only 1 patient who went on to joint replacement 13 years after osteotomy. Young patients with moderate disease are considered candidates for this procedure.

Arthrodesis

Arthrodesis is indicated in patients with disabling arthritis who cannot undergo joint replacement. Most patient have either previous or ongoing sepsis of their knee. In addition, severely immunocompromised patients may be best treated with arthrodesis rather than joint replacement. Houghton and Dickson[27] reported a series of 11 arthrodeses performed over an 11-year period. The preoperative motion was only 31 degrees. The technique used cross-screw fixation with 6.5-mm cancellous screws. Cast immobilization was used. We have had little experience with this technique, but advocate it for severely ill or infected patients.

Total Knee Replacement

Disabling arthropathy is the end result of repeated bleeds into the knee. Today with coagulation factor administration and close hematological surveillance, total knee replacement (total knee arthroplasty [TKA]) is the best treatment for disabling knee arthritis.[10,59,72] Despite the overall success of TKA in alleviating pain[20] and improving function, complications have been reported with greater frequency than typically seen with patients undergoing TKA for other arthritic conditions, particularly in patients who are seropositive for HIV.[36]

Angular deformity is common in advanced stages of arthropathy. Extensive joint erosions and synovial cysts can create bone stock deficiency. Epiphyseal overgrowth may require the use of a custom prosthesis (Fig. 58–6). The diaphysis may be narrow, requiring the necessity that extramedullary instrumentation be available. The severe arthrofibrosis may make the exposure difficult. A quadriceps snip or turndown may be used. The patella is always resurfaced, but the bone stock may be deficient. Patellec-tomy is an option if reconstruction cannot be obtained. Almost all patients are reconstructed with a posterior stabilized implant, and occasionally a constrained device is used (Fig. 58–7).

Perioperative bleeding complications can be kept to a minimum by aggressive factor administration. Our protocol is to keep a 100% factor level by continuous infusion for at least 1 week after surgery. Figgie and colleagues[17] reported complications in six of seven patients who had factor levels less than 80%. Goldberg and associates[21] experienced few complications in 13 TKAs when factor levels were maintained at 100%. Lachiewicz and coworkers[33] followed a similar protocol and noted only 1 postoperative bleed in 24 TKAs.

Prosthetic loosening has been suggested to be a problem in the hemophiliac population undergoing TKA. Thomason and colleagues[66] reported a high rate of loosening in 23 knees at 7.5 years' follow-up. It is likely that poor cement technique in the periarticular osteoporotic hemophiliac bone was responsible for this. Our own series of 51 TKAs did not show any long-term problems with loosening (Fig. 58–8).[2] Lachiewicz and coworkers[33] reported only 8 incomplete radiolucencies in 24 knees.

Postoperative stiffness that can compromise knee function is a common problem in patients undergoing TKA for hemophilia. The preoperative range of motion and flexion contracture influence the postoperative result. Lachiewicz and coworkers[33] noted 14 of 24 knees required a manipulation. Karthaus and Novakova[29] performed a manipulation in 7 of 11 TKAs. In our series, 32% required manipulation. Stiffness after TKA is a function of the long-term scarring, severe deformity, and limited preoperative motion in the hemophilia population. Given our favorable results with TKA, we currently counsel patients with hemophilia to consider TKA before contractures and stiffness arise.

Since the association of hemophilia and HIV was reported in 1984, the advisability of performing TKA in HIV-positive hemophiliacs has been controversial. Kjaergaard-Anderson and coworkers[31] reported a 44% mortality after TKA and concluded that joint replacement should be offered to HIV-negative patients only. Thomason and associates[66] reported that out of 15 patients undergoing TKA who were followed for 7.5 years, 7 HIV-positive patients died from AIDS-related complications. Ragni and coworkers[50] noted that 9 of 10 HIV-positive hemophiliacs with CD4 counts less than 200 cells/μL became infected. Norian and associates[42] reported on 53 TKAs and noted 7 failures from infection.

More recent studies have been more positive. Greene and colleagues[22] found the risk of infection in 30 HIV-positive patients to be only slightly higher if the CD4 count was greater than 400 cells/μL. Weidel and coworkers[72] noted a 10.4% infection rate when the CD4 count was less than 200 cells/μL. Our initial study of 26 TKAs in 15 hemophiliacs showed no loosening or infections on follow-up at 4.4 years.[68] Follow-up of this population showed that despite 82% of the patients being HIV-positive, with 7 of 26 having CD4 counts less than 200 cells/μL, there were no infections. Four patients died during the follow-up period, but death was due to hepatitis rather than HIV disease.

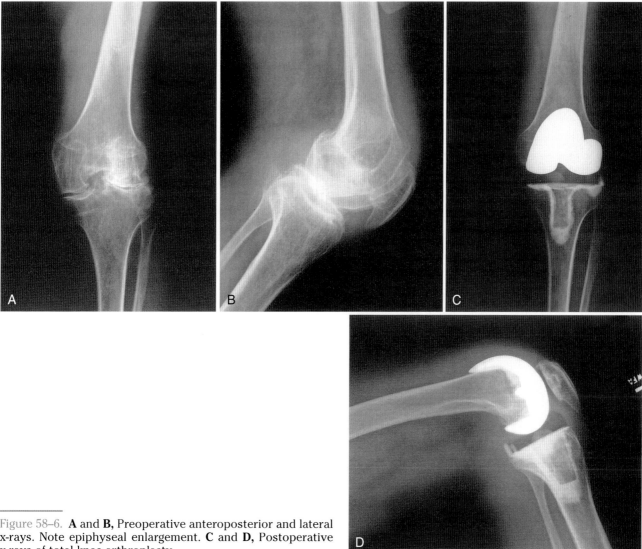

Figure 58–6. **A** and **B**, Preoperative anteroposterior and lateral x-rays. Note epiphyseal enlargement. **C** and **D**, Postoperative x-rays of total knee arthroplasty.

Successful treatment of hemophiliacs with TKA is predicated on a comprehensive care plan at a hemophilia treatment center. The development of potent, new anti-retroviral agents, including protease inhibitors, has led to a more favorable history of HIV disease. Immune function can be improved, prolonging the AIDS-free survival period. The use of combinations of highly active anti-retroviral therapies has been found to decrease the incidence of opportunistic infections by 73%. A 49% decrease in the death rate has been reported compared with data from 1994.

Our protocol is to consider all patients with hemophilia who have CD4 counts greater than 200 cells/μL. Patients cannot have a history of an opportunistic infection. Inhibitors are a relative contraindication, although today with recombinant factor these patients may be treated as well. Standing radiographs are obtained. Because many patients have severe deformity and bone loss, careful pre-operative planning is necessary. Most implants inserted were posterior cruciate substituting. Occasionally a con-strained device with wedges or stems is necessary.

All patients receive prophylactic antibiotics. If there is bilateral disease, we prefer simultaneous bilateral TKA to reduce factor costs and improve rehabilitation. Arthro-plasty is performed under tourniquet; the tourniquet is released before closure. All patients are at the 100% factor level. This level is maintained for at least 1 week, then reduced to 75% for the next 1 to 2 weeks. Patients receive factor before physical therapy on discharge for 2 months. Continuous passive motion machines are not used. The average hospitalization is 10 days. TKA in hemophiliacs is an acceptable procedure with durable, functional results.

PIGMENTED VILLONODULAR SYNOVITIS

Pigmented villonodular synovitis (PVNS) is a proliferative disease of synovial joints and tendon sheaths. It is believed to be a benign synovial neoplasm with the potential for local recurrence.[51] In young adults, PVNS is found most commonly in the knee and is virtually always monarthric.

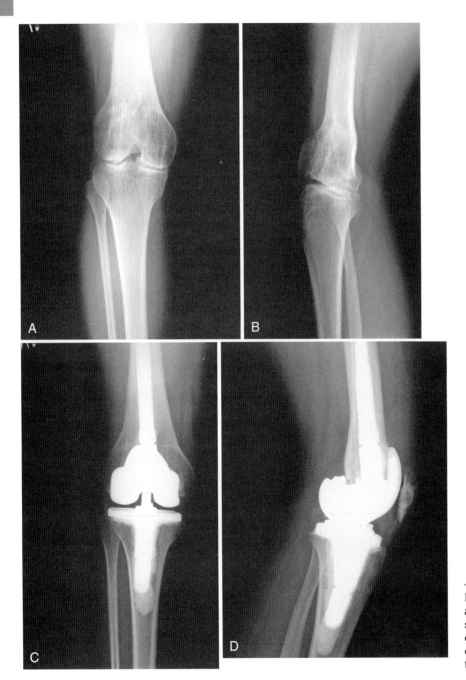

Figure 58–7. **A** and **B,** Preoperative anteroposterior and lateral x-rays show severe anteroposterior deficiency. **C** and **D,** Postoperative x-rays of reconstruction with constrained total knee arthroplasty.

Lesions in the hand generally occur in older patients and present as a firm, nodular mass, called *giant cell tumor of tendon sheath*.[51] PVNS in the knee may occur as a single nodule, a cluster of synovial nodules, or as a diffuse, boggy proliferative synovitis (Fig. 58–9). The most common clinical presentation in the knee is a painless or mildly painful effusion, although a nodule can mimic a loose body, a torn meniscus, or patellofemoral disease.[18] PVNS frequently involves the posterior compartment, presenting with a popliteal cyst.[18,51] Typically the onset of swelling is insidious, with the degree of swelling often out of proportion to the relatively modest discomfort.

The synovial fluid in PVNS may appear normal, but is brownish red in about half of cases owing to the contained hemosiderin,[18] similar to hemophilia. The synovium itself may be diffusely or focally pigmented, but does not have to be.[18,51] Brown color is partially attributable to hemosiderin, scavenged from areas of microscopic hemorrhage, and partially due to yellow pigment within the lipid-laden macrophages that are found throughout the nodules. Histologically, PVNS appears as nodular lesions, composed predominantly of polyhedral, collagen-producing cells and histiocytic foam cells, with varying numbers of multinucleated giant cells. Hyperplastic synovial villi often are adjacent or over the nodules, giving rise to the impression of a proliferative synovitis, particularly in the diffuse form of the disease. Microscopically, inflammation is not a prominent feature, however.[51] The subsynovial nodules may erode through the synovium and into the joint. Extra-articular disease and bursal involvement also

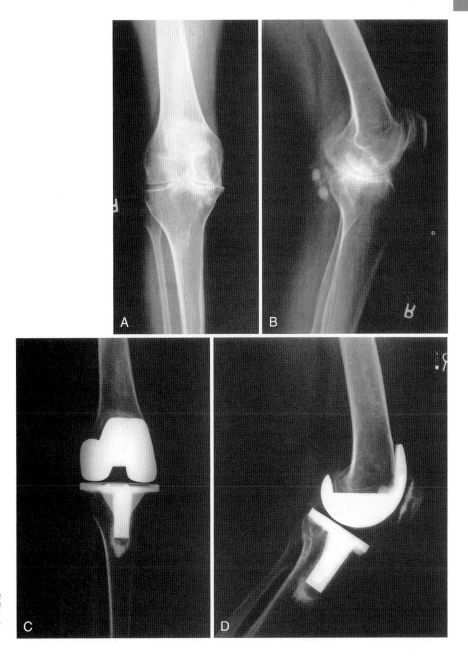

Figure 58–8. **A** and **B,** Preoperative anteroposterior and lateral x-rays of stage 4 hemophilia. **C** and **D,** X-rays at 14 years' follow-up.

occur frequently.[9] Malignant PVNS has been reported rarely.[3]

Plain radiographs of the knee are often normal or show only soft-tissue swelling. When PVNS involves a joint with a tight, firmly applied fibrous capsule, such as the hip or the ankle, cystic erosions, surrounded by minimal or no sclerosis, often are seen at the time of presentation, and degenerative changes occur early in the course of the disease.[8] In the knee, the suprapatellar pouch can expand considerably before there are significant symptoms or the patient seeks treatment. Consequently, bone erosion is less common at the time of presentation, the joint spaces are well maintained, and degenerative changes generally occur later. PVNS does not calcify. MRI is helpful in initial diagnosis, defining the extent of disease, and in the detection of recurrence.[8,9,18,48] Typically, there are voids or areas

of low signal in the central portions of the proliferative nodules on T1-weighted and T2-weighted images, largely resulting from the contained hemosiderin (Fig. 58–10). Increased signal is seen in the areas of synovitis at the periphery of the nodules.[8,48] As with plain radiographs, relatively little bone involvement is seen on MRI of the knee.[8]

Treatment of PVNS is surgical. Open and arthroscopic synovectomy have been employed. Our current recommendation is for the arthroscopic procedure because the stiffness, discomfort, and length of hospitalization are considerably less, and greater motion generally is achieved after an arthroscopic procedure. Recurrences always can be treated by open synovectomy, if required. The rate of recurrence after synovectomy approaches 20%, with diffuse lesions much more prone to recurrence.[12,45,77]

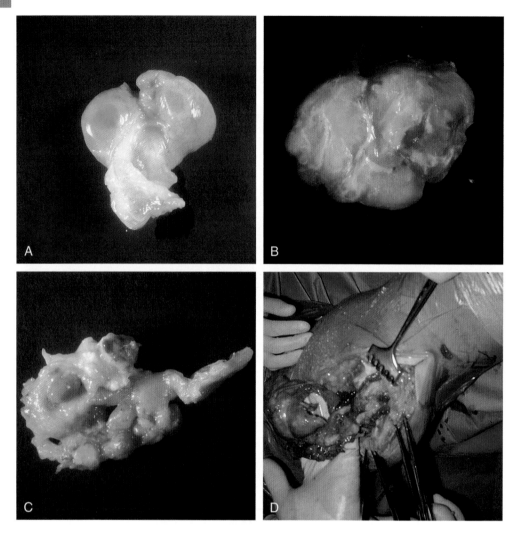

Figure 58–9. Pigmented villonodular synovitis/giant cell tumor of tendon sheath. **A,** Loose body. **B,** Localized nodule (gross appearance, cross-section). **C,** Localized aggregate of multiple nodules. **D,** Diffuse type throughout the joint. (From Vigorita VJ: The synovium. In Vigorita VJ, Ghelman B: Orthopaedic Pathology. Philadelphia, Lippincott/Williams & Wilkins, 1999.)

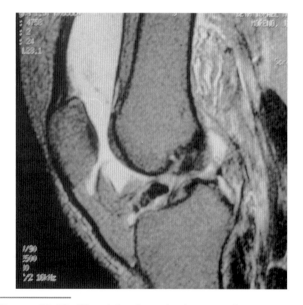

Figure 58–10. T2-weighted sagittal magnetic resonance image demonstrates areas of signal void anterior to the anterior cruciate ligament and adjacent to the anterior border of the tibial plateau caused by hemosiderin deposition. Notice the large effusion in the suprapatellar bursa.

Localized PVNS usually can be treated successfully with limited synovectomy alone.[12,45,77] Diffuse disease is best treated by total synovectomy, including the posterior compartment.[12,45,77] Partial synovectomy often is followed by recurrence rates on the order of 50%, independent of the histologic grading of the disease. Because of the high risk of recurrence, combined treatment by synovectomy and radiation therapy, either with external-beam or intra-articular injection of radioisotope, has been employed.[4,9,30,58] Good clinical results have been reported in 86% to 93% of patients,[4,9] although recurrence of disease has not been eliminated completely. Although no significant complications have been reported after radiation for PVNS, as with hemophilia, we prefer arthroscopic synovectomy when possible because the long-term effects of radiation on articular cartilage are uncertain. We have employed adjuvant radiation in the treatment of recurrences, however, especially when the complete resection of recurrent disease was doubtful. When degenerative disease from PVNS becomes sufficiently symptomatic, TKA is the procedure of choice. In contrast to other arthritides, we routinely perform a formal synovectomy at the time of TKA, removing the villonodular tissue to prevent further recurrences.

References

1. Arnold WD, Hilgartner MW: Hemophilic arthropathy. J Bone Joint Surg Am 59:287, 1977.
2. Arsht SJ, Dungy DS, Unger AS, et al: Total knee replacement for advanced hemophilic arthropathy: A long term follow-up study. Presented at American Association of Orthopaedic Surgeons annual meeting, New Orleans, 2003.
3. Bertoni F, Unni KK, Beabout JW, et al: Malignant giant cell tumor of the tendon sheaths and joints (malignant pigmented villonodular synovitis). Am J Pathol 21:153, 1997.
4. Blanco CE, Leon HO, Guthrie TB: Combined partial arthroscopic synovectomy and radiation therapy for diffuse pigmented villonodular synovitis of the knee. Arthroscopy 5:527, 2001.
5. Boonjunwetwat D, Thaiarte N: Hemophiliacs bone pseudotumors. J Med Assoc Thai 82:89, 1999.
6. Brettler DB, Forsberg AD, O'Connell FD, et al: A long-term study of hemophilic arthropathy of the knee joint on a program of factor VIII replacement given at time of each hemarthrosis. Am J Hematol 18:13, 1985.
7. Caviglia HA, Perez-Bianco R, Galatro G, et al: Extensor supracondylar femoral osteotomy as treatment for flexed haemophilic knee. Haemphilia 5:28, 1999.
8. Cheng XG, You YH, Liu W, et al: MRI features of pigmented villonodular synovitis (PVNS). Clin Rheumatol 1:31, 2004.
9. Chin KR, Barr SJ, Winalski C, et al: Treatment of advanced primary and recurrent pigmented villonodular synovitis of the knee. J Bone Joint Surg Am 84:2192, 2002.
10. Cohen I, Heim M, Martinowitz U, et al: Orthopaedic outcome of total knee replacement in haemophilia A. Haemophilia 6:104, 2000.
11. Dawson TM, Ryan PRJ, Street AM, et al: Yttrium synovectomy in hemophilic arthropathy. Br J Rheumatol 33:351, 1994.
12. DePonti A, Sansone V, Malchere M: Results of arthroscopic treatment of pigmented villonodular synovitis of the knee. Arthroscopy 6:602, 2003.
13. Djourdjev BA, Pavlova AK: Intensive rehabilitation of a knee joint in hemophilic patients—a preliminary study. Folia Med 44:40, 2002.
14. Dobon M, Lucia JF, Aguilar C, et al: Value of magnetic resonance imaging for the diagnosis and follow-up of haemophilic arthropathy. Hemophilia 9:76, 2003.
15. Eichhoff HH, Koch W, Raderschadt G, et al: Arthroscopy for chronic hemophilic synovitis. Orthop 343:58, 1997.
16. Fernandez-Palazzi F, Visco R, Boadas A, et al: Intra-articular hyaluronic acid in the treatment of haemophilic chronic arthropathy. Hemophilia 8:375, 2002.
17. Figgie MP, Goldberg VM, Figgie HE III, et al: Total knee arthroplasty for the treatment of chronic hemophilic arthropathy. Clin Orthop 248:98, 1989.
18. Flandry F, Hughston JC, McCann SB, et al: Diagnostic features of diffuse pigmented villonodular synovitis of the knee. Clin Orthop 298:212, 1994.
19. Gilbert MS, Radomisli TE: Therapeutic options in the management of hemophilic synovitis. Clin Orthop 343:88, 1997.
20. Goddard NJ, Rodriguez-Merchan EC, Weidel JD: Total knee replacement in haemophilia. Haemophilia 8:382, 2002.
21. Goldberg VM, Heiple KG, Figgie HE, et al: Total knee arthroplasty for the treatment of chronic hemophilic arthropathy. J Bone Joint Surg Am 63:695, 1981.
22. Greene WB, DeGnore LT, White GC: Orthopaedic procedures and prognosis in hemophilic patients who are seropositive for the human immunodeficiency virus. J Bone Joint Surg Am 72:2, 1990.
23. Greene WB, McMillan CW, Warren MW: Prophylactic transfusion for hypertrophic synovitis in children with hemophilia. Clin Orthop 343:19, 1997.
24. Greene WB, Yankaskas BC, Guilford WB: Roentgenographic classifications of hemophilic arthropathy. J Bone Joint Surg Am 71:237, 1989.
25. Heim M, Horoszowski H, Lieberman L, et al: Methods and results of radionucleotide synovectomies. In Gilbert MS, Greene WB (eds): Musculoskeletal Problems in Hemophilia. New York, National Hemophilia Foundation, 1990, p 98.
26. Holdredge S, Isaacson J: Open synovectomy of the knee in hemophilia. In Gilbert MS, Green WB (eds): Musculoskeletal Problems in Hemophilia. New York, National Hemophilia Foundation, 1990, p 87.
27. Houghton GR, Dickson RA: Lower limb arthrodesis in hemophilia. J Bone Joint Surg Br 60:143, 1978.
28. Johnson RP, Bobbitt DP: Five stages of joint disintegration compared with range of motion in hemophilia. Clin Orthop 201:36, 1985.
29. Karthaus RP, Novakova IRO: Total knee replacement in hemophilic arthropathy. J Bone Joint Surg Br 70:382, 1988.
30. Kat S, Kutz R, Elbracht T, et al: Radiosynovectomy in pigmented villonodular synovitis. Nuklearmedizin 7:209, 2000.
31. Kjaergaard-Anderson P, Christiansen SE, Ingerslev J, et al: Total knee arthroplasty in classic hemophilia. Clin Orthop 256:137, 1990.
32. Klein K, Aland C, Kim H, et al: Long term follow-up of arthroscopic synovectomy for chronic hemophilic synovitis. Arthroscopy (NY) 3:231, 1987.
33. Lachiewicz PF, Inglis A, Insall JN, et al: Total knee arthroplasty in hemophilia. J Bone Joint Surg Am 67:1361, 1985.
34. Lang L: Dynasplint for knee flexion contratures. In Gilbert MS, Greene WB (eds): Musculoskeletal Problems in Hemophilia. New York, National Hemophilia Foundation, 1990, p 83.
35. Limbird T, Dennis S: Arthroscope synovectomy and continuous passive motion (CPM) in hemophiliac patients. Arthroscopy (NY) 3:72, 1987.
36. Magone JB, Dennis DA, Weis LD: Total knee arthroplasty in chronic haemophilic arthropathy. Orthopaedics 9:653, 1986.
37. McCullough NC, Enis JE, Lovitt J, et al: Synovectomy or total replacement of the knee in hemophilia. J Bone Joint Surg Am 61:69, 1979.
38. Merchan ECR, Magallon M, Martin-Villar J, et al: Long term follow-up of hemophilic arthropathy treated by Au-198 radiation synovectomy. Int Orthop 17:120, 1993.
39. Molho P, Verrier P, Stieltjes N, et al: A retrospective study on chemical and radioactive synovectomy in severe haemophilic patients with recurrent haemarthrosis. Haemophilia 5:115, 1999.
40. Montane I, McCollough N, Chun-Yet Lian E: Synovectomy of the knee for hemophilic arthropathy. J Bone Joint Surg Am 68:210, 1986.
41. Nilsson IM, Berntorp E, Lofqvist T, et al: Twenty-five years' experience of prophylactic treatment in severe haemophilia A and B. J Intern Med 232:25, 1992.
42. Norian JM, Ries MD, Karp S, et al: Total knee arthroplasty in hemophilic arthropathy. J Bone Joint Surg Am 84:1138, 2002.
43. Nuss R, Kilcoyne RF, Geraghty S, et al: Utility of magnetic resonance imaging for management of hemophiliac arthropathy in children. J Pediatr 123:388, 1998.
44. O'Connell FD: Open surgical synovectomy of the knee in hemophilia: A long term follow-up. In Gilbert MS, Greene WB (eds): Musculoskeletal Problems in Hemophilia. New York, National Hemophilia Foundation, 1990, p 91.
45. Ogilvie-Harris DJ, McLean J, Zarnett ME: Pigmented villonodular synovitis of the knee: The results of total arthroscopic synovectomy, partial arthroscopic synovectomy, and arthroscopic local excision. J Bone Joint Surg Am 74:119, 1992.
46. Pettersson H, Ahlberg A, Nilsson IM: A radiographic classification of hemophilic arthropathy. Clin Orthop 149:152, 1980.
47. Pirich C, Schwamesis E, Bernecker P, et al: Influence of radiation synovectomy on articular cartilage, synovial thickness and enhancement as evidenced by MRI in patients with chronic synovitis. J Nucl Med 40:1277, 1999.
48. Poletti SC, Gates HS 3rd, Martinez SM, Richardson WJ: The use of magnetic resonance imaging in the diagnosis of pigmented villonodular synovitis. Orthopedics 13:185, 1990.
49. Post M, Watta G, Telfer M: Synovectomy in hemophilic arthropathy. Clin Orthop 202:139, 1986.
50. Ragni MV, Crossett LS, Herndon JH: Postoperative infection following orthopaedic surgery in human immunodeficiency virus-infected hemophiliacs with CD4 counts < 200/mm. J Arthroplasty 10:716, 1995.
51. Rao S, Vigorita VJ: Pigmented villonodular synovitis (giant cell tumor of the tendon sheath and synovial membrane): A review of eighty-one cases. J Bone Joint Surg Am 66:76, 1984.
52. Ribbans WJ, Giangrande P, Beeton: Conservative treatment of hemarthrosis for prevention of hemophilic synovitis. Clin Orthop 343:12, 1997.
53. Rodriguez-Merchan EC: Pathogenesis, early diagnosis, and prophylaxis for chronic hemophilic synovitis. Clin Orthop 343:6, 1997.
54. Rodriguez-Merchan EC, Magallon M, Galindo E: Joint debridement for haemophilic arthropathy of the knee. Int Orthop 18:135, 1994.

55. Rodriguez-Merchan EC, Weidel JD: General principles and indications of synoviorthesis (medical synovectomy) in haemophilia. Hemophilia 2:6, 2001.

56. Roosendal G, Vianen ME, Wenting MJG, et al: Iron deposits and catabolic properties of synovial tissue from patients with haemophilia. J Bone Joint Surg Br 80:540, 1998.

57. Selvilla J, Alvarez MT, Canales M, et al: Therapeutic embolization and surgical excision of haemophilic pseudotumor. Hemophilia 5:360, 1999.

58. Shabat S, Kollender Y, Merimsky O, et al: The use of surgery and yttrium 90 in the management of extensive and diffuse pigmented villonodular synovitis of large joints. Rheumatology 41:1113, 2002.

59. Sheth DS, Oldfield D, Ambrose C, et al: Total knee arthroplasty in hemophilic arthropathy. J Arthroplasty 19:56, 2004.

60. Silva M, Luck JV, Siegel ME: 32P chromic phosphorus radio-synovectomy for chronic haemophilic synovitis. Haemophilia 2:40, 2001.

61. Stein H, Duthie RB: The pathogenesis of chronic haemopihilic arthropathy. J Bone Joint Surg Br 63:601, 1989.

62. Stein H, Dickson RA: Reverse dynamic slings for knee flexion contractures in the hemophiliac. J Bone Joint Surg Am 57:282, 1975.

63. Storti E, Ascari E: Surgical and chemical synovectomy. Ann N Y Acad Sci 240:316, 1994.

64. Tamurian RM, Spencer EE, Wojtys EM: The role of arthroscopic synovectomy in the management of hemarthrosis in hemophilia patients: Financial perspectives. Arthroscopy 18:789, 2002.

65. Teigland JC, Tjonnfjord GE, Evensen SA, et al: Synovectomy for haemophiliac arthropathy: 6-21 years follow-up in 16 patients. J Intern Med 235:239, 1994.

66. Thomason HC III, Wilson FC, Lachiewicz PF, et al: Knee arthroplasty in hemophilic arthropathy. Clin Orthop 360:169, 1999.

67. Trieb K, Panotopoulos J, Hartl H, et al: Outcome of osteotomies for the treatment of haemophilic arthropathy of the knee. Langenbaeks Arch Surg 389:209, 2004.

68. Unger AS, Kessler CM, Lewis RJ: Total knee arthroplasty in human immunodeficiency virus-infected hemophilics. J Arthroplasty 10:448, 1995.

69. Wallny T, Brackmann HH, Semper H: Intra-articular hyaluronic acid in the treatment of haemophilic arthropathy of the knee: Clinical, radiological and sonographic assessment. Hemophilia 6:566, 2000.

70. Wallny T, Saker A, Hoffman P, et al: Long-term follow-up after osteotomy for haemophilic arthropathy of the knee. Haemophilia 9:69, 2003.

71. Weidel J: Arthroscopic synovectomy of the knee in hemophilia. Clin Orthop 328:46, 1996.

72. Weidel J, Luck J, Gilbert M: Total knee arthroplasty in patients with hemophilia: Evaluation of ling-term results. In Gilbert MS, Green WB (eds): Musculoskeletal Problems in Hemophilia. New York, National Hemophilia Foundation, 1990, p 152.

73. Wilkins RM, Weidel JD: Septic arthritis of the knee in a hemophiliac. J Bone Joint Surg Am 65:267, 1983.

74. Wilson DJ, McLardy-Smith PD, Woodham CH, et al: Diagnostic ultrasound in haemophilia. J Bone Joint Surg Br 69:103, 1987.

75. Yulish BS, Lieberman JM, Strabdjord SE, et al: Hemophilic arthropathy: Assessment with MR imaging. Radiology 164:759, 1987.

76. Zuckerman J, Solomon G, Shortkroff, et al: Principles of radiation synovectomy. In Gilbert MS, Greene WB (eds): Musculoskeletal Problems in Hemophilia. New York, National Hemophilia Foundation, 1990, p 93.

77. Zvijac JE, Lau AC, Hechtman KS, et al: Arthroscopic treatment of pigmented villonodular synovitis of the knee. Arthroscopy 15:613, 1999.

CHAPTER 59

HIV Infection and Its Relationship to Knee Disorders

Alison Selleck • Henry Masur

When caring for patients infected with human immuno-deficiency virus (HIV), orthopedic surgeons need to be familiar with the complex nature of HIV infection to make rational decisions regarding diagnosis and treatment of both HIV-related and HIV-unrelated orthopedic and rheumatic conditions. In addition, they must be knowledge-able about modes of transmission of HIV and universal precautions to protect patients, colleagues, and themselves from exposure. In the event of exposure, they need to be familiar with the risk of transmission associated with certain events, as well as the current recommendations for postexposure chemoprophylaxis to make informed decisions regarding prophylaxis treatment. Finally, all health care providers should be familiar with and open to discussing HIV prevention with both HIV-infected and HIV-uninfected patients because every encounter with a health care provider can have an impact on patient understanding and behavior.

The Centers for Disease Control and Prevention (CDC) estimates that between 650,000 and 900,000 people are living with HIV infection in the United States.[34] Many of these individuals are asymptomatic; that is, they have HIV infection but do not have the clinical or laboratory criteria to meet the definition of acquired immunodeficiency syndrome (AIDS). As of 2002, there had been 877,275 reported patients with AIDS in the United States. Of these, over 500,000 had died.[34] Moreover, the estimated annual rate of new infections in this country is approximately 40,000 per year.[27,34] Although these statistics are striking, there is some encouraging news. In general, HIV-infected individuals in developed countries are living longer than in previous years. The age-adjusted death rate from HIV infection in the United States dropped an estimated 42% from 1996 to 1997 and has decreased slightly in subsequent years.[34] This decline in mortality can be attributed to the use of potent combination antiretroviral medications, establishment of guidelines for the management of antiretroviral therapy, treatment and prophylaxis of opportunistic infections, establishment of prevention programs, and increasing expertise in the care of HIV-infected individuals. Worldwide, the epidemic continues to grow, with over 42 million individuals infected throughout the world. There are more than 5 million new cases and 3 million deaths each year globally.

Given that the epidemic continues to spread and that people infected with HIV are living longer, nearly all practicing physicians will encounter patients with HIV in their practice. Natural history studies indicate that untreated HIV-infected individuals often live about 8 to 12 years from the time of initial infection to their first major AIDS manifestation.[1,92] From their first AIDS manifestation, AIDS patients live for 1 to 2 years if untreated. With the use of potent antiretroviral regimens and prophylaxis for opportunistic infections, many individuals currently infected with HIV are living longer and healthier lives.[26,47] They are participating in activities for fitness and recreation, as well as in competitive high-school, college, and professional sports. Furthermore, weight training to build lean muscle mass is considered a standard component of treatment and prevention of wasting syndrome and lipodystrophy in HIV-infected individuals. Consequently, in addition to HIV-related musculoskeletal conditions, these patients experience trauma and degenerative processes just like their uninfected counterparts. Thus, careful evaluation and familiarity with the complex nature of HIV infection will help ensure accurate assessment and appropriate treatment of HIV-infected individuals with orthopedic and rheumatic conditions. Orthopedists need to also recognize that the population of patients whom they may see with HIV infection will include individuals infected by homosexual and heterosexual activity, individuals infected by intravenous drug abuse, and individuals infected domestically and abroad. In short, the possibility of HIV infection needs to be considered in the entire range of patient populations.

HIV VIROLOGY

Human T-cell lymphotropic virus type I (HTLV-I), HTLV-II, and HTLV-III (HIV-1 and HIV-2) are the four known human retroviruses. HIV-1 is by far the most important retrovirus of humans currently known and has been established as the causative agent of AIDS. HIV-2 causes a similar, but milder disease, primarily in western Africa. Retroviruses are a group of RNA viruses that produce reverse transcriptase, an enzyme that converts viral RNA to proviral DNA. This proviral DNA is then integrated into the chromosomal DNA of the host cell.

The hallmark of HIV disease is a profound immunodeficiency resulting primarily from a progressive quantitative and qualitative deficiency of CD4$^+$ helper T lymphocytes.[62] This subset of CD4$^+$ helper T cells is defined by the presence of the CD4$^+$ T-lymphocyte molecule on its surface. Monocytes, macrophages, and follicular dendritic cells express the CD4$^+$ molecule on their surface as well. This CD4$^+$ molecule, together with coreceptors, serves as the primary receptor for HIV. Although a number of both direct and indirect mechanisms that contribute to CD4+ T-lymphocyte depletion and dysfunction have been identified in vitro, the manner in which HIV infection results in a progressive decline in CD4+ T-lymphocyte counts and immune function remains unclear.

HIV infection is persistent and associated with an extended period during which the usual clinical features of the disease are not apparent. Infection stimulates an immune response to HIV that initially appears to hinder viral replication but fails to eradicate the virus.[2,42,59,66] Without therapy, nearly all infected individuals ultimately experience a progressive deterioration in immune function that results in susceptibility to HIV-related complications and opportunistic infections.[47,49,62] Current potent combination antiretroviral therapy has been shown to slow the decline in immune function.[47]

CLINICAL MANIFESTATIONS OF HIV INFECTION

The clinical manifestations of HIV infection include (1) an acute syndrome associated with primary infection, (2) a prolonged asymptomatic state, and (3) a period of profound immunosuppression during which clinical manifestations occur. Natural history studies of HIV infection in individuals not receiving antiretroviral therapy or prophylaxis for Pneumocystis jiroveci pneumonia (PCP) indicate that the average time from initial infection to an AIDS-defining diagnosis is about 10 years and the time from an AIDS-defining diagnosis to death is about 1 year, although significant variation exists.[1,92] In contrast, patients receiving potent antiretroviral combinations and aggressive prophylaxis and treatment of opportunistic infections are living longer.[26,28,47] Some have been clinically and immunologically stable for over a decade.

With few exceptions, the level of CD4+ T lymphocytes in blood decreases gradually and progressively in untreated HIV-infected individuals. The rate of decline in CD4+ T-lymphocyte counts and the absolute viral burden have been shown to correlate with the time to development of clinical manifestations.[87] Patients often remain asymptomatic during this progressive decline. Active viral replication and progressive immunological impairment occur throughout the course of HIV infection in most patients, even during the clinically latent stage.[92] CD4+ T-lymphocyte dysfunction has been demonstrated in patients early in the course of infection, even when the CD4+ T-lymphocyte count is in the low-normal range. Immunological activation by HIV appears to cause this qualitative dysfunction. Most AIDS-defining opportunistic infections and malignancies occur in the advanced stage of disease. Some manifestations, such as tuberculosis, bacterial respiratory infections, and lymphoma, can occur at all stages of HIV infection.

Three basic mechanisms are thought to underlie the production of disease in HIV infection: depletion and functional impairment of CD4+ T-lymphocyte counts resulting in susceptibility to opportunistic infections and malignancies; development of immune complex–mediated events such as glomerulonephritis and thrombocytopenia; and damage to specific organs such as the heart, brain, peripheral nerves, and lungs because of direct or indirect retroviral effects. The time frame in which these events unfold and the precise disease manifestation in an individual are highly variable, impossible to predict, and presumably the result of a complex interaction between viral factors and host defense mechanisms. Viral factors include size of the inoculum, strain-specific virulence, and viral replicative accuracy and efficiency. Host factors that may predispose to disease progression, such as age at the time of infection, route of transmission, sex, ethnicity, and coinfection with other infectious agents, are less defined and remain to be conclusively determined for all patient groups.

Primary HIV Infection

It is estimated that 50% to 70% of individuals infected with HIV experience an acute clinical syndrome approximately 3 to 6 weeks after the acquisition of infection. The syndrome is usually similar to acute infectious mononucleosis.[43,46,52,54,76,113] Clinical manifestations may include generalized symptoms such as fever, fatigue, malaise, pharyngitis, headache, photophobia, myalgias, anorexia, nausea, vomiting, and diarrhea, as well as neurological complications such as meningitis, encephalitis, peripheral neuropathy, and myelopathy. Findings may include a morbilliform rash, mucocutaneous ulcerations, thrush, generalized lymphadenopathy, hepatosplenomegaly, elevated transaminase levels, and leukopenia with atypical lymphocytes. Arthralgias, but not usually arthritis, can be a prominent aspect of primary infection. The severity and constellation of manifestations vary. The illness is self-limited, with resolution of symptoms within days to weeks. Seroconversion documented by enzyme-linked immunosorbent assay (ELISA) and verified by Western blot analysis occurs within 3 to 12 weeks after the acquisition of HIV in 99% of exposed persons.[67,76] Viremia can be detected by polymerase chain reaction (PCR) RNA or branched DNA assays 4 to 7 days after the acquisition of infection and thus is the best approach to early identification of the infection. Well-documented cases of seroconversion more than 12 weeks after infection are extremely rare.

The clinical manifestations of acute HIV syndrome coincide with a rapid rise in the plasma level of viral RNA and p24 antigen, widespread dissemination of virus, and a drop in the CD4+ T-lymphocyte count.[53] The associated immunodeficiency at this stage results from both reduced numbers and functional impairment of CD4+ T lymphocytes and can be accompanied by opportunistic infections. An immune response subsequently develops and leads to a decrease in the plasma level of viral RNA, an increase in the CD4+ T-lymphocyte count, and gradual resolution of symptoms. In most patients, the CD4+ T-lymphocyte count remains mildly depressed for a period before progressively declining to more markedly abnormal levels. In some patients, the CD4+ T-lymphocyte count returns to the normal range, although some qualitative dysfunction remains. A small percentage of patients manifest fulminant immunological and clinical deterioration after primary infection and may die within 1 to 2 years of acquiring HIV infection. However, in the majority of patients, primary infection is followed by a prolonged period of clinical latency.

Asymptomatic Infection

The asymptomatic stage of HIV infection is referred to as clinical latency. Active viral replication continues during this asymptomatic period. Although viral loads in many patients, particularly those taking potent antiretroviral combinations, may be determined to be below the level of detection in the blood with currently available tests, it has been shown that the virus is still replicating in other reservoirs such as lymphoid tissue.[94]

The rate of disease progression is directly correlated with HIV RNA levels. In most cases, a patient with high levels of HIV RNA will progress to symptomatic disease faster than will a patient with low levels of HIV RNA.[13] Although the length of time from initial infection to development of clinical disease varies greatly, the median time is approximately 10 years in the absence of antiretroviral therapy or PCP prophylaxis. Multiple studies have shown that progression to AIDS, the frequency of opportunistic infections, and survival correlate directly with CD4+ T-lymphocyte counts.[14,20,83,96,108]

The term "long-term survivor" refers to the rare individual who has been infected with HIV for 10 or more years and whose CD4+ T-lymphocyte counts have remained in the normal range despite lack of antiretroviral therapy. These patients generally have a low viral burden.

Early Symptomatic Disease, AIDS, and Opportunistic Infections

Once the CD4+ T-lymphocyte count falls below 500 cells/mm^3, signs and symptoms of clinical illness often begin to develop. Common clinical features of early symptomatic disease include vulvovaginal and oropharyngeal candidiasis (thrush), oral hairy leukoplakia, persistent generalized lymphadenopathy, reactivation herpes zoster (shingles), recurrent herpes simplex, aphthous ulcers, molluscum contagiosum, condyloma acuminatum, and thrombocytopenia. Individuals may also experience constitutional symptoms such as persistent fever to 38.5° C or diarrhea lasting more than 1 month. The occurrence of these events in an otherwise asymptomatic individual should prompt consideration of underlying HIV infection.

Opportunistic infections are generally encountered when the CD4+ T-lymphocyte count declines below 200 cells/μL. Many of the organisms that cause opportunistic infections, such as P. jiroveci, Mycobacterium avium complex (MAC), and cytomegalovirus (CMV), are ubiquitous in nature and do not ordinarily cause disease in the absence of a compromised immune system. Opportunis-

tic infections can also be caused by common bacterial and mycobacterial pathogens. Such infections are the leading cause of morbidity and mortality in HIV-infected individuals who are not receiving drug therapies. With the development of more effective management of HIV and more aggressive treatment and prophylaxis of opportunistic infections, the clinical spectrum of disease caused by opportunistic organisms will continue to change.

The median time from the onset of severe immunosuppression (CD4+ T-lymphocyte count <200 cells/mm^3) to an AIDS-defining diagnosis (by 1987 criteria) is 12 to 18 months in persons not receiving antiretroviral therapy.[49,73] Studies have shown that in patients receiving monotherapy with zidovudine (AZT), this time frame was delayed by 9 to 10 months.[60] For patients adherent to potent combination regimens, the time frame has been delayed even further. As noted earlier, some patients have been clinically and immunologically stable for over a decade. In 1993, the CDC revised the AIDS surveillance case definition to include all HIV-infected individuals with a CD4+ T-lymphocyte count of less than 200 cells/μL. In addition, recurrent bacterial pneumonia, invasive cervical cancer, and pulmonary tuberculosis were added to the 1987 list of AIDS-defining illness. The major AIDS-defining diagnosis as well as the major identifiable cause of death in patients with AIDS is PCP. The risk of infection with P. jiroveci is inversely correlated with CD4+ T-lymphocyte counts. PCP is most frequently encountered in patients with CD4+ T-lymphocyte counts of less than 200 cells/μL and in those who have had a previous episode of PCP. PCP prophylaxis is recommended in any HIV-infected individual who has experienced a previous episode of PCP or has a CD4+ T-lymphocyte count of less than 200 cells/μL, oral candidiasis, or unexplained fevers for more than 2 weeks.[32]

The most common opportunistic bacterial infection encountered in HIV-infected persons is disseminated mycobacterial infection, particularly with MAC. Infection with MAC is a late complication of HIV infection and is usually seen when CD4+ T-lymphocyte counts drop below 100/μL. Other common opportunistic infections encountered in advanced stages of HIV infection include toxoplasmosis, CMV retinitis and colitis, Mycobacterium tuberculosis, and superficial and systemic fungal infections.

TRANSMISSION OF HIV

HIV is transmitted between humans by the exchange of body fluids via three principal routes: sexual contact, parenteral inoculation, and vertical transmission from an infected mother to her child. Body fluids identified as potentially significant sources of HIV exposure include blood, semen (including pre-ejaculatory fluid), vaginal secretions, breast milk, cerebrospinal fluid, synovial fluid, pleural fluid, peritoneal fluid, pericardial fluid, amniotic fluid, and any body fluid containing blood.[18,84] Body fluids considered to represent minimal risk for transmission of HIV include feces, nasal secretions, sputum, saliva, sweat, tears, urine, and vomitus, unless contaminated with visible blood. The quantity of virus isolated from a body fluid varies by site and stage of HIV infection. Viral burden in blood and other fluids is highest during acute infection before seroconversion.[42,59,66] However, even when the circulating viremia is quantitatively high, HIV has not been shown to be transmitted by casual contact or by insect vectors such as mosquitoes.

Sexual Transmission

Throughout the world, the predominant mode of HIV transmission is through sexual contact. Historically, homosexual contact has accounted for the preponderance of sexual transmission in developed countries. In developing countries, most sexual transmission of HIV is through heterosexual contact. In the United States, aggressive educational programs targeting high-risk behavior in homosexual men resulted in an increase in "safer sex" practices and a decline in the incidence of new cases for a period. However, there are disturbing trends indicating a rise in unsafe sexual practices among homosexual men. On the other hand, the incidence of new cases of AIDS contracted through heterosexual contact is increasing in the United States, particularly among women, African Americans, and teens and young adults.[23]

Regardless of the mode of sexual contact, it is evident that both behavioral and biological factors contribute to the transmission of HIV infection.[30] Transmission of HIV is strongly associated with receptive anal intercourse. Even when intact, the thin, fragile rectal mucosa offers little protection against infection from deposited semen. Moreover, anal intercourse, as well as other sexual practices involving the rectum such as "fisting" and insertion of objects, traumatizes the rectal mucosa, thereby increasing the likelihood of infection during receptive anal intercourse.

HIV can be transmitted to either partner through vaginal intercourse, but there is an estimated 20-fold greater chance of transmission of HIV from a man to a woman than from a woman to a man by this means. This greater risk in women is thought to be due in part to the prolonged exposure to infected seminal fluid by the vaginal, cervical, and endometrial mucosa. Transmission of HIV is also closely associated with genital ulceration. Important cofactors in the transmission of HIV include infection with herpes simplex virus, *Treponema pallidum* (syphilis), and *Haemophilus ducreyi* (chancroid).[30,71] Similarly, genital inflammatory conditions such as cervicitis, urethritis, and epididymitis associated with gonorrhea and chlamydia have been linked to the transmission of HIV. Although oral sex appears to be a less efficient mode of transmission of HIV, it is a misperception that oral sex is a form of "safe sex." HIV transmission has been reported as resulting solely from receptive fellatio and insertive cunnilingus. The risk appears to be increased by the presence of oral ulcerations and gum bleeding.

Alcohol consumption and drug use have been associated with the transmission of HIV as well. The disinhibition and poor judgment that accompany alcohol and drug use often lead to unsafe sexual behavior. Other important risk factors for infection include the number of sexual contacts, sex with a prostitute, being a prostitute, being a sex partner of an infected person, being a sex partner of an intravenous drug user, and having a history of other sexually transmitted diseases, particularly ulcerative genital disease.[71]

Parenteral Transmission and Intravenous Drug Use

HIV infection in intravenous drug users is highly prevalent throughout the world. Risk factors for HIV infection in intravenous drug users include the frequency of injection, the number of persons with whom needles are shared, anonymous sharing of needles and other paraphernalia, cocaine use, and the use of injection drugs in geographic locations with a high prevalence of HIV infection, such as inner-city areas.[39] This population appears to be functioning as the primary reservoir for the rapid spread of HIV infection into the heterosexual population throughout the world.[24,26,34,80,97]

Although the risk of infection is highest with direct sharing of needles, the sharing of drug paraphernalia, such as syringes, water, "spoons" and "cookers" (used to dissolve drugs in water and to heat drug solutions), and "cottons" (small pieces of cotton or cigarette filters used to filter out particles that could block the needle), can also increase the risk of transmission. Street sellers of syringes and needles often repackage and sell them as "sterile." Needle or syringe sharing for any use, including skin popping and injecting anabolic steroids, can put one at risk for HIV and other blood-borne infections such as hepatitis B and C. Athletes have transmitted HIV to each other by sharing syringes for injection of illicit drugs designed to enhance performance.

Parenteral Transmission and Blood Products

Currently, blood products almost never transmit HIV infection in the United States. Only three to five cases of blood product–related HIV infection occur per year in the United States. However, transmission of HIV infection by transfusion of blood products was a major problem in the United States from the late 1970s until 1985, when a serological test for HIV was developed. Unfortunately, the use of pooled clotting factor had already resulted in widespread infection among hemophiliacs. In general, persons with factor VIII deficiency (hemophilia A) have greater factor requirements than do those with factor IX deficiency (hemophilia B, Christmas disease) and hence have a higher prevalence of HIV infection.[38]

From data obtained in the early 1990s, it has been estimated that routine screening fails to detect HIV infection in 1 per 450,000 to 660,000 blood donations.[77] Measures such as testing donated blood for HIV, syphilis, and hepatitis B and C, as well as excluding high-risk donors based on self-reported risk factors, are effective in reducing the risk. The majority of false-negative results are attributed to donation during the several-week "window period" when the donor is infectious but before HIV antibodies are detectable. In 1995, the U.S. Food and Drug Administration recommended that all donated blood and plasma also be screened for HIV-1 p24 antigen. Consequently, the risk of transmission from a single donation of blood is thought to be even smaller than previously estimated. Although p24 antigen testing is very specific, it has failed to detect infection in a few cases in which HIV PCR testing was positive. It is anticipated that molecular testing of donated blood will further decrease the risk of transmission. Currently, donated blood is screened for both HIV-1 and HIV-2 antibodies. There have been no reported cases of transmission of HIV-2 (via donated blood) in the United States to date. However, individuals who receive transfusions in developing countries that do not screen their blood are at high risk.

Transmission rates in hemophiliacs have been further reduced by the heat treatment of blood products and the development of recombinant factor. Similarly, because the virus is either inactivated or removed during processing, hyperimmune gamma globulin, hepatitis B immune globulin, plasma-derived hepatitis B vaccine, and Rh_0 immune globulin have not been associated with HIV transmission. Nonetheless, in many developing countries, blood transfusions remain an important source of ongoing transmission because of lack of serological screening as a result of economic and technical constraints.

Occupational Transmission of HIV

Parenteral transmission of HIV is a major concern for health care workers.[36,55,56,70] Surgeons should recognize that there have been no verified cases in which a surgeon has acquired HIV in the operating room, either in the United States or abroad. All well-verified cases of occupationally acquired HIV infection have involved exposure to blood, bloody body fluids, or laboratory HIV cultures. The majority of exposures have resulted from needlestick injuries or cuts. The results of several large studies suggest that the risk of transmission from an infected source with the usual needlestick injury (hollow-bore needle, in contrast to a solid-bore suture needle) is approximately 1 per 300, or 0.3%.[63,69] A retrospective case-control study of occupational HIV infection reported that an increased risk of seroconversion after percutaneous exposure to HIV-infected blood is associated with exposure involving a deep injury; a relatively large quantity of blood, such as with a device visibly contaminated with the patient's blood; or a procedure with a needle placed directly in a vein or artery.[16] In addition, an increased risk of seroconversion is associated with exposure to blood from patients with high viral loads. Presumably, this increased risk is due to the higher titer of HIV in the blood, as well as to the presence of more virulent strains of virus. On the other hand, a decreased risk of seroconversion was associated with AZT postexposure prophylaxis.[16] In simulated needlesticks, the use of gloves appears to decrease the amount of blood transferred.[81] Finally, a temporal rela-

tionship between implementation of universal precautions and decrease in percutaneous and nonparenteral exposure has been shown.[9,51]

Although seroconversion has been noted after mucocutaneous exposure to infected blood, the efficiency of transmission by mucocutaneous exposure is substantially less than with percutaneous needle injury. The risk of seroconversion after mucous membrane exposure has been estimated to be 0.09%.[23] The few documented mucocutaneous exposures involved transmission through mucous membranes or abraded skin. There have been no documented transmissions through intact skin.[55,63] Factors that might be associated with nonsexual mucocutaneous transmission of HIV include exposure to an unusually large volume of blood, prolonged contact, and a potential portal of entry, such as mucocutaneous abrasions.[55]

As of 2001, 57 cases of occupationally acquired HIV infection in health care workers in the United States had been confirmed.[33,34] An additional 133 health care workers have been classified as having possible occupationally acquired HIV. In these cases, the health care workers have a history of occupational exposure to blood, other body fluids, or HIV-infected laboratory material and report no other identifiable risk factors for HIV infection but do not have documentation of a negative HIV test result before the exposure. Of the 57 confirmed cases, nurses and laboratory technicians have been highly represented, and all transmissions involve blood or bloody body fluid, except for 3 involving laboratory workers exposed to HIV cultures. Of these 54 confirmed cases, 46 were associated with percutaneous exposure, 5 with mucous membrane exposure, and 2 with both percutaneous and mucous membrane exposure. In one case the route of exposure was unknown. The source specimen was blood in 49 cases, bloody pleural fluid in 1 case, unspecified fluid in 1 case, and concentrated virus stock in 3 cases.

Thus far, there have been no confirmed cases of occupationally acquired HIV infection in surgeons or in any personnel after percutaneous exposure with a suture needle. In an anonymous seroprevalence survey of 3420 orthopedic surgeons, 39% of respondents reported percutaneous exposure to patient blood, usually involving a suture needle. Seventy-five percent of these respondents practiced in an area with a relatively high prevalence of HIV infection. A total of 0.8% reported one or more injuries from a sharp object involving an HIV-infected patient during the previous year. Another 3.2% reported a percutaneous injury at some point during their career from a patient known to have HIV infection or AIDS. No cases of occupational infection were identified[115]; however, considerable underreporting of occupational percutaneous injury exists.

In a survey of adults reported with AIDS through 2002, 24,844 had been employed in health care, which represents 5.1% of cases.[34] This number included 122 surgeons. As noted, none for whom information was available appeared to have acquired HIV infection occupationally. Of the 57 health care workers who have been documented to have seroconverted after an occupational exposure, 48 had percutaneous injuries, 5 had mucocutaneous exposure, and 2 had both percutaneous and mucocutaneous exposure. Thus, almost all cases result from a known exposure. Another 139 health care workers had HIV infection in which no exposure was reported. They appear to have been infected by sex or needle sharing. There have been no documented cases of occupationally acquired HIV between December 2001 and December 2002. Orthopedic procedures, in general, have been shown to have a relatively low percutaneous injury rate when compared with other surgical subspecialty procedures. In one observational study, total knee replacement and open reduction plus internal fixation of the hip were shown to have percutaneous exposure rates of 8% and 7%, respectively. All other orthopedic procedures were shown to have a combined percutaneous exposure rate of 2%.[114] The incidence of skin and mucous membrane contact with blood has been estimated to be 16.7 contacts per 100 orthopedic procedures.[115] Hand contact has been most closely associated with the duration of the procedure, whereas body contact has been associated with the estimated blood loss.[116]

Universal precautions recommended by the CDC to protect health care workers from contact with potentially infected body fluids emphasize barrier techniques to prevent skin and mucous membrane exposure to blood and other body fluids.[17,21] The major criticism of barrier precautions is that they often fail to prevent injuries with sharp instruments (e.g., needlestick punctures, cuts), which are the source of more than 80% of confirmed cases of occupationally acquired HIV infection.[38] Nonetheless, as noted earlier, the use of gloves appears to decrease the amount of blood transferred in simulated needlesticks, whereas the implementation of universal precautions has been temporally related to a decrease in the frequency of needlesticks.[9,81] In 1992, the U.S. Occupational Safety and Health Administration (OSHA) established mandatory regulations requiring national standards for the prevention of occupational exposure to hepatitis B and HIV, including guidelines for disposal of sharp instruments, such as not recapping needles and using designated boxes. A review of the circumstances of reported exposures suggests that the risk of transmission could have been decreased or prevented if universal precautions and OSHA guidelines had been followed. This observation is supported by Tokars et al in their observational study of percutaneous injuries during surgery, in which injuries often occurred when fingers were used instead of instruments to hold tissue or suture needles during suturing or when instruments were being handled by a coworker.[114]

Although exposure to HIV is a significant concern for health care workers, exposure to other pathogens such as hepatitis B and C, *M. tuberculosis*, and less commonly, HTLV-I and HTLV-II should also be cause for concern. In fact, the risk for infection with hepatitis B and C virus after percutaneous injury ranges from 2% to 40% and from 3% to 10%, respectively, as compared with 0.3% for HIV.[55] It has been projected that of the approximately 1000 health care workers infected with hepatitis B in 1994, 22 will die as a result of infection.[104] Consequently, it is advisable for all health care workers to be vaccinated for hepatitis B. Moreover, hepatitis C, the most common chronic bloodborne infection in the United States, results in chronic infection in 75% to 85% of infected individuals.[31] There is no vaccine available for hepatitis C.

In addition to protecting health care workers from HIV and other blood-borne pathogens, universal precautions protect patients from infected health care personnel, especially those performing invasive procedures.[51] Few controversies involving HIV infection have generated as much media or public sector commentary as the highly publicized incident of HIV transmission from a Florida dentist to at least six of his patients over a decade ago.[25,40] Documentation that the dentist was the source of infection was based on the lack of alternative substantive risk factors in several of his patients, the fact that all patients underwent multiple procedures, including extractions after onset of the dentist's symptomatic disease, and genetic analysis of HIV strains. Although it is evident that the dentist was the source of infection in these patients, the mechanism of transmission remains unclear.

Lot et al reported a case of probable transmission of HIV from an orthopedic surgeon to a patient in France.[79] After HIV infection was diagnosed in the surgeon in 1995, serological tests were obtained from 983 patients of the infected surgeon. One patient tested positive. This patient, a 67-year-old woman, had no other identifiable risk factors for HIV exposure. She tested negative for HIV before placement of a total hip prosthesis with a bone graft. She subsequently underwent hip aspiration and removal of the prosthesis by the same surgeon. This woman received two units of packed red blood cells after the third procedure. However, the donor of the bone graft and both units of blood tested negative for HIV infection. The patient had no reported sexual exposure to HIV. In addition, the surgeon reported a high frequency of intraoperative injury. Molecular analysis indicated that the viral sequences obtained from the surgeon and patient were closely related.[11] The patient did undergo noninvasive tooth whitening in Indonesia, where HIV infection is prevalent, and the mechanism and date of transmission could not be definitively established. It appears as though the most likely source of infection was the surgeon.[56]

It has been estimated that the average risk of transmission of HIV from a surgeon to a patient as a result of percutaneous injury during an invasive procedure is 2.4 to 24 per million.[10,34,99] All numerical estimates of risk are hypothetical. Thus, although rare, the risk of provider-to-patient transmission of HIV during invasive procedures does exist.

The CDC issued guidelines for the prevention of transmission of HIV and hepatitis B by health care workers who perform exposure-prone invasive procedures.[31] In general, these guidelines advocate the use of universal precautions, voluntary testing for HIV and hepatitis B and C in health care workers who perform exposure-prone procedures, and counseling of infected workers who perform such procedures. The responsibility for developing and implementing such guidelines has been delegated to the state level.

Transmission Issues in Surgery

Given their prolonged and repeated exposure to potentially large volumes of blood, surgeons' concerns about possible occupational acquisition of HIV infection are understandable. However, studies have documented that nurses, followed by house staff and operating room nurses and technicians, are at greatest risk for occupational sharp instrument injuries,[85] the type of injury most likely to be associated with transmission of HIV infection. Factors that may influence the risk of HIV transmission during surgery include the skill and training level of the surgeon, the surgical procedure being performed, the volume and duration of blood exposure during the procedure, the number of procedures performed, and conditions under which the procedure is performed—that is, emergency versus elective.[7] Practices undertaken to reduce the risk of exposure to HIV and other blood-borne pathogens include restriction of operating room personnel, double-gloving, use of protective eyewear and appropriate garment shields, and minimization of sharp instrument use.[7,98]

Although HIV-1 has been demonstrated to remain viable in the cool vapors and aerosols produced by several common surgical power instruments, the significance of this exposure as a potential risk for transmission of HIV infection to surgeons during procedures is unknown.[72] Interestingly, no infectious HIV was detected in aerosols generated by electrocautery or manual wound irrigation syringes. Serological surveys of orthopedic surgeons have not yet identified any infected physicians who appear to have acquired HIV infection through occupational exposure.[7] It is conceivable that in the future surgeons will be identified who have been infected with HIV as a consequence of the practice of their profession. However, based on current knowledge of infection rates and inefficiency of HIV transmission, such an event is likely to be a rare occurrence.

Transmission and Sports

No cases of HIV transmission have been documented to date during participation in athletic activities. The risk of transmission during sports participation is estimated to be extremely low, and it would be expected to occur only after direct body contact with blood, presumably by mucous membranes or open skin. There appears to be no measurable risk of HIV transmission through sports activities when bleeding does not occur.[34] Transmission of both HIV and hepatitis B and C can occur by sharing razors, toothbrushes, and needles used to administer anabolic steroids; such activities involve blood or saliva exposure to mucous membranes or parenteral injections.

In their joint position statement on HIV and other blood-borne pathogens in sports, the American Medical Society for Sports Medicine and the American Academy of Sports Medicine maintain that sports medicine practitioners should play a role in the education of infected and uninfected athletes, their families, and the sports community regarding disease transmission and prevention.[4] Athletes should be advised that it is their responsibility to report wounds and injuries in a timely manner. If an athlete is bleeding, sports participation should be interrupted. After the wound stops bleeding and has been antiseptically cleaned and securely bandaged, participation may be resumed. Universal precautions and basic principles of hygiene should be observed. In addition, the position statement asserts that sports medicine practitioners should be knowledgeable about management issues involving HIV-infected athletes and should maintain the confidentiality of HIV-infected athletes.

VERTICAL TRANSMISSION

Although HIV infection can be transmitted from an infected mother to her fetus throughout pregnancy, most transmissions occur at or near delivery. AZT alone and nevirapine alone have been shown to significantly reduce the rate of perinatal transmission.[41] Consequently, all pregnant women should be tested for HIV infection. In addition, all HIV-infected women should be counseled about the risks and benefits of antiretroviral therapy for both the mother and the infant.[117] Current practice is to treat and promote the mother's health as the first priority. To this end, pregnant women should receive multiple-drug combinations designed to reduce the mother's circulating HIV RNA levels to less than 50 copies/μL, with avoidance of teratogenic drugs such as efavirenz, if possible.

TESTING

All patients should consider undergoing HIV testing if they have engaged in any activity that would put them at risk. Individuals who should especially undergo HIV testing include (1) persons with current or past sexually transmitted disease; (2) those in known high-risk groups (intravenous drug users, gay and bisexual men, hemophiliacs, regular sexual partners of persons in these categories, and partners of persons with known HIV infection); (3) those in lower-risk categories (prostitutes, persons who received blood products from 1977 to May 1985, and heterosexual persons with at least one sex partner in the past 12 months or noncompliance with condom use in the past 6 months); (4) those who consider themselves at risk or who request the test; (5) pregnant women; (6) those with active tuberculosis; (7) those with occupational exposure (both recipient and source); (8) patients aged 15 to 54 years admitted to hospitals where the seroprevalence exceeds 1% or AIDS case rates exceed 1 per 1000 discharges; (9) health care workers who perform exposure-prone invasive procedures, depending on institutional policies; (10) blood, semen, and organ donors; and (11) patients with clinical or laboratory findings suggestive of HIV infection.[8]

The diagnosis of HIV infection is most often based on antibodies to the virus detected by ELISA and confirmed by Western blot. Criteria for a positive HIV test are a positive ELISA result followed by a positive Western blot result. A positive Western blot result requires the identification of antibodies to two of the following viral proteins: p24, gp41, and gp120/160. The accuracy of HIV serology is excellent, with a reported sensitivity of 99.3% and a specificity of 99.7%.[22]

Antibody to HIV usually appears 3 to 12 weeks after primary infection but may occasionally take as long as 6 months to appear. False-negative results occur most frequently in recently infected persons before seroconversion. The newer, more sensitive antibody tests reduce the typical window period to 3 to 4 weeks. False-negative test results have also been reported in individuals with agammaglobulinemia, in individuals infected with strains showing little genetic homology with HIV-1, and in those who remain persistently seronegative because of an "atypical host response." The most common cause of an apparent false-positive test result is vaccination with experimental HIV-1 vaccines.[8]

Indeterminate results may occur in an HIV-infected individual who either is in the process of seroconversion or has advanced HIV infection with decreased titers of antibodies. Indeterminate results also occur in uninfected individuals who have cross-reacting alloantibodies from pregnancy, blood transfusions, or organ transplantation; in individuals who have autoantibodies as seen with collagen vascular disease, autoimmune diseases, and malignancy; or in recipients of experimental HIV-1 vaccines. An individual infected with HIV-2 may have a positive or indeterminate result on Western blot for HIV-1. Repeat testing at 3 and 6 months is generally advocated for individuals with indeterminate test results.

Additional methods for establishing HIV infection include HIV DNA and RNA PCR and viral culture of peripheral blood mononuclear cells. These tests are used for diagnostic purposes in special circumstances.

Direct viral tests may be useful in individuals with indeterminate tests, for virological monitoring in therapeutic trials, and for HIV detection when routine serological tests are likely to be misleading. If there is high suspicion of acute HIV infection and the ELISA and western blot results have not yet become positive, an RNA PCR test can be helpful. Acutely infected patients almost always have more than 100,000 copies/μL. Low valves—less than 5000 copies/μL—should be viewed with suspicion; they are likely to be false positives. Quantitative HIV RNA (viral load) assay is also useful for predicting progression and for therapeutic monitoring. In fact, it has been shown that HIV RNA levels are the most important measure of therapeutic response.[87] Viral burden testing does not test immune function, nor does it detect viral burden in compartments other than blood (lymph nodes, central nervous system, genital secretions). CD4+ T-lymphocyte count testing, on the other hand, determines immunocompetence and serves as an independent predictor of prognosis. The viral load should be obtained only at times of clinical stability and with the same laboratory and technology.

Informed consent is an important issue with regard to HIV testing. It is required by law in most states and recommended in all other states. HIV testing has the potential to significantly affect an individual's life. A person who tests positive must cope with the diagnosis of an incurable disease. Such a person may experience depression, anxiety, and isolation, as well as changing family and personal relationships. Furthermore, a person may face discrimination from insurance carriers, health care workers, employers, and coworkers. Consequently, both pretest and post-test counseling for all individuals receiving HIV testing should be provided. Almost universally, documented patient consent is required before HIV testing. However, some states permit testing of the source without consent in cases of occupational exposure of health care workers. In addition, testing of all blood, bone marrow, semen, and organ donors is mandatory.

TREATMENT OF HIV INFECTION

Management of Antiretroviral Drugs

The explosion of information regarding HIV, the increasing number of antiretroviral medications, the development of resistance to these medications, and the long-term survival of many patients with HIV has led to increasing complexity in the treatment of HIV-infected individuals. This complexity has necessitated the formalization of guidelines for the management of antiretroviral agents, management and prophylaxis of opportunistic infections, and management of occupational exposure to HIV and recommendations for postexposure prophylaxis.[1,23,27,34] These guidelines are prepared by a panel of leading experts in the field of HIV care and the U.S. Department of Health and Human Services. They are frequently updated and readily available on-line (www.aidsinfo.nih.gov).[35,37,92] Antiretroviral therapies are medically complex and associated with a significant number of side effects and drug interactions, which can complicate both physician management and patient adherence. Although the guidelines recommend that management of HIV-infected individuals be supervised by a physician experienced in HIV care, nearly all physicians will participate in the care of HIV-infected individuals at some time and thus should be familiar with the principles set forth by the guidelines. They should be particularly aware that whenever new drugs are prescribed, drug interactions require expert management by an experienced clinician.

Preoperative Evaluation

No formal guidelines have been established for the preoperative evaluation of HIV-infected patients. In general, consultation with a clinician experienced in the care of HIV-infected individuals is appropriate. In addition to potential opportunistic infections, patients with HIV infection are predisposed to a variety of organ system deficiencies. Thrombocytopenia, anemia, and leukopenia because of bone marrow suppression from antiretroviral medications or infiltration by opportunistic pathogens or HIV or as a result of an autoimmune phenomenon are common. Renal insufficiency from HIV nephropathy, drug toxicity, and various other causes are frequently encountered. Patients infected with HIV often have elevated liver enzymes because of medications or chronic infection with hepatitis B or C. Adrenal insufficiency in HIV infection is well documented. Moreover, HIV-infected individuals are predisposed to dilated cardiomyopathy as a result of HIV itself.[5,26,47] They are predisposed to cerebrovascular and cardiovascular disease by HIV and/or by antiretroviral drugs. More and more patients in the 30- to 40-year age range have severe coronary artery disease.[95] Finally, protease inhibitors, a common class of antiretroviral medications, have been associated with glucose intolerance and diabetes, as well as dyslipidemia.

If patients are receiving antiretroviral drugs, they must consult with the prescribing physician before starting or stopping antiretroviral drugs. Orthopedists must recognize two major issues. First, if antiretroviral drugs are not taken as prescribed and fully absorbed with expected pharmacokinetics, viral resistance can occur as a result of the suboptimal management. This resistance will limit patient treatment options for life. Poor absorption in the perioperative period or discontinuation without consideration of pharmacokinetics (i.e., the long half-life of efavirenz as opposed to the short half-life of nucleosides) can rapidly lead to viral drug resistance. Second, dramatic and life-threatening interactions can occur between antiretroviral agents and a wide array of drugs, largely those metabolized by the hepatic cytochrome P-450 system, but occasionally involving other mechanisms as well. Interactions of lopinavir-ritonavir or efavirenz with warfarin, digoxin, anticonvulsants, and antibiotics are well documented. Orthopedists should obtain an appropriate consultation before starting or stopping any medications if a patient is receiving antiretroviral agents.

Management of Occupational Exposure to HIV and Recommendations for Postexposure Prophylaxis

Many experts suggest that all health care workers consider the pros and cons of postexposure prophylaxis before an occupational exposure occurs so that they may be better prepared to take immediate action and to cope with the anxiety of decision making and the uncertainty of outcome. All known and suspected exposures should be reported, regardless of how small the perceived risk, because the collective data continue to provide much of our understanding regarding transmission risk. The Public Health Service recommendations[33] for postexposure prophylaxis are based on an algorithm that stratifies the risk of transmission according to the type and degree of exposure, as well as the likelihood of infectivity of the source.

There is considerable variation in opinion about what antiretroviral regimen to use after exposure. The CDC has advocated basing the number of antiretroviral drugs on the relative risk posed by the exposure. Their guidelines have recommended giving fewer drugs to patients with less intense exposure. Other experts advocate an "all or none" policy; that is, if it is determined that postexposure prophylaxis is needed, a potent regimen similar to that recommended for HIV-infected patients infected by the more usual routes should be given. In the absence of data confirming the results of these different approaches, it is impossible to be dogmatic about an optimal approach. Most authorities would agree, however, on the following:

- Start postexposure prophylaxis as soon as possible after exposure—if possible, within hours of the exposure and certainly within 72 to 96 hours.
- Use a highly potent regimen that is not likely to lead to viral resistance.
- Reassess after 48 to 72 hours to be certain that the facts of the case warrant prophylaxis.
- Reassess after 48 to 72 hours to make certain that the drugs chosen are appropriate given the source of virus.
- Monitor the health care provider carefully for tolerance and adherence; health care providers have a poor record of completing a full 4-week regimen.
- Continue for a minimum of 4 weeks of therapy.
- Retest the health care worker at 4, 12, and 24 weeks to determine whether HIV infection has occurred.

HIV INFECTION AND MUSCULOSKELETAL DISEASE

Nearly 75% of HIV-infected individuals report musculoskeletal symptoms.[74] Infectious, inflammatory, and neoplastic processes are all represented in the spectrum of rheumatic manifestations of HIV disease. The frequency and type of processes clinically manifested appear to be a function of the patient's level of immunosuppression and primary risk factor for HIV infection. Infectious and neoplastic complications are frequently seen in patients with late-stage infection,[69,103] who commonly, though not exclusively, have intravenous drug use as their risk factor for HIV infection.[91] In contrast, reactive rheumatological processes can occur in persons with early or late symptomatic disease[90,102] and are reported more consistently in those with HIV infection acquired through homosexual activity.[15]

Musculoskeletal Infections

From their retrospective cohort study and literature review of musculoskeletal infections in patients with HIV disease, Vassilopoulos et al estimated the incidence to be 0.3% to 3.5%.[119] Septic arthritis, osteomyelitis, pyomyositis, avascular necrosis, and bursitis are the most common orthopedic infectious complications seen in patients with HIV infection.[57,69,89-91,119] Infection occurs with conventional or atypical bacteria, fungi, or other opportunistic organisms. The diagnosis depends on isolation of the infecting organism from synovial fluid, bone, muscle, or blood. Despite the low incidence, HIV-infected individuals with musculoskeletal infections experience significant morbidity and mortality.[119]

In addition, a resurgence of tuberculosis has paralleled the emergence of the HIV epidemic. M. tuberculosis has increasingly been associated with infectious musculoskeletal disorders in HIV-infected patients. Classic Pott's disease still occurs. Tuberculosis appears to be a very aggressive disease associated with frequent dissemination, multidrug resistance, and high mortality in patients with HIV infection. Consequently, orthopedic surgeons must be aware that pulmonary disease may coexist and must take appropriate respiratory isolation precautions to prevent the spread of infection to other patients and health care workers.

Septic arthritis is usually monoarticular, with the knee[69] and hip[91] most commonly involved. Unusual sites of joint infection, including the sternoclavicular and sacroiliac joints and the intervertebral disks, have been described in intravenous drug users.[74] Infection of the joint occurs via hematogenous spread or direct extension from an adjacent soft-tissue or bone infection. Polyarticular involvement is generally seen in the setting of disseminated disease.

Staphylococcus aureus and *Candida albicans* are the most frequently isolated causes of septic arthritis and osteomyelitis.[69,90,91] In addition to a variety of conventional bacterial organisms, several uncommon organisms have been isolated as well, including fungi, *M. tuberculosis*, and atypical mycobacteria.[101] Clinically, septic arthritis caused by *S. aureus* is manifested similarly in both seropositive and seronegative patients. Erythema, effusion, and tenderness are usually noted on examination. Although atypical organisms such as fungi and mycobacteria often result in a chronic infectious arthritis in seronegative individuals, an acute or subacute infectious arthritic process may ensue in seropositive patients.[74]

Even though effusion is often present, synovial fluid cultures may frequently be negative despite the presence of organisms on Gram stain, wet mount, or acid-fast bacillus smears.[69] Blood cultures may be helpful in definitively establishing a microbiological diagnosis, although discordant blood and joint culture results have been reported.[44,82] Synovial biopsies may be necessary to isolate fungi and mycobacteria from joints. Imaging studies, such as serial radiograms and/or radionuclide bone scans, should be performed in patients with septic arthritis to eliminate the possibility of coexistent osteomyelitis.[74] In addition, septic bursitis caused by *S. aureus* has been reported in a number of patients with HIV infection.[119]

Although the relationship between HIV risk factors and the incidence of septic arthritis has yet to be clearly defined, it appears as though septic arthritis occurs more frequently in patients with intravenous drug use and hemophilia as risk factors.[90,91] The degree of immunosuppression does not appear to be a contributing factor for infection with pathogens commonly introduced via needles. However, infection with opportunistic pathogens tends to occur in patients with more advanced HIV disease and CD4+ T-lymphocyte count of less than 100. One study revealed a median CD4+ T-lymphocyte count of 241 in a group of seropositive patients with septic arthritis.[119]

The most commonly isolated pathogens in osteomyelitis are *S. aureus* and atypical *Mycobacterium* species.[119] Hirsch et al reported that the rate of infection with atypical mycobacteria and *M. tuberculosis* was 676-fold and 35-fold higher, respectively, in HIV-infected patients than in the general population.[65] Generally, fungal osteomyelitis is uncommon, but when it does occur, it is hematogenously spread and thus often develops in more than one bone.[103]

In patients with osteomyelitis, bone biopsy is usually required to establish the diagnosis. In addition, osteomyelitis is associated with a high mortality rate in HIV-positive patients, probably because of their immunocompromised state. Osteomyelitis is more frequently seen in advanced HIV disease, with a median CD4+ T-lymphocyte count of 41 documented in one study.[119]

Bacillary angiomatosis associated with disseminated *Bartonella henselae* has been reported to cause lytic bone lesions.[6,64,118] This clinical syndrome is characterized by subcutaneous nodules and osteolytic lesions that are typically culture negative on biopsy and aspirate samples. Electron microscopy and histopathological examination of vascular soft tissue may verify the presence of *B. henselae*.

Once primarily seen in tropical climates, pyomyositis appears to be associated with advanced HIV infection in temperate climates. By far the most common organism identified in HIV-infected individuals is *S. aureus*.[45,119] Other organisms reported include *Streptococcus* and *Salmonella* species, as well as *Toxoplasma gondii*, *Cryptococcus neoformans*, MAC, and microsporidia.[74,119]

Noninfectious Inflammatory Conditions of the Joints

Inflammatory musculoskeletal complications, particularly arthritis, arthralgia, and myalgia, are common in HIV infection.[15] Arthralgias are the most common musculoskeletal manifestations seen during the course of HIV infection[90] and can be present in approximately 35% to 40% of patients.[50,102] Three primary types of arthritis have been described in association with HIV infection: reactive arthritis (Reiter's syndrome), psoriatic arthritis, and HIV-associated arthritis.

Arthrocentesis is necessary in HIV-infected patients with subacute and chronic arthritis before attributing such arthritides to a noninfectious cause. As discussed earlier, synovial biopsies are sometimes necessary for isolation of fungi and mycobacteria.[74] Identification of such organisms is particularly important for both initiating appropriate therapy and avoiding the inappropriate use of immunosuppressive agents (e.g., methotrexate) in patients who are already immunocompromised.

As noted earlier, the most common musculoskeletal manifestation seen during the course of HIV infection is arthralgia.[90] Diffuse arthralgias may be seen in the setting of acute primary infection, as well as at other times during the course of HIV infection. The large joints, such as the knee, shoulder, and elbow, are most commonly involved. Symptoms are usually of moderate intensity and intermittent, but rarely, they can be extremely severe and debilitating. Often the clinical examination is without evidence of inflammatory signs.[3] Simple analgesics are generally adequate for treatment of arthralgia in HIV-infected individuals.

Reiter's syndrome is reported as a common rheumatological syndrome in HIV infection, although the true association with HIV infection remains unclear. The signs and symptoms are similar to those of idiopathic Reiter's syndrome and consist of asymmetric oligoarthritis of the large joints (knees, shoulders, and ankles). Inflammation of the Achilles tendon, plantar fascia, and anterior and posterior tibial tendons is common. Patients may have gait disturbances secondary to these enthesopathies combined with multidigit dactylitis of the toes.[74]

The classic triad of arthritis, urethritis, and conjunctivitis is seen in a much smaller proportion of patients. Urethritis has been found in 59% of HIV-infected individuals with Reiter's syndrome, conjunctivitis in 47%, keratoderma blennorrhagicum in 25%, and circinate balanitis in 29%.[74] Organisms such as *Salmonella typhimurium*, *Shigella flexneri*, *Campylobacter fetus*, *Ureaplasma urealyticum*, and *Yersinia* species have been found in less than a third of HIV-infected patients with reactive arthritis. However, an antecedent culture-negative diarrheal illness often precedes the onset of Reiter's syndrome and reactive arthritis in HIV-infected patients.[74] In a patient with a Reiter syndrome–like arthritis but lacking the other defining features, it may be more appropriate to classify the patient as having nonspecific reactive arthritis.

The signs and symptoms of Reiter's syndrome can occur before the onset of clinical immunodeficiency. Given the possible association of Reiter's syndrome with HIV infection, physicians examining a patient with Reiter's syndrome or reactive arthritis should inquire about HIV risk factors. Both noninfected and HIV-infected white North American patients with Reiter's syndrome have high HLA-B27 seropositivity. In contrast, in a cohort of 13 African American patients with Reiter's syndrome and HIV infection, no HLA-B27 seropositivity was found. This finding may reflect the low prevalence of HLA-B27 in African American people in general.[74]

HIV-associated arthritis is an oligoarthritis that primarily involves the knees and ankles. It is characterized by brief episodes of debilitating pain. The peak intensity occurs within 1 to 4 weeks and often remits within 6 weeks to 6 months. Intense pain may necessitate the use of narcotics, nonsteroidal anti-inflammatory drugs (NSAIDs), and intra-articular corticosteroids. Arthrocentesis reveals fluid that is noninflammatory. Synovial biopsy reveals a chronic mononuclear infiltrate. The antecedent infections, mucocutaneous lesions, and ophthalmological and urogenital features commonly seen with Reiter's syndrome and psoriatic arthritis are not associated with these patients. Rheumatological markers (HLA-B27, rheumatoid factor, antinuclear antibodies) and bacterial and viral cultures are negative in these patients as well. The pathophysiology is unknown; however, a direct viral infection, immune complex deposition in the joint, and a form of reactive arthritis have been proposed as possible mechanisms.[3,74,93]

Psoriasis and psoriatic arthritis are reported more frequently in HIV-infected individuals than in the general population. Psoriatic arthritis may precede, occur concomitantly, or follow the clinical onset of AIDS. It is frequently an asymmetric, polyarticular disease that can be accompanied by enthesopathy and dactylitis. The clinical course is variable, ranging from mild to rapidly progressive and deforming.[45] Psoriatic arthritis may occur alone or in conjunction with psoriatic skin lesions. Various types of psoriatic skin lesions, including vulgaris, guttate, seborrheic, pustular, and exfoliative erythroderma forms, have been described in both HIV-positive and HIV-negative individuals.

Painful articular syndrome involves the acute onset of painful arthralgias in up to three joints. The physical examination is not suggestive of synovitis. The pain usually resolves within 24 hours, but narcotics may be required because NSAIDs often do not adequately control the pain. This syndrome appears to be unique to HIV-infected patients. Avascular necrosis has been reported in HIV-infected patients and should be considered in the differential diagnosis.[74,112] Other considerations include infections with parvovirus B19 and hepatitis C.

Some of these syndromes have been associated with the institution of antiretroviral therapy. These "immune reconstitution syndromes" occur within weeks or months after the initiation of antiretroviral therapy. They may represent an enhanced inflammatory response to latent microorganisms or to nonviable antigens. After appropriate diagnostic evaluation to rule out active infection, these syndromes are managed symptomatically with anti-inflammatory agents, sometimes including corticosteroids. Peripheral sensory neuropathy is common in HIV-infected individuals. HIV-related axonal degeneration or nerve destruction because of the antiretroviral agents stavudine (d4T) and didanosine (ddI) are the most common causes. Isoniazid, dapsone, and CMV cause similar syndromes. Peripheral neuropathy may lead to gait disturbance with subsequent mechanical derangement of weightbearing joints over time.

Avascular Necrosis

Avascular necrosis of one or more joints will develop in approximately 4.5% of patients with HIV infection. It has been recognized most often in the hip but has been described in almost every joint. Some patients have unilateral disease; others have bilateral disease involving many different joints.

If patients with HIV infection are scanned, silent lesions consistent with avascular necrosis can be found.[61,75] These lesions do not necessarily fit the paradigm that might have been expected from experience with other patient populations, such as those with hemoglobinopathies (e.g., sickle cell disease) or those receiving chronic steroid therapy. These lesions may not progress to structural collapse and pain within a few weeks or months; however, in a substantial number of these patients, such lesions do progress and cause considerable dysfunction and pain necessitating joint replacement.

What causes aseptic necrosis is not clear. In several cases, pathological examination of the head of the femur has not demonstrated any unusual findings. HIV infection and antiretroviral therapy may each have roles in promoting the lesions. Epidemiological studies have associated the occurrence of such lesions with vigorous activity, yet such activities may simply cause the ultimate damage after the initial weakening of the substrate that brought the patient to medical attention. These lesions have also been linked to previous corticosteroid use. It is conceivable that HIV-infected patients who receive corticosteroids, especially those who are taking antiretroviral agents that increase the area under the curve for corticosteroids, may be predisposed to avascular necrosis.

Hip replacement has been performed in dozens of patients with HIV-related avascular necrosis, with good results. There is no known way to prevent this complication.

Osteoporosis

An increasing amount of literature is documenting osteoporosis in patients with HIV infection.[12,48,57,68,109,111] Whether the osteoporosis is related to HIV infection or to antiretroviral drug therapy is not clear. At this juncture, there has been no evidence for an increased incidence of pathological fractures as a result of documented osteoporosis. The obvious concern is that if the demineralization is not reversed, such fractures will occur.

Bone Transplantation

HIV infection of bone is well documented,[13,86,199] and reports of transmission of HIV infection in bone transplant recipients[19,105] highlight the concern that every precaution be taken to avoid this devastating complication. The primary safeguards against potential transmission of HIV by bone allograft are screening and testing of patients.[78] The freezing step in bone tissue banking probably results in further reduction of the risk of transmission.[13,105] Techniques designed to minimize requirements for blood transfusion during operative procedures include intraoperative autologous transfusion and postoperative blood salvage,[106] both of which may serve to further minimize the risk of parenteral HIV transmission.

Neoplastic Complications

Kaposi's sarcoma, the most common neoplasm reported in adults with HIV infection, can be present at any stage of HIV disease. Sites of involvement include the skin and viscera, as well as bone and muscle. Lesions may be asymptomatic or painful. Computed tomography (CT) may reveal osteolytic bone lesions that may be associated with periosteal reaction and an overlying soft-tissue mass.[110] Bone scans and plain films may be negative. Early bone changes may be best detected with magnetic resonance imaging (MRI). Muscle involvement may be seen on MRI as well.

Non-Hodgkin's lymphoma, the second most frequent tumor found in adults with AIDS, is the most common tumor in children with AIDS. The central nervous system and the gastrointestinal tract are the most frequent sites of involvement, although bone and muscle involvement is fairly common as well. Patients with bone involvement may suffer pain and pathological fractures, whereas patients with muscle involvement may complain of painful swelling, which may mimic pyomyositis or thrombophlebitis. Plain films and CT of bone lesions may reveal osteolytic lesions with cortical destruction, sclerosis, indistinct transition zones, periosteal reaction, pathological fractures, and an associated soft-tissue mass.[110]

Although non-Hodgkin's lymphoma and Kaposi's sarcoma are well described in patients with HIV infection, reports of the occurrence of malignant plasma cell tumors are relatively uncommon.[58,88] Historically, multiple myeloma and extramedullary plasmacytomas are diseases associated with an older population and are extraordinarily rare in young persons. Their detection in young adults with HIV infection suggests that these tumors may represent another complication of HIV disease.

SUMMARY

Virtually all physicians, including orthopedic surgeons, will encounter individuals with HIV infection in their practice of medicine. Orthopedic surgeons need to be familiar with the risk of acquiring HIV from needlesticks, other surgical accidents, and blood transfusions, as well as the principles of risk reduction to ensure the safety of both patients and the entire health care team. Moreover, individuals infected with HIV are living longer, healthier, and more active lives. Consequently, orthopedists need to be aware of the possibility that their patients may have orthopedic complications not only because of HIV, but also independent of HIV infection. Thus, individuals with HIV infection deserve the same careful diagnostic and therapeutic management as uninfected patients. Finally, nearly all practicing physicians will encounter patients who are at risk for acquiring HIV infection, likely to be HIV infected, or in whom HIV infection is already diagnosed but is not being adequately treated. In such situations, frank discussion about prevention of transmission and testing, as well as referral to an HIV specialist when indicated, may contribute to the overall health of the individual and efforts to stem the tide of the HIV epidemic.

References

1. Alcabes P, Munoz A, Vlahov D, et al: Incubation period of human immunodeficiency virus. Epidemiol Rev 15:303-318, 1993.
2. Allain JP, Laurian Y, Paul DA, et al: Long-term evaluation of HIV antigen and antibodies to p24 and gp41 in patients with hemophilia. Potential clinical importance. N Engl J Med 317:1114-1121, 1987.
3. Alpiner N: Rehabilitation in joint and connective tissue diseases. 1. Systemic diseases. Arch Phys Med Rehabil 76:S32-S40, 1995.
4. American Medical Society for Sports Medicine (AMSSM) and the American Academy of Sports Medicine (AASM): Human immunodeficiency virus (HIV) and other blood-borne pathogens in sports. Joint position statement. Am J Sports Med 26:510-514, 1995.
5. Barbaro G, Di Lorenzo G, Grisorio B, et al: Incidence of dilated cardiomyopathy and detection of HIV in myocardial cells of HIV-positive patients. Gruppo Italiano per lo Studio Cardiologico dei Pazienti Affetti da AIDS. N Engl J Med 339:1093-1099, 1998.
6. Baron AL, Steinbach LS, LeBoit PE, et al: Osteolytic lesions and bacillary angiomatosis in HIV infection: Radiologic differentiation from AIDS-related Kaposi's sarcoma. Radiology 177:77-81, 1990.
7. Bartlett JG: HIV infection and surgeons. Curr Probl Surg 29:197-280, 1992.

8. Bartlett J: Medical Management of HIV Infection. Baltimore, Johns Hopkins University, 1998.

9. Beekmann SE, Vlahov D, Koziol DE, et al: Temporal association between implementation of universal precautions and a sustained, progressive decrease in percutaneous exposures to blood. Clin Infect Dis 18:562-569, 1994.

10. Bell DM, Shapiro CN, Ciesielski CA, et al: Preventing bloodborne pathogen transmission from health-care workers to patients. The CDC perspective. Surg Clin North Am 75:1189-1203, 1995.

11. Blanchard A, Ferris S, Chamaret S, et al: Molecular evidence for nosocomial transmission of human immunodeficiency virus from a surgeon to one of his patients. J Virol 72:4537-4540, 1998.

12. Brown TT, Ruppe MD, Kassner R, et al: Reduced bone mineral density in human immunodeficiency virus–infected patients and its association with increased central adiposity and postload hyperglycemia. J Clin Endocrinol Metab 89:1200-1206, 2004.

13. Buck BE, Resnick L, Shah SM, et al: Human immunodeficiency virus cultured from bone. Implications for transplantation. Clin Orthop 251:249-253, 1990.

14. Burcham J, Marmor M, Dubin N, et al: CD4% is the best predictor of development of AIDS in a cohort of HIV-infected homosexual men. AIDS 5:365-372, 1991.

15. Buskila D, Gladman D: Musculoskeletal manifestations of infection with human immunodeficiency virus. Rev Infect Dis 12:223-235, 1990.

16. Cardo DM, Culver DH, Ciesielski CA, et al: A case-control study of HIV seroconversion in health care workers after percutaneous exposure. Centers for Disease Control and Prevention Needlestick Surveillance Group. N Engl J Med 337:1485-1490, 1997.

17. Centers for Disease Control and Prevention: Recommendations for prevention of HIV transmission in health-care settings. MMWR Morb Mortal Wkly Rep 36(S2), 1987.

18. Centers for Disease Control and Prevention: Update: Universal precautions for prevention of transmission of human immunodeficiency virus, hepatitis B virus, and·other blood borne pathogens in health-care settings. MMWR Morb Mortal Wkly Rep 37(24):377-382, 387-388, 1988.

19. Centers for Disease Control and Prevention: Transmission of HIV through bone transplantation: Case report and public health recommendations. MMWR Morb Mortal Wkly Rep 37(39):597-599, 1988.

20. Centers for Disease Control and Prevention: Guidelines for prophylaxis against *Pneumocystis carinii* pneumonia for persons infected with HIV. MMWR Morb Mortal Wkly Rep 38(Suppl 5):1-19, 1989.

21. Centers for Disease Control and Prevention: Guidelines for prevention of transmission of human immunodeficiency virus and hepatitis B virus to health-care and public-safety workers. MMWR Morb Mortal Wkly Rep 38(Suppl 6):1-37, 1989.

22. Centers for Disease Control and Prevention: Update: Serologic testing for HIV-1 antibody—United States, 1988 and 1989. MMWR Morb Mortal Wkly Rep 39(22):380-383, 1990.

23. Centers for Disease Control and Prevention: Current trends in preliminary analysis: HIV serosurvey of orthopedic surgeons, 1991. MMWR Morb Mortal Wkly Rep 40(19):309-312, 1991.

24. Centers for Disease Control and Prevention: The HIV/AIDS epidemic: The first ten years. MMWR Morb Mortal Wkly Rep 40:357, 1991.

25. Centers for Disease Control and Prevention: Update: Transmission of HIV infection during invasive dental procedure—Florida. MMWR Morb Mortal Wkly Rep 40(23):377-381, 1991.

26. Centers for Disease Control and Prevention: Update: Trends in AIDS incidence, deaths, and prevalence—United States, 1996. MMWR Morb Mortal Wkly Rep 46(8):165-173, 1997.

27. Centers for Disease Control and Prevention: CDC Update: Combating Complacency in HIV. Prevention. http://www.cdc.gov/nchstp/hiv-aids/pubs/facts/combat.htm. Updated July 1998.

28. Centers for Disease Control and Prevention: Management of possible sexual, injecting drug use, or other nonoccupational exposure to HIV, including considerations related to antiretroviral therapy, 1998 (accessed at www.hivatis.org.).

29. Centers for Disease Control and Prevention: Preventing occupational HIV transmission to health care workers. http://www.cdc.gov/nchstp/hiv-aids. Updated October 1998.

30. Centers for Disease Control and Prevention: HIV prevention through early detection and treatment of other sexually transmitted diseases—United States. Recommendations of the Advisory Committeee for HIV and STD Prevention. MMWR Recomm Rep 47(RR-12):1-24, 1998.

31. Centers for Disease Control and Prevention: Recommendations for prevention and control of hepatitis C virus infection (HCV) and HCV-related chronic disease. MMWR Recomm Rep 47(RR-19):1-39, 1998.

32. Centers for Disease Control and Prevention: 1999 USPHS/IDSA guidelines for the prevention of opportunistic infections in persons infected with human immunodeficiency virus. MMWR Recomm Rep 48(RR-10):1-59, 61-66, 1999.

33. Centers for Disease Control and Prevention: Updated U.S. Public Health Service guidelines for the management of occupational exposures to HBV, HCV, and HIV and recommendations for postexposure prophylaxis. MMWR Recomm Rep 50(RR-11):1-42, 2001.

34. Centers for Disease Control and Prevention: HIV/AIDS Surveillance Report: Cases of HIV Infection and AIDS in the United States. MMWR 14:1–40, 2002.

35. Centers for Disease Control and Prevention: Guidelines for the use of antiretroviral agents in HIV-infected adults and adolescents, 2004 (accessed at wwwhivatisorg).

36. Centers for Disease Control and Prevention: Issues in Health Care Settings, 2004 (accessed at wwwhivatisorg).

37. Centers for Disease Control and Prevention: National AIDS Clearinghouse, 2004 (accessed at www.cdcnac.org).

38. Chaisson R: Epidemiology of human immunodeficiency virus and acquired immunodeficiency syndrome. In Gorabach S (ed): Infectious Diseases. Philadelphia, WB Saunders, 1992, p 912.

39. Chin J: Global estimates of AIDS cases and HIV infections: 1990. AIDS 4(Suppl 1):S277-S283, 1990.

40. Ciesielski C, Marianos D, Ou CY, et al: Transmission of human immunodeficiency virus in a dental practice. Ann Intern Med 116:798-805, 1992.

41. Connor EM, Sperling RS, Gelber R, et al: Reduction of maternal-infant transmission of human immunodeficiency virus type 1 with zidovudine treatment. Pediatric AIDS Clinical Trials Group Protocol 076 Study Group. N Engl J Med 331:1173-1180, 1994.

42. Coombs RW, Collier AC, Allain JP, et al: Plasma viremia in human immunodeficiency virus infection. N Engl J Med 321:1626-1631, 1989.

43. Cooper DA, Gold J, Maclean P, et al: Acute AIDS retrovirus infection. Definition of a clinical illness associated with seroconversion. Lancet 1:537-540, 1985.

44. Crawfurd EJ, Baird PR: An orthopaedic presentation of AIDS: Brief report. J Bone Joint Surg Br 69:672-673, 1987.

45. Cuellar ML: HIV infection–associated inflammatory musculoskeletal disorders. Rheum Dis Clin North Am 24:403-421, 1998.

46. Denning DW, Anderson J, Rudge P, et al: Acute myelopathy associated with primary infection with human immunodeficiency virus. Br Med J (Clin Res Ed) 294:143-144, 1987.

47. Detels R, Munoz A, McFarlane G, et al: Effectiveness of potent antiretroviral therapy on time to AIDS and death in men with known HIV infection duration. Multicenter AIDS Cohort Study Investigators. JAMA 280:1497-1503, 1998.

48. Dolan SE, Huang JS, Killilea KM, et al: Reduced bone density in HIV-infected women. AIDS 18:475-483, 2004.

49. Enger C, Graham N, Peng Y, et al: Survival from early, intermediate, and late stages of HIV infection. JAMA 275:1329-1334, 1996.

50. Espinoza LR, Jara LJ, Espinoza CG, et al: There is an association between human immunodeficiency virus infection and spondyloarthropathies. Rheum Dis Clin North Am 18:257-266, 1992.

51. Fahey BJ, Koziol DE, Banks SM, et al: Frequency of nonparenteral occupational exposures to blood and body fluids before and after universal precautions training. Am J Med 90:145-153, 1991.

52. Farthing C, Gazzard B: Acute illnesses associated with HTLV-III seroconversion. Lancet 1:935-936, 1985.

53. Fauci AS, Pantaleo G, Stanley S, et al: Immunopathogenic mechanisms of HIV infection. Ann Intern Med 124:654-663, 1996.

54. Fox R, Eldred LJ, Fuchs EJ, et al: Clinical manifestations of acute infection with human immunodeficiency virus in a cohort of gay men. AIDS 1:35-38, 1987.

55. Gerberding JL: Management of occupational exposures to blood-borne viruses. N Engl J Med 332:444-451, 1995.

56. Gerberding J: Provider-to-patient HIV transmission: How to keep it exceedingly rare. Ann Intern Med 130:64-65, 1999.

57. Glesby MJ: Bone disorders in human immunodeficiency virus infection. Clin Infect Dis 37(Suppl 2):S91-S95, 2003.

58. Gold JE, Schwam L, Castella A, et al: Malignant plasma cell tumors in human immunodeficiency virus–infected patients. Cancer 66:363-368, 1990.

59. Goudsmit J, de Wolf F, Paul DA, et al: Expression of human immunodeficiency virus antigen (HIV-Ag) in serum and cerebrospinal fluid during acute and chronic infection. Lancet 2:177-180, 1986.

60. Graham NM, Zeger SL, Park LP, et al: Effect of zidovudine and Pneumocystis carinii pneumonia prophylaxis on progression of HIV-1 infection to AIDS. The Multicenter AIDS Cohort Study. Lancet 338:265-269, 1991.

61. Gutierrez F, Padilla S, Ortega E, et al: Avascular necrosis of the bone in HIV-infected patients: Incidence and associated factors. AIDS 16:481-483, 2002.

62. Haynes BF, Pantaleo G, Fauci AS: Toward an understanding of the correlates of protective immunity to HIV infection. Science 271:324-328, 1996.

63. Henderson DK, Fahey BJ, Willy M, et al: Risk for occupational transmission of human immunodeficiency virus type 1 (HIV-1) associated with clinical exposures. A prospective evaluation. Ann Intern Med 113:740-746, 1990.

64. Herts BR, Rafii M, Spiegel G: Soft-tissue and osseous lesions caused by bacillary angiomatosis: Unusual manifestations of cat-scratch fever in patients with AIDS. AJR Am J Roentgenol 157:1249-1251, 1991.

65. Hirsch R, Miller SM, Kazi S, et al: Human immunodeficiency virus–associated atypical mycobacterial skeletal infections. Semin Arthritis Rheum 25:347-356, 1996.

66. Ho DD, Moudgil T, Alam M. Quantitation of human immunodeficiency virus type 1 in the blood of infected persons. N Engl J Med 321:1621-1625, 1989.

67. Ho DD, Sarngadharan MG, Resnick L, et al: Primary human T-lymphotropic virus type III infection. Ann Intern Med 103:880-883, 1985.

68. Hoy J: Osteopenia in a randomized, multicenter study of protease inhibitor (PI) substitution in patients with the lipodystrophy syndrome and well-controlled HIV viremia [abstract 208]. Presented at the Seventh Conference on Retrovirus and Opportunistic Infections, San Francisco, 2000.

69. Hughes RA, Rowe IF, Shanson D, et al: Septic bone, joint and muscle lesions associated with human immunodeficiency virus infection. Br J Rheumatol 31:381-388, 1992.

70. Ippolito G, Puro V, De Carli G: The risk of occupational human immunodeficiency virus infection in health care workers. Italian Multicenter Study. The Italian Study Group on Occupational Risk of HIV infection. Arch Intern Med 153:1451-1458, 1993.

71. Johnson AM, Laga M: Heterosexual transmission of HIV. AIDS 2(Suppl 1):S49-S56, 1988.

72. Johnson GK, Robinson WS: Human immunodeficiency virus-1 (HIV-1) in the vapors of surgical power instruments. J Med Virol 33:47-50, 1991.

73. Karon JM, Buehler JW, Byers RH, et al: Projections of the number of persons diagnosed with AIDS and the number of immunosuppressed HIV-infected persons, United States, 1992-1994. MMWR Recomm Rep 41(RR-18):1-29, 1992.

74. Kaye BR: Rheumatologic manifestations of HIV infections. Clin Rev Allergy Immunol 14:385-416, 1996.

75. Keruly J, Chaisson R, Moore R: Increasing incidence of avascular necrosis of the hip in HIV-infected patients [letter]. J Acquir Immune Defic Syndr 28:101-102, 2001.

76. Kessler HA, Blaauw B, Spear J, et al: Diagnosis of human immunodeficiency virus infection in seronegative homosexuals presenting with an acute viral syndrome. JAMA 258:1196-1199, 1987.

77. Lackritz EM, Satten GA, Aberle-Grasse J, et al: Estimated risk of transmission of the human immunodeficiency virus by screened blood in the United States. N Engl J Med 333:1721-1725, 1995.

78. La Prairie AJ, Gross M: A simplified protocol for banking bone from surgical donors requiring a 90-day quarantine and an HIV-1 antibody test. Can J Surg 34:41-48, 1991.

79. Lot F, Seguier JC, Fegueux S, et al: Probable transmission of HIV from an orthopedic surgeon to a patient in France. Ann Intern Med 130:1-6, 1999.

80. Mann JM: AIDS—the second decade: A global perspective. J Infect Dis 165:245-250, 1992.

81. Mast ST, Woolwine JD, Gerberding JL: Efficacy of gloves in reducing blood volumes transferred during simulated needlestick injury. J Infect Dis 168:1589-1592, 1993.

82. Masters DL, Lentino JR: Cervical osteomyelitis related to Nocardia asteroides. J Infect Dis 149:824-825, 1984.

83. Masur H, Ognibene FP, Yarchoan R, et al: CD4 counts as predictors of opportunistic pneumonias in human immunodeficiency virus (HIV) infection. Ann Intern Med 111:223-231, 1989.

84. Matava MJ, Horgan M: Serial quantification of the human immunodeficiency virus in an arthroscopic effluent. Arthroscopy 13:739-742, 1997.

85. McCormick RD, Meisch MG, Ircink FG, et al: Epidemiology of hospital sharps injuries: A 14-year prospective study in the pre-AIDS and AIDS eras. Am J Med 91(3B):301S-307S, 1991.

86. Mellert W, Kleinschmidt A, Schmidt J, et al: Infection of human fibroblasts and osteoblast-like cells with HIV-1. AIDS 4:527-535, 1990.

87. Mellors JW, Munoz A, Giorgi JV, et al: Plasma viral load and CD4+ lymphocytes as prognostic markers of HIV-1 infection. Ann Intern Med 126:946-954, 1997.

88. Meyers SA, Kuhlman JE, Fishman EK: Kaposi sarcoma involving bone: CT demonstration in a patient with AIDS. J Comput Assist Tomogr 14:161-162, 1990.

89. Miller KD, Masur H, Jones EC, et al: High prevalence of osteonecrosis of the femoral head in HIV-infected adults. Ann Intern Med 137:17-25, 2002.

90. Munoz F: Rheumatic manifestations in 556 patients with human immunodeficiency virus infection. Semin Arthritis Rheum 21:30, 1991.

91. Munoz F: Osteoarticular infection associated with the human immunodeficiency virus. Clin Exp Rheumatol 9:489, 1991.

92. Niu MT, Stein DS, Schnittman SM: Primary human immunodeficiency virus type 1 infection: Review of pathogenesis and early treatment intervention in humans and animal retrovirus infections. J Infect Dis 168:1490-1501, 1993.

93. Oh TH, Brander VA, Hinderer SR, et al: Rehabilitation in joint and connective tissue diseases. 2. Inflammatory and degenerative spine diseases. Arch Phys Med Rehabil 76(5 Spec No):S41-S46, 1995.

94. Pantaleo G, Graziosi C, Demarest JF, et al: HIV infection is active and progressive in lymphoid tissue during the clinically latent stage of disease. Nature 362:355-358, 1993.

95. Paton P, Tabib A, Loire R, et al: Coronary artery lesions and human immunodeficiency virus infection. Res Virol 144:225-231, 1993.

96. Polis MA, Masur H: Predicting the progression to AIDS. Am J Med 89:701-705, 1990.

97. Quinn TC: The epidemiology of AIDS: A decade of experience. Curr Clin Top Infect Dis 11:61-93, 1991.

98. Raahave D, Bremmelgaard A: New operative technique to reduce surgeons' risk of HIV infection. J Hosp Infect 18(Suppl A):177-183, 1991.

99. Robert LM, Chamberland ME, Cleveland JL, et al: Investigations of patients of health care workers infected with HIV. The Centers for Disease Control and Prevention database. Ann Intern Med 122:653-657, 1995.

100. Roder W, Muller H, Muller WE, et al: HIV infection in human bone. J Bone Joint Surg Br 74:179-180, 1992.

101. Rowe IF: HIV- and AIDS-related musculoskeletal problems. Curr Opin Rheumatol 2:642-647, 1990.

102. Rowe IF: Arthritis in the acquired immunodeficiency syndrome and other viral infections. Curr Opin Rheumatol 3:621-627, 1991.

103. Sabbagh M, Meyer O, De Bandt M, et al: Bone manifestations associated with acquired immunodeficiency syndrome (AIDS). Ann Med Interne (Paris) 143:50-56, 1992.

104. Shapiro CN: Occupational risk of infection with hepatitis B and hepatitis C virus. Surg Clin North Am 75:1047-1056, 1995.

105. Simonds RJ, Holmberg SD, Hurwitz RL, et al: Transmission of human immunodeficiency virus type 1 from a seronegative organ and tissue donor. N Engl J Med 326:726-732, 1992.

106. Slagis SV, Benjamin JB, Volz RG, et al: Postoperative blood salvage in total hip and knee arthroplasty. A randomised controlled trial. J Bone Joint Surg Br 73:591-594, 1991.

107. Surveillance of Health Care Workers with AIDS, 2004 (accessed at www.cdc.gov/niosh-chartbook/appendix/ap-a-18.html).

108. Taylor JM, Fahey JL, Detels R, et al: CD4 percentage, CD4 number, and CD4:CD8 ratio in HIV infection: Which to choose and how to use. J Acquir Immune Defic Syndr 2:114-124, 1989.

109. Tebas P: Accelerated bone mineral loss in HIV-infected patients receiving patient antiretroviral therapy [abstract 207]. Presented at the Seventh Conference on Retrovirus and Opportunistic Infections, San Francisco, 2000.

110. Tehranzadeh J, O'Malley P, Rafii M: The spectrum of osteoarticular and soft tissue changes in patients with human immunodeficiency virus (HIV) infection. Crit Rev Diagn Imaging 37:305-347, 1996.

111. Thomas J, Doherty SM: HIV infection—a risk factor for osteoporosis. J Acquir Immune Defic Syndr 33:281-291, 2003.

112. Timpone J: Avascular necrosis in HIV+ patients a potential link to protease inhibitors [abstract 680]. Presented at the Sixth Conference on Retroviruses and Opportunistic Infections, Chicago, January 31-February 4, 1999.

113. Tindall B, Barker S, Donovan B, et al: Characterization of the acute clinical illness associated with human immunodeficiency virus infection. Arch Intern Med 148:945-949, 1988.

114. Tokars JI, Bell DM, Culver DH, et al: Percutaneous injuries during surgical procedures. JAMA 267:2899-2904, 1992.

115. Tokars JI, Chamberland ME, Schable CA, et al: A survey of occupational blood contact and HIV infection among orthopedic surgeons. The American Academy of Orthopaedic Surgeons Serosurvey Study Committee. JAMA 268:489-494, 1992.

116. Tokars JI, Marcus R, Culver DH, et al: Surveillance of HIV infection and zidovudine use among health care workers after occupational exposure to HIV-infected blood. The CDC Cooperative Needlestick Surveillance Group. Ann Intern Med 118:913-919, 1993.

117. U.S. Public Health Service Task Force recommendations for the use of antiretroviral drugs in pregnant women infected with HIV-1 for maternal health and for reducing perinatal HIV-1 transmission in the United States, 2004 (accessed at www.hivatis.org).

118. van der Wouw PA, Hadderingh RJ, Reiss P, et al: Disseminated cat-scratch disease in a patient with AIDS. AIDS 3:751-753, 1989.

119. Vassilopoulos D, Chalasani P, Jurado RL, et al: Musculoskeletal infections in patients with human immunodeficiency virus infection. Medicine (Baltimore) 76:284-294, 1997.

CHAPTER 60

Anesthesia for Knee Surgery

Richard Brull • Nigel E. Sharrock

This chapter outlines the anesthetic techniques for the most common types of knee surgery performed in modern orthopedic practice, with particular emphasis on the benefits of regional anesthesia (RA) and the challenges of ambulatory surgery. Anesthetic considerations specific to surgery about the knee, including implications of the tourniquet and deep vein thrombosis (DVT), are also addressed. Finally, the conflict of RA in the setting of perioperative anticoagulation is discussed.

ANESTHETIC TECHNIQUES FOR KNEE SURGERY

General Anesthesia

General anesthesia (GA) is the time-tested standard for safe and effective surgical anesthesia. GA offers several advantages over RA. Importantly, GA affords a 100% success rate, in contrast to RA, which carries an inherent failure rate even in experienced hands.[104] More anesthesiologists are familiar with providing GA than RA,[136] GA can be performed faster than RA, and the technical skills needed to administer GA are easier to acquire than those for RA. It follows that GA is the most widely used anesthetic technique for ambulatory surgery, with sustained popularity among patients, surgeons, and anesthesiologists alike.[149] However, GA is widely recognized to result in more postoperative pain and more postoperative nausea and vomiting (PONV) than RA is.[88] Newer short-acting general anesthetic agents culminate in significantly fewer adverse effects,[113] shorter recovery time in the hospital,[110] and improved patient satisfaction[41] in comparison to older agents.

Regional Anesthesia

RA for knee surgery includes central neuraxial blockade (CNB), specifically, epidural and spinal anesthesia, as well as peripheral nerve blockade (PNB). One of the principal advantages of RA is the dual capacity for dense surgical anesthesia and long-lasting, opioid-sparing postoperative analgesia. All RA techniques for knee surgery are associated with numerous benefits when compared with GA, as described later. The choice of RA technique is oftentimes determined by patient factors, such as patient preference and comorbid conditions (e.g., obesity),[25] as well as by extraneous factors, such as surgeon preference, time constraints, availability of a "block room," anesthetic personnel, and perceived liability risk. When GA is not strictly indicated by patient- and/or surgery-related factors, RA alone or in combination with GA should be considered. RA combined with GA effectively spares intraoperative opioid requirements (and avoids their unwanted adverse effects), enables faster emergence,[158] and affords postoperative analgesia superior to that of GA alone. Importantly, one contraindication to performing RA is an unconscious patient who cannot communicate symptoms of an improperly positioned (e.g., intraneural) needle. Therefore, when a combination of GA and RA is planned, GA should be induced after CNB or PNB is established.

CENTRAL NEURAXIAL BLOCKADE

Both spinal and epidural anesthesia provide excellent surgical anesthesia for knee surgery. Most anesthesiologists are well versed in spinal and epidural anesthesia, and these CNB techniques are often easier to perform and afford greater reliability than is the case with PNB. In a recent systematic review of 141 clinical trials comparing postoperative morbidity and mortality after CNB or GA, overall mortality was reduced by a third in patients allocated to CNB, and CNB reduced the odds of DVT by 44%, pulmonary embolism by 55%, transfusion requirements by 50%, pneumonia by 39%, and respiratory depression by 59%.[121] Specifically, the reduction in relative risk for in-hospital mortality after TKA approaches 85% with epidural anesthesia as compared with GA.[129] Furthermore, continuous and/or patient-controlled epidural analgesia after major knee surgery decreases postoperative pain and, importantly, facilitates rehabilitation and hastens convalescence[13,159] when compared with traditional intravenous morphine patient-controlled analgesia.

Major complications of CNB include hypotension and bradycardia as a result of blockade of sympathetic nerve fibers and, rarely, epidural abscess and spinal hematoma (see "Anticoagulation and Regional Anesthesia," later). Post–dural puncture headache (PDPH) is a benign, often severe postural fronto-occipital headache stemming from dural puncture and, presumably, consequent leakage of cerebrospinal fluid. The reported incidence of PDPH after accidental dural puncture with a large-diameter (e.g., 17 to 18 gauge) epidural needle for epidural anesthesia is as high as 80%,[29,30] whereas the incidence of PDPH after intentional dural puncture with a small-diameter (22 to 27 gauge) spinal needle for spinal anesthesia is as high as

37%.[44] Important disadvantages of CNB techniques include anesthesia of the nonoperative limb, which can delay ambulation, as well as urinary retention.

Spinal anesthesia is increasingly being performed for ambulatory knee surgery ever since the introduction of small pencil-point tip needles (e.g., Whitacre), which have resulted in a much lower incidence of PDPH than noted with traditional cutting tip needles (e.g., Quincke).[57] The needle of choice for spinal anesthesia at our home institution is a 27-gauge Whitacre needle, which bears an incidence of PDPH ranging from 0% to 0.5%.[24,93,124] In addition, the side port of the Whitacre needle enables local anesthetic to be directed toward the site of surgery in an attempt to anesthetize only the ipsilateral nerve roots, thus sparing the nonoperative limb.[42]

Combined spinal-epidural anesthesia is an ideal technique for major knee surgery that combines the benefits of spinal and epidural anesthesia: reliable, rapid-onset, dense surgical anesthesia conferred by the spinal dose of local anesthetic and the flexibility to administer supplemental local anesthetic as necessary via the epidural catheter for prolonged intraoperative anesthesia and/or excellent postoperative analgesia.

PERIPHERAL NERVE BLOCKADE

PNB avoids the unwanted adverse effects of GA and CNB and allows for targeted unilateral blockade of the operative limb and thus earlier postoperative ambulation. For ambulatory knee surgery, PNB results in less postoperative pain, decreased PONV, shorter postoperative stay in the postanesthesia care unit, and greater patient satisfaction than GA does.[75,156] For major knee surgery, the analgesic effects of single-injection PNB with a long-acting local anesthetic (e.g., bupivacaine with epinephrine) can last up to 18 hours postoperatively,[27,50] with opioid-sparing effects for up to 36 hours postoperatively.[2]

Continuous PNB has gained tremendous popularity in recent years because continuous perineural infusion of dilute long-acting local anesthetic solution via an indwelling catheter can significantly prolong postoperative analgesia[95] and, importantly, facilitate rehabilitation after major knee surgery[13,135,159] since opioid-related adverse effects are spared.[95] Continuous PNB catheters are inserted much like epidural catheters; that is, a 20-gauge catheter is inserted alongside the target nerve via a 17- or 18-gauge introducer (e.g., Touhy) needle.

Major knee surgery is accompanied by moderate to severe pain[9] that often mandates hospital admission for postoperative parenteral analgesics. With the ongoing shift away from costly perioperative hospital admission toward ambulatory surgery, providing safe and effective postoperative analgesia to outpatients undergoing major knee surgery is a challenging endeavor. The advent of disposable elastometric balloon pumps and portable programmable mechanical pumps has enabled the use of continuous PNB at home[14] and has thus shortened postoperative hospital admission or obviated the need for admission altogether.[85] Indeed, recent reports favor the feasibility, efficacy, and safety of continuous PNB at home after major knee surgery.[20,40,84]

The most commonly used technique for nerve localization during PNB is peripheral nerve stimulation. Peripheral nerve stimulation involves the use of a special stimulating needle that has an insulated sheath along the needle shaft while the needle tip is uninsulated. A 1.5-mA, 2-Hz current is applied to the stimulating needle with a nerve stimulator. Anatomic landmarks identify the point of needle insertion, and the needle is advanced until an appropriate motor response (muscle twitch corresponding to the desired peripheral nerve) is obtained. Before injection of local anesthetic, the location of the needle tip is carefully adjusted to maintain the desired motor twitch while the electrical current is reduced below 0.5 mA, which conventionally designates close approximation of the needle tip to the nerve. After aspiration to exclude intravascular placement, a predetermined dose of local anesthetic (usually 30 mL for large peripheral nerves) is injected incrementally, all the while maintaining verbal communication with the patient to ensure the absence of intense pain or paresthesias during injection, both of which suggest intraneural needle placement and mandate immediate cessation and needle relocation. More recently, ultrasonography for nerve localization has been the subject of fervent interest among anesthesiologists worldwide because ultrasound guidance affords real-time visualization of the needle tip, the nerve, and the local anesthetic injectate.[18] The theoretical benefit of ultrasound-guided nerve localization is safety because vascular structures are easily identified and avoided and the risk of intraneural or intravascular injection of local anesthetic is diminished significantly. A reduction in anesthesia-related complications coupled with deflated ultrasonographic equipment costs will, it is hoped, broaden the use of ultrasound for PNB in the near future. Nonetheless, there have been no studies to date that definitively demonstrate fewer complications or an improved rate of success with the use of ultrasonography as opposed to peripheral nerve stimulation for lower extremity PNB.

PNB requires an in-depth knowledge of functional anatomy as well as technical skill for safe and successful performance. The knee joint is innervated by the femoral (L2-L4 ventral rami), obturator (L2-L4 ventral rami), and sciatic (L4-S3 rami) nerves. Structures adjacent to the knee are innervated by these three nerves, as well as by the lateral femoral cutaneous nerve of the thigh (L2-L3 ventral rami). Thus, for complete surgical anesthesia of the knee, blockade of all four nerves is required. The most commonly performed PNB techniques for knee surgery are discussed in the following paragraphs.

The femoral, obturator, and lateral femoral cutaneous nerves can be blocked simultaneously by using a single-injection technique described by Winnie et al as the "3-in-1" block.[160] The efficacy of the 3-in-1 block is based on the presumption that the femoral, obturator, and lateral femoral cutaneous nerves travel together in a continuous fascia-enclosed space and that a large volume of local anesthetic injected into this compartment will spread to anesthetize all three nerves. In practice, however, blockade of all three nerves has been difficult to achieve with the 3-in-1 technique, with the obturator nerve most commonly being missed.[87,107] Each of the femoral, obturator, and lateral femoral cutaneous nerves can be blocked individually with more targeted approaches, but these techniques are time consuming and not commonly used for knee surgery. Because the femoral nerve predominantly innervates the knee joint and is therefore the primary target for the 3-in-1 block, most anesthesiologists, including the present authors, use the term femoral nerve block (FNB) interchangeably with 3-in-1 block. For the purposes of this chapter, FNB refers to the 3-in-1 block. FNB is performed with the patient positioned supine. An insulated needle is inserted perpendicular to the skin at a point 2 cm below the inguinal ligament and 1 cm lateral to the femoral artery pulsation. The needle is advanced until contraction of the quadriceps muscle (so-called patella twitch) is elicited with a nerve stimulator, followed by injection of local anesthetic.

The entire lumbar plexus (L1-L4 ventral rami) can be reliably anesthetized by a single injection via a posterior approach with the patient in the lateral decubitus position, as described by Winnie et al[161] and Chayen et al.[19] An insulated needle is inserted approximately 5 cm lateral to the L4-L5 spinous interspace and advanced to encounter the lumbar plexus in between the psoas and quadratum lumborum muscles. Contraction of the quadriceps or thigh adductors is elicited with a nerve stimulator. However, similar to the 3-in-1 block, the lumbar plexus block (LPB) spares the sciatic distribution. LPB is reportedly associated with a 1% incidence of major complications, including cardiac arrest, total spinal anesthesia, and seizures.[4]

For knee surgery, the sciatic nerve (L4-S3) can be blocked with a variety of approaches, the most common of which is termed the classic posterior approach of Labat.[35] With the patient positioned semiprone and the operative side uppermost, a line is drawn between the greater trochanter of the femur and the posterior superior iliac spine. A second line is drawn between the greater trochanter of the femur and the sacral hiatus. A tangential line extending from the midpoint of the first line to its intersection with the second line identifies the point of needle insertion. An insulated needle is inserted and advanced until plantar flexion (tibial branch of the sciatic nerve) or dorsiflexion (common peroneal branch of the sciatic nerve) is elicited with a nerve stimulator. Alternatively, when the patient cannot be placed semiprone (e.g., trauma), the anterior approach to sciatic nerve blockade is performed at the level of the lesser trochanter of the femur.[94] Two disadvantages of the anterior approach to sciatic nerve blockade are sparing of the posterior cutaneous nerve of the thigh, which is implicated in tourniquet pain, and difficulty placing a catheter for continuous PNB.

Local Anesthetics

Local anesthetic preparations vary with respect to the duration of blockade and should be selected according to the anticipated duration of surgery and requirements for postoperative analgesia. The following local anesthetic preparations are recommended for surgical anesthesia: chloroprocaine for short-duration blockade (<1 hour),

lidocaine or mepivacaine for medium-duration blockade (1 to 3 hours), and bupivacaine or ropivacaine for prolonged blockade (2 to 4 hours) or continuous PNB.[28]

Anesthesia for Knee Arthroscopy

Knee arthroscopy is a minimally invasive procedure that is typically performed electively on an ambulatory basis. Characteristics of the ideal anesthetic for outpatient knee arthroscopy include rapid onset, rapid offset, good operating conditions, effective postoperative analgesia, few adverse effects, early discharge, and high patient satisfaction. However, patient expectations and comorbid conditions, as well as the skill and experience of the surgeon and anesthesiologist, may preclude achievement of the optimal anesthetic.[68] Short-acting general anesthetic agents (propofol, desflurane, remifentanil) offer rapid induction and emergence, which contribute to an efficient perioperative environment and facilitate discharge from the hospital.[31,101] Moreover, the laryngeal mask airway has revolutionized airway management for GA during ambulatory surgery such that endotracheal intubation and its implications (muscle paralysis, hemodynamic fluctuations associated with laryngoscopy, and sore throat) are often avoided.

Knee arthroscopy is also well suited for RA techniques because RA results in less postoperative pain and PONV than GA does, both of which are the predominant reasons for delayed discharge from the hospital after ambulatory surgery.[22] Indeed, RA has been shown to provide more rapid discharge,[108,109] superior perioperative resource utilization,[75] and improved patient satisfaction[75] when compared with short-acting GA for ambulatory knee arthroscopy. Appropriate RA techniques for outpatients undergoing knee arthroscopy include spinal[6,7] or epidural[101,102,108] anesthesia, combined spinal-epidural anesthesia,[145] combined femoral-sciatic nerve block,[15,123] FNB with intravenous sedation,[10] and local anesthesia of the knee (intra-articular injection) with intravenous sedation.[45,73,74,128] Despite the many aforementioned benefits of RA, there are limitations to each CNB and PNB technique. For example, management of PDPH on an outpatient basis can be complex. Similarly, slow regression of CNB and consequent urinary retention may limit the use of spinal and epidural anesthesia in the ambulatory setting. Moreover, there is no ideal local anesthetic solution for spinal anesthesia for outpatient knee arthroscopy. The short-acting local anesthetic lidocaine is associated with a high incidence of transient neurological symptoms, specifically, back pain radiating to the buttocks and thighs that lasts for several days.[112] The incidence of such symptoms after knee arthroscopy is as high as 31% and 22% with 5% hyperbaric[63] and 2% isobaric[89] lidocaine, respectively. Transient neurological symptoms typically respond well to nonsteroidal anti-inflammatory drugs (NSAIDs). It is noted that these symptoms are relatively uncommon following epidural anesthesia. Long-acting local anesthetics (e.g., bupivacaine) are not associated with transient neurological symptoms[47] but are less suitable for knee arthroscopy because of delayed recovery of motor function after surgery. Attempts to decrease the dose of bupivacaine and/or add intrathecal opioid culminate in suboptimal anesthesia and excessive adverse effects (vomiting, pruritus, urinary retention), respectively.[7,54] Moreover, attempts to provide unilateral spinal anesthesia appear to be overly time consuming for routine use.[15,42] Spinal anesthesia and combined femoral-sciatic nerve block have each been demonstrated to shorten the length of stay in the postanesthesia care unit in comparison to short-acting GA,[16,17] but prolonged lower extremity paralysis may ultimately delay discharge home.

Finally, a myriad of agents, either alone or in combination, has been shown to reduce pain after knee arthroscopy when injected intra-articularly. These agents include local anesthetics (e.g., bupivacaine),[100] opioids (e.g., morphine),[52,137,138] NSAIDs (e.g., ketorolac),[23,51,117] glucocorticoids (e.g., methylprednisolone),[83,115,116] N-methyl-D-aspartic acid (NMDA) receptor antagonists (e.g., ketamine),[32] α_2-adrenergic receptor agonists (e.g., clonidine),[79,118] anticholinesterases (e.g., neostigmine),[32,165] and even saline.[122] The intra-articular preparation administered to patients at our home institution after knee arthroscopy is composed of 10 mL of 0.25% bupivacaine with 1 : 300,000 epinephrine and 5 mg morphine.

Anesthesia for Anterior Cruciate Ligament Reconstruction

Complex anterior cruciate ligament reconstruction surgery is increasingly being performed on an outpatient basis and is greatly facilitated by RA techniques, including spinal, epidural, and combined spinal-epidural anesthesia or combined femoral-sciatic nerve block for surgical anesthesia. Alternatively, FNB or combined femoral-sciatic nerve block can be used for excellent postoperative analgesia after ambulatory anterior cruciate ligament reconstruction performed under GA,[36] thus allowing patients to bypass the postanesthesia care unit with reliable same-day discharge from the hospital.[156,157]

Anesthesia for Total Knee Arthroplasty

The anesthetic technique influences clinical outcome most notably after TKA. When compared with GA, epidural anesthesia reduces the incidence of distal and proximal DVT by approximately 20% and 50%, respectively (see "Deep Vein Thrombosis," later). With the introduction of epidural anesthesia and analgesia for TKA at our home institution, in-hospital mortality declined from 0.44% to 0.07% over the subsequent 10 years[129]—a dramatic testimony to the effect of anesthesia on outcome after TKA. Moreover, epidural anesthesia facilitates bilateral sequential one-stage TKA with very low perioperative morbidity and mortality.[111] Alternatively, combined LPB–sciatic nerve block has been used for surgical anesthesia for TKA with a high degree of patient satisfaction; however, this method is associated with an unacceptably high rate of conversion to GA as a result of insufficient

anesthesia.[92] The ideal postoperative analgesic regimen to control the moderate to severe pain that follows TKA[9] is controversial. Epidural analgesia, single-injection FNB, and continuous catheter-based FNB have each been demonstrated to improve pain control[2,13,37,62,114,127,152,153,159] and facilitate rehabilitation[13,152,159] after TKA when compared with systemic analgesia. Interestingly, sciatic afferents (i.e., posterior aspect of the knee) do not appear to contribute significantly to pain after TKA.[2] In one study that compared single-injection FNB with continuous catheter FNB for postoperative analgesia after TKA, little or no additional benefit was achieved by the placement of a catheter as opposed to the single-injection technique.[62] Patients undergoing TKA at our home institution receive patient-controlled epidural analgesia combined with single-injection FNB; this combination has recently been demonstrated to significantly reduce pain during the first 3 postoperative days and facilitate rehabilitation when compared with patient-controlled epidural analgesia alone after TKA.[163]

Anesthesia for Fractures about the Knee

Fractures in and around the knee create a number of perioperative complexities for the anesthesiologist. These include, but are not limited to, multiply injured patients, blood loss, fat embolism (see "Fat Embolism," later), full stomach, and anticoagulation. FNB and LPB provide excellent pain control for distal femoral and patellar fractures. Tibial fractures may be complicated by compartment syndrome, thus rendering sciatic nerve block precarious (see "Compartment Syndrome," later).

ANESTHETIC CONSIDERATIONS FOR KNEE SURGERY

Perioperative Bleeding

Blood loss can be significant after TKA (average, 1500 mL),[91] major ligament reconstruction, and trauma surgery about the knee. Blood conservation strategies for TKA include preoperative erythropoietin and autologous blood donation,[26] meticulous surgical technique, induced hypotension,[80] acute normovolemic hemodilution,[106] red cell salvage,[58,142] and administration of antifibrinolytics such as tranexamic acid.[8,59,60,150] The majority of blood loss associated with TKA occurs after surgery; therefore, the use of an intraoperative tourniquet does not appear to influence blood transfusion requirements (see the next section).

Tourniquet

Intraoperative tourniquet use can cause multiple physiological insults of special interest to the anesthesiologist, most notably, cardiovascular and metabolic derangements.

Thigh tourniquet application (inflation) causes an increase in circulating blood volume that is manifested as a transient rise in mean arterial pressure (MAP), central venous pressure (CVP), and systemic vascular resistance (SVR).[49,81] Although most patients can tolerate these hemodynamic alterations, an acute increase in preload and afterload can cause patients with significant cardiac disease (e.g., congestive heart failure) to decompensate. Moreover, tourniquet application becomes increasingly painful over time, as manifested by a 30% rise in systolic or diastolic blood pressure about 45 to 60 minutes after inflation (so-called tourniquet hypertension).[82,146,147] Tourniquet hypertension can be blunted by RA techniques, but it is classically difficult to treat under inhalational GA.[146,147] NMDA receptor antagonists such as ketamine[126] and dextromethorphan[164] have recently shown promise in treating tourniquet hypertension under GA, thus suggesting a central sensitization mechanism behind this phenomenon.

On removal (deflation) of the tourniquet, a transient decline in MAP, CVP, SVR, and core body temperature ensues.[49,81] The observed reduction in SVR exceeds that of MAP such that cardiac output and, correspondingly, oxygen consumption (VO_2), are significantly increased after tourniquet deflation.[49] An increase in $PaCO_2$ and lactate is also observed because of entry of hypercapnic blood (metabolic acidosis) into the systemic circulation from the ischemic leg,[49] as manifested by a rise in end-tidal CO_2 in a mechanically ventilated patient or by a brisk, transient increase in ventilation in a spontaneously breathing patient.[11] Indeed, tourniquet deflation has been associated with acute pulmonary edema[105] and even cardiac arrest.[48] Finally, systemic levels of fibrinopeptide A, a hematological marker of thrombosis, abruptly increase within seconds of tourniquet deflation.[130]

Well-documented injury to the nerves,[103,125,133,155] muscles,[1] and blood vessels[86] underneath the tourniquet is probably related to both inflation pressure and the duration of inflation.[81] It is recommended that the tourniquet be deflated every 90 to 120 minutes to minimize the risk for postoperative neuropraxia.[125] Tourniquet use is contraindicated in patients with previous arterial reconstruction in the leg because of the risk for graft thrombosis. The risk of arterial injury in patients with calcified femoral vessels is unclear.[77] Nevertheless, it may be preferable to operate without a tourniquet in patients with known peripheral vascular disease. In these situations, bleeding can be minimized by using other aforementioned blood conservation strategies.

Recent prospective randomized controlled trials demonstrate improved outcome when a tourniquet is not used for TKA. When compared with TKA performed with a tourniquet, the absence of a tourniquet does not prolong operating time or increase total blood loss and may reduce postoperative pain, superficial wound infections, and the incidence of DVT, as well as facilitate the achievement of postoperative rehabilitation milestones.[1,151] If a tourniquet must be used for TKA, early tourniquet release (i.e., before closure of the quadriceps mechanism) results in less postoperative pain and earlier straight-leg raising, with similar operating time and total blood loss, than conventional tourniquet deflation does after wound closure and band-

aging.[5] Emerging data such are these may limit tourniquet use for major knee surgery in the future.

Deep Vein Thrombosis

Postoperative DVT has been reported to occur in up to 88% of patients after TKA and proximal DVT in up to 20% of patients after TKA.[55,61,90,96,132,140,141] The anesthetic technique can profoundly affect the incidence of DVT associated with TKA. In studies comparing the rate of DVT associated with epidural anesthesia or GA for TKA, the relative risk for DVT is reportedly reduced up to 69% after epidural anesthesia versus GA.[78,131,159] The incidence of pulmonary embolism is reduced by up to a third with epidural anesthesia versus GA for TKA.[131,159] Whether the protective effect of epidural anesthesia occurs during or immediately after surgery is unknown. Hematological markers of thrombosis and fibrinolysis do not differ between patients who undergo TKA with epidural anesthesia or GA,[130] thus suggesting that the effect of epidural anesthesia may occur in the postoperative period rather than during surgery. Moreover, tourniquet use probably blunts much of the hemodynamic benefits of epidural anesthesia in the operative limb. One possible mechanism whereby epidural anesthesia may decrease DVT rates is by enhancing lower extremity venous blood flow postoperatively[99] and perhaps "washing out" the thrombogenic load accumulated during surgery. Additionally, epidural analgesia facilitates postoperative rehabilitation after TKA,[13,135,159] which may indirectly prevent DVT formation.

No trials have compared the incidence of DVT after spinal anesthesia versus either GA or epidural anesthesia for TKA. However, both epidural anesthesia and spinal anesthesia prevent DVT after total hip arthroplasty when compared with GA[34]; thus, it is probable that spinal anesthesia also confers a benefit over GA for TKA. The physiological effects of spinal anesthesia are similar to those of epidural anesthesia. The one disadvantage of spinal anesthesia is the inability to provide prolonged postoperative analgesia, for the early ambulation facilitated by epidural analgesia may well prevent or retard DVT formation.

Because of concern for spinal hematoma when using low-molecular-weight heparin (LMWH) in the setting of epidural anesthesia (see "Anticoagulation and Regional Anesthesia," later), our home institution uses a multimodal approach to DVT prophylaxis[98] with efficacy rates rivaling those of thromboprophylaxis with LMWH,[162] all the while providing optimal analgesia and reducing the risk of bleeding. Our multimodal approach includes epidural anesthesia and analgesia, warfarin or aspirin, pneumatic compression stockings,[55,154] and early rehabilitation.

Fat Embolism Syndrome

Fat embolism occurs ubiquitously during major joint replacement surgery because intramedullary reaming and implantation of cemented prostheses pressurize the medullary cavity, thereby forcing fat, accompanied by clot and air, into the venous circulation. Using transesophageal echocardiography, fat emboli can be detected in the right ventricle in 90% of patients during intramedullary instrumentation.[21] These emboli may traverse the pulmonary vasculature and be detected as microemboli by transcranial Doppler.[46,119] Although the majority of fat emboli are subclinical,[21] fat embolism can readily cause right ventricular outflow tract obstruction, cardiovascular collapse, and less commonly, severe multisystem failure, which is termed fat embolism syndrome (FES) and characterized primarily by mental status changes, respiratory insufficiency, and petechial rash.[12,53] Mortality associated with FES is reportedly as high as 20%.[12,120] The presence of a thigh tourniquet does not prevent fat embolization[38]; indeed, FES is well documented after TKA.[64,76] Management of acute fat embolism includes resuscitation with intravenous crystalloid (or colloid) and epinephrine. Treatment of FES is mainly supportive. Effort should be directed at prevention and early detection, such as surgical venting of the femoral shaft, use of uncemented prostheses, and invasive monitoring and transesophageal echocardiography for high-risk patients, especially those with pulmonary hypertension or a patent foramen ovale (up to 34% of the population).[56]

Compartment Syndrome

Bleeding or swelling inside a closed fascial compartment can lead to catastrophic neurovascular compromise. Compartment syndrome most commonly occurs in the anterior compartment of the leg after tibial fracture, high tibial osteotomy, or complex knee replacement surgery. Early diagnosis is essential to enable fasciotomy and prevent further neuromuscular damage. Epidural analgesia and long-acting PNB can obscure the pain associated with compartment syndrome, thereby interfering with the examination of neuromuscular function and potentially delaying the diagnosis. Thus, whenever a likelihood of postoperative compartment syndrome exists, epidural analgesia and/or long-acting PNB (specifically, sciatic nerve block) are inadvisable.

ANTICOAGULATION AND REGIONAL ANESTHESIA

In the perioperative management of patients undergoing major knee surgery, two mutually exclusive interventions—thromboprophylaxis and RA—are of undisputed value. Controversy arises, however, when the administration of one of these valuable interventions purportedly precludes that of the other. This historic conflict primarily involves CNB techniques and the risk of spinal hematoma in an anticoagulated patient. Indeed, one important advantage of PNB is that PNB techniques are performed safely in an anticoagulated patient. The true incidence of spinal hematoma after CNB is unknown but is theoretically estimated to be less than 1 in 220,000 spinal anesthetics and less than 1 in 150,000 epidural anesthetics in patients without specific risk factors.[143] Symptoms of spinal hematoma include severe radicular back pain, progression of numbness or weakness, and bowel and bladder dysfunction, which usually develop 48 to 72 hours after spinal or epidural anesthesia. A delay in the diagnosis and surgical decompression of a spinal hematoma may lead to irreversible spinal cord ischemia. Factors believed to predispose to spinal hematoma include traumatic insertion of the spinal or epidural needle, thrombocytopenia, anticoagulation, and manipulation or removal of the epidural catheter.[67]

Adjusted-dose warfarin is the most commonly used pharmacological thromboprophylaxis regimen for patients undergoing TKA in the United States.[3] Although no definitive data exist regarding the administration of CNB and warfarin thromboprophylaxis, it is widely accepted among anesthesiologists that CNB should be deferred until the international normalized ratio (INR) is at least subtherapeutic,[97,144] if not normal.[65,134,139] In addition, case series data suggest that 30% to 60% of all clinically important spinal hematomas occur after epidural catheter removal.[144] Because indwelling epidural catheter manipulation may predispose to spinal hematoma, it has been recommended that epidural catheters be removed under the same conditions present during insertion[148]; therefore, catheter removal is often deferred until the INR has normalized. However, the safety of removing epidural catheters in anticoagulated patients is clouded by the unreliability of INR measurements as a reflection of anticoagulation on initiation or termination of warfarin therapy. During the initiation of warfarin therapy, the INR primarily reflects the rapid depletion of factor VII, yet the therapeutic effect of warfarin is most dependent on the reduction in factors II and X. Therefore, an elevated INR measured early after the initiation of warfarin therapy may falsely indicate therapeutic anticoagulation. Conversely, early after the discontinuation of warfarin therapy, factors II and X may not have recovered sufficiently for normal coagulation despite adequate factor VII activity and thus a low INR. Consequently, an INR less than 1.5 does not guarantee satisfactory coagulation in patients in whom warfarin therapy has recently been terminated.[39,72] Moreover, the concurrent use of common analgesics (e.g., aspirin, NSAIDs) that affect hemostasis may increase the degree of anticoagulation without affecting the INR, thus limiting the utility of the measured INR when considering the timing for epidural catheter removal.

The ongoing controversy regarding anticoagulation and CNB peaked after the introduction of LMWH in the United States, which resulted in an abrupt increase in the number of spinal hematomas reported to the U.S. Food and Drug Administration (FDA). In 1997, the FDA advised against the performance of CNB in patients who had received LMWH within 12 hours and that the use of LMWH in patients with an epidural catheter in place is hazardous.[43] Subsequently, much discussion surrounding the dose and timing of LMWH administration in relation to the insertion and withdrawal of an epidural catheter[66,69-71] ultimately culminated in the publication of safe practice guidelines by the American Society of Regional Anesthesia (ASRA).[72] However, despite best efforts to schedule epidural catheter withdrawal according to the most recent LMWH injection, catheters may dislodge spontaneously at any time. Notwithstanding the practice guidelines published by ASRA, it is the authors' opinion that the risk of spinal hematoma predominantly stems from spinal or epidural needle insertion rather than epidural catheter withdrawal.

At our home institution we limit the use of perioperative LMWH; instead, warfarin or aspirin is administered as part of a multimodal regimen after TKA,[98] and the epidural catheter is removed 48 to 72 hours after surgery irrespective of the measured INR. When LMWH is used for thromboprophylaxis after TKA, combined femoral-sciatic nerve block should be considered for postoperative analgesia. Combined single-injection femoral-sciatic nerve block offers advantages in pain control, perioperative blood loss, rehabilitation, and patient satisfaction comparable to epidural analgesia after TKA,[33] without the risk of spinal hematoma.

SUMMARY

RA is often an advantageous alternative to GA for surgical procedures about the knee. With careful attention to technique, both CNB and PNB are reliably performed with very high success rates and few major complications. Versatile applications of PNB, including continuous catheter-based techniques, provide prolonged postoperative analgesia, early rehabilitation, and excellent patient satisfaction. A safe and successful RA program requires a supportive infrastructure, informed patients, and vigilant personnel, including dedicated acute pain specialists. Detailed knowledge of the indications and limitations of RA is important for surgeons and anesthesiologists alike who are considering CNB and PNB techniques for their patients undergoing knee surgery.

References

1. Abdel-Salam A, Eyres KS: Effects of tourniquet during total knee arthroplasty. A prospective randomised study. J Bone Joint Surg Br 77:250-253, 1995.
2. Allen HW, Liu SS, Ware PD, et al: Peripheral nerve blocks improve analgesia after total knee replacement surgery. Anesth Analg 87:93-97, 1998.
3. Anderson FA Jr, Hirsh J, White K, Fitzgerald RH Jr: Temporal trends in prevention of venous thromboembolism following primary total hip or knee arthroplasty 1996-2001: Findings from the Hip and Knee Registry. Chest 124(6 Suppl):349S-356S, 2003.
4. Auroy Y, Benhamou D, Bargues L, et al: Major complications of regional anesthesia in France: The SOS Regional Anesthesia Hotline Service. Anesthesiology 97:1274-1280, 2002.
5. Barwell J, Anderson G, Hassan A, Rawlings I: The effects of early tourniquet release during total knee arthroplasty: A prospective randomized double-blind study. J Bone Joint Surg Br 79:265-268, 1997.
6. Ben David B, Maryanovsky M, Gurevitch A, et al: A comparison of minidose lidocaine-fentanyl and conventional-dose lidocaine spinal anesthesia. Anesth Analg 91:865-870, 2000.
7. Ben David B, Solomon E, Levin H, et al: Intrathecal fentanyl with small-dose dilute bupivacaine: Better anesthesia without prolonging recovery. Anesth Analg 85:560-565, 1997.
8. Benoni G, Fredin H: Fibrinolytic inhibition with tranexamic acid reduces blood loss and blood transfusion after knee arthroplasty:

A prospective, randomised, double-blind study of 86 patients. J Bone Joint Surg Br 78:434-440, 1996.
9. Bonica J: Postoperative pain. In Bonica J (ed): The Management of Pain, 2nd ed. Philadelphia, Lea & Febiger, 1990, pp 461-480.
10. Bonicalzi V, Gallino M: Comparison of two regional anesthetic techniques for knee arthroscopy. Arthroscopy 11:207-212, 1995.
11. Bourke DL, Silberberg MS, Ortega R, Willock MM: Respiratory responses associated with release of intraoperative tourniquets. Anesth Analg 69:541-544, 1989.
12. Bulger EM, Smith DG, Maier RV, Jurkovich GJ: Fat embolism syndrome. A 10-year review. Arch Surg 132:435-439, 1997.
13. Capdevila X, Barthelet Y, Biboulet P, et al: Effects of perioperative analgesic technique on the surgical outcome and duration of rehabilitation after major knee surgery. Anesthesiology 91:8-15, 1999.
14. Capdevila X, Macaire P, Aknin P, et al: Patient-controlled perineural analgesia after ambulatory orthopedic surgery: A comparison of electronic versus elastomeric pumps. Anesth Analg 96:414-417, 2003.
15. Cappelleri G, Casati A, Fanelli G, et al: Unilateral spinal anesthesia or combined sciatic-femoral nerve block for day-case knee arthroscopy. A prospective, randomized comparison. Minerva Anestesiol 66:131-136, 2000.
16. Casati A, Cappelleri G, Aldegheri G, et al: Total intravenous anesthesia, spinal anesthesia or combined sciatic-femoral nerve block for outpatient knee arthroscopy. Minerva Anestesiol 70:493-502, 2004.
17. Casati A, Cappelleri G, Berti M, et al: Randomized comparison of remifentanil-propofol with a sciatic-femoral nerve block for outpatient knee arthroscopy. Eur J Anaesthesiol 19:109-114, 2002.
18. Chan VW: Nerve localization—seek but not so easy to find? Reg Anesth Pain Med 27:245-248, 2002.
19. Chayen D, Nathan H, Chayen M: The psoas compartment block. Anesthesiology 45:95-99, 1976.
20. Chelly JE, Delaunay L, Williams B, Borghi B: Outpatient lower extremity infusions. Best Pract Res Clin Anaesthesiol 16:311-320, 2002.
21. Christie J, Robinson CM, Pell AC, et al: Transcardiac echocardiography during invasive intramedullary procedures. J Bone Joint Surg Br 77:450-455, 1995.
22. Chung F, Mezei G: Factors contributing to a prolonged stay after ambulatory surgery. Anesth Analg 89:1352-1359, 1999.
23. Convery PN, Milligan KR, Quinn P, et al: Low-dose intra-articular ketorolac for pain relief following arthroscopy of the knee joint. Anaesthesia 53:1125-1129, 1998.
24. Corbey MP, Bach AB, Lech K, Frorup AM: Grading of severity of postdural puncture headache after 27-gauge Quincke and Whitacre needles. Acta Anaesthesiol Scand 41:779-784, 1997.
25. Cotter JT, Nielsen KC, Guller U, et al: Increased body mass index and ASA physical status IV are risk factors for block failure in ambulatory surgery—an analysis of 9,342 blocks. Can J Anaesth 51:810-816, 2004.
26. Couvret C, Laffon M, Baud A, et al: A restrictive use of both autologous donation and recombinant human erythropoietin is an efficient policy for primary total hip or knee arthroplasty. Anesth Analg 99:262-271, 2004.
27. Coventry DM, Todd JG: Alkalinisation of bupivacaine for sciatic nerve blockade. Anaesthesia 44:467-470, 1989.
28. Covino B, Wildsmith J: Clinical pharmacology of local anesthetic agents. In Cousins MJ, Bridenbaugh PO (eds): Neural Blockade in Clinical Anesthesia and Management of Pain, 3rd ed. Philadelphia, JB Lippincott, 1998, pp 97-128.
29. Craft JB, Epstein BS, Coakley CS: Prophylaxis of dural-puncture headache with epidural saline. Anesth Analg 52:228-231, 1973.
30. Crawford JS: The prevention of headache consequent upon dural puncture. Br J Anaesth 44:598-600, 1972.
31. Dahl V, Gierloff C, Omland E, Raeder JC: Spinal, epidural or propofol anaesthesia for out-patient knee arthroscopy? Acta Anaesthesiol Scand 41:1341-1345, 1997.
32. Dal D, Tetik O, Altunkaya H, et al: The efficacy of intra-articular ketamine for postoperative analgesia in outpatient arthroscopic surgery. Arthroscopy 20:300-305, 2004.
33. Davies AF, Segar EP, Murdoch J, et al: Epidural infusion or combined femoral and sciatic nerve blocks as perioperative analgesia for knee arthroplasty. Br J Anaesth 93:368-374, 2004.

34. Davis FM, Laurenson VG, et al: Deep vein thrombosis after total hip replacement. A comparison between spinal and general anaesthesia. J Bone Joint Surg Br 71:181-185, 1989.

35. Dilger JA: Lower extremity nerve blocks. Anesthesiol Clin North Am 18:319-340, 2000.

36. Edkin BS, McCarty EC, Spindler KP, Flanagan JF: Analgesia with femoral nerve block for anterior cruciate ligament reconstruction. Clin Orthop 369:289-295, 1999.

37. Edwards ND, Wright EM: Continuous low-dose 3-in-1 nerve blockade for postoperative pain relief after total knee replacement. Anesth Analg 75:265-267, 1992.

38. Enneking FK: Cardiac arrest during total knee replacement using a long-stem prosthesis. J Clin Anesth 7:253-263, 1995.

39. Enneking FK, Benzon H: Oral anticoagulants and regional anesthesia: A perspective. Reg Anesth Pain Med 23:140-145, 1998.

40. Enneking FK, Ilfeld BM: Major surgery in the ambulatory environment: Continuous catheters and home infusions. Best Pract Res Clin Anaesthesiol 16:285-294, 2002.

41. Epple J, Kubitz J, Schmidt H, et al: Comparative analysis of costs of total intravenous anaesthesia with propofol and remifentanil vs. balanced anaesthesia with isoflurane and fentanyl. Eur J Anaesthesiol 18:20-28, 2001.

42. Fanelli G, Borghi B, Casati A, et al: Unilateral bupivacaine spinal anesthesia for outpatient knee arthroscopy. Italian Study Group on Unilateral Spinal Anesthesia. Can J Anaesth 47:746-751, 2000.

43. FDA public health advisory: Reports of epidural or spinal hematomas with the concurrent use of low molecular weight heparin and spinal/epidural anesthesia or spinal puncture. U.S. Department of Health and Human Resources, 1997.

44. Flaatten H, Raeder J: Spinal anaesthesia for outpatient surgery. Anaesthesia 40:1108-1111, 1985.

45. Forssblad M, Weidenhielm L: Knee arthroscopy in local versus general anaesthesia. The incidence of rearthroscopy. Knee Surg Sports Traumatol Arthrosc 7:323-326, 1999.

46. Forteza AM, Koch S, Romano JG, et al: Transcranial Doppler detection of fat emboli. Stroke 30:2687-2691, 1999.

47. Freedman JM, Li DK, Drasner K, et al: Transient neurologic symptoms after spinal anesthesia: An epidemiologic study of 1,863 patients. Anesthesiology 89:633-641, 1998.

48. Gielen M: Cardiac arrest after tourniquet release. Can J Anaesth 38:541, 1991.

49. Girardis M, Milesi S, Donato S, et al: The hemodynamic and metabolic effects of tourniquet application during knee surgery. Anesth Analg 91:727-731, 2000.

50. Greengrass RA, Klein SM, D'Ercole FJ, et al: Lumbar plexus and sciatic nerve block for knee arthroplasty: Comparison of ropivacaine and bupivacaine. Can J Anaesth 45:1094-1096, 1998.

51. Gupta A, Axelsson K, Allvin R, et al: Postoperative pain following knee arthroscopy: The effects of intra-articular ketorolac and/or morphine. Reg Anesth Pain Med 24:225-230, 1999.

52. Gupta A, Bodin L, Holmstrom B, Berggren L: A systematic review of the peripheral analgesic effects of intraarticular morphine. Anesth Analg 93:761-770, 2001.

53. Gurd AR, Wilson RI: The fat embolism syndrome. J Bone Joint Surg Br 56:408-416, 1974.

54. Gurkan Y, Canatay H, Ozdamar D, et al: Spinal anesthesia for arthroscopic knee surgery. Acta Anaesthesiol Scand 48:513-517, 2004.

55. Haas SB, Insall JN, Scuderi GR, et al: Pneumatic sequential-compression boots compared with aspirin prophylaxis of deep-vein thrombosis after total knee arthroplasty. J Bone Joint Surg Am 72:27-31, 1990.

56. Hagen PT, Scholz DG, Edwards WD: Incidence and size of patent foramen ovale during the first 10 decades of life: An autopsy study of 965 normal hearts. Mayo Clin Proc 59:17-20, 1984.

57. Halpern S, Preston R: Postdural puncture headache and spinal needle design. Metaanalyses Anesthesiol 81:1376-1383, 1994.

58. Heddle NM, Brox WT, Klama LN, et al: A randomized trial on the efficacy of an autologous blood drainage and transfusion device in patients undergoing elective knee arthroplasty. Transfusion 32:742-746, 1992.

59. Hiippala S, Strid L, Wennerstrand M, et al: Tranexamic acid (Cyklokapron) reduces perioperative blood loss associated with total knee arthroplasty. Br J Anaesth 74:534-537, 1995.

60. Hiippala ST, Strid LJ, Wennerstrand MI, et al: Tranexamic acid radically decreases blood loss and transfusions associated with total knee arthroplasty. Anesth Analg 84:839-844, 1997.

61. Hirsh J: Prevention of venous thrombosis in patients undergoing major orthopaedic surgical procedures. Acta Chir Scand Suppl 556:30-35, 1990.

62. Hirst GC, Lang SA, Dust WN, et al: Femoral nerve block. Single injection versus continuous infusion for total knee arthroplasty. Reg Anesth 21:292-297, 1996.

63. Hodgson PS, Liu SS, Batra MS, et al: Procaine compared with lidocaine for incidence of transient neurologic symptoms. Reg Anesth Pain Med 25:218-222, 2000.

64. Hofmann S, Hopf R, Huemer G, et al: [Modified surgical technique for the reduction of bone marrow spilling in knee endoprosthesis.] Orthopade 24:144-150, 1995.

65. Horlocker TT: When to remove a spinal or epidural catheter in an anticoagulated patient. Reg Anesth 18:264-265, 1993.

66. Horlocker TT: Low molecular weight heparin and neuraxial anesthesia. Thromb Res 101:V141-V154, 2001.

67. Horlocker TT: Thromboprophylaxis and neuraxial anesthesia. Orthopedics 26:s243-s249, 2003.

68. Horlocker TT, Hebl JR: Anesthesia for outpatient knee arthroscopy: Is there an optimal technique? Reg Anesth Pain Med 28:58-63, 2003.

69. Horlocker TT, Heit JA: Low molecular weight heparin: Biochemistry, pharmacology, perioperative prophylaxis regimens, and guidelines for regional anesthetic management. Anesth Analg 85:874-885, 1997.

70. Horlocker TT, Wedel DJ: Neuraxial block and low-molecular-weight heparin: Balancing perioperative analgesia and thromboprophylaxis. Reg Anesth Pain Med 23:164-177, 1998.

71. Horlocker TT, Wedel DJ: Spinal and epidural blockade and perioperative low molecular weight heparin: Smooth sailing on the Titanic. Anesth Analg 86:1153-1156, 1998.

72. Horlocker TT, Wedel DJ, Benzon H, et al: Regional anesthesia in the anticoagulated patient: Defining the risks. Reg Anesth Pain Med 29:1-12, 2004.

73. Hultin J, Hamberg P, Stenstrom A: Knee arthroscopy using local anesthesia. Arthroscopy 8:239-241, 1992.

74. Jacobson E, Forssblad M, Rosenberg J, et al: Can local anesthesia be recommended for routine use in elective knee arthroscopy? A comparison between local, spinal, and general anesthesia. Arthroscopy 16:183-190, 2000.

75. Jankowski CJ, Hebl JR, Stuart MJ, et al: A comparison of psoas compartment block and general anesthesia for outpatient knee arthroscopy. Anesth Analg 97:1003-1009, 2003.

76. Jenkins K, Chung F, Wennberg R, et al: Fat embolism syndrome and elective knee arthroplasty. Can J Anaesth 49:19-24, 2002.

77. Jeyaseelan S, Stevenson TM, Pfitzner J: Tourniquet failure and arterial calcification. Case report and theoretical dangers. Anaesthesia 36:48-50, 1981.

78. Jorgensen LN, Rasmussen LS, Nielsen PT, et al: Antithrombotic efficacy of continuous extradural analgesia after knee replacement. Br J Anaesth 66:8-12, 1991.

79. Joshi W, Reuben SS, Kilaru PR, et al: Postoperative analgesia for outpatient arthroscopic knee surgery with intraarticular clonidine and/or morphine. Anesth Analg 90:1102-1106, 2000.

80. Juelsgaard P, Larsen UT, Sorensen JV, et al: Hypotensive epidural anesthesia in total knee replacement without tourniquet: Reduced blood loss and transfusion. Reg Anesth Pain Med 26:105-110, 2001.

81. Kam PC, Kavanagh R, Yoong FF: The arterial tourniquet: Pathophysiological consequences and anaesthetic implications. Anaesthesia 56:534-545, 2001.

82. Kaufman RD, Walts LF: Tourniquet-induced hypertension. Br J Anaesth 54:333-336, 1982.

83. Kizilkaya M, Yildirim OS, Dogan N, et al: Analgesic effects of intraarticular sufentanil and sufentanil plus methylprednisolone after arthroscopic knee surgery. Anesth Analg 98:1062-1065, 2004.

84. Klein SM, Buckenmaier CC III: Ambulatory surgery with long acting regional anesthesia. Minerva Anestesiol 68:833-841, 2002.

85. Klein SM, Greengrass RA, Grant SA, et al: Ambulatory surgery for multi-ligament knee reconstruction with continuous dual catheter peripheral nerve blockade. Can J Anaesth 48:375-378, 2001.

86. Kumar SN, Chapman JA, Rawlins I: Vascular injuries in total knee arthroplasty. A review of the problem with special reference to the possible effects of the tourniquet. J Arthroplasty 13:211-216, 1998.

87. Lang SA, Yip RW, Chang PC, Gerard MA: The femoral 3-in-1 block revisited. J Clin Anesth 5:292-296, 1993.

88. Larsson S, Lundberg D: A prospective survey of postoperative nausea and vomiting with special regard to incidence and relations to patient characteristics, anesthetic routines and surgical procedures. Acta Anaesthesiol Scand 39:539-545, 1995.

89. Liguori GA, Zayas VM, Chisholm MF: Transient neurologic symptoms after spinal anesthesia with mepivacaine and lidocaine. Anesthesiology 88:619-623, 1998.

90. Lotke PA, Ecker ML, Alavi A, Berkowitz H: Indications for the treatment of deep venous thrombosis following total knee replacement. J Bone Joint Surg Am 66:202-208, 1984.

91. Lotke PA, Faralli VJ, Orenstein EM, Ecker ML: Blood loss after total knee replacement. Effects of tourniquet release and continuous passive motion. J Bone Joint Surg Am 73:1037-1040, 1991.

92. Luber MJ, Greengrass R, Vail TP: Patient satisfaction and effectiveness of lumbar plexus and sciatic nerve block for total knee arthroplasty. J Arthroplasty 16:17-21, 2001.

93. Lynch J, Kasper SM, Strick K, et al: The use of Quincke and Whitacre 27-gauge needles in orthopedic patients: Incidence of failed spinal anesthesia and postdural puncture headache. Anesth Analg 79:124-128, 1994.

94. Magora F, Pessachovitch B, Shoham I: Sciatic nerve block by the anterior approach for operations on the lower extremity. Br J Anaesth 46:121-123, 1974.

95. Matheny JM, Hanks GA, Rung GW, et al: A comparison of patient-controlled analgesia and continuous lumbar plexus block after anterior cruciate ligament reconstruction. Arthroscopy 9:87-90, 1993.

96. McKenna R, Bachmann F, Kaushal SP, Galante JO: Thromboembolic disease in patients undergoing total knee replacement. J Bone Joint Surg Am 58:928-932, 1976.

97. Millar FA, Mackenzie A, Hutchison G, Bannister J: Hemostasis-altering drugs and central neural block. A survey of anesthetic practice in Scotland and the United Kingdom. Reg Anesth 21:529-533, 1996.

98. Miric A, Lombardi P, Sculco TP: Deep vein thrombosis prophylaxis: A comprehensive approach for total hip and total knee arthroplasty patient populations. Am J Orthop 29:269-274, 2000.

99. Modig J, Malmberg P, Karlstrom G: Effect of epidural versus general anaesthesia on calf blood flow. Acta Anaesthesiol Scand 24:305-309, 1980.

100. Moiniche S, Mikkelsen S, Wetterslev J, Dahl JB: A systematic review of intra-articular local anesthesia for postoperative pain relief after arthroscopic knee surgery. Reg Anesth Pain Med 24:430-437, 1999.

101. Mulroy MF, Larkin KL, Hodgson PS, et al: A comparison of spinal, epidural, and general anesthesia for outpatient knee arthroscopy. Anesth Analg 91:860-864, 2000.

102. Neal JM, Deck JJ, Kopacz DJ, Lewis MA: Hospital discharge after ambulatory knee arthroscopy: A comparison of epidural 2-chloroprocaine versus lidocaine. Reg Anesth Pain Med 26:35-40, 2001.

103. Newman RJ: Metabolic effects of tourniquet ischaemia studied by nuclear magnetic resonance spectroscopy. J Bone Joint Surg Br 66:434-440, 1984.

104. Nielsen KC, Steele S M: Outcome after regional anaesthesia in the ambulatory setting—is it really worth it? Best Pract Res Clin Anaesthesiol 16:145-157, 2002.

105. O'Leary AM, Veall G, Butler P, Anderson GH: Acute pulmonary oedema after tourniquet release. Can J Anaesth 37:826-827, 1990.

106. Olsfanger D, Fredman B, Goldstein B, et al: Acute normovolaemic haemodilution decreases postoperative allogeneic blood transfusion after total knee replacement. Br J Anaesth 79:317-321, 1997.

107. Parkinson SK, Mueller JB, Little WL, Bailey SL: Extent of blockade with various approaches to the lumbar plexus. Anesth Analg 68:243-248, 1989.

108. Parnass SM, McCarthy RJ, Bach BR Jr, et al: Beneficial im-pact of epidural anesthesia on recovery after outpatient arthroscopy. Arthroscopy 9:91-95, 1993.

109. Patel NJ, Flashburg MH, Paskin S, Grossman R: A regional anesthetic technique compared to general anesthesia for outpatient knee arthroscopy. Anesth Analg 65:185-187, 1986.

110. Pavlin DJ, Rapp SE, Polissar NL, et al: Factors affecting discharge time in adult outpatients. Anesth Analg 87:816-826, 1998.

111. Pavone V, Johnson T, Saulog PS, et al: Perioperative morbidity in bilateral one-stage total knee replacements. Clin Orthop 421:155-161, 2004.

112. Pollock JE: Transient neurologic symptoms: Etiology, risk factors, and management. Reg Anesth Pain Med 27:581-586, 2002.

113. Prabhu A, Chung F: Anaesthetic strategies towards developments in day care surgery. Eur J Anaesthesiol Suppl 23:36-42, 2001.

114. Raj PP, Knarr DC, Vigdorth E, et al: Comparison of continuous epidural infusion of a local anesthetic and administration of systemic narcotics in the management of pain after total knee replacement surgery. Anesth Analg 66:401-406, 1987.

115. Rasmussen S, Larsen AS, Thomsen ST, Kehlet H: Intra-articular glucocorticoid, bupivacaine and morphine reduces pain, inflammatory response and convalescence after arthroscopic meniscectomy. Pain 78:131-134, 1998.

116. Rasmussen S, Lorentzen JS, Larsen AS, et al: Combined intra-articular glucocorticoid, bupivacaine and morphine reduces pain and convalescence after diagnostic knee arthroscopy. Acta Orthop Scand 73:175-178, 2002.

117. Reuben SS, Connelly NR: Postoperative analgesia for outpatient arthroscopic knee surgery with intraarticular bupivacaine and ketorolac. Anesth Analg 80:1154-1157, 1995.

118. Reuben SS, Connelly NR: Postoperative analgesia for outpatient arthroscopic knee surgery with intraarticular clonidine. Anesth Analg 88:729-733, 1999.

119. Riding G, Daly K, Hutchinson S, et al: Paradoxical cerebral embolisation. An explanation for fat embolism syndrome. J Bone Joint Surg Br 86:95-98, 2004.

120. Robert JH, Hoffmeyer P, Broquet PE, et al: Fat embolism syndrome. Orthop Rev 22:567-571, 1993.

121. Rodgers A, Walker N, Schug S, et al: Reduction of postoperative mortality and morbidity with epidural or spinal anaesthesia: Results from overview of randomised trials. BMJ 321:1493, 2000.

122. Rosseland LA, Helgesen KG, Breivik H, Stubhaug A: Moderate-to-severe pain after knee arthroscopy is relieved by intraarticular saline: A randomized controlled trial. Anesth Analg 98:1546-1551, 2004.

123. Sansone V, De Ponti A, Fanelli G, Agostoni M: Combined sciatic and femoral nerve block for knee arthroscopy: 4 years' experience. Arch Orthop Trauma Surg 119:163-167, 1999.

124. Santanen U, Rautoma P, Luurila H, et al: Comparison of 27-gauge (0.41-mm) Whitacre and Quincke spinal needles with respect to post–dural puncture headache and non–dural puncture headache. Acta Anaesthesiol Scand 48:474-479, 2004.

125. Sapega AA, Heppenstall RB, Chance B, et al: Optimizing tourniquet application and release times in extremity surgery. A biochemical and ultrastructural study. J Bone Joint Surg Am 67:303-314, 1985.

126. Satsumae T, Yamaguchi H, Sakaguchi M, et al: Preoperative small-dose ketamine prevented tourniquet-induced arterial pressure increase in orthopedic patients under general anesthesia. Anesth Analg 92:1286-1289, 2001.

127. Serpell MG, Millar FA, Thomson MF: Comparison of lumbar plexus block versus conventional opioid analgesia after total knee replacement. Anaesthesia 46:275-277, 1991.

128. Shapiro MS, Safran MR, Crockett H, Finerman GA: Local anesthesia for knee arthroscopy. Efficacy and cost benefits. Am J Sports Med 23:50-53, 1995.

129. Sharrock NE, Cazan MG, Hargett MJ, et al: Changes in mortality after total hip and knee arthroplasty over a ten-year period. Anesth Analg 80:242-248, 1995.

130. Sharrock NE, Go G, Williams-Russo P, et al: Comparison of extradural and general anaesthesia on the fibrinolytic response to total knee arthroplasty. Br J Anaesth 79:29-34, 1997.

131. Sharrock NE, Haas SB, Hargett MJ, et al: Effects of epidural anesthesia on the incidence of deep-vein thrombosis after total knee arthroplasty. J Bone Joint Surg Am 73:502-506, 1991.

132. Sharrock NE, Hargett MJ, Urquhart B, et al: Factors affecting deep vein thrombosis rate following total knee arthroplasty under epidural anesthesia. J Arthroplasty 8:133-139, 1993.

133. Shaw JA, Murray DG: The relationship between tourniquet pressure and underlying soft-tissue pressure in the thigh. J Bone Joint Surg Am 64:1148-1152, 1982.

134. Silverman SM: Epidural anesthesia and anticoagulation. Anesthesiology 79:204-205, 1993.

135. Singelyn FJ, Deyaert M, Joris D, et al: Effects of intravenous patient-controlled analgesia with morphine, continuous epidural analgesia, and continuous three-in-one block on postoperative pain and knee rehabilitation after unilateral total knee arthroplasty. Anesth Analg 87:88-92, 1998.

136. Smith MP, Sprung J, Zura A, et al: A survey of exposure to regional anesthesia techniques in American anesthesia residency training programs. Reg Anesth Pain Med 24:11-16, 1999.

137. Soderlund A, Boreus LO, Westman L, et al: A comparison of 50, 100 and 200 mg of intra-articular pethidine during knee joint surgery, a controlled study with evidence for local demethylation to norpethidine. Pain 80:229-238, 1999.

138. Stein C, Comisel K, Haimerl E, et al: Analgesic effect of intraarticular morphine after arthroscopic knee surgery. N Engl J Med 325:1123-1126, 1991.

139. Stevens DS: Epidural hematoma: Was catheter removed during complete anticoagulation? Anesth Analg 75:863-864, 1992.

140. Stringer MD, Steadman CA, Hedges AR, et al: Deep vein thrombosis after elective knee surgery. An incidence study in 312 patients. J Bone Joint Surg Br 71:492-497, 1989.

141. Stulberg BN, Insall JN, Williams GW, Ghelman B: Deep-vein thrombosis following total knee replacement. An analysis of six hundred and thirty-eight arthroplasties. J Bone Joint Surg Am 66:194-201, 1984.

142. Thomas D, Wareham K, Cohen D, Hutchings H: Autologous blood transfusion in total knee replacement surgery. Br J Anaesth 86:669-673, 2001.

143. Tryba M: [Epidural regional anesthesia and low molecular heparin: Pro.] Anasthesiol Intensivmed Notfallmed Schmerzther 28:179-181, 1993.

144. Tryba M: European practice guidelines: Thromboembolism prophylaxis and regional anesthesia. Reg Anesth Pain Med 23:178-182, 1998.

145. Urmey WF, Stanton J, Peterson M, Sharrock NE: Combined spinal-epidural anesthesia for outpatient surgery. Dose-response characteristics of intrathecal isobaric lidocaine using a 27-gauge Whitacre spinal needle. Anesthesiology 83:528-534, 1995.

146. Valli H, Rosenberg PH: Effects of three anaesthesia methods on haemodynamic responses connected with the use of thigh tourniquet in orthopaedic patients. Acta Anaesthesiol Scand 29:142-147, 1985.

147. Valli H, Rosenberg PH, Kytta J, Nurminen M: Arterial hypertension associated with the use of a tourniquet with either general or regional anaesthesia. Acta Anaesthesiol Scand 31:279-283, 1987.

148. Vandermeulen EP, Van Aken H, Vermylen J: Anticoagulants and spinal-epidural anesthesia. Anesth Analg 79:1165-1177, 1994.

149. van Vlymen JM, White PF: Outpatient anesthesia. In Miller RD (ed): Anesthesia, 5th ed. Philadelphia, Churchill Livingstone, 2000, pp 22-23.

150. Veien M, Sorensen JV, Madsen F, Juelsgaard P: Tranexamic acid given intraoperatively reduces blood loss after total knee replacement: A randomized, controlled study. Acta Anaesthesiol Scand 46:1206-1211, 2002.

151. Wakankar HM, Nicholl JE, Koka R, D'Arcy JC: The tourniquet in total knee arthroplasty. A prospective, randomised study. J. Bone Joint Surg Br 81:30-33, 1999.

152. Wang H, Boctor B, Verner J: The effect of single-injection femoral nerve block on rehabilitation and length of hospital stay after total knee replacement. Reg Anesth Pain Med 27:139-144, 2002.

153. Weller R, Rosenblum M, Conard P, Gross JB: Comparison of epidural and patient-controlled intravenous morphine following joint replacement surgery. Can J Anaesth 38:582-586, 1991.

154. Westrich GH, Sculco TP: Prophylaxis against deep venous thrombosis after total knee arthroplasty. Pneumatic plantar compression and aspirin compared with aspirin alone. J Bone Joint Surg Am 78:826-834, 1996.

155. Wilgis EF: Observations on the effects of tourniquet ischemia. J Bone Joint Surg Am 53:1343-1346, 1971.

156. Williams BA, Kentor ML, Vogt MT, et al: Femoral-sciatic nerve blocks for complex outpatient knee surgery are associated with less postoperative pain before same-day discharge: A review of 1,200 consecutive cases from the period 1996-1999. Anesthesiology 98:1206-1213, 2003.

157. Williams BA, Kentor ML, Vogt MT, et al: Economics of nerve block pain management after anterior cruciate ligament reconstruction: Potential hospital cost savings via associated postanesthesia care unit bypass and same-day discharge. Anesthesiology 100:697-706, 2004.

158. Williams BA, Kentor ML, Williams JP, et al: Process analysis in outpatient knee surgery: Effects of regional and general anesthesia on anesthesia-controlled time. Anesthesiology 93:529-538, 2000.

159. Williams-Russo P, Sharrock NE, Haas SB, et al: Randomized trial of epidural versus general anesthesia: Outcomes after primary total knee replacement. Clin Orthop 331:199-208, 1996.

160. Winnie AP, Ramamurthy S, Durrani Z: The inguinal paravascular technic of lumbar plexus anesthesia: The "3-in-1 block." Anesth Analg 52:989-996, 1973.

161. Winnie AP, Ramamurthy S, Durrani Z, Radonjic R: Plexus blocks for lower extremity surgery: New answers to old problems. Anesth Rev 1:1-6, 1974.

162. Woolson ST, Robinson RK, Khan NQ, et al: Deep venous thrombosis prophylaxis for knee replacement: Warfarin and pneumatic compression. Am J Orthop 27:299-304, 1998.

163. Ya Deau JT, Cahill JB, Zawadsky MW, et al: Effects of femoral nerve blockade in conjunction with epidural analgesia after total knee arthroplasty. Anesth Analg (in press).

164. Yamashita S, Yamaguchi H, Hisajima Y, et al: Preoperative oral dextromethorphan attenuated tourniquet-induced arterial blood pressure and heart rate increases in knee cruciate ligament reconstruction patients under general anesthesia. Anesth Analg 98:994-998, 2004.

165. Yang LC, Chen LM, Wang CJ, Buerkle H: Postoperative analgesia by intra-articular neostigmine in patients undergoing knee arthroscopy. Anesthesiology 88:334-339, 1998.

CHAPTER 61

Reflex Sympathetic Dystrophy of the Knee: Complex Regional Pain Syndrome

Michael A. Mont • Phillip S. Ragland

Reflex sympathetic dystrophy (RSD) is an uncommon condition that occasionally affects the knee. It can be a multisystem disorder, but it usually is confined to one extremity. RSD of the knee is inadequately understood and difficult to treat. Various reports describe an incidence ranging from 0.5% to 2% after total knee arthroplasties.[6] It occurs more commonly after minor injuries and minor surgical procedures, such as arthroscopy.[8,9,16,43,51,52,55] This condition presents with a variety of signs and symptoms, so in addition to being rare, these conditions are difficult to diagnose (Table 61–1). The one major hallmark of RSD is pain out of proportion to the injury. This pain can be quite difficult to eradicate. There are a multitude of methods to treat this disease, which range from non-operative to operative. Physicians should be aware of this difficult-to-diagnose condition because it seems that early treatment allows for the fastest recovery and greater success for patients. This chapter focuses on the different diagnostic methods for this condition with the range of treatment options used.

DEFINITIONS, PATHOPHYSIOLOGY, AND PATHOLOGY

RSD is a painful disorder that typically denotes patients who have pain out of proportion to their inciting injury. It is a condition of uncertain etiology that was first described in 1864 by Mitchell, who termed this group of disorders *causalgia*.[31] Other names for this disease have included *disuse osteoporosis, algodystrophy, Sudeck's atrophy*, and more recently *complex regional pain syndrome* (CRPS). The International Association for the Study of Pain (IASP) has recommended that *CRPS* replace the term *RSD*.[18,54] *CRPS type I* and *CRPS type II* are terms for RSD and causalgia (Table 61–2). As stated, the exact etiology of this disorder is unknown, but multiple investigators have confirmed that it is mediated by a disorder of the autonomic nervous system.[28,31,38] The typical normal physiologic pain stimulus enters via the afferent nerve fibers into the central nervous system. In affected patients, instead of the pain dissipating, a vicious cycle of continuing symptoms occurs. Various authors have described the pathophysiology to include altered blood supply, altered afferent nerve fibers, pathological muscle fibers, and other physiological changes (Table 61–3), which may occur in the setting of a patient with a genetic or psychological predisposition to this problem.[28,31,34,38] Pathologi-

cally, in a study by van der Laan and coauthors,[58] an examination was made of the muscle and nerve tissue of eight patients who had an above-knee amputation for non-functional limb in patients with a known diagnosis of RSD. They analyzed muscle and nerve fibers under light and electron microscopy and found small changes in afferent sensory fibers and in the nerve tissue, with decreased type 1 fibers and atrophic fibers in the gastrocnemius and soleus muscle tissue. These authors concluded that there were no tremendous hallmarks of this disease, but the histological changes were similar to patients with diabetes mellitus. It is beyond the scope of this chapter to describe further the possible pathophysiological mechanisms for this ill-defined disorder, and readers are referred to various references for further discussion.[28,31,34,38,44]

DIAGNOSIS

The diagnosis of RSD of the knee should be based on symptoms alone according to the IASP. A constellation of symptoms with varying degrees of expression has been described for this syndrome, which sometimes can be confirmed only with special tests, such as radiographs, bone scanning, thermography, and a positive response to a lumbar sympathetic block.

The clinical diagnosis encompasses a wide variety of signs and symptoms with the hallmark pain out of proportion to the inciting injury. The following symptoms have been found to be associated with RSD: allodynia, hyperesthesia, edema, vasomotor changes, pain with a burning quality, pseudomotor changes, joint stiffness, and a temperature difference between the extremities. The physician may not be concerned with any one of these symptoms in a specific patient, but knowledge of the full array of symptoms can be an alert, if the symptoms are persisting for a longer than expected time after an injury or procedure. Other causes of these symptoms need to be ruled out, such as persistent injury, anatomic problems, or infection, which all can masquerade as RSD. Typically, to make this diagnosis, a patient would have to have at least four of the above-mentioned symptoms with further testing to confirm the diagnosis.

CRPS traditionally has been divided into three stages for the upper extremity that describe clinical features and radiographic findings over a time course from 0 to 12 months. This type of staging may not be as relevant to treatment and prognosis for the lower extremity.

Table 61–1. Stages of Complex Regional Pain Syndrome

STAGE	USUAL TIME COURSE (mo)	CLINICAL FEATURES	RADIOGRAPHIC FINDINGS
Acute	0-3	Warm, red, edematous extremity; aching, burning pain; intolerance to cold; altered sweat pattern; joint stiffness without any significant effusion; hyperesthetic skin; no fixed joint contractures	Normal plain radiographs; may have abnormal uptake of imaging agent on bone scan
Dystrophic	3-6	Cool, cyanotic, edematous extremity; shiny, hyperesthetic skin; fixed contractures; fibrotic changes occur in the synovium	Subchondral osteopenia; patellar and medial femoral condyle osteopenia on sunrise view; may have abnormal uptake of imaging agent on bone scan
Atrophic	6-12	Loss of hair, nails, skin folds; fixed contractures; muscle wasting	Bone demineralization

From Hogan J, Hurwitz SR: Treatment of complex regional pain syndrome of the lower extremity. J Am Acad Orthop Surg 10:282, 2002.

Table 61–2. Complex Regional Pain Syndrome (CRPS) Diagnostic Criteria

CRPS Type I
Presence of an initiating noxious event or a cause of immobilization
Continuing pain, allodynia, or hyperalgesia in which the pain is disproportionate to any inciting event
Evidence at some time of edema, changes in skin blood flow (skin color changes, skin temperature changes >1.1°C difference from the homologous body part), or abnormal sudomotor activity in the region of pain
Diagnosis excluded by the existence of conditions that otherwise would account for the degree of pain and dysfunction

CRPS Type II
Presence of continuing pain, allodynia, or hyperalgesia after a nerve injury, not limited to the distribution of the injured nerve
Evidence at some time of edema, changes in skin blood flow (skin color changes, skin temperature changes >1.1°C), or abnormal sudomotor activity in the region of pain
Diagnosis excluded by the existence of conditions that otherwise would account for the degree of pain and dysfunction.

Adapted from Merskey H, Bogduk N: Classification of Chronic Pain. Seattle, IASP Press, 1994.

According to the IASP Classification Committee, there are various clinical criteria for making the diagnosis of CRPS, after other conditions that would account for the symptoms have been excluded,[18] including persistent pain out of proportion to an inciting event and periods of edema and changes in skin blood flow (color or temperature differences compared with contralateral side). This committee recommended an evaluation of diagnostic criteria as further published information becomes available.

In a study by Perez and coworkers,[42] various clinical instruments were assessed to see which, if any, could predict the presence or absence of CRPS I in 66 patients affected. They found that measured pain, temperature, volume, and range of motion can be used as diagnostic indicators for this syndrome. More studies such as this one are needed to refine further the appropriate diagnostic methods and help guide early and successful treatment.

The diagnosis may be confirmed by a positive response (even if temporary) to a lumbar sympathetic block. This type of block also is useful for treatment of this disease. More recently, lumbar sympathetic block has not been believed to be necessary for diagnosis. Various other tests to diagnose this disease are described next.

OTHER DIAGNOSTIC TESTS

Radiographs

Standard radiographs may not be diagnostic, but often a patient's symptoms coincide with osteopenia, or patchy osteopenia of the knee may alert the physician. Radiographs should include standard anteroposterior and lateral views. In addition, sunrise or Merchant views of the patella should be obtained because osteopenia of the patella has been found to be the most common x-ray finding in this disorder. Diffuse osteopenia only rarely occurs.

Thermography

Thermography has been used in the past, whereby a difference in the temperature of the affected extremity of greater than 1.1°C can be shown clearly on thermograms. Because of the availability of other temperature measurement devices, such as skin temperature probes, these tests are presently not used often. Infrared computer-assisted videothermography was useful in a study of 13 patients and might allow for monitoring during therapeutic interventions.[29] Transcutaneous oxygen tension measurements were not found to be useful in patients with CRPS I in one study.[12]

Bone Scanning

Technetium-99m bone scan is a nonspecific test that when typically positive shows high asymmetric uptake in the extremity that is involved.[56] This test has a low specificity and in one study had a sensitivity of only 50%.[57] In a study assessing the interobserver reproducibility of interpreta-

Table 61–3. Postulated Pathophysiological Mechanisms

MECHANISM	DESCRIPTION
Aberrant healing	Exaggerated and persistent inflammatory response is present Local release of substance P, CGRP, bradykinin, leukotrienes, histamine, prostaglandins, and serotonin into the damaged tissues may result in vasodilation and increased vascular permeability[31]
Disuse	Physiological changes associated with not using a body part are present, including swelling (dependent edema), cold (decreased blood flow), and trophic changes (decreased blood flow) Immobilizing a rodent limb with casting for several weeks results in significant allodynia (pain caused by non-noxious stimulation) and changes within the dorsal horn similar to changes caused by peripheral nerve injury[34,52] After uncomplicated orthopedic surgery and casting, a study showed that most patients postoperatively experience CRPS symptoms and signs, which resolve with time and physical therapy[9]
Myofascial	Tight spastic muscles may be involved primarily or secondarily in the symptoms of some CRPS patients On examination, 61% of CRPS patients had evidence of trigger points in the proximal musculature that reproduced CRPS signs and symptoms when palpated[42]
Peripheral somatic nerve	In CRPS type II, as with any other peripheral neuropathic pain, it is presumed that abnormal ectopic impulses develop at the site of injury and adjacent to the dorsal root ganglia In CRPS type I, abnormal somatic nerve function may be present even if EMG and NCV are normal; EMG and NCV measure only large fiber function and cannot test small fiber function. In addition, they do not assess neurotransmitter/neuropeptide alterations within the peripheral nervous system
Spinal cord	Abnormal impulses from peripheral nerve result in abnormal sensitivity of dorsal horn neurons
Brain	All pain ultimately is perceived in the brain Autonomic nervous system has a central nervous system component that, when stimulated, results in peripheral dysautonomic signs Alterations in the thalamus have been shown in PET of CRPS patients[3]

CGRP, calcitonin gene-related peptide; CRPS, complex regional pain syndrome; EMG, electromyogram; NCV, nerve conduction velocity; PET, positron emission tomography.
Adapted from Merskey H, Bogduk N: Classification of Chronic Pain. Seattle, IASP Press, 1994.

tion of bone scans from 10 patients, 54 nuclear medicine physicians were able to agree on perfectly normal or obviously focal scans. There was less interobserver agreement with mildly increased activity scans. This study calls into question the use of this test as a diagnostic modality.[57]

Magnetic Resonance Imaging

MRI has been used as a diagnostic method for staging patients with RSD, but it has not been found to be highly sensitive or specific for this disorder. In a study by Graif and associates,[27] the overall sensitivity for diagnosis with typical criteria was only 60%. If an effusion was added as a diagnostic criterion, the sensitivity for diagnosing RSD increased to 91%.

Sympathetic Blockade Tests

Any test that represses the sympathetic system and can relieve symptoms can confirm the diagnosis. These tests can include direct sympathetic blocks, but confirmation can be obtained indirectly by epidural anesthesia, which represses the lumbar sympathetic system as well. Sympathetic blockade classically has been considered a hallmark for the diagnosis of RSD. More recently, studies have not used this test as the *sine qua non* for diagnosis. Because the IASP Classification Committee does not consider the sympathetic nervous system as the single or major underlying cause of this disorder, and they use only clinical symptoms

for diagnostic criteria, blockade cannot be considered the diagnostic gold standard. Nevertheless, we continue to use these modalities as important diagnostic and treatment methods. We believe that if there is no response to sympathetic blockade (no decrease in pain symptoms), another diagnosis should be considered.

TREATMENT METHODS

In a review article, Ghai and Dureja[22] defined five primary goals for managing patients with CRPS: (1) perform a comprehensive diagnostic evaluation, (2) be prompt and aggressive in treatment interventions, (3) assess and reassess the patient's clinical and psychological status, (4) be consistently supportive, and (5) strive for the maximal amount of pain relief and functional improvement. These are important goals for this difficult-to-treat disorder.

The various initial treatment methods for RSD of the knee include progressive mobilization and physical therapy methods, various analgesic medications, anti-inflammatory medications and vasodilators, psychological support, and other physical therapy maneuvers.[28] A multimodality approach should be used to decrease pain and restore function. When these methods fail, single or multiple lumbar sympathetic blocks combined with all modalities can be used. Sympathectomy or implantable spinal cord pumps can be considered only as a last resort.

It is important to realize that invasive knee procedures in patients with RSD typically increase their symptoms. All procedures on the knee should be avoided if possible. If surgery is absolutely necessary, one should use intraoperative epidural blocks and continue postoperatively with epidural blocks.

Oral Medication Pain Control

The first method to treat patients is to gain pain control. Sometimes simply giving the patient appropriate analgesics can allow the patient to proceed with physical therapy methods. Often, various medications are necessary. We have used a "triple cocktail," which includes anti-inflammatories, vasodilators, and benzodiazepines (as muscle relaxants), successfully. This triple cocktail is used in combination with opioid narcotic analgesic medications.

Neurontin (gabapentin) has been used commonly for the treatment of RSD of the knee. The drug dose is titrated upward in serial incremental steps until pain relief is obtained or side effects are observed. A randomized, double-blind, placebo-controlled crossover study of gabapentin and placebo included 58 patients.[59] The study found only a mild effect on pain in CRPS type I. The investigators concluded that a subpopulation of patients may benefit from gabapentin. Mellick and Mellick[37] reported that gabapentin relieved pain in a series of six patients with CRPS type I.

Some authors have advocated the use of bisphosphonates. In one study of 15 cases of RSD (two of the knee), pamidronate was found to be efficacious.[11] These findings are still preliminary, however, and further work is necessary to define the role of these agents. In a study by Manicourt and coworkers,[36] an oral dose of 40 mg of alendronate was markedly effective in 19 patients with CRPS I (RSD) of the lower extremity compared with 20 placebo-treated patients. The authors believed that alendronate might relieve pain by effects on nociceptive primary afferents in bone, pain-associated changes in the spinal cord, and possibly a central mechanism.

Corticosteroids given orally for 12 weeks at dosages of 80 mg/day of prednisone have been found to be beneficial in the short-term.[7,50] We do not advocate long-term use of corticosteroids. Various agents that have not been found to be effective in the treatment of RSD include tricyclic antidepressants, calcitonin, β-blockers, and oral sympatholytic agents, such as prazosin and phenoxybenzamine.[1,5,23,24,45,50]

Intravenous Medication

Pamidronate was studied by Robinson and associates[48] in 27 patients (14 treated, 13 placebo) who received 60 mg intravenously as a single dose. Pamidronate was found to be efficacious in many patients, although the treatment response varied.

The use of intravenous administration of subanesthetic ketamine was studied in 33 patients with CRPS type I by Correll and colleagues.[10] There was 76% complete pain relief after one infusion (25 patients). Repeated ketamine infusions led to longer lasting relief. Side effects included

hallucinations in a few patients. This treatment modality seems promising, although more research is needed to establish safety and efficacy guidelines for this method.

In another study, 27 patients with CRPS (8 with lower extremity involvement) were treated with intravenous lidocaine and methylprednisolone.[41] The investigators found that four of eight patients had symptomatic improvement.

Topical Agents

Lidocaine patches have been used for various painful conditions around the knee, although there are few published reports of their use for knee RSD.[2,15,19,49] One small study applied transdermal clonidine patches for various skin sensitivity problems; this offers potential as a possible modality for use in RSD.[13]

Early Mobilization and Physical Therapy

One of the goals or the mainstay of treatment is to obtain adequate pain relief and mobilize the patient as soon as possible. All efforts should be directed first toward maintaining motion of the knee and second toward developing strength. Any of various multiple physical therapy modalities can be used to produce these results. No studies have reviewed the efficacy of different physical therapy modalities for RSD of the knee.

We have used techniques that stress moving the knee and avoiding immobilization of the knee. One technique involves manipulation under anesthesia performed by the surgeon in conjunction with sympathetic blockade. The physical therapist should avoid aggressive passive manipulation, however. Desensitization techniques with modalities such as transcutaneous electrical stimulation may be efficacious, but have been shown to be useful only in a small study of pediatric patients.[3]

Psychological Counseling

If RSD is long-standing, it may be appropriate to counsel patients about this disease, and if it tremendously affects their lives, patients may need to seek further psychological counseling and support.[26,34,38] Patients need to understand the importance of controlling their pain and gradually making their knee or extremity more functional with physical therapy. They need to realize that this is not a simple process, but may require more invasive methods to gain control of symptoms.

Intravenous Regional Sympathetic Blocks

Not only are lumbar sympathetic blocks a major diagnostic method, but also they are often the mainstay of treatment. Typically, patients obtain pain relief at least temporarily from a lumbar sympathetic block, and one to six of these procedures can be performed.[14,46] Physical therapy and other modalities should be combined immediately with successful sympathetic blocks. The medication used most commonly is bretylium. In one study, the authors advocated mixing clonidine, 1 µg/kg, with 0.5% lidocaine with the block.[47] They obtained pain relief in five of seven patients with four to six blocks. Two patients had plateaus, but these patients had persistent anatomic lesions. These procedures are well tolerated. In another study by Cameron and associates,[6] 29 patients were treated with lumbar sympathetic blocks with local anesthetics, and only 13 patients (45%) had complete resolution of their symptoms. Three of the patients who failed to achieve resolution had a history of symptoms for more than 2 years. O'Brien and colleagues[39] used frequent sympathetic blocks (up to 30) on an outpatient basis for treatment of symptomatic knee patients. We prefer indwelling, more prolonged blockade (see next section).

Regional Anesthesia

An indwelling epidural block with bupivacaine for several days and narcotics while treating patients with various functional rehabilitation modalities can be efficacious.[20,21] In one study, intravenous regional anesthesia using lidocaine 0.5% and methylprednisolone was used.[20] The investigators reported tremendous relief in patients who had failed analgesic medications, psychological counseling, and physical therapy methods.

We use epidural blocks rather than sympathetic blocks because the epidural can be left in place for 1 week with other modalities. A sympathetic block may offer only transient relief of symptoms. An indwelling block avoids the need for repeated procedures and allows the patient to obtain pain-free various physical therapy modalities and knee manipulations as necessary. We advocate treatment modalities that maintain a 90 degree or more flexion arc.

Some words of caution are useful for hospitalization with epidural anesthesia. Complications of this treatment modality include hypotension and urinary retention. Nevertheless, this method has become the mainstay method of treatment at our institution.

Spinal Cord Stimulation

Various spinal stimulators and pumps have been used in patients with RSD of the knee.[4,25,53] There are few published reports concerning the efficacy of these devices. A meta-analysis of the use of these devices concluded that more trials were needed to confirm whether spinal cord stimulation is an effective treatment for CRPS type I.[35] Forouzantan and coworkers[17] reported that spinal cord stimulation improved health status in most patients with CRPS type I at 6 months, 1 year, and 2 years after implantation in 36 patients. Similar results were reported in a 2-year follow-up study of 36 patients treated with spinal cord stimulation and physical therapy.[32]

Sympathectomy

When lumbar sympathetic blocks are found to relieve pain temporarily, but symptoms persistently recur, sympathectomy may be considered. This procedure has been reported to be successful after repeated lumbar sympathetic blocks have provided some relief, but patients continue to have symptoms; patients should have at least one trial of an inpatient epidural admission before contemplating this procedure. This is a surgical procedure, although chemical sympathectomies also can be performed. The treatment results can vary, and symptoms may recur weeks to months later. In addition, some patients may end up with painful thighs after the procedure; this complication is called the *postsympathectomy syndrome*. Sympathectomy is a drastic technique to be used for a severely afflicted patient with few other treatment choices.

Amputation

Some clinicians have advocated amputation for patients with recalcitrant severe disease. Amputation is not a definitive solution, however. In one study of patients with below-knee amputation, 2 of 164 patients had persistent pain in their stump consistent with RSD.[30]

SURGICAL PROCEDURES AND EXPLORATION

We discourage the use of any invasive surgical procedures, even in the setting of intra-articular pathology. The first attempts should be made at obtaining pain control. The orthopedic surgeon may combine manipulations under anesthesia with epidurals that are maintained for treatment of stiff knees. Intra-articular surgery should be considered only after pain is well controlled. Procedures should be performed in a setting where an indwelling block is maintained for several days after the procedure.

PROGNOSIS

Results of treatment have varied.[33] Katz and Hungerford[31] described the treatment of 36 patients and found that they had a successful treatment in 64% within 1 year. Some patients required lumbar sympathetic blocks. These investigators believed that they had the best results in patients diagnosed early. These results were confirmed by Ogilvie-Harris, who studied 19 patients in 1987.[40] They followed the patients for an average of 3.4 years. The patients who went from diagnosis to treatment in less than 6 months did better, but none of these patients were normal as evaluated by objective measurements, such as a Cybex-II dynamometer. In a study by O'Brien and associates,[39] 60 patients who had RSD after arthroscopy procedures were evaluated at follow-up of 2 years. Fifty-five of the patients

(92%) had reasonable resolution of their symptoms with sympathetic blockade.[39] In contradistinction to the previous studies, these authors did not find that the time of onset to the initiation of treatment affected outcome. The prognosis was based more on a persistent anatomic lesion that continued to act as a painful stimulus. In patients in whom there were no anatomic lesions or lesions that had been treated reasonably successfully, 29 of 36 had complete resolution of symptoms (81%). Only 5 of 24 patients who had persistent anatomic lesions (21%) had complete resolution of their symptoms, however. These authors advocated that it was important to establish the precise diagnosis before performing surgery on the knee, including any type of arthroscopy.

SUMMARY

RSD of the knee is an uncommon disorder of the knee, occurring in approximately 1% to 2% of patients after knee surgical procedures. The etiology and pathophysiology of this syndrome are not clearly understood. It is important to lessen the morbidity by diagnosing the syndrome by an array of clinical signs as early as possible. The clinician can institute methods of treatment, including pain control with various rehabilitative methods, as soon as possible. When these methods fail, various more invasive treatment modalities are available. Epidural and lumbar sympathetic blocks can be used in combination with physical therapy. Various spinal pumps, sympathectomy, or amputation should used only as a final choice for severely afflicted patients who are recalcitrant to treatment. Well-controlled, prospective, randomized studies that have assessed the efficacy of various treatment modalities are lacking. In the future, it is hoped that larger and probably necessarily multicenter prospective studies will support the most appropriate modalities to treat these patients.

References

1. Abram SE, Lightfoot RW: Treatment of long-standing causalgia with prazosin. Reg Anesth 6:79, 1981.
2. Argoff CE, Galer BS, Jensen MP, et al: Effectiveness of the lidocaine patch 5% on pain qualities in three chronic pain states: Assessment with the Neuropathic Pain Scale. Curr Med Res Opin 20(Suppl 2):21, 2004.
3. Ashwad S, Tomasi L, Neumann M, Schneider S: Reflex sympathy dystrophy syndrome in children. Pediatr Neurol 4:28, 1988.
4. Barolet G, Schartzman R, Woo R: Epidural spinal cord stimulation in the management of reflex sympathetic dystrophy. Stereotact Funct Neurosurg 53:29, 1989.
5. Bickerstaff DR, Kanis JA: The use of nasal calcitonin in the treatment of post-traumatic algodystrophy. Br J Rheumatol 30:291, 1991.
6. Cameron HO, Park YS, Krestown M: Reflex sympathetic dystrophy following total knee replacement. Contemp Orthop 29:279, 1994.
7. Christensen K, Jensen EM, Noer I: The reflex sympathetic dystrophy syndrome response to treatment with systemic corticosteroids. Acta Chir Scand 148:653, 1982.
8. Cooper DE, DeLee JC: Reflex sympathetic dystrophy of the knee. J Am Acad Orthop Surg 2:79, 1994.
9. Cooper DE, DeLee JC, Ramamurthy S: Reflex sympathetic dystrophy of the knee. J Bone Joint Surg Am 71:365, 1989.
10. Correll GE, Maleki J, Gracely EJ, et al: Subanesthetic ketamine infusion therapy: A retrospective analysis of a novel therapeutic approach to complex regional pain syndrome. Pain Med 5:263, 2004.
11. Cortet B, Flipo RM, Coquerelle P, et al: Treatment of severe, recalcitrant reflex sympathetic dystrophy: Assessment of efficacy and safety of the second generation biphosphonate pamindronate. Clin Rheum 16:51, 1997.
12. Daviet JC, Dudognon P, Preux PM, et al: Reliability of transcutaneous oxygen tension measurements on back of the hand and complex regional pain syndrome after stroke. Arch Phys Med Rehabil 85:1102, 2004.
13. Davis KD, Treede RD, Raja SN, et al: Topical application of clonidine relieves hyperalgesia in patients with sympathetically maintained pain. Pain 47:309, 1991.
14. Dellemijn PJI, Fields HL, Allen RR, et al: The interpretation of pain relief and sensory changes following sympathetic block. Brain 17:1475, 1994.
15. Devers A, Galer BS: Topical lidocaine patch relieves a variety of neuropathic pain conditions: An open label experience. Clin J Pain 16(3):205-208, 2000.
16. Ficat RP, Hungerford DS: Disorders of the Patello-femoral Joint. Baltimore, Williams & Wilkins, 1977, pp 149-169.
17. Fourouzantan T, Kemler MA, Weber WE, et al: Spinal cord stimulation in complex regional pain syndrome: Cervical and lumbar devices are comparably effective. Br J Anaesth 92:348, 2004.
18. Galer BS, Bruehl S, Harden RN: IASP diagnostic criteria for complex regional pain syndrome: A preliminary empirical validation study. Clin J Pain 14:48, 1998.
19. Galer BS, Gammaitoni AR, Oleka N, et al: Use of the lidocaine patch 5% in reducing intensity of various pain qualities reported by patients with low-back pain. Curr Med Res Opin 20(Suppl 2):5, 2004.
20. Galer BS, Harle J, Rowbotham MC: Response to intravenous lidocaine infusion predicts subsequent response to oral mexiletine: A prospective study. J Pain Symptom Manage 12:161, 1996.
21. Galer BS, Miller KV, Rowbotham MC: Response to intravenous lidocaine infusion differs based on clinical diagnosis and site of nervous system injury. Neurology 43:1233, 1993.
22. Ghai B, Dureja GP: Complex regional pain syndrome: A review. J Postgrad Med 50:300, 2004.
23. Ghostine SY, Comair YG, Turner DM, et al: Phenoxybenzamine in the treatment of causalgia: Report of 40 cases. J Neurosurg 60:1263, 1984.
24. Gobelet C, Waldburger M, Meier JL: The effect of adding calcitonin to physical treatment of reflex sympathetic dystrophy. Pain 48:171, 1992.
25. Goodman R, Brisman R: Treatment of lower extremity reflex sympathetic dystrophy with continuous intrathecal morphine infusion. Appl Neurophysiol 50:425, 1987.
26. Grabow TS, Christo PJ, Raja SN: Complex regional pain syndrome: Diagnostic controversies, psychological dysfunction, and emerging concepts. Adv Psychosom Med 25:89, 2004.
27. Graif M, Schweitzer ME, Marks B, et al: Synovial effusion in reflex sympathetic dystrophy: An additional sign for diagnosing and staging. Skeletal Radiol 27:262, 1998.
28. Hogan CJ, Hurwitz SR: Treatment of complex regional pain syndrome of the lower extremity. J Am Acad Orthop Surg 10:281, 2002.
29. Huygen FJ, Niehof S, Klein J, Zijlstra FJ: Computer-assisted skin videothermography is a highly sensitive quality tool in the diagnosis and monitoring of complex regional pain syndrome type I. Eur J Appl Physiol 91:516, 2004.
30. Isakov E, Susak Z, Korzets A: Reflex sympathetic dystrophy of the stump in below-knee amputees. Clin J Pain 8:270, 1992.
31. Katz MM, Hungerford DS: Reflex sympathetic dystrophy affecting the knee. J Bone Joint Surg Br 69:797, 1987.
32. Kemler MA, DeVet HC, Barendse GA, et al: The effect of spinal cord stimulation in patients with chronic regional sympathetic dystrophy: Two years follow-up of the randomized controlled trial. Ann Neurol 55:13, 2004.
33. Kingery WS: A critical review of controlled clinical trials for peripheral neuropathic pain and complex regional pain syndromes. Pain 73:123, 1997.
34. Lynch ME: Psychological aspects of reflex sympathetic dystrophy: A review of the adult and paediatric literature. Pain 49:337, 1992.

35. Mailis-Gagnon A, Furlan AD, Sandoval JA, Taylor R: Spinal cord stimulation for chronic pain. Cochrane Database Syst Rev 3:CD003783, 2004.

36. Manicourt DH, Brasseur JP, Boutsen Y, et al: Role of alendronate in therapy for posttraumatic complex regional pain syndrome type I of the lower extremity. Arthritis Rheum 50:3690, 2004.

37. Mellick GA, Mellick LB: Reflex sympathetic dystrophy treated with gabapentin. Arch Phys Med Rehabil 78:98, 1997.

38. Miller RL: Reflex sympathetic dystrophy. Orthop Nurs 22:91, 2003.

39. O'Brien SJ, Ngeow J, Gibne MA, et al: Reflex sympathetic dystrophy of the knee: Causes, diagnosis, and treatment. Am J Sports Med 23:655, 1995.

40. Ogilvie-Harris DJ, Roscoe M: Reflex sympathetic dystrophy of the knee. J Bone Joint Surg Br 69(5):804-806, 1987.

41. Papadopoulos GS, Xenakis TA, Arnaoutoglou E, et al: The treatment of reflex sympathetic dystrophy in a 9 year-old boy with long-standing symptoms. J Min Anestesiol 67:659, 2001.

42. Perez RS, Keiszer G, Bezemer PD, et al: Predictive value of symptom level measurements for complex regional pain syndrome type I. Eur J Pain 9:49, 2005.

43. Poehling GG, Pollock FE, Koman LA: Reflex sympathetic dystrophy of the knee after sensory nerve injury. Arthroscopy 4:31, 1988.

44. Poplawski ZJ, Wiley AM, Murray JF: Post-traumatic dystrophy of the extremities. J Bone Joint Surg Am 65:642, 1983.

45. Prough DS, McLeskey CH, Poehling GG, et al: Efficacy of oral nifedipine in the treatment of reflex sympathetic dystrophy. Anesthesiology 62:769, 1985.

46. Raja SR: Nerve blocks in the evaluation of chronic pain: A plea for caution in their use and interpretation. Anesthesiology 86:4, 1997.

47. Reuben SS, Sklar J: Intravenous regional anesthesia with clonidine in the management of complex regional pain syndrome of the knee. J Clin Anesth 14:87, 2003.

48. Robinson JN, Sandom J, Chapman PT: Efficacy of pamidronate in complex regional pain syndrome type I. Pain Med 5:276, 2004.

49. Rowbotham MC, Davies PJ, Verkempinck CM, et al: Lidocaine patch: Double-blind controlled study of a new treatment method for postherpetic neuralgia. Pain 65:39, 1996.

50. Scadding JW, Wall PD, Parry W, et al: Clinical trial of propranolol in post-traumatic neuralgia. Pain 14:283, 1982.

51. Sherman OH, Fox JM, Snyder SJ, et al: Arthroscopy—"no problem surgery": An analysis of complications in two thousand six hunderd and forty cases. J Bone Joint Surg Am 68:256, 1986.

52. Small NC: Complications in arthroscopic surgery performed by experienced arthroscopists. Arthroscopy 4:215, 1988.

53. Stangl JA, Loeser JD: Intraspinal opioid infusion therapy in the treatment of chronic nonmalignant pain. Curr Rev Pain 1:353, 1997.

54. Stanton-Hicks M, Baron R, Boas R: Consensus report—complex regional syndromes: Guidelines for therapy. Clin J Pain 14:155, 1998.

55. Tanelian DT: Reflex sympathetic dystrophy: A reevaluation of the literature. Pain Forum 5:247, 1996.

56. Teasdall RD, Koman A, Wessinger P, et al: Reflex sympathetic dystrophy of the foot and ankle. Foot Ankle Clin 3:485, 1998.

57. Tondeur M, Sand A, Ham H: Interobserver reproducibility in the interpretation of bone scans from patients suspected of having reflex sympathetic dystrophy. Clin Nucl Med 30:4, 2005.

58. van der Laan L, ter Laak HJ, Gabreels-Festen A, et al: Complex regional pain syndrome type I: Pathology of skeletal muscle and peripheral nerves. Neurology 51:20, 1998.

59. van de Vusse AC, Stomp-van den Berg SG, Kessels AH, Weber WE: Randomized controlled trial of gabapentin in complex regional pain syndrome type I. BMC Neurol 4(1):13, 2004.

60. Veldman PH, Reynen HM, Arntz IE, et al: Signs and symptoms of reflex sympathetic dystrophy: Prospective study of 829 patients. Lancet 342:1012, 1993.

CHAPTER 62

Partial Denervation for the Treatment of Painful Neuromas Complicating Total Knee Replacement

A. Lee Dellon • Michael A. Mont

Successful management of knee pain is critical to the practice of most orthopedic surgeons. Nonoperative treatment of knee pain of musculoskeletal origin is part of the daily practice of most orthopedic surgeons. Operative approaches to the treatment of knee pain have been described extensively and range from relatively less invasive procedures, such as arthroscopy and the correction of patellofemoral tracking, to high tibial osteotomies, Maquet's procedure, and total knee replacement. Management of persistent knee pain after the aforementioned approaches has provided less than satisfactory results; it is perplexing, time-consuming, and usually frustrating for the orthopedic surgeon. This chapter provides an algorithm for the care of patients with persistent knee pain.

For a patient to perceive pain, there must be a neural pathway for transmission of the impulses generated from the injured tissues. This concept is easily accepted for the skin, where a direct injury may disrupt, crush, or stretch a nerve that innervates a piece of skin. Although the mechanisms to be discussed were introduced for upper extremity pain in the 1980s and 1990s, their application to knee pain was initiated more recently. An analogy is helpful to provide the theoretical framework for the lower extremity application.

If after an injury to the dorsoradial aspect of the distal forearm a patient complained of pain in that region, and physical examination suggested that the musculoskeletal system was intact, and radiographic imaging showed no abnormalities, a neuroma or compression of the radial sensory nerve would be the likely source of pain. If the anatomic variations of that region of skin were considered carefully, the differential diagnosis would be expanded to consider an injury to the lateral antebrachial cutaneous nerve, which overlaps with the radial sensory nerve in 75% of people.[37] Similarly, if a ganglion were removed from the dorsal aspect of the wrist, and the postoperative incision were painful and remained painful, it would raise the possibility of a neuroma of a branch of these same two cutaneous nerves. If the patient's pain after ganglion removal were deeper and became worse with wrist flexion and extension, however, a nerve pathway that involved the dorsal wrist capsule would need to be considered in the cause of the pain. The terminal branch of the posterior interosseous nerve innervates the dorsal wrist capsule and in particular the scapholunate ligament.[17] A neuroma of this nerve may have resulted when the ganglion was excised from a portion of this ligament. If the patient's pain did not resolve with therapy, steroid massage, or steroid injection, and if pain limited hand function, successful treatment could be achieved by appropriate treatment of the involved nerve. To determine the involved nerve, nerve blocks would be used to identify the source of pain as coming from either one or both cutaneous nerves or the nerve that innervates the wrist joint or all three. For a cutaneous neuroma, the treatment must include resection of the neuroma or at least interruption of its neural pathway because the neuroma can be a source of pain.[44] For the dorsoradial aspect of the hand, the appropriate treatment is to transfer the proximal end of the cutaneous nerve into a proximal large muscle, such as the brachioradialis.[39] For the dorsal wrist, a partial (dorsal) wrist denervation is indicated.[6]

Why has it taken so long for this approach, proven successful for management of upper extremity pain, to be applied to the lower extremity? The reason almost certainly is related to continuing misconceptions about neuroma formation and treatment and to lack of information about innervation of joints and ligaments. For the knee in particular, there was until more recently an absence of any accepted anatomic basis about innervation of the knee joint. Before describing the neuroanatomy of the knee region, however, a review of the pathophysiology of neuroma formation and of the treatment of the painful neuroma is in order.

PATHOPHYSIOLOGY OF NEUROMA FORMATION

In the peripheral nervous system, the response to division of a peripheral nerve has been well documented. That response involves degeneration of the distal axons, survival of the distal Schwann's cells, sprouting of the proximal nerve fibers (because this is the physiologic response of the cell bodies located in the dorsal root ganglion), and production of nerve growth factor by the distal (denervated) Schwann's cells. This response results in the proximal axon sprouts regenerating distally toward the chemotactic gradient of nerve growth factor. These sprouts track along the basement, where fibronectin, type I collagen, and laminin also attract the sprouts.[8,40] There is currently no available biological tool to prevent this cascade of events. Without destruction of the dorsal root ganglion, neuroma formation always occurs.

One of the most common misconceptions about management of a painful neuroma is that resection of the neuroma always results in another painful neuroma. Based on the neurophysiology just presented, it is clear that resection of a painful neuroma always results in an attempt by the nerve to regenerate. A recurrent painful neuroma results if that regeneration is allowed to occur into an area of movement, frequent contact, trauma, or scar. A recurrent painful neuroma does not occur if the proximal end is allowed to regenerate into a peaceful area (e.g., innervated muscle away from an area of contact or trauma). Another suitable area into which to put the proximal end of the nerve after neuroma resection is a large area containing fat, which is also away from contact points. A common example is when the sural nerve is harvested for nerve grafting, and the proximal end of the nerve is allowed to lie in the popliteal fossa. A recurrent painful neuroma does not occur if the proximal end of the nerve is permitted to regenerate into a appropriate end organ. An example is the type of regeneration that occurs when a nerve is divided and then reconstructed either with a nerve repair or a nerve graft; the nerve regenerates into its own distal territory.

TREATMENT OF A PAINFUL NEUROMA

Management of a painful neuroma can be done successfully if the following three steps are followed:
1. Identify the correct peripheral nerve that is the source of the pain; this requires careful clinical evaluation, understanding of anomalous innervation, and diagnostic nerve blocks.[37,38]
2. Resect the end-bulb neuroma because it is the source of spontaneous C-fiber and A-delta fiber activity that signals pain, and it is mechanosensitive and chemosensitive.[44]
3. Relocate the proximal nerve into a site that is away from joint movement, away from nerve growth factor stimulation, and away from usual physical contact points; intramuscular placement has proved to be a successful strategy.[11,14]

Studies in monkeys have shown that when the proximal nerve sprouts into an environment of innervated muscle, and when that muscle is chosen to have minimal excursion, classic end-bulb neuromas do not form.[41] Clinically, this approach has proved successful for the upper and lower extremities—the radial sensory and lateral antebrachial cutaneous nerves into the brachioradialis muscle,[39] the palmar cutaneous branch of the median nerve into the pronator quadratus muscle,[20] the plantar digital nerves into the foot intrinsic muscles,[7] and the superficial and deep peroneal nerves into the anterolateral compartment muscles.[9] For neuromas related to nerves that innervate joints, resection of the neuroma or the peripheral nerve in an area proximal to the joint usually allows the resected proximal end of the nerve to lie in an internervous plane, and direct muscle implantation is

not needed. Examples are the anterior and posterior interosseous nerves in the forearm.[6,8,13]

HISTORY OF PARTIAL JOINT DENERVATION IN THE EXTREMITIES

In 1966, Wilhelm[54] published, in German, his approach to the treatment of persistent wrist joint pain. This concept became available to non–German-reading surgeons in 1977, when Buck-Gramcko[3] reviewed the German-speaking people's experience with 313 patients. With an 80% follow-up that exceeded 2 years, their results included excellent results in 69% of 195 patients. This was a complex review, including results from many surgeons, with 10 separate nerves being resected circumferentially about the wrist during a total wrist denervation. Many patients had "incomplete" or partial denervations done based on local anesthetic blocks. The patient population included patients who had persistent pain after forearm or wrist fractures, advanced arthritis, carpal instability, and severe sprains. Poorest results were in patients with unstable wrists, who later required fusions.

In 1978, Dellon and Seif[17] published a description of the innervation of the dorsal wrist capsule by the terminal branch of the posterior interosseous nerve. This nerve could be identified easily over the distal dorsal forearm, proximal to the wrist. This publication implied that if wrist pain, regardless of its cause, could be isolated to neural transmission along this nerve pathway, that pathway alone could be interrupted, eliminating wrist pain—a partial, rather than a total, approach to wrist denervation. This hypothesis was tested in 29 patients studied between July 1981 and June 1984.[6] Pain in these patients was caused by wrist fracture ($n = 8$), carpal instability ($n = 4$), arthritis ($n = 3$), severe wrist sprain ($n = 10$), and dorsal ganglionectomy ($n = 4$). Range of wrist motion and grip strength were measured, an anesthetic block of the posterior interosseous nerve was done, and the range of motion and grip strength were repeated (Fig. 62–1). For the patient to be considered a surgical candidate, pain relief, increased range of motion, and increased grip strength had to be present. The results were that 90% of the patients achieved pain relief and improved wrist function; 83% returned to work. Failure occurred in three of the four patients with carpal instability, who required a subsequent wrist fusion. Three patients had reflex sympathetic dystrophy after their wrist fracture; two of these patients previously had had Darrach's procedures, and two had had a carpal tunnel decompression. Two of the reflex sympathetic dystrophy patients had subjective improvement after partial dorsal wrist denervation and had improved range of motion, but none of the three returned to work. The conclusions were that partial joint denervation was effective in relieving pain and improving function in selected patients, that total joint denervation was not necessary, and that structural instability was a contraindication to joint denervation.

Logically, there would be a group of patients for whom anterior wrist pain could be treated by a partial volar wrist denervation procedure. In 1984, Dellon and colleagues,[13]

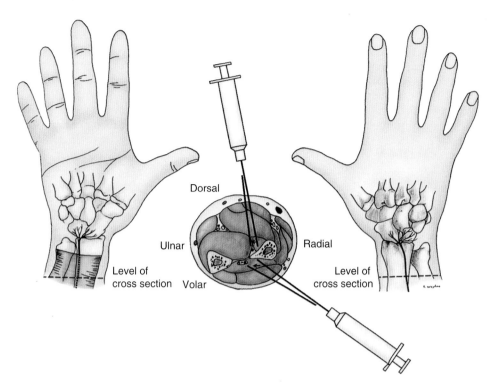

Figure 62–1. Local anesthetic nerve block. To identify the nerve that is the neural transmission route for the pain signal, it is essential to block a specific nerve with a local anesthetic. Relief of pain with either a regional or an intra-articular block is not sufficient to identify the individual nerves that may be rejected in a partial joint denervation. This type of block is illustrated here for the wrist, where either the anterior or the posterior interosseous nerves can be blocked. Many patients have either a dorsal or a volar injury in the wrist, and a single nerve may be the source of pain. For some problems, such as a triangular fibrocartilage tear, it may be necessary to block both of these nerves to obtain pain relief. This same approach must be used in the knee to identify individual components of pain arising from the medial or the lateral retinacular nerve or both.

after basic anatomic dissections to identify the terminal branch of the anterior interosseous nerve distal to the pronator quadratus muscle, attempted partial volar wrist denervation in a small group of patients. From April 1982 through March 1984, there were 11 patients with persistent volar wrist pain; 9 had work-related injuries, and 2 were involved in motor vehicle accidents. Each patient had good relief of pain, increased wrist range of motion, and increased grip strength after a block of the anterior interosseous nerve (see Fig. 62–1). At a mean follow-up of 12.8 months (range 4 to 24 months), all patients had good to excellent relief of their pain. Four patients had returned to their regular job, three returned to "light duty" jobs, and four were in vocational rehabilitation. The conclusions were that partial joint denervation was effective in relieving pain and improving function in selected patients and that total joint denervation was not necessary.

In 1993, Dellon and Horner[10] reviewed experience in 51 patients treated for wrist pain with partial denervation. Overall, there was a 98% improvement for pain, with the visual analog scale level decreasing in all patients between 6 and 8 points out of 10. Improved range of motion occurred in 60% of the whole group. No patients with carpal instability were included in this more recent group.

Currently, partial wrist denervation is an accepted procedure for patients (1) whose wrist pain persists after at least 6 months of nonoperative management; (2) who

have no carpal instability; and (3) who respond appropriately with decreased pain and increased motion after specific local anesthetic blocks of selected, identifiable, peripheral nerves. Before the lessons learned in upper extremity joint denervation can be applied to the lower extremity, it is essential to identify the specific nerves that mediate pain from the knee region.

CUTANEOUS INNERVATION OF THE KNEE REGION

Virtually all anatomy books agree on the presence of the saphenous nerve innervating the infrapatellar region. The saphenous nerve originates medially, from the femoral nerve, and descends in the medial thigh through the adductor canal to emerge around the sartorius muscle or through the sartorius muscle. The infrapatellar branch divides from the femoral nerve variably: in the proximal third of the thigh (17.6%), in the middle third of the thigh (58.8%), and in the distal third of the thigh (23.5%).[26] In 86% of people, there are two saphenous nerve branches in Hunter's canal.[26] In this situation, the more anterior of the two branches becomes the infrapatellar branch of the saphenous nerve, which when it enters the medial knee region is about 4 mm in width and begins to branch as it approaches the anterior midline. It always crosses the leg below the patella and usually has branches from below the patella to below the tibial tuberosity. The infrapatellar branch of the saphenous nerve innervates the anterior midline of the region below the patella and the lateral region below the patella. It does not innervate the skin covering the patella (Figs. 62–2 and 62–3). It may send branches into the distal anterior knee joint capsule.[26]

The skin covering the patella is innervated by the medial cutaneous nerve of the thigh. This is a better name

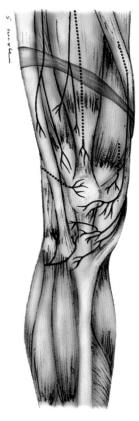

Figure 62–2. Anterior view of innervation of the knee region: medial cutaneous nerve of the thigh, medial retinacular nerve, infrapatellar branch of the saphenous nerve, lateral retinacular nerve, lateral femoral cutaneous nerve, anterior femoral cutaneous nerve, innervation of the prepatellar bursal structures, and innervation of the proximal tibiofibular joint. The dotted lines are innervation of the knee joint.

for this nerve than the anterior or medial femoral cutaneous nerve because this nerve almost always branches from the saphenous nerve and travels as a separate branch, superficial to (39.1%), through (30.4%), or deep to (30.5%) the sartorius, to emerge in the region of the femoral condyle, lying in the superficial subcutaneous plane.[26] This nerve may range in size from 0.6 to 1.1 mm, and there may be more than one branch. Its branches often lie directly over the medial retinacular nerve, and a local anesthetic block in this region blocks both nerves (see Figs. 62–2 and 62–3).

It is unclear as to whether the obturator nerve contributes branches to one or both of the branches of the saphenous nerve. The obturator nerve's sensory branches enter into the complex of nerves within the adductor canal and do not emerge as a single identifiable branch in this distal thigh or knee region. Branches of the obturator nerve do participate in the innervation of the posterior knee capsule (Fig. 62–4).

The distal saphenous nerve theoretically begins distal to the infrapatellar branch of the saphenous nerve. Usually it has a separate branch in the thigh, or it may be the continuation of the saphenous nerve after the infrapatellar branch. Most often, regardless of its origin, in the region distal to the tibial tuberosity, the distal saphenous nerve gives off one or more transverse branches, which may become a source of pain from long anterior or medial incisions. The terminal skin innervated by the distal saphenous nerve includes the medial dorsum of the foot, and a region posterior to the medial malleolus (see Figs. 62–2 and 62–3).

The anterior femoral cutaneous nerve originates from the femoral nerve in the groin region and terminates at the patellar region. It has many small (<1 mm) branches in this region, and there is usually not an identifiable neuroma of this nerve (see Fig. 62–2).

The medial femoral cutaneous nerve probably does not exist as such. The territories shown for it are best considered from a surgical anatomy point of view as being supplied by either the anterior femoral cutaneous nerve or the medial cutaneous nerve of the thigh.

The lateral femoral cutaneous nerve begins at the hip region as a continuation of the L1 and L2 nerve roots. It has a branch that innervates the lateral buttock and a branch that innervates the lateral thigh skin extending to the level of the lateral knee. At the level of the inguinal ligament, the lateral femoral cutaneous nerve is 3 to 7 mm in size. At the lateral knee region, it has terminal branches

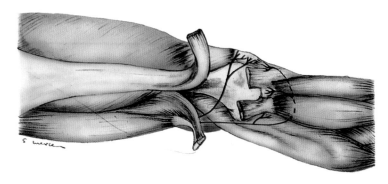

Figure 62–3. Lateral view of innervation of the knee region: the biceps femoris and the iliotibial tract have been divided and reflected; the lateral retinacular nerve innervating the lateral knee joint structures after arising from the sciatic nerve; the innervation of the proximal tibiofibular joint, from the common peroneal nerve.

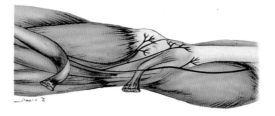

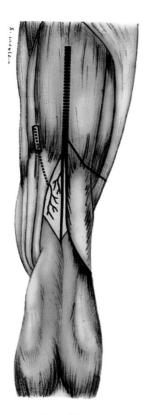

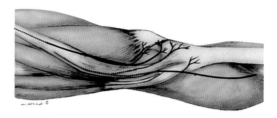

Figure 62–4. Posterior view of innervation of the knee joint: lateral retinacular nerve arising from the sciatic nerve. The posterior knee capsule is innervated from branches of the obturator nerve coming through the adductor canal and from branches of the sciatic nerve.

Figure 62–5. Medial view of innervation of the knee region. The sartorius muscle *(top)* has been divided and reflected *(bottom)*. The medial retinacular nerve continues distally after innervating the vastus medialis to enter the medial knee joint structures. The saphenous nerve and its branches are unlabeled.

only, which are usually too small to identify. Although pain can be referred to the knee from compression of the lateral femoral cutaneous nerve at the hip, direct injury to the knee or surgery in the knee region almost never causes a neuroma of this nerve. Lateral knee skin pain is almost always due to a neuroma of the medial cutaneous nerve of the thigh or the infrapatellar branch of the saphenous nerve (see Fig. 62–2).

INNERVATION OF THE KNEE JOINT

The innervation of the human knee joint has been described by Ruedinger (1857),[51] Druner (1927),[18] Jeletsky (1931),[30] Gardner (1948),[24] Wilhelm (1958),[53] Kennedy and coworkers (1982),[33] and Wojtys and associates (1990).[55] None of these descriptions were from a large number of fresh human cadavers, and none provided detailed anatomic drawings sufficient to permit surgical approaches to these nerves. Clarification of nomenclature was required. A study was reported in 1994 by Horner and Dellon[26] and serves as the basis for the following description and nomenclature. In that study, 45 fresh cadaveric adult knees were dissected using loupe magnification. The following description is based on that study and supplemented by clinical and operative experience over 4 years.

The lateral retinacular nerve is consistently present. It arises directly from the sciatic nerve, proximal to the popliteal fossa, and continues laterally to go beneath the biceps femoris tendon to reach the lateral retinacular structures. The lateral retinacular nerve lies beneath the lateral retinaculum. At this level, it exists as two or three 1-mm branches, entering into the deeper structures of the knee joint. It always is accompanied by the recurrent lateral geniculate vessel and always is just distal to the vastus lateralis muscle. It is immediately superficial to the synovial structures of the knee joint (Fig. 62–5; see Figs. 62–2 and 62–4).

The medial retinacular nerve is consistently present. It arises from the branch of the femoral nerve that innervates the vastus medialis muscle. It exits from beneath the distal posterior aspect of the vastus medialis and travels anteriorly to innervate the medial retinacular structures in 90%, whereas in the other 10%, it exits through the muscle to innervate the medial retinacular structures.[26] The medial retinacular nerve lies beneath the medial retinaculum and at this level exists as two or three 1-mm branches, entering into the deeper structures of the knee joint. It always is accompanied by the recurrent medial geniculate vessels and always is just distal to the vastus medialis muscle. It is immediately superficial to the synovial structures of the knee joint (see Figs. 62–2 and 62–3).

Nerves to the prepatellar bursal structures arise from the terminal branches of femoral nerves that innervate the vastus intermedius muscle. These continue distal to the muscle, lying on the anteromedial side of the distal femur, to enter into the prepatellar bursa and its surrounding structures. There is no unique name given to these nerve branches, which are approximately 1 mm each in diameter (see Fig. 62–2).

Nerves to the posterior knee capsule arise from the sciatic nerve over a 2-cm distance and widely innervate the posterior knee structures. There is no unique name given to these nerve branches, which are less than 1 mm each in diameter (see Fig. 62–4). Druner[18] observed in 1927 that the posterior knee capsule received branches from the obturator nerve through Hunter's canal. The confluence of these branches with the branches from the sciatic nerve was named the popliteal plexus by Ruedinger.[51]

INNERVATION OF THE PROXIMAL TIBIOFIBULAR JOINT

Although it is clear that the proximal tibiofibular joint is not part of the true knee joint, pain from the proximal tibiofibular joint may accompany knee pain in a patient's complaints. It is crucial to be able to discern the difference between these two joints and appreciate the separate source of innervation of the proximal tibiofibular joint from the true knee joint.

The common peroneal branch of the sciatic nerve gives the branches that innervate the proximal tibiofibular joint. These branches do not have a unique name. There is one branch that arises proximal to the fibular head and one or two that arise just distal to the fibular head. These branches are quite small, generally less than 1 mm in diameter, and require loupe magnification to identify. They travel into the structures between the fibular head and Gerdy's tubercle of the tibia (see Figs. 62–2, 62–4, and 62–5).

Immediately adjacent to these two small nerves are motor branches that innervate the tibialis anterior muscle. They cannot be distinguished morphologically. It is crucial to use intraoperative electrical stimulation to identify the motor branches of the tibial nerve. To be most correct, it is crucial to stimulate the nerve fiber believed to innervate this joint and ensure that it is not a motor nerve by showing that it does not cause a muscle contraction before it is cut.

RATIONALE FOR DENERVATION FOR PERSISTENT PAIN AFTER TOTAL KNEE ARTHROPLASTY

Nerve injury has been associated with virtually all orthopedic lower extremity procedures, from relatively "simple" procedures such as arthroscopy or arthrotomy,[1,5,27,35,52,56] to total joint replacement.[25,26] These reports have described injury to well-known peripheral nerves, such as the sciatic, common peroneal, femoral, saphenous, and posterior tibial. The treatment of these nerve injuries varies from the conservative "observation," when nerve compression is thought to be the cause, to resection of individual small cutaneous nerves when they can be

identified, to indwelling spinal catheters or lumbar sympathetic blocks for the treatment of major pain, such as reflex sympathetic dystrophy.[21,31,32,49,50]

Pain after total knee replacement may have a structural or biomechanical cause, such as malalignment or loosening, or may have a medical cause, such as infection. When these possibilities have been evaluated carefully by traditional orthopedic approaches, it is plausible that the persistent pain may be of neural origin (Table 62–1). As with any incision anywhere on the body, a cutaneous nerve may become entrapped in the scar or may have been divided during the surgery. A cutaneous neuroma should be treated according to the rationale given previously for a peripheral nerve in the upper extremity. The rationale of treating pain arising from the knee joint itself after a total knee arthroplasty may seem to involve a contradiction: How can a joint that has been surgically removed be a source of pain?

When it is accepted that there are identifiable nerves to the knee joint structures, just as there are to the wrist joint, it becomes clear that some of these nerves must be transected in every total knee replacement during the process of removing the necessary bone. What happens to the proximal end of these normal nerves after the surgery? Most probably, related to the degree of traction that occurs during the procedure, they retract into proximal tissues and form their neuromas in a quiet region (i.e., they form a nonpainful neuroma). This is most likely the explanation for the excellent results that occur in greater than 97% of patients having total knee replacement.[23] It is hypothesized that the cause of the deep knee pain in 1% to 3% of total knee replacement patients who have persistent pain is the nerves supplying the knee joint. These nerves (i.e., the medial and lateral retinacular nerves) are most likely transected during the procedure and become adherent to the capsule that forms around the implant. If this is true, postoperative range of motion of the knee stimulates these nerves through stretch/traction, eliciting a neural response that the brain interprets as a painful knee.[15] In one of the first denervation operations, the lateral retinacular nerve was followed down to the capsule and resected with a portion of the capsule. The pathology report showed a true neuroma (Fig. 62–6). As described subsequently, this approach is *not* recommended because a synovial leak developed in this patient, requiring reoperation. Nevertheless, the specimen obtained at that time supported this rationale.

Table 62–1. Indications for Knee Denervation

Persistent pain for at least 6 mo after a knee procedure or an injury that was not relieved by nonsteroidal anti-inflammatory drugs
Absence of active synovitis, knee joint effusion, or infection
Absence of radiographic evidence of bony or implant problems
Absence of mechanical reasons that could account for the pain (e.g., ligamentous instability—laxity in the mediolateral or anteroposterior plane >0.5 cm)

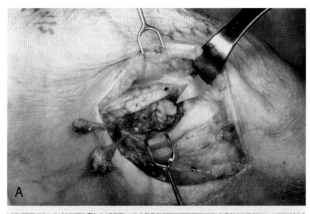

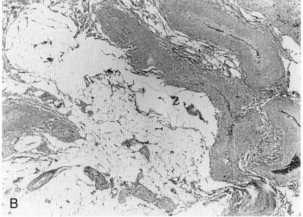

Figure 62–6. Neuroma formation on the lateral retinacular nerve after total knee replacement. **A,** The intraoperative appearance of the neuromas on branches of the lateral retinacular nerve in a patient with persistent pain after a total knee replacement. **B,** The histological appearance of the specimen, which shows a true neuroma. (Hematoxylin and eosin stain, 1 × 25.)

DIAGNOSIS OF KNEE PAIN OF NEURAL ORIGIN

In general, each patient must have every musculoskeletal problem treated to the highest level. Denervating a joint cannot restore structural integrity. Conversely, restoring structural integrity does not always relieve pain. Although modern radiographic imaging can identify small defects in ligaments, menisci, and cartilage, they cannot identify the small nerves that innervate the knee joints and the surrounding skin.

Knee pain in the presence of a relatively normal physical examination of the musculoskeletal system, in the presence of normal x-rays and a normal MRI, and even in the presence of a relatively normal or "negative" arthroscopy should be considered of neural origin. The diagnosis must be made based on nerve blocks.

The first step in deciding which nerves to block is to listen to the patient's complaints. Try to decide whether the complaints are just related to the knee joint or also involve the skin. Crucial historical points include learning whether there was any direct injury to the knee itself (i.e., a fall during which the knee hit the floor or an

object). A previous surgery, such as a knee replacement procedure, satisfies this historical point, as does a previous arthroscopy. Any previous surgery in the knee region may have resulted in a neuroma of one of its cutaneous nerves. The patient may indicate that bedclothes or clothing is painful or disturbing when it touches the knee. These historical points implicate a cutaneous nerve. At the same time, complaints related to knee function (i.e., kneeling, walking, and climbing steps) suggest that nerves innervating the knee structures are implicated in the pain mechanism. The patient should be asked to give a numerical value to the level of the pain, using a rating scale from 0 (no pain) to 10 (the worst pain they ever had). If possible, a formal visual analog scale should be used. In general, to be considered a candidate for surgery, the pain level should be 5 or higher.

The physical examination must attempt to locate the source of the trigger zones that identify the site of the involved nerve and the site for the nerve block. First, the examiner locates areas of decreased sensation to a moving-touch stimulus at the patellar and infrapatellar areas by touching these areas bilaterally. Next, the examiner begins distally over the pretibial region and works toward the tibial tuberosity, pressing deeply to identify sites where cutaneous nerves may be sending impulses from a neuroma. Even if no incision touches this area, in an operation requiring as much retraction and dissection as a total knee replacement, it is conceivable that cutaneous nerves may have become scarred at these relatively remote sites. Sites of cutaneous neuromas most commonly are noted near a transverse distal saphenous nerve branch, at the infrapatellar branch of the saphenous nerve just medial to the tibial tuberosity, and at the medial cutaneous nerve of the thigh just medial to the patella (Fig. 62–7). The final area for a painful cutaneous neuroma is in the anterior scar proximal to the patella. Often the scar is depressed where the skin is adherent to the quadriceps tendon.

Involvement of the joint afferents in the pain syndrome can be identified during the physical examination. Deep pressure just distal to the femoral condyles and posterior to the patella reveal these nerves, which are sufficiently thickened from scar tissue that they become palpable.

Pain related to the innervation of the proximal tibiofibular joint can be identified by pressure just anterior to the fibular head. Historically, these patients usually have had a high tibial osteotomy, a Maquet procedure, or a fibular fracture. There may be an associated compression of the common peroneal nerve at the fibular head. This compression can be found during the physical examination by gentle pressure of this nerve against the fibular head (this is not usually painful), by identifying weakness in the muscles innervated by this nerve (weakness of the extensor hallucis longus often is the first to be detected), and by observing abnormal sensibility in the distribution of the superficial or deep peroneal nerves. The physical examination has not been useful in identifying problems with innervation of the posterior knee joint capsule.

A diagnostic nerve block is not an intra-articular block. Anesthetic injected into the knee joint diffuses to many different areas. It is unclear from an intra-articular anesthetic injection which nerve has been blocked.

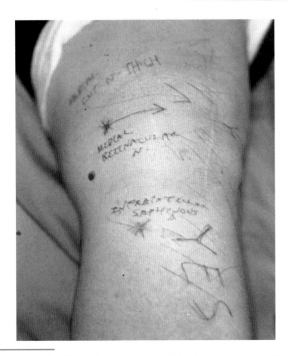

Figure 62–7. Clinical evaluation of the knee preoperatively. Abnormal areas of skin sensibility have been roughly estimated by crosshatched lines on the skin. These territories suggest that the medial cutaneous nerve of the thigh and the intrapatellar branch of the saphenous nerve are involved in the pain mechanism, directing the examination to find the Tinel's sign locations or trigger spots for the neuromas. These are denoted by inked asterisks on the skin, to help with intraoperative localization.

Based on the anatomic descriptions given previously, it is possible to block specifically the individual nerves that may be the source of pain. The only overlap of these nerves is in the intersection in a superficial and deep plane of the medial cutaneous nerve of the thigh and the medial retinacular nerve. If the skin of the patellar region is reduced, dysesthetic, or painful, in addition to the complaints of deep medial joint pain related to the medial retinacular nerve, there must be a cutaneous nerve involved as well. Most commonly, both of these nerves are involved in the painful knee.

The block should be done using aseptic technique. An iodine-containing skin preparation is preferred. We use 1% lidocaine and 0.5% bupivacaine, each without epinephrine; 5 mL of a 1:1 mixture of these two anesthetics is used. Each of the identified cutaneous and joint afferents is blocked, usually all at the same time. If for some reason it is difficult to identify the contributing sites, the medial side can be blocked, then later during the same office visit or at a second office visit, the lateral side can be blocked. This block may be needed especially if the patient's complaints are localized to the distal anterior knee joint region or to the "whole knee." Another example of a patient who may require more than one period of anesthetic administration is one who has a "reflex sympathetic dystrophy" of the knee. If the nerve to the proximal tibiofibular joint is to be blocked, the common peroneal nerve should not be blocked because this would interfere

with the patient's ambulation. To block the nerve to the proximal tibiofibular joint, a local anesthetic should be injected adjacent to the anterior region of the fibular head.

After the anesthetic block, the patient must have knee function stressed. At about 15 minutes after the block, the patient should be asked to climb a flight of steps, walk in the hall, or kneel on a padded chair. During this time, he or she should be accompanied by a relative or a member of the office staff. Observations should be recorded for the office chart. The patient should give a numerical assessment of the pain level, preferably on a visual analog scale. If there is residual pain, its location should be identified, and, if necessary, another nerve block should be done, with the knee function and pain score being repeated.

OPERATIVE TECHNIQUE

The patient is interviewed and examined in the induction area before surgery. The surgery is done on an outpatient basis, but depending on the medical situation, an overnight stay in the hospital may be justified. The exact sites of pain are marked with indelible ink, to aid in making the incision in the operating room. Typically, there is a 3- to 5-cm incision over the medial knee (to approach the medial cutaneous nerve of the thigh and the medial retinacular nerves); a similar one over the lateral knee (to approach the lateral retinacular nerve); and a third incision about 3 cm distal to the medial incision, which is used to identify the infrapatellar branch of the saphenous nerve. When one long medial incision is made, there seems to be higher postoperative incidence of bruising or hematoma formation. A neuroma is not resected, but rather a segment of nerve, which pathologically may show fibrosis, is resected. This is technically a denervation rather than a neuroma resection. If the pathology report indicates that a normal nerve has been removed, this is acceptable. The patient receives 1 g of a cephalosporin drug intravenously in the induction area (another drug is used if there is a penicillin allergy history).

Knee denervation surgery should be considered peripheral nerve surgery and, as such, employ bipolar coagulation and loupe magnification. A microscope is not needed. The patient is placed supine on the operating table. The surgery should be done in a bloodless field; a pneumatic tourniquet should be used. The patient is placed under spinal or general anesthesia. Unless just one nerve is to be resected, local anesthesia is not sufficient to remove the discomfort of the upper thigh tourniquet plus anesthetize the incision site. Depending on the patient's size and systolic pressure, the tourniquet is inflated to 300 mm Hg or 350 mm Hg after removing most of the blood from the leg with an Ace bandage. Because a guide to identifying the nerves is the blood in the vessels that accompany the nerve, it is suggested that the leg not be exsanguinated completely. We prefer to cauterize extensively during the surgery, close each incision, dress the leg with a dressing that includes a tightly applied Ace bandage, and then let down the tourniquet. The Ace bandage is removed after half an hour in the recovery room, before the patient is

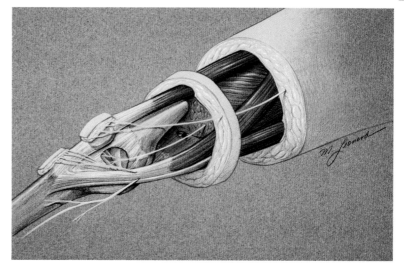

Figure 62–8. Three-dimensional view of anatomy of the innervation of the medial knee. Note the differing relationships of the medial nerves to the skin of the patellar and infrapatellar regions at the knee level and at the level below the knee. Note also the medial retinacular nerve traveling through the muscle of the vastus medialis to enter the knee joint structures beneath the medial retinaculum, in a location that places it immediately below the medial cutaneous nerve of the thigh.

discharged. Alternatively the tourniquet can be let down at the completion of the procedure, hemostasis obtained, local anesthetic instilled, and the wounds closed.

During the medial dissection about the knee, the leg is externally rotated at the hip with the knee flexed, "froglegged." During the lateral dissection, the knee is flexed, the leg is internally rotated, and the hip is flexed, bringing the knee up off the operating table.

Medially the incision is deepened into the subcutaneous tissue, looking for the medial cutaneous nerve of the thigh over the site of the marking where the medial retinacular nerve is expected to be found. In the superficial subcutaneous plane, a search is made for any small blood vessels going from posterior to anterior, not from proximal to distal. The soft tissues are spread with the scissors, which causes the nerve to be identified by its relatively stable position. When the structure suspected to be the medial cutaneous nerve of the thigh is identified, it is dissected proximally. If the structure is the nerve and not connective tissue, it can be followed proximally. As it approaches the longitudinal incision that was used for the knee replacement, 1 cm of the nerve is resected distally, and it is submitted to the pathology department. A true neuroma is not resected, but rather a segment of the nerve is. The proximal end is turned, a widow is created in the fascia of the vastus medialis, and the nerve is implanted loose for a 2-cm length into the muscle. A suture is not needed. Bupivacaine is instilled into the implantation site at this time (Figs. 62–8 to 62–10).

The medial retinacular nerve is identified through the same incision used for the medial cutaneous nerve of the thigh by incising the fascia transversely just distal to the vastus medialis muscle. In this area, the recurrent medial geniculate vessel should be present. The nerve accompanies this vessel, and at this level the nerve already has branched. The bipolar coagulator is used to dissect and cauterize anteriorly and distally until all the structures accompanying these vessels can be dissected proximally toward their origin from beneath the vastus medialis muscle. There may be significant scarring in this region from the previous joint replacement surgery. The proximal end is followed, and it is noted that a clear neurovascular

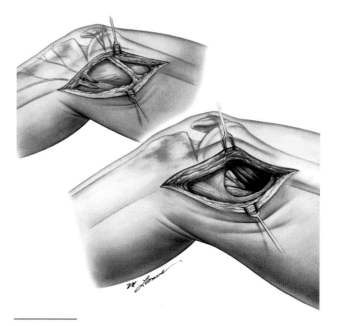

Figure 62–9. Operative approach to medial knee denervation. An incision is made medially at the knee, the medial retinaculum is approached, and the medial retinacular nerve is identified at this level. A segment is rejected, with the proximal level of resection lying beneath or within the vastus medialis muscle.

pedicle is identified. This is cauterized at the level at which it lies completely beneath the muscle, and the distal segment is submitted to pathology. A true neuroma is not resected, the joint capsule around the implant is not identified, and the implant is not exposed during the dissection. A biopsy specimen of the synovium is not obtained. The medial retinaculum is closed with figure-eight, No. 4-0 absorbable polyglycolic acid sutures. Bupivacaine is instilled, and the wound is closed with No. 4-0 absorbable suture in the dermis and interrupted and continuous No. 5-0 nylon in the skin (see Figs. 62–8 to 62–10).

A new incision is made to identify the infrapatellar branch of the saphenous nerve. This nerve is deep to the

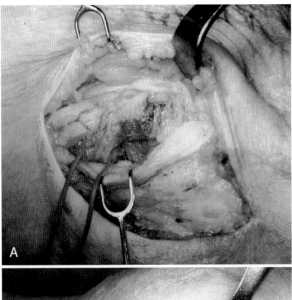

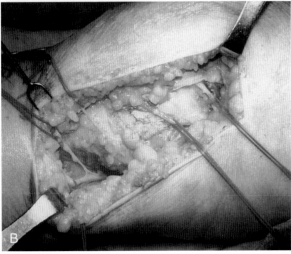

Figure 62–10. Intraoperative view during knee denervation. **A,** Lateral retinacular nerve. **B,** Medial retinacular nerve.

subcutaneous tissue, lying on the deep fascia, and accompanied by a vein. The nerve may be pulled on to reveal dimpling of the skin in the region of the painful incision from the knee replacement. The nerve is dissected far proximally, where it extends along a tunnel to have a relationship with the sartorius muscle. The distal 2 cm of the nerve is resected and submitted to pathology. A neuroma is not resected. A long curved clamp facilitates the dissection that creates a tunnel into the sartorius muscle. The proximal end of the nerve is turned and implanted into the sartorius muscle tunnel for a length of about 2 cm. The nerve does not need to be sutured into the muscle. Bupivacaine is instilled into the wound, and it is closed as described earlier (see Figs. 62–8 to 62–10).

If there is a more distal pain trigger zone medially, and it cannot be reached through the same incision as one used to resect the infrapatellar branch of the saphenous nerve, a third incision should be made to identify the transverse, distal branch of the saphenous nerve. This branch is located in the deep subcutaneous tissue, often on the periosteum. There is an accompanying small vessel. The

proximal dissection leads to the saphenous vein and terminal branch of the saphenous nerve. These are left intact.

The lateral retinacular nerve is identified through a 3- to 5-cm incision made laterally at the knee centered over the tender point marked preoperatively. The incision is deepened down to the lateral retinaculum. The iliotibial band is incised longitudinally with a scalpel beginning just over the distal end of the vastus lateralis and extended distally until just past the recurrent geniculate vessels, which are apparent in the underlying tissues. The nerve accompanies this vessel; at this level, the nerve already has branched. If a previous lateral release has been done during the knee replacement surgery, this area may be extensively scarred. The small nerve branches may not be seen. The bipolar coagulator is used to dissect and cauterize anteriorly and distally until all the structures accompanying the geniculate vessels have been dissected proximally toward their origin from beneath the iliotibial band and the biceps tendon. This dissection is facilitated by placing a double hook into the iliotibial band and retracting laterally. The proximal end is followed, and a clear neurovascular pedicle is identified originating from the popliteal fossa. This pedicle is cauterized at the level at which it lies completely deep to the iliotibial band and where the proximal end can be cauterized adequately. The distal segment is resected and submitted to pathology. A true neuroma is not resected, the joint capsule around the implant is not identified, and the implant is not exposed during the dissection. A biopsy specimen of the synovium is not obtained. The lateral retinaculum is closed with three figure-eight, No. 4-0 absorbable polyglycolic acid sutures. Bupivacaine is instilled, and the wound is closed with No. 4-0 absorbable suture in the dermis and interrupted with continuous No. 5-0 nylon in the skin (Figs. 62–11 and 62–12; see Fig. 62–10).

The innervation of the proximal tibiofibular joint is identified through an approach that requires a formal neurolysis of the common peroneal nerve at the fibular head. A 6-cm incision is made over the fibular head, obliquely, deepened into the subcutaneous tissue, and the lateral cutaneous nerve of the calf, if present, is preserved. The common peroneal nerve is palpated, the deep fascia covering is opened, and the common peroneal nerve is identified. It is followed anteriorly toward the fascia overlying the peroneus longus muscle. This fascia is slit transversely anteriorly, proximally, and distally. The muscle is elevated, and any deep bands are divided. The common peroneal nerve is gently separated from all surrounding tissues, and using microsurgical dissecting instruments, the branches in and around the fibular head are separated from the fat, doing a fascicular dissection. At times, to identify these branches, an intrafascicular dissection is required. A disposable nerve stimulator is set on the lowest setting, and the gastrocnemius or peroneus muscle is stimulated as a positive control. Then the individual fascicles are stimulated to identify those to the tibialis anterior. The one to three small fascicles (<1 mm) that do not stimulate a muscle contraction are presumed to be the fascicles that innervate the proximal tibiofibular joint. These are resected and submitted to pathology. For intraoperative electrical stimulation to work, oxygen must be present in the nerve. This portion of the procedure should be done

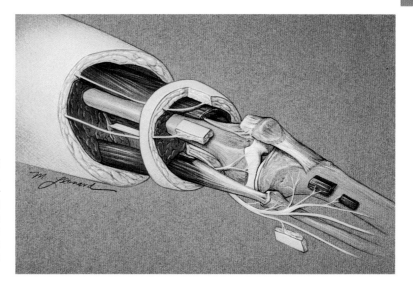

Figure 62–11. Three-dimensional view of anatomy of the innervation of the lateral knee. Note the lateral retinacular nerve arising posteriorly from the sciatic nerve and entering the region from beneath the biceps femoris. This nerve enters the lateral knee structures deep to the lateral retinaculum. Note the innervation of the proximal tibiofibular joint arising from the common peroneal nerve.

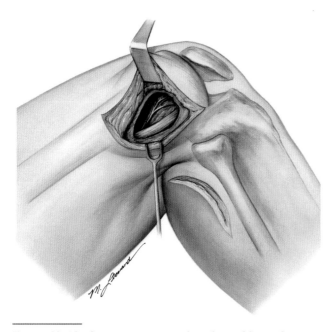

Figure 62–12. Operative approach to lateral knee denervation. An incision is made laterally at the knee; the iliotibial band is approached and incised just distal to the vastus lateralis. The lateral retinacular nerve is identified at this level. A segment is rejected, with the proximal level of resection lying in the popliteal fossa.

first, before the tourniquet time has exceeded 0.5 hour. Bupivacaine is instilled just into the skin edges so that peroneal motor function is not lost in the recovery room. The deep fascial structures are not sutured to prevent peroneal nerve entrapment. The skin is closed as described earlier (Fig. 62–13; see Figs. 62–11 and 62–12).

If the anterior femoral cutaneous nerve or the nerve that innervates the prepatellar bursa must be approached, the existing scar is opened, and the dissection is carried out. The superficial cutaneous nerve is small and may not be identified directly. Rather, the deep-scarred tissue down to the quadriceps tendon is rejected as a block of tissue and dissected proximally; at that point, a small nerve twig may

be identified. The entire scar is submitted to pathology. In this instance of a small nerve twig, it is rejected back into the fat in this region. If a clearly identifiable nerve is present, it should be turned and implanted into the adjacent quadriceps muscle. If necessary, the dissection can be carried deeper with a muscle-splitting incision down to the femur. In the fat at this level, and accompanied by a vessel, one or more small nerves go distally into the bursal region. These nerves are rejected and submitted to pathology, allowing their proximal ends to lie within the quadriceps muscles. Bupivacaine is instilled, and the skin is closed, usually with a separate set of sutures to pull some fat between the skin closure and quadriceps.

POSTOPERATIVE CARE

An excellent postoperative strategy is to encourage water walking in a heated pool for weeks 2 through 4 postoperatively. Beginning about postoperative week 3, a steroid cream is prescribed to massage into each scar. A 0.1% form of betamethasone is effective. This cream loosens the scar from the surrounding tissues and helps to desensitize the skin that has been denervated. For some patients, the denervated skin territory presents a problem as the adjacent intact normal nerves regenerate (collateral sprouting), restoring sensation to these areas.

Most patients know that their original pain is either gone or different by the time of their first office visit and are happy with their result even at 3 weeks. It takes 6 weeks, however, for some patients to recover from the firmness and pain of the postoperative chemical inflammation from the fat oils, especially in the obese medial thigh area. Most patients resume full activity by 3 months after surgery.

COMPLICATIONS

The most common complication is postoperative bruising, with some swelling about the knee. Bruising is present in

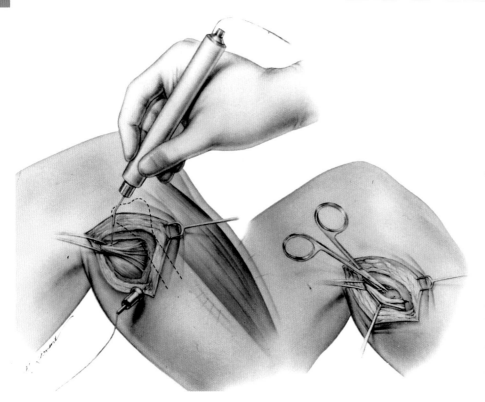

Figure 62–13. Intraoperative electrical stimulation to identify the innervation of the proximal tibiofibular joint. The common peroneal nerve is exposed and decompressed beneath the peroneus longus muscle. After a microdissection of the deep peroneal nerve, electrical stimulation identifies small fascicles that cause muscle twitches. The first two or three small fascicles that do not cause a muscle contraction are the innervation of the proximal tibiofibular joint, and these are rejected.

about 40% of patients. It is treated with topical moist heat three times a day. It resolves during the first 2 weeks.

A chemical inflammation related to the oil from the fat cells causes a postoperative appearance similar to a cellulitis in about 10% of the patients. These patients are given an extra week of oral antibiotics; they apply warm compresses to the region three times a day and, if they are not intolerant of nonsteroidals, are given an anti-inflammatory medication.

Two patients have had to be taken back to surgery to drain a hematoma during postoperative week 2, and one had to be taken back to surgery to have a local infection drained. These procedures were done by their own orthopedic surgeon after the patients had returned to their own geographic area. No patient has had to be taken back to surgery acutely for bleeding.

Postoperative stiffness or limited range of motion of the knee that was present before the knee denervation was not considered a postoperative complication. Preoperative stiffness usually represented arthrofibrosis related to the initial injury or surgery and was not anticipated to be improved. Patients must be made aware preoperatively that denervation usually does not change knee range of motion.

A frequent postoperative problem associated with resection of cutaneous nerves is the hypersensitivity that results owing to collateral sprouting from adjacent normal nerves. This is a normal process by which the uninjured adjacent nerve responds to the nerve growth factor released by the Schwann's cells in the distal degenerated nerve fibers. The sprouting normal axons generate neural impulses that often are interpreted as recurrent pain. This is an area in which preoperative discussion with patients is crucial to helping them understand postoperatively that

this is expected and is not recurrence of the preexisting pain. It is self-limited. Gentle desensitization resolves the problem over 3 to 6 weeks. Water walking or a hot tub is helpful, as is wearing long pants and touching the area. A neuropathic pain medication, such as amitriptyline (Elavil) or gabapentin (Neurontin), may be helpful. A narcotic pain medication and the topical application of steroid cream to the scars are indicated during this time. Frequent office visits and reassurance are crucial elements to success during this early healing phase.

One patient had to be taken back to surgery at 3 weeks after denervation to have draining synovial fluid corrected by oversewing the joint capsule. This was the only patient in whom there was an attempt to resect the neuroma in which the retinacular nerve entered the joint capsule (see Fig. 62–6). This approach is not recommended (i.e., a denervation, not a neuroma resection, is done at surgery).

The most disturbing complication is persistent knee pain. This is almost never the same pain that existed preoperatively, but rather pain in an area that was not approached. A patient who has a medial approach only to the knee joint may have lateral pain, or a patient who has a medial and a lateral approach to the knee joint may have pain persist in the proximal tibiofibular joint. This problem occurred in almost 10% of the patients in the early series, requiring a second operation to remove another nerve. This problem now is reduced to about 5% of patients. Some patients require a second operation because of anatomic variations.

No patient has developed a Charcot joint after this operation. Because a total knee replacement creates a totally denervated joint anyway, it is not logical to be concerned that this partial knee denervation will create one. Even when partial knee denervation is done for persistent knee pain in a patient who has had knee surgery but still retains his or her own knee, a Charcot joint does not result because this is a partial knee denervation. Nevertheless, this is a frequently asked question about a potential postoperative complication. It is supportive of this position for the knee to note that in 13 years of postoperative follow-up after wrist denervation, a Charcot joint was not observed.[3]

RESULTS OF PARTIAL KNEE DENERVATION

In 1993, the results of treatment of pain of neural origin after total knee replacement were presented to the American Academy of Orthopaedic Surgeons and later published. That initial experience comprised just 15 patients.[15] Each patient had had pain for at least 6 months after the arthroplasty. All patients were improved subjectively after selective denervation at a mean follow-up of 15 months (range 9 to 19 months). Knee Society objective scores improved from a mean of 55 points (range 30 to 60 points) to a mean of 90 points (range 80 to 100 points).

The first 70 patients having a knee denervation with this approach were reported in 1995 by Dellon and colleagues.[16] The indications for knee denervation are given in Table 62–1. There were 46 men and 24 women. Mean age was 57 years (range 23 to 78 years). They previously had had a mean of 3.1 surgical procedures on their painful knee (range 0 to 11 procedures). The number of nerves resected varied with the individual patient's pain pattern; one patient had six different nerves resected, and five patients had just one nerve resected. Twenty-six patients had three nerves resected, and 22 patients had four nerves resected. Twenty-eight patients had just the medial side denervated, 5 patients had just the lateral side denervated, and 37 patients had medial and lateral knee denervations. The most commonly resected nerve was the infrapatellar branch of the saphenous nerve. Open resected nerves included the medial retinacular nerve,[55] the medial cutaneous nerve of the thigh,[38] and the lateral retinacular nerve.[32] The proximal tibiofibular joint was denervated 13 times. Follow-up after the knee denervation procedure was a minimum of 12 months (range 12 to 36 months). Of the 70 patients, 31 had a total knee replacement, 32 had previous knee injury, and 7 had a previous high tibial osteotomy or Maquet's procedure. All candidates were referred for knee denervation only after all traditional approaches for treatment had been exhausted. Each patient in the series had at least a 5-point reduction in their pain level after a local anesthetic block of specific nerve. The results showed that 86% of patients were satisfied with the denervation as judged by direct questioning and a reduction in their preoperative pain visual analog score of 5 or more points. The average Knee Society score improved from 51 points (range 40 to 62 points) to 82 points (range 50 to 100 points; $p < 0.01$). Of 26 patients followed for a minimum of 24 months, 85% had 5-point pain score reductions, and 77% had Knee Society objective scores greater than 80 points ($p < 0.01$). In general,

the patients' results at 6 months mirrored the results at 2 years. In 1998, a group of 15 knee denervations were reported by members of this group[36] with similar results.

In the years since this chapter was first included in this book, we have had experience with another 400 patients requiring partial knee denervation (Table 62–2). This experience includes patients who have had more than 10 previous knee surgeries, some with more than 15 previous procedures (Table 62–3). One of these patients had a previous knee fusion. Many patients have had peripheral nerve or spinal stimulators placed to treat their chronic pain. Many patients are on long-term high-dose narcotics, often taken with non-narcotic neuropathic pain medication, muscle relaxants, and sleep medications. Even these difficult, discouraged, and often suicidal patients can be helped. In general, the present trend is to be able to identify more nerves contributing to the overall painful knee than before, enabling more involved nerves to be resected at the initial knee denervation (Table 62–4). There is still a small group requiring a second denervation, and a rare individual who requires a third denervation as more nerves or anomalous innervation to the knee joint is identified. Causes for poor results are listed in Table 62–5. Careful counseling is needed in the presence of a patient advocate or family member because these patients are not likely to understand all that is said in the examining room. Their response to local anesthetic blocks is crucial to their

Table 62–2. Indications for Partial Knee Denervation: 1993-1998

Total knee arthroplasty	255
Knee injury	89
Total patients	*344*

Table 62–3. Results of Partial Knee Denervation: 1993-1998

Excellent	70%
Good	20%
Improved	5%
No change (poor)	5%
Worse	0%

Table 62–4. Number of Nerves Removed in Partial Knee Denervation: 1993-1998

NO. NERVES	NO. PATIENTS	%
1	0	0
2	66	19
3	44	13
4	89	26
5	37	11
6	108	31
Total patients	*344*	*100%*

Table 62–5. Causes for Poor Results in Partial Knee Denervation: 1993-1998

CAUSE	NO. PATIENTS	%
Alzheimer's disease	5	29
Drug abuse (addiction)	3	18
Workers' compensation	9	53
Total patients	*17*	*100%*

management. An agreement usually is made with these patients that after the partial knee denervation procedure is done, and they have recovered they will go through detoxification before any consideration is given to a repeat surgical procedure. There is hope for even these difficult patients. The experience now extends to younger patients with knee injuries from sports or martial arts, who have significant radiographic evidence of degenerative joint disease but who are "too young" for even hemiarthroplasty. Partial joint denervation is an excellent alternative for this group of patients. Some patients who have had such a difficult time either with the surgery required for a total knee replacement or with the rehabilitation do not have the same procedure done on the contralateral side, despite significant osteoarthritis. Partial joint denervation is an excellent alternative for this group of patients. Nahabedian and coauthors[47,48] described similar results with this technique in selected patients.

CONCLUSION

Partial knee denervation is more than a surgical procedure. It is an approach to the patient with knee pain that should be used increasingly in the orthopedic community. When knee pain can be understood as persisting from neural origin after the musculoskeletal system has been adequately treated, a new dimension will open to patients previously thought to be beyond our reach.

References

1. Abram LJ, Froimson AI: Saphenous nerve injury: An unusual arthroscopic complication. Am J Sports Med 18:41, 1991.
2. Aszman OC, Dellon AL, Birely B, et al: Innervation of the human shoulder joint and its implication for surgery. Clin Orthop 330:202, 1996.
3. Buck-Gramcko D: Denervation of the wrist joint. J Hand Surg 2:54, 1977.
4. Bosley RC: Total acromionectomy: A twenty-year review. J Bone Joint Surg Am 73:961, 1991.
5. Chambers GH: The prepatellar nerve: A cause of suboptimal results in knee arthrotomy. Clin Orthop 182:157, 1977.
6. Dellon AL: Partial dorsal wrist denervation: Resection of distal posterior interosseous nerve. J Hand Surg 10:527, 1985.
7. Dellon AL: Treatment of recurrent metatarsalgia by neuroma resection and muscle implantation: Case report and algorithm for management of Morton's "neuroma." Microsurgery 10:256, 1989.
8. Dellon AL: Somatosensory Testing and Rehabilitation. Bethesda, MD, American Occupational Therapy Association, 1997.
9. Dellon AL, Aszmann OC: Treatment of dorsal foot neuromas by translocation of nerves into the anterolateral compartment. Foot Ankle 19:700, 1998.
10. Dellon AL, Horner G: Partial wrist denervation. In Marsh J (ed): Current Therapy in Plastic Surgery: The Wrist. Philadelphia, JB Lippincott, 1993, pp 252-261.
11. Dellon AL, Mackinnon SE: Treatment of the painful neuroma by neuroma resection and muscle implantation. Plast Reconstr Surg 77:427, 1986.
12. Dellon AL, Mackinnon SE: Human ulnar neuropathy at the elbow: Clinical, electrical and morphometric correlation. J Reconstr Microsurg 4:179, 1988.
13. Dellon AL, Mackinnon SE, Daneshvar A: Terminal branch of anterior interosseous nerve as source of wrist pain. J Hand Surg 9:316, 1984.
14. Dellon AL, Mackinnon SE, Pestronk A: Implantation of sensory nerve into muscle: Preliminary clinical and experimental observation on neuroma formation. Ann Plast Surg 12:30, 1984.
15. Dellon AL, Mont MA, Hungerford DS: Partial denervation for treatment of persistent pain after total knee arthroplasty. Clin Orthop 316:145, 1995.
16. Dellon AL, Mont MA, Mullick T, et al: Partial denervation for persistent neuroma pain around the knee. Clin Orthop 329:216, 1966.
17. Dellon AL, Seif SS: Neuroma of the posterior interosseous nerve simulating a recurrent ganglion: Case report and anatomical dissection relating the posterior interosseous nerve to the carpus and etiology of dorsal ganglion pain. J Hand Surg 3:326, 1978.
18. Druner L: Ueber die Beteiligung des nervus obtutatorius an der Innervation des Knieglenks. AF Anat U Entwick 82:388, 1927.
19. Ellman H: Arthroscopic subacromial decompression for chronic impingement: Two to five year results. J Bone Joint Surg Br 73:395, 1991.
20. Evans GRD, Dellon AL: Implantation of the palmar cutaneous branch of the median nerve into the pronator quadratus for treatment of painful neuroma. J Hand Surg 19:203, 1994.
21. Finterbush A: Reflex sympathetic dystrophy of the patellofemoral joint. Orthop Rev 20:877, 1991.
22. Fulkerson JP, Gossling HR: Anatomy of the knee joint lateral retinaculum. Clin Orthop 153:183, 1980.
23. Fulkerson JP, Tennant R, Javin JS, et al: Histological evidence of retinacular nerve injury associated with patellofemoral malalignment. Clin Orthop 197:196, 1985.
24. Gardner E: The innervation of the knee joint. Anat Rec 101:109, 1948.
25. Gardner E: The innervation of the shoulder joint. Anat Rec 102:1, 1948.
26. Horner G, Dellon AL: Innervation of the human knee joint and implication for surgery. Clin Orthop 301:221, 1994.
27. Huckle JR: Meniscectomy: A benign procedure? A long-term follow-up. Can J Surg 8:254, 1965.
28. Hungerford DS, Krackow KA, Kenna RV: Clinical experience with the PCA prosthesis with and without cement. In Hungerford DS, Krackow KA, Denna RV (eds): Total Knee Arthroplasty: A Comprehensive Approach. Baltimore, Williams & Wilkins, 1984, pp 127-130.
29. Insall JN, Dorr LD, Scott RS, et al: Rationale of the Knee Society clinical rating system. Clin Orthop 248:13, 1989.
30. Jeletsky AG: On the innervation of the capsule and epiphysis of the knee joint. Vestn Khir 22:74, 1931.
31. Katz MM, Hungerford DS: Reflex sympathetic dystrophy affecting the knee. J Bone Joint Surg Br 69:797, 1987.
32. Katz MM, Hungerford DS, Krackow KA, et al: Reflex sympathetic dystrophy as a cause of poor results following total knee arthroplasty. J Arthrosc 1:117, 1986.
33. Kennedy JC, Alexander IJ, Hayes KC: Nerve supply to the human knee and its functional importance. Am J Sports Med 10:329, 1982.
34. Krackow KA, Maar DC, Mont MA, et al: Surgical decompression for peroneal nerve palsy after total knee arthroplasty. Clin Orthop 292:223, 1993.
35. Krompinger WJ, Fulkerson JP: Lateral retinacular release for intractable lateral pain. Clin Orthop 179:191, 1983.
36. Lewallen DG: Neurovascular injury associated with hip arthroplasty. J Bone Joint Surg Am 79:1870, 1997.

37. Mackinnon SE, Dellon AL: Overlap of lateral antebrachial cutaneous nerve and superficial sensory branch of the radial nerve. J Hand Surg 10:522, 1985.

38. Mackinnon SE, Dellon AL: Experimental study of chronic nerve compression: Clinical implications. Clin Hand Surg 2:639, 1986.

39. Mackinnon SE, Dellon AL: Results of treatment of recurrent dorsoradial wrist neuromas. Ann Plast Surg 19:54, 1987.

40. Mackinnon SE, Dellon AL: Surgery of the Peripheral Nerve. New York, Thieme, 1988.

41. Mackinnon SE, Dellon AL, Hudson AR, et al: Alteration of neuroma by manipulation of neural microenvironment. Plast Reconstr Surg 76:345, 1985.

42. Mackinnon SE, Dellon AL, Hudson AR, et al: A primate model for chronic nerve compression. J Reconstr Microsurg 1:185, 1985.

43. Mackinnon SE, Dellon AL, Hudson AR, et al: Histopathology of compression of the superficial radial nerve in the forearm. J Hand Surg 11:206, 1986.

44. Meyer RA, Raja SN, Campbell JN, et al: Neural activity originating from a neuroma in the baboon. Brain Res 325:255, 1985.

45. Mont MA, Dellon AL, Chen F, et al: Operative treatment of peroneal nerve palsy. J Bone Joint Surg Am 78:863, 1996.

46. Mori Y, Fujimoto A, Okumo H, et al: Lateral retinacular release in adolescent patellofemoral disorders: Its relationship to peripheral nerve injury in the lateral retinaculum. Bull Hosp Joint Dis Orthop Inst 51:218, 1981.

47. Nahabedian MY, Johnson CA: Operative management of neuromatous knee pain: Patient selection and outcome. Ann Plast Surg 46:15, 2001.

48. Nahabedian MY, Mont MA, Hungerford DS: Selective denervation of the knee. Am J Knee Surg 11:175, 1998.

49. Ogilvie-Harris DJ, Marin R: Reflex sympathetic dystrophy of the knee. J Bone Joint Surg Br 69:804, 1987.

50. Poehling GG, Pollock FE Jr, Koman LA: Reflex sympathetic dystrophy of the knee after sensory nerve injury. Arthroscopy 4:31, 1988.

51. Ruedinger N: Die Gelenknerven des Mennschlichen Koerpers. Erlangen, Ferdinand Inke, 1857.

52. Swanson AJG: The incidence of prepatellar neuropathy following medial meniscectomy. Clin Orthop 181:151, 1983.

53. Wilhelm A: Zur Innervation der Gelenke der Oberen Extremitaet. Z Anat Entwicklungsgesch 120:331, 1958.

54. Wilhelm A: Die Gelenksdenervation und ihre anatomischen Grundlagen: Ein neues Behandlungsprinzip in der Handcirurgie. Hefte Unfallheilk 86:100, 1966.

55. Wojtys EM, Beaman DN, Glover RA, et al: Innervation of the human knee joint by substance P fibers. Arthroscopy 6:254, 1990.

56. Worth RM, Kettelkamp DB, Defalque RJ, et al: Saphenous nerve entrapment: A cause of medial knee pain. Am J Sports Med 12: 80, 1984.

57. Wrete M: The innervation of the shoulder joint in man. Acta Anat (Basel) 7:173, 1949.

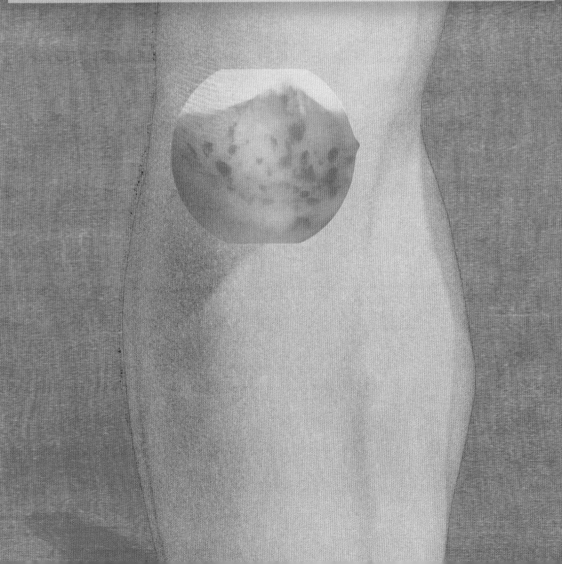

SECTION VIII

Plastic Surgery

CHAPTER 63

Soft-Tissue Healing

Susan Craig Scott • Robert Siskind Reiffel

A patient who is to undergo total knee arthroplasty is focused on relief of pain and increased mobility, major quality-of-life issues that the operation reliably provides. Considerations of soft-tissue healing are not ordinarily present in the patient's mind at the time of initial evaluation. That there might be difficulty with soft-tissue healing may well be the farthest thing from a patient's thoughts. It is not unusual for a physician who introduces the subject of wound healing to be met with surprise, disbelief, or even suspicion. Only those who have had difficulty with soft-tissue healing in the past are even aware that healing might be an issue. Unfortunately, patients who are likely to have difficulty with soft-tissue healing are not limited to those with difficulty in the past.

Responsibility for assessing both the condition of the soft tissues as well as systemic and local factors that might cause difficulty with healing lies with the treating physician. In the past 30 to 40 years encompassing the modern era of total knee replacement, our knowledge of these wound-compromising factors has allowed us to predict with some degree of accuracy those who might have trouble and what we might do preoperatively, intraoperatively and postoperatively to maximize healing. This chapter is a summary of our current knowledge and approach to soft-tissue healing. A basic understanding of the biochemical and cellular processes of wound healing helps us appreciate the complexity of a process that we sometimes take for granted. In addition, in exploring factors that influence wound healing, we can better realize at what points interruption of normal healing might occur. Last, steps that might be taken before and after surgery to favorably influence the wound-healing process become clear if we know where normal healing might go wrong.

Uncomplicated wound healing is a beautiful and precise series of events. A troublesome wound can cause significant disability and prolonged recovery and result in prosthesis loss, amputation, and in extreme circumstances, death. In the last decade there has been an explosion of research and information about the biochemical aspects of healing, chemoattractants, cytokines, growth factors, and recombinant DNA technology, all of which hold promise for furthering our understanding of soft-tissue healing. Although this exciting research has not yet led to acceleration of the normal healing of a wound in a healthy patient, it shows great promise in treating difficult wounds, as this chapter will outline. The normal healing phases will be described, and factors that might enhance these phases in a wound that is healing poorly will be identified.

HISTORY

As long as there have been medical writings, attention has been directed to wound healing and attempts to enhance and accelerate it. The use of plant extracts, even bread mold, in healing is at least 2000 years old by written record.[6,37] Both the Edwin Smith Surgical Papyrus from 3000 to 2500 BC and the Ebers Papyrus describe certain of the earliest known wound manipulations—splinting and honey—to influence outcome.[4,12] Among the contributions of Hypocrates, who lived around 400 BC, was his insistence on cleanliness and irrigation of wounds with boiled water.[6] In addition, his prescient emphasis on documentation and accurate recording of events is a primary characteristic of good medical practice to this day. Hypocrates' scholarship was followed 300 years later by the Roman Celcus and about 100 years after that by Galen, whose work on wounded gladiators of Asia Minor led to his understanding of the venous and arterial systems, wound care dressings, and meticulous follow-up.[6] Descartes wrote the first western physiology text, and Ambrose Pare deserves credit for one of the most significant contributions to our approach today, his emphasis on gentle handling of tissues and on the harmful effects of trauma on tissue.[18,30] This concept, crucial in the present day in the handling of all surgical wounds, such as avoidance of crushing clamps and prolonged vigorous retraction, is all the more remarkable because it was introduced into a medical world in which wounds were being treated with boiling oil and "laudable pus" was the ideal. Pare insisted that careful tissue handling was the first step to uncomplicated tissue healing, a point we will emphasize.

The late 19th and early 20th centuries saw rapid progress in our understanding of the causes of healing difficulties; Joseph Lister's practical acceptance of Pasteur's germ theory of infection, controversial at the time, bore fruit in his description of aseptic technique and the use of carbolic acid as a topical disinfectant in hospitals where infection was rampant.[6] His practical application of this sound principle, coupled with the discovery of antibiotics, sulfanilamide in the late 1930s and penicillin soon after, which resulted in Alexander Fleming's shared Nobel Prize in 1945, put in place the last essential component of normal wound healing, control of infection, as the second half of the 20th century began.[6,10]

The latter part of the 20th century has seen dramatic technological advances, as well as advances in molecular biology, biochemistry, and immunology. At the same time, our surgical techniques and scholarship have produced real replacements for knees, hips, wrists, and elbows and functional replacements for kidneys, lungs, and even, for short periods, hearts. There is no limit to our ingenuity and to what the confluence of this ingenuity and adequate resources coupled with need might produce. Our challenge remains to follow where these advances lead without losing sight of the basic precepts that brought us here.

PHASES OF WOUND HEALING

Wound healing may be separated chronologically into three phases. Although these phases overlap, the events that predominate in each phase are different and together produce the strong, substantial, protective, resilient endpoint that we called the healed wound.

Phase of Inflammation

Initiation of the inflammatory phase of healing may be nonspecific—infection, laceration, or trauma—but the surgical wound is the inciting factor that we deal with here. The very first component of the inflammatory phase, vasoconstriction, occurs even before the wound is closed. Lasting roughly 10 minutes, this phase is followed rapidly by vasodilatation, whose purpose is to allow the influx of cellular elements that are responsible for cleaning debris from the wound in preparation for the structural events that result in wound closure. An influx of platelets is followed by polymorphonuclear leukocytes, lymphocytes, and macrophages. Vascular permeability increases dramatically at the wound site, most likely moderated by histamine. These cellular events, especially the influx of platelets, result in the release of multiple factors—cytokines, platelet-derived factors, complement, and possibly even prostaglandins—that enhance the local cellular response in preparation for healing.

The elements of this first healing phase result in local control, hemostasis, protection against infection, and preparation for the series of structural events that will ultimately close the soft tissue in a healed wound.

Fibroblastic Proliferative Phase

The cellular elements and chemotactants that rapidly accumulate in the wound during the first phase of healing prepare the wound for the migration of fibroblasts, which are the primary synthesizers of collagen, the substance responsible for the healed wound's strength and durability.

This second phase of healing begins at about 48 hours after wounding. Fibroblasts climb along the fibrin matrix that has been deposited during the inflammatory phase of platelet aggregation and hemostasis. This crucially important matrix can be interfered with and can be a cause of wound-healing delay.[57] As fibroblasts migrate in and provide the predominant cell type present in the healing wound at about day 5, they produce ground substance, a gel-like combination of hyaluronic acid and chondroitin 4-sulfate, the glycosaminoglycans. This substrate will act as a matrix for the collagen fibrils synthesized most rapidly during the first few days of wound healing. This first collagen synthesized—tropocollagen—is converted to collagen fibrils, which assume structural and biochemical integrity and on which wound strength is based; it is in the first 3 or so weeks after healing that we see the most rapid rise in wound strength gains.[41] Collagen homeostasis is reached at about 3 weeks as collagen synthesis and degradation rates approach one another; this stage leads to the last and most prolonged phase of wound healing, the phase of remodeling or the phase of collagen maturation.

Wound Maturation Phase

In this last phase, the cellular elements producing collagen within the wound are markedly diminished; the collagen fibrils deposited become dramatically more organized and structured in response to a variety of factors, including local mechanical demands. The water content of the wound, along with measurable ground substance, diminishes and is manifested as local induration. The amount of type III collagen, initially present in large amounts, is reduced and replaced by type I collagen as the tissue strength–providing elements much more closely approach the elements that give strength to normal skin. Stronger collagen cross-links create mechanical resistance to disruption in the now-maturing wound. This process continues for many months, even years after the initiating event.[46,47]

Cellular Elements of Healing

Specific cellular elements in wound healing are responsible for stimulation of fibroblasts, for ingrowth of new and essential blood vessels, and for clearing out debris in preparation for healing. Some medical illnesses, certain medications, and even environmental factors can challenge the ability of these cellular elements to perform their essential functions.

T lymphocytes produce a sustained response to injury in the wound. They generate local influences on the vascular endothelial lining in preparation for regrowth of new vessels. In addition, they produce fibroblast-activating factor, which encourages and regulates fibroblastic activity in the healing wound. T-cell depletion at the time that a wound occurs can significantly deter breaking strength in the healing wound.[3,48]

Macrophages migrate into the healing wound and are activated as they participate in the initial inflammatory phase. These cells remain in the wound much longer than other responders, such as polymorphonuclear leukocytes, and release cytokines responsible for angiogenesis and for stimulating fibroblast proliferation.[40] In fact, studies support significant loss of the essential early functions of fibroplasia and debris clearance if the accumulation or availability of macrophages or their active migration into a wound is interfered with.[69]

FACTORS THAT AFFECT WOUND HEALING

With a clear understanding of the normal unfolding of events from wounding to a strong stable healed wound, a variety of factors that have some bearing on tissue healing, which are ever present in patients and might be manipulated to benefit or deter tissue healing, can now be examined for the role that they play before, during, and after surgery.

In the practical reality of the day-to-day care of a surgical patient, environmental and physical factors, patient-related factors, and nutrition-related factors, as well as factors related to underlying medical illnesses, can all affect the progress of wound healing. A thorough understanding of the role that such factors play in wound healing helps the physician avoid healing difficulties, encourages patient participation in recovery, and mitigates the effects when healing does not progress as expected.

Scarring and Tissue Perfusion

Adequate levels of PO_2 in the healing wound are essential. The oxygen delivery system, by which inspired oxygen traverses the pulmonary vessels, binds to hemoglobin, and is subsequently released in response to tissue demands, can be subject to breakdown at several points.[35] Local scarring, irradiated tissue, diabetes, and chronic exposure to cigarette smoke can all interfere with the ability of small vessels to provide sufficient oxygen to the healing wound. Even local swelling or increased tissue pressure such as that created by a hematoma can so reduce perfusion that ischemia results.[62] Preparation for surgery requires attention to all of the aforementioned factors. At the molecular level, collagen synthesis by fibroblasts will not occur if tissue oxygenation is not adequate.

The mechanism by which the destructive effect of tissue ischemia occurs, whether the result of poor perfusion, radiation injury, or even small-vessel disease such as seen in diabetes mellitus, is believed to be the production of oxygen free radicals; these free radicals may even be a factor in aging skin and its loss of elasticity. Free radicals are in fact cytotoxic to cells, both to cell membranes and to their internal components.[42,72] In addition, free radicals can disrupt protein components such as enzymes and cause collagen to degrade prematurely.[65] Minimizing free radical production by ensuring adequate tissue oxygenation is one way of minimizing or even reversing these detrimental effects.

When local factors dramatically reduce wound perfusion and create severe local ischemia, the only solution is a dramatic increase in local tissue oxygenation or the local blood supply. One option for treating this situation is the use of hyperbaric oxygenation therapy. This mode of therapy increases the partial pressure of oxygen in plasma

by subjecting the patient and the wound to an atmosphere of 100% oxygen at twice normal atmospheric pressure at sea level.[73] This creates an elevated PO_2 level in the arterioles, thereby forcing increased amounts of oxygen into compromised tissue (Fig. 63–1). For this treatment to be effective there must be no local infection, nor should there be any local perfusion problems. Most notably, hyperbaric oxygenation therapy is not effective in the presence of frank tissue necrosis; the requirement for specialized equipment is an additional factor in this choice of treatment. Currently, tissue that is severely ischemic in the postoperative period is treated by local or distant flap transfer, which allows removal of tissue with circulatory compromise and the introduction of healthy, well-vascularized tissue providing oxygen delivery so that healing may progress.[43]

Cigarette Smoking

Although cigarette smoking has an unhealthy effect on virtually every organ system of the body, the detrimental effects on wound healing can be manifested in the postoperative period as unfortunately progressing wound ischemia and marginal necrosis. Absorbed nicotine and its breakdown product cotinine have an inhibiting effect on capillary circulation and cause necrosis of skin margins to an unpredictable degree. Moreover, in a cigarette smoker the addition of even a small degree of overzealous traction may cause wound compromise because the effect is additive with the peripheral circulatory effect of inhaled cigarette smoke. In addition, the carbon monoxide contained in cigarette smoke forms carboxyhemoglobin; this form of hemoglobin shifts the oxygen dissociation curve to the left, which makes oxygen release to ischemic tissue more difficult.[17,23,36,58] This twofold effect of cigarette smoking on tissue oxygenation puts a patient who smokes at risk for wound-healing difficulties; although there is no hard evidence regarding a well-defined preoperative period of discontinuation of smoking that would ensure uncompromised healing, we insist on at least 3 weeks' abstention from smoking or from exposure to second-hand smoke and require such abstention until skin sutures are removed in the postoperative period. Cigarette smokers are required to sign an additional consent form in our practice (Fig. 63–2).

Diabetes Mellitus

The fact that a diabetic patient is prone to a variety of secondary vascular, neurological, and wound-healing difficulties is well known to surgeons. However, the concept of small-vessel occlusive disease as the primary reason for these secondary illnesses, as well as for the wound-healing difficulties sometimes experienced by diabetic patients, has not been borne out in multiple studies of ischemia in the diabetic wound; other factors seem to play a larger role.[39]

Diabetic patients have increased blood viscosity secondary to a stiffer, less deformable red blood cell, thus

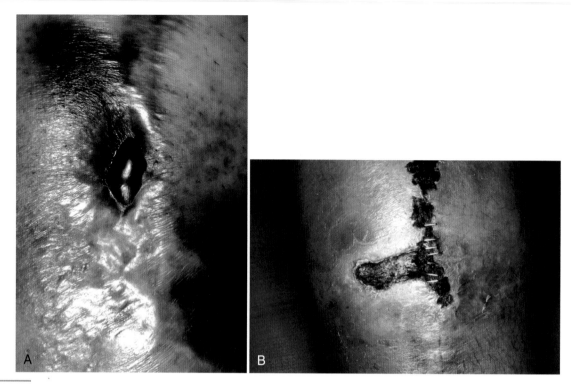

Figure 63–1. **A,** Circulation present but compromised; hyperbaric O_2 therapy is indicated. **B,** An eschar indicates full-thickness tissue loss with no circulation; hyperbaric O_2 therapy is contraindicated.

CONSENT FOR SURGICAL PROCEDURES FOR SMOKERS

Patient _____   Age _____

Dr. _____ and her staff have advised me that I must not smoke or use nicotine substitutes for a **minimum** of three weeks before surgery and after my surgery.

It has been explained to me that the risks of surgery are much greater for smokers, and even if I am refraining from the use of nicotine for three weeks before and after surgery, I may still experience the effects of nicotine in my bloodstream.

There is a greater risk in smokers of bad scarring, hematoma formation, intraoperative bleeding, poor or delayed healing, hair loss, sloughing of the skin (skin loss), infection, increased or prolonged bruising, and hyperpigmentation.

I ACKNOWLEDGE THAT I HAVE READ AND FULLY UNDERSTAND THE ABOVE CONSENT TO OPERATION AND THAT THE RISKS HAVE BEEN FULLY EXPLAINED TO ME, AND I WISH TO PROCEED WITH SURGERY.

Patient signature _____   Date _____

Figure 63–2. Consent form used for patients who smoke cigarettes.

making it more difficult for the red cells to pass through the tiny capillaries supplying oxygen to local tissue.[63]

The high serum glucose in a poorly controlled diabetic patient shifts the hemoglobin dissociation curve and inhibits oxygen delivery to the capillaries, thereby causing lower tissue PO_2 and resulting in impaired healing.[9]

Last, the tibial and peroneal arteries in a diabetic patient seem to be particularly prone to atherosclerotic peripheral vascular disease.[45] Preventive measures regarding these vulnerable patients include preoperative vascular examination of the lower extremities with palpation of the peripheral pulses and further evaluation if abnormalities are noted, meticulous control of serum glucose in the perioperative period, and avoidance of extremity edema and the local compounding of a diabetic's rheological changes that edema increases.

Anemia

The evidence regarding anemia as a contributing factor in the failure of wounds to heal is inconclusive. Hemoglobinopathies and extreme drops in hematocrit, both of which can compromise delivery of oxygen, have not been proved to cause compromise in soft-tissue healing.[2,24,31,60]

Radiation Therapy

Ionizing radiation causes injury not just to the target tissue but also to the tissue that surrounds the target. Radiation was at one time used to aid in wound healing and to treat scar formation and for keloid control in particular; there are patients today who have had such exposure (Fig. 63–3). The damage caused by ionizing radiation is permanent, progressive, and irreversible. Radiation causes an obliterative endarteritis that results in local tissue ischemia and permanent difficulty with wound healing, with normal wound contracture, and even with the formation of healthy granulation tissue. There is some evidence that these healing difficulties in irradiated tissue are caused by collateral damage to local fibroblasts and their proliferation, on which tissue healing is dependent.[21,22,61]

Corticosteroids

It becomes obvious from a discussion of the phases of wound healing that corticosteroids, which inhibit fibrin

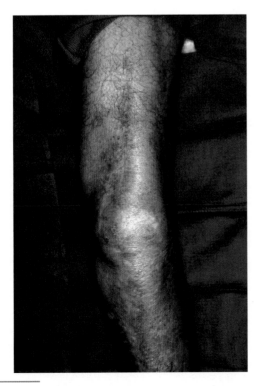

Figure 63–3. Radiation therapy in childhood caused profound scarring; tissue must be replaced by well-vascularized coverage.

synthesis, macrophage migration, wound contracture, and the events that lead to the formation and ingrowth of new blood vessels, are responsible for the poor progression in wound healing that we see in patients receiving corticosteroid therapy. Early and late effects, including loss of tensile strength and failure to gain strength in the healing wound, can both be attributed to steroid intake.

The effect of steroids on wound healing can be minimized by the administration of vitamin A either topically or orally. Collagen deposition and increase in wound strength, as well as functional macrophage support, are documented effects of oral vitamin A in a steroid-dependent patient.[14,25,26]

Aspirin/Nonsteroidal Medications

Many prospective total knee replacement patients take nonsteroidal medication for pain relief, and a large number of adults are taking one or more aspirin tablets per day as a cardioprotective regimen. There is some evidence that collagen synthesis is inhibited by normal therapeutic dosages of these medications, even in the normal population, and discontinuation of these medications in the perioperative and postoperative period is recommended, in part because of this effect.[33]

Chemotherapeutic Agents

Medications used to fight cancer inhibit wound healing. Although there is variation in the category and mechanism of action of this group of drugs, they are all designed to target rapidly dividing cells in some fashion. None are selective enough to protect healing tissue while continuing antineoplastic activity elsewhere, and it is recommended, when possible, that the perioperative period provide a break in administration of chemotherapeutic agents. The harmful effects seem to be most evident in the early phases of wound healing; a 2-week postoperative delay in administration can mitigate these harmful effects.[15,16]

Age

It is unclear whether advancing age alone inhibits wound healing. There is ample anecdotal evidence that whereas very young patients heal with scars that remain hyperemic and indurated for prolonged periods, older patients seem much less prone to this type of healing, a fact that is to their advantage when incisions are placed in cosmetically obvious areas such as the face.[1,11,19,34,71] There is certainly no evidence that the final results of wound healing in terms of ultimate closure and tensile strength are inhibited or influenced by age. It may simply be that aging produces a slowing in the processes that lead to wound healing and that a more protracted course of collagen synthesis and cross-linking is quite normal in an older patient.

Nutrition

Nutritional factors play a role in wound healing; a serum protein level below 2 g/dL is indicative of severe nutritional deficiency and can result in a very prolonged inflammatory phase and impaired fibroplasia.[51,54,68] Nutritional factors seem to be most important in the early phases of wound healing when the local inflammatory response and early fibroplasia are most active. In fact, only when profound malnutrition is present are the phases of wound healing impaired. Although it is most unlikely to encounter this problem in today's surgical environment, many elderly patients are at least mildly deficient in one or more vitamins essential to healing; obtaining a nutrition consultation plus supplementing these patients with certain essential elements is an excellent idea.

VITAMIN C

An essential element of wound healing, vitamin C, is required for maintenance of tissue integrity in a normal healthy patient.[50] Even a completely healed wound will lose strength over time if vitamin C intake is not adequate. Ascorbic acid is an absolute requirement for the normal synthesis of collagen, so stable structural elements, including the vessel wall, skin integrity, and the type III collagen of healing tissue, are affected when vitamin C intake is deficient. A truly vitamin C–deficient wound can be separated with only the smallest amount of manual pressure, and hemorrhage from weakened capillaries is common. Rarely seen today, vitamin C deficiency is easily remedied when recognized.[7]

ZINC

Zinc is a trace element present in all human tissue and is required in virtually every enzymic reaction. Administration of exogenous zinc increases the rate of wound healing only when there is a zinc deficiency; the surgeon may encounter deficiencies of this trace element in patients with chronic alcoholism, cirrhosis, and gastrointestinal absorption problems such as short-bowel syndrome. Zinc is required in such minute amounts for normal healing that only a dramatic loss of absorptive surface will produce a deficiency; in such instances, zinc administration can rapidly and markedly accelerate healing when provided as a supplement.[38,53]

Delay in the early phases of wound healing has been demonstrated in animal studies of zinc deficiency; compromise in both the cellular and humeral immune systems occurs as well.[55,56]

VITAMIN E

Vitamin E, tocopherol, has achieved almost mythical properties in our popular culture for preserving healthy tissue, particularly for minimizing scar overhealing and keloid formation. The best evidence for vitamin E's beneficial effect indicates that it is a membrane-stabilizing antioxidant that counters the damaging, cumulative effect of preoperative irradiation on wounds; in large doses, vitamin E has an inhibitory effect on wound healing that can be reversed by vitamin A.[67]

Several studies demonstrating a beneficial effect of vitamin E supplementation in lowering the risk for coronary artery disease have made this vitamin an extremely popular supplement.[59] It should, however, be discontinued before surgery because of its inhibiting effect on platelet adhesion.[28,64] In addition, there is evidence that supplementing a normal diet with vitamin E can cause impaired collagen synthesis and impaired wound healing.[13]

Mechanical Stress of Healing

All healing tissue responds to mechanical stress. Expanded tissue gains strength, and its collagen is more precisely oriented to resist disruption than nonexpanded tissue is. More specifically, forces on a healing wound, depending on their magnitude and direction, will affect the orientation, the amount, and the strength of collagen fibers that create healing. The benefits of controlled passive motion on the postoperative wound are not just a rapid and early gain in range of motion. Provided that swelling is controlled, hematoma and the potential for wound necrosis are avoided, and stress across the wound is gradual, the benefit in both short- and long-term wound healing is evident.[20,70]

Skin Closure

An assessment of the available and commonly used wound closure materials is appropriate at this point.

The purpose of closure is to provide sufficient local support for the evolution of wound healing and strength gain for enough time that the mechanical support afforded by suture is no longer needed. Primary suturing of a wound provides skin closure as a temporary barrier between contamination from the skin surface and the outside world and replicates the function of the skin as an organ. To this end, an evaluation of closure techniques and materials is in order.

A variety of options exist to effect skin closure: staples, skin sutures, skin tape, and skin glue, all of which will coapt the skin margins appropriately. As they contribute to wound healing, sutures also have a number of less desirable effects. By penetrating local intact skin to a variable degree, sutures introduce an additional source of local contamination. When tied tightly, sutures can impede local blood supply, and if left in place for a long period, cosmetically unsatisfactory cutaneous marks or "railroad tracks" can be the result (Fig. 63–4).

Suturing of a wound can be accomplished with material that is braided or monofilament, permanent or nonpermanent. Closure can also be achieved with skin staples,

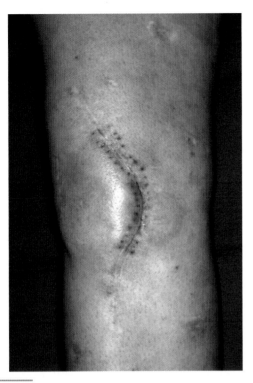

Figure 63–4. Cutaneous sutures in place for 3 weeks epithelialize along suture tracks; permanent scarring results.

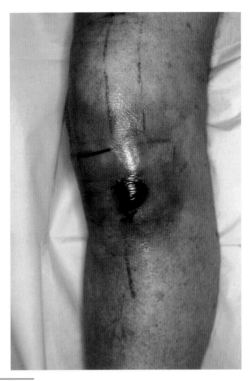

Figure 63–5. Partial-thickness skin circulatory compromise is indicated by skin blistering.

which are stainless steel and smooth surfaced. Skin tape made of a variety of materials—plastic, fabric, paper—is bonded to an adhesive and applied to dry skin where appropriate.

Several important facts are known regarding the materials that we use for skin closure. First, there is excellent evidence that stapled wounds provide superior resistance to infection when compared with sutured wounds. Particularly at lower levels of bacterial contamination, skin staples have a lower infection rate than even the least reactive nonabsorbable suture, monofilament nylon.[29,66]

Second, skin tapes used to close a wound that is dry (but not when continuous oozing loosens the tape) seem to provide the greatest resistance to infection, especially from surface contamination, when compared with other closure techniques.[8] Perfect skin edge-to-edge coaptation is essential for uneventful wound healing. Although manual suturing is perhaps best suited to compensate for the inequalities in skin thickness that give rise to surface overlap or override, if the deep tissues are accurately approximated, skin staples appear to be an excellent choice for skin closure in total knee arthroplasty. Concern regarding compressive ischemia between the legs of the skin staples is unfounded.

SKIN HEALING

Faced with the possible loss of skin coverage and the need to promote healing and provide a barrier, surgeons dealing with wound problems about the knee have the added concern of protecting the prosthesis from infection.

There are several steps involved in assessing the progress of healing; determining tissue viability and therefore the propensity for healing is essential. Tissue whose blood supply is clearly compromised is treated differently from tissue in which viability is questionable or marginal or is robustly adequate. In the postoperative period, cutaneous blistering of the skin is an indication of superficial loss (Fig. 63–5).

Care of the Wound

The largest organ in the body, the skin, has certain nutritional and metabolic requirements and physical characteristics that must be respected and supported if optimal healing is desired. Therefore, a discussion regarding treatment of a nonhealing surgical wound must begin with an analysis of the cause of the healing problem. The final common denominator for most wound-healing issues is insufficient blood flow at the cellular level. There must be sufficient circulation to provide for routine cellular metabolic requirements and, in addition, for the added demands of both tissue repair and bacterial defense. Therefore, factors such as anemia, malnutrition, circulatory inadequacy from large- or small-vessel disease, hypotension with vasoconstriction, cigarette smoking, and other issues must be recognized in the preoperative period. Certainly, they must be addressed if wound-healing problems occur.

Prevention of problems before they occur is frequently easier to accomplish than treating established complications. Proper tissue handling leaves the skin flaps and wound edges better able to meet the demands of the healing process. Numerous factors can damage skin or fat cells: excessive traction during wound exposure; the use of cutting cautery, which damages cells on either side of the tissue that it actually cuts; or even excessively tight sutures or staples, which not only pull the skin flaps tighter but can also constrict and damage the tissue contained within the suture. In areas of good tissue perfusion, such as the head and neck, the issues just outlined seem to not play as crucial a role as in the anterior surface of the knee, where circulatory compromise is a greater risk. However, when other factors coexist, adding avoidable surgical trauma to the existing biological condition is a recipe for trouble.

Although we try our best to thoroughly clean the skin in preparation for surgery, bacterial contamination at the time of surgery is inevitable in every operation. It is impossible to achieve absolute sterility, no mater what type of preparation is performed. The key to limiting infection is reducing the bacterial inoculum to a size that the tissue can handle. For ordinary tissue, this has been calculated to be 10^5 organisms of typical cutaneous variety. In preparing to create a surgical wound we have two major methods of minimizing the risk of infection and the wound-healing compromise that would result: eliminating local bacteria and improving tissue resistance.

With regard to the first method, the type of preparation used to lower the surface bacterial count matters. The skin is typically colonized by numerous gram-positive bacteria; they live on the surface and extend down hair follicles. Therefore, the skin preparation should be chosen in such a manner as to remove the skin oils and dead outer layer, as well as target the type of bacteria resident. In addition, the time that it takes to achieve bacterial death, the duration of action, and the potential for allergies and skin irritation are important issues to consider.

Painting a topical solution on the skin surface does not fully remove the skin oils or dead cells, and to this end a surgical scrub is preferred. Some agents, such as chlorhexidine gluconate with alcohol (Hibiclens and others), are more effective against routine skin flora than povidone-iodine (Betadine) is. The alcohol contained in the former is toxic to the cornea, thus making it contraindicated on the face. However, 3.0% chloroxylenol (Technicare) is more effective, longer lasting, and less irritating than both Hibiclens and Betadine and for that reason can be used anywhere.

Improving tissue resistance by definition means preserving the nutrient circulation by limiting tissue damage with gentle handling, proper planning of incisions to minimize ischemia, the use of prophylactic antibiotics, and limiting the amount of foreign material left in the wound, of which sutures are a prime example. The presence of sutures in tissue can reduce the ability of skin to fight bacteria by a factor of 10^3.

SKIN HEALING COMPROMISE

Once a wound shows characteristics of poor healing, an evaluation of the factor or factors that have compromised

the area must be made. Both a common and a treatable problem around the knee is a hematoma beneath the skin flaps. Large bone cuts have been made and moderate subcutaneous dissection has been accomplished. Collections of blood are toxic to the overlying dermis and cause pressure necrosis from beneath. After the first 12 to 24 hours and lasting as long as 2 weeks, the blood clot remains a gelatinous mass that cannot be evacuated by a drain, no matter the size, or by an aspiration needle. During that early postoperative interval, if a significant hematoma is recognized, it must be drained and irrigated in the operating room. If not done, topical treatment will not be sufficient to halt and reverse the process of progressive tissue loss. Usually by about 2 weeks the hematoma has begun to liquefy, with a soft spot forming that can be palpated and successfully aspirated on one or more occasions. Although this approach is recommended in other anatomic areas, needle aspiration must be approached with great caution in total joint replacement. Any hematoma sufficient to require drainage or cause circulatory compromise should be drained under sterile conditions in the operating room. Drainage is an important factor in removing the underlying offending material while treating the surface effects. Small hematomas that cause no skin compromise can be left to resorb on their own.

The pattern of skin involvement may also provide clues regarding the cause of skin distress. If there is discoloration of the skin on only one side of the incision, a circulatory problem of that particular flap is present. If redness, swelling, or discoloration is observed on both sides of the incision, a more general problem is probably present, such as a hematoma, an infection, or both.

Tight dressings can impede lymphatic and/or venous blood flow. Especially when combined with absence of the pumping action provided by the lower leg muscles during ambulation, edema can develop. Right-sided heart failure can also contribute to the problem. Edema reduces cellular nutrition, thereby compromising healing, and causes increased postoperative scarring and fibrin deposition.

Next, a closer look at the wound itself will provide clues about the cause and extent of the problem. A wound that is bluish but still retains some capillary refill indicates that the epidermis has been compromised but the underlying dermis, which contains the capillaries and small arterioles, still has some viability. If the color is brown, gray, or black and the wound is hard, necrosis, a full-thickness injury, has occurred. It is important to assess, as closely as possible, the depth of the tissue compromised, for the functions of the different skin and soft tissue layers that are in jeopardy are different and dictate the need to substitute for them or replace them completely.

The several layers of the skin each have a particular function. The purpose of the epidermis is to keep the underlying organism clean and moist in the dry, hostile outside environment. Bacteria and other pathogens are to be kept out. Flexibility is to be allowed. Epidermal cells start off as a living layer at the dermoepidermal junction, where they replicate and begin a 6-week migration up to the surface. By the time that the journey is complete, they have formed a flat, dry, dead, flexible layer. Epidermal cells extend deep into the dermis along adnexal structures such as hair follicles, which extend down into the dermis and often into subcutaneous fat. If the epidermal layer has been lost but the dermis is preserved, assuming that no further loss of tissue occurs, a new epidermal layer will regenerate. A functional layer will usually develop within about 2 weeks, although it can take 6 weeks for a mature layer to form that is able to withstand the usual traumas of daily life.

If epidermis is lost, a substitute for its function must be provided until it regenerates: a moist environment that simulates the isotonic properties of normal tissue and prevents bacterial colonization. Various agents are available for this purpose. In choosing which to use, one must consider effectiveness, ease of use, cost, and any ancillary requirements, such as treatment or prevention of infection.

The simplest and least expensive type of treatment is petrolatum (Vaseline and others). If antibiotic prophylaxis or treatment is also desired, a topical antibiotic ointment may be used. The type of ointment depends on assessment of the organisms identified or suspected, as well as a history of patient allergies. Bacitracin is effective against *Staphylococcus aureus*; Neosporin contains bacitracin as well as neomycin and polymyxin, thereby adding a measure of gram-negative coverage. However, cutaneous allergies to either bacitracin or Neosporin are quite common and are manifested as a macular rash in the area of application. Another agent, mupirocin (Bactroban) is effective against a wide range of gram-positive bacteria, including methicillin-resistant *S. aureus*, as well as certain gram-negative bacteria; Bactroban has the added benefit of rare allergenicity.

The aforementioned agents are useful for wounds that have exhibited a healing problem, as well as for treatment of all routine surgical wounds. The purpose of the epidermis is to keep the underlying dermis protected and moist. When an incision is made, the epidermis in the line of the incision is discontinuous and is lost. Using an ointment on the incision can hasten the growth of epidermal cells across the healing incision. The wound can be safely washed with soap and water once or twice daily to remove any debris and old ointment and then dried thoroughly. A fresh layer of ointment and a dry, sterile dressing should be applied. Getting a wound wet as in washing is not equivalent to leaving it wet, so wet bandages, waterproof tape, and similar items should absolutely be avoided because maceration may well occur and cause skin breakdown, which will lead to infection.

Another alternative to the treatment of superficial skin loss involves the use of an aloe vera–based agent called Carrasyn Gel, which has been shown to increase the rate of skin cell growth and decrease the rate of bacterial growth. It has been compared with Silvadene, which is highly effective in preventing bacterial growth; Silvadene, however, slows skin cell growth. Salicylic acid cream increases skin cell growth but does not fight bacteria. Carrasyn requires two or three dressing changes per day, but is highly effective.

A number of hydrogel products are currently available for use in wound care. Some are thicker and easier to handle. However, none have been shown to increase the rate of skin cell growth or decrease the rate of bacterial growth when compared with other modalities.

If the wound is draining, the use of an absorptive layer can remove exudates, limit maceration, and remove potentially toxic enzymes. Calcium or sodium alginate dressing (Sorbsan and others) can be placed in the wound after cleaning with saline and covered with dry gauze. It absorbs drainage and is changed daily, or even less frequently, depending on the amount of drainage.

Hydrofiber dressings such as Aquacel also absorb many times their weight in exudates. Such dressings have the advantage of ease of use because they do not fragment on removal. Aquacel AG is silver impregnated and highly effective against even antibiotic-resistant bacteria. It is used until the infection resolves, at which time Aquacel (minus silver) is again used.

A second silver-containing product is Acticoat, a gauze-type dressing that releases silver into an infected wound, thereby combating even drug-resistant bacteria; in most cases, however, it is not as absorptive as the alginates or hydrofibers.

The next decision that must be made is how to handle necrotic tissue. If the wound is pink or red but capillary refill is present, the underlying dermis is probably viable. In this situation, the topical remedies mentioned earlier will usually stabilize the situation until the wound re-epithelializes. However, if the wound surface appears brown or even black, a deeper loss of tissue is indicated. Necrotic tissue is dead and cannot heal or fight infection; in fact, it can be a nidus for bacterial growth.

Provided that the margins have not separated, small areas of eschar or tissue necrosis can be left in place. As soon as the edges begin to separate, however, the potential for bacterial invasion is introduced, and the necrotic tissue must be immediately dealt with.

The problem that usually arises is deciding what tissue is viable and what is going to die. Radical early débridement may unnecessarily sacrifice tissue that would otherwise survive. Wet-to-dry dressings do adhere to necrotic tissue and mechanically remove it; moreover, in the process such dressings may damage fragile healthy tissue and are frequently painful. Concentrated solutions of Betadine or hydrogen peroxide are extremely toxic to fragile cells and should also be avoided. They may be used for cleaning crusted material, but should then be irrigated away thoroughly with saline.

Several types of enzymatic débriding agents are in current use. The papain-urea preparations (Accuzyme, Gladase) use the proteolytic enzyme action of papain combined with the denaturant effect of urea to digest and remove only nonviable protein. Panafil is a combination of papain-urea and chlorophyll and helps control odor in heavily draining wounds. Heavy metal ions such as lead, silver, and mercury inactivate the protein and should be avoided, along with hydrogen peroxide and Betadine, when using any of these products.

When iodine's antibacterial properties are desired, a product containing iodine is recommended—Iodosorb gel not only provides the antibiotic properties of that chemical but also absorbs many times its own weight in exudate. Iodosorb can be combined with a papain-urea cream to provide the benefits of both medications. This product is rinsed with saline and changed once or twice daily, depending on the amount of drainage.

An alternative débriding agent, collagenase (Santyl), digests and removes necrotic collagen. It is also affected by heavy metal ions and is deactivated by detergents and any pH other than neutral. It is used once or twice daily and can be mixed with topical antibacterials such as Bactroban, Neosporin, or polymyxin B–bacitracin. The affected area must be rinsed with saline before application of the ointment to ensure that all traces of loosened material have been removed and the pH has been restored to neutral. Occasional patients will manifest an allergic reaction to one or the other débriding agent, which requires a change or discontinuation of treatment.

The appearance of granulation tissue is an excellent sign because it indicates that necrotic tissue is gone; granulation tissue, which is rich in blood supply, may be contaminated but is rarely infected. The treating surgeon must also be aware that systemic antibiotics do not usually penetrate granulation tissue, so topical antibiotics are essential for local bacterial control.

Growth Factors

A complete discussion of the topical treatment of healing wounds must include a discussion of cytokines, or polypeptides whose function is to facilitate the cellular, biochemical, and mechanical stages of normal wound healing and to regulate many of these processes.[44] Among these cytokines are growth factors, which have been explored as topical applications to the open wound to aid in healing. The nomenclature of growth factors is confusing; some are named for the cell from which they are derived, some for the cell that is their target, or in some cases even for the function for which they are responsible. Growth factors are large polypeptides that function to facilitate the various stages of wound healing. Certain growth factors encourage angiogenesis, others are responsible for cell mitosis, and still others influence the cellular elements in surrounding soft tissue to mobilize in response to injury.

The literature over the last decade contains many studies using growth factors to aid in wound healing; the evidence for their use to benefit normal wound healing in terms of either speed of healing, strength gain, or ultimate satisfactory cosmesis is conflicting.[5,32,49] Some clinical trials support evidence for more rapid shrinkage of an opened wound where growth factors are applied, whereas other evidence indicates that the ultimate outcome regarding time to closure and breaking strength is unaffected. Thinking of these agents as an early step in influencing more rapid wound closure is useful because evidence exists to support their importance in aiding closure of difficult wounds. More recently there is some evidence that growth factors can influence events in disorders of healing skin, such as keloid and hypertrophic scar formation.[27,52,74] Whether this information will ultimately lead to topical agents that accelerate wound healing, in addition to agents that are useful adjuncts to the basic surgical principles of

adequate débridement and edema control in local wound care, is hoped but not yet ensured.

References

1. Ashcroft GS, Horan MA, Ferguson MWJ: The effects of ageing on cutaneous wound healing in mammals. J Anat 187:1, 1995.
2. Bains JW, Crawford DT, Ketchum AS: Effect of chronic anemia on wound tensile strength: Correlation with blood volume, total red cell volume and proteins. Ann Surg 164:243, 1966.
3. Barbal A: Immune aspects of wound repair. Clin Plast Surg 17:433, 1990.
4. Breasted JH: The Edwin Smith Surgical Papyrus. Chicago, University of Chicago Press, 1930.
5. Brown GL, et al: Enhancement of wound healing by topical treatment with epidermal growth factor. N Engl J Med 321:76, 1989.
6. Brown H: Wound healing research through the ages. In Cohen IK, Diegelmann RF, Lindblad WJ (eds): Wound Healing: Biochemical and Clinical Aspects. Philadelphia, WB Saunders, 1992, pp 5, 9, 11, 14.
7. Burns JL, Mancoll JS, Phillips LG: Impairments to wound healing. Clin Plast Surg 30:49, 2003.
8. Conolly WB, Hunt TK, Zederfelot B, et al: Clinical comparison of surgical wounds closed by suture and adhesive tapes. Am J Surg 117:318, 1969.
9. Ditzel J: Changes in red cell oxygen release capacity in diabetes mellitus. Fed Proc 38:2484, 1979.
10. Dolmain CE: Alexander Fleming. In Gillespie CC (ed): Dictionary of Scientific Biography, vol V. New York, Charles Scribner & Sons, 1972, pp 28-31.
11. Eaglstein WH: Wound healing and aging. Dermatol Clin 4:481, 1986.
12. Ebbell B: The Papyrus Ebers. The Greatest Egyptian Medical Document. London, Oxford University Press, 1937.
13. Ehrlich P, Tarver H, Hunt TK: Inhibitory effect of vitamin E on collagen synthesis and wound repair. Ann Surg 175:235, 1972.
14. Ehrlich P, Tarver H, Hunt TK: The effects of vitamin A and glucocorticoids upon repair and collagen synthesis. Ann Surg 177:22, 1973.
15. Falcone RE, Nappi JF: Chemotherapy and wound healing. Surg Clin North Am 64:779, 1984.
16. Ferguson MK: The effect of anti-neoplastic agents on wound healing. Surg Gynecol Obstet 154:421, 1982.
17. Forrest CR, Pang CY, Lindsay WK: Dose and time effects of nicotine treatment on the capillary blood flow and viability of random pattern skin flaps in the rat. Br J Plast Surg 40:295, 1987.
18. Garrison FH: An Introduction to the History of Medicine. Philadelphia, WB Saunders, 1929, pp 92-101.
19. Gerstein AD, Phillips TJ, Rogers GS, Gilchrest BA: Wound healing and aging. Dermatol Clin 11:749, 1993.
20. Gibson T, Kenedi RM: Biomechanical properties of skin. Surg Clin North Am 47:279, 1967.
21. Grant RA, Cox RW, Kent CM: The effects of gamma irradiation on the structure and reactivity of mature and cross linked-collagen fibers. J Anat 115:29, 1973.
22. Grillo HC: Derivation of fibroblasts in the healing wound. Arch Surg 88:2181, 1964.
23. Guyton AC, Hall JE (eds): Textbook of Medical Physiology, 10th ed. Philadelphia, WB Saunders, 2000, pp 469-470.
24. Heughan C, Grislis G, Hunt TK: The effect of anemia on wound healing. Ann Surg 179:163, 1974.
25. Hunt TK: Vitamin A and wound healing. J Am Acad Dermatol 15:817, 1986.
26. Hunt TK, Ehrlich HP, Garcia JA, Dunphy TE: Effect of vitamin A on reversing the inhibitory effect of cortisone on healing of open wounds in animals and man. Ann Surg 170:633, 1969.
27. Igarashi A, Nashiro K. Kikuchi K, et al: Connective tissue growth factor gene expression in tissue sections from localized scleroderma, keloid, and other fibrotic skin disorders. J Invest Dermatol 106:729, 1996.
28. Jandak JM, Richardson PD: Alphatocopherol, an effective inhibitor of platelet adhesion. Blood 73:141, 1989.

29. Johnson A, Rodeheaver GT, Durand LS, et al: Automatic disposable stapling devices for wound closure. Ann Emerg Med 10:631, 1981.

30. Johnson T: The Works of That Famous Chirurgion Ambrose Parey. London, R Cotes & W Du-Gaard, 1649.

31. Jonsson K, Jensen JA, Goodson WH 3rd, et al: Tissue oxygenation, anemia, and perfusion in relation to wound healing in surgical patients. Ann Surg 214:605, 1991.

32. Knighton DR, et al: Classification and treatment of chronic non-healing wounds. Successful treatment with autologous platelet-derived wound healing factors (PDWHF). Ann Surg 204:322, 1986.

33. Kulick MI: An vitro-in vivo investigation of the effect of non-steroidal anti-inflammatory agents on collagen synthesis. Presented at the 71st Annual Clinical Congress of the American College of Surgeons, 1987, Chicago.

34. Lau HC, Granick MS, Aisner AM, Solomon MP: Wound care in the elderly patient. Surg Clin North Am 74:441, 1994.

35. LaVan FB, Hunt TK: Oxygen and wound healing. Clin Plast Surg 17:463, 1990.

36. Lawrence WT, Murphy RC, Robson MC, Heggers JP: The detrimental effect of cigarette smoking on flap survival: An experimental study in the rat. Br J Plast Surg 37:216, 1984.

37. Lecture in Chinese traditional medicine. Gangzhou (Canton), China, Zuong Cho School of Chinese Traditional Medicine, May 1984.

38. Lee PWR, Green MA, Long WB 3rd, Gull W: Zinc and wound healing. Surg Gyncol Obstet 143:549, 1976.

39. LeGerfo FW, Coffman JD: Vascular and microvascular disease of the foot in diabetes: Implications for foot care. N Engl J Med 311:1615, 1984.

40. Leibovich SJ, Ross R: The role of the macrophage in wound repair: A study with hydrocortisone and antimacrophage serum. Am J Pathol 78:71, 1975.

41. Madden JW, Peacock EE: Studies on the biology of collagen during wound healing. III. Dynamic metabolism of scar collagen and remodeling of dermal wounds. Ann Surg 174:511, 1971.

42. Manson PN, Anthenelli RM, Im MJ, et al: The role of oxygen free radicals in ischemic tissue injury in island skin flaps. Ann Surg 198:87, 1983.

43. Mathes SJ, Feng L-J, Hunt TK: Coverage of the infected wound. Ann Surg 198:420, 1983.

44. McGrath MH: Peptide growth factors in wound healing. Clin Plast Surg 17:421, 1990.

45. Morain WD, Colen LB: Wound healing in diabetes mellitus. Clin Plast Surg 17:494, 1990.

46. Peacock EE: Symposium on biological control of scar tissue. Plast Reconstr Surg 41:8, 1968.

47. Peacock EE: Collagenolysis: The other side of the equation. World J Surg 4:297, 1980.

48. Peterson JM, Barbul A, Breslin RJ, et al: Significance of T-lympho-cytes in wound healing. Surgery 102:300, 1987.

49. Pierce GJ, et al: In vivo incisional wound healing augmented by platelet-derived growth factor and recombinant C-sis gene homod-imeric proteins. J Exp Med 167:974, 1988.

50. Pirani CL, Levenson SM: Effect of vitamin C deficiency on healed wounds. Proc Soc Exp Biol Med 82:95, 1953.

51. Pollack SV: Wound healing: A review. III. Nutritional factors affecting wound healing. J Dermatol Surg Oncol 5:615, 1979.

52. Polo M, Smith PD, Kim YJ, et al: Effect of TGF-β2 on proliferative scar fibroblast kinetics. Ann Plast Surg 43:185, 1999.

53. Pories WJ, Henzel JH, Rob CG, Strain WH: Acceleration of healing with zinc sulfate. Ann Surg 165:432, 1967.

54. Powanda MC, Moyer ED: Plasma proteins and wound healing. Surg Gynecol Obstet 153:749, 1981.

55. Prasad AS: Clinical manifestations of zinc deficiency. Annu Rev Nutr 5:341, 1985.

56. Prasad AS: Zinc and growth in development and the spectrum of human zinc deficiency J Am Coll Nutr 7:377, 1988.

57. Prockop DJ, Kivirikko KI, Tuderman L, Guzman NA: The biosynthesis of collagen and its disorders (first of two parts). N Engl J Med 301:13, 1979.

58. Rees TD, Liverett DM, Guy GL: The effect of cigarette smoking on skin flap survival in the facelift patient. Plast Reconstr Surg 73:911, 1984.

59. Rimm EB, Stampfer MJ, Ascherio A, et al: Vitamin E consumption and the risk of coronary disease in men. N Engl J Med 328:1450, 1993.

60. Rohrich RJ, Robinson JB: Wound healing. Select Read Plast Surg 9(3):10, 1999.

61. Rudolph R, Vande Berg J, Schneider JA, et al: Slowed growth of cultured fibroblasts from human radiation wounds. Plast Reconstr Surg 82:669, 1988.

62. Silver IA: Oxygen tension and epithelialization. In Maibach HI, Rovee DT (eds): Epidermal Wound Healing. Chicago, Year Book, 1972, p 291.

63. Simpson LO: Intrinsic stiffening of red blood cells as the fundamental cause of diabetic nephropathy and microangiopathy: A new hypothesis. Nephron 39:344, 1985.

64. Steiner M: Influence of vitamin E on platelet function in humans. J Am Coll Nutr 10:466, 1991.

65. Stephens FO, Hunt TK: Effective changes in inspired oxygen and carbon dioxide tensions on wound tensile strength. Ann Surg 173:515, 1971.

66. Stillman RM, Marino CA, Seligman SJ: Skin staples in potentially contaminated wounds. Arch Surg 119:821, 1984.

67. Taren DL, Chvapil M, Weber CW: Increasing the breaking strength of wounds exposed to pre-operative irradiation using vitamin E supplementation. Int J Vitam Nutr Res 57:133, 1987.

68. Temple WJ, Voitk AJ, Snelling CF, Crispin JS: Effect of nutrition, diet and suture material on long term wound healing. Ann Surg 182:93, 1975.

69. Thakral KK, Goodson WH, Hunt TK: Stimulation of wound blood vessel growth by wound macrophages. J Surg Res 26:430, 1979.

70. Timmenga EJF, et al: The effect of mechanical stress on healing skin wounds: An experimental study in rabbits using tissue expansion. Br J Plast Surg 44:514, 1991.

71. Van de Kerkhof PC, Van Bergen B, Spruijt K, Kuiper JP: Age related changes in wound healing. Clin Exp Dermatol 19:369, 1994.

72. White MJ, Heckler FR: Oxygen free radicals and wound healing. Clin Plast Surg 17:473, 1990.

73. Zamboni WA, Browder LK, Martinez J: Hyperbaric oxygen and wound healing. Clin Plast Surg 20:69, 2003.

74. Zhou L-J, Ono I, Kaneko F: Role of transforming growth factor-β in fibroblasts derived from normal and hypertrophic scarred skin. Arch Dermatol Res 289:646, 1997.

CHAPTER 64

The Problem Wound: Coverage Options

Susan Craig Scott

In assessing our approach to soft-tissue healing in patients who are candidates for total knee arthroplasty, ideal circumstances allow sufficient preoperative planning to provide optimal skin conditions for wound healing. Such planning involves, in addition to assessing factors in the patient's history that might inhibit healing, manipulation of the operative area in an attempt to ensure primary healing.

LOCAL SOFT-TISSUE MANIPULATION

Certain patients have multiple existing incisions or other local conditions that might portend primary wound-healing difficulties after total knee arthroplasty (Fig. 64–1). Anticipating which patients might have healing difficulties allows us to plan preoperatively for primary healing and provide healthy soft-tissue coverage; consequently, wound compromise is avoided, and the long months of recovery, delay in motion gains, and other complications that occur when healing fails to progress as expected are avoided. In these patients we will use either a sham incision, tissue expansion, or pre–joint replacement or simultaneous free flap coverage.

Sham Incision

A sham incision creates the skin and subcutaneous tissue incision for total knee arthroplasty; this incision is then closed. The usefulness of this approach is that it informs us regarding the health and vascularity of local tissue. If the sham incision heals primarily, we can anticipate no wound complications when the joint is replaced. The sham acts as a kind of delay; by interrupting the blood supply that traverses the incision and increasing demand from the periphery, we anticipate a local response, which augments the existing supply. In fact, the primary benefit of the sham incision is its effect on local tissue in stimulating increased blood supply.

The sham incision, and probably tissue expansion as well, makes use of the delay phenomenon to increase tissue survival. Despite some controversy regarding the actual mechanism for effecting delay, there is no doubt that delay works when planned with care. When a surgical wound is incised with a plan to delay, hypertrophy and reorganization of vessels along the axis of the delayed tissue occur and result in improved surviving length.[2] Whether the success of the delay technique is due to ingrowth in response to ischemia, enlargement of existing vessels, or possibly conditioning of tissue to ischemia is unknown.[7] One week is sufficient time for the delay phenomenon to occur; longer time provides no advantage in the number or size of improved vasculature.[16,18]

The indication for a sham incision is a situation wherein the likelihood of primary healing is good, but some question remains regarding the health and vascularity of the local soft tissue. The disadvantage of this approach is the potential for tissue loss in the wound created by the sham incision. Although it is certainly preferable to have tissue loss occur in the knee before placement of a prosthesis, the surgeon is now faced with addressing a nonhealing wound in a patient who has yet to undergo total knee arthroplasty. In an attempt to avoid this situation, to provide adequate soft-tissue coverage, and to increase vascular supply to the skin over the knee in situations of marginal supply before joint replacement, tissue expansion has in our hands proved to be an excellent technique (Fig. 64–2). Our indications for its use have evolved over the last decade, as have our contraindications. We now find that this coordinated approach is an excellent solution in selected patients.

Soft-Tissue Expansion

The tissue expander is inserted about 8 weeks before the planned total knee arthroplasty. To insert the expander, a pocket is created in the area and adjacent to the area of questionable blood supply; as large an expander as can be accommodated by the space is inserted. The expander is completely buried, as is its access port. Weekly or biweekly injections follow until adequate expansion is achieved.

The access port to the tissue expander is always placed proximally, and injections are carried out with a needle no larger than 23 gauge. The expander tubing and port will be surrounded by a well-vascularized pseudocapsule, and this capsule will generate a small amount of fluid. If the port is placed distal to the expander in a dependent position, there may be leakage around the needle insertion site for a prolonged period when weekly injections are performed.

When inserting the expander, the planned arthroplasty incision is drawn. In a proximal section of this incision, a 1.5-inch-long segment is selected as the access incision. A large amount, 250 to 350 mL, of very dilute lidocaine is injected to create a plane by hydrodissection, and the pocket to receive the expander follows this plane.

The expander is removed at the time of total knee arthroplasty; at closure, the expander pocket is always

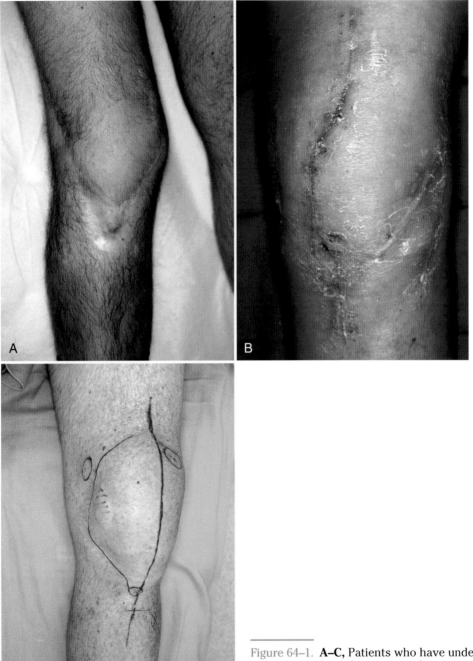

Figure 64–1. **A–C,** Patients who have undergone multiple previous surgical procedures through a variety of incisions may be at risk for healing compromise after total knee arthroplasty.

drained separately with a large-bore drain. This drain is removed when it returns less than 20 mL per shift. When the expander is removed, it is critically important to keep the capsular attachment at the perimeter of the expander pocket in continuity with the anterior and posterior capsular surfaces because this region is the source of the plentiful vessels in the vascular layer of the pseudocapsule.

It is our preference to place one or more rectangular expanders, oriented longitudinally, on the anterior aspect of the knee. Tissue expanders are available in a wide variety of shapes and sizes.

THE PROBLEM WOUND

Skin Grafting

When full-thickness tissue has been lost, meticulous wound care after débridement will provide a bed that is satisfactory for the least complex form of coverage, skin grafting. This approach is used when the joint capsule is completely intact and there is no threat of prosthesis exposure.

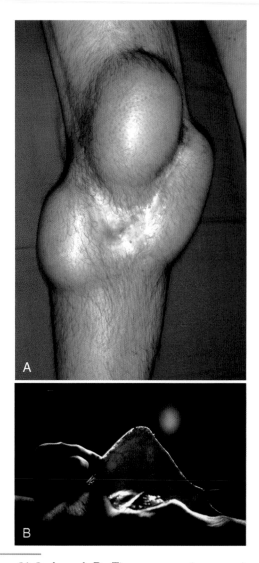

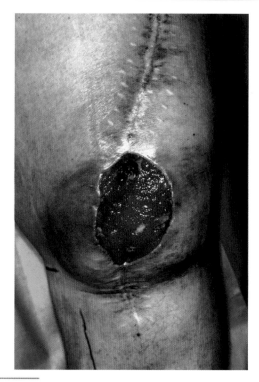

Figure 64–3. A healthy bed with excellent vascularity will support a split-thickness skin graft.

Figure 64–2. **A** and **B**, Tissue expansion can improve the local blood supply in patients with potential healing compromise.

Skin grafting removes a dermal-epidermal layer of skin from a donor site and applies it to a suitably prepared recipient bed. The bed must have appropriate vascularity to allow the skin graft to survive initially by serum imbibition for 48 hours, after which the skin graft is penetrated by ingrowth of vascular channels; by about day 5 or 6 after grafting, circulation is reestablished.[1,4,5] The bed on which the graft is placed must be free of infection with excellent hemostasis (Fig. 64–3). Once in place, the graft must be well fixed with suture, a compressive dressing, or the application of V.A.C.* Stability will allow revascularization.

At about 5 days the skin graft dressing may be removed and dependence of the limb gradually initiated. Topical ointment should be applied to the graft until all crusted

areas are gone, whether in the interstices or at the perimeter of the grafted area. Depending on thickness, the graft in the long term is likely to be dry and to require some assistance with moisturizing because its limited thickness does not bring with it any lubricating glands normally located in the deep dermis or subdermis to maintain adequate surface moisture.

The skin graft donor site ordinarily heals by secondary intention and must be protected from trauma and invasion of bacteria until healing occurs. It may be dressed with Xeroform and allowed to air-dry, or it may be dressed with an occlusive dressing, as the surgeon prefers. There is some evidence that occlusion until the donor site heals is more comfortable for the patient. Once the donor site has epithelialized, long-term effects such as pruritus, sensitivity, pigment changes, and even scar hypertrophy may occur. These conditions are ordinarily self-limited, but if persistently troublesome, they may be addressed with antipruritics, antihistamines, lubricants, or silicon sheeting such as Mepiform or Cica-Care (Fig. 64–4).

When tissue loss is more extensive than simply skin and subcutaneous tissue, when the prosthesis is exposed or at significant risk of exposure, or when skin only is lost in a situation of incomplete joint capsuler closure, as is sometimes the case, more robust coverage that brings with it its own vascular supply and is relatively independent of local tissue conditions is the treatment of choice. This option includes local rotation flaps composed of skin and muscle, muscle alone, skin and fascia, or fascia alone. The location and precise coverage requirements of the recipient bed determine the choice of coverage. These tissues are most expeditiously raised as either a pedicle that is rotated or an island that is transposed into position, as

*Vacuum-assisted closure, also called negative-pressure wound therapy, is a method of wound treatment that applies continuous adjustable negative pressure (suction) to a wound surface transmitted through a sealed sponge dressing. Once suction is applied, the sponge dressing is firmly fixed in place.

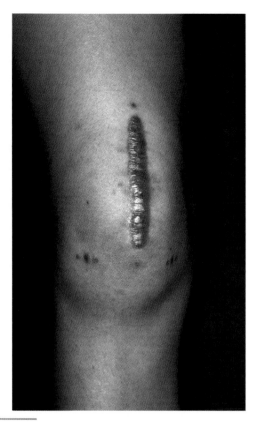

Figure 64–4. Scar hypertrophy will respond to the application of topical silicone sheeting.

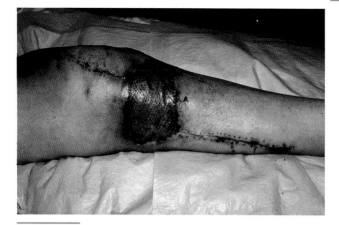

Figure 64–5. The gastrocnemius muscle flap provides reliable soft-tissue coverage when needed.

required. In a multiply operated knee, the surgeon may face a situation in which there is no suitable local donor site. In such cases a free flap of muscle and skin or muscle alone from a distant part of the body is the solution of choice.

Muscle and Myocutaneous Flaps

The workhorse local muscle or myocutaneous flap for coverage of defects about the knee is the gastrocnemius muscle. The most superficial muscle layer of the posterior region of the calf, this muscle has a medial and a lateral head, each of which is usually supplied by an independent artery.[14] Each head of the muscle originates on its respective posterior surface of the femoral condyle, the medial head originating medially and the lateral head laterally. The medial head is usually the longer of the two heads and extends farther distal from its origin than the lateral head does; the two heads are divided by a median raphe, which also marks a clear division of their separate vascular territories. The raphe transitions to the musculotendinous junction as the gastrocnemius contributes to the broad, substantial Achilles tendon. Each gastrocnemius muscle head is a type II flap anatomically, with a single arterial pedicle providing blood supply supported by at least one secondary pedicle from the posterior tibial and peroneal arteries.[19] The medial and lateral heads are supplied by the medial and lateral sural arteries, respec-

tively. The arteries arise at (60%) or above (32%) the joint line of the knee.[17] Most commonly, the medial sural artery arises slightly more proximally than the lateral artery; there are few, if any arterial communications between the medial and lateral heads within or across the median raphe.[19] Because of this independent and very reliable blood supply, each head can be taken separately with or without overlying skin for coverage. Each sural artery has a 6- to 8-cm course before it penetrates the deep surface of the muscle and then arborizes and divides within that muscle.

This muscle provides a number of perforators to the skin overlying the muscle and distal to it and can be taken with a sizable skin paddle when needed. The perforators are located just off the midline of the posterior of the calf. The first of those over the medial head is approximately at the level of the tibial plateau, the next is about 3 cm lower, and the last perforating branch is close to but above the musculotendinous insertion into the Achilles tendon.[3,6,20] Provided that these perforators are identified and protected, a medial gastrocnemius flap can be harvested with overlying skin to within 5 cm of the medial malleolus with continuous Doppler assessment of perforators to verify viability as the flap is manipulated.[8] The arc of rotation of the medial gastrocnemius muscle flap allows coverage of the proximal third of the tibia, the medial knee joint, the tibial tubercle, and the patella (Fig. 64–5). When taken as an extended flap with overlying skin, coverage can be achieved from the middle third of the tibia to the suprapatellar region. If more extensive reach is needed, the muscle origin can be taken down from behind the medial femoral condyle. This technique provides adequate release if there is any tension on the closure and can add almost 2 cm of flap advancement if needed. If the required coverage is deficient in width rather than length, the deep muscle surface can be incised through its fascia and the muscle spread to increase its width of coverage.[13]

The lateral head of the gastrocnemius is shorter than the medial head and can be used to cover the lateral knee joint and the lateral aspect of the fibula; it, too, can be taken with overlying skin, while carefully identifying the perforators, to provide more extensive coverage. Proximal dissection and transposition must be done with great care because the peroneal nerve is in a vulnerable subcutaneous position as it comes around the head the fibula.[13]

The major drawback to the use of a gastrocnemius myocutaneous flap is the cosmetic deformity that is created at the donor site. Some patients have a thick superficial and deep adipose layer over the muscle, which adds to the significant donor deformity when this flap is used and can result in a sizable disparity in thickness between the flap and skin edges in the thin recipient area of the anterior aspect of the knee, which is often lacking in subcutaneous fat. We prefer to address this issue by a thorough discussion with the patient before surgery, by transposing muscle only when possible, by elevating skin margins in the recipient area and tucking the flap margin beneath, and of course by meticulous repair of the donor site.

Fascial and Fasciocutaneous Flaps

Our understanding of the blood supply to the skin and subcutaneous tissues of the leg is a direct result of original work by Pontén, Haertsch, and Cormack and Lamberty, whose descriptions of blood supply and fascial organization outlined the essential foundation for the more recent development of fasciocutaneous flaps for knee coverage.[6,9,15] Expansion of our understanding of these flaps and their clinical application is due primarily to Hallock's elegant and original descriptions of fasciocutaneous flap procedures.[10,11] Varied flap design allows satisfactory coverage while minimizing the cosmetic deformity resulting from harvesting the gastrocnemius muscle and overlying skin. Carefully designed, these flaps can provide hardy coverage of the exposed knee joint and a satisfactory bed for skin grafting. Only the reliability of their vascular pedicle, which is not present in all patients and must be meticulously defined, prevents them from being adapted universally as the most satisfactory local coverage option about the knee joint.

The fasciocutaneous system of the lower extremity has been clearly outlined in several studies.[12,21,22] This system, similar in concept to the system of angiosomes, which informs our understanding of musculocutaneous flaps, allows harvest and transposition of a variety of thin flaps in the lower extremity. Although the basis for this work is almost 25 years old, clinical application is still evolving as our experience grows and their reliability is reinforced.

Several local fasciocutaneous flaps may be used to cover the variety of defects seen around the knee. Among these flaps is the posterior calf fasciocutaneous flap supplied directly by the descending cutaneous branch of the popliteal artery, called the median sural artery by Cormack and Lamberty.[6] When the artery is present, this fascial or fasciocutaneous flap extends from the popliteal crease to the junction of the middle and distal thirds of the posterior aspect of the calf. Harvest of the flap requires careful preoperative Doppler outlining of the vascular supply because as in about a third of cases the aforementioned artery is small or absent.[21] This flap is available for thin coverage about the knee or as a free flap donor for distant sites.

The second fasciocutaneous flap coverage option in this area is the saphenous fasciocutaneous flap. The saphenous artery, a branch of the descending genicular artery from the femoral artery, supplies the skin of the medial aspect of the thigh and the superior anteromedial aspect of the leg. It is very reliably present, although its superficial subcutaneous course below the insertion of the sartorius muscle, to which it lies deep, makes it vulnerable to injury in the course of joint replacement surgery, particularly if wound-healing complications follow. In addition, the artery, its fasciocutaneous course, and its cutaneous perforators must be dissected with meticulous care before flap incision because adequate anterior perforators are present in only about 45% of dissections.[21]

Our evolving knowledge and experience with subcutaneous and fascial blood supply make these flaps possible for local coverage of the knee.

Free Flap Coverage

When local tissue has been used in previous surgical procedures or has been treated in a way that would not provide for adequate local healing, a flap from a distant part of the body is used for coverage of full-thickness defects in which there is threatened exposure of the joint or prosthesis. Although more than one potential donor site can be used for free flap coverage of the knee, local requirements mean that a flap of adequate dimension to cover the exposed area and allow excision of compromised soft tissue is required. In ideal circumstances, the flap must bring with it a pedicle of adequate length to allow a vascular anastomosis outside the area of immediate surgical involvement.

Patients requiring free flap coverage of wounds about the knee have often been hospitalized for a period. Not infrequently, more conservative wound care approaches have been tried for a number of weeks and have been unsuccessful. There may have been one or more attempts at coverage, perhaps with skin graft or a local flap, that were not successful. Patients approach total knee arthroplasty with the expectation that within a few short weeks after surgery they will be fully ambulatory and able to resume a normal life. There is always a great deal of disappointment and frustration involved in these relatively rare instances when healing does not progress as expected. When healing problems occur, our approach is one of watchful waiting, provided that we have full control of local tissue conditions, there is no infection, and most important, there is no threat of exposure of the prosthesis. When such is the case, we are extremely aggressive in our approach.

When distant tissue coverage is required, our preferred donor site to cover the anterior of the knee is the latissimus dorsi muscle with its lengthy thoracodorsal pedicle (Fig. 64–6). The flap offers several advantages over other choices. First, the latissimus dorsi muscle is broad and relatively flat and provides an excellent and large surface area of coverage. Second, the blood supply to this flap, the tho-

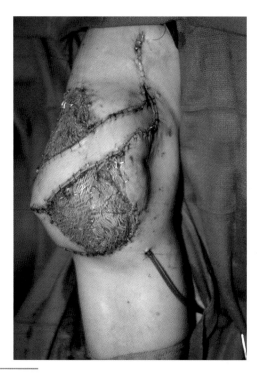

Figure 64–6. Free myocutaneous flap coverage is the ideal solution when local coverage is not available.

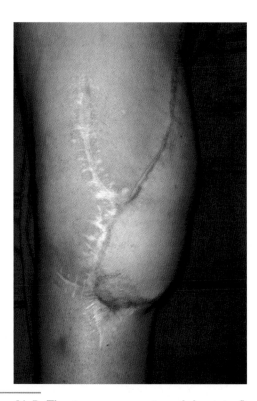

Figure 64–7. The transverse rectus abdominis flap provides thin suitable coverage in selected patients.

racodorsal artery, is extremely reliable. It is a terminal branch of the subscapular artery, which originates from the axillary artery. The length of the thoracodorsal pedicle can be as long as 10 cm, thus allowing its anastomosis to be placed quite proximal to the knee. In our hands, the preferred recipient vessel is the descending genicular branch of the superficial femoral artery, which is commonly found after exposing Hunter's canal, with one or two accompanying veins. When this vessel is not satisfactory, an end-to-side juncture with the superficial femoral artery and/or the superficial femoral vein can be created via this exposure. Third, use of this particular muscle allows for a two-team approach. The flap can be dissected from the back on the side opposite the involved knee by one team while the second team exposes and prepares the recipient vessels.

The only real liability with this choice of donor is the other side of its size advantage: although it provides wide, relatively thin coverage, in some patients it can be quite bulky in this recipient area of limited anatomic dimension.

Other coverage donor site options include the transverse rectus abdominis muscle flap (Fig. 64–7) and one of several smaller muscle flaps, such as the gracilis.

References

1. Birch J, Branemark PI: The vascularization of a free full thickness skin graft. Scand J Plast Reconstr Surg 3:1, 1969.
2. Callegari PR, Taylor GT, Caddy CM, et al: An anatomic review of the delay phenomenon: I Experimental studies. Plast Reconstr Surg 89:397, 1992.
3. Cavadas PC, Sanz-Gimenez-Rico JR, Gutierrez-de la Camara A, et al: The medial sural artery perforator free flap. Plast Reconstr Surg 108:1611, discussion 1616, 2001.
4. Converse JM, Ballantyne DL Jr: Distribution of diphosphopyridine nucleotide diaphorase in rat skin autograft and homografts. Plast Reconstr Surg 30:415, 1962.
5. Converse JM, Rapaport FT: The vascularization of skin autografts and homografts; an experimental study in man. Ann Surg 143:306, 1956.
6. Cormack GC, Lamberty BGH: The Arterial Anatomy of Skin Flaps. Edinburgh, Churchill Livingstone, 1986, pp 225, 235.
7. Dhar SC, Taylor GI: The delay phenomenon: The story unfolds. Plast Reconstr Surg 104:2079, 1999.
8. Dibbell DG Edstron LE: The gastrocnemius myocutaneous flap. Clin Plast Surg 7:45, 1980.
9. Haertsch PA: The blood supply to the skin of the leg: A post mortem investigation. Br J Plast Surg 34:470, 1981.
10. Hallock GG: Local knee random fasciocutaneous flaps. Ann Plast Surg 23:289-296, 1989.
11. Hallock GG: Lower extremity muscle perforator flaps for lower extremity reconstruction. Plast Reconstr Surg 114:1128, 2004.
12. Hollier L, Sharma S, Babigumira E, et al: Versatility of the sural fasciocutaneous flap in the coverage of lower extremity wounds. Plast Reconstr Surg 110:1673, 2002.
13. Mathes SJ, Nahai F: Clinical Applications for Muscle and Myocutaneous Flaps. St. Louis, CV Mosby, 1982, p 546.
14. Merten SL, Rome PD, Stern HS, et al: The "extended pedicle" gastrocnemius free muscle flap. Plast Reconstr Surg 112:204, 2003.
15. Pontén B: The fasciocutaneous flap: Its use in soft tissue defects of the lower leg. Br J Plast Surg 34:215, 1981.
16. Restifo RJ, Syed SA, Ward BA, et al: Surgical delay in TRAM flap breast reconstruction: A comparison of 7- and 14-day delay periods. Ann Plast Surg 38: 330, 1997.
17. Salmon M: Arteries of the muscles of extremities and trunk. In Taylor GI, Razaboni RM (eds): Anatomic Studies Book I. St. Louis, Quality Medical Publishing, 1994.

18. Seitchuk MW, Kahn S: The effects of delay on the circulatory efficiency of pedicled tissue. Plast Reconstr Surg 33:16, 1964.

19. Taylor GI, Pan WR: Angiosomes of the leg: Anatomic study and clinical implications. Plast Reconstr Surg 102:599, 1998.

20. Taylor GI, Tempest M, Salmon M: Arteries of the Skin. London, Churchill Livingstone, 1988, p 61.

21. Waton RL, Rothkopf DM: Fasciocutaneous flaps about the knee. In Hallock GG (ed): Fasciocutaneous Flaps. Boston, Blackwell Scientific, 1992.

22. Whetzel TP, Barnard MA, Stokes RB: Arterial fasciocutaneous vascular territories of the lower leg. Plast Reconstr Surg 100:1172, 1997.

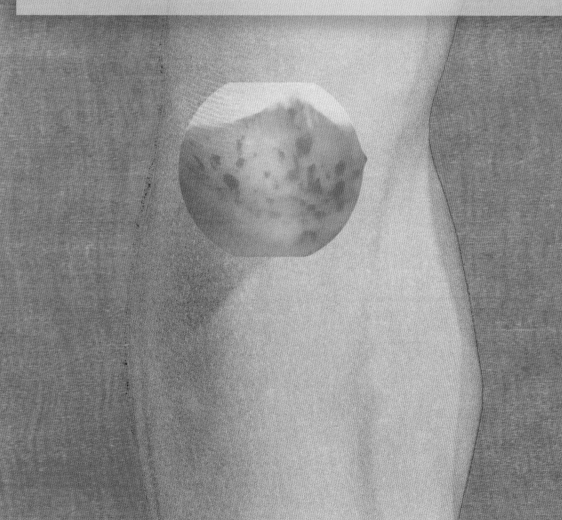

SECTION IX

Fractures about the Knee

CHAPTER 65

Distal Femur Fractures

Eric M. Lindvall • Anthony Infante • Roy Sanders

ANATOMY

General Anatomy

The distal femur extends for approximately the distal third of the femur.[23,28,70] It begins as the canal gradually widens and the cortices thin and continues distally to the joint line. The supracondylar region (distal metaphysis) flares medially greater than laterally in the coronal plane and broadens laterally greater than medially in the sagittal plane. The anterior and distal trochlear groove allows patellar articulation with the distal end of the femur. The intercondylar notch is posteriorly based and houses the cruciate ligaments.

An axial cut through the distal articular surface reveals a trapezoidal shape with the greatest dimension located posteriorly in a lateral-to-medial direction and the narrowest dimension located medially in an anterior-to-posterior direction. The medial side slopes approximately 25 degrees in a posteromedial-to-anterolateral direction. The lateral side slopes approximately 15 degrees in a posterolateral-to-anteromedial direction (Fig. 65–1).[55] The shaft lies in the anterior two-thirds of the condyles in the sagittal plane and slightly lateral with a 9-degree valgus orientation in the coronal plane.[28,55,61,87]

The joint capsule has greater space anteriorly than posteriorly and extends more than 2 cm proximal to the superior pole of the patella along the anterior aspect of the distal femur. Posteriorly, the joint space extends only to the condyle-shaft junction.

The articular surface involves the entire medial and lateral condyles and is thickest along the distal articular curvature and within the trochlear groove, the regions with the highest contact pressure. Anteriorly, the articular cartilage extends more proximally on the lateral condyle than on the medial condyle.

The critical nervous and arterial anatomy of the distal end of the femur includes the sciatic nerve and femoral artery. The femoral artery proceeds distally beneath the sartorius to lie between the adductors and the vastus medialis before entering the adductor canal. It then courses posteriorly through the adductor hiatus and into the popliteal fossa, where it changes name and becomes the popliteal artery until its trifurcation. The sciatic nerve lies posterior in the thigh between the long head of the biceps femoris and the semimembranosus. It then divides into the tibial and common peroneal branches before it emerges from the popliteal fossa.

Radiographic Anatomy

The anteroposterior (AP) radiograph demonstrates the 9-degree valgus angle created between the femoral shaft and the distal joint line. It also shows the greater medial condyle flare but does not reveal the trapezoidal shape as seen on an axial computed tomography (CT) image. The lateral radiograph demonstrates an anterior curvilinear sclerotic line representing the trochlear groove and a convergent posterior sclerotic line representing the intercondylar notch (Blumensatt's line), both of which end as they meet distally (Fig. 65–2). In addition, a true lateral radiograph of the knee allows identification of the medial femoral condyle as it articulates with the concave medial tibial plateau and the lateral femoral condyle as it articulates with the convex lateral tibial plateau (Fig. 63–2). Flexion of the knee during the AP radiograph allows visualization of the intercondylar notch.

Surface Anatomy

Palpation of the distal femur demonstrates a medial prominence, the adductor tubercle, which allows for muscle and ligament attachment. A lesser lateral prominence slightly more proximal represents the lateral tubercle. With the knee in the extended position, the inferior pole of the patella corresponds to the level of the tibiofemoral joint line. Approximately two to three fingerbreadths proximal to the superior pole of the patella is the proximal extension of the suprapatellar pouch. Four fingerbreadths proximal to the adductor tubercle corresponds to the level where the femoral artery traverses from the anterior half of the femur to the posterior half.

INCIDENCE AND ETIOLOGY

The incidence of supracondylar femoral fractures has a bimodal distribution—young adult patients with higher-energy injuries and elderly patients with lower-energy injuries.[3,23,38,86] It is typically the result of an external force, but the amount of force required to cause the fracture can vary significantly and is dependent on bone quality. In a 2000 report on 2165 distal femoral fractures, the distribution of such fractures was found to be bimodal and occur in young men and elderly women.[47] Lower-energy

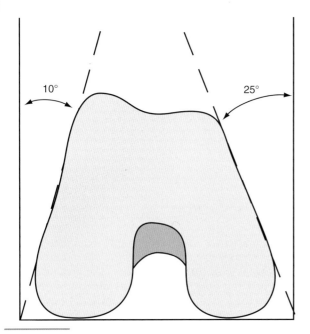

Figure 65–1. Diagram depicting the trapezoidal shape of the distal end of the femur. The 10-degree slope is shown laterally, and the 25-degree slope is shown medially.

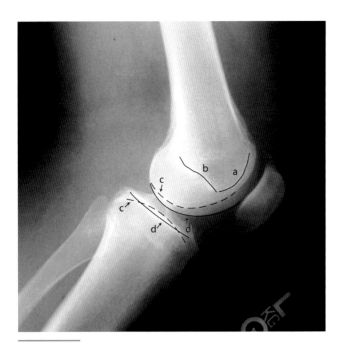

Figure 65–2. Lateral radiograph of the knee showing (a) the trochlear groove, (b) the intercondylar notch (Blumensaat's line), (c) the lateral distal femoral condylar articular surface with the matching lateral tibial convex surface, and (d) the medial femoral condylar articular surface with the matching medial tibial concave surface.

injuries are generally the result of ground-level falls or torsional injuries in patients with osteopenic or osteoporotic bone. Periprosthetic fractures are usually low-energy injuries and are encountered most commonly in the elderly as a result of disuse osteopenia, osteoporosis, and/or stress shielding around a prosthetic device or other

metallic implant. A stress riser is created in the transition area between the prosthesis and routine bone. Examples include the area distal to a hip stem, proximal to a short supracondylar nail, and proximal to a total knee prosthesis.

Paraplegics and quadriplegics also have weakened bone and, because of the resultant osteopenia and frequent contractures, are at increased risk for distal femoral fractures through falls from a wheelchair or transfer of the patient.

The amount of energy required to cause a supracondylar or distal femoral fracture in young patients without any existing bone pathology is usually significant and is often seen in conjunction with other associated fractures.[4,6,8,14,81] Knee ligament injuries and intra-articular pathology have also been reported in approximately 20% to 70% of ipsilateral femoral fractures.[6,14,81] Motor vehicle or motorcycle accidents, falls from heights, pedestrian versus auto accidents, or other heavy industrial accidents are common mechanisms of injury.[47]

CLASSIFICATION

A number of classification systems have been proposed for fractures of the distal femur. Neer and associates initially described a classification system in 1967 that divided fractures into three main categories—minimal displacement, condylar displacement from the shaft, and supracondylar or shaft comminution.[57] Seinsheimer later published a more detailed system.[70] The Swiss Arbeitsgemeinschaft für Osteosynthesefragen/Association for the Study of Internal Fixation (AO/ASIF) group has since developed a comprehensive fracture classification scheme that has become accepted in the trauma community—type A, extra-articular; type B, unicondylar; and type C, bicondylar (Fig. 65–3). This classification is further subdivided by the degree of comminution.[56] The Orthopaedic Trauma Association (OTA) has also developed a similar detailed and well-accepted classification system that encompasses the entire axial skeleton.[19]

DIAGNOSIS

History and Physical Examination

As with any traumatized patient, a complete history and detailed physical examination should be conducted. The preinjury level of function and additional medical conditions should be recorded because such knowledge will aid in determining whether conservative or operative treatment should be performed. The mechanism of injury must also be ascertained to help determine the severity of the injury and other associated injuries. The physical examination should include a detailed evaluation of the entire limb and other extremities to rule out ipsilateral and associated fractures.[8] The skin must be circumferentially inspected for open wounds, and a detailed neurological and vascular examination of the entire extremity should be documented. Higher-energy injuries can result in

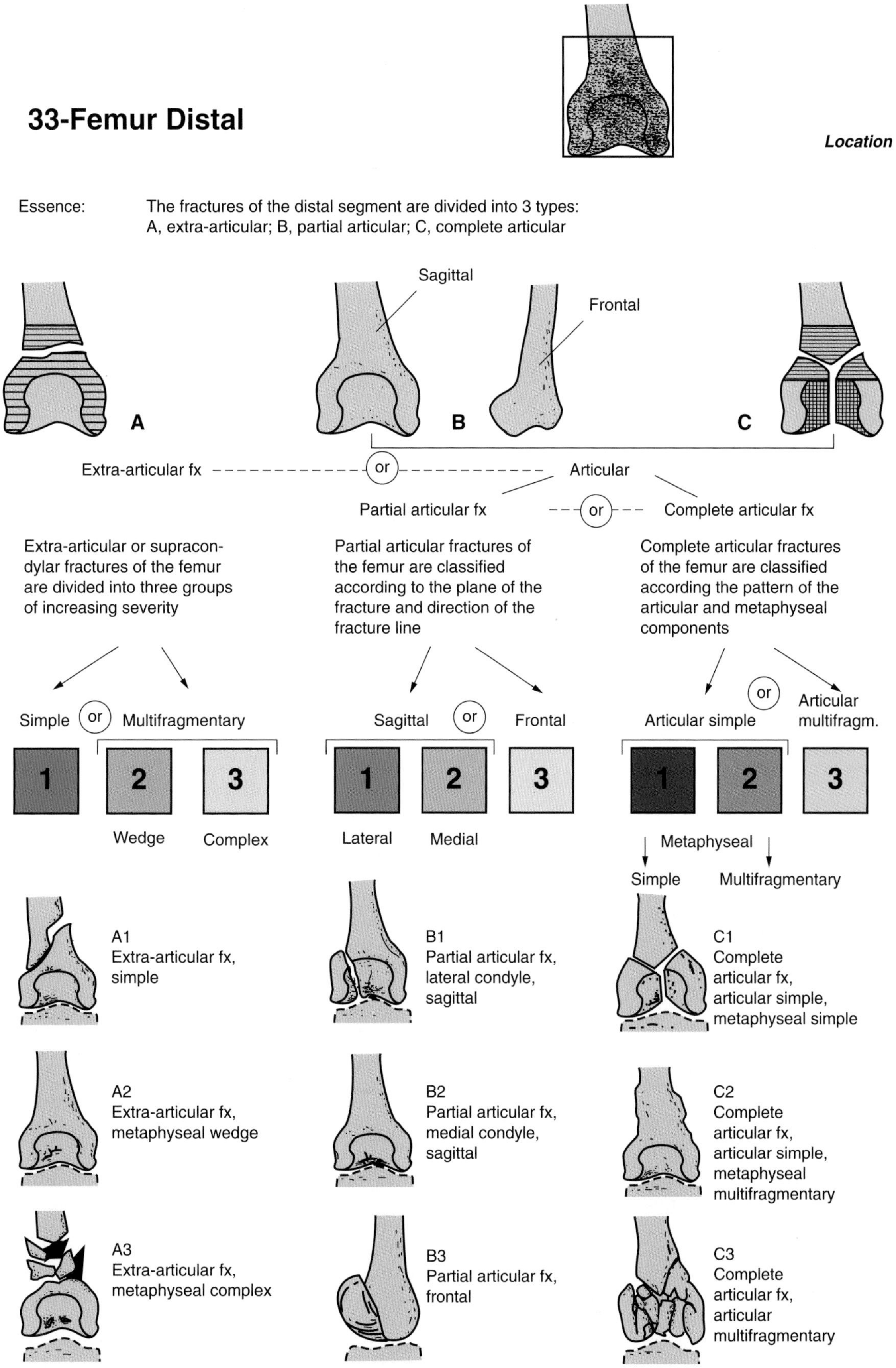

33-Femur Distal

Location

Essence: The fractures of the distal segment are divided into 3 types:
A, extra-articular; B, partial articular; C, complete articular

A

B

Sagittal

Frontal

C

Extra-articular fx – – – – – – – – – – – or – – – – – – – – – – – Articular

Partial articular fx – – – or – – – Complete articular fx

Extra-articular or supracon-dylar fractures of the femur are divided into three groups of increasing severity	Partial articular fractures of the femur are classified according to the plane of the fracture and direction of the fracture line	Complete articular fractures of the femur are classified according the pattern of the articular and metaphyseal components

Simple (or) Multifragmentary

Sagittal (or) Frontal

Articular simple (or) Articular multifragm.

1   **2**   **3**

Wedge   Complex

1   **2**   **3**

Lateral   Medial

1   **2**   **3**

Metaphyseal

Simple   Multifragmentary

A1
Extra-articular fx,
simple

B1
Partial articular fx,
lateral condyle,
sagittal

C1
Complete
articular fx,
articular simple,
metaphyseal simple

A2
Extra-articular fx,
metaphyseal wedge

B2
Partial articular fx,
medial condyle,
sagittal

C2
Complete
articular fx,
articular simple,
metaphyseal
multifragmentary

A3
Extra-articular fx,
metaphyseal complex

B3
Partial articular fx,
frontal

C3
Complete
articular fx,
articular
multifragmentary

Figure 65–3. AO/ASIF classification. (From Müller ME, Nazarian S, Koch P, Schatzker: The Comprehensive Classification of Fractures of Long Bones. Bern, Switzerland, M.E. Müller Foundation, 1995.)

laceration or rupture of the quadriceps tendon, the femoral artery as it exits the adductor hiatus, the popliteal artery, and knee ligaments.[4,6,81] The knee joint itself should be evaluated for an effusion because an effusion will often represent a radiographically unnoticed intercondylar split, an associated tibial plateau or patella fracture, and/or anterior or posterior cruciate ligament rupture.

In higher-energy fractures, the ankle-brachial index should be documented even if palpable pulses are present. A ratio less than 0.9 has been shown to correlate with a high incidence of arterial injuries, whereas ratios greater than 0.9 have not required vascular intervention. If abnormal, angiography and vascular surgery consultation should be performed.[37,51]

Radiographic Examination

As with any fracture, orthogonal views (AP and lateral) are indicated. Both knee and femur radiographs are necessary to fully evaluate the fracture and the entire femoral shaft. A traction radiograph may be helpful to better delineate all fracture fragments. Knee views will better diagnose intra-articular extension or comminution and associated patellar or tibial plateau fractures. Coronal condylar fractures (the so-called Hoffa fragment) seen in the lateral view must not be missed because the presence of such coronal splits will influence the selection of fixation devices.[4,30] Femoral shaft radiographs will determine the proximal extent of the fracture, segmental fracture patterns, or possibly ipsilateral femoral neck fractures. If femoral neck involvement is at all suspected, dedicated hip radiographs must be obtained because intraoperative discovery of this associated fracture can lead to different instrumentation and patient positioning. CT is indicated for comminuted fractures or if absolute certainty of all fracture lines cannot be gained from plain radiographs. Once all fracture planes are determined, more optimal fixation can then be applied. The authors routinely obtain CT scans when planning definitive internal fixation.

MANAGEMENT

Conservative versus Operative Management

Nonoperative management should be reserved for patients who are too debilitated and/or bedridden or who have prohibitive medical comorbid conditions. Other indications for conservative treatment may include nondisplaced, incomplete, and/or avulsion fractures. These situations are extremely rare.

The overwhelming majority of distal femoral fractures should be treated surgically. Operative stabilization allows increased mobility and early knee range of motion. The goals of surgical treatment are to reduce the joint anatomically, restore condyle-shaft alignment, and provide fracture stability to permit uneventful fracture healing and regain early knee range of motion.

Surgical Approaches

Lateral. The lateral approach, the most commonly used approach for supracondylar and distal femoral fractures, is an extension of the lateral approach to the femoral shaft. The patient is positioned supine and the incision begins along the midlateral aspect of the thigh and extends distally to the lateral femoral epicondyle. If joint visualization is necessary, the incision is extended distally and curved anteriorly toward the midportion of the patellar tendon. The iliotibial band is then incised in line with the skin incision. Distally, the joint capsule is incised as distal as necessary, and medial subluxation of the patella will allow intercondylar inspection. Proximally, the fascia of the vastus lateralis is incised and the muscle is dissected in a distal-to-proximal direction from the lateral intermuscular septum and posterior fascia, with ligation of any perforating arteries that are encountered. The muscle is then retracted anteriorly to expose the distal femoral shaft. The periosteum should be carefully preserved and no medial dissection should be performed to avoid devascularization of the fracture fragments.

Alternative Exposures

Medial. The medial approach is less commonly used because essentially all anatomically designed plates have been created for the lateral aspect of the distal femur. If necessary, however, the medial approach also offers adequate distal femur exposure. The incision is made along the medial aspect of the distal femur, just anterior to the sartorius, while avoiding the saphenous vein. The fascia is incised in line with the skin incision to expose the vastus medialis. The vastus medialis fascia is then incised at the medial intermuscular septum. As with the lateral approach, the muscle is dissected in a distal-to-proximal direction off the fascia (medial intermuscular septum), and any perforating arteries encountered are ligated. The muscle is retracted anteriorly to expose the medial aspect of the distal femur. The femoral artery remains posterior and proximal to the dissection. This approach may be useful for isolated medial condylar fractures or for corrective distal femur osteotomies.

Anteromedial and Anterolateral. The anteromedial and anterolateral approaches are rarely used because of additional adhesions that are created by dissection through the vastus intermedius. The adhesions often lead to decreased knee range of motion, and therefore these approaches should be reserved for fractures that do not extend into the midshaft of the femur or that do not already have a large open wound through this region.

The anteromedial approach involves dissection between the rectus femoris and vastus medialis. The fascia is incised over this palpable interval, and the distal portion of the incision includes the medial border of the patellar tendon to facilitate later closure. The vastus intermedius is then visualized, and splitting these fibers longitudinally allows exposure of the distal femur. The anterolateral approach involves dissection between the rectus femoris and vastus lateralis. Separation of these two muscles exposes the vastus intermedius. As with the anteromedial approach, the vastus intermedius must now be split longitudinally to allow visualization of the distal femoral shaft.

Anterior. The anterior approach requires a midline incision and a parapatellar arthrotomy. It allows excellent joint exposure but also requires separation of the vastus intermedius as the approach is extended proximally from the knee joint. A variation of the anterior approach described as the "swashbuckler" also allows for excellent joint exposure and is basically a lateral approach with an anteriorly placed incision.[75] Other variations of the aforementioned standard approaches have also been described.[52,58]

IMPLANTS—DESIGN AND FUNCTION

Numerous implants have been described and designed for supracondylar and distal femoral fractures. Implant types include short and long retrograde nails, various fixed-angled devices, and standard compression and buttress plates. Specific examples include the Zickel, GSH, and standard retrograde nails; the AO angled blade plate; the dynamic condylar screw; the condylar buttress plate; and more recently, locked plates.*

Intramedullary nails are available as shorter-length nails with multiple holes for interlocking or as longer "retrograde" nails that typically provide only two or three distal locking options. If sufficient distal bone is available, retrograde nailing is an excellent fixation option, especially for extra-articular fractures.

Plates initially consisted of a condylar buttress-type plate and standard compression plates. The AO angled blade plate and condylar compression screw were the early forms of "fixed"-angle devices, with the condylar compression screw allowing an additional degree of freedom and therefore easier insertion. Although the 95-degree angled blade plate does not anatomically match the medial distal femoral angle (99 degrees), the design allows for slight overbending of the plate to create compression of the opposite medial cortex. As the blade is inserted parallel to the joint line, the femoral shaft is reduced to the plate, which causes the "preloaded" plate to compress the opposite cortex. The 95-degree condylar compression screw, however, is extremely rigid and can therefore create a slight varus deformity if inserted improperly.

Currently, additional fixed-angle devices have become available in the form of anatomically designed plates that have locking screw technology and can be inserted either through a traditional open approach or percutaneously.[17,41] The locking plate design also creates a 95-degree angle between the distal screws and the plate. Proper insertion is achieved with the distal screws parallel to the joint line followed by reduction of the femoral shaft to the plate.[20,65] The advantage of locked plates over the traditional angled blade plate is seen with intercondylar split fractures. Insertion of an angled blade generates significantly more force

than does insertion of a threaded locked screw and can therefore displace an undisplaced or previously reduced and compressed intercondylar split. In addition, rotational freedom during insertion is present with locked plates, as with the condylar screw, while gaining the advantage of a fixed-angle device. Newer anatomically designed locking plates may also allow for variable-angle locked screws that are inserted at the surgeon's preferred angle and then locked to the plate once fully seated.

In cases of extreme osteopenia, osteoporosis, tumor, or other conditions with poor bone quality, a second medial implant has also been described to add to construct stability.[26,35,48,49,64] The addition of bone cement has likewise been advocated in similar situations to achieve increased screw purchase.[5,77] With the advent of modern locking plate technology, the need for adjunctive medial fixation or cement augmentation has essentially been eliminated.

The choice of implant is dependent on the location of the fracture, the fracture pattern, existing hardware, bone quality, and surgeon preference.

TREATMENT

Initially, as with all fractures, splinting and immobilization were favored over internal fixation. In the 1940s and 1950s, internal fixation was reported, but without overwhelming success.[1,79,85] As technology advanced and techniques improved, success rates with internal fixation began to increase. The Swiss AO group in 1958 defined the goals of open reduction and internal fixation as follows: (1) anatomic reduction, (2) preservation of the blood supply, (3) stable internal fixation, and (4) early mobilization.[54] Wenzl and Schatzker began documenting improved results with the AO principles and showed open reduction and internal fixation to be superior to conservative management.[66-68,84] Other authors soon reported similar findings.[11,27,52,58,72,73,76] Today, though slightly modified, the AO principles are still being used and the results of surgical treatment remain superior to those of nonoperative management for displaced fractures.

Conservative Treatment

Conservative management of distal femoral and supracondylar fractures has fallen out of favor as surgical techniques, implant designs, and rehabilitation protocols have continued to progress and yield outcomes superior to those of nonoperative treatment.* Certain situations, however, still require nonoperative management, and it is therefore necessary to remain familiar with the conservative treatment options.

For patients with low-energy, extra-articular, nondisplaced fractures who either refuse or cannot medically tolerate a surgical procedure, cast bracing or casting is recommended. Non-weightbearing must be enforced until

---

*References 24, 29, 33, 54, 63, 65, 69, 71, 73, 90.

*References 11, 27, 52, 57, 58, 66-68, 72, 73, 76, 84.

adequate healing is achieved to avoid creating a deformity or unstable fracture. Knee joint stiffness typically becomes problematic with longer than 6 weeks of immobilization.[21]

Special attention must be paid to the skin condition during casting or bracing. Paraplegics and quadriplegics also present a treatment challenge because skin breakdown can occur without warning and lead to further setbacks.

Operative Management

Operative stabilization of low-energy, nondisplaced, or minimally displaced fractures is similar to operative stabilization of displaced or high-energy fractures, but usually with less difficulty in achieving anatomic alignment. For extra-articular fractures, anatomic reduction is less important than anatomic alignment. Intra-articular fractures, however, should undergo anatomic reduction to decrease the chance of later arthritis. The more distal the fracture and the greater the mechanism of injury, the more the likelihood of an unrecognized intra-articular split. Depending on the location of the fracture, either an intramedullary device or a plate is typically used to achieve fracture stability. The ideal implant would be inserted with minimal dissection and allow immediate knee range of motion and early weightbearing.

High-energy injuries involving the distal femur are frequently comminuted and have significant intra-articular involvement (Fig. 65–4A-D). If the fracture is an open fracture, adequate initial débridement must be performed, followed by thorough irrigation and either temporary or definitive stabilization. If temporary stabilization is chosen, a spanning external fixator can be used with the pins for the fixator placed away from the region of future definitive fixation. Two pins are typically inserted either anteriorly or laterally into the femur and two pins into the proximal end of the tibia, with the frame then spanning the knee joint (Fig. 65–5). If the soft tissues appear stable and the appropriate studies and implants are available, definitive fixation may be performed at the time of initial débridement. When significant intra-articular comminution warrants a CT scan, a staged approach must be adopted if the CT scan is not available prior to the initial open fracture débridement. The distal femur has better soft-tissue coverage than the tibia, so plate application can be safely performed as the initial surgical treatment unless significant soft-tissue loss and/or excessive gross contamination is present. If tissue transfer is required for bone or plate coverage, or for both, initial spanning external fixation would be more appropriate. Intravenous antibiotic coverage based on the type and degree of soft-tissue wounds is necessary, as in all long-bone open fractures. Initial bone grafting of open fractures is not recommended because of the increased risk of infection, although the literature mostly pertains to open tibia rather than open femur fractures. Intraoperative techniques that can assist in achieving adequate length or fracture reduction include manual traction, application of the AO femoral distractor, and use of the AO articulating tensioning device.

Operative Treatment: General Principle

Regardless of whether a plate or nail is chosen to stabilize an intra-articular distal femoral fracture, the following principles must be adhere to:
1. Achieving anatomic reduction with isolated lag screw fixation of the articular surface
2. Maximizing distal fragment fixation
3. Obtaining correct coronal and sagittal plane alignment (5 to 7 degrees valgus)
4. Obtaining correct leg length
5. Obtaining correct leg rotation
6. Achieving stable proximal fragment fixation
7. Preserving fracture fragment viability by avoiding periosteal stripping and medial dissection

Intramedullary Devices

Once the "personality" of the fracture has been defined, the surgeon can then decide on the most appropriate implant. The authors find retrograde nailing useful for extra-articular fractures with a distal fragment of sufficient length to allow stable distal fixation. Occasionally, a fracture with extensive femoral shaft extension and simple intra-articular involvement can be managed effectively with lag screws and a retrograde nail. If a retrograde intramedullary nail is selected, an anterior incision is made over the patellar tendon and a medial miniarthrotomy performed on the medial border of the tendon. The entry point in the trochlear groove must be accurately placed to avoid injury to the anterior cruciate ligament and patella. Ideally, the entry point should cheat a few millimeters medial to center on the AP view and at the intersection of Blumensaat's line and the sclerotic line representing the femoral notch on the lateral view.[10] If the nail is inserted in the center and not directed slightly lateral to remain in line with the anatomic femoral axis, a varus deformity will result when the nail enters the isthmus of the femoral canal. Because there is no canal fit in the metaphyseal flare of the distal femur, it is easy to create an angular deformity during nail insertion. A flexion or extension deformity can also be created if reduction in the sagittal plane is not obtained and maintained before reaming and insertion of the nail. Vigilance is required to avoid malalignment. It is important to understand that the nail will not reduce the fracture in this situation.

Early treatment of supracondylar femoral fractures with a retrograde intramedullary device was reported by Zickel and associates in 1977.[90] Difficulty was noted in achieving stability in patients with intra-articular comminution. A subsequent report by Zickel and colleagues showed improved results with the Zickel nail, but half the patients with intra-articular fractures did not regain more than 90 degrees of knee motion.[91]

Antegrade nailing of supracondylar femoral fractures has also been reported as a successful procedure.[8,44] Its effectiveness is limited with intercondylar fractures unless adjunctive fixation is used.[44,78] Adequate distal fragment length is necessary to achieve stable distal fixation.

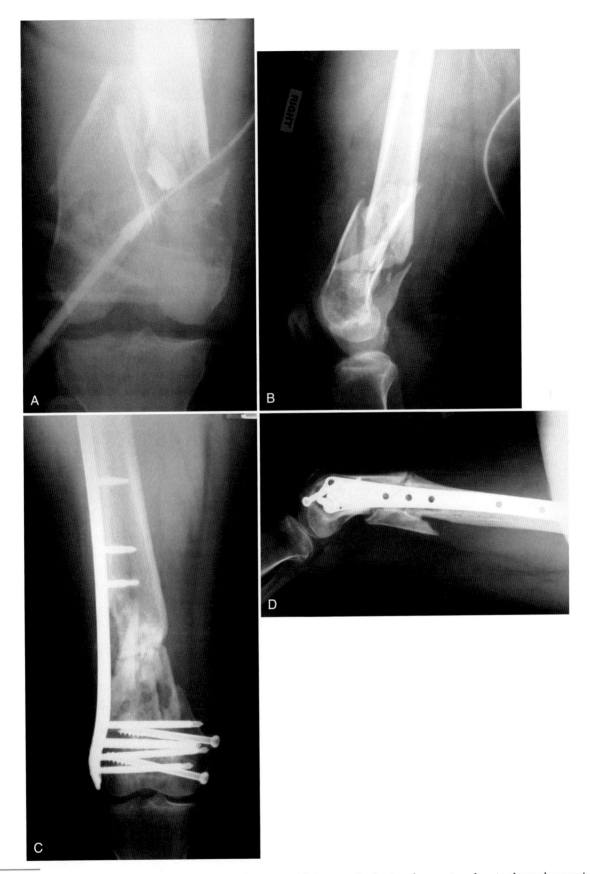

Figure 65–4. Radiographs depicting a high-energy fracture with intra-articular involvement and metaphyseal comminution (**A** and **B**) and a healed fracture with lag screws for intra-articular fractures and a plate spanning the fracture zone (**C** and **D**).

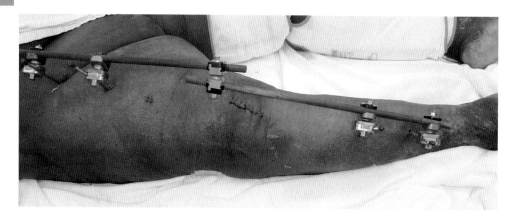

Figure 65–5. Photograph demonstrating a temporary spanning external fixator for an open fracture of the distal end of the femur.

Tornetta and Tiburzi achieved a 100% union rate with antegrade nailing of supracondylar femoral fractures but reported a 50% incidence of valgus malunion in patients in whom nailing was performed in the lateral position.[78] Dominquez and associates also noted successful results with antegrade nailing of distal femoral fractures and had only 1 nonunion in a series of 20 fractures.[15]

Retrograde nailing continues to be more popular than antegrade nailing because it appears to be easier to control the distal fragments. The so-called supracondylar nail was inserted through the knee joint and not the condyles.[29] Lucas and colleagues reported union of all 25 fractures in their series with use of the GSH nail, although 4 fractures did require bone grafting.[45] Danziger and associates also demonstrated successful treatment with the GSH nail, with all but 1 of 16 fractures healing in their series.[12] Iannacone and associates, however, reported four nonunions, five delayed unions, and four stress nail fatigue fractures in 41 patients.[32] During their series, the nail was changed from an initial 11-mm nail with 6.4-mm locking screws to 12- and 13-mm nails with 5.0-mm locking screws. All device failures were noted with the 11-mm nail. In a series of fractures in elderly patients that involved the supracondylar region, Janzing and coauthors reported 89% good or excellent results with use of the GSH nail.[34] They did comment, however, on poor fixation distally with locking screws in osteoporotic bone.

Mechanical testing to evaluate various fixation constructs has been reported. Firoozbaksh and associates tested retrograde nailing versus DCS plate fixation in a synthetic bone model.[18] The DCS plate was found to be stiffer in lateral bending and torsion, but no significant difference was found with respect to bending stiffness in varus and flexion. Because the most common clinical forms of failure occurred in varus and flexion, both devices were deemed biomechanically adequate fixation for these fractures.[18] Koval and coworkers compared a short retrograde nail, an antegrade nail, and a DCS plate in a cadaveric model.[40] They demonstrated the antegrade nail to be the least stable and recommended use of the DCS plate when maximum stiffness is desired. In a comparison of a locked intramedullary nail and the 95-degree angled plate, David and associates also concluded that the plate provided greater stiffness.[13] Ito and colleagues similarly compared the 95-degree angled plate with both the GSH and AO supracondylar nail and concluded that the

nails were inferior in torsion and varus loading.[33] With respect to specific nail comparison, Voor and associates compared fatigue testing on 5- and 12-hole supracondylar nails and found better fatigue strength in 5-hole nails because of fewer stress risers and therefore recommended their use.[80] More recently, biomechanical comparisons of modern retrograde nails have even been reported.[31] The authors routinely use long retrograde nails when treating these fractures. Long nails allow the fit in the femoral diaphysis to assist with proximal fixation and alignment and avoid the need for interlocking screws in the femoral diaphysis.

Plates

Plate insertion requires knowledge of the femoral condylar anatomy in the coronal, sagittal, and axial planes. Although most distal femoral or supracondylar plates are anatomically designed, they still require correct placement to achieve anatomically aligned reduction. The need for double plating and intramedullary plating for medially comminuted fractures has essentially been eliminated with the advent of locked plating.[45,83,92] The locked plate has replaced the traditional condylar plates and, to a large extent, the condylar screw and blade plate (Fig. 65–6).[42,43,45,62,69,74] Four locked screws distally have been shown to be equivalent in fixation to the standard blade of a 95-degree blade plate.[39] The locked plates can be inserted percutaneously and thus allow easier insertion, as well as enhanced stability, especially in comminuted fractures of both the medial and lateral columns (Fig. 65–7).[83] The locked plate must be correctly placed on the distal end of the femur to allow precise placement of the locked screws because the angle of screw insertion is not variable and the screws will lock into the plate only at the predetermined angle. Once the correct plate location is achieved in the AP and lateral views, the appropriate femoral length and alignment must be restored before proximal plate fixation.[36,88] As with intramedullary nailing, flexion or extension deformities can occur and are often difficult to assess intraoperatively if an external locking handle of the plate partially obstructs a fluoroscopic image.[43] Provisional fixation of the plate both distally and proximally is encouraged to avoid extensive revision of screw or plate

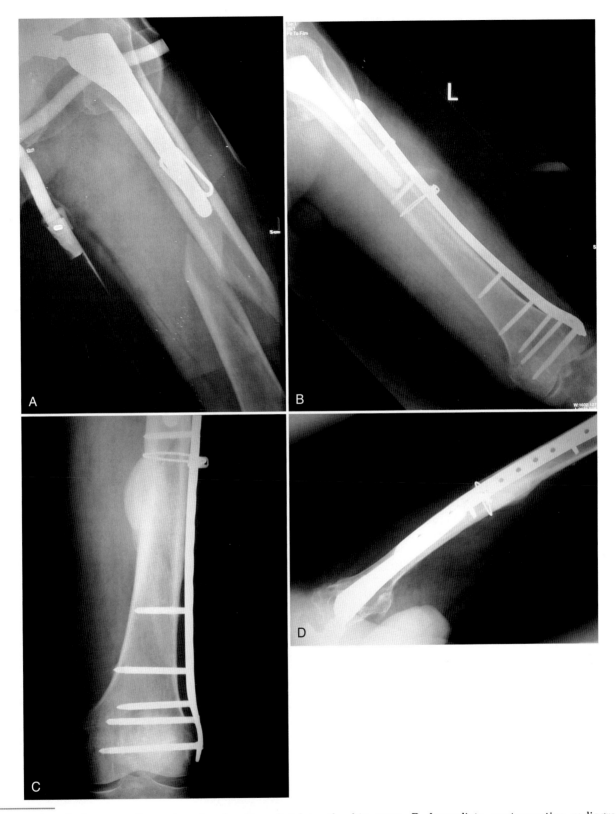

Figure 65–6. **A**, Injury radiographs of a fracture distal to the hip stem. **B**, Immediate postoperative radiograph. **C** and **D**, Healed radiographs with callus formation at the fracture site. The fracture site was exposed only proximally for cerclage wiring and left undisturbed more distally.

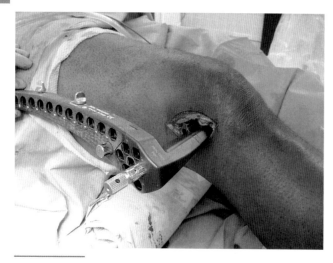

Figure 65–7. Photograph demonstrating percutaneous insertion of a locked plate on the distal end of the femur with a guide for insertion of screws (L.I.S.S., Synthes, Paoli, PA).

placement should adjustments be necessary. If the plate is fixed distally first, a small amount of anterior or posterior plate angulation will translate into an increasing amount of plate-shaft mismatch as one progresses proximally. A flexion or extension deformity will therefore result as one reduces the plate to the shaft. To avoid extensive intraoperative revision, a single initial locked screw can be inserted distally without seating the head to allow rotational freedom of the plate. Once appropriate length is restored through gentle manual traction or the use of a femoral distractor, the plate can be fixed proximally to the shaft. The distal screw is then seated and locked to achieve rotational control. If adjustments are required, distal screw revision is simplified because only a single screw needs to be removed. The surgeon must be extremely vigilant to avoid plate malposition or fracture malalignment.

Plate fixation of the distal femur with a condylar screw, angled blade plate, or lateral condylar buttress plate is a well-established procedure described in detail elsewhere.[1,7,50,60,63,71,79,84] Fixation of intra-articular distal femoral fractures with a DCS plate has been compared with nonoperative treatment in elderly patients and shown to result in fewer malunions, fewer nonunions, and a decrease in complications such as respiratory infections, deep vein thrombosis, and pressure sores.[9] Other forms of plate fixation have also provided satisfactory results.[1,7,50,60,84] Wenzl documented the first series of supracondylar femoral fractures stabilized with the angled blade plate and reported 73.5% good to excellent results.[84] Indirect reduction, pioneered by Mast and associates,[48] has changed fracture fixation techniques and continues to evolve. The lateral condylar buttress plate and angled blade plate combined with indirect reduction techniques have provided 84% to 87% good to excellent results in treating supracondylar femoral fractures with intra-articular comminution.[7,60] Malunion and nonunion have been shown to often be the result of bone loss, severe osteoporosis, and/or medial column comminution.[2] Because of medial comminution, osteoporosis, and/or

bone loss, double plating, intramedullary plating, bone grafting, and the use of bone cement are some of the techniques described to add additional medial stability and avoid varus collapse or fixation failure.[5,26,35,48,49,64,77]

The locked plated construct, even in osteoporotic bone, has been shown to provide enhanced stability and rarely requires additional fixation.[16,22,46,74,83,92] Locked plating has evolved as an extension of indirect reduction techniques, and the early results appear to be better than those of traditional techniques.[42,43,69,83] Weight and Collinge reported on 22 patients with unstable distal femoral fractures (AO/OTA types A2, A3, C2, and C3) stabilized with percutaneous locked plating and documented a 100% union rate.[83] All fractures healed without need for bone grafting, and no hardware failures were noted. Average knee range of motion was 5 to 114 degrees. Kregor and colleagues also documented similar results in 103 distal femoral fractures stabilized with percutaneous locked plating.[43] They reported a 93% union rate after the initial procedure and average knee motion of 1 to 109 degrees. Only 1 of 68 closed fractures required later bone grafting, whereas 6 of 35 open fractures needed later bone grafting (because of bone loss) to eventually achieve union in all fractures. Of importance was the fact that no fracture sustained loss of distal fixation. Schutz and associates also reported early healing in 37 of 40 patients treated with locked percutaneous plating of the distal femur.[69]

COMPLICATIONS

Complications of nonoperative treatment include skin breakdown from casting, stiffness from prolonged immobilization, malunion, and nonunion. Skin breakdown often occurs in patients who are bedridden and may not be surgical candidates. Knee stiffness is seen more frequently in nonoperatively treated patients than in operatively stabilized patients because early motion will occur through the fracture site and therefore lengthier immobilization is required. Malunion is also more common with closed treatment because achieving fracture stability is more difficult without internal fixation (Fig. 63–8A and B).[9] Although nonunion can also occur, some bedridden patients fare better with nonunion than with a postoperative infection or wound complication. Other complications with conservative care include deep vein thrombosis, respiratory infections, and pressure sores.[9]

Infection remains the most significant complication of operative treatment (Fig. 63–9). Although the infection rate was previously reported to be as high as 20%, advances in surgical technique, patient selection, and perioperative antibiotic therapy have continued to decrease infection rates to below 7%.[7,11,43,57,59,60,63,72,83] Factors that contribute to an increased risk for infection include open fractures, high-energy trauma, lengthy and extensive surgical dissection, and inadequate surgical stabilization.[28]

Mast and associates pioneered the technique of indirect reduction and biological, balanced, stable internal fixation.[48] Bolhofner et al and Ostrum and Geel have applied these concepts and reported much improved results when

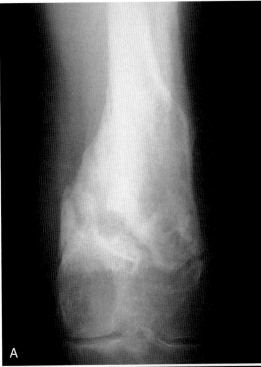

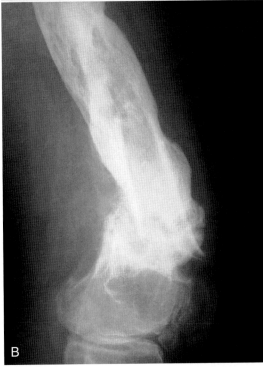

Figure 65–8. **A and B**, Radiographs showing malunion of a supracondylar femoral fracture treated 12 years earlier by skeletal traction.

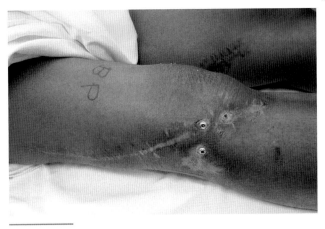

Figure 65–9. Clinical photograph revealing exposed hardware with active drainage from wounds.

prophylaxis and appropriate antibiotic administration, followed by initial immediate surgical wound irrigation and débridement. Controversy still exists regarding the number of débridement sessions required and the timing of wound closure. These issues must be individualized by the surgeon and should take into account the mechanism of injury, the quality of local tissue at the time of initial surgery, and the presence or absence of any gross contamination. Once the tissues are judged to be healthy and clean, definitive wound closure should be performed. The sooner the traumatized region can resume its previous biological environment, the sooner the healing process can occur. Ostermann and associates demonstrated decreased infection rates in open fractures when antibiotic polymethylmethacrylate beads were inserted into the fracture zone, but no prospective, randomized study has evaluated the routine use of beads in open distal femoral fractures.[59] The senior author uses beads routinely in high-energy open fractures with bone loss. These beads not only provide high local concentrations of antibiotic but also make subsequent bone grafting easier by "keeping the space open."

Nonunion is a possible complication of any fracture and initially occurred in 10% to 19% of patients in the early reports of open reduction and internal fixation of supracondylar femoral fractures (Fig. 63–10A and B).[53,57,72,89] The current literature has demonstrated a significant improvement in the nonunion rate of operatively stabilized supracondylar femoral fractures, and it is now reported to be between 0% and 5%.[23,42,43,57,68,83,84,89] Two recent studies have documented successful treatment of distal femoral nonunion with union rates of 95% to 100%.[25,82] Haidukewych and associates reported on distal femoral nonunion in 22 patients and achieved union in 21 with repeat open reduction and internal fixation and bone grafting.[25] Achieving stable fixation of the distal fragment was critical to successful union. Autogenous bone grafting was used in the vast majority of cases. Wang and Weng documented a 100% union rate in 13 distal femoral nonunions treated with cortical strut allografting, autogenous bone grafting, and internal fixation with angled blade plates and intramedullary nails.[82]

compared with the older techniques described in the literature.[7,60] More recent techniques involving percutaneous locked plating have also decreased infection rates to 0% to 3%.[43,83]

Open fracture management continues to improve. The tenets of open fracture care include immediate tetanus

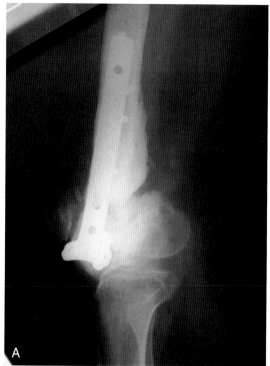

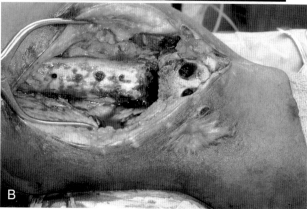

Figure 65–10. **A,** Radiograph of fracture nonunion and hardware migration. **B,** Intraoperative photograph demonstrating fracture nonunion and enlarged screw holes secondary to loosening and bone absorption.

Malunion is another complication and was initially seen most commonly in fractures with significant medial comminution treated with conventional nonlocking plates. Traditional plating techniques have been associated with malunion greater than 5 degrees in the frontal plane in as many as 26% of patients.[88] Newer plating techniques with anatomically designed locked plates also initially resulted in higher than expected rates of malunion greater than 5 degrees in the frontal plane, with rates reported to be as high as 20%.[69] Percutaneous techniques require vigilance to avoid plate malposition and fracture malalignment. With more experience and greater understanding of the newer implants, percutaneous locked plating continues to improve and most recently has resulted in malunion rates as low as 4.5% to 6%.[42,83]

SUMMARY AND FUTURE DIRECTIONS

Internal fixation techniques for distal femoral fractures continue to evolve. More biologically friendly plating techniques using locked screw technology for improved mechanical performance and percutaneous plate insertion and screw targeting for preservation of fracture vascularity have improved union rates and essentially eliminated varus collapse and the need for bone grafting. Newer-generation locking plates offer polyaxial locking screws in conjunction with fixed locking screws. Such "hybrid plate" technology will offer even more versatility in achieving maximal distal fragment fixation. The role of orthobiological agents remains undefined.

References

1. Altenberg AR, Shorkey RL: Blade-plate fixation in nonunion and in complicated fractures of the supracondylar region of the femur. J Bone Joint Surg Am 31:312, 1949.
2. Althausen PL, Lee MA, Finkemeier CG, et al: Operative stabilization of supracondylar femur fractures above total knee arthroplasty: A comparison of four treatment methods. J Arthroplasty 18:834, 2003.
3. Arneson TJ, Melton LJ, Lewallen DG, et al: Epidemiology of diaphyseal and distal femoral fractures in Rochester, Minnesota, 1965-1984. Clin Orthop 234:188, 1988.
4. Baker BJ, Escobedo EM, Nork SE, et al: Hoffa fracture: A common association with high-energy supracondylar fracture of the distal femur. AJR Am J Roentgenol 178:994, 2002.
5. Benum P: The use of cement as an adjunct to internal fixation of supracondylar fractures of osteoporotic femurs. Acta Orthop Scand 48:52, 1977.
6. Blacksin MF, Zurlo JV, Levy AS: Internal derangement of the knee after ipsilateral femoral shaft fracture: MR imaging findings. Skeletal Radiol 27:434, 1998.
7. Bolhofner BR, Carmen B, Clifford P: The results of open reduction and internal fixation of distal femur fractures using a biological (indirect) reduction technique. J Orthop Trauma 10:372, 1996.
8. Butler MS, Brumback RJ, Ellison TS, et al: Interlocking intramedullary nailing for ipsilateral fractures of the femoral shaft and distal part of the femur. J Bone Joint Surg Am 73:1492, 1991.
9. Butt MS, Krikler SR, Ali MS: Displaced fractures of the distal femur in elderly patients. J Bone Joint Surg Am 77:110, 1995.
10. Carmack DB, Moed BR, Kingston C, et al: Identification of the optimal intercondylar starting point for retrograde femoral nailing: An anatomic study. J Trauma 55:692, 2003.
11. Chiron HS, Casey P: Fractures of the distal third of the femur treated by internal fixation. Clin Orthop 100:160, 1974.
12. Danziger M, Caucci D, Zechner SB, et al: Treatment of intercondylar and supracondylar distal femur fractures using the GSH supracondylar nail. Am J Orthop 8:684, 1995.
13. David SM, Harrow ME, Peindl RD, et al: Comparative biomechanical analysis of supracondylar femur fracture fixation: Locked intramedullary nail versus 95 degree angled plate. J Orthop Trauma 11:344, 1997.
14. Dickson KF, Galland MW, Barrack RL, et al: Magnetic resonance imaging of the knee after ipsilateral femur fracture. J Orthop Trauma 16:567, 2002.
15. Dominquez I, Moro Rodriquez E, DePedro Moro JA, et al: Antegrade nailing for fractures of the distal femur. Clin Orthop 350:74, 1998.
16. Egol KA, Kubiak EN, Fulkerson E, et al: Biomechanics of locked plates and screws. J Orthop Trauma 18:488, 2004.
17. Farouk O, Krettek C, Miclau T, et al: The minimal invasive plate osteosynthesis: Is percutaneous plating biologically superior to the traditional technique? J Orthop Trauma 13:401, 1999.
18. Firoozbaksh K, Behzadi K, DeCoster TA, et al: Mechanics of retrograde nail versus plate fixation for supracondylar femur fractures. J Orthop Trauma 9:152, 1995.

19. Fracture and dislocation compendium. Orthopaedic Trauma Association Committee for Coding and Classification. J Orthop Trauma 10(Suppl 1):v, 1, 1996.

20. Frigg R, Appenzeller A, Christensen R, et al: The development of the distal femur Less Invasive Stabilization System (LISS). Injury 32(Suppl 3):SC24, 2001.

21. Gausewitz S, Hohl M: The significance of early motion in the treatment of tibial plateau fractures. Clin Orthop 202:135, 1986.

22. Gautier E, Sommer C: Guidelines for the clinical application of the LCP. Injury 32(Suppl 2):B63, 2003.

23. Giles JB, DeLee JC, Heckman J et al: Supracondylar-intercondylar fractures of the femur treated with a supracondylar plate and lag screw. J Bone Joint Surg Am 64:864, 1982.

24. Goesling T, Frenk A, Appenzeller A, et al: LISS plate: Design, mechanical and biomechanical characteristics. Injury 34 (Suppl 1):A11, 2003.

25. Haidukewych GJ, Berry DJ, Jacofsky DJ, et al: Treatment of supracondylar nonunions with open reduction and internal fixation. Am J Orthop 32:564, 2003.

26. Hall MF: Two-plane fixation of acute supracondylar and intracondylar fractures of the femur. South Med J 71:1474, 1978.

27. Healy WL, Brooker AF: Distal femoral fractures: Comparison of open and closed methods of treatment. Clin Orthop 174:166, 1983.

28. Helfet DL, Lorich DG: Fractures of the distal femur. In Browner BD, Jupiter JB, Levine AM, Trafton PG (eds): Skeletal Trauma, vol 2, 2nd ed. Philadelphia, WB Saunders, 1997, p 2033.

29. Henry S, Trager S, Green S, et al: Management of supracondylar fractures of the femur with the GSH supracondylar nail. Contemp Orthop 22:631, 1991.

30. Holmes SM, Bomback D, Baumgaertner MR: Coronal fractures of the femoral condyle: A brief report of five cases. J Orthop Trauma 18:316, 2004.

31. Hora N, Markel DC, Haynes A, et al: Biomechanical analysis of supracondylar femoral fractures fixed with modern retrograde intramedullary nails. J Orthop Trauma 13:539, 1999.

32. Iannacone WM, Bennett FS, DeLong WG, et al: Initial experience with the treatment of supracondylar femoral fractures using the supracondylar intramedullary nail: A preliminary report. J Orthop Trauma 8:322, 1994.

33. Ito K, Grass R, Zwipp H: Internal fixation of supracondylar femur fractures: Comparative biomechanical performance of the 95-degree angled blade and retrograde nails. J Orthop Trauma 12:259, 1998.

34. Janzing HM, Stockman B, Van Damme G, et al: The retrograde intramedullary nail: Prospective experience in patients older than sixty-five years. J Orthop Trauma 12:330, 1998.

35. Jazrawi LM, Kummer FJ, Simon JA, et al: New technique for treatment of unstable distal femur fractures by locked double plating: Case report and biomechanical evaluation. J Trauma 48:87, 2000.

36. Karunakar MA, Kellam JF, Zehnter MK, et al: Avoiding malunion with 95-degree fixed-angle distal femoral implants. J Orthop Trauma 18:443, 2004.

37. Klineberg EO, Crites BM, Flinn WR, et al: The role of arteriography in assessing popliteal artery injury in knee dislocation. J Trauma 56:786, 2004.

38. Kolmert L, Wulff K: Epidemiology and treatment of distal femoral fractures in adults. Acta Orthop Scand 53:957, 1982.

39. Koval KJ, Hoehl JJ, Kummer FJ, et al: Distal femoral fixation: A biomechanical comparison of the standard condylar buttress plate, a locked buttress plate, and the 95 degree blade plate. J Orthop Trauma 11:521, 1997.

40. Koval KJ, Kummer FJ, Bharam S, et al: Distal femoral fixation: A laboratory comparison of the 95 degree plate, antegrade and retrograde inserted reamed intramedullary nails. J Orthop Trauma 10: 378, 1996.

41. Kregor PJ: Distal femur fractures with complex articular involvement: Management by articular exposure and submuscular fixation. Orthop Clin North Am 33:153, 2002.

42. Kregor PJ, Stannard J, Zlowodski M, et al: Distal femoral fracture fixation utilizing the Less Invasive Stabilization System (LISS): The technique and early results. Injury 32:SC32, 2001.

43. Kregor PJ, Stannard JA, Zlowodski M, et al: Treatment of distal femur fractures using the less invasive stabilization system: Surgical experience and early clinical results in 103 fractures. J Orthop Trauma 18:509, 2004.

44. Leung KS, Shen WY, So WS, et al: Interlocking intramedullary nailing for supracondylar and intercondylar fractures of the distal part of the femur. J Bone Joint Surg Am 73:332, 1991.

45. Lucas SE, Seligson D, Henry SL: Intramedullary supracondylar nailing of femoral fractures: A preliminary report of the GSH supracondylar nail. Clin Orthop 296:200, 1993.

46. Marti A, Fankhauser C, Frenk A, et al: Biomechanical evaluation of the less invasive stabilization system for internal fixation of distal femur fractures. J Orthop Trauma 5:482, 2001.

47. Martinet O, Cordey J, Harder Y et al: The epidemiology of fractures of the distal femur. Injury 31(Suppl 3):SC62, 2000.

48. Mast J, Jakob R, Ganz R: Planning and Reduction Techniques in Fracture Surgery. New York, Springer-Verlag, 1989.

49. Matelic TM, Monroe MT, Mast JW: The use of endosteal substitution in the treatment of recalcitrant nonunions of the femur: Report of seven cases. J Orthop Trauma 10:1, 1996.

50. Merchan EC, Maestu PR, Blanco RP: Blade-plating of closed displaced supracondylar fractures of the distal femur with the AO system. J Trauma 32:174, 1992.

51. Mills WJ, Barei DP, McNair P: The value of the ankle-brachial index for diagnosing arterial injury after knee dislocation: A prospective study. J Trauma 56:1261, 2004.

52. Mize RD, Bucholz RW, Grogan DP: Surgical treatment of distal, comminuted fractures of the distal end of the femur. J Bone Joint Surg Am 64:871, 1982.

53. Moore T, Watson T, Green S, et al: Complications of surgically treated supracondylar fractures of the femur. J Trauma 27:402, 1987.

54. Müller ME, Allgower M, Schneider R, Willenegger H: Manual of Internal Fixation, 3rd ed. New York, Springer-Verlag, 1991.

55. Müller ME, Allgower M, Schneider R, Willenegger H: Insertion of the plates into the distal femur. In Manual of Internal Fixation, 3rd ed. New York, Springer-Verlag, 1995, p 266.

56. Müller ME, Nazarian S, Koch P, et al: The Comprehensive Classification of Fractures of Long Bones. New York, Springer-Verlag, 1990, p 116.

57. Neer CS, Grantham SA, Shelton ML: Supracondylar fracture of the adult femur. J Bone Joint Surg Am 49:591, 1967.

58. Olerud S: Operative treatment of supracondylar fractures of the femur: Technique and results in fifteen cases. J Bone Joint Surg Am 54:1015, 1972.

59. Ostermann PA, Seligson D, Henry SL: Local antibiotic therapy for severe open fractures. A review of 1085 consecutive cases. J Bone Joint Surg Br 77:93, 1995.

60. Ostrum RF, Geel C: Indirect reduction and internal fixation of supracondylar femur fractures without bone graft. J Orthop Trauma 9:278, 1995.

61. Paley D, Herzenberg JE, Tetsworth K, et al: Deformity planning for frontal and sagittal plane corrective osteotomies. Orthop Clin North Am 25:426, 1994.

62. Ricci AR, Yue JJ, Taffet R, et al: Less invasive stabilization system for treatment of distal femur fractures. Am J Orthop 33:250, 2004.

63. Sanders R, Regazzoni P, Reudi T: Treatment of supracondylar-intraarticular fractures of the femur using the dynamic condylar screw. J Orthop Trauma 3:214, 1989.

64. Sanders RW, Swiontkowski M, Rosen H, et al: Complex fractures and malunions of the distal femur: Results of treatment with double plates. J Bone Joint Surg Am 73:341, 1991.

65. Schandelmaier P, Partenheimer A, Koenemann B, et al: Distal femoral fractures and LISS stabilization. Injury 32(Suppl 3):SC55, 2001.

66. Schatzker J: Fractures of the distal femur revisited. Clin Orthop 347:43, 1998.

67. Schatzker J, Horne G, Waddell J: The Toronto experience with the supracondylar fracture of the femur, 1966-1972. Injury 6:113, 1975.

68. Schatzker J, Lambert DC: Supracondylar fractures of the distal femur. Clin Orthop 138:77, 1979.

69. Schutz M, Muller M, Krettek C, et al: Minimally invasive fracture stabilization of distal femoral fractures with the LISS: A prospective multicenter study. Results of a clinical study with special emphasis on difficult cases. Injury 32(Suppl 3):SC48, 2001.

70. Seinsheimer F III: Fractures of the distal femur. Clin Orthop 153:169, 1980.

71. Shewring DJ, Meggitt BF: Fractures of the distal femur treated with the AO dynamic condylar screw. J Bone Joint Surg Am 74:122, 1992.

72. Siliski JM, Mahring M, Hofer HP: Supracondylar-intercondylar fractures of the femur: Treatment by internal fixation. J Bone Joint Surg Am 71:95, 1989.

73. Slatis P, Ryoppy S, Huttinen V: AO osteosynthesis of fractures of the distal third of the femur. Acta Orthop Scand 42:162, 1971.

74. Sommer C, Gautier E, Muller M, et al: First clinical results of the locking compression plate (LCP). Injury 34(Suppl 2):B43, 2003.

75. Starr AJ, Jones AL, Reinert CM: The "swashbuckler." A modified anterior approach for fractures of the distal femur. J Orthop Trauma 13:138, 1999.

76. Stewart MJ, Sisk TD, Wallace SL: Fractures of the distal third of the femur: A comparison of methods of treatment. J Bone Joint Surg Am 48:784, 1966.

77. Struhl S, Szporn MN, Cobelli NJ, et al: Cemented internal fixation for supracondylar femur fractures in osteoporotic patients. J Orthop Trauma 4:151, 1990.

78. Tornetta P, Tiburzi D: Antegrade interlocked nailing of distal femoral fractures after gunshot wounds. J Orthop Trauma 8:220, 1994.

79. Unmansky AL: Blade-plate internal fixation for fracture of the distal end of the femur. Bull Hosp Jt Dis 9:18, 1948.

80. Voor MJ, Verst DA, Mladsi SW, et al: Fatigue properties of a twelve-hole versus a five-hole intramedullary supracondylar nail. J Orthop Trauma 11:98, 1997.

81. Walling AK, Seradge H, Spiegel PG: Injuries to the knee ligaments with fractures of the femur. J Bone Joint Surg Am 64:1324, 1982.

82. Wang JW, Weng LH: Treatment of distal femoral nonunion with internal fixation, cortical allograft struts, and autogenous bone-grafting. J Bone Joint Surg Am 85:564, 2003.

83. Weight M, Collinge C: Early results of the Less Invasive Stabilization System for mechanically unstable fractures of the distal femur (AO/OTA types A2, A3, C2, and C3). J Orthop Trauma 18:503, 2004.

84. Wenzl H: [Results in 112 surgically treated distal femoral fractures.] Hefte Unfallheilkd 120:15, 1975.

85. White EH, Russin LA: Supracondylar fractures of the femur treated by internal fixation with immediate knee motion. Am J Surg 22:801, 1956.

86. Yang, RS, Liu HG, Liu TK: Supracondylar fractures of the femur. J Trauma 30:315, 1990.

87. Yoshoika Y, Siu D, Cooke DV: The anatomy and functional axes of the femur. J Bone Joint Surg Am 69:873, 1987.

88. Zehnter MK, Marchesi DG, Burch H, et al: Alignment of supracondylar/intercondylar fractures of the femur after internal fixation by AO/ASIF technique. J Orthop Trauma 6:318, 1992.

89. Zickel RE: Nonunions of fractures of the proximal and distal thirds of the shaft of the femur. Instr Course Lect 37:173, 1988.

90. Zickel RE, Fietti VG, Lawsing JF, et al: A new intramedullary fixation device for the distal third of the femur. Clin Orthop 125:185, 1977.

91. Zickel RE, Hobeika P, Robbins DS: Zickel supracondylar nails for fractures of the distal end of the femur. Clin Orthop 212:79, 1986.

92. Zlowodski M, Williamson S, Cole PA, et al: Biomechanical evaluation of the Less Invasive Stabilization System, angled blade plate, and retrograde intramedullary nail for the internal fixation of distal femur fractures. J Orthop Trauma 18:494, 2004.

CHAPTER 66

Tibial Plateau Fractures

David J. Jacofsky • George J. Haidukewych

Fractures of the tibial plateau represent only 1% to 2% of all fractures but account for approximately 8% of fractures occurring in the elderly.[18] As our understanding of the importance of soft-tissue injury has evolved concurrently with the evolution of internal fixation devices and techniques, management of these difficult injuries has slowly shifted from primarily a nonoperative course to one of restoration of the articular surface with internal or external fixation and early motion, when possible. Additionally, new classification systems and clinical outcome data have dramatically improved our ability to understand and manage these fractures.

Articular fractures of the proximal end of the tibia not only involve the articular cartilage itself but can also involve the epiphysis, metaphysis, and in more severe injuries, the diaphysis as well. At times, associated injuries of the tibial spine, tibial tuberosity, menisci, and ligamentous structures can make management of these injuries all the more difficult. Furthermore, to the frustration of orthopedic traumatologists, even anatomic reduction of high-energy injuries often results in the development of post-traumatic arthritis because of damage to the chondral surface.

RELEVANT ANATOMY

The proximal surface of the tibia contains the medial and the lateral tibial plateaus, which are separated by the intercondylar tibial eminences. The articular cartilage on the lateral plateau is slightly thicker than that on the medial side. The lateral tibial plateau is convex in the sagittal plane and nearly flat to slightly convex in the coronal plane. The medial tibial plateau is larger than the lateral plateau and is gently concave in both the sagittal and coronal planes. In the frontal plane, the tibial articular surface forms an angle of approximately 3 degrees of varus with the long axis of the tibia. This varus, as well as the slight difference in cartilaginous thickness between the medial and lateral plateaus, results in the lateral plateau being slightly higher than the medial plateau. This difference is further exacerbated by the convexity of the lateral side and the concavity of the medial side. Such knowledge is extremely important during placement of screws from the lateral to the medial side of the proximal end of the tibia because if not cognizant of this anatomy, one can easily place a subchondral lateral screw through the articular cartilage of the lower medial side.

Between the plateaus lies a nonarticular area that contains the anterior and posterior tibial spines. The anterior spine is more medial and lies just posterior to the insertion of the anterior cruciate ligament (ACL). This area is often comminuted in high-energy injuries involving the tibial plateau, and though nonarticular, it is important to restore the general width of the intercondylar eminence to appropriately restore the anatomic width of the proximal end of the tibia as a whole. In a normal knee, load is predominantly borne on the medial side. Consequently, the trabecular bone on the medial tibial condyle is stronger and more sclerotic than that on the lateral side, perhaps the reason why lateral-sided fractures are far more common, except in higher-energy injuries.

The medial and lateral menisci are both semilunar, triangular-shaped fibrocartilage that rest between the femoral condyles and the tibial plateaus. They serve an important function in load sharing by protecting the articular cartilage from up to 60% of the load encountered by the knee.[20] The lateral meniscus is larger than the medial meniscus and covers a larger percentage of the lateral plateau. The intermeniscal ligament anteriorly connects the anterior horns of the two menisci, and the menisci are attached peripherally by the coronary ligaments to the peripheral rim of their respective tibial plateaus. The anterior attachment of the lateral meniscus is slightly posterior to that of the medial meniscus. It is important to recognize the normal anatomy of these structures because they are often damaged and require repair in the management of tibial plateau fractures.

MECHANISM OF INJURY

The predominant pattern producing tibial plateau fractures is a varus or valgus stress with concomitant axial loading. This combination may be seen with low-energy injuries, such as falls from a standing height, or with high-energy injuries, such as motor vehicle accidents. Isolated valgus or varus loading tends to cause an isolated lateral or medial injury, respectively. The more an axial load predominates, the more likely a patient is to sustain a bicondylar injury. The lateral plateau is involved in 55% to 70% of cases, with medial plateau or bicondylar involvement occurring in 10% to 30% of cases.[18] Simple central depression–type injuries are often the result of low-energy injuries in elderly patients with osteoporotic bone, and conversely, bicondylar fractures with axial loading and shearing injuries tend to be seen in high-energy injuries in younger patients.

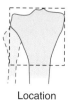

Location

Essence:

The fractures of the distal segment are divided into 3 Types:
A extra-articular, B partial articular, C complete articular

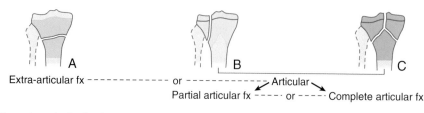

Extra-articular fx - - - - - - - - - - - or - - - - - - - - - - -> Articular
                                    Partial articular fx - - - - or - - - - Complete articular fx

The extra-articular fx of Tibia/Fibula proximal are subdivided into avulsion fx involving the major ligaments, into metaphyseal simple and metaphyseal multifragmentary fractures

The partial articular fx of Tibia/Fibula proximal are classified on the basis of the severity of the articular lesion

Complete articular fx of the Tibia/Fibula proximal are classified according to the pattern of the articular and metaphyseal components

avulsion or metaphyseal

| 1 | 2 | 3 |

simple   multifragm

pure split or depression

| 1 | 2 | 3 |

pure   +split

articular simple or articular multifrag.

| 1 | 2 | 3 |

↓ metaphyseal ↓
simple   multifragm.

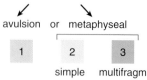

A1
Extra-articular fx, avulsion

A2
Extra-articular fx, metaphyseal simple

A3
Extra-articular fx, metaphyseal multifragmentary

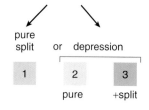

B1
Partial articular fx, pure split

B2
Partial articular fx, pure depression

B3
Partial articular fx, split-depression

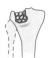

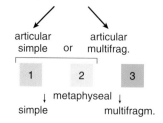

C1
Complete articular fx, articular simple, metaphyseal simple

C2
Complete articular fx, articular simple, metaphyseal multifragmentary

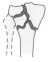

C3
Complete articular fx, articular multifragmentary

Figure 66–1. The AO/ASIF classification. (From Müller ME, Nazarian S, Koch P, Schatzker J: The Comprehensive Classification of Fractures of Long Bones. Bern, Switzerland, M.E. Müller Foundation, 1995.)

CLASSIFICATION

Comprehensive anatomic classifications such as the AO classification or the Orthopaedic Trauma Association classification may be useful for research purposes (Fig. 66–1). However, they are somewhat cumbersome and may be difficult for surgeons to use for clinical communication. The most commonly used classification system in clinical practice is the Schatzker classification system (Fig. 66–2).[19]

In the Schatzker classification system, a type I injury is a "pure" split fracture of the lateral tibial plateau. It is typically seen in young patients with strong cancellous bone,

and by definition there is no associated articular depression. With significant displacement, it is frequently associated with a peripheral tear of the lateral meniscus. Type II fractures are combined split-depression fractures of the lateral tibial plateau. Similar to a type I injury, this injury is most commonly caused by a lateral bending force combined with axial loading. Type III fractures, the most common fracture pattern in Schatzker's series (accounting for 36% of injuries), are pure depression fractures of the lateral plateau and are primarily seen in elderly osteoporotic individuals sustaining lower-energy injuries. The type IV fracture pattern is a fracture of the medial tibial plateau. Because the medial plateau is stronger than the

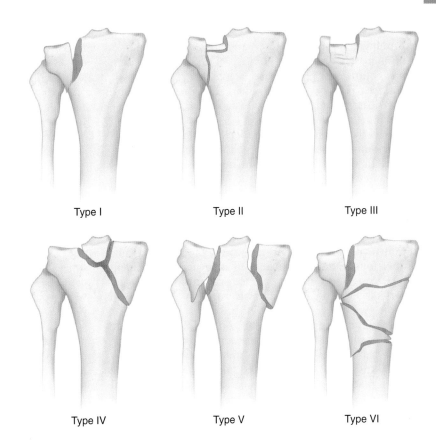

Type I

Type II

Type III

Type IV

Type V

Type VI

Figure 66–2. The Schatzker classification.

lateral side, these fractures are typically secondary to higher-energy injuries and, as such, have commonly associated ligamentous soft-tissue damage. Type V injuries are bicondylar fractures involving both the medial and lateral plateaus and are often the result of a pure axial load applied while the knee is in full extension, such as may be seen in a driver pressing on the brake before impact during a motor vehicle accident. Type VI injuries are the highest-energy injuries; they involve both the medial and lateral plateaus and are associated with metaphyseal/diaphyseal dissociation.

Experienced surgeons know that it is the status of the soft tissues and the classification of the soft-tissue envelope injury that are as important, if not more important, than the underlying osseous injury. The Tscherne classification of soft-tissue damage in closed fractures is an excellent means by which surgeons can evaluate associated soft-tissue injuries.[16] A grade 0 injury results from indirect trauma and is associated with negligible soft-tissue damage. A grade I injury typically results from low or moderate energy and is identified by superficial abrasions or overlying contusions. In grade II injuries, significant muscle contusion and possible deep contaminated abrasions may be seen. Grade II injuries may be the result of a "bumper strike" and are often associated with marked fracture comminution. The highest grade in the classification system is grade III soft-tissue injury, which is frequently associated with extensive crushing of soft tissues and subcutaneous degloving. There may be concomitant arterial injury. Patients with compartment syndrome automatically fall into the grade III category.

CLINICAL EVALUATION

History

The type of knee injury that has occurred can usually be inferred from a thorough patient history. Establishing the magnitude and direction of the force that was applied to the knee, when possible, is extremely helpful. The force from high-velocity motor vehicle accidents will certainly create a different and often more obvious injury pattern than will the noncontact injuries that may occur with sudden stops or pivoting movements during sports. In polytraumatized patients, especially those with high-energy injuries to the lower extremities, the physician must expect and exclude knee injuries. Oftentimes, these polytraumatized patients are unable to give any history at all because they may have closed head injury, be intubated, or suffer distracting injuries. The time at which the injury occurred can be of paramount importance in the event of vascular injury or impending compartment syndrome.

Physical Examination

Clearly, in a polytraumatized patient, primary advanced trauma life support survey protocols and examination to stabilize the patient should be undertaken. During the secondary survey, the entire skeleton should be examined as indicated, and if a tibial plateau fracture is present, it is mandatory that the entire affected limb be examined fully.

Careful circumferential inspection to rule out open fractures is mandatory, and visual inspection can reveal abrasions, contusions, or early fracture blisters that must be considered because they may markedly alter the recommended surgical management. Visual inspection may also reveal an effusion or hemarthrosis.

Although examination of the ligaments and menisci is of paramount importance, it is typically too painful for the patient in the acute setting and needs to be performed under anesthesia. Likewise, without the concomitant use of fluoroscopy, it is difficult to determine whether fracture or ligamentous insufficiency has led to perceived instability on physical examination.

One cannot overemphasize the importance of a complete neurological and vascular examination. Knee dislocations leading to vascular or neurological injury in association with tibial plateau fractures have been reported to spontaneously reduce and may be missed without careful examination. If pulses are not equal on palpation, arteriography may be performed.[15] Use of the "ankle-brachial index" to compare blood pressure in the arm and ankle can help further evaluate the vascular status of the limb. Neurological injury, most commonly in the form of peroneal nerve palsy, is not uncommon.[19] Careful motor and sensory evaluation of the lower part of the leg must be undertaken arduously.

Careful evaluation for compartment syndrome should be performed in all patients with tibial fractures. The index of suspicion should be high for Shitake type 4, 5, and 6, but compartment syndrome can also occur in "simpler" fractures associated with high-energy injury. Patients who are at risk for compartment syndrome should be monitored carefully for at least the first 24 to 48 hours after injury and for a similar period after each closed reduction or surgical intervention. If any question about compartment syndrome exists as a result of clinical evaluation, compartment pressures should be measured and fasciotomies performed.

Imaging Studies

Radiographs should be obtained after all acute knee injuries. The standard knee trauma series should include an anteroposterior, lateral, and patellar tangential view. Oblique radiographs can be extremely helpful in diagnosing minimally displaced fractures of the proximal end of the tibia. Alignment, the presence of bony injury, and the details of the soft tissue should all be examined on radiographs. Stress radiographs may occasionally be helpful to better define the severity and stability of tibial plateau fractures and associated collateral ligament injuries. However, the authors find them rarely helpful. Moreover, stress radiographs have not been shown to increase diagnostic accuracy over examination under anesthesia and/or arthroscopy.

Computed tomography (CT) is perhaps the most valuable test because it helps to both rule out the possibility of occult plateau fractures that are missed on plain radio-graphs and define the nature of these complex intra-articular fractures. Surgical planning of tibial plateau fractures is largely aided by two-dimensional and, occasionally, three-dimensional reconstructions from CT scans. CT, however, is an adjuvant test that should be performed with, and not in place of plain radiographs. Soft-tissue structures such as the menisci and the collateral ligaments are poorly visualized on a CT scan. Magnetic resonance imaging (MRI) is superior for determining the status of such structures.

The use of MRI in the evaluation of acute knee injuries continues to improve and evolve. The sensitivity and specificity of MRI for meniscal and cruciate ligament injury are greater than 90% when correlated with arthroscopic or intraoperative findings.[5] MRI should not be used indiscriminately in place of a careful clinical evaluation and routine plain films and CT scanning. Its benefit in tibial plateau fractures lies largely in exclusion of significant meniscal tears or ligamentous injuries in patients who would otherwise be treated nonoperatively or in a percutaneous fashion such that these injuries would then perhaps be missed. Studies in which MRI was performed on tibial plateau fractures showed associated soft-tissue injuries in greater than 45% of patients.[11] The role of MRI in the preoperative evaluation of these injuries remains undefined.

Angiography

Angiography is indicated when the vascularity of the lower part of the leg is in question. Asymmetric distal pulses or an ankle-brachial index below 0.9 should prompt angiographic examination.[15] It is important to recognize that if a leg is obviously ischemic, angiography may be helpful in localizing the injured area, but it must not delay vascular exploration and subsequent revascularization to the point that viability of the limb will potentially be compromised. "On the table" angiography by the vascular team in the operating room while spanning external fixation is being performed may help expedite the overall care of the patient in such circumstances. Prolonged ischemia may cause a "reperfusion" compartment syndrome after perfusion is restored. "Prophylactic" fasciotomies may be indicated.

MANAGEMENT

Initial Management

In all tibial plateau fractures, the status of the soft tissues is of paramount importance in determining the timing of internal fixation. Patients with higher-energy injuries and significant soft-tissue damage should typically undergo temporizing knee-spanning external fixation, a period in a splint until the soft tissues have recovered to a state where a surgical incision can safely be made. Surgical incisions made through acutely traumatized tissue portend a high rate of wound dehiscence, wound infection, and subsequent soft-tissue complications. It is not uncommon in

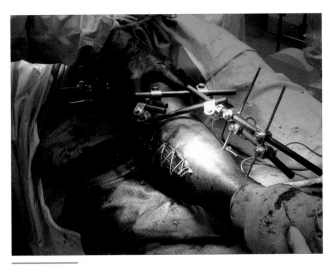

Figure 66–3. Clinical postoperative photograph taken in the operating room after a patient with a tibial plateau fracture and compartment syndrome underwent fasciotomies and spanning external fixation.

higher-energy injuries for it to take several weeks for the soft-tissue envelope to become amenable to surgical intervention. At times, it may be estimated by an experienced physician that the soft-tissue envelope will not become amenable to surgical incision for more than 3 to 4 weeks. In such situations, methods other than formal internal fixation will probably need to be used. Delayed definitive internal fixation with the use of temporizing spanning external fixation (Fig. 66–3) has markedly decreased the rate of complications in this difficult patient population. Lower-energy injuries, such as those seen after a simple fall that results in a depression fracture in an osteoporotic patient, may often be fixed in relatively short order because the associated soft-tissue injury is minor. Obviously, surgeon judgment is paramount in evaluating the character of the osseous and soft-tissue injury.

Nonoperative Management

Although no clear-cut guidelines have been established across all patient ages and activity levels regarding what is acceptable to treat nonoperatively, some general rules can be applied. Articular step-off of less than 3 mm or condylar widening of less than 5 mm tends to have an acceptably low rate of adverse long-term effects if treated nonoperatively. Function deteriorates, however, with varus tilt, whereas mild valgus tilt up to 5 degrees is generally well tolerated.[8] Nonoperative management would be poorly advised if a tibial plateau fracture was associated with varus or valgus instability in a fully extended knee joint. Age alone is not an absolute contraindication to surgical management because older patients do well functionally with proper treatment.[10] However, surgeons must clearly use their judgment about the expectations, functional demands, medical comorbid conditions, and surgical risks of the specific patient being treated when making a decision regarding the most appropriate intervention. The goal of nonoperative treatment is still to allow early

range of motion to include full extension and 120 degrees of flexion. It is known that permanent knee stiffness will probably develop if fractures treated nonoperatively are immobilized for longer than 6 weeks.[6]

Nonoperative management can include a period of traction and/or casting, followed by early range of motion in either a cast brace or a functional brace. Cast brace treatment of minimally displaced unicondylar fractures tends to yield good results, but outcomes are far less predictable with bicondylar fractures.[2] In general, nonoperative treatment is typically reserved for stable, well-aligned, minimally displaced fractures or fractures in patients with prohibitive medical comorbidity.

Operative Management

SCHATZKER TYPE I

A displaced wedge or split fracture of the lateral plateau will be unstable and in most cases is an absolute indication for open reduction and internal fixation. In general, reduction may be achieved by applying a varus force manually or by using a laterally based femoral distractor, or reduction may be performed with the use of a large "King-Tong" or pelvic-type reduction forceps placed percutaneously through small stab incisions (Fig. 66–4). Clamps that are curved may be beneficial in protecting the soft tissues around the anterior face of the tibia from becoming crushed during compression of the fracture. It is important to note that if compression of the fracture site appears to be difficult in that the fracture seems to require significant force to completely close down, the lateral meniscus may be incarcerated in this fracture fragment and either arthroscopic or open removal of the meniscus from the fracture site must be undertaken. It is possible to place so much force on the reduction forceps that the meniscus will simply be crushed within the trabecular bone and the fracture will appear reduced under fluoroscopy. If the split does not "close down" easily, a "mini-open," arthroscopic, or formal open reduction is indicated.

Fixation is typically accomplished with two or three large cannulated screws inserted percutaneously. As with all fractures, the screws should be placed perpendicular to the major fracture lines to achieve compression of the fracture without displacing it when the screws are tightened.[12,14]

In general, two to three solitary lag screws are adequate for fixation,[13] although an antiglide plate or a buttress plate may be necessary in patients with poor bone quality, especially in the face of a vertically oriented condylar fracture. A gentle varus-valgus stress under "live" fluoroscopy can help determine whether screw fixation alone is adequate. If instability is noted and the screws "toggle," buttress plate fixation is indicated.

SCHATZKER TYPE II

Schatzker type II injuries are more difficult to treat than type I injuries because of the associated joint depression

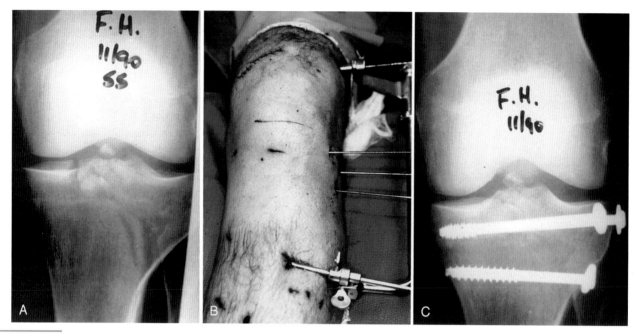

Figure 66–4. Schatzker type I tibial plateau fracture in a 30-year-old man who fell from a ladder. **A,** Preoperative antero-posterior radiograph. **B,** Intraoperative photograph showing a femoral distractor being used to obtain indirect reduction, with guide wires for the cannulated screws in place. **C,** Postoperative anteroposterior radiograph showing anatomic reduction of the tibial plateau.

and, at times, more severe instability than seen with a simple split fracture of the lateral condyle (Fig. 66–5). Minimally invasive techniques such as arthroscopically assisted fixation are rarely indicated, but at times they may be feasible when the lateral cortical disruption is either nondisplaced or minimally displaced and the peripheral rim of cortical bone laterally is functionally competent. In this situation, arthroscopically assisted reduction of the joint surface can be performed. The arthroscope is placed in the joint and a hole is drilled in the medial face of the tibia through a stab incision in a location that will allow curved or straight bone tamps to reach the area of the depressed lateral plateau. An ACL drill guide may be helpful to precisely position the drill. Bone graft or a bone graft substitute can then be impacted or injected through the tunnel from the medial aspect of the tibia to beneath the area of reduced subchondral bone. The arthroscope can assist in determining when appropriate reduction has been achieved. Over-reduction by 0.5 to 1 mm may be beneficial because subsidence occurs in most cases despite the best efforts of the surgeon. Newer, injectable bioresorbable cement may help alleviate this problem, but long-term data are not yet available. After articular reduction has been achieved, multiple 3.5-mm screws may be placed just under the subchondral bone to help prevent settling and fracture of the lateral condyle. Smaller-diameter screws can be placed in close proximity to subchondral bone in so-called raft fashion.

More commonly, however, open reduction with internal fixation is required for most type II injuries. In this situation, the authors prefer a straight lateral parapatellar arthrotomy to allow improved visualization of the joint line. The lateral aspect of the joint may be visualized either through a submeniscal approach or by splitting the inter-

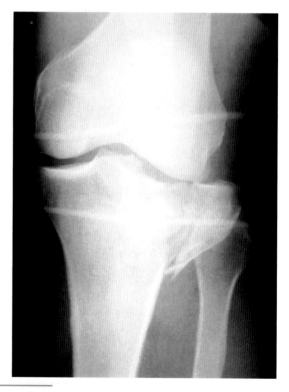

Figure 66–5. Anteroposterior radiograph of a patient with a Schatzker type II tibial plateau fracture.

meniscal and anterior coronary ligaments of the lateral meniscus and reflecting the lateral meniscus posteriorly to expose the lateral side of the joint. In most cases a plate is required, and as such, the distal aspect of the lateral parapatellar arthrotomy at the lateral aspect of the tibial

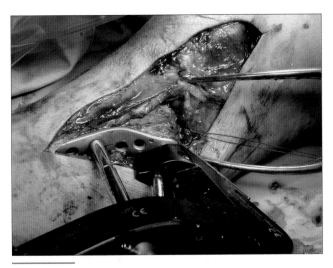

Figure 66–6. Intraoperative clinical photograph of a lateral submeniscal exposure with placement of a lateral submuscular plate.

tubercle can typically be extended laterally and inferiorly to dissect the anterior compartment muscles extraperiosteally from the proximal end of the tibia and allow placement of either a traditional or a percutaneous plate. For simpler fracture patterns requiring a plate, a laterally based submeniscal approach may be adequate (Fig. 66–6). It is important to not strip all the musculature from the lateral condylar fragment, but rather strip only what is required to allow placement of the plate. The fracture itself will actually act as access to the subchondral and posterior regions of the lateral plateau in that reduction and grafting can be performed through a fracture line that has been "booked open." A femoral distractor is often helpful for visualizing the joint space and allowing enough space to be created so that the joint line that is depressed can be elevated without competing with the lateral femoral condyle. Flexion of the knee to force femoral rollback posteriorly also assists with reduction of the joint, especially anteriorly and centrally.

After the fracture has been "booked open," the joint line is reduced with an impactor. The impactor is used to scrape metaphyseal cancellous bone from beneath the articular fragments such that the articular fragments are reduced indirectly with this metaphyseal cancellous bone. Placing the impactor directly on subchondral bone, though tempting, can often lead to complete cracking of incompletely cracked articular cartilage as a result of overzealous force. Additionally, this metaphyseal cancellous bone makes excellent autograft for the subchondral grafting portion of the procedure. Once the depressed articular surface has been anatomically elevated under direct vision, additional graft material can be placed in the defect that typically remains inferior to the area that has been reduced. Grafting can be performed with autograft but is commonly performed with allograft or a bone graft substitute, as discussed later. The split condyle is then reduced and held with a large reduction clamp. Fixation of the condyles should be achieved with a periarticular buttress plate. Newer locked plates may have advantages

in osteoporotic bone, but in general they are reserved for more unstable injuries.

SCHATZKER TYPE III

Type III fractures of the lateral plateau are pure depression fractures usually found in osteoporotic patients after sustaining a valgus stress; however, they can occur as a result of athletic trauma in younger individuals. Valgus instability of greater than 5 to 8 degrees in a patient without significant preexisting arthritis is typically an indication for surgical intervention.

Treatment of this injury in general is now performed with arthroscopic or fluoroscopic assistance in a percutaneous fashion (Fig. 66–7 through Fig. 66–11). The arthroscope is placed in the joint as previously described for type II injuries. A cortical window is made distally on the medial or lateral face of the metadiaphysis to allow percutaneous bone tamps to be placed through a tunnel to reduce the depressed fracture fragments under arthroscopic visualization. The location of this window can best be determined by the location of the depression needing to be accessed, which is best determined with a CT scan. Very anterior depressions are typically best managed through a medial corticotomy, whereas posterolateral depressions are often best managed from the distal aspect of the lateral tibial metaphysis. An ACL drill guide can be used to more accurately place the tunnel. After the tunnel is then completely packed with graft, screws are placed across the joint just under subchondral bone to prevent collapse of the elevated joint surface.

SCHATZKER TYPE IV

Nonoperative management of type IV injuries has been associated with a high incidence of varus malunion and is indicated only for nondisplaced stable injuries.[3,4] In general, however, because of the fact that these injuries are typically caused by very high energy, nondisplaced fractures of the medial plateau are exceedingly rare. It is extremely important to remember that these fractures are often associated with disruption of the lateral collateral ligament complex and, as such, should often be thought of as fracture-dislocation variants of knee dislocations. Therefore, neurovascular examination as previously described is of the utmost importance. It is the magnitude of the soft-tissue injuries associated with medial plateau fractures that portend the higher complication rates and the poorer prognosis, more so than the osseous injury itself.

Because these fractures are typically displaced and comminuted to some degree, open reduction plus internal fixation is generally the preferred method of treatment. One cannot, however, overemphasize the importance of delaying definitive open reduction and internal fixation in the face of a high-energy fracture. Temporizing spanning external fixation until the soft-tissue envelope has recovered adequately is recommended to minimize complications. In general, definitive surgery is carried out through

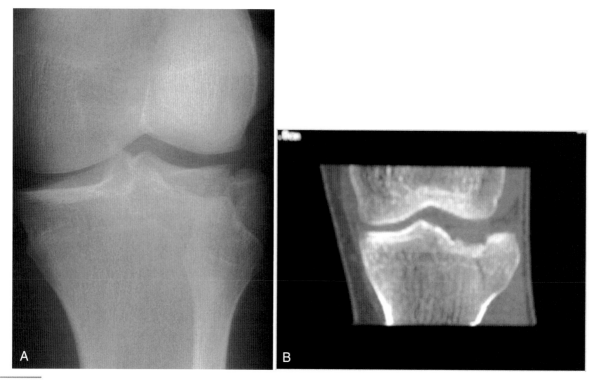

Figure 66–7. **A** and **B,** Preoperative two-dimensional coronal reconstruction of a Schatzker type III tibial plateau fracture amenable to percutaneous treatment.

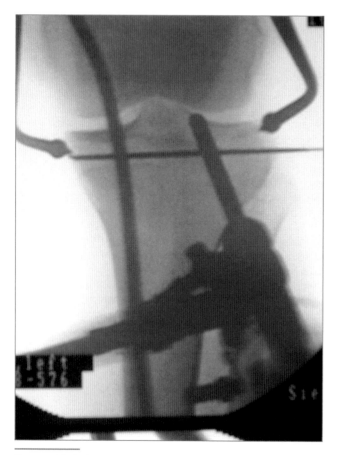

Figure 66–8. Intraoperative fluoroscopic image of reduction of the "cortical rim" and placement of the arthroscope.

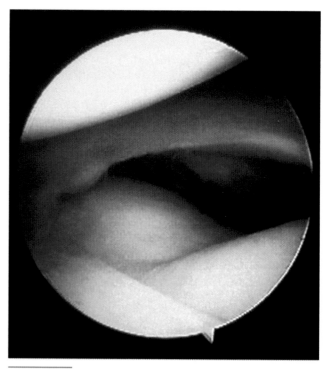

Figure 66–9. Intra-articular view through the arthroscope of the articular depression present before reduction of the articular surface.

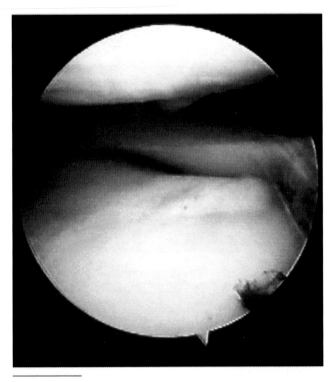

Figure 66–10. Intra-articular view through the arthroscope of the articular surface after reduction.

a medial parapatellar arthrotomy, and after adequate reduction, fixation is achieved with a plate and screws. The plate is typically placed medially, and exposure of an isolated medial condylar fracture requires elevation of the pes anserinus and the superficial medial collateral ligament in an extraperiosteal fashion. Some authors advocate placing the plate superficial to this complex, and fixation can occasionally be performed in such a manner if the condylar split is near the location of the incision and the entire exposure can be accomplished by "booking open" the fracture. Placing the plate outside the superficial medial collateral ligament complex does help preserve the vascularity to the area of the fracture but also, in theory, may lead to increased wound-healing complications because the flap that is created will be subcutaneous in nature (Figs. 66–12 and 66–13).

In the rare situation of an isolated posteromedial fracture fragment, a posteromedial incision may be adequate for reduction and fixation. The complexity of the posteromedial fragment as determined by CT scan will best establish whether a single medially based plate will be adequate. A significant posteromedial fragment that is separate and displaced from the medial condyle proper may require a second posteromedial incision and placement of a posteromedial buttress plate to prevent displacement and subsidence of the posteromedial fragment, which can lead to posterior subluxation of the medial femoral condyle, subsequent instability, and poor results.[7]

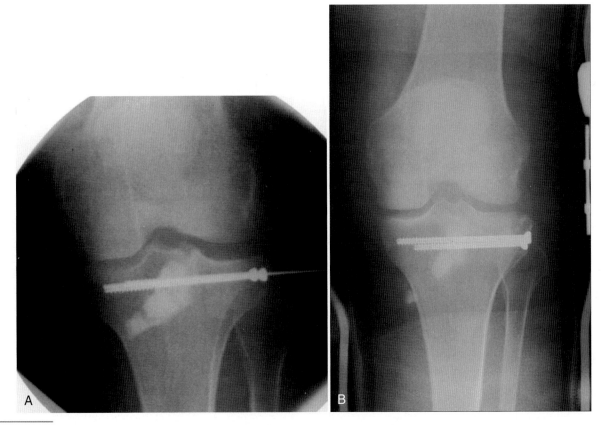

Figure 66–11. **A,** Intraoperative anteroposterior radiograph of a reduction achieved through a metaphyseal tunnel that was "back-filled" with calcium sulfate cement. **B,** Anteroposterior radiograph of the same patient 6 weeks after surgery showing resorption of the calcium sulfate cement.

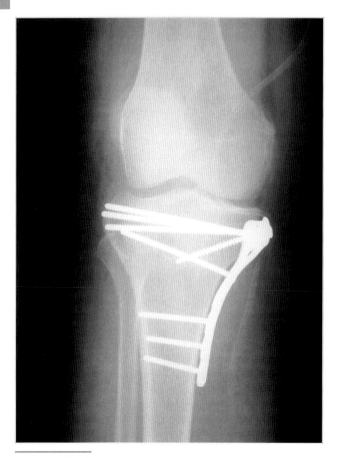

Figure 66–12. Anteroposterior radiograph after open reduction and internal fixation of a Schatzker type IV tibial plateau fracture with a medial buttress plate.

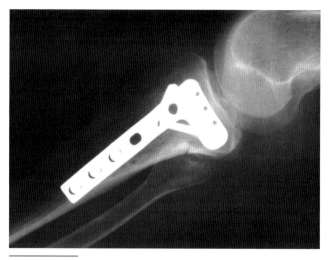

Figure 66–13. Lateral radiograph after open reduction and internal fixation of a Schatzker type IV tibial plateau fracture with a medial buttress plate.

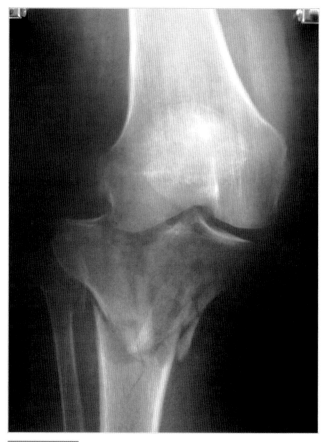

Figure 66–14. Anteroposterior radiograph of a Schatzker type VI tibial plateau fracture.

SCHATZKER TYPES V AND VI

All type V and type VI injuries are high-energy injuries. Both are bicondylar tibial plateau fractures, with type VI injury being complicated by metadiaphyseal dissociation and, often, shaft extension (Figs. 66–14 and 66–15).

These injuries should always be considered high-energy injuries, and as such, immediate definitive incision and internal fixation are generally contraindicated. Temporizing spanning external fixation, as well as fasciotomies when indicated for compartment syndrome, is typically the mainstay of initial treatment (Fig. 66–16). As previously discussed, definitive internal fixation should be carried out only when the soft-tissue envelope has recovered to the point where such fixation is safe and reasonable, typically 7 to 10 days after injury but, in more severe injuries, weeks later.

Open reduction plus internal fixation of these injuries generally requires a standard parapatellar arthrotomy. One can split the intermeniscal ligament centrally and then the coronary ligaments peripherally so that the menisci can be tagged and lifted to expose and visualize both condylar surfaces. Traditionally, plating both condyles had been required for most of these bicondylar injuries. However, if the medial condylar component is large and relatively "simple," a laterally based locked plate may be adequate

for maintenance of medial reduction (Fig. 66–17). The early data are encouraging; however, long-term data on the ability of laterally based locked plates to maintain reduction of the medial side are still unavailable.[11] Locked screws in a plate prevent screw toggle and can therefore

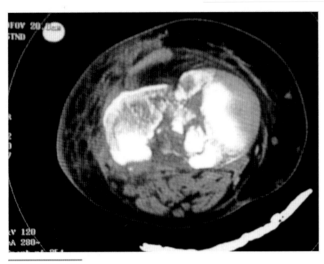

Figure 66–15. Axial computed tomographic scan of a Schatzker type VI tibial plateau fracture showing a split of the condyles and comminution in the region of the tibial spines.

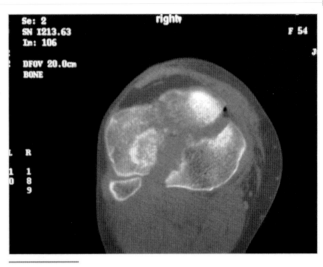

Figure 66–17. Axial computed tomographic scan showing a large posteromedial fracture fragment in a Schatzker type VI tibial plateau fracture.

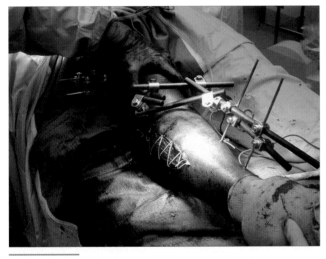

Figure 66–16. Clinical postoperative photograph taken in the operating room after a patient with a tibial plateau fracture and compartment syndrome underwent fasciotomies and spanning external fixation.

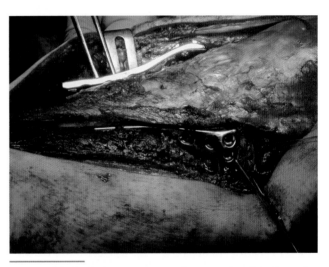

Figure 66–18. Intraoperative photograph showing the exposure for double platting through a midline incision. Note that the medial plate should be placed superficial to the superficial medial collateral ligament.

prevent varus collapse of coronally unstable fractures without the need for adjuvant medial plating. This concept, of course, depends on a medial condylar fragment of sufficient size to be able to be "controlled" with laterally inserted screws. The biological advantage of avoiding double plating and the inevitable soft-tissue dissection necessary for double plating is intuitive. Gentle "varus-valgus" stress testing under "live" fluoroscopy can assist the surgeon in deciding whether a lateral locking plate is "sufficient" fixation. If double plating is to be performed, it is recommended that the medial plate be placed superficial to the superficial medial collateral ligament and pes anserinus to prevent what has become to be known as "the dead bone sandwich," which results from stripping of both the lateral and medial aspects of the tibial metaphysis (Figs. 66–18 and 66–19).

In general, CT scans to evaluate the complexity of the medial condylar component can help determine whether a lateral locked plate will suffice or whether a medial plate will be necessary. Typically, the more complex the medial fracture, the more likely a medial plate will be needed. For the posteromedial fragment, a posteromedial approach and plating are necessary for adequate stability.

In patients whose soft-tissue envelope the surgeon deems will not be amenable to formal open reduction and internal fixation within 14 to 21 days or in those with a markedly comminuted metaphysis and minimal involvement of the articular surfaces, hybrid or fine-wire external fixation may be the best option (Fig. 66–20). Multiple percutaneous screws can be placed to lag large fragments at the joint, and fine wires and/or half-pins can be placed proximally to achieve adequate proximal fixation. It is

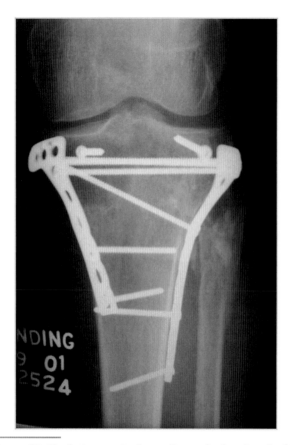

Figure 66–19. Anteroposterior radiograph showing double plating in the same patient seen in Figure 64-18.

important to remember that wires and half-pins should be placed at least 15 mm distal to the joint line to prevent penetration of the synovial capsular reflections and thereby lead to intra-articular hardware and possible septic arthritis.[1] Olive wires can be helpful for achieving and maintaining reduction. Additionally, external fixation can be used definitively in patients with extensive meta-diaphyseal comminution, especially those with associated significant soft-tissue injury (Fig. 66–21).

OPEN FRACTURES

Open fractures of the tibial plateau require emergency irrigation and débridement. Spanning external fixation is very useful in this setting. Extensions of incisions to expose and débride the fracture and/or fasciotomy incisions should be undertaken with consideration for the location of future incisions that will probably be needed for the reconstruction. General principles of open fracture management apply, and definitive internal fixation, when indicated, should commence only after the soft-tissue envelope permits and the wounds are deemed to be "clean." Grossly contaminated wounds may require multiple débridement to achieve this end. When using temporizing external fixators, pins should be placed well away from the area of planned future incisions to avoid potential bacterial contamination and infection.

ORTHOBIOLOGICAL AGENTS

Injectable resorbable cement has begun to gain popularity, especially for percutaneous injection of contained defects in periarticular areas. Watson reported a series of eight comminuted tibial plateau or tibial pilon fractures in 2004 treated with calcium sulfate injectable cement. Although one with a large defect required additional grafting, the other seven healed. At 3 months, over 90% of the graft was resorbed radiographically. The same technique has been used for distal radius fractures in an effort to assist with stability by percutaneous grafting after closed reduction or external fixation. Russell et al and others have reported similar findings in prospective, randomized trials, even showing calcium phosphate cement to be superior to autograft impaction for subchondral support in tibial plateau fractures. Such agents avoid the donor site morbidity associated with autografts and the risk of disease transmission associated with allografts.

COMPLICATIONS

Infection

Deep infections in tibial plateau fractures often result from surgical procedures performed through tenuous soft-tissue envelopes with subsequent poor wound healing and bacterial colonization. Superficial wound infections that occur early should be aggressively treated with antibiotics, and surgeons should have a low threshold for surgical débridement. Deep infections may require irrigation and débridement with arthrotomy and irrigation of the knee joint as well. Stable implants are typically retained if the fracture has not yet united, and it may be beneficial, when an organism has been isolated, to orally medicate patients until union has occurred. Hardware can subsequently be removed as indicated. Loose hardware should be removed. Consultation and comanagement with an infectious disease specialist and a plastic surgeon may be beneficial.

Arthrofibrosis

Stiffness is one of the most common complications after tibial plateau fractures, especially in more severe injuries. The best treatment is prevention, which can be achieved through early range of motion. Early range of motion requires that the surgeon obtain as stable fixation as possible. Closed manipulation in conjunction with arthroscopic lysis of adhesions in appropriately chosen patients who do not respond to physical therapy may be performed, but one must be cautious with manipulation in patients with existing fractures, and the authors find that such treatment is rarely indicated. It may be preferable, after fracture union has been achieved, to consider open lysis of adhesions, with or without quadricepsplasty, followed by physical therapy with epidural anesthesia.

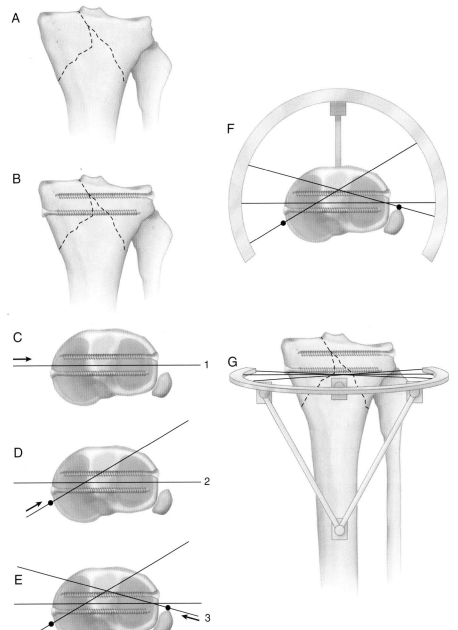

Figure 66–20. Technique for reduction and fixation of a Schatzker type V tibial plateau fracture with cannulated screws and a hybrid external fixator. **A,** Reduction is obtained via open or closed methods and held with a reduction clamp. **B,** Cannulated screws are placed to hold the articular reduction. **C,** A smooth guide wire for the external fixator is placed in the coronal plane, at least 14 mm distal to the joint line. **D,** The second wire, with a bead or olive, is passed posteromedially to anterolaterally. **E,** A third wire, also beaded, is passed posterolaterally to anteromedially. **F,** The wires are appropriately tensioned and fixed to the ring. An optional half-pin can be placed from the anterior to the posterior aspect and attached to the ring for increased stability. **G,** Half-pins are inserted into the tibial shaft, and the distal pins are connected to the ring with the appropriate clamps and bars.

Post-traumatic Complications

The articular cartilage and meniscal damage that occurs at the time of tibial plateau fracture predisposes the joint to arthrosis, often regardless of the adequacy of the surgeon's reduction.[9] Honkonen reported that 44% of his patients had arthrosis at a mean of 7.6 years after injury. In patients who underwent total meniscectomy on the affected plateau, this percentage rose to 74%. However, it is difficult to determine whether it was the meniscectomy or perhaps the increased magnitude of the injury causing the meniscal pathology that led to this change. The best prognosis was seen in patients with normal or slight valgus limb alignment and an intact meniscus on the affected side. It is important to remember, however, that many studies have found little correlation between radiographic arthrosis and clinical symptoms.[14,17] Corrective osteotomy, total knee arthroplasty, unicompartmental arthroplasty, and arthrodesis are potentially viable options for the management of symptomatic post-traumatic arthritis that is refractory to conservative management. Decision making is based on the underlying pathology, patient age, and activity. A full discussion of reconstructive options is beyond the scope of this chapter.

Nonunion

Nonunion of tibial plateau fractures is relatively rare. It is typically associated with open fractures or higher-energy

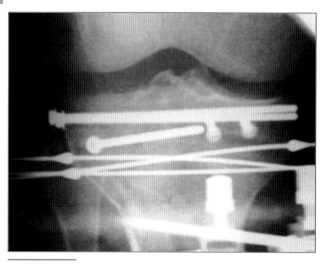

Figure 66–21. Anteroposterior radiograph of a patient with a Schatzker type VI tibial plateau fracture. Extensive metaphyseal comminution and a "simple" articular fracture are seen. A fine wire fixator and lag screw fixation at the subchondral region were used in this patient because of significant soft-tissue injury.

injuries with significant soft-tissue damage. In patients who appear to be acutely at risk for nonunion secondary to significant bone loss or a poor soft-tissue envelope, bone grafting can be performed at the time of the index definitive procedure if feasible. If, however, healing appears to be delayed in the postoperative course, early bone grafting should be performed. If nonunion has led to fixation failure, revision of this fixation is typically indicated.

CONCLUSIONS

Tibial plateau fractures are severe injuries that continue to pose a significant challenge to even the most highly trained orthopedic traumatologists. To the frustration of many surgeons, the injuries sustained by the cartilage may cause the development of arthrosis, even when a "perfect" postoperative radiograph is obtained. Minimally invasive treatment modalities and locked plating technologies have continued to evolve, and these advances, as well as the development of improved bone graft substitutes that may minimize articular loss of reduction, may translate into improvements in outcome. Our recognition of the importance of the soft-tissue envelope in higher-energy injuries

and our understanding of the use of temporizing external fixation before definitive internal fixation have markedly reduced the complication rate in the management of these injuries.

References

1. DeCoster TA, Crawford MK, Kraut MA: Safe extracapsular placement of proximal tibia transfixation pins. J Orthop Trauma 13:236-240, 1999.
2. DeCoster TA, Nepola JV, el-Khoury GY: Cast brace treatment of proximal tibia fractures. A 10-year follow-up study. Clin Orthop 231:196-204, 1988.
3. Delamarter R, Hohl M: The cast brace and tibial plateau fractures. Clin Orthop 242:26-31, 1989.
4. Drennan DB, Locker FG, Maylahn D: Fractures of the tibial plateau: Treatment by closed reduction and spica cast. J Bone Joint Surg Am 61:989-995, 1979.
5. Fischer SP, Fox JM, Del Pizzo W, et al: Accuracy of diagnoses from magnetic resonance imaging of the knee. A multicenter analysis of 1014 patients. J Bone Joint Surg Am 73:2-10, 1991.
6. Gausewitz S, Hohl M: The significance of early motion in the treatment of tibial plateau fractures. Clin Orthop 202:135-138, 1986.
7. Georgiadis GM: Combined anterior and posterior approaches for complex tibial plateau fractures. J Bone Joint Surg Br 76:285-289, 1994.
8. Honkonen SE: Indications for surgical treatment of tibial condyle fractures. Clin Orthop 302:199-205, 1994.
9. Honkonen SE: Degenerative arthritis after tibial plateau fractures. J Orthop Trauma 9:273-277, 1995.
10. Houben PF, van der Linden ES, van den Wildenberg FA, Stapert JW: Functional and radiological outcome after intra-articular tibial plateau fractures. Injury 28:459-462, 1997.
11. Kode L, Lieberman JM, Motta AO, et al: Evaluation of tibial plateau fractures: Efficacy of MR imaging compared with CT. AJR Am J Roentgenol 163:141-147, 1994.
12. Koval KJ, Helfet DL: Tibial plateau fractures: Evaluation and treatment. J Am Acad Orthop Surg 3:86-94, 1995.
13. Koval K, Polatsch D, Kummer FJ, et al: Split fractures of the lateral tibial plateau: Evaluation of three fixation methods. J Orthop Trauma 10:304-308, 1996.
14. Koval K, Sanders R, Borrelli J, et al: Indirect reduction and percutaneous screw fixation of displaced tibial plateau fractures. J Orthop Trauma 6:340-346, 1992.
15. Lynch K, Johansen K: Can Doppler pressure measurement replace "exclusion" arteriography in the diagnosis of occult extremity arterial trauma? Ann Surg 214:737-741, 1991.
16. Oesteren HJ, Tscherne H: Pathophysiology in classification of soft tissue injuries associated with fractures. In Tscherne H, Gotzen L (eds): Fractures with Soft Tissue Injuries. New York, Springer-Verlag, 1984, pp 1-9.
17. Roberts JM: Fractures of the condyles of the tibia: An anatomical and clinical end-result study of 100 cases. J Bone Joint Surg 50:1505-1521, 1968.
18. Ruth J: Fractures of the tibial plateau. Am J Knee Surg 14:125-128, 2001.
19. Schatzker J, McBroom R: Tibial plateau fractures: The Toronto experience, 1968-1975. Clin Orthop 138:94-104, 1979.
20. Walker PS, Erkman MJ: The role of the menisci in force transmission across the knee. Clin Orthop 109:184-192, 1975.

CHAPTER 67

Fractures of the Patella

Nathan M. Melton • Frank Liporace • Thomas DiPasquale

HISTORICAL PERSPECTIVE

Until the 19th century, extension splinting was used to treat the vast majority of patella fractures. The final results were often poor, and patients generally incurred permanent disability. Physicians' interest in other means of treatment was obvious. Malgaigne designed the first external fixator in 1843, named the "*griffe métallique*" (metal claw) (Fig. 67–1). It was a simple design consisting of two pairs of curved, pointed hooks connected to sliding plates attached to a compressive screw. The device was initially used for widely displaced patella fractures by Malgaigne to reapproximate the extensor mechanism, but it was Cucuel and Rigaud who later modified the technique by pressing the hooks into bony fragments, thereby essentially becoming the first use of an external fixator.[23] Lister and Cameron in 1877 began treating patella fractures by open arthrotomy and interfragmentary wiring. This technique was initially met with scorn by the rest of the world, until improved results were verified independently by Dennis. With the advance of antiseptic surgery, open procedures became much more popular by eliminating the great risk to life and limb. Two options appeared, open wiring and patellectomy, but stable constructs were difficult to obtain. Numerous materials were used, such as various wire, gut suture, xenograft (kangaroo), allograft (Achilles), nails, screws, and inlay grafts.[28] One of the greatest advances then occurred in the 1950s, when the anterior tension band principle was reported and then recommended by the Arbeitsgemeinschaft für Osteosynthesefragen/Association for the Study of Internal Fixation (AO/ASIF).[53] It was a stable construct that unlike previous ones, allowed for early range of motion. Treatment has progressed to the point that there are three options when discussing operative intervention: internal fixation and partial and complete patellectomy.

Despite its relatively small size, a suboptimally treated patella fracture may result in significant long-term sequelae. Complications such as residual joint stiffness, quadriceps weakness, painful post-traumatic arthritis, or a combination of all three are not uncommon. Because of the wide range of injuries to the patella, treatment options vary considerably. Yet the goals of treatment remain constant and are of paramount importance: restoring the functional integrity of the extensor mechanism and maintaining or restoring the articular surface of the patella.

ANATOMY OF THE PATELLA

Bony Architecture

The patella is the largest sesamoid bone and has a "rounded triangular" shape, with its most distal aspect anteroinferiorly termed the apex and its proximal portion termed the basis.[10]

The articular surface of the patella is composed of seven facets divided by several bony ridges (Fig. 67–2). A large vertical ridge separates the lateral and medial facets, and a smaller vertical ridge medially defines the odd facet, a small narrow strip of articular surface. Two additional horizontal ridges create superior, intermediate, and inferior facets.[59]

Variance in the size and shape of the patellar facets was characterized and classified by Wiberg[94] into three main types:

- Type I: The medial and lateral facets are both concave and roughly equal in size.
- Type II: The medial, concave facet is smaller than the lateral facet.
- Type III: The medial facet is smaller than the lateral facet but is convex shaped.

Baumgartl[6] further characterized the patellar facets into three additional types: type II-III, a small, flat medial facet; type IV, a very small, steeply sloped medial facet with a medial ridge present; and type V (Jaegerhut patella), no medial facet or vertical ridge. These classification schemes essentially describe the relative constancy of the lateral facet with varying degrees of medial patellar facet dysplasia.

One particularly important point regarding the bony architecture of the patella is that the proximal three-fourths of the patella is covered with thick articular cartilage and the distal fourth (the distal pole) is entirely extra-articular. This anatomic peculiarity becomes clinically important when treating certain types of patellar fractures.[25]

Blood Supply

The arterial blood supply to the patella is derived mainly from the peripatellar plexus, which receives contributions from six separate arteries (Fig. 67–3). This plexus helps

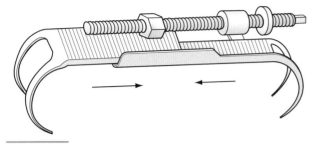

Figure 67–1. The griffe métallique used by Malgaine in 1843 for patella fractures was the first external fixator. (Redrawn from Browner B, Levine A, Jupiter J, Trafton P [eds]: Skeletal Trauma, 3rd ed. Philadelphia, WB Saunders, 2003, p 18.)

preserve the vascularity of fracture fragments even in comminuted patellar fractures (Fig. 67–4). The supreme geniculate artery branches from the superficial femoral artery at the level of the adductor canal. Four geniculate arteries originate from the popliteal artery. The superolateral geniculate is the most superior of the four and joins the peripatellar plexus at its most superior point. The superomedial geniculate artery branches from the popliteal artery just above the joint line and enters the plexus at the midpoint of the patella on the medial side. The inferolateral geniculate arises from the popliteal artery just below the joint line and courses anteriorly adjacent to the lateral meniscus. It proceeds superiorly to join the plexus. The inferomedial geniculate is the most inferior of the four vessels and originates from the popliteal artery. It courses anteriorly 2 cm below the joint line and then proceeds superiorly to join the plexus. The final branch

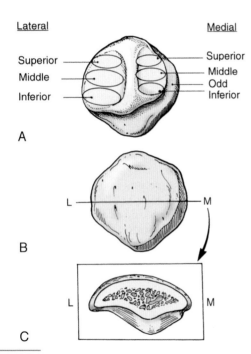

Figure 67–2. **A,** The seven patellar facets. **B,** The anterior surface. **C,** Cross-section of a Wiberg II patella. (From Scuderi G: The Patella. New York, Springer-Verlag, 1995.)

contributing to the peripatellar plexus is the recurrent anterior tibial artery, which is a branch of the anterior tibial artery at the point where the vessel penetrates the interosseous membrane 1 cm below the proximal tibiofibular joint. It then courses superiorly to join the plexus.[73] Despite the symmetric appearance of the peripatellar plexus, Scapinelli[66] demonstrated that the functional blood supply to the patella is from the distal to the proximal aspect.[75]

ANATOMY AND BIOMECHANICS OF THE EXTENSOR MECHANISM

Muscular Anatomy

The extensor mechanism, of which the patella is an integral component, consists of the quadriceps mechanism, the patellar retinaculum, and the patellar tendon. The quadriceps consists of four separate muscles: the rectus femoris, vastus medialis, vastus lateralis, and vastus intermedius. The tendons of these four muscles blend distally into a complex insertion into the patella (Fig. 67–5).[59]

The rectus femoris muscle occupies the most central and superficial position in the quadriceps.[2] Its muscle fibers run somewhat medially in relation to the shaft of the femur, with a 7- to 10-degree angle between the two.[47]

The vastus medialis consists of two parts. A more proximal portion, the vastus medialis longus, attaches to the patella at an angle between 15 and 18 degrees. The more distal portion, the vastus medialis obliquus, attaches to the patella at an angle between 50 and 55 degrees.[47] The oblique orientation of the muscle fibers and the short tendinous attachment of the vastus medialis contribute to the importance of the vastus medialis as a dynamic stabilizing force for patellar tracking.

The vastus lateralis attaches to the patella more proximally than the vastus medialis does, at a more vertical angle of approximately 30 degrees. Its most medial fibers insert into the superolateral aspect of the patella, and the lateral fibers traverse past the patella, where they contribute to the lateral retinaculum and fuse with the iliotibial tract.[47]

The vastus intermedius lies deep to the other three muscles, with most of its fibers attaching directly into the superior aspect of the patella.

The fascia lata over the anterior aspect of the knee combines with the aponeurosis of both the vastus medialis and the vastus lateralis to form the retinaculum, which inserts directly on either side of the proximal end of the tibia. Thickenings of the capsule, which connect the medial and lateral edges of the patella to their corresponding epicondyles, are termed the patellofemoral ligaments, which complete the retinaculum. The patellar retinaculum performs two important functions: stabilization of the patella and, along with the iliotibial band, secondary knee extension.[10,59]

The patellar tendon, a stout, flat structure measuring approximately 5 cm in length, is formed primarily by a continuation of the central fibers of the rectus femoris and inserts into the tibial tubercle. Blending with the patellar

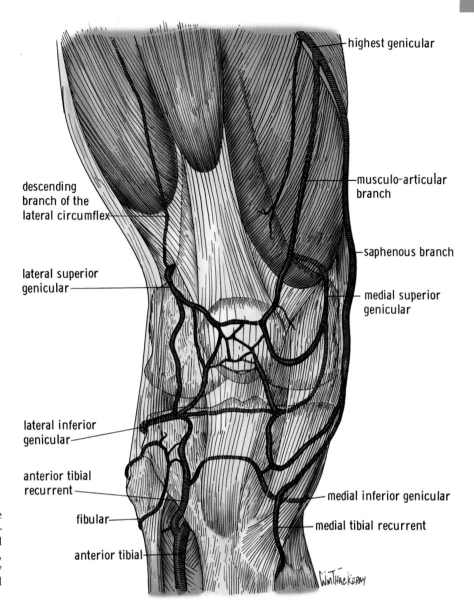

highest genicular

musculo-articular
branch

saphenous branch

medial superior
genicular

descending
branch of the
lateral circumflex

lateral superior
genicular

lateral inferior
genicular

anterior tibial
recurrent

fibular

anterior tibial

medial inferior genicular

medial tibial recurrent

Figure 67–3. Anastomosis at the front of the knee formed by genicular branches from the popliteal artery and descending branches, which connect the femoral artery proximally with the popliteal and anterior tibial arteries distally.

tendon on either side are fascial expansions of the iliotibial band and patellar retinaculum.

Biomechanics

The patella has three functions: increase the strength of the quadriceps, act as a protective shield for the femoral condyles, and less importantly, when absent, change the cosmetic appearance of the knee.[85] The most important function is its mechanical role in increasing the strength of the extensor mechanism. The patella, by virtue of its thickness, displaces the tendon away from the center of rotation of the knee, thereby increasing its moment arm, which increases the force of knee extension by as much as 50%, depending on the angle of the knee (Fig. 67–6). Numerous clinical studies have documented up to a 50% decrease in isokinetic strength after patellectomy.[21,22,57,84,91]

During initial extension from a fully flexed position, the patella serves as a mechanical link between the quadriceps and the patellar tendon. This link allows for torque generated from the quadriceps to be transferred to the tibia. The torque generated is considerable, ranging from four up to eight times body weight in athletes.[38] As extension progresses to 135 degrees, the patella engages the intercondylar notch. At this angle, the patellar contact surface on the femur is occupied by both the patella and the quadriceps tendon proximally. As extension progresses, the contact area of the quadriceps tendon on the femur decreases progressively until at 45 degrees, the patella is the only portion of the extensor mechanism to contact the femur. It is during the terminal portion of extension that the increased moment arm of the patella becomes important because it requires twice as much torque to extend the knee the final 15 degrees as it does to extend it from a maximally flexed position up to 15 degrees.[47]

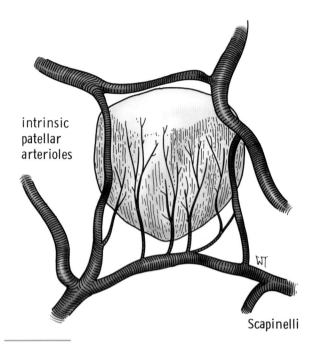

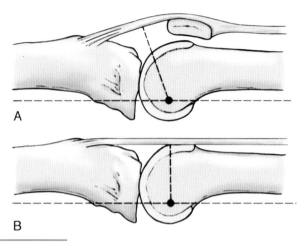

Figure 67–6. In **A,** the patella increases the effective moment arm. In **B,** after patellectomy, the moment arm is decreased, thereby diminishing extensor force. (From Sanders R: Patella fractures and extensor mechanism injuries. In Browner B [ed]: Skeletal Trauma. Philadelphia, WB Saunders, 1992.)

Figure 67–4. Vascular circle around the patella, which according to Scapinelli,[66] supplies the patella by nutrient arteries that enter predominantly at the inferior pole. The genicular arteries and their branches lie in the most superficial layer of the deep fascia.

Because of the high torque generated by the extensor mechanism and the convex configuration of the patella, compressive force on the patella is quite high, ranging from 3.3 times body weight with stair climbing up to 7.6 times body weight while squatting.[50] Although patellofemoral force is generally less than tibiofemoral force with weightbearing and knee motion, because of the smaller contact area of the patellofemoral joint, it has been estimated that the contact stress on the patellofemoral joint is higher than on any other major weightbearing joint.[17]

The contact area between the patella and femur changes in location and extent during range of motion. The patella centers within the trochlear groove at around 20 degrees of flexion. As flexion continues, the contact area on the patella, a horizontal band across both condyles, moves proximally and reaches a maximum at 90 degrees of flexion. Beyond 90 degrees, the contact area separates into two discrete areas of contact on the patellar facets.[3,35] As the contact area moves proximally on the patella, the contact area on the trochlea moves more distally with increasing flexion (Fig. 67–7).

DIAGNOSIS

Fractures of the patella are relatively common injuries and account for approximately 1% of all skeletal fractures.[10] The patella is prone to injury by virtue of its anterior location, the large force generated through it, and the minimal amount of overlying soft tissue protecting it from direct trauma. Fractures of the patella may be direct, indirect, or a combination. Direct injuries involve a blow to the anterior aspect of the knee and may be either low energy, as sustained from a fall, or high energy, as from a motor vehicle accident. Indirect trauma occurs with a violent contraction of the quadriceps while the knee is bent, which literally pulls the patella apart and concomitantly

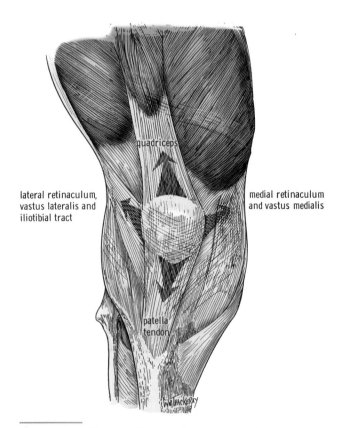

Figure 67–5. The patella is anchored and stabilized to the knee by four structures in a cruciform fashion: the patellar tendon inferiorly, the quadriceps tendon superiorly, and the retinaculum medially and laterally.

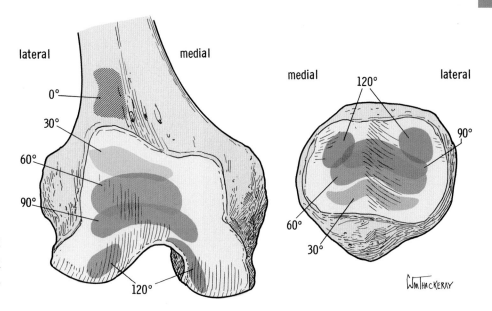

lateral   medial

medial   120°   lateral

0°
30°
60°
90°
120°

90°

60°

30°

Figure 67–7. Patellofemoral contact zones. (From Aglietti P, Insall JN, Walker PS, et al: A new patella prosthesis. Clin Orthop 107:175, 1975.)

disrupts the patellar retinacular portion of the extensor mechanism. Previous classification systems for fractures of the patella were based on the mechanism of injury, with transverse fractures being the result of indirect trauma and comminuted fractures being the result of direct injury.[92] It is now evident that some types of patella fractures can be caused by either mechanism and that other factors, such as the patient age, degree of knee flexion, extent of osteoporosis, and energy absorbed by the patella, can influence the sustained fracture pattern. In many instances, it is difficult to reconstruct the events leading to injury, and most likely it is a combination of direct force, muscle contraction, and joint collapse that results in fracture.[1]

Historical information obtained from the patient usually includes a direct blow to the anterior aspect of the knee, a fall from a height, or a near fall with strong contraction of the quadriceps on a loaded, flexed knee. The onset of anterior pain, acute effusion of the knee, and an inability or limited ability to walk after the fall are also important clinical indicators of injury to the extensor mechanism. Other essential information that should be obtained includes the presence of pain at other sites, especially if the accident involved a high-energy mechanism such as a motor vehicle crash.

Physical examination should include inspection of the skin for abrasions, contusions, and lacerations. If there is any question whether a laceration is an open fracture or communicates with the knee joint, sterile aspiration of the knee followed by infusion of saline with methylene blue dye and local anesthetic will quickly determine joint or bone contamination if infused fluid exits from the wound. Additionally, local anesthetic in the knee may facilitate a more complete examination. The knee should be palpated gently for determination of any skeletal defects, the size of the effusion, or any ligamentous instability. If the history or examination raises suspicion for other orthopedic injuries, especially on the ipsilateral limb, these should be examined as well. Competence of the extensor mechanism should be tested by determining the patient's ability to perform a straight-leg raise or extend the partially flexed knee against gravity.

RADIOGRAPHY

Plain radiography is usually all that is required to confirm an injury to the patella or extensor mechanism. On occasion, more subtle injuries such as osteochondral fractures or partial disruption of the extensor mechanism will require more specialized studies such as computed tomography or magnetic resonance imaging. Appropriate standard plain radiographic views include an adequate anteroposterior (AP) and lateral view of the knee and a tangential view of the patellofemoral joint. The AP view should be performed on a 14 × 17-inch cassette to evaluate the distal end of the femur and proximal end of the tibia for concomitant injuries. The AP view should be evaluated for the position of the patella in the midline within the femoral sulcus, the height of the patella in relation to its distal pole, and the profile of the femoral condyles.

Occasionally, a bipartite or tripartite patella can be mistaken for a fracture.[51] This normal variant is caused by separate ossification centers of the patella that fail to fuse. It is usually located on the superolateral aspect of the patella, is generally bilateral, and requires no treatment. It is not associated with focal bony tenderness or compromise of extensor mechanism function. Comparative x-ray films of the contralateral knee may be obtained to confirm the diagnosis.

A lateral view of the knee will clearly define a transverse or comminuted patellar fracture. Other, more subtle information can be obtained with less obvious injuries or fracture patterns. The lateral view should include a good profile of the tibial tubercle to detect an avulsion from this site. Additionally, the position of the patella and its relationship to the femur should be observed. The most reliable indicator of the height of the patella is the Insall-Salvati ratio, which compares the length of the patella with the length the patellar tendon. A normal ratio is 1.02 (±0.13); a ratio less than 1.0 may indicate a patellar tendon rupture.[18,41] The relationship of the distal pole of the patella to the distal physeal scar remnant (Blumen-

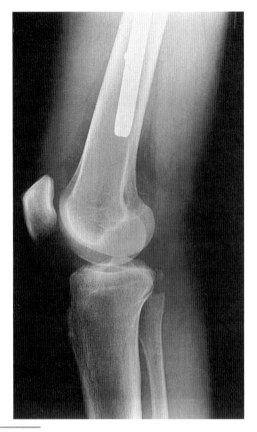

Figure 67–8. Lateral radiograph of a previously undiagnosed patella fracture in a multiply injured patient.

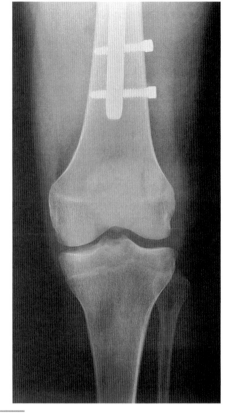

Figure 67–9. An anteroposterior radiograph of the patient in Figure 65-8 more clearly identifies the patella fracture.

saat's line) can also be compared to look for disruption of the extensor mechanism.[60]

The tangential view of the patellofemoral joint is helpful in identifying osteochondral fractures as well as marginal or vertical fractures that may not be readily apparent on the AP or lateral views of the knee (Figs. 67–8 to 67–12). The Merchant view is the most practical projection in trauma evaluation because of the lack of participation required by the patient and the supine passive positioning of the limb at 45 degrees of flexion.[52]

PATELLA FRACTURE CLASSIFICATION

Patella fractures can be classified by the degree of displacement, the fracture pattern, the proposed mechanism of injury, or a combination of two or more of these descriptors. With the wide variability in patella fracture patterns, no single classification system has been effective in stratifying fracture patterns and their respective outcomes.[8,10,74] Because of this difficulty, most authors have reported long-term results according to the type of treatment as opposed to the type of fracture.[8,10,11,19,48,54,74,87]

Displaced patella fractures are defined as fractures with greater than 3 mm between fracture fragments and/or articular incongruity greater than 2 mm.[8,10,51,74] Because of the articular step-off, these fractures are usually treated operatively.

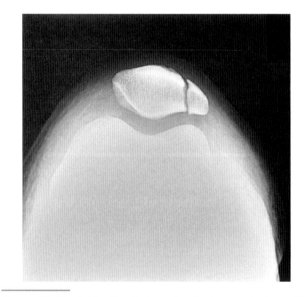

Figure 67–10. A Merchant view clearly demonstrates a displaced longitudinal fracture.

Classification by mechanism of injury is based on a direct blow, such as from a fall or motor vehicle accident, or on an indirect mechanism, such as occurs with violent quadriceps contraction on a loaded flexed knee. As stated previously, the mechanism of injury may not be readily

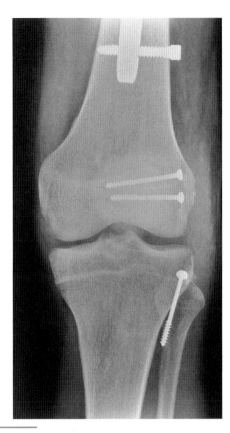

Figure 67–11. Postoperative radiograph of the patella repaired with cancellous screws.

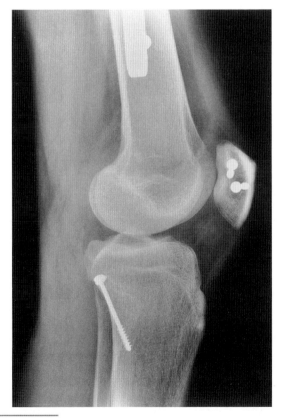

Figure 67–12. Lateral postoperative radiograph of screw fixation.

determined, and varied fracture patterns may occur with the same injury mechanism.[85]

Fracture classification by the configuration of the fracture line or lines provides the most useful information to the surgeon, especially when it includes characterization of the degree of displacement associated with the fracture pattern. Described fracture patterns of the patella include transverse, vertical, stellate (comminuted), apical or marginal, and osteochondral. In addition, sleeve fractures with a large portion of the distal fragment being articular cartilage can occur in skeletally immature patients (Fig. 67–13).

NONOPERATIVE TREATMENT

Successful nonoperative treatment of patella fractures depends most of all on a relative lack of displacement or separation between fragments, lack of articular incongruity, and the integrity of the extensor mechanism. Longitudinal fractures are best suited for nonoperative management because the pull of the intact extensor mechanism is parallel to the fracture, thereby helping prevent displacement (Fig. 67–14). Nonoperative treatment should provide good to excellent results in more than 90% of patella fractures.[10] Relative indications for nonoperative treatment include elderly low-demand patients with significant osteopenia, thus making stable fixation impossible, and patients for whom general or regional anesthesia is contraindicated because of preexisting medical conditions.

Nonoperative treatment consists of the application of a well-padded cylinder cast or long-leg cast in nearly full extension for 4 to 6 weeks, with weightbearing to tolerance for longitudinal fractures and partial weightbearing for nondisplaced transverse fractures. Patients are encouraged to perform straight-leg raises in the cast to maintain some quadriceps muscle strength. If patient reliability and compliance are not a concern, a hinged knee brace locked in extension may be substituted for the cylinder cast. Extension is maintained until fracture consolidation is evident on radiographs, at which time gentle, active range-of-motion exercises may be implemented.

OPERATIVE TREATMENT

Operative treatment of patella fractures is indicated for displacement between fragments of 3 mm or more or for articular incongruity or step-off greater than 2 mm.[25] The goals of surgical treatment are to obtain accurate reduction of the fracture and provide stable fixation or repair to facilitate early range of motion of the knee.

Surgical techniques can be divided into three main categories: internal fixation, partial patellectomy with reattachment of the extensor mechanism to the remaining patella, and total patellectomy. On occasion, it is possible to combine internal fixation with partial patellectomy techniques to preserve more patellar bone within the extensor mechanism.

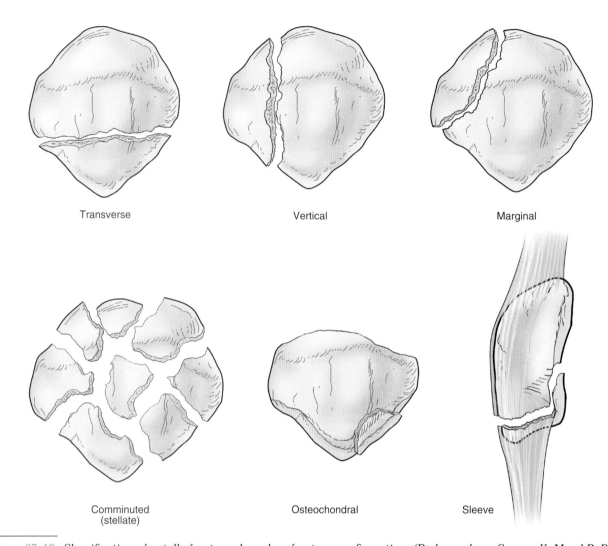

Transverse   Vertical   Marginal

Comminuted
(stellate)   Osteochondral   Sleeve

Figure 67–13. Classification of patella fractures based on fracture configuration. (Redrawn from Cramer K, Moed B: Patellar fractures: Contemporary approach to treatment. J Am Acad Orthop Surg 5:323, 1997.)

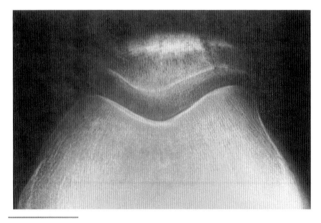

Figure 67–14. Merchant view demonstrating maintenance of articular congruity after closed treatment of this longitudinal patella fracture.

Surgical exposure, preferably under tourniquet control, can be achieved through either a transverse or vertical skin incision. We prefer the more utilitarian vertical incision, which provides excellent exposure for any of the surgical techniques performed, and it can be used later with little concern for soft-tissue problems should additional surgical procedures on the knee be necessary.[88] In the event of an open patella fracture, the laceration should be incorporated into the skin incision if possible. After adequate exposure of the fracture, the joint should be evaluated for articular damage to the patella and femur. Additionally, the retinacular and proximal and distal soft-tissue attachments to the patella should be assessed before selecting the definitive surgical repair technique. Small comminuted bone fragments, especially those with no soft-tissue attachment, should be removed before attempted reduction. During reduction, the articular surface must be accessible for palpation and direct visualization to assess the quality of reduction. Additional exposure may be necessary and can be achieved by extending the arthrotomy vertically through a preexisting retinacular tear. Intra-

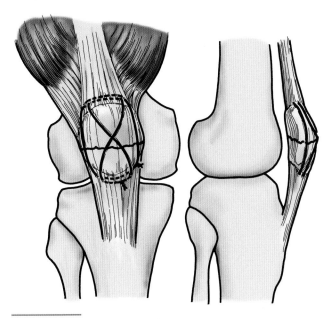

Figure 67–15. Tension cerclage of patellar fractures.

operative radiographs may be required to assess the articular reduction.

Internal Fixation

A variety of techniques have been described for stabilization of displaced patella fractures: wires in a cerclage or tension band configuration, screw fixation, and a combination of these methods. Of historical interest, initial wiring techniques involved circumferential cerclage of the patella, followed by cast treatment in extension for 4 to 6 weeks.[4,10,49,73] Magnuson[49] and Payr[56] advocated the use of a wire passed through two vertical, longitudinal drill holes. Anderson suggested the use of equatorial circumferential wiring.[4] The early wiring techniques were less than optimal for treatment of these fractures because of the inability to start early motion postoperatively, lack of compression at the articular surface, and the risk of displacement if tensile force was placed on the construct. Others have advocated screw fixation for transverse or longitudinal fractures.[27,67,78]

The ASIF has popularized the technique of tension band cerclage of the patella, with or without the addition of longitudinal Kirschner wires. This method is ideal for transverse patellar fractures because it allows immediate range of motion postoperatively. Two stainless steel 18-gauge wires (1.2 mm) are inserted anteriorly through the quadriceps and patellar tendons, with one placed in a figure-of-eight fashion and the other in a cerclage configuration (Figs. 67–15 and 67–16). Tightening of the wires overreduces the transverse fracture, but when the knee is flexed, the pressure of the femoral condyles against the patella transforms the tension into interfragmentary compression. Two twisting sites for the wires have been shown to provide greater compression.[68] Additionally, in a biomechanical study by Scilaris et al, less displacement was shown through cyclic loading with the use of 1.0-mm steel braided cable than with 1.0-mm monofilament wire. This method can be augmented with two parallel 2-mm Kirschner wires placed longitudinally through the patella, which helps prevent tilting of the distal fragment (Figs. 67–17 and 67–18).[69] This same technique has been used for comminuted patella fractures. A variation of the tension band technique, according to Lotke and Ecker,[48] is to use a tension band construct with the wire placed through longitudinal drill holes in the patella (Fig. 67–19). To minimize the risk for subsequent hardware irritation, No. 5 nonabsorbable polyester sutures may be substituted for the stainless steel wires used in tension

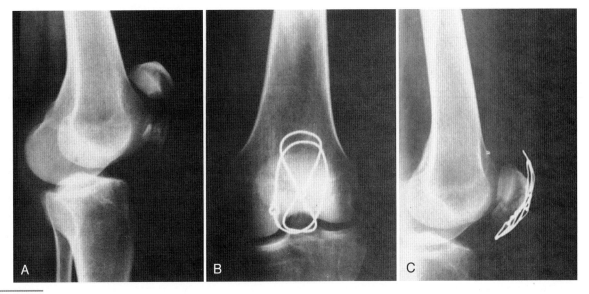

Figure 67–16. **A,** Transverse fracture of the patella with some distal fragment comminution. **B** and **C,** Treatment by tension band cerclage with two wires; after 1 month, the fracture showed good healing, with a little step on the articular surface.

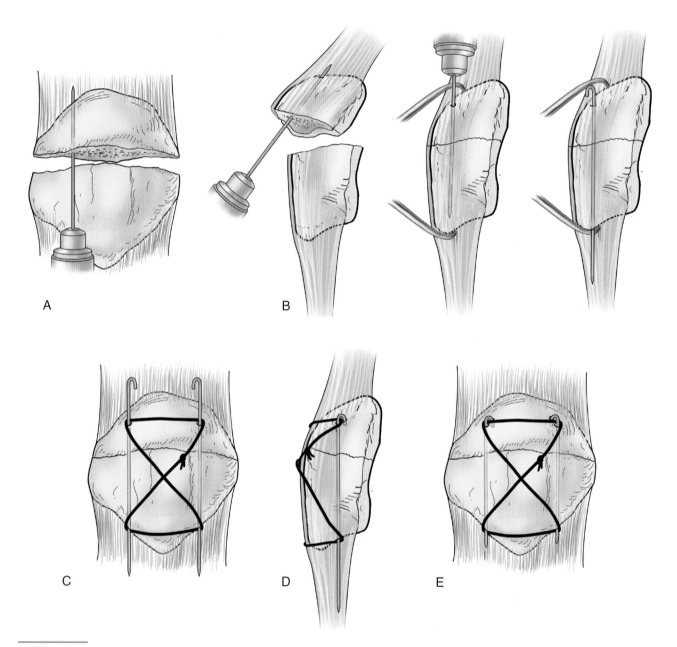

Figure 67–17. The tension band technique for patella fractures. **A,** Kirschner wires are placed retrograde in a distal-to-proximal direction to the fracture's edge of the proximal fragment. **B,** The fracture is reduced and held with bone clamps while the Kirschner wires are advanced distally across the fracture site. **C,** A figure-of-eight tension band wire is passed around the Kirschner wires and tightened. **D** and **E** The Kirschner wires are countersunk proximally, and excess wire is removed distally. (Redrawn from Scuderi G: The Patella. New York, Springer-Verlag, 1995.)

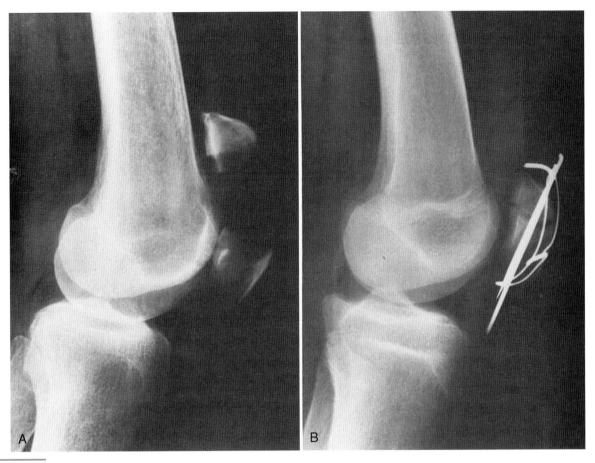

Figure 67–18. **A,** Transverse fracture of the patella. **B,** Treatment with modified tension cerclage. The K-pins were too long and had to be removed at 3 months after secure healing of the fracture. (From Aglietti P, Scarfi G: Trattamento chirurgico delle fratture di rotula. Arch Putti 30:301, 1980.)

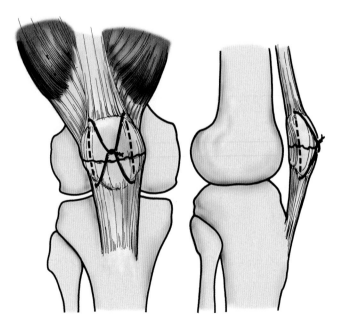

Figure 67–19. Internal fixation of a transverse fracture of the patella according to the method of Lotke and Ecker.

banding the patella (Fig. 67–20). Sutures alone are more prone to failure than wires and may require cast immobilization. Nonabsorbable suture placed in a cerclage fashion may be used for internal fixation of the sleeve fracture of the patella seen most often in the pediatric population (Fig. 67–21).[82]

Cannulated screws with a tension band wire placed through the screws have also been reported to provide excellent fracture fixation. This technique is very similar to the ASIF tension band technique, with 3.5-mm cannulated screws being substituted for the Kirschner wires. Care must be taken to avoid protruding the threads of the screws beyond the far cortex, which may lead to early wire failure (Fig. 67–22).[17]

Internal fixation with 3.5- to 4.5-mm-diameter screws may also be used for fixation of patella fractures. With simple transverse or displaced longitudinal fractures in patients with good bone stock, two parallel screws placed across the fracture in a lag technique may be all that is required (Fig. 67–23). Additionally, screw fixation or additional Kirschner wires may be used to convert more comminuted fracture patterns into those that are amenable to tension band fixation (Fig. 67–24).[25] A comminuted central portion of the patella, not amenable to fixation, may be removed and the remaining fragments fixed with screw fixation (Fig. 67–25).

The knee is typically mobilized early, with no cast needed. Intraoperative assessment of fixation construct stability is critical in guiding the surgeon to the appropriate progression of range of motion postoperatively. Typically, the incision is allowed to "rest" for a few days with a period of immobilization in full extension in a hinged knee brace with drop locks. Initiation of range of motion is then based on the intraoperative range of motion that maintained a stable construct. This, of course, will differ from patient to patient. For example, in a more elderly patient with poor bone stock, the authors typically begin motion from 0 to 30 degrees for 2 weeks, 0 to 60 degrees for 2 weeks, 0 to 90 degrees for 2 weeks, and then motion as tolerated. In contrast, a younger patient with excellent bone stock and outstanding fixation stability will not need such restrictions. Surgeon judgment is paramount in prescribing the appropriate rehabilitation regimen. Cast immobilization is reserved only for fractures in which construct stability is marginal and additional external immobilization may prevent catastrophic construct failure. Casts may also be useful in demented, noncompliant, or mentally retarded patients.

A biomechanical study comparing the strength of four different fixation techniques (circumferential wiring, tension band wiring, modified tension band over K-wires, and the Lotke and Ecker technique) in the treatment of simulated transverse fractures and retinacular disruption identified the circumferential wiring method as providing the weakest fixation, with up to 20 mm of displacement with tension stress. The tension band wiring method

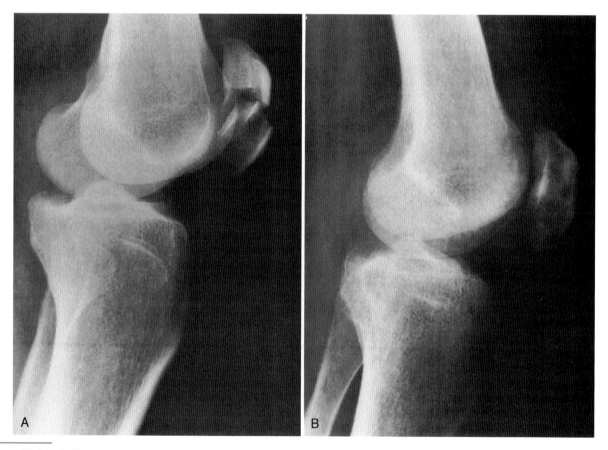

Figure 67–20. **A,** Transverse patella fracture treated by traditional circumferential cerclage with suture fixation. **B,** Good result after 6 weeks of cast immobilization.

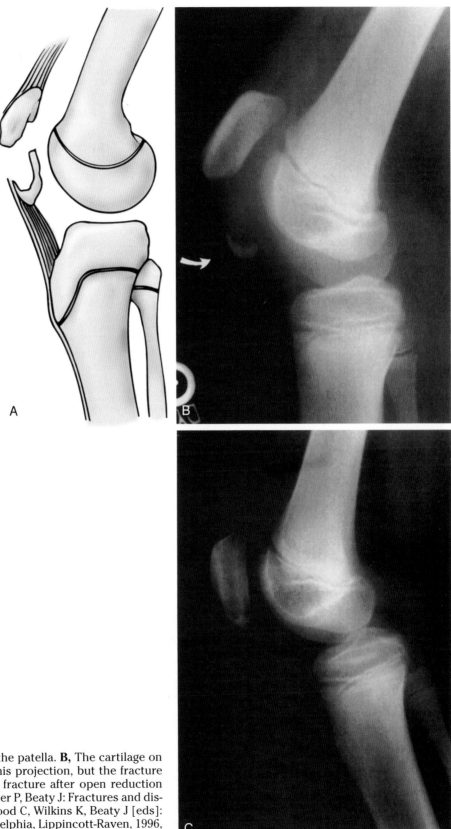

Figure 67–21. **A,** Sleeve fracture of the patella. **B,** The cartilage on the distal fragment is not seen in this projection, but the fracture fragment is evident. **C,** The healed fracture after open reduction and internal fixation. (From Sponseller P, Beaty J: Fractures and dislocations about the knee. In Rockwood C, Wilkins K, Beaty J [eds]: Fractures in Children, 4th ed. Philadelphia, Lippincott-Raven, 1996, p 1287.)

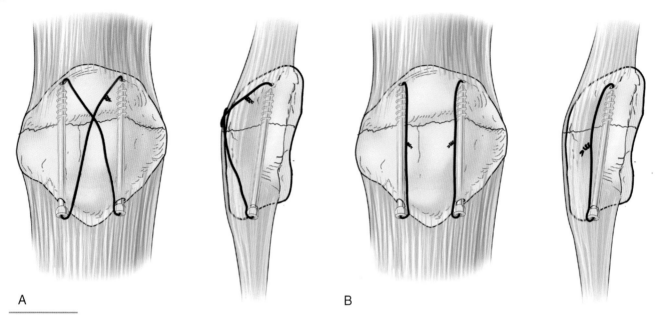

Figure 67–22. **A,** Cannulated screws augmented with a figure-of-eight tension band anteriorly. Note that the threads of the screw do not cross the fracture site. **B,** The separate tension bands are applied vertically. (Redrawn from Cramer K, Moed B: Patellar fractures: Contemporary approach to treatment. J Am Acad Orthop Surg 5:323, 1997.)

showed improved stability, with only 2.5 mm of displacement. The addition of Kirschner wires to modify the tension band technique further improved fracture stability. Surprisingly, the technique of Lotke and Ecker showed fracture stability similar to that of the modified tension band method, with less than 1 mm of maximum displacement at the fracture site.[15] It was concluded that the combination of transosseous fixation and tension band principles offers the best results. More recently, Carpenter et al compared the modified tension band technique with the tension band technique incorporated into cannulated

screws and screws alone in a simulated leg extension model. Their results demonstrated that the anterior tension band with incorporated cannulated screws failed at higher loads (mean, 732 N) than did screws alone (mean, 554 N) or the standard modified tension band (mean, 395 N). Additionally, the modified tension band allowed more fracture displacement under tension stress than the other two methods did.[17]

Clinical studies published to date have reported the best results with tension band wiring for internal fixation, with 86% of patients achieving excellent or good outcomes.[8,9,45]

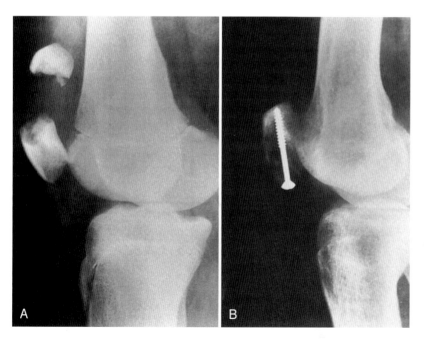

Figure 67–23. **A,** Transverse fracture of the upper third of the patella. **B,** Treatment with a screw; a good result is seen at 1 year. (From Aglietti P, Scarfi G: Trattamento chirurgico delle fratture di rotula. Arch Putti 30:301, 1980.)

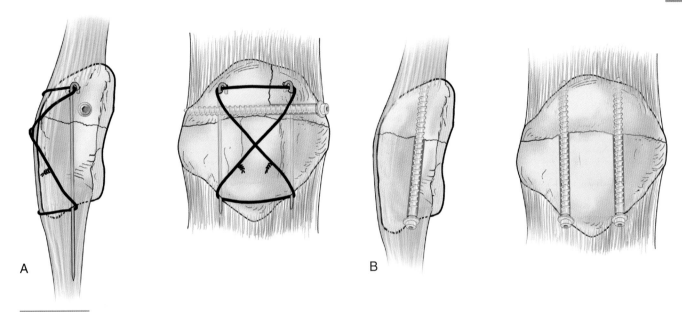

Figure 67–24. **A,** A transverse screw converts this comminuted fracture into a simple transverse fracture. **B,** Lag screws without tension band augmentation. (Redrawn from Cramer K, Moed B: Patella fractures: Contemporary approach to treatment. J Am Acad Orthop Surg 5:323, 1997.)

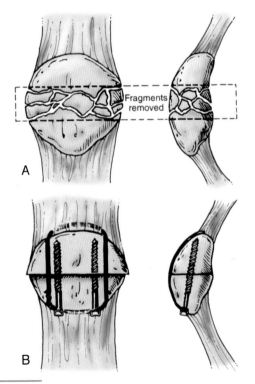

Figure 67–25. **A,** The comminuted fragments are removed, and the fracture surfaces are cut evenly, with subsequent reduction and fixation with screws plus wire cerclage in **B.** (From Scuderi G: The Patella. New York, Springer Verlag, 1995.)

Bostman et al[9] reported significantly better results with the modified tension band technique than with circumferential wiring, partial patellectomy, or screw fixation. Data regarding the results of surgical treatment should be interpreted with caution, however, because most surgical results have been reported by the method of surgical treatment rather than by the actual type of fracture treated.[8,10,11,19,48,54,87]

Our preferred treatment of the vast majority of fractures amenable to internal fixation is the modified tension band over Kirschner wires or through cannulated screws, with selected use of an additional circumferential wire or suture for more comminuted fractures.

Partial Patellectomy

Partial patellectomy is indicated when the amount of patellar comminution prevents secure fixation of all fracture fragments. Retention of as much congruous articular surface as possible is desirable; therefore, internal fixation of larger fragments with screws or Kirschner wires may help minimize the amount of bone lost with partial patellectomy and extensor mechanism repair.[25]

After adequate exposure, unsalvageable comminuted fragments are removed while preserving as much soft tissue as possible. Longitudinal drill holes are placed through the remaining patella to serve as tunnels for the tendon sutures. It is imperative that the holes be placed near the articular surface so that the patella does not tilt abnormally. A tendon-grasping, locking, nonabsorbable suture is placed through the tendon, passed through the bone tunnels, and tied over the bony bridge. An overlapping repair of the retinacular tears is then performed (Figs. 67–26 and 67–27). If protection of the repair is deemed necessary for immediate postoperative motion, the repair may be protected by a cable or wire passed through the tibial tubercle distally and just proximal to the superior aspect of the patella.[58] Postoperatively, partial weightbearing in full extension is allowed, with range-of-motion exercises dependent on the security of the repair and/or

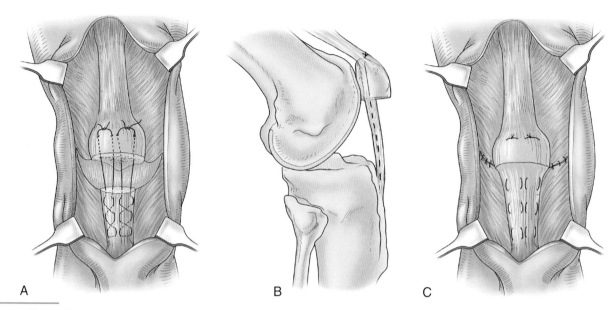

Figure 67–26. Technique of partial patellectomy. Note the placement of the patellar tendon at the articular surface of the remaining patella. (Redrawn from Cramer K, Moed B: Patellar fractures: Contemporary approach to treatment. J Am Acad Orthop Surg 5:323, 1997.)

the use of a load-sharing wire or cable. Extension splinting for ambulation is continued for 4 to 6 weeks, at which time quadriceps strengthening may commence.

The clinical results after partial patellectomy are favorable, with studies reporting good or excellent results in 78% to 86% of patients.[8-10,64] Other reports have demonstrated comparable results between partial patellectomy and internal fixation.[9,10,55] Bostrom et al[10] reported on a group of patients with transverse patellar fractures and inferior pole comminution. Of these patients, 88% treated by partial patellectomy had good to excellent results, as compared with 74% treated by internal fixation. Given this information, partial patellectomy should be considered if

adequate internal fixation of a comminuted fracture cannot be achieved. Most reports of partial patellectomy involve predominantly distal pole fractures that to a large extent are extra-articular.[8,55,64] The results of proximal pole excision and tendon repair have not been reported to date.

Total Patellectomy

Total patellectomy is rarely required and should be reserved for instances in which the comminution is so extensive that it is impossible to retain any congruous

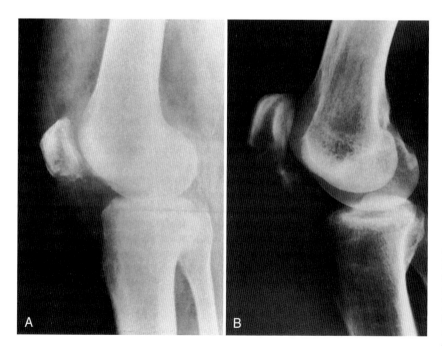

Figure 67–27. **A,** Distal patellar fracture of the apex. **B,** Treatment by partial patellectomy. A good result is evident at 1 year. (From Aglietti P, Scarfi G: Trattamento chirurgico delle fratture di rotula. Arch Putti 30:301, 1980.)

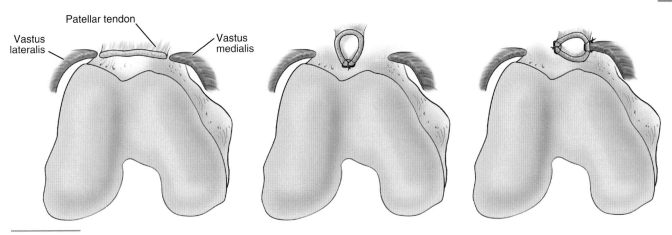

Figure 67–28. Compere's technique for patellectomy (see text). Ossification will occur within the tube.

fragments for articulation with the femur. Function after patellectomy is usually compromised, and for that reason it should be considered a salvage operation when no other surgical alternatives exist. The point at which bone retention is futile and total patellectomy is indicated has not been determined. Saltzman et al[64] were unable to show a correlation between the clinical outcome and the size of the retained fragment of patella. Pandey et al[55] believed that retention of even a small fragment of bone may provide a biomechanical advantage over total patellectomy.

If complete patellectomy is necessary, it is important to restore normal tension within the extensor mechanism after repair to minimize the loss of the biomechanical advantage generated by the patella. The extensor mechanism is effectively lengthened by patellectomy; therefore, some form of tissue imbrication is necessary to avoid a significant extensor lag.[65] After resection of all loose bone fragments with retention of as much soft tissue as possible, repair of the extensor mechanism can be performed with multiple tendon-grasping, nonabsorbable sutures. The retinacular disruption should also be repaired to restore the appropriate tension of the extensor mechanism. It is important that 80 to 90 degrees of flexion be possible on the operating table without placing undue tension on the repair. In the event that inadequate soft tissue is available for a primary repair or for soft-tissue augmentation, it may be necessary to perform an inverted V-plasty of the quadriceps tendon to fill the defect.[76] Postoperatively, the leg is kept in extension for 2 to 3 weeks to allow adequate soft-tissue healing. After this period of immobilization, a rehabilitation program is initiated.

If the soft tissues permit, our preferred method of total patellectomy is that described by Compere et al (Fig. 67–28),[24] which maintains the continuity and tubularizes the extensor mechanism after patellar excision. Frequently, ossification will occur within the tubularized patella tendon and create a "pseudopatella" that will enhance the mechanical advantage of the extensor mechanism.

The results after complete patellectomy have generally been inferior to those after partial patellectomy or internal fixation. Before the advent of tension band fixation, poor reconstructive methods (usually a simple cerclage wire) and results may have justified total excision of the patella.[14,28] Numerous studies have reported poor outcomes after total patellectomy when compared with those after partial excision or internal fixation. Sutton et al[84] compared total patellectomy with partial patellectomy in terms of quadriceps strength and functional ability. Their results revealed a 49% reduction in extensor mechanism strength with total excision. Functionally, patients lacked the ability to support their weight on the affected leg with stair climbing after total excision. Long-term follow-up on patellectomy patients has also demonstrated less than optimal results. Einola et al[32] reported on 28 patients monitored for an average of 7.5 years after excision, with only 6 having a good result. A common finding was persistent quadriceps atrophy, along with pain and weakness in the knee during activity. Scott[70] reported similar long-term results, with only 4 of 71 patients satisfied with their outcome. More than half these patients experienced weakness, and 90% experienced pain with activity. Atrophy of the quadriceps was a consistent finding. Sorensen[80] thought that attempts to salvage some patella was usually indicated, given the poor functional outcome of patients after total excision. Patients complained of pain and giving way of the affected knee with running and stair climbing. Additionally, no patients regained full quadriceps strength after patellectomy.

COMPLICATIONS OF OPERATIVE TREATMENT

Loss of Knee Motion

Decreased range of motion after treatment of patellar fractures is probably the most common complication encountered. The motion lost is usually in the terminal degrees of flexion and is well tolerated by most patients.[25] With the advent of tension band techniques, early range of motion is permitted, which usually results in a functional range of motion after fracture healing. In the event that some symptomatic stiffness results after fracture healing, an intense physical therapy program may help improve the functional range of motion. In rare instances, manipulation of the knee under anesthesia, with or without arthroscopic lysis of adhesions, may be required if a prolonged therapy program fails to yield beneficial results. We try to determine the need for further intervention at 3 months postoperatively because the fracture has typically united by this time and more aggressive attempts to gain motion may be considered without risking failure of internal fixation. The indications and timing for these interventions are not clearly delineated in the literature.

Infection

Infection rates after operative treatment of patella fractures have ranged from 3% to 10%.[8,39,79] Because of their superficial location, patella fractures are often accompanied by varying degrees of soft-tissue injury ranging from superficial abrasions to frank, open fractures. For open fractures, internal fixation should accompany emergency débridement and irrigation to reduce further soft-tissue damage and minimize the risk for infection. For closed injuries, some consideration can be given to postponing definitive fracture fixation until the soft tissues have had a chance to heal. Regardless of the timing of the definitive fracture fixation, careful handling of the soft tissue is mandatory to minimize the risk for infection. Superficial postoperative infections may be managed by a brief period of immobilization and antibiotic therapy until the infection resolves. Deep infection requires more aggressive treatment, including serial open débridement and irrigations, with definitive wound closure delayed until the wound is clean. If the fracture has not yet healed, stable internal fixation devices should be retained if possible. If persistent infection is present after fracture healing has occurred, hardware removal in addition to débridement and irrigation should be performed.

Loss of Reduction

The incidence of loss of operative reduction or loss of internal fixation of patella fractures has ranged from 0% to 20% in the literature.[8,39,79] Smith studied early complications of operative fixation in 51 fractures available for their study, with 49 of them treated with modified tension band wiring. Of the 11 failures (displacement >2 mm), 5 were attributed to errors in technique, with either the wire being placed in a circular fashion and not allowing for an effective tension band construct or the wire not being threaded posterior to the K-wires. Inadequate fixation as well as extensive comminution, patient noncompliance with activity and weightbearing restrictions, and early mobilization for constructs not amenable to early motion may contribute to loss of reduction.[45,79] If the resulting displacement or incongruity is minimal, a period of immobilization may be attempted in an effort to salvage the operation and allow the fracture to heal. If on the other hand the loss of reduction is too great or the extensor

mechanism has been compromised, reoperation is indicated.

Delayed Union and Nonunion

With the advent of new surgical fixation methods, delayed union and nonunion have become extremely uncommon. Carpenter et al[17] reported a nonunion rate of less than 1% after operative reduction and fixation. If delayed union is diagnosed, a period of immobilization may allow the fracture to consolidate. If a fracture fails to unite after a period of immobilization, consideration should be given to a repeated attempt at rigid fixation with autogenous bone grafting. In a report describing their operative revision of patellar nonunion, Weber and Cech[93] achieved a subsequent 100% union rate with the use of standard fixation techniques.

For neglected nonunion with wide separation between the fragments, an attempt should be made to reconstruct the extensor mechanism. If the nonunion is long-standing, it may be necessary to perform a quadriceps-plasty to mobilize a shortened, contracted quadriceps tendon before fracture fixation.[37]

Osteoarthrosis

Degeneration of the patellofemoral joint after patella fracture has several causes. Some are a direct result of the injury, and others are iatrogenic. First, articular damage may occur at the time of injury, and despite successful restoration of the articular surface, post-traumatic arthrosis may develop. Second, exuberant callus formation after apparent successful treatment (operative or nonoperative) of a comminuted patella fracture may also lead to patellofemoral joint degeneration.[65] Third, inadequate restoration of the articular surface has been defined as a source of subsequent joint degeneration. Fourth, improper placement plus repair of the patellar tendon on the patellar remnant after partial patellectomy has been shown to lead to patellofemoral arthritis.[31] Long-term follow-up studies of patients after patella fracture have demonstrated an increased incidence of radiographic degeneration when compared with the uninvolved knee.[37,80]

Hardware Irritation

Although irritation of the soft tissues by the underlying hardware is not a true complication of treatment, it occurs often enough to warrant mentioning, and patients should be counseled preoperatively of the possible need for hardware removal after fracture healing. Two studies[39,79] have quoted a 15% incidence of soft-tissue irritation from retained hardware that necessitated removal. Hardware removal should be done on an elective basis after complete fracture healing and restoration of knee motion.

SPECIAL CIRCUMSTANCES

Patella Fractures after Anterior Cruciate Ligament Reconstruction

Patella fracture after anterior cruciate ligament (ACL) reconstruction is a relatively rare occurrence, with a reported incidence of between 0.23% and 1.3%.[83,90] The mechanism is most commonly a direct fall on the harvested patella; however, there have been cases of fracture from no direct trauma.

Harvesting techniques and the shape of the graft are of considerable interest. A cadaver study by DuMontier et al compared the ultimate tensile strength of patellae after ACL harvest with three different shapes of grafts (circular, triangular, and rectangular). They found no significant difference in ultimate tensile strength or the method in which the patellae failed.[29] Other considerations include precise instruments. In Viola and Vianello's series of 1320 ACL reconstructions, three postoperative patella fractures occurred, all of them transverse. They thought that a contributing factor was the switch from a 7-mm saw blade to a 9-mm saw blade because the increased travel of the blade could create a greater horizontal stress riser.[90] Daluge et al discussed a technique in which they obtained autograft with curets from the tibial tubercle origin of the graft, as well as collected reaming material from the tibial and femoral tunnels. They then packed this autograft into the patella graft site and closed the deep retinacular fascia over the top of the patella graft site. Their conclusion was that primary bone grafting of the graft donor site is a relatively simple endeavor and could decrease the risk for a stress riser once the graft is incorporated.[26]

Most fractures after ACL reconstruction are usually transverse horizontal fractures with often little comminution. Their fixation is relatively straightforward with lag screws, tension band wiring, or combination wiring through lag screws. A small subset of fractures after ACL reconstruction are vertical fractures. Special attention must be paid to avoid placing inferior screws across the graft site with a lag technique. Doing so may cause fracture distraction proximally because of the loss of cortical contact inferiorly as a result of bone loss.

Patella Fractures after Total Knee Arthroplasty

Fracture of the patella is rare after total knee replacement. The reported incidence of patella fractures after patellar resurfacing has ranged from 0.33% to as high as 6.3% in one series.[16,36]

A multitude of risk factors for patella fracture after total knee arthroplasty have been compiled in the literature, and they have been categorized into patient-related factors, implant design factors, and surgical technique factors (Box 67–1).[46]

Excessive body weight and an increased activity level have been associated with an increased incidence of patel-

Box 67-1. Risk Factors for Patella Fracture after Total Knee Arthroplasty

Patient Factors
Osteoporosis
Rheumatoid arthritis
Male sex
Overactivity
Excessive knee motion

Implant Design Factors
Patellar replacement/nonreplacement
Central peg
Cementless implants
Posterior cruciate ligament–substituting prosthesis
Inset design
Polyethylene osteolysis

Technical Factors
Excessive resection
Inadequate resection
Anterior patella perforation
Revision surgery
Cement use
Malalignment
Patella subluxation/dislocation
Patella blood supply disruption

lar fracture.[30,40,86] Excessive postoperative flexion has also been associated with patella fractures in some series,[2,40] and others have found no relationship between range of motion and fracture.[77] Osteoporotic bone secondary to rheumatoid arthritis and long-term steroid use have also been identified as risk factors for fracture.[71] Although little can be done surgically to alter these patient-related risk factors for fracture, knowledge of their presence should alert the surgeon to avoid further compromising the success of patellar resurfacing by means of careful surgical technique and implant selection decisions.

The design of the component can also influence the risk for patella fracture. Patellar buttons with a central peg are believed to result in more frequent fractures, especially if the anterior cortex of the patella is perforated.[13,16,71] The type of fixation used for the patella has likewise been implicated, with some authors believing that the use of cementless pegs increases the incidence of fracture and others believing that the thermal effects of polymerizing bone cement may increase the risk for patellar fracture.[20] Patellar components that are designed to be inset within the periphery of the patella have also been associated with so-called rim fractures of the peripheral portion of the patella.[46] Insall and Dethmers[40] believe that excessive knee motion and increased activity postoperatively place patients at risk for patella fracture, but this in effect is a testament to the success of the total knee arthroplasty.

The goal of patellar resurfacing is to re-create the original dimensions of the patella after prosthetic replacement. Any deviation from this technique increases the risk for patellar fracture. Excessive bone resection may predispose the thin bone to fracture by virtue of its inability to withstand the physiological strains placed on it. The same also applies to asymmetric resurfacing, with the thin portion at risk for failure.[61,71,86] Conversely, inadequate bone resection may thicken the patellofemoral joint excessively, which may lead to patellar fracture through increased contact force.[5,12,86] If the appropriate femoral and tibial rotation is not achieved, maltracking of the patella may occur, which will increase the force on the patellofemoral joint and potentially lead to subluxation and/or fracture.[33,77] Additionally, anterior placement of the femur may increase the force across the patellofemoral joint and potentially lead to fracture.

The other iatrogenic risk factor for patella fracture is circulatory embarrassment to the patella as a result of the surgical exposure and correction of patellofemoral maltracking by lateral retinacular release. Avascular necrosis of the patella has been reported after ligation of the superior lateral geniculate artery, especially when associated with a medial arthrotomy.[13,20,43,72] However, other authors have disputed this claim.[42,62,63] Despite the controversy, it is recommended that an attempt be made to spare the superior lateral geniculate artery during lateral release if at all possible, with the understanding that good patellofemoral tracking should take precedence over conservation of this vessel. It is difficult to stratify the many risk factors associated with periprosthetic patella fracture in terms of their relative contribution to this complication.

Figgie et al,[33] in their review of 36 patella fractures after condylar total knee arthroplasty, concluded that the most serious contributing factor to patella fracture was the overall alignment of the prosthesis. Malalignment also had a major impact on the severity of the fracture and on the prognosis of the patella fracture after treatment.

Classification of periprosthetic patellar fractures has also been confusing, with many systems having been developed to help guide treatment and predict prognosis. Fractures may be classified by mechanism of injury, such as direct, indirect, or stress fractures with no identifiable injury. Insall and Haas[42] differentiated patella fractures by configuration of the fracture: horizontal, vertical, and comminuted. They also categorized periprosthetic fractures into traumatic injuries, which were often displaced (Fig. 67–29) and required operative intervention, and fatigue fractures (Figs. 67–30 and 67–31), which are best treated with a period of decreased motion or activity until asymptomatic. Perhaps the most useful classification system in terms of guiding treatment is that described by Goldberg et al,[34] which attempts to account for the patellar fracture pattern and any concomitant extensor mechanism pathology (Fig. 67–32).[44]

Type I fractures are marginal fractures with no extension into the implant-bone interface and no extensor mechanism injury. Type II fractures are characterized by either disruption of the extensor mechanism or disruption

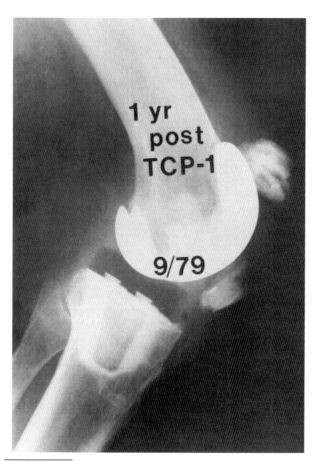

Figure 67–29. Post-traumatic vertical fracture of the patella requiring open reduction.

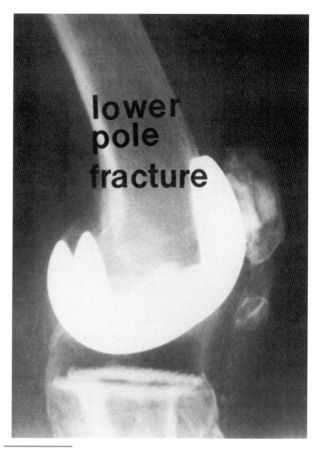

Figure 67–30. Vertical fatigue fracture of the patella. In contradistinction to traumatic fractures, this type usually heals spontaneously, as occurred in this case.

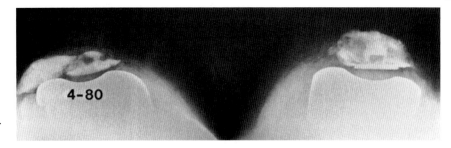

Figure 67–31. Horizontal fatigue fracture of the patella.

of the implant-bone interface. Type III injuries involve the inferior pole of the patella, with subtype III-A having disruption of the patellar tendon and subtype III-B having an intact patellar tendon. Type IV fractures are those associated with patellofemoral dislocation.

Management of periprosthetic patellar fractures must be guided by a number of factors, and it is important to evaluate all components of the arthroplasty to optimize treatment results. As Figgie et al[33] concluded in their review, the overall alignment of the arthroplasty is critical, and failure to address such alignment may compromise the results of periprosthetic patella fracture treatment.

Patella fractures after total knee arthroplasty can often be treated nonoperatively if no significant displacement or extensor lag exists. Fractures that are marginal and have no extension into the bone-implant interface or disruption of the extensor mechanism (type I) can be successfully treated by a period of bracing or casting until fracture consolidation occurs (see Fig. 67–25). Even comminuted fractures with little displacement and an intact prosthesis and extensor mechanism can be treated without surgical intervention. If component loosening has occurred, it may be prudent to allow the fracture to consolidate before attempting component revision, as opposed to attempting both in the acute setting.[81] Grossly loose or free-floating implants may require removal to prevent further damage to the joint or extensor mechanism. Fractures that involve disruption of the extensor mechanism (types II and III-B) mandate surgical repair to minimize the functional disability of a permanent extensor lag. Patellar fractures with significant displacement should also be treated by open reduction and internal fixation.[3,12,34,36] Standard tension band wiring with supplemental Kirschner wires or screws is not always possible because of osteopenic bone, poor

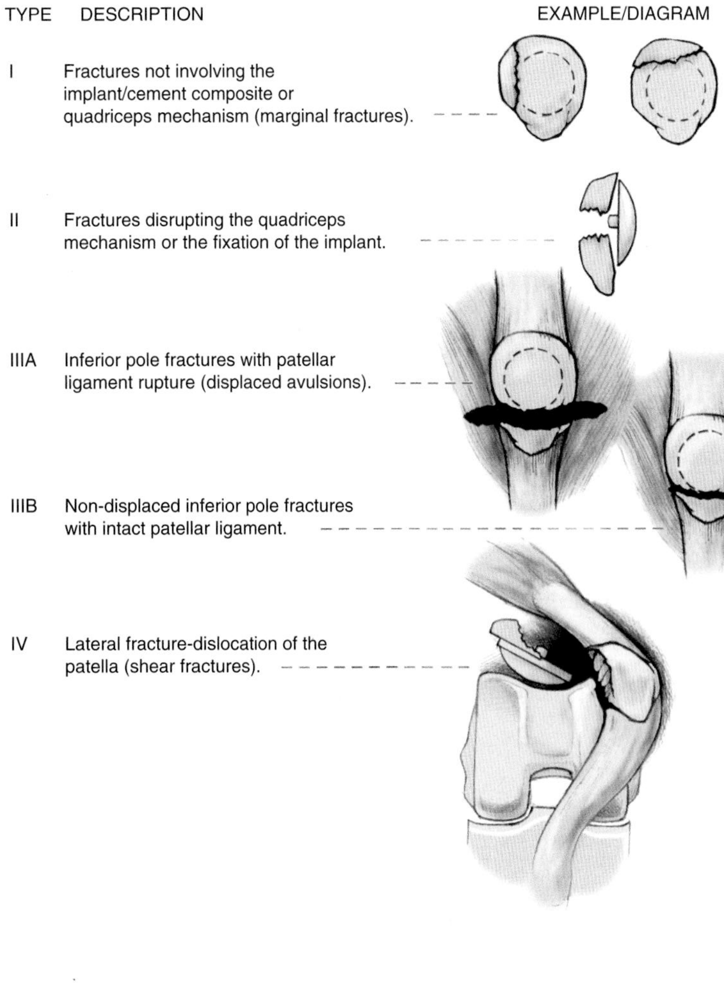

TYPE	DESCRIPTION	EXAMPLE/DIAGRAM
I	Fractures not involving the implant/cement composite or quadriceps mechanism (marginal fractures).	
II	Fractures disrupting the quadriceps mechanism or the fixation of the implant.	
IIIA	Inferior pole fractures with patellar ligament rupture (displaced avulsions).	
IIIB	Non-displaced inferior pole fractures with intact patellar ligament.	
IV	Lateral fracture-dislocation of the patella (shear fractures).	

Figure 67–32. Goldberg's classification[34] of patella fractures after total knee arthroplasty. (From Kolessar D, Rand J: Extensor mechanism problems following total knee arthroplasty. In Morrey B [ed]: Reconstructive Surgery of the Joints, 2nd ed. New York, Churchill Livingstone, 1996.)

capacity to heal, and the presence of a patellar component, so cerclage wiring may be the only surgical option. As a result of the compromised fixation, early postoperative motion may not be possible.[83] If surgical repair of a patella fracture is not possible and resurfacing of the patellar remnant is not technically feasible, patelloplasty (partial patellectomy without resurfacing) is much more preferable than total patellectomy. Conserving a portion of the patella helps maintain the biomechanical advantage of the extensor mechanism and also minimizes the risk for tendon rupture and the total knee arthroplasty instability sometimes seen after total patellectomy.[7,89]

In summary, for patella fractures after total knee arthroplasty, many of these injuries do well without surgery despite an unusual radiographic appearance. Operative decision making is guided by the integrity of the extensor mechanism, the fixation status of the patellar component, and the displacement of the fracture.

ACKNOWLEDGMENT

Special thanks to Patricia T. Simmons.

References

1. Aglietti P, Buzzi B: Fractures of the patella. In Insall J (ed): Surgery of the Knee, 2nd ed. New York, Churchill Livingstone, 1993.
2. Aglietti P, Buzzi B, Gaudanzi A: Patellofemoral functional results and complications with the posterior stabilized total condylar prosthesis. J Arthroplasty 3:17, 1988.
3. Aglietti P, Insall J, Walker P, et al: A new patellar prosthesis. Clin Orthop 180:158, 1981.
4. Anderson L: Fractures. In Crenshaw DI (ed): Campbell's Operative Orthopaedics, 5th ed. St Louis, CV Mosby, 1971.
5. Barnes C, Scott R: Patellofemoral complications of total knee replacement. Instr Course Lect 42:304, 1993.
6. Baumgartl F: Das Kniegelenk. Berlin, Springer-Verlag, 1964.
7. Bayne O, Cameron H: Total knee arthroplasty following patellectomy. Clin Orthop 186:112, 1984.
8. Bostman O, Kivilvoto O, Nirhama J: Comminuted displaced fractures of the patella. Injury 13:196, 1981.
9. Bostman O, Kivilvoto O, Santavirta S, et al: Fractures of the patella treated by operation. Arch Orthop Trauma Surg 102:78, 1983.
10. Bostrom A: Fracture of the patella: A study of 422 patellar fractures. Acta Orthop Scand 143:1, 1972.
11. Bostrom A: Longitudinal fractures of the patella. Rec Surg Traumatol 14:136, 1974.
12. Brick G, Scott R: The patellofemoral component of total knee arthroplasty. Clin Orthop 231:163, 1988.
13. Brick G, Scott R: Blood supply to the patella: Significance in total knee arthroplasty. J Arthroplasty 4:75, 1989.
14. Brooke J: The treatment of fractured patella by excision: A study of morphology and function. Br J Surg 24:733, 1936.
15. Buzzi R, Aglietti P: Fratture transversali di rotulz: Valutazione sperementale del metodo di fissazione interna di Lotke e Ecker. Arch Putti 37:283, 1989.
16. Cameron H, Fedorkow D: The patella in total knee arthroplasty. Clin Orthop 165:197, 1982.
17. Carpenter J, Kasman R, Matthews L: Patella fractures. Instr Course Lect 43:97, 1994.
18. Carson W, James S, Larson R, et al: Patellofemoral disorders: II— Radiographic examination. Clin Orthop 185:178, 1984.
19. Chiroff R: A new technique for the treatment of comminuted transverse fractures of the patella. Surg Gynecol Obstet 79:909, 1977.
20. Clayton M, Thirupathi R: Patellar complications after total condylar arthroplasty. Clin Orthop 170:152, 1982.
21. Coffer H: Mechanical function of the patella. J Bone Joint Surg Am 53:1551, 1971.
22. Coffer H: Patellobiomechanics. Clin Orthop 144:51, 1979.
23. Colton C: The history of fracture treatment. In Browner B, Levine A, Jupiter J, Trafton P (eds): Skeletal Trauma, 3rd ed. Philadelphia, WB Saunders, 2003.
24. Compere C, Hill J, Lewinnek G, et al: A new method of patellectomy for patellofemoral arthritis. J Bone Joint Surg Am 61:714, 1979.
25. Cramer K, Moed B: Patellar fractures: Contemporary approach to treatment. J Am Acad Orthop Surg 5:323, 1997.
26. Daluga D, Johnson C, Bach B: Primary bone grafting following graft procurement for anterior cruciate ligament insufficiency. J Arthroscopy 6:3:205, 1990.
27. De Palma AF: Diseases of the Knee. Philadelphia, JB Lippincott, 1954.
28. Dobbie R, Ryerson S: The treatment of fractured patella by excision. Am J Surg 55:339, 1942.
29. DuMonteir T, Metcalf M, Simonian P, Larson R: Patella fracture after anterior cruciate ligament reconstruction with the patella tendon. Am J Knee Surg 14:9, 2001.
30. Dupont J, Baker S: Complications of patellofemoral resurfacing in total knee arthroplasty. Orthop Trans 6:369, 1982.
31. Duthie H, Hutchinson J: The results of partial and total excision of the patella. J Bone Joint Surg Br 40:75, 1958.
32. Einola S, Aho A, Kallio P: Patellectomy after fracture. Acta Orthop Scand 47:441, 1976.
33. Figgie H, Goldberg V, Figgie M, et al: The effect of alignment on fractures of the patella after condylar total knee arthroplasty. J Bone Joint Surg Am 71:1031, 1989.
34. Goldberg V, Figgie H, Inglis A, et al: Patella fracture type and prognosis in condylar total knee arthroplasty. Clin Orthop 236:115, 1988.
35. Goodfellow J, Hungerford D, Woods C: Patellofemoral joint mechanics and pathology of chondromalacia-patella. J Bone Joint Surg Br 59:291, 1976.
36. Grace J, Sim F: Fracture of the patella after total knee arthroplasty. Clin Orthop 230:168, 1988.
37. Hesketh K: Experiences with the Thompson quadriceps-plasty. J Bone Joint Surg Br 45:491, 1963.
38. Huberti H, Hayes W, Stone J, et al: Force ratios in the quadriceps tendon and ligamentum patella. J Orthop Res 2:49, 1984.
39. Hung L, Chan K, Chow Y, et al: Fractured patella: Operative treatment using the tension band principle. Injury 16:343, 1985.
40. Insall J, Dethmers D: Revision of total knee arthroplasty. Clin Orthop 170:123, 1982.
41. Insall J, Goldberg V, Salvati E: Recurrent dislocation of the high riding patella. Clin Orthop 88:67, 1972.
42. Insall J, Haas S: Complications of total knee arthroplasty. In Insall J (ed): Surgery of the Knee, 2nd ed. New York, Churchill Livingstone, 1993.
43. Kayler D, Lyttle D: Surgical interruption of patellar blood supply by total knee arthroplasty. Clin Orthop 229:221, 1988.
44. Kolessar D, Rand J: Extensor mechanism problems following total knee arthroplasty. In Morrey B (ed): Reconstructive Surgery of the Joints, 2nd ed. New York, Churchill Livingstone, 1996.
45. Levack B, Flannagan J, Hobbs S: Results of surgical treatment of patella fractures. J Bone Joint Surg Br 67:416, 1985.
46. Lewis P, Rorabeck C: Periprosthetic fractures. In Engh G (ed): Revision Total Knee Arthroplasty. Philadelphia, Williams & Wilkins, 1997.
47. Lieb F, Perry J: Quadriceps function. J Bone Joint Surg Am 50:1535, 1968.
48. Lotke P, Ecker M: Transverse fractures of the patella. Clin Orthop 158:180, 1981.
49. Magnuson P: Fractures, 2nd ed. Philadelphia, JB Lippincott, 1933.
50. Matthews L, Sanstegard D, Henke J: Load-bearing characteristics of the patellofemoral joint. Acta Orthop Scand 48:511, 1977.
51. McMaster P: Fractures of the patella. Clin Orthop 4:24, 1953.
52. Merchant A, Mercer R, Jacobsen R, et al: Roentgenographic analysis of patellofemoral congruence. J Bone Joint Surg Am 56:1391, 1974.
53. Müller M, Allgöwer R, Schneider R, Willinegger H: Maual of Internal Fixation. Techniques Recommended by the AO Group. Berlin, Springer-Verlag, 1979.
54. Nummi J: Operative treatment of patella fractures. Acta Orthop Scand 42:437, 1971.

55. Pandey A, Pandey S, Pandey P: Results of partial patellectomy. Acta Orthop Trauma Surg 110:246, 1991.
56. Payr E: Zur operativen Behandlung der Kniegelenksteife nach langdauernder Ruhigstellung. Zentralbl Chir 44:809, 1917.
57. Peeples R, Margo M: Function after patellectomy. Clin Orthop 132:180, 1978.
58. Perry C, McCarthy J, Kain C, et al: Patellar fixation protected with a load-sharing cable: A mechanical and clinical study. J Orthop Trauma 2:234, 1988.
59. Reider B, Marshall J, Kostin B, et al: The anterior aspect of the knee joint. J Bone Joint Surg Am 63:351, 1981.
60. Resneck D, Niwayama G: Disorders of Bone and Joint Disorders, 2nd ed. Philadelphia, WB Saunders, 1988.
61. Reuben J, McDonald C, Woodward P, et al: Effect of patella thickness on patella strain following total knee arthroplasty. J Arthroplasty 6:251, 1991.
62. Ritter M, Campbell E: Postoperative patellar complications with or without lateral release during total knee arthroplasty. Clin Orthop 219:163, 1987.
63. Ritter M, Keating E, Faris P: Clinical roentgenographic and scintigraphic results after interruption of the superior lateral genicular artery during total knee arthroplasty. Clin Orthop 248:145, 1989.
64. Saltzman C, Goulet J, McClellan R, et al: Results of treatment of displaced patella fractures by partial patellectomy. J Bone Joint Surg Am 72:1279, 1990.
65. Sanders R: Patella fractures and extensor mechanism injuries. In Browner B (ed): Skeletal Trauma, Philadelphia, WB Saunders, 1992.
66. Scapinelli R: Blood supply of the human patella. J Bone Joint Surg Br 3:563, 1967.
67. Schatzker J, Tile M: The Rationale of Operative Fracture Care. New York, Springer-Verlag, 1987.
68. Schauwecker R: The Practice of Osteosynthesis. Stuttgart, Germany, Georg Thieme, 1974.
69. Scilaris T, Grantham J, Prayson M, et al: Biomechanical comparison of fixation methods in transverse patella fractures. J Orthop Trauma 12:5:356, 1998.
70. Scott J: Fractures of the patella. J Bone Joint Surg Br 31:76, 1949.
71. Scott R: Duopatellar total knee replacement: The Brigham experience. Orthop Clin North Am 13:89, 1982.
72. Scucki G, Scharf S, Meltzer L, et al: The relationship of lateral release to patella viability in total knee arthroplasty. J Arthroplasty 2:209, 1987.
73. Scuderi G: The Patella. New York, Springer-Verlag, 1995.
74. Seligo W: Fractures of the patella. Reconstr Surg Traumatol 12:1281, 1971.
75. Shim S, Leung G: Blood supply of the knee joint: A microangiographic study in children and adults. Clin Orthop 208:119, 1986.
76. Shorbe H, Dobson C: Patellectomy. J Bone Joint Surg Am 40:1281, 1958.
77. Sirrison A, Noble J, Harding K: Complications of the Altenborough knee replacement. J Bone Joint Surg Br 68:100, 1986.
78. Smillie IS: Injuries of the Knee Joint, 4th ed. Edinburgh, Churchill Livingstone, 1970.
79. Smith S, Cramer K, Kargus D, et al: Early complications in the operative treatment of patella fractures. J Orthop Trauma 11:183, 1997.
80. Sorensen K: The later prognosis after fracture of the patella. Acta Orthop Scand 47:441, 1976.
81. Spitzer A, Vince K: Patella considerations in total knee replacement. In Scuderi G (ed): The Patella, New York, Springer-Verlag, 1995.
82. Sponseller P, Beaty J: Fractures and dislocations about the knee. In Rockwood C, Wilkins K, Beaty J (eds): Fractures in Children, 4th ed. Philadelphia, JB Lippincott, 1996, p 1287.
83. Stein D, Hunt S, Rosen J, Sherman O: The incidence and outcome of patella fractures after anterior cruciate ligament reconstruction. J Arthroscopy 18:6:578, 2002.
84. Sutton F, Thompson C, Lipke J, et al: The effect of patellectomy on knee function. J Bone Joint Surg Am 58:537, 1976.
85. Templeman D: Fractures of the patella. In Gustilo RB, Kyle RF, Templeman DC (eds): Fractures and Dislocations. St Louis, CV Mosby, 1993.
86. Thompson F, Hood R, Insall J: Patella fractures in total knee arthroplasty. Orthop Trans 5:490, 1981.
87. Thompson J: Comminuted fractures of the patella. J Bone Joint Surg Am 17:431, 1935.
88. Vince K, Cameron H: Total knee arthroplasty following patellectomy. Clin Orthop 186:112, 1984.
89. Vince K, McPherson E: The patella in total knee arthroplasty. Orthop Clin North Am 23:675, 1992.
90. Viola R, Vianello R: Three cases of patella fracture in 1320 ACL reconstructions with bone–patella tendon–bone autograft. J Arthroscopy 15:93, 1999.
91. Watkins M, Harris B, Wender S: Effect of patellectomy on the function of the quadriceps and hamstrings. J Bone Joint Surg Am 65:390, 1983.
92. Watson-Jones R: Fractures and Joint Injuries. Baltimore, Williams & Wilkins, 1952.
93. Weber B, Cech O: Pseudarthrosis. New York, Grune & Stratton, 1976.
94. Wiberg G: Roentgenographic and anatomic studies of the patellofemoral joint. Acta Orthop Scand 12:319, 1941.

CHAPTER 68

Treatment of Periprosthetic Fractures around a Total Knee Arthroplasty

George J. Haidukewych • *Steven Lyons* • *Tom Bernasek*

Periprosthetic fractures remain problematic complications after total knee arthroplasty. The number of knee arthroplasties performed worldwide continues to increase, and with the ever-growing elderly population, the number of periprosthetic fractures will continue to increase as well. Decision making regarding the management of these fractures is divided according to whether the fracture has occurred in the femur or the tibia and whether the arthroplasty is loose or well fixed. Fractures of the distal end of the femur above a well-fixed arthroplasty are typically treated with some form of internal fixation. The use of fixed-angled, locked, percutaneously inserted plates has revolutionized the treatment of these fractures. Early clinical and biomechanical data are encouraging. For loose implants, revision is typically considered. Bony defects, areas of osteolysis, osteopenia, and short periarticular fragments all pose challenges to a successful revision arthroplasty in this setting. In elderly patients, distal femoral replacement "tumor prostheses" are often required to reconstruct massive bony defects. Attention to specific technical details is necessary for a successful result, and surgeons undertaking such reconstructions should be experienced in both arthroplasty and fracture management techniques.

Over 200,000 primary knee arthroplasties are performed annually in the United States, and this number continues to increase. It is estimated that 0.3% to 2.5% of patients will sustain a periprosthetic fracture as a complication of total knee arthroplasty.[1,11,31] Patient-specific risk factors such as rheumatoid arthritis, osteolysis, osteopenic bone, and frequent falls, common in the elderly population, and technique-specific risk factors such as anterior femoral cortical notching have all been implicated as potential causes of periprosthetic fractures. The economic impact as well as disability associated with these fractures is substantial; therefore, having an effective strategy to manage these challenging injuries is important. Typically, fractures occur in the supracondylar area of the femur above a well-fixed total knee arthroplasty (Fig. 68–1).[1,2,11,18,24,31] Fractures of the tibia are much less common and are frequently associated with implant loosening.[1,11,12,17] Decision making regarding the treatment of periprosthetic fractures around a total knee arthroplasty is divided according to whether the fracture has occurred in the distal end of the femur or the proximal end of the tibia and whether the implant is well fixed or loose. In general, patients with fractures around loose implants are considered candidates for revision total knee arthroplasty, whereas fractures around well-fixed implants are candidates for open reduction and internal fixation. Various methods of internal fixation have been described for the treatment of these injuries.[2,5,18,24,31,33] There has been recent enthusiasm for minimally invasive osteosynthesis of these injuries with the use of locked plates. Revision arthroplasty in this setting can be very demanding with a unique set of technical challenges. The purpose of this chapter is to review the decision making, contemporary techniques, and potential complications of the management of periprosthetic fractures of the femur and tibia around a total knee arthroplasty. Periprosthetic fractures of the patella are discussed in Chapter 67.

PATIENT EVALUATION

Patients with fractures around asymptomatic, well-fixed implants do not usually require an infection workup. However, in patients with a loose implant or a history of prefracture knee pain, routine preoperative evaluation of these patients should include a complete blood count with manual differential, sedimentation rate, C-reactive protein serology, and knee aspiration to exclude occult infection. Medical optimization for these frequently frail elderly patients is recommended.

Adequate radiographs are necessary to evaluate the fixation status of the arthroplasty and the amount and quality of remaining periarticular bone stock. The history and physical examination should focus on prefracture knee symptoms such as pain, instability, and stiffness. If available, the operative notes from the original arthroplasty should be obtained. This is especially important if isolated component revision is contemplated. Older implant designs may not offer varying degrees of constraint, augmentation, polyethylene insert sizes, and other factors, and thus compatibility issues may necessitate complete arthroplasty revision. Previous incisions and the status of the soft tissues should be circumferentially evaluated. The neurovascular status of the limb should be carefully documented.

SUPRACONDYLAR PERIPROSTHETIC FRACTURES—OPEN REDUCTION AND INTERNAL FIXATION

The most common clinical situation that the orthopedic surgeon will encounter is a supracondylar femoral fracture

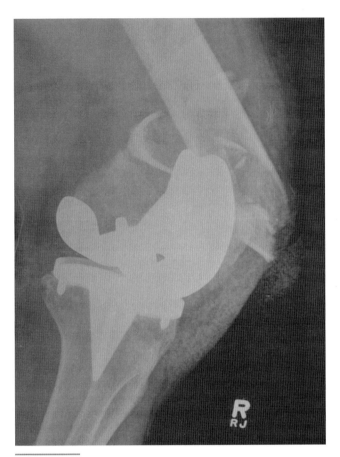

Figure 68–1. Displaced comminuted periprosthetic distal femoral fracture

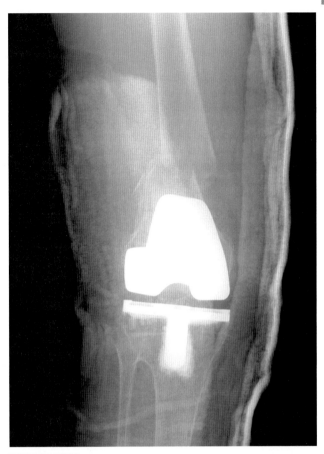

Figure 68–2. Anteroposterior view of a typical distal femoral periprosthetic fracture above a well-fixed total knee arthroplasty.

above a well-fixed, well-functioning, total knee arthroplasty in an elderly patient (Figs. 68–2 and 68–3).[1,11] Minimally displaced, stable fractures and those impacted in good alignment may be candidates for nonoperative treatment. In the authors' experience, however, these situations are quite rare. Long-leg casting with or without incorporation of a hip guide brace to control leg rotation is recommended. Close radiographic follow-up is indicated with early surgical intervention if fracture instability is noted. Prolonged attempts at managing unstable fractures with casting may result in further erosion of distal bone stock and potentially compromise the success of any future reconstruction.

The goals of treatment of these injuries include obtaining bony union; maintaining correct limb alignment, length, and rotation; and avoiding complications. Surgical challenges to achieving these goals include the often short, osteopenic distal bony fragments, fracture comminution, areas of osteolysis, and parts of the femoral component that can make obtaining stable distal fixation difficult, such as lugs, boxes, and stems. Such fractures usually require an internal fixation device that provides coronal plane stability to avoid the deformity, typically varus collapse, that can occur during the healing process. In the past, devices such as the 95-degree angled blade plate and dynamic condylar screw have been used with mixed results.[1-3,5,8,18,31,33] Because of the extremely distal nature

of these fractures, often the blade of the blade plate or the lag screw of the dynamic condylar screw must be inserted more proximally to avoid portions of the femoral component, and thus distal fixation is often suboptimal. The traditional condylar buttress plate offers more freedom of angulation of distal screws but provides no coronal plane stability. Unacceptable rates of varus collapse have been reported when this device is used for unstable fractures.[8,10]

Intramedullary nailing has been used successfully in many series to manage these fractures and offers the advantage of soft-tissue–friendly, minimally invasive stability for complex periprosthetic fractures.[1,5,11,18,19,20] Challenges to successful union with intramedullary techniques include the marginal distal fixation provided by locking screws for the typically comminuted, osteopenic distal bony fragments (Figs. 68–4 and 68–5). Additionally, intramedullary nailing is not practical with implants that substitute for the posterior cruciate ligament because the femoral housing precludes access to the intramedullary canal. The authors currently reserve intramedullary techniques for fractures above cruciate-retaining designs with sufficient distal bone to allow purchase with a minimum of two distal locking screws. Furthermore, recent biomechanical evidence suggests that in the presence of medial comminution, retrograde intramedullary nails may be

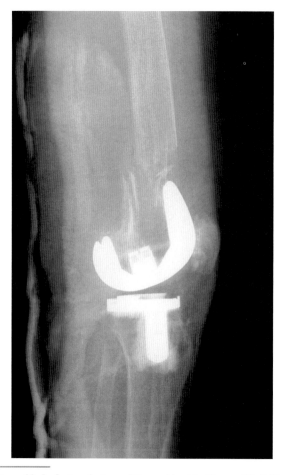

Figure 68–3. Lateral view of the patient in Figure 66–2. Note the fracture at the level of the anterior femoral flange, the most common fracture location.

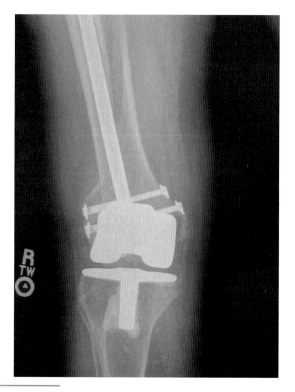

Figure 68–4. Loss of fixation after retrograde nailing because of inadequate distal fixation.

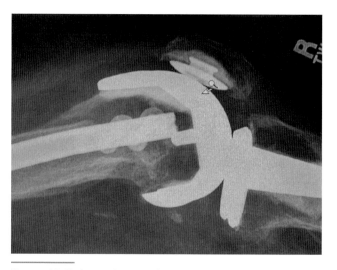

Figure 68–5. Lateral view of the patient in Figure 66–4.

mechanically more stable than laterally placed locking plates.[4] Occasionally, antegrade femoral nailing can be used for periprosthetic distal femoral fractures as well, provided that a sufficiently long distal fragment is present. In the authors' experience, such fractures are extremely rare. The main challenge with antegrade techniques is obtaining appropriate alignment and stable distal fixation. Additionally, with antegrade techniques, an area of high stress concentration is created between the distal end of the nail and the femoral component.

Recently, locking plate technology has gained popularity for the management of complex periarticular fractures about the knee.[7,16,21,23-26,28,30,34,35] Threads on the screw heads are threaded into corresponding threads in the plate holes, thereby forming a fixed-angle construct and providing coronal plane stability.[15] These devices have been used with excellent results for the management of complex periarticular injuries and have an excellent track record for providing reliable distal fixation. Additionally, such devices allow multiple locked screws to be placed around and between portions of the femoral component to improve distal fixation (Figs. 68–6 to 68–8).[16,38] Recently, Kregor et al reported a series of 38 periprosthetic fractures treated with the Less Invasive Stabilization System (LISS) device (Synthes, Paoli, PA).[24,25] There were only two failures (5%). One patient required revision knee arthroplasty and one required bone grafting to achieve solid union. Ultimately, 37 of 38 fractures (97%) healed. Medical and orthopedic complications were uncommon. Leaving metaphyseal comminution undisturbed, thereby preserving vascularity to the fragments, is critical to predictable healing with this technique.

In addition to providing excellent mechanical stability, several locked plating designs also offer the added theoretic biological advantage of allowing percutaneous

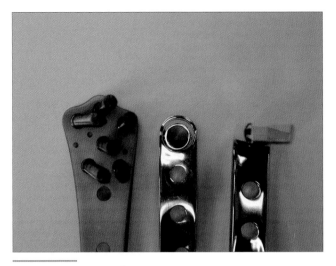

Figure 68–6. "En face" view of a locked plate, a dynamic condylar screw, and a blade plate. The versatility and superior ability to obtain distal fixation with the locked plate are obvious.

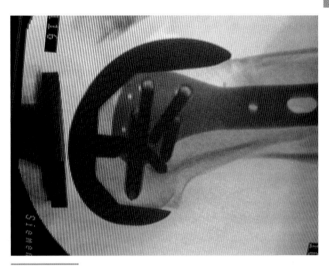

Figure 68–8. Internal fixation with the PolyAx device (DePuy, Warsaw, IN), which allows angled polyaxial screws and fixed-angle locking screws as well.

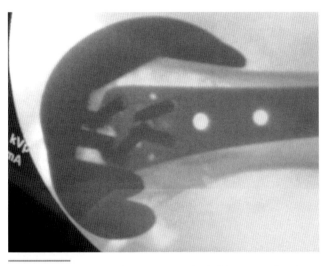

Figure 68–7. Internal fixation with the LISS device (Synthes, Paoli, PA). Note the positioning of the screws around distal obstacles such as femoral lugs.

PERCUTANEOUS TECHNIQUE OF OPEN REDUCTION AND INTERNAL FIXATION OF THE DISTAL END OF THE FEMUR USING LOCKED PLATING DESIGNS

The patient is positioned supine on a radiolucent table, and intravenous antibiotics are administered. Excellent muscle relaxation and fluoroscopic images are essential. Preparing both legs in the operative field can make it easier to obtain a lateral view of the fractured extremity by lifting the normal extremity out of the C-arm beam (Fig. 68–9). A lateral incision is made at the flare of the lateral condyle. A plate of appropriate length is then inserted in a submuscular, extraperiosteal fashion under fluoroscopic control. The plate is positioned as distal as possible on the distal fragment and provisionally held with a guide pin. It is critical to place this guide pin parallel to the knee joint to ensure excellent alignment. Limb length and rotation are then adjusted, and a second guide pin is placed proximally into the femoral shaft. Leaving metaphyseal comminution undisturbed by "bridging" this area is critical to the success of this technique. A combination of gentle manual traction and placement of a small bump under the fracture site can assist with closed reduction, the most difficult portion of the procedure. There is a strong tendency for the distal fragment to tip into hyperextension because of pull of the gastrocnemius muscles (Figs. 68–10 to 68–15). With first-generation locking plates, it is critical to have the plate positioned accurately and have all aspects of the reduction complete before placing any locking screws. These screws will not "pull" the plate down to bone, nor will they allow fine adjustments in alignment once they are inserted. Newer locking plate designs offer "hybrid" fixation that allows the surgeon a choice of either locked, traditional unlocked, or polyaxial angled locked screws (PolyAx, DePuy, Warsaw, IN). Distal fixation should be optimized by placing as

insertion.[23] Such insertion minimizes the need for additional large incisions around the knee and potentially minimizes the soft-tissue complications and stiffness associated with the traditional exposures used for open reduction and internal fixation.[16] When percutaneous techniques are used, vigilance is required to avoid malalignment, typically valgus deformity and hyperextension of the distal fragment.[16] Many commercially available locked plating designs offer the surgeon the option of either open or percutaneous insertion. When possible, the authors perform the internal fixation percutaneously to take advantage of the mechanical stability provided by these devices, as well as the theoretic biological advantages that percutaneous insertion allows.[12]

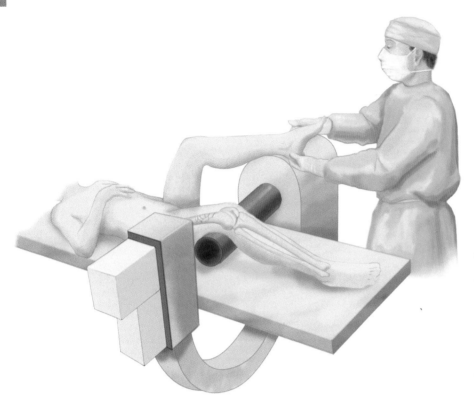

Figure 68–9. Patient positioning with the fluoroscope from the opposite side and inclusion of both lower extremities in the surgical draping. Such positioning allows simple lifting of the well leg to obtain a true lateral view. (By permission of Mayo Foundation for medical education and research. All rights reserved.)

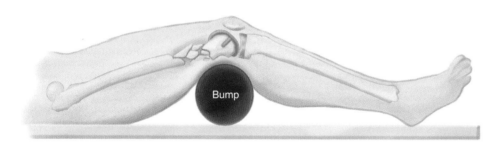

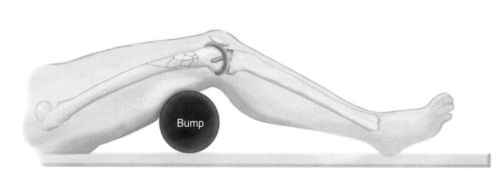

Figure 68–10. Use of a bump to assist in avoiding hyperextension of the distal fragment. A more proximal bump location allows the distal fragment to flex into the appropriate position. Often, multiple attempts with bumps of various sizes and positions are necessary to "learn" which will reduce the fracture best.

many distal screws as possible. Typically, screws can pass just posterior to the anterior flange of the femoral component or just above the "box" of a posterior stabilized housing. The authors currently attempt to use all distal screws and at least four proximal screws. Fracture stability is assessed by intraoperatively testing flexion and varus/valgus stability under live fluoroscopy. The wound is closed in a routine layered fashion over a suction drain. Generally, a hinged knee brace is used postoperatively and knee motion is started when the wound is dry. Toe-touch weightbearing is maintained until healing is evident, typically 10 to 12 weeks (Fig. 68–16).

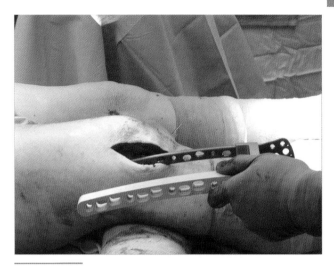

Figure 68–12. Clinical photograph of percutaneous plating.

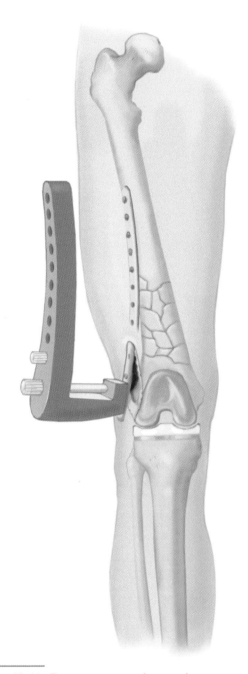

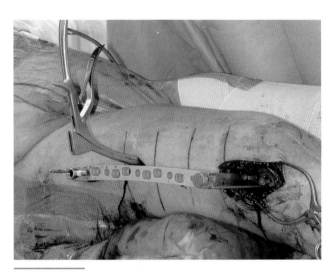

Figure 68–13. Use of percutaneous clamps for reduction and an aiming arm to target percutaneous screws.

Figure 68–11. Percutaneous, submuscular, extraperiosteal insertion of a locked plate. (By permission of Mayo Foundation for medical education and research. All rights reserved.)

PERIPROSTHETIC TIBIAL FRACTURES—OPEN REDUCTION AND INTERNAL FIXATION

Periprosthetic fractures of the proximal end of the tibia are very rare, and no specific incidence has been reported. Felix et al[13] reported on 102 periprosthetic tibial fractures below a total knee arthroplasty. Eighty-three fractures occurred postoperatively and 19 occurred intraoperatively. They developed a treatment-based classification system in

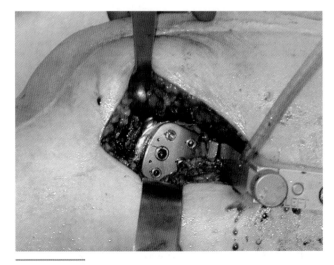

Figure 68–14. Clinical photograph demonstrating the minimally invasive nature of the internal fixation.

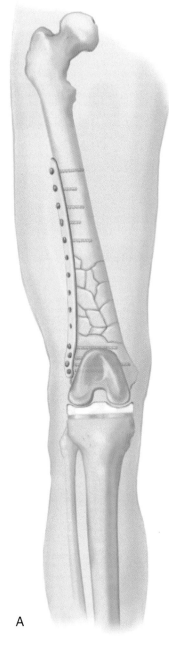

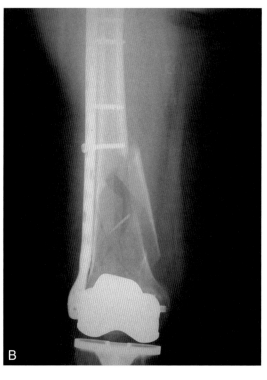

A

B

Figure 68–15. **A** and **B,** "Bridge plating" leaving the metaphyseal comminution undisturbed, thereby preserving its vascularity. (By permission of Mayo Foundation for medical education and research. All rights reserved.)

which fractures were classified into four types based on the location of the fracture and the fixation status of the implant. Type A fractures occurred around implants that were radiographically well fixed, type B occurred in those that were radiographically loose, and type C fractures occurred intraoperatively. Type I fractures occurred at the tibial plateau, type II were located adjacent to the prosthetic stem, type III occurred distal to the prosthetic stem, and Type IV involved the tibial tubercle. Type I fractures were the most common, accounting for 61 fractures. Type II fractures were the second most common, accounting for 22 fractures. Only 17 fractures occurred distal to the prosthetic stem. Most proximal fractures were associated with a loose prosthesis, and these were managed successfully with revision surgery, typically involving stems to bypass the deficient bone. Fractures around a stable implant were managed successfully by the standard principles for tibial

fracture management. No large series has evaluated the outcomes of open reduction and internal fixation of periprosthetic fractures of the tibia below a total knee arthroplasty. Therefore, treatment of fractures of the tibia below a total knee arthroplasty is dictated by the location and stability of the fracture and the fixation status of the implant.[1,8,11,13,17,31] For example, closed reduction and casting may be very successful for spiral, "boot top"–type distal tibial fractures; however, a comminuted midshaft, same-level tibial-fibular fracture would probably be very difficult to manage nonoperatively.

Fractures of the tibia remote from the arthroplasty can often be managed by closed reduction and casting if appropriate alignment can be obtained. The tibial component obviously precludes the use of routine locked intramedullary nails, and therefore plating may be the best choice for unstable fractures with a healthy soft-tissue

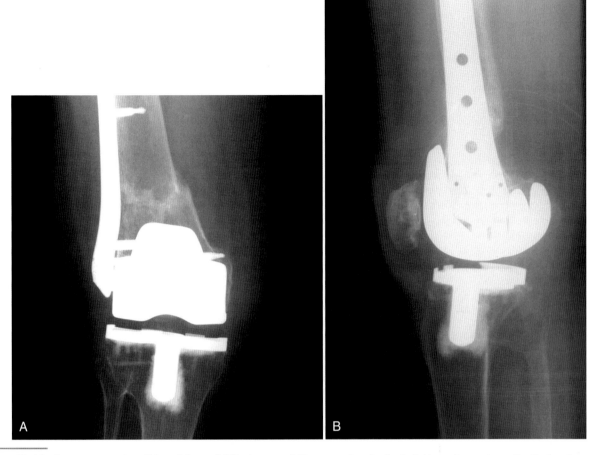

Figure 68–16. Anteroposterior (**A**) and lateral (**B**) views at follow-up after locked plating of a periprosthetic fracture. Note the slight valgus malalignment. Careful vigilance and fluoroscopic scrutiny is necessary to avoid malalignment when using percutaneous techniques.

envelope. Contemporary locked plate technology allows long, fixed-angle plates to be applied percutaneously, thus minimizing soft-tissue dissection and the potential disastrous risk of wound infection. Additionally, excellent proximal fixation can be obtained with multiple locked screws placed around stems or keels of the tibial component.[7]

Fractures of the proximal end of the tibia in contact with the tibial component are typically associated with loosening of the tibial component and are usually managed with revision arthroplasty in which the deficient proximal bone is bypassed with an intramedullary stem.[1,11,13] The use of metal augmentation or structural bone grafting may be required if insufficient host bone support for the tibial component is available.

The use of external fixation is discouraged because of concern for pin site sepsis and potential contamination of the total knee arthroplasty. When external fixation is unavoidable, meticulous pin site care and extreme vigilance are recommended to minimize pin site infections. Because of this concern, the authors currently reserve the use of external fixation as a last resort when treating these injuries.

THE ROLE OF REVISION ARTHROPLASTY

The need for revision total knee arthroplasty secondary to a periprosthetic fracture has become less common in the authors' practices with the advent of improved internal fixation devices such as locked plates. Typically, revision arthroplasty is reserved for fractures around a loose prosthesis, fractures with inadequate bone stock to allow for stable internal fixation, or recalcitrant supracondylar nonunion that requires resection and implantation of a so-called tumor prosthesis. Surgeons who treat periprosthetic fractures around a total knee arthroplasty must have the expertise and technical support to be able to perform long-stemmed revision total knee arthroplasty because one is often unable to determine which reconstructive option is necessary until the fracture has been exposed in the operating room. Bony defects secondary to comminution, multiple previous procedures, the presence of broken hardware, and the presence of deformity may all present technical challenges to a successful outcome.

Revision Arthroplasty for Supracondylar Fracture of the Distal End of the Femur

Revision total knee arthroplasty with intramedullary femoral stems that engage the diaphysis and simultaneously stabilize the fracture can be performed. Cemented stems may be used, but care must be taken to prevent extrusion of cement into the fracture site. Allograft struts with cerclage wiring can be used to reinforce the stability provided by a long-stemmed prosthesis. It is very unusual, however, to have distal femoral bone stock that is inadequate for internal fixation yet adequate for formal revision. The ideal indication for long-stemmed revision total knee arthroplasty would be the presence of adequate bone stock in the face of a supracondylar fracture with a grossly loose femoral component.[1,11] Most of the clinical data evaluating the outcomes of a simultaneous revision arthroplasty with intramedullary stem fixation of a supracondylar fracture have been gathered from the treatment of distal femoral nonunion in this situation. Kress et al[27] reported a small series of nonunions about the knee treated successfully with revision and uncemented femoral stems with bone grafting. Union was achieved in 6 months.

Distal femoral replacement "tumor prostheses" have been used for salvage of failed internal fixation of supracondylar periprosthetic femoral fractures. The long-term results of the kinematic rotating-hinge prosthesis for oncological resections about the knee have been good, with a 10-year survivorship of approximately 90%.[36] As their success becomes more predictable, the indications for such "megaprostheses" are expanding. Elderly patients with refractory periprosthetic supracondylar nonunion or those with acute fractures and bone stock inadequate for internal fixation are reasonable candidates for megaprostheses. Davila et al reported a small series of supracondylar distal femoral nonunions treated with a megaprosthesis in elderly patients. They have shown that a cemented megaprosthesis in this patient population permits early ambulation and return to activities of daily living.[9] Freedman and colleagues performed distal femoral replacement in five elderly patients with acute fractures and reported four good results and one poor result secondary to infection. The four patients with good results regained ambulation in less than 1 month and had an average arc of motion of 99 degrees. All patients had some degree of extension lag.[14]

For a younger, active patient, an allograft prosthetic composite may be a better alternative. Distal femoral reconstruction with an allograft prosthetic composite to provide a biological interface can help restore bone stock and potentially make future revision easier.[11,16] Kraay et al reported a series of allograft prosthetic reconstructions for the treatment of supracondylar fractures in patients with total knee arthroplasties. At a minimum 2-year follow-up, the mean Knee Society score was 71 and the mean arc of motion was 96 degrees. All femoral components were well fixed at follow-up. The results of this study indicate that large segmental distal femoral allograft prosthetic composites can be a reasonable treatment method in this setting.[22]

Revision Arthroplasty for Periprosthetic Fractures of the Tibia

Periprosthetic fractures of the tibia associated with total knee arthroplasty are extremely uncommon. Tibial fractures associated with loose components are best treated with revision arthroplasty, frequently with the use of a long stem to bypass the fracture.[1,11,13] Often, these fractures are associated with extensive osteolysis and may therefore require structural or morselized bone grafting, the use of metal wedges, or in the most severe cases, a proximal tibial megaprosthesis or allograft prosthetic composite. Maximizing host bone support is critical for a good result. The largest series of periprosthetic tibial fractures around loose prostheses was reported by Rand and Coventry.[32] In their series all 15 knees had varus axial malalignment when compared with a control group. Similar studies have confirmed that varus malalignment may be a potential risk factor for periprosthetic tibial fractures.[29,37] Specific technical considerations include careful soft-tissue dissection and retraction to minimize soft-tissue trauma to the already compromised skin flaps. It is important that surgeons undertaking these reconstructions be experienced in revision arthroplasty techniques and fracture management techniques to achieve a successful outcome.

CONCLUSIONS

Periprosthetic fractures around total knee arthroplasty remain difficult injuries to treat. With the ever-growing elderly population, the incidence of these fractures will increase. Decision making regarding open reduction and internal fixation or revision arthroplasty is based on the fixation status of the implant, the remaining bone quality, the physiological age of the patient, and the location and stability of the fracture. Recent advances in locked plate technology show promise for improved fixation of such complex fractures with minimal additional soft-tissue trauma. More data are needed to fully define the role of this exciting new technology alongside traditional techniques of internal fixation of these fractures. Revision arthroplasty frequently requires modular distal femoral replacement, metal or allograft augmentation of bone deficiency, and long stems to bypass deficient bone. These reconstructions are demanding and are fraught with complications. Attention to specific technical details is essential for a successful result.

References

1. Ayers DC: Supracondylar fractures of the distal femur proximal to a total knee replacement. Instruct Course Lect 46:197-203, 1997.
2. Ayers DC, Dennis DA, Johanson NA, Pelligrini VD Jr: Common complications of total knee arthroplasty. J Bone Joint Surg Am 79:278-311, 1997.
3. Bolhofner BR, Carmen B, Clifford P: The results of open reduction and internal fixation of distal femur fractures using a biologic (indirect) reduction technique. J Orthop Trauma 10:372-377, 1996.

4. Bong MR, Egol KA, Koval KJ, et al: Comparison of the LISS and a retrograde inserted supracondylar intramedullary nail for fixation of a periprosthetic distal femur fracture proximal to a total knee arthroplasty. Presented at the 18th Annual Meeting of the Orthopaedic Trauma Association, October 2002, Toronto.

5. Chen F, Mont MA, Bachner RS: Management of ipsilateral supracondylar femur fractures following total knee arthroplasty. J Arthroplasty 9:521-526, 1994.

6. Clatworthy MG, Ballance J, Brick GW, et al: The use of structural allograft for uncontained defects in revision total knee arthroplasty: A minimum five year review. J Bone Joint Surg Am 83:404-411, 2001.

7. Cole PA, Kregor PJ: Prospective clinical trial of the less invasive stabilization system (LISS) for proximal tibia fractures. Presented at the 16th Annual Meeting of the Orthopaedic Trauma Association, 2000 San Antonio, TX.

8. Cordeiro EN, Costa RC, Carazzab JG, et al: Periprosthetic fractures in patients with total knee arthroplasties. Clin Orthop 252:182-189, 1990.

9. Davila J, Malkani A, Paiso JM: Supracondylar distal femoral nonunions treated with a megaprosthesis in elderly patients: A report of two cases. J Orthop Trauma 15:574-578, 2001.

10. Davison BL: Varus collapse of comminuted distal femur fractures after ORIF with a lateral condylar buttress plate. Am J Orthop 32:27-30, 2003.

11. Engh GA, Ammeen DJ: Periprosthetic fractures adjacent to total knee implants: Treatment and clinical results. Instruct Course Lect 47:437-448, 1998.

12. Farouk O, Krettek C, Miclau T, et al: Minimally invasive plate osteosynthesis: Does percutaneous plating disrupt femoral blood supply less than the traditional technique? J Orthop Trauma 13:401-406, 1999.

13. Felix N, Stuart M, Hanssen A: Periprosthetic fractures of the tibia associated with total knee arthroplasty. Clin Orthop 345:113-124, 1997.

14. Freedman DL, Hak DJ, Johnson EE, et al: Total knee arthroplasty including a modular distal femoral component in elderly patients with acute fracture or nonunion. J Orthop Trauma 9:231-237, 1995.

15. Frigg R, Appenzeller A, Christensen R, et al: The development of the distal femur Less Invasive Stabilization System (LISS). Injury 32:SC24-SC31, 2001.

16. Haidukewych GJ: Innovations in locking plate technology for orthopedic trauma. J Am Acad Orthop Surg 12:205-212, 2004.

17. Healy WL: Tibial fractures below total knee arthroplasty. In Insall JN, Scott WN, Scuderi GR (eds): Current Concepts in Primary and Revision Total Knee Arthroplasty. Philadelphia, Lippincott-Raven, 1996, pp 163-167.

18. Healy WL, Siliski JM, Incavo SJ: Operative treatment of distal femoral fractures proximal to total knee replacements. J Bone Joint Surg Am 75:27-34, 1993.

19. Henry SL: Management of supracondylar fractures proximal to total knee arthroplasty with the GSH supracondylar nail. Contemp Orthop 31:231-238, 1995.

20. Henry SL, Busconi B, Gold S, et al: Management of supracondylar femur fractures proximal to total knee prostheses with the GSH supracondylar intramedullary nail. Orthop Trans 19:153, 1995.

21. Koval KJ, Hoehl JJ, Kummer FJ, Simon JA: Distal femoral fixation: A biomechanical comparison of the standard condylar buttress plate, a locked buttress plate, and the 95-degree blade plate. J Orthop Trauma 11:521-524, 1997.

22. Kraay MJ, Goldberg VM, Figgie MP, Figgie HE III: Distal femoral replacement with allograft/prosthetic reconstruction for treatment of supracondylar fractures in patients with total knee arthroplasty. J Arthroplasty 7:7-16, 1992.

23. Kregor PJ: Distal femur fractures with complex articular involvement. Management by articular exposure and submuscular fixation. Orthop Clin North Am 33:153-175, 2002.

24. Kregor PJ, Haidukewych GJ, Sims S: Locked plate internal fixation of supracondylar fractures above a total knee arthroplasty. Unpublished data.

25. Kregor PJ, Hughes JL, Cole PA: Fixation of distal femoral fractures above total knee arthroplasty utilizing the Less Invasive Stabilization System (LISS). Injury 32:SC64-SC75, 2001.

26. Kregor PJ, Stannard J, Zlowodzki M, et al: Distal femoral fracture fixation utilizing the Less Invasive Stabilization System (LISS): The technique and early results. Injury 32:SC32-SC47, 2001.

27. Kress K, Scuderi GR, Windsor RE, et al: Treatment of nonunion about the knee utilizing custom total knee arthroplasty with press-fit intramedullary stems. J Arthroplasty 8:49-55, 1993.

28. Krettek C, Müller M, Miclau T: Evolution of minimally invasive plate osteosynthesis (MIPO) in the femur. Injury 32:SC14-SC23, 2001.

29. Lotke PA, Ecker ML: Influence of positioning of the prosthesis in total knee replacement. J Bone Joint Surg Am 59:77-79, 1977.

30. Marti A, Fankhauser C, Frenk A, et al: Biomechanical evaluation of the less invasive stabilization system for the internal fixation of distal femur fractures. J Orthop Trauma 15:482-487, 2001.

31. Mulvey TJ, et al: Complications associated with total knee arthroplasty. In Pellici PM, Tria AJ, Garvin KL (eds): Orthopedic Knowledge Update. Rosemont, IL, American Academy of Orthopaedic Surgeons, 2000, pp 323-327.

32. Rand JA, Coventry MB: Stress fractures after total knee arthroplasty. J Bone Joint Surg Am 62:226-232, 1980.

33. Sanders R, Regazzoni P, Ruedi TP: Treatment of supracondylar-intracondylar fractures of the femur using the dynamic condylar screw. J Orthop Trauma 3:214-222, 1989.

34. Schandelmaier P, Partenheimer A, Koenemann B, et al: Distal femoral fractures and LISS stabilization. Injury 32:SC55-SC63, 2001.

35. Schütz M, Müller M, Krettek C, et al: Minimally invasive fracture stabilization of distal femoral fractures with the LISS: A prospective multicenter study. Results of a clinical study with special emphasis on difficult cases. Injury 32:SC48-SC54, 2001.

36. Ward G: Five to ten year results of custom endoprosthetic replacement for tumors of the distal femur in complications of limb salvage surgery: Prevention, management, outcome. Presented at the Sixth International Symposium on Limb Salvage, 1991.

37. Wilson FC, Venters GC: Results of knee replacement with the Walldius prosthesis: An interim report. Clin Orthop 120:39-46, 1976.

38. Zlowodzki M, Williamson RS, Zardiackas LD, Kregor PJ: Biomechanical evaluation of the less invasive stabilization system, angled blade plate, and retrograde intramedullary nail for the fixation of distal femur fractures: An osteoporotic cadaveric model. Presented at the 18th Annual Meeting of the Orthopaedic Trauma Association, October 2002, Toronto.

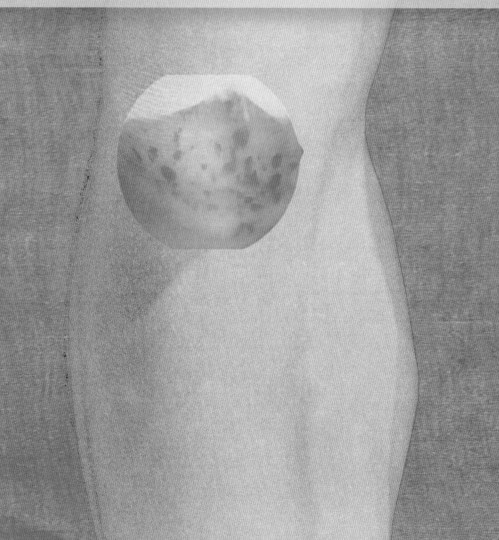

CHAPTER 69

Normal Knee Embryology and Development

James G. Jarvis • Hans K. Uhthoff

The term *embryology* infers the study of embryos. Today, embryology generally refers to the entire period of prenatal development, however, and includes the study of embryos and fetuses. Although prenatal development is more rapid than postnatal development and results in striking changes, the developmental mechanisms of the two periods are the same. "Embryology provides a mechanism to help understand the causes of variations in human structure. It illuminates gross anatomy and explains how both normal relations and abnormalities develop."[19]

OVERVIEW OF EMBRYOLOGY

Prenatal development consists of four sequential stages:
1. *Gametogenesis.* Gametogenesis is the process of formation and development of specialized generative cells called *gametes,* which unite at fertilization to form a single cell called a *zygote.*
2. *Early embryonic period (weeks 1 and 2).* The early embryonic phase encompasses the 2-week period from fertilization to implantation of the embryo during which the zygote repeatedly divides. During week 2, the amniotic cavity and trilaminar embryonic disk are formed. The early embryo usually is aborted if a lethal or serious genetic defect is present, although, at this time, the early embryo is less susceptible to teratogens than during the remainder of the embryonic period.
3. *Embryo (weeks 3 to 8).* Week 3 is the first week of organogenesis. The trilaminar embryonic disk develops, somites begin to form, and the neuroplate closes to form a neural tube (Fig. 69–1).[36] At week 4, the limb buds become recognizable, and the somites differentiate into three segments. The dematome becomes skin, the myotome becomes muscle, and the sclerotome becomes cartilage and bone. Serious defects in limb development may originate at this time (Fig. 69–2).[35] By week 8, the basic organ systems are complete.
4. *Fetus (week 8 to term).* The first half of the fetal period is characterized by rapid growth and changes in body proportions. The lower limbs become proportionate, and most bones ossify. During the second half of gestation, growth continues, and body proportions become more infant-like (see Fig. 69–2).

TIMING AND STAGING OF DEVELOPMENT

Gestational age based on the date of the mother's last menstrual period overestimates the actual gestational age by more than 2 weeks. To estimate age more accurately, embryos are staged according to the method of Streeter.[38] This system, a derivative of the Carnegie Embryonic Staging System, divides the embryonic period into 23 stages based on clearly defined details of either external form or the development of structures.[25,26,38] The maturity of older embryos and fetuses is based on measurement of the crown-rump length.[27]

NORMAL SEQUENTIAL EMBRYOLOGICAL DEVELOPMENT OF THE KNEE*

Week 6

Figure 69–3 shows an embryo 6 weeks old, Streeter stage 17. The cartilaginous anlagen of femur and tibia are separated by cells of uniform density—the future femorotibial joint. Early evidence of cavitation in the otherwise homogeneous, uniform interzone is easily recognizable.

Week 7

Figure 69–4 shows an embryo 7 weeks old, Streeter stage 19. Already at this stage, the lateral femoral condyle and the medial femoral condyle are well formed. The lateral collateral ligament spans from the femur to the fibular head, and the medial collateral ligament connects the femur to the tibia.

*Note: All specimens are from spontaneous abortions because no therapeutic abortions are permitted in our Catholic institution.

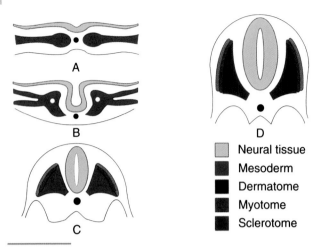

Figure 69–1. **A-D,** Trilaminar disk. The neural tube closes. The mesoderm differentiates into dermatome, myotome, and sclerotome. (From Staheli L: Growth. In: Practice of Pediatric Orthopedics. Philadelphia, Lippincott Williams & Wilkins, 2001.)

Week 8

Figure 69–5 shows an embryo 8 weeks old, Streeter stage 23. Cavitation has progressed, and various cavities have become confluent. The cavity reaches between the patella and femur, but does not extend yet into the future site of the suprapatellar bursa. The posterior cruciate ligament already is composed of dense collagenous tissue. Between femur and tibia, the three-layer arrangement of the interzone becomes apparent; both cartilaginous anlagen are covered by a dense layer of cells having round nuclei. The intermediate layer is less dense.

Week 10

Figure 69–6 shows a fetus 10 weeks old. Between the medial femoral condyle and tibia, the medial meniscus can be seen. A small plica connects the midpart of the medial

		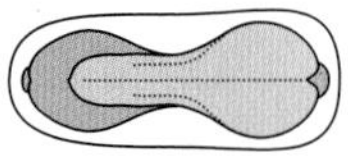	Trilaminar notochord			Neural plate
		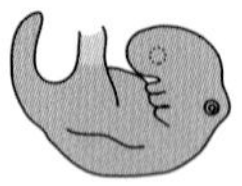	Limb buds	Sclerotomes	Somites	Neural tube
		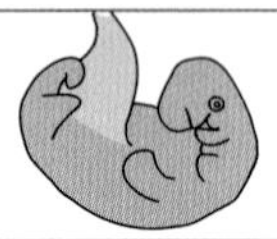	Hand plate	Mesenchyme condenses	Premuscle	
	12	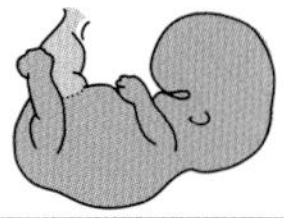	Digits	Chondrification	Fusion myotomes	
	17	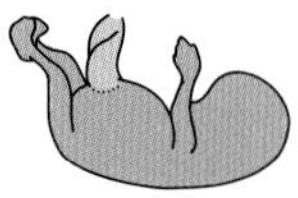	Limbs rotate	Early ossification	Differentiation	
	23	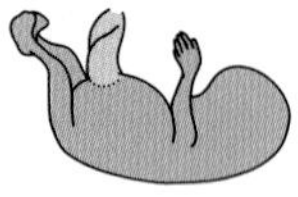	Fingers separate		Definite muscles	Cord equals vertebral length
12	156	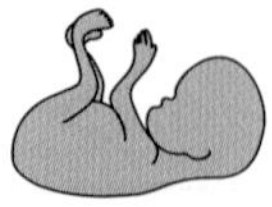	Sex determined	Ossification spreading		
16	112	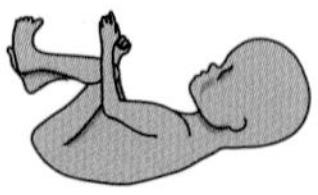	Face human	Joint cavities	Spontaneous activity	
20 40	160– 350	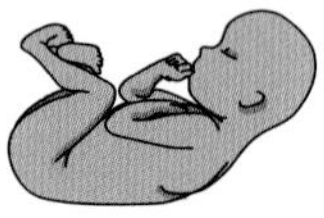	Body more proportional			Myelin sheath forms; cord ends L3

Figure 69–2. Prenatal development. This chart summarizes musculoskeletal development during embryonic and fetal life. (From Staheli L: Growth. In Practice of Pediatric Orthopedics. Philadelphia, Lippincott Williams & Wilkins, 2001.)

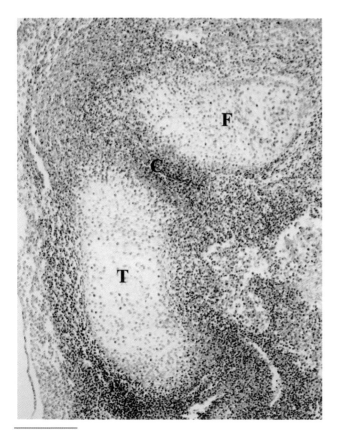

Figure 69–3. Embryo 117N, 6 weeks old, Streeter stage 17. Sagittal section (see text). C, cavitation; F, femur; T, tibia. (Goldner ×100.)

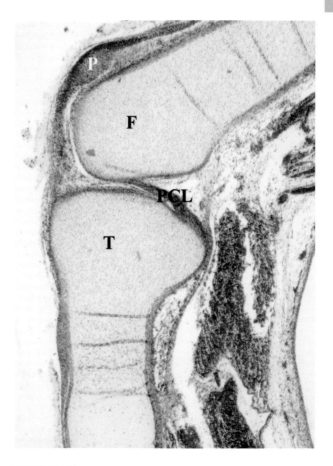

Figure 69–5. Embryo 50N, 8 weeks old, Streeter stage 23. Sagittal section (see text). F, femur; P, patella; PCL, posterior cruciate ligament; T, tibia. (Goldner ×100.)

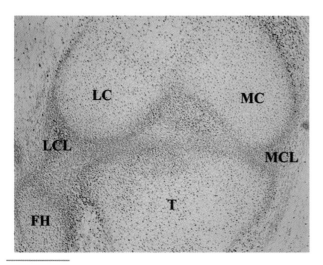

Figure 69–4. Embryo 123N, 7 weeks old, Streeter stage 19. Frontal section (see text). FH, fibular head; LC, lateral femoral condyle; LCL, lateral collateral ligament; MC, medial femoral condyle; MCL, medial collateral ligament; T, tibia. (Azan ×100.)

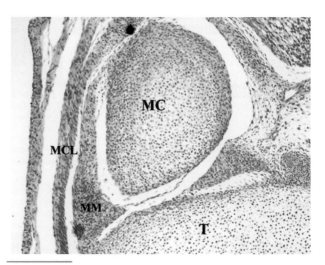

Figure 69–6. Fetus HHF2, 10 weeks old. Frontal, slightly oblique section going through the posterior part of the medial compartment (see text). MC, medial femoral condyle; MCL, medial collateral ligament; MM, medial meniscus; T, tibia. (Azan ×100.)

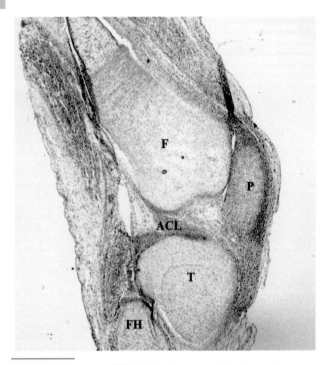

Figure 69–7. Fetus HKSAG3, 10 weeks old. Sagittal section (see text). ACL, anterior cruciate ligament; F, femur; FH, fibular head; T, tibia. (Goldner ×20.)

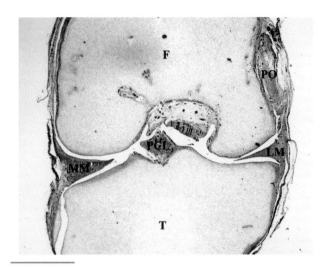

Figure 69–8. Fetus HK24F, 12.5 weeks old. Frontal section (see text). F, femur; LM, lateral meniscus; MM, medial meniscus; PCL, posterior cruciate ligament; PO, popliteus muscle; T, tibia. (Goldner ×20.)

meniscus with the medial femoral condyle. The medial meniscus is not attached to the medial collateral ligament.

Figure 69–7 also shows a fetus 10 weeks old. Not only the femur, tibia, and fibular head, but also the anterior cruciate ligament are seen in the figure. At this stage, no vascular channels are present in the epiphyses.

Week 12.5

Figure 69–8 shows a fetus 12.5 weeks old. A dense layer of cells covers the articular surfaces of the femur and tibia. Lateral to the lateral femoral condyle, the popliteus muscle is seen. Both menisci are well formed. Vessels are present at their periphery. Vascular channels are present in the femoral epiphysis. The posterior cruciate ligament inserts into the tibia.

Week 15.5

Figure 69–9 shows a fetus 15.5 weeks old. The much longer lateral facet of the patella helps to distinguish it from the medial facet. The lateral retinaculum is much denser than the medial retinaculum.

Week 16.5

Figure 69–10 shows a fetus 16.5 weeks old. The ossification processes that started in the diaphyses of the femur

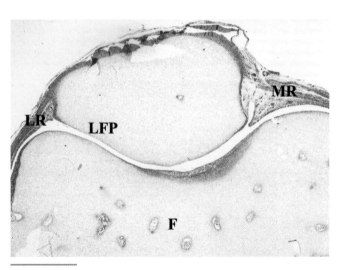

Figure 69–9. Fetus 130N, HKFr, 15.5 weeks old. Frontal section going through the patellofemoral joint (see text). F, femur; LFP, lateral facet of the patella; LR, lateral retinaculum; MR, medial retinaculum. (Azan ×20.)

and tibia are progressing toward the metaphyses. At this stage, blood vessels still cross the growth plate. The suprapatellar bursa extends under the quadriceps muscle. The posterior cruciate ligament originates in the intercondylar fossa and the infrapatellar fat pad.

Week 18

Figure 69–11 shows a fetus 18 weeks old. The formation of the tibial tuberosity (TT) that had started at 14 weeks has continued to separate this apophysis from the tibial epiphysis as a result of an advancing ingrowth of vessels.

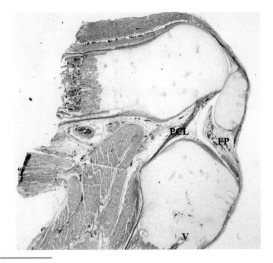

Figure 69–10. Fetus 147N, HKSag, 16.5 weeks old. Sagittal section (see text). FP, infrapatellar fat pad; PCL, posterior cruciate ligament; V, blood vessels. (Goldner ×5.)

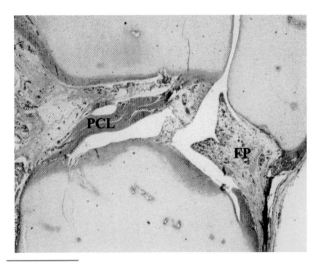

Figure 69–12. Fetus 28N, 19 weeks old. Sagittal section (see text). FP, fat pad; PCL, posterior cruciate ligament. (Goldner ×20.)

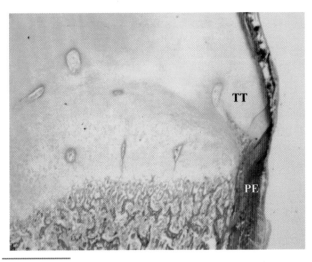

Figure 69–11. Fetus 73N, 18 weeks old. Sagittal section (see text). PE, periosteum; TT, tibial tuberosity. (Goldner ×20.)

A thick periosteum (PE) spans from the tuberosity to the tibial metaphysis.

Week 19

Figure 69–12 shows a fetus 19 weeks old. Intra-articular tissues at the level of the intercondylar notch are visible in the figure. The fat pad is well developed. The posterior cruciate ligament is extra-articular.

Week 20

Figure 69–13 shows a fetus 20 weeks old. Although vessels are seen at the periphery of the medial meniscus

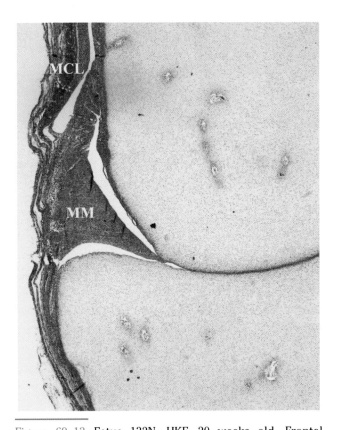

Figure 69–13. Fetus 132N, HKF, 20 weeks old. Frontal section of the medial compartment (see text). MCL, medial collateral ligament; MM, medial meniscus. (Azan ×20.)

(MM), no vascular structures can be identified at its inner border. A cleft between the medial meniscus and medial collateral ligament (MCL) is visible.

Figure 69–14 also shows a fetus 20 weeks old. The enchondral ossification of the tibia has almost reached its final destination between the metaphysis and epiphysis.

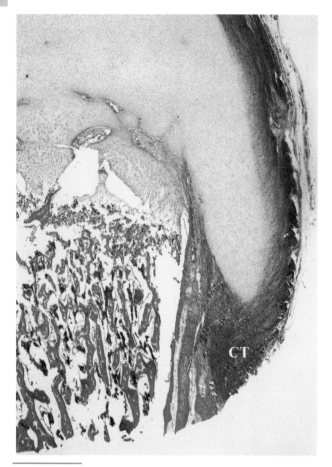

Figure 69–14. Fetus 116N, 20 weeks old. Sagittal section at the level of the tibial tuberosity (see text). CT, collagenous tissue. (Azan ×20.)

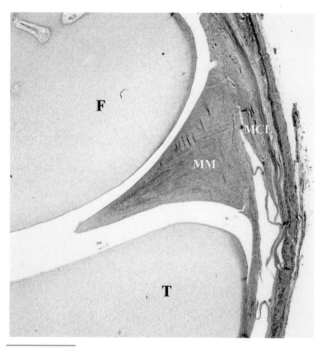

Figure 69–15. Fetus A10917, term. Frontal section showing the medial meniscus (see text). F, femur; MCL, medial collateral ligament; MM, medial meniscus; T, tibia. (Goldner ×20.)

Ossification of the tibial tuberosity occurs late and is a postnatal event.[24,32] Strong collagenous tissue binds this apophysis to the periosteum of the tibia.

Week 40 (Full-Term)

Figure 69–15 shows a term fetus. Rich vascularity is present at the base of the meniscus. The meniscus is separated from the medial collateral ligament.

Week 19.5

Figure 69–16 shows a fetus 19.5 weeks old. This fetus presented with a bilateral (congenital) dislocation of the knee accompanied by rotation. Not only is the knee in hyperextension, but also the tibia is displaced anteriorly; it rides on the anterior surface of the femur. The joint cavity barely reaches under the patella. Despite more than 200 serial sections, we could not detect a cruciate ligament going from femur to tibia. An unusually strong component of fibrous tissue was noted in the quadriceps muscle.

EMBRYOLOGICAL DEVELOPMENT OF VARIANTS AND SPECIFIC ABNORMALITIES

Discoid Lateral Meniscus

Discoid lateral meniscus initially was believed to be a failure of the embryological degeneration of the center of the meniscus[34]; however, this subsequently was shown not to be the case.[13] It is now known that the lateral meniscus is semilunar in shape from its earliest development.[9,14,30] Although some discoid menisci (Wrisberg type 1) may be due to abnormal meniscal attachments, because discoid menisci have been reported in very young children, the condition is likely the result of early development.[1,21]

Congenital Dislocation of the Knee

First described in the early 1800s,[4,29] congenital dislocation of the knee now can be diagnosed in the prenatal period using ultrasound.[6] Although congenital dislocation is seen frequently in association with other hereditary conditions (e.g., Larsen's syndrome), it is not believed to be genetic.[5,12,15,17] Uhthoff and Ogata[41] reported congenital dislocation in a fetus of 19.5 weeks' gestation (see Fig. 69–16).

Multiple etiological theories involving intrauterine events have been proposed, including abnormal fetal position of hyperextension,[33] congenital absence of the cruci-

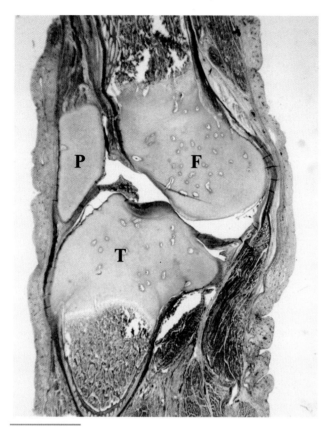

Figure 69–16. Fetus 71N, 19.5 weeks old. Sagittal section (see text). F, femur; P, patella; T, tibia. (Azan × 5.)

ate ligaments,[15] fibrosis of quadriceps,[18] and intrauterine ischemia causing compartment syndrome–like fibrosis.[7] It has not always been possible to separate cause and effect, but these findings are most likely to be secondary adaptive changes.[41]

Bipartite Patella

Bipartite patella is a phenomenon of secondary ossification and probably a postnatal event.

Synovial Plica

The embryonic knee is partitioned into suprapatellar, medial, and lateral compartments by synovial septa. Synovial plicae are regarded as remnants of the divisions between these compartments that were present in the knee during embryological development.[28] Although more typically seen in adults than children, residual synovial plicae have been noted in the fetus between 11 and 20 weeks of gestation (see Fig. 69–6).[23]

The suprapatellar plica can be explained as a septum between the suprapatellar bursa and the patellofemoral cavitation. The infrapatellar plica may be considered a septum of the medial and lateral femorotibial cavitations. The mediopatellar plica is not a remnant of a septum of a

distinct compartment present during the developmental stage, but probably constitutes a remnant of mesenchymal tissue owing to developmental circumstances.[23]

Patellofemoral Instability and Congenital Dislocation of the Patella

Recurrent dislocation of the patella usually is due to lateral malalignment of the quadriceps mechanism. Associated contributing factors, including ligamentous laxity, lateral soft-tissue contractures, external tibial torsion, shallow intercondylar notch of the femur, patella alta, and vastus medialis insufficiency, play a role, but mainly develop in the postnatal period.

In congenital dislocation of the patella, the patella is dislocated at birth, and there is usually deformity of the knee. Although the condition has been reported within families,[20] it also is seen in association with other conditions, most notably, arthrogryposis and Down syndrome.[16] Stanisavljevic and colleagues[37] suggested dislocation occurs during the first trimester as a result of failure of medial rotation of the myotome that contains the quadriceps mechanism.

Both patellar retinacula can be recognized in the fetus by 9.5 weeks. The lateral retinaculum is dense and fibrous, whereas the medial retinaculum is loosely arranged. The patella is not completely centered in the femoral groove and tends to ride more laterally. These two features may predispose to lateral tracking or dislocation of the patella or both (see Fig. 69–9).[8,41]

Congenital Absence of the Anterior Cruciate Ligament

Although typically described in association with congenital dislocation of the knee, congenital absence of the anterior cruciate ligament also has been reported as an isolated finding.[2,10] Associations with other abnormalities include congenital short femur,[2,11] congenital absence of the meniscus,[39] congenital ring menisci,[3,22] and thrombocytopenic absent radius syndrome.[31,40]

References

1. Barnes CL, McCarthy RE, Vander Schilden JL, et al: Discoid lateral meniscus in a young child: Case report and review of the literature. J Pediatr Orthop 8:707, 1988.
2. Barrett GR, Tomasin JD: Bilateral congenital absence of the anterior cruciate ligament. Orthopedics 11:431, 1988.
3. Basmajian JV: A ring-shaped medial semi-lunar cartilage. J Bone Joint Surg Br 34:638, 1952.
4. Bensahel H, Dal Monte A, Hjelmstedt A, et al: Congenital dislocation of the knee. J Pediatr Orthop Am 9(2):174-177, 1989.
5. Curtis B, Fisher R: Congenital hyperextension with anterior subluxation of the knee: Surgical treatment and long-term observation. J Bone Joint Surg Am 51(2):255-269, 1969.
6. Elchalal U, Ben Itzhak I, Ben-Meir G, et al: Antenatal diagnosis of congenital dislocation of the knee: A case report. Am J Perinatol 10:194, 1993.

7. Ferris B, Aichroth P: The treatment of congenital knee dislocation: A review of nineteen knees. Clin Orthop 216:135, 1987.

8. Finnegan M, Uhthoff H: The development of the knee. In Uhthoff HK: The Embryology of the Human Locomotor System. New York, Springer-Verlag, 1990, pp. 129-140.

9. Gardner E, O'Rahilly R: The early development of the knee joint in staged human embryos. J Anat 102:289-299, 1968.

10. Johansson E, Aparisi T: Congenital absence of the cruciate ligaments: A case report and review of the literature. Clin Orthop 162:108, 1982.

11. Johansson E, Aparisi T: Missing cruciate ligament in congenital short femur. J Bone Joint Surg Am 65:1109, 1983.

12. Johnson E, Audell R, Oppenheim WL: Congenital dislocation of the knee. J Pediatr Orthop 7:194, 1987.

13. Kaplan E: The embyology of the menisci of the knee joint. Bull Hosp Joint Dis 16(2):111-124, 1955.

14. Kaplan E: Discoid lateral meniscus of the knee joint: Nature, mechanism, and operative treatment. J Bone Joint Surg Am 39:77, 1957.

15. Katz M, Grogono J, Soper K: The etiology and treatment of congenital dislocation of the knee. J Bone Joint Surg Br 49:112, 1967.

16. McCall RE, Lessenberry HB: Bilateral congenital dislocation of the patella. J Pediatr Orthop 7:100, 1987.

17. McFarland B: Congenital dislocation of the knee. J Bone Joint Surg 11:281, 1929.

18. Middleton D: The pathology of congenital recurvatum. Br J Surg 22:696, 1935.

19. Moore KL, Persaud TVN: The Developing Human—Clinically Oriented Embryology, 6th ed. Philadelphia, WB Saunders, 1998.

20. Mumford EB: Congenital dislocation of the patella: Case report with a history of four generations. J Bone Joint Surg 29:1083, 1947.

21. Nathan P, Cole S: Discoid meniscus: A clinical and pathologic study. Clin Orthop 64:107, 1969.

22. Noble J: Congenital absence of the anterior cruciate ligament associated with a ring meniscus: Report of a case. J Bone Joint Surg Am 57:1165, 1975.

23. Ogata S, Uhthoff HK: The development of synovial plicae in human knee joints: An embryologic study. Arthroscopy 6:315, 1990.

24. Ogden JA, Southwick WO: Osgood-Schlatter's disease and tibial tuberosity development. Clin Orthop 116:180, 1976.

25. O'Rahilly R: Early human development and the chief sources of information on staged human embryos. Eur J Obstet Gynecol Reprod Biol 9:273, 1979.

26. O'Rahilly R, Muller F: Developmental Stages in Human Embryos. Washington, DC, Carnegie Institute of Washington, 1987.

27. Patten BM: Human Embryology. New York, McGraw-Hill, 1953.

28. Pipkin G: Knee injuries: The role of the suprapatellar plica and suprapatellar bursa in simulating internal derangements. Clin Orthop 74:161, 1971.

29. Rechmann L: Beitrag zur Therapie der kongenitalen Luxation des Kniegelenkes. Arch Orthop Unfallchir 13:227, 1914.

30. Ross J, Tough I, English T: Congenital discoid cartilage: Report of a case of discoid medial cartilage with an embryological note. J Bone Joint Surg Br 40:262, 1958.

31. Schoenecker PL, Cohn AK, Sedgwick WG, et al: Dysplasia of the knee associated with the syndrome of thrombocytopenia and absent radius. J Bone Joint Surg Am 66(3):421-427, 1984.

32. Shapiro F: Epiphyseal disorders of the knee. In Pediatric Orthopedic Deformities—Basic Science, Diagnosis, and Treatment. San Diego, Academic Press, 2001, pp 462-516.

33. Shattock S: Genu recurvatum on a foetus at term. Trans Pathol Soc Lond 42:280, 1891.

34. Smillie I: The congenital discoid meniscus. J Bone Joint Surg Br 30:671, 1948.

35. Staheli L: Fundamentals of Pediatric Orthopedics. Philadelphia, Lippincott-Raven, 1998.

36. Staheli L: Practice of Pediatric Orthopedics. Philadelphia, Lippincott Williams & Wilkins, 2001.

37. Stanisavljevic S, Zemenick G, Miller D: Congenital, irreducible, permanent lateral dislocation of the patella. Clin Orthop 116:190, 1976.

38. Streeter GH: Developmental Horizons in Human Embryos. Washington, DC, Carnegie Institution of Washington, 1951.

39. Tolo VT: Congenital absence of the menisci and cruciate ligaments of the knee: A case report. J Bone Joint Surg Am 63:1022, 1981.

40. Torode IP, Gillespie R: Anteroposterior instability of the knee: A sign of congenital limb deficiency. J Pediatr Orthop 3:467, 1983.

41. Uhthoff HK, Ogata S: Early intrauterine presence of congenital dislocation of the knee. J Pediatr Orthop 14:254, 1994.

CHAPTER 70

Congenital Deformities of the Knee

Charles E. Johnston II

Congenital deformities of the knee include hyperextension and flexion deformities, present at birth, whose severity at first glance may appear to be incompatible with functional ambulation. With the exception of patellar dislocation, which may not be apparent at birth, these deformities differ from acquired or developmental angular, torsional, or internal derangement problems in that they are usually obvious in the newborn or toddler. Once the diagnosis is made and the overall prognosis defined, rational early treatment can significantly improve the outlook for functional ambulation. The purpose of this chapter is to describe and review the latest treatment options for these relatively rare, but dramatic congenital knee abnormalities.

CONGENITAL DISLOCATION OF THE KNEE

Few orthopedic birth abnormalities are as dramatic and obvious as congenital dislocation of the knee (CDK) (Fig. 70–1A). Those unfamiliar with the deformity may describe the extremity as having "the knee on backwards" because of the unstable excessive hyperextension combined with an element of angular deformity. CDK is rare, about 100 times less common than congenital hip dislocation.[27] Even if the milder form of congenital hyperextension deformity is included as CDK, the incidence is still less than 1 per 1000.[8] It can be diagnosed prenatally by ultrasound.[15]

Clinically, the hyperextension deformity is unmistakable, with the femoral condyles often being prominent on the posterior distal aspect of the thigh. The foot may be positioned at the baby's face or shoulders, and this marked hyperflexion of the hip (Fig. 70–1B), reflecting the positioning in utero,[44] raises the suspicion of concomitant congenital hip instability. Radiographically, the relationship between the distal femur and proximal tibia should be determined on a *true lateral* view of the knee to define the joint as *hyperextended, subluxated,* or *dislocated* (Fig. 70–2). Next, the degree of passive flexion of the knee is important for determining the prognosis because it may be immediately apparent that the knee will flex and reduce with gentle stretching of the quadriceps, in which case the deformity is classified clinically as grade 1 congenital hyperextension.[10,35] On the other hand, any flexion of the knee may be impossible, and the tibia, which is anteriorly translated in the resting position, may subluxate laterally on the femur when more vigorous flexion is attempted, indicative of a grade 3, irreducible dislocation (Fig. 70–3).

The latter is always associated with significant quadriceps fibrosis and shortening, which has been considered by some as the main cause of the deformity.[39] An intermediate degree of contracture, grade 2 subluxation, may be noted when the knee will not flex beyond neutral extension but the femoral and tibial epiphyses are in contact and do not subluxate readily when flexion is attempted.

Equally important at the initial evaluation is the search for associated anomalies and syndromes. Ipsilateral hip dysplasia and clubfoot are present 70% and 50% of the time, respectively,[5,28] and other anomalies of the upper extremity, face, and gastrointestinal and genitourinary systems are not uncommon. Bilateral CDK is almost always *syndromic*, most commonly associated with laxity syndromes such as Larsen's, Beals', or Ehlers-Danlos syndrome. Neurological conditions, such as arthrogryposis or spinal dysraphism, may be associated with bilateral CDK or may be characterized by one extended (dislocated) knee and one with a flexion deformity. Whether isolated or syndromic, abnormal fetal positioning is probably the common mechanical etiology. Lack of movement because of neuromuscular conditions (e.g., arthrogryposis) or hyperlaxity can easily be invoked as causative once the abnormal position (see Fig. 70–1B) occurs, with quadriceps fibrosis and atrophy developing when the knee cannot move and the muscle shortens in the extended position. Hypoplasia of the patella and contracture of the iliotibial (IT) band probably result from the same lack of joint and muscle movement.

Ligamentous laxity with elongation, insufficiency, or absence of the cruciate ligaments has long been known as a complicating feature of CDK,[4,10,31,45] although it is downplayed in importance in some reports.[5,50] The author has observed that cruciate absence is actually typical of bilateral, syndromic cases (see Fig. 70–3D) and probably should be addressed as part of the comprehensive surgical management (discussed later). Conversely, *isolated* CDK (with or without ipsilateral hip or foot deformity) is often *unilateral*, and once reduced the knee is relatively stable (anterior cruciate ligament [ACL] present) and thus can been termed "stiff" CDK as opposed to the "lax" syndromic variety.

Other pathological findings in grade 3 CDK include anterior subluxation of the posterolateral and posteromedial structures, including the hamstring tendons and the IT band, because of the chronic hyperextension and anterior translation of the tibia on the femur (Fig. 70–4).[5,10,28,59] The suprapatellar pouch may be atrophic or obliterated, with adhesions between the hypoplastic patella and the femur and IT band. All these intra-

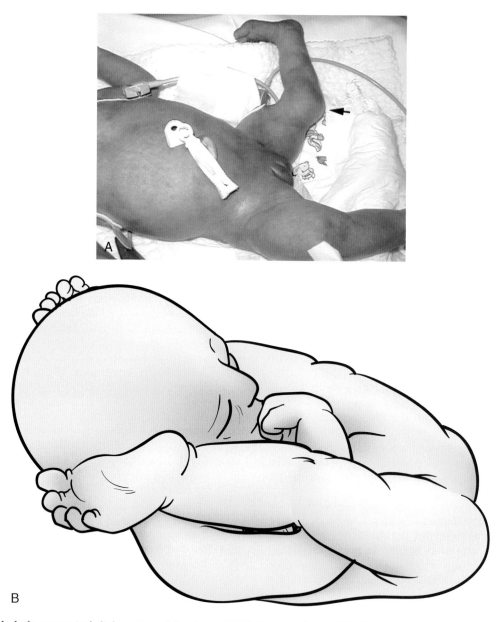

Figure 70–1. **A,** Left congenital dislocation of the knee (CDK) in a newborn. The femoral condyles in the popliteal fossa are prominent *(arrow)*. **B,** Typical intrauterine position associated with CDK: hyperflexion of the hips with hyperextended knees. (Redrawn from Niebauer JJ, King D: Congenital dislocation of the knee. J Bone Joint Surg Am 42:207, 1960.)

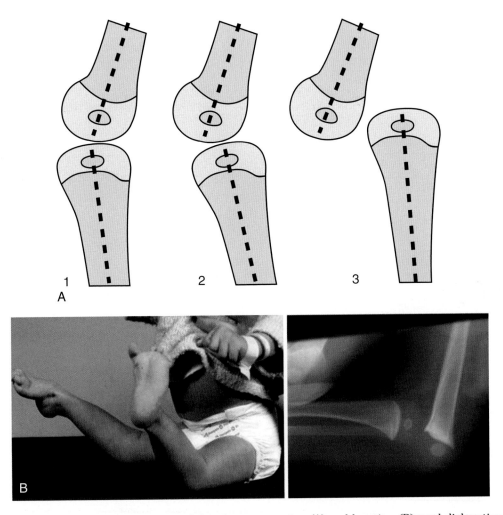

Figure 70–2. **A,** Degrees of congenital knee instability: hyperextension (A), subluxation (B), and dislocation (C). **B,** Clinical and radiographic views of a grade 3 dislocation.

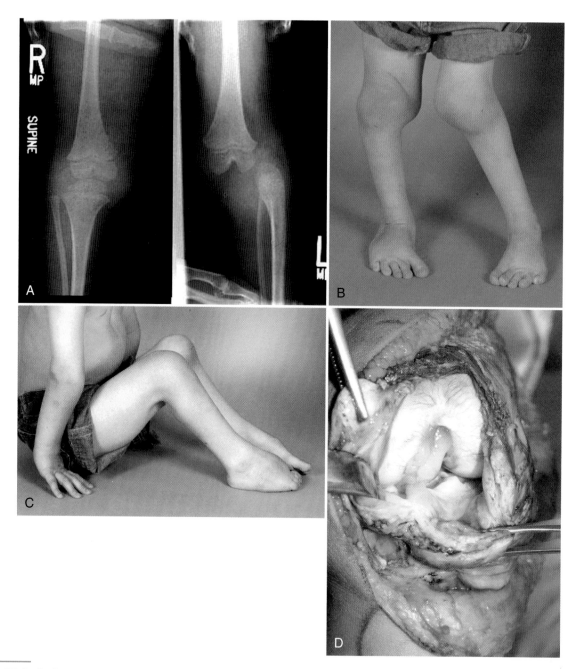

Figure 70–3. **A,** Anteroposterior radiographs of a 3-year-old boy with Larsen's syndrome and bilateral congenital dislocation of the knee. **B,** Clinical appearance, with grade 3 dislocation on the *left*. **C,** The right knee reduces with flexion and is thus grade 1 (see Fig. 68-11). **D,** The anterior cruciate ligament is congenitally absent.

articular abnormalities need to be addressed surgically in irreducible CDK.

Treatment—Nonoperative

Nonoperative treatment should begin as soon as possible in infancy. After determining the radiographic position (see Fig. 70–2A), initial flexibility of the quadriceps contracture is assessed by applying gentle traction to the tibia and attempting flexion of the knee.[32] The tibia, if anteriorly located, engages the distal end of the femur and translates posteriorly with traction, and as the knee is flexed, a stable articulation can be palpated. In simple hyperextension cases, this may be readily achievable and can usually be maintained with an anterior plaster slab or a long-leg cast. The latter is actually more difficult to apply in an infant and maintain reduction. Obviously, forceful manipulation is contraindicated because of the risk of pressure damage to cartilaginous epiphyses or fracture-separation of the proximal tibial physis (Fig. 70–5).[54] Serial manipu-

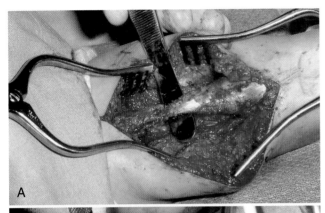

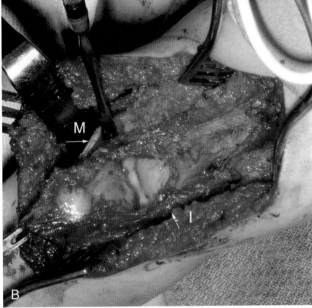

Figure 70–4. **A,** Contracted quadriceps tendon before V-Y lengthening (not recommended) during open reduction. The hip is to the *right*. **B,** The medial hamstrings (M) and IT band (I) are both subluxated anterior to the distal end of the femur (note the physis). The patella has been reflected distally with the quadriceps tendon.

lation and splinting in increasing flexion proceed until the knee will flex more than 90 degrees, at which time a removable plastic splint can be used to maintain reduction while allowing some active motion. Alternatively, if the patient also has ipsilateral congenital dislocation of the hip, the knee can be maintained in a Pavlik harness while the hip is simultaneously addressed.[32]

In knees with more severe quadriceps contracture preventing effective gradual flexion, femoral nerve block or botulinum toxin (Botox) can be effective. Botox injection of the quadriceps has the added advantage of longer-term paralysis of the quadriceps, thereby allowing gradual stretching to occur even when the initial flexibility seems unfavorable for nonoperative reduction (Fig. 70–6). A trial of nonoperative management, with or without adjunctive neuromuscular blockade, is appropriate initial treatment in infants up to 12 months of age.

Treatment—Surgical

Surgical treatment is indicated for patients not responding to nonoperative means and has been advocated for infants as early as 6 months of age.[4,5] Although it may be argued that earlier reduction of the knee provides maximum potential for remodeling of the articular surfaces, patients as old as 4 years have had successful initial reduction, and patients as old as 16 years have had late gross instability with reducible, but recurrent dislocation addressed. In view of the current use of femoral shortening to achieve reduction (see the next section), the earliest age for surgery should be when the surgeon thinks that the femur is robust enough to achieve meaningful internal fixation to stabilize a shortening osteotomy.

REDUCTION/FLEXION WITH FEMORAL SHORTENING

Classic surgical treatment of CDK has invariably used extensive V-Y quadriceps tendon lengthening (Fig. 70–7; see also Fig. 70–4) to gain flexion and hence reduction of the joint. Outcomes of such lengthening are poorly documented in many series, with simple documentation of reduction and reporting of passive range of motion being about all that is recorded. Since many patients have other anomalies and comorbid conditions affecting the outcome, the functional results *of the knees themselves* have rarely been reported. In truth, the extensive lengthening invariably leads to weakness and extensor lag, whereas the extensive dissection required to obtain such length produces additional fibrosis that limits flexion. Finally, wound healing over the anterior knee surface may be compromised because of the ischemia produced by flexion stretching the contracted anterior skin (see Fig. 70–7C).

In addition to the quadricepsplasty, arthrotomy must be performed to mobilize the anteriorly subluxated medial and lateral periarticular structures and allow them to relocate to their normal anatomic position as the knee is flexed (see Fig. 70–4B). However, once the knee is reduced in flexion, the redundant posterior capsule resulting from that maneuver has rarely been addressed (by capsulorrhaphy), thus inviting redislocation into the same incompetent posterior space. The *irrationality* of this oversight can easily be appreciated if one considers that late open reduction of congenital hip dislocation would *never* be completed without performing capsulorrhaphy to obliterate a potential space into which the femoral head could redislocate. Thus, if the ACL is also congenitally absent in a CDK reduced without capsulorrhaphy, it is hardly surprising that chronic hyperlaxity/instability of the knee at a minimum and frank redislocation at the other extreme would be the common outcome of knees treated by such a historical approach, especially if flexion is limited by a scarred, fibrotic quadriceps muscle that has been extensively dissected.

As a result, V-Y quadricepsplasty should be abandoned in favor of femoral shortening to minimize quadriceps dissection and weakening (Fig. 70–8). Acute femoral short-

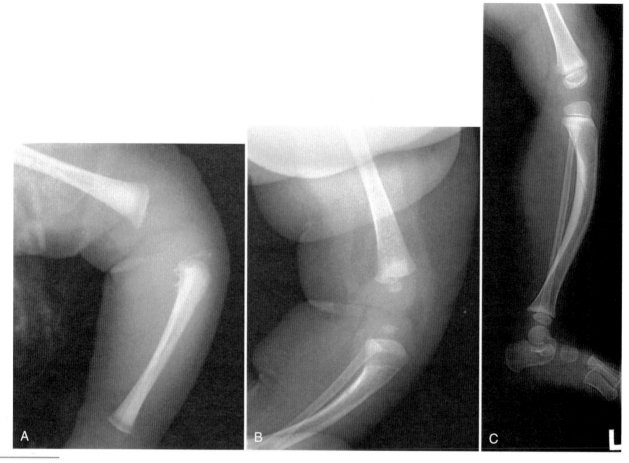

Figure 70–5. **A,** Fracture-separation of the proximal tibial epiphysis in a 2-week-old infant initially with a hyperextended knee. **B,** Healed fracture at the age of 4 months. The limb was splinted in the degree of flexion obtained in **A. C,** Residual antecurvatum deformity with otherwise normal growth of the tibia, age 3.

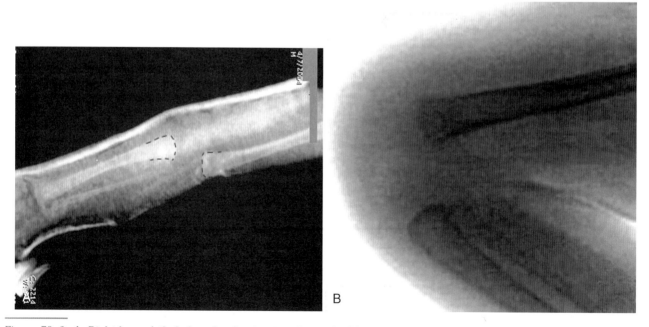

Figure 70–6. **A,** Right knee, failed closed reduction in a 2-month-old. **B,** Botox was injected twice at 1-month intervals and daily manipulations carried out. Two months later, full flexion/reduction was achieved.

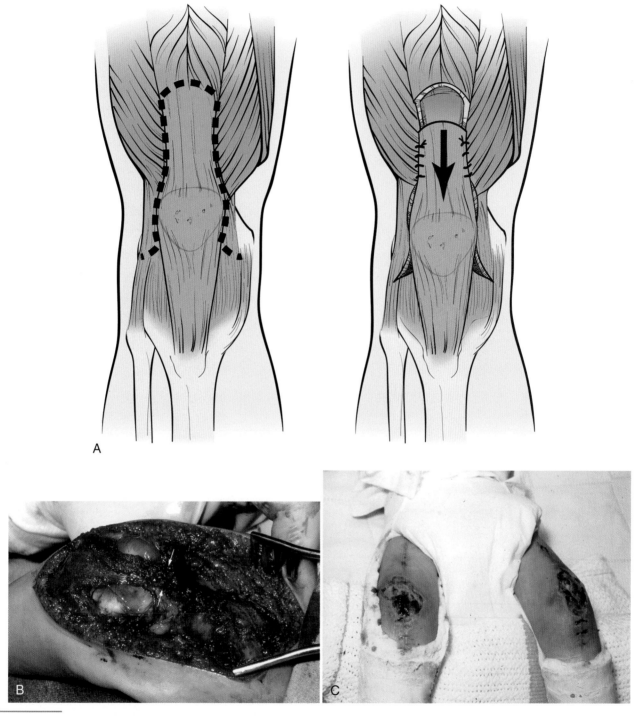

Figure 70–7. **A,** Classic V-Y quadricepsplasty.[10] **B,** The resulting "repair" of the quadriceps tendon (*arrows*) is tenuous at best because of the extensive lengthening required to gain knee reduction (same patient as Fig. 70–4). **C,** Wound dehiscence/slough as a result of skin necrosis from knee flexion.

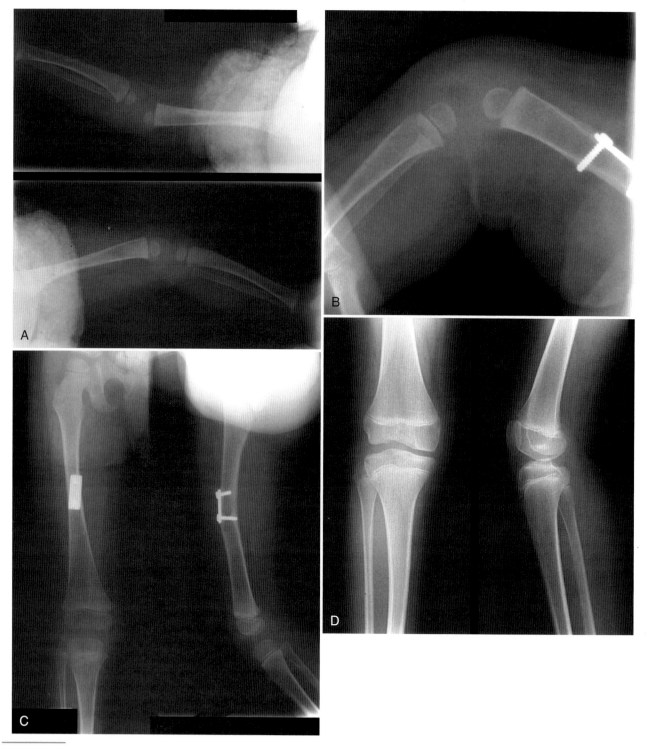

Figure 70–8. **A,** Lateral radiographs of a 6-month-old female with persistent subluxation and inadequate flexion. **B,** Four months after limited open reduction (no quadriceps tendon lengthening) and femoral shortening. **C,** Three years post-operatively. **D,** Twelve years postoperatively. Range of motion is 5 to 70 degrees of flexion, with normal quadriceps strength. Note the hypoplastic patella. She is completely asymptomatic other than the limited flexion.

ening decompresses the anterior skin and allows knee flexion without surgical lengthening of the muscle. The operative procedure begins with a lateral parapatellar arthrotomy incision that is extended proximally along the lateral aspect of the femur to allow mobilization of the distal contracted lateral tissues (IT band, released

from its distal insertion, and vastus lateralis, released from the intermuscular septum) and provide subperiosteal access to the supracondylar region for bone shortening (Fig. 70–9). The quadriceps tendon, patella, and patellar tendon are mobilized as a continuous longitudinal structure via a medial arthrotomy to allow sharp dissection/

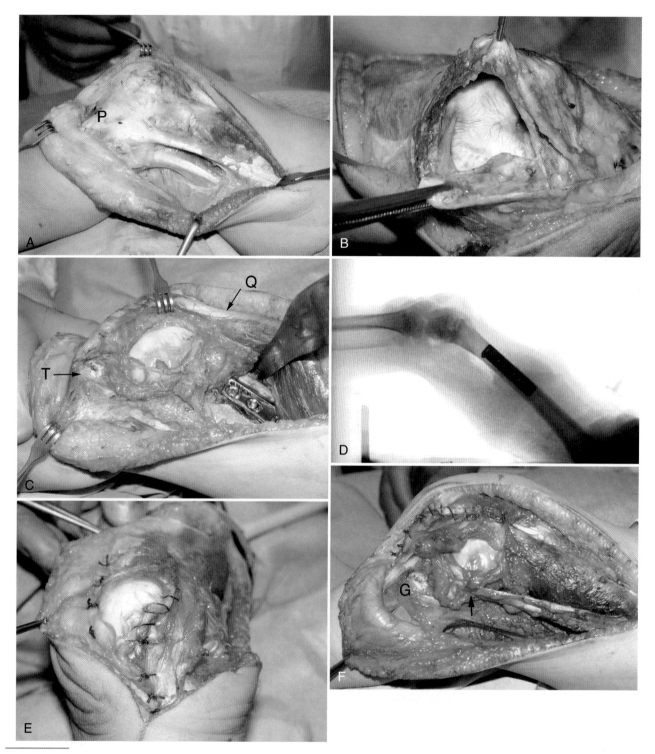

Figure 70–9. **A,** Lateral knee/distal femoral exposure. The tibia is dislocated posterolaterally (same patient as in Fig. 70–3, left knee). The iliotibial band and biceps are seen before release of the former from its insertion. Anteriorly, the patellar tendon is marked. **B,** Medial arthrotomy. The vastus medialis and medial retinaculum are being separated from the quadriceps tendon (inferior clamp). **C,** The femur has been shortened and plated. The tibia (T) now reduces under direct vision. The quadriceps mechanism (Q) is in continuity. **D,** Intraoperative radiograph confirming reduction. **E,** Anterior view of advancement/imbrication of the vastus medialis to hold the patella centralized (medialis to the right). **F,** Lateral view of the imbrication. No attempt has been made to close the lateral arthrotomy. The vastus lateralis covers the plate. Posterolateral capsulorrhaphy has been performed deep to the iliotibial band, which has been reattached to the posterolateral condyle *(arrow)*—re-attachment to Gerdy's tubercle (G) is both impossible and contraindicated.

elevation of the medial periarticular structures (pes tendons), which are subluxated anteriorly. The intercondylar notch is inspected for the presence or absence of the ACL. Once the femur is acutely shortened and plated—usually around 2.0 to 2.5 cm is removed—the knee will generally reduce with flexion, and the only repair necessary is stabilization of the patellar mechanism in the intercondylar groove, typically by medial imbrication and advancement of the vastus medialis obliquus (see Fig. 70–9E and F). The lateral "release" is repaired only to the extent of covering the internal fixation.

Capsulorrhaphy is performed at the posterolateral corner of the lateral femoral condyle by bluntly dissecting the capsule, with the knee flexed, from the more superficial tissues with an elevator. The dissection is simplified once the IT band and vastus lateralis have been released and mobilized. The lateral half of the posterior capsule is imbricated proximal to the distal edges after the excision of 1 to 1.5 cm of redundant patulous capsule. Shortening

of the hamstrings[4,5,28] may be done in conjunction with the capsulorrhaphy (and ACL reconstruction, if necessary—see the next section), but should *not* be considered a replacement for it.

The posteromedial capsulorrhaphy is performed through a separate 3- to 4-cm incision behind the medial femoral condyle (Fig. 70–10). This incision can be located by placing a blunt instrument from inside the arthrotomy to the posteromedial corner and then cutting down on the instrument tenting the skin. The redundant capsule is dissected free of superficial tissue with the knee flexed, a segment is excised, and the imbrication is performed (see Fig. 70–10B and C). After medial/lateral capsulorrhaphy, the knee should lack 30 degrees or more of full extension—the patient will eventually "stretch" this iatrogenic flexion contracture in 4 to 6 months.

At this point the knee must be assessed for ligamentous instability, especially anterior drawer with the knee flexed (the posterior capsulorrhaphy should prevent significant

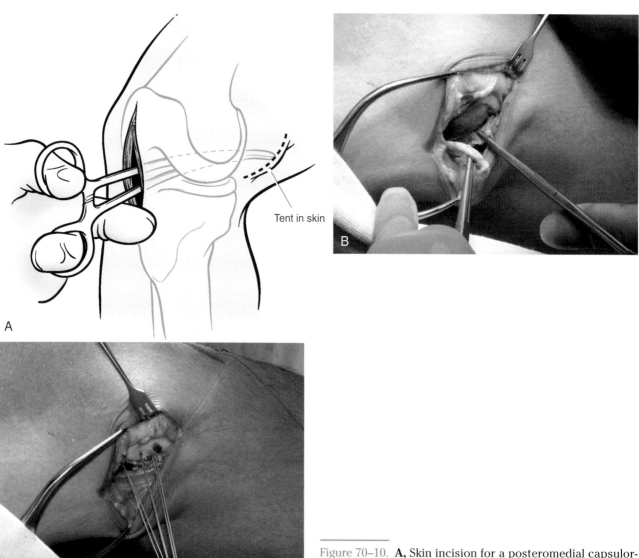

Figure 70–10. **A,** Skin incision for a posteromedial capsulorrhaphy. **B,** Excision of redundant capsule (in the clamp). **C,** Completed capsulorrhaphy.

drawer in maximum extension). The surgeon must decide whether the ACL should be reconstructed if congenitally absent or severely attenuated. If anterior drawer is unacceptable, the ligament should be reconstructed, if not during this procedure, as a staged procedure later. If ACL competence is satisfactory, the wounds are closed and the knee placed in a cast in 45 to 60 degrees of flexion for 8 weeks, followed by gradual active range-of-motion exercises with full extension limited by a brace for the first 4 months.

ANTERIOR CRUCIATE LIGAMENT RECONSTRUCTION

The issue of ACL reconstruction in a young child is controversial, to say the least, but in an unpublished review of 22 knees (14 patients) treated at Texas Scottish Rite Hospital for Children with up to 15 years' follow-up, the 9 knees that underwent reduction by V-Y quadricepsplasty with no ligament reconstruction were uniformly unstable; quadriceps strength was poor, and the patients required full-time bracing and/or resorted to assistive devices (crutches, wheelchair) for community ambulation. Eight of these nine unsatisfactory knees were in patients with laxity syndromes (predominantly Larsen's). The instability was dramatic in that unbraced knees dislocated in the extended position (Fig. 70–11) and even with bracing were still unstable, although they were usually capable of weightbearing. As a result of this review, an attempt to reconstruct an ACL-deficient knee in the laxity syndrome group seems justified in an effort to improve the uniformly unacceptable results of the earlier cases.

Although historically there has been reluctance to attempt intra-articular ACL reconstruction in children because of fear of physeal injury producing deformity and growth arrest from transphyseal procedures, these concerns are gradually relenting as both clinical and experimental studies have shown that this risk may be overplayed. Options include both transphyseal and physeal-sparing techniques. Although drilling an anchoring hole across any physis potentially risks injury, the practice of placing smooth pins across physes for periarticular and physeal trauma is well accepted, especially if the fixation is temporary. Logically, a smooth, centrally placed hole across a physis that is filled with a nonosseous (e.g., tendon) material is no more likely to produce growth disturbance than temporary pin fixation is by virtue of being an "interposition" material. Both animal[23,56] and clinical studies[47] using the hamstrings, IT band, or patellar tendon for transphyseal ligament reconstruction have demonstrated knee stability without limb length or angular deformity.

The pes anserinus tendons are conveniently used for ACL reconstruction by either physis-sparing or physis-crossing techniques.[2,36,47,49] The tendon or tendons are left attached at their insertion, detached proximally in the posteromedial aspect of the thigh, pulled distally and rerouted superficially over the anterior tibial surface, passed under the transverse meniscal ligament to penetrate the knee joint, and then passed through the intercondylar notch

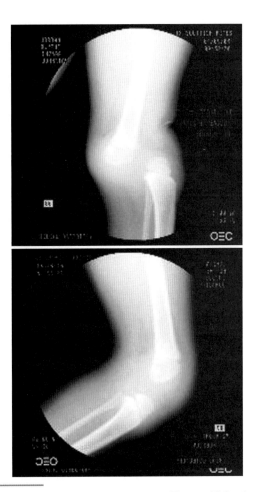

Figure 70–11. Right knee, patient in Figure 68-3, showing dislocation in extension and reduction in flexion.

and "over the top" of the lateral femoral condyle to be anchored to bone and the lateral intermuscular septum (Fig. 70–12A). To place such an ACL substitution closer to anatomic position, the tendon or tendons may be passed through a transphyseal drill hole exiting the tibial articular surface at the normal ACL insertion point (Fig. 70–12B). A 6-mm drill hole has proved technically adequate and noninjurious, with the tendons again anchored over the top of the lateral femoral condyle after traversing the notch. In either technique, care in drilling/passing tendons near the *tibial tubercle* is most important because this part of the physis seems most vulnerable. For the same reason, use of the patellar tendon as a ligament substitution is *not* recommended because of dissection near this portion of the physis. Several small series[2,36,49] have reported restoration of stability—documented by KT-1000 instrumentation, improvement in the Lachman test, and return to the previous level of sport—without physeal injury in immature patients monitored for up to 5 years.

The author has used the IT band transfer rerouted through the intercondylar notch, as described by Insall.[26,53,60] It is readily detached from Gerdy's tubercle during the approach described for open reduction of the knee (see Figs. 70–9 and 70–12C) and mobilized proximally; it is then passed antegrade "over the top" of the

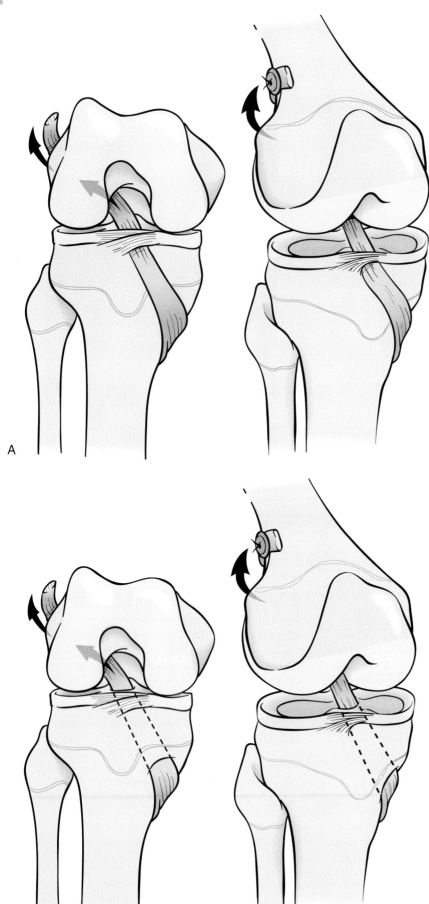

Figure 70–12. **A,** Complete physeal-sparing anterior cruciate ligament (ACL) reconstruction using the pes tendon or tendons. No drill holes cross any physes. **B,** Transtibial physis reconstruction using the pes tendon or tendons.

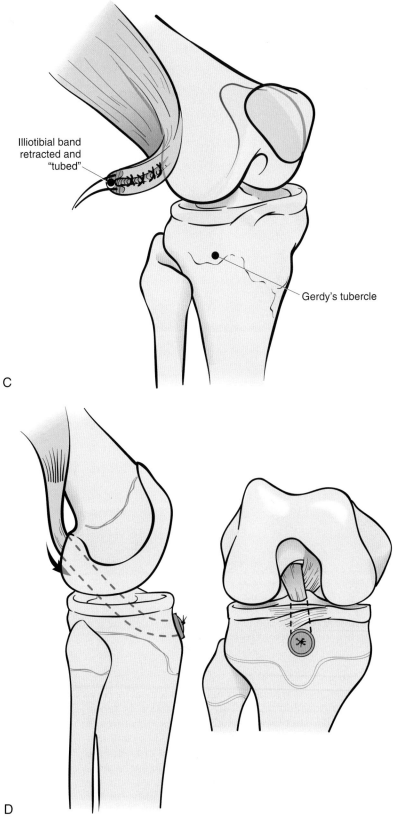

Illiotibial band
retracted and
"tubed"

Gerdy's tubercle

C

Figure 70–12, cont'd. **C** and **D,** Insall-type
reconstruction using the iliotibial (IT) band
rerouted antegrade "over the top" of the
femoral condyle and anchored within the
proximal tibial epiphysis (physeal sparing).   D

(Figure continues)

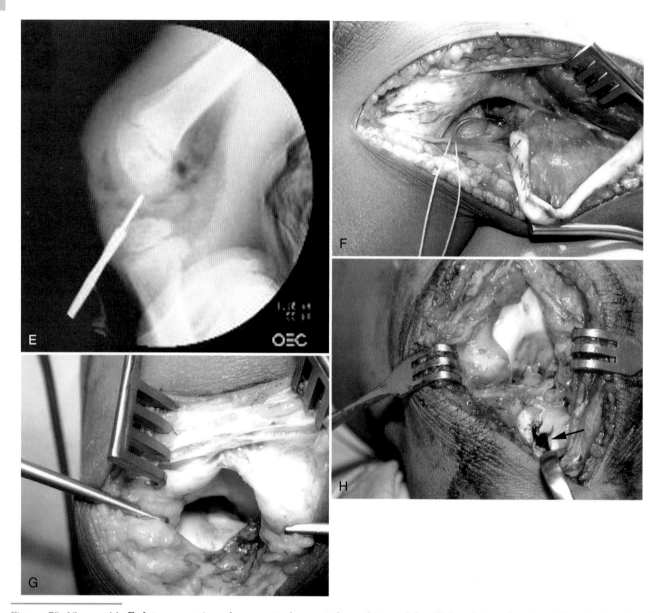

Figure 70–12, cont'd. **E,** Intraoperative placement of an epiphyseal tunnel for IT band transfer. A guide wire is placed entirely within the epiphysis, followed by a cannulated drill. **F,** Tubed IT band tendon ready for rerouting "over the top" of the lateral femoral condyle. **G,** Congenital absence of the ACL. **H,** The transferred IT band has been anchored in the epiphyseal hole *(arrow)* created in **E.**

lateral femoral condyle and through the notch before completing the capsulorrhaphy. The tubed tendon is subsequently anchored in the proximal end of the tibia through a drill hole *within the epiphysis* (see Fig. 70–12D) and tensioned before wound closure with the tibia in maximum posterior drawer and suture tied over a button on the anterior tibial skin or, alternatively, over a suture staple in the tibial metaphysis. The drill hole should be placed under radiographic control to minimize the possibility of oblique transphyseal placement, and the tunnel must include the ossification center to provide tendon-to-bone anchorage. Alternative transphyseal placement through a more vertical, centrally placed tunnel can be attempted if sufficient length of tendon is available. Postoperative care is exactly the same as for the knee reduction procedure.

The advantage of the Insall technique, as opposed to other ACL substitution procedures in which the IT band is left attached at its insertion and rerouted as a passive restraint,[40,43] is that the transferred IT band is less likely to attenuate because it is an *active* transfer where only the insertion of the tendon is being rerouted. The structure being transferred is also arguably one of the deforming forces maintaining the CDK in the first place, and thus rerouting of it should be beneficial. It will be dissected and mobilized as part of the open reduction/shortening procedure in any event. The disadvantage of this transfer remains the possibility of physeal injury at the proximal end of the tibia, the feared complication that has restrained the use of transphyseal ACL substitution except in adolescents nearing skeletal maturity. Indeed, three knees in two children *younger than 5 years* have undergone this reconstruction simultaneously with the index open reduction procedure, with one physeal arrest (Fig. 70–13). This complication occurred in the first of bilateral reconstructions in a boy with Larsen's syndrome in whom surgery was performed at the age of 18 months. He underwent the identical procedure on the second knee at age 3, with no physeal injury apparent at 9 years' follow-up. A varus-flexion deformity eventually developed in the first side and was corrected uneventfully by a simple open wedge proximal tibia osteotomy at the age of 12. Both knees are painless and stable, with 0 to 120 degrees range of motion and normal quadriceps strength (see Fig. 70–13). The third knee (in a second child with fibular hemimelia) in the series is stable and painless, and the patient actively runs and plays with the use of a Syme

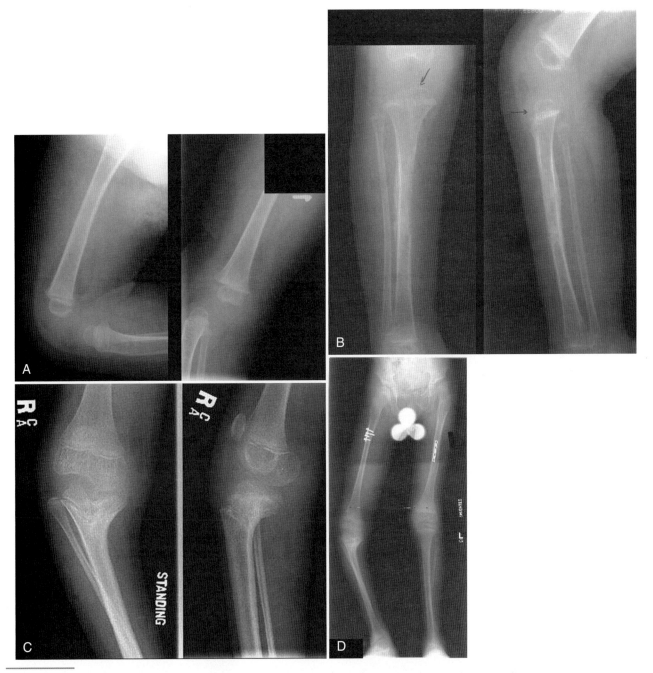

Figure 70–13. **A,** Radiographs of an unstable right knee in an 18-month-old boy with Larsen's syndrome after closed reduction of congenital dislocation of the knee. **B,** Five months after anterior cruciate ligament reconstruction using the iliotibial band (tunnel visible in the epiphysis). A tibial diaphyseal bone graft had been harvested previously for a cervical fusion. **C** and **D,** At age 12, a flexion/varus deformity has developed and was subsequently corrected by osteotomy. No deformity is seen in the left knee, which had an identical procedure performed at age 3.

amputation prosthesis on the operated side. Other investigators[43] have reported satisfactory stability without physeal injury in older children (age 12 years) with this technique.

Summary—Congenital Dislocation of the Knee

This imposing birth deformity should no longer present a disabling or unreconstructible problem as a result of joint instability and quadriceps insufficiency. Early treatment (newborn) often succeeds in gaining closed reduction,[50] and with the use of adjunctive nerve block or Botox, even grade 3 dislocations can be successfully reduced nonoperatively. Late reduction (after walking age) via femoral shortening, to minimize quadriceps weakening and scarring by extensive dissection, and *early* ACL reconstruction, either simultaneous with the open reduction or staged, in syndromic knees can still provide a stable and functional outcome if the treatment approach as described in this chapter is effectively applied. Although transphyseal ACL reconstruction will remain controversial, especially in children younger than 5 years of age undergoing CDK reduction, the author is convinced that at least a physeal-sparing reconstruction is indicated to provide a functional knee in a patient with perhaps other syndromic orthopedic disabilities as well. The stability provided by early ACL reconstruction is *invaluable* to the function of such syndromic patients, and should a physeal growth disturbance occur, it can always be reconstructed later by appropriate osteotomy and/or lengthening.

CONGENITAL DISLOCATION OF THE PATELLA

Patellofemoral instability is a common and well-known problem familiar to all orthopedists. The term describes a continuum of deformities that in the severest form is *congenital dislocation* of the patella, which should be defined as a laterally displaced, hypoplastic patella present at birth, diagnosed by age 10, associated with a flexion contracture of the knee and a valgus and external rotation deformity of the leg, and basically irreducible ("fixed" dislocation) by closed means.[16,57] The continuum or grades of congenital patella dislocation and dysplasia are also described as *recurrent*, *habitual*, or *obligatory* dislocation,[14] where the patella is sometimes reducible in extension but unstable in flexion and resumes its laterally displaced position as the knee is flexed (Fig. 70–14) because of a variety of soft-tissue contractures and/or a deficient lateral femoral condyle. Regardless, an attempt to discuss all grades and types of patellofemoral instability, such as those associated with adolescence, including developmental, rotational ("miserable malalignment"), and possibly traumatic causes, is a monumental task fraught with confusing terms and a myriad of treatment approaches. Thus, this chapter will limit discussion to the aforementioned irreducible or obligatory congenital lesion.

Clinical Features

Goldthwait[20] first described the surgical treatment of a "permanent" dislocation of the patella in 1899, whereas

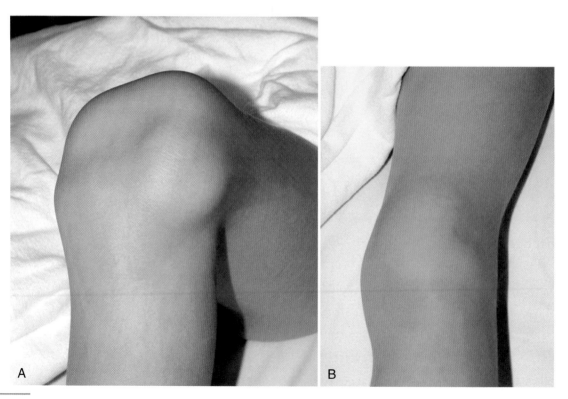

Figure 70–14. **A,** Obligatory patellar dislocation when the knee is flexed in a 5-year-old. **B,** Reduction in extension.

Conn[9] described release of the contracted lateral soft tissues and advancement of the vastus medialis in 1925. However, the true etiology and pathoanatomy of a dislocated patella were probably not described until Stanisavljevic et al in 1976 described failure of internal rotation of the quadriceps myotome in the fetus.[57] They noted that the laterally placed thigh structures normally rotate internally in the first trimester of fetal development and that when this rotation fails to occur, the patella remains laterally displaced on the lateral femoral condyle, and the entire quadriceps mechanism remains rotated anterolaterally. The actual diagnosis of this condition may be delayed because of an inability to palpate the true position of the patella in a newborn or young child and an inability to document its position radiographically until later. Normal ossification of the patella occurs around age 3, but it is often delayed further when the patella is hypoplastic as in congenital dislocation.

Diagnosis of the condition may not occur until the child is evaluated for a disability of the leg, including delayed weightbearing.[17,37] There may be a valgus and flexion deformity, external tibial torsion with seemingly lateral instability during weightbearing, and an empty intercondylar space at the anterior distal aspect of the femur when the knee is flexed. As already noted, the patella may not be palpable because of its hypoplasia and fixation to the lateral femoral condyle—thus it is mistaken for the latter structure. Quadriceps insufficiency, denoted by an extension lag (and thus the flexion contracture deformity), may be the most obvious physical finding suggesting the diagnosis in an infant. In contrast, in patients with less quadriceps insufficiency and a mobile patella reducible in extension, lateral dislocation of the patella with flexion will confirm the diagnosis (see Fig. 70–14). It may be possible to demonstrate an inability to extend the knee against resistance from a flexed position when the patella is dislocated, whereas strength tested in extension, when the patella is more normally positioned, is nearly normal. Depending on the degree of quadriceps dysfunction, the child may do relatively well in the first decade, only to begin falling or have increasing relative weakness or loss of the ability to keep up with peers as increasing body size overstresses the quadriceps mechanism. This scenario is often seen in patients with syndromic associations underlying their patellar dislocation, such as Down's, Rubinstein-Taybi, or nail-patella syndrome. It may be necessary to resort to computed tomography, magnetic resonance imaging, or rarely, open exploration to make the diagnosis in some cases.[17]

Treatment

Treatment of congenital dislocation of the patella is surgical because this dislocation is by definition irreducible or unstable. The goal is to realign the quadriceps mechanism and place the patella in the intercondylar groove, thereby balancing the muscle insertions so that the reduction is stable and the groove, which is congenitally hypoplastic because of anterior flattening of the lateral femoral condyle, will deepen as normal patella tracking ensues.[14]

The classic procedure involves the concepts of Judet and Stanisavljevic in dissecting the vastus lateralis from the lateral intermuscular septum from its origin to its insertion and subperiosteally rotating the entire quadriceps muscle mass medially.[30,57] Thus, the skin incision basically extends from the greater trochanter to the lateral parapatellar area and, if infrapatellar realignment is necessary, distally to just beyond the tibial tubercle (Fig. 70–15). Distally in the thigh, the lateral retinaculum and muscle insertions are abnormally contracted and must be divided to free the patella from these tethering structures (see Fig. 70–15C), which actually produce the flexion deformity by being displaced posterior to the axis of knee motion. Transversely dividing the IT band corrects the external tibial rotation, genu valgum, and knee flexion deformity. Lengthening the quadriceps tendon by Z- or V-Y–plasty has been advocated, if necessary, to remedy the obligatory dislocation caused by quadriceps contracture.[14] Femoral shortening, as described in the previous section on CDK, may be a better solution if the quadriceps is that severely contracted. The biceps may also require division to completely reduce the tibial subluxation/valgus.[14] Once the patella and quadriceps can be centralized, medial imbrication is necessary to maintain the reduction. A medial arthrotomy is performed to mobilize the vastus medialis insertion, which is then advanced distally and laterally to maintain centralization of the patella (see Figs. 70–9E and F). There is no need to close or otherwise repair the large lateral retinacular defect, although some authors have described excising the fascia lata and using it as a graft to cover the defect and close the joint.

The final step is to realign the patellar tendon insertion if it remains too lateral. The classic Goldthwait transfer of the lateral half of the patellar tendon, split longitudinally from the medial half, sharply dissected from its insertion, and passed medially under the intact medial portion to be reattached to bone/periosteum for distal medial advancement, is generally used in immature patients for this purpose.[20] Other authors prefer complete release and reinsertion of the entire patellar tendon,[14,34] although the risk of tibial tubercle physeal injury[22] or excessive patellofemoral joint compression[38] may be increased by this method. Before closure, the knee is ranged to ascertain whether either the suprapatellar or infrapatellar imbrications are too tight and preventing passive flexion to at least 45 degrees. Alternatively, if the patella continues to dislocate laterally, additional proximal lateral release (see later) and/or revision of the medial imbrication is indicated. In the most severe cases, semitendinosus transfer[3,14] may be added as an additional checkrein to continued lateral subluxation. Normally, 6 to 8 weeks of cast immobilization in slight flexion is required to achieve stability after the medial imbrication and Goldthwait and Dewar procedures, followed by vigorous rehabilitation.

Often, the aforementioned extensive quadriceps dissection plus mobilization into the proximal aspect of the thigh is unnecessary. Although it may seem logical to perform this dissection to completely address the pathoanatomy, in point of fact the dissection can often be limited to the distal third of the thigh, thus avoiding filleting the thigh from the trochanter to the knee to rotate the entire quadriceps. The author has found that a com-

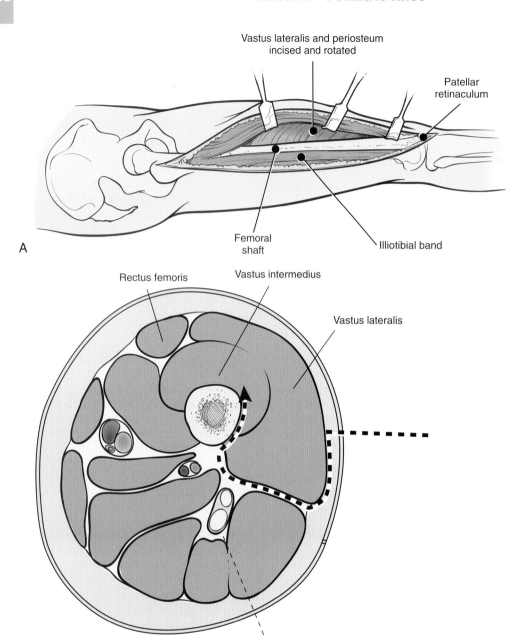

Vastus lateralis and periosteum
incised and rotated

Patellar
retinaculum

Femoral
shaft

Illiotibial band

A

Rectus femoris

Vastus intermedius

Vastus lateralis

Sciatic nerve

B

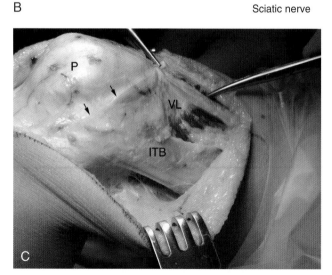

P

VL

ITB

C

Figure 70–15. **A,** Incision and mobilization of the vastus lateralis, intermedius, and rectus for Judet/Stanisavljevic quadricepsplasty. **B,** Dissection posterior to the vastus lateralis with subperiosteal mobilization of the vastus lateralis and intermedius. **C,** Abnormal lateral insertions of the vastus lateralis (VL) and iliotibial band (ITB) into the patella retinaculum (P).

petent and adequately tensioned medial imbrication is quite stable, even if there appears to be some persistent lateralization of the proximal thigh musculature. If intraoperative stability through 45 to 60 degrees of flexion is documented, additional dissection of the intermuscular septum proximally is unnecessary. Furthermore, early range-of-motion exercises can be started after allowing 2 to 3 weeks for wound healing if the medial imbrication is competent and the patella stable. Similar experiences have been reported.[17]

Results/Commentary

Unfortunately, the results of quadriceps realignment are not that well documented. A 10% incidence of recurrent dislocation is reported[16,21,29] at an average of 5 years after surgery, and extension lag is generally improved, though not always in the more severe arthrogrypotic or skeletal dysplasia patients.[34] Other complications include medial dislocation—presumably from overzealous vastus medialis advancement—and peroneal nerve palsy.[21,29] In patients with Down's syndrome, in which patellar instability occurs in 5% to 8% of affected persons and includes both fixed persistent dislocation and frank obligatory instability, the indication for patellar stabilization has been questioned because of the frequent absence of symptoms or functional deficit.[13,58] Operative treatment for patients with poor function secondary to instability has been reported to be successful in up to 86% of patients[38] and in patients monitored for up to 15 years,[13] although most series are small and have short follow-up. Readers can draw their own conclusions concerning the effectiveness of patellar stabilization in this group of patients with notorious laxity and consequent risk of recurrence.

Since the main indication for patellar stabilization surgery is the *local* functional deficit caused by the impaired quadriceps function and the flexion–valgus–external rotation deformity, any outcome that improves the extension lag, gait instability, and overall function with a range of knee motion compatible with normal activities—arguably 0 to 90 degrees of motion—should be considered worthwhile, even if a repeat operation is necessary at a later date to deal with recurrence. Ultimately, it is assumed that chronic patellar dislocation, fixed or recurrent/obligatory, will degenerate into significant painful arthritis, at which time other reconstructive procedures, including patellectomy or total knee arthroplasty, may not be attractive because of long-standing quadriceps and periarticular soft-tissue laxity/insufficiency. Thus, surgical reduction of congenital patellar dislocation with *any* functional impairment should always be attempted except in cases such as Down's syndrome, where symptoms and long-term disability are documented to *not* occur with significant frequency.

FLEXION DEFORMITY OF THE KNEE

A knee flexion contracture (KFC) of up to 45 degrees is a normal finding in a neonate, with further flexion to 160

degrees—the normal intrauterine position of the knee at term—also being possible. As long as quadriceps function is normal and there are no other neurologic or dysmorphic features, this congenital contracture gradually resolves in the first few months of life. By the age of 6 months, a significant amount of fixed knee flexion (45 degrees or more), with or without limitation of further flexion, will probably have been noted if there is a local or syndromic condition affecting the extremity. In general, such a knee deformity would be a manifestation of one of the underlying conditions in Box 70–1, which would probably have been recognized because of other orthopedic deformities or syndromic features.

Establishing the associated diagnosis underlying the knee flexion deformity has important prognostic and therapeutic value. In conditions in which femoral-tibial extension is blocked is by intrinsic bony deformity (e.g., skeletal dysplasia), early soft-tissue release is probably of little value to increase extension, and thus correction by osteotomy or growth manipulation will be considered and probably delayed until technical considerations and ambulatory status indicate treatment. On the other hand, in the soft-tissue contracture syndromes, early aggressive treatment may be important to prevent the development of secondary joint deformity precluding full extension and irreversible quadriceps dysfunction, which will impede ambulatory capability. Finally, treatment of the knee in patients with limb reduction anomalies (femoral deficiency, tibial hemimelia) is dictated by overall function, knee stability, *limb length* considerations, and whether the involvement is unilateral or bilateral. This section will focus on the soft-tissue "webbing" syndromes, where early reconstructive knee surgery may be of benefit, whereas the skeletal dysplasias and limb reduction anomalies, which require a combination of angular and growth manipulations of the entire extremity, will not be discussed further here.

Box 70-1. Conditions Associated with Congenital Knee Flexion Deformity

Localized Dysplasia Affecting the Extremity Only
Congenital femoral deficiency
Tibial hemimelia types 1a, 1b
Congenital quadriceps/patellar tendon dysplasia
Congenital dislocation (fixed) of the patella

Syndromes with Soft-Tissue Contracture
Arthrogryposis
Popliteal pterygium syndrome
Escobar's (multiple pterygium) syndrome
Beals' syndrome (congenital contractural arachnodactyly)
Paralytic (sacral agenesis, myelodysplasia)

Skeletal Dysplasia with Bony Flexion Deformity
Diastrophic dysplasia
Metatropic dysplasia
Miscellaneous skeletal dysplasias

Correcting a congenital KFC—indeed *any* significant KFC—is often a frustrating and complication-riddled proposition. The decision to proceed must involve an overall evaluation of the prognosis for functional ambulation, with appreciation of the extent of involvement of the ipsilateral hip and foot, as well as any neurodevelopmental implications for function. A KFC exceeding 30 degrees alters gait adversely because of overstressing of the quadriceps.[51] It is often problematic to determine the pretreatment status of the quadriceps when a significant KFC is present. Furthermore, significant hip flexion deformity or severe equinus may have to be corrected simultaneously, or else these uncorrected deformities will induce recurrent knee flexion to maintain overall sagittal alignment for upright posture. The *absolute* prerequisite for KFC treatment is identification of a *functional quadriceps*, without which any extension obtained through treatment will certainly be lost as the unopposed forces producing the original contracture persist.

Pterygium Syndromes

These congenital syndromic deformities produce soft-tissue webbing on the flexion side of various joints. The popliteal pterygium syndrome (also known as facial-genital-popliteal syndrome) includes, besides the popliteal web restricting extension, cleft lip and palate, intraoral webbing sometimes requiring surgical release to open the mouth, intercrural webs distorting the external genitalia, and finger and toe syndactyly with nail abnormalities (Fig. 70–16). Patients have normal intelligence and development. In multiple pterygium (Escobar's) syndrome, webs occur across every flexion area, with particular involvement of the neck (85%) and popliteal (60%) areas and less common involvement of the axilla, antecubital area, and fingers. Severe kyphoscoliosis and short stature (adult height, 135 cm) are typical of patients with Escobar's syndrome, who may also show little abnormality at birth and then the webs "develop" with growth. In arthrogryposis and Beals' syndrome (Fig. 70–17), multiple joints are typically involved, with stiffness, lack of active motion, and absence of flexion creases noted especially in classic arthrogryposis. In sacral agenesis and myelodysplasia, lack of motion is also obvious and is related to the neurological deficit of spinal cord origin.

Pathoanatomy

The hallmark of popliteal pterygia is extension of a fibrous band from the ischium to the calcaneus, with a subcutaneous cord (the calcaneo-ischiadicus muscle) and the sciatic nerve or one of its divisions (usually the tibial) intimately adherent within the web (Fig. 70–18). There is often a longitudinal skin marking of a lighter color outlining the path of the subcutaneous cord. The cord is covered by a tent of muscle or fascia that fills the web and connects to the medial and lateral intramuscular septa of the thigh and leg. Abnormal muscle bellies and aberrant nerve paths piercing the pterygium fascia should be expected in any surgical dissection.

Obstacles to correction of a pterygium contracture include the calcaneo-ischial cord, which is not generally flexible and intuitively invites excision, usually with a Z-plasty of the skin; the shortness of the sciatic or tibial nerve division accompanying the cord,[24,46] which of course cannot be stretched acutely; and intra-articular incongruity secondary to flattening of the femoral condyles because of persistence of growth in flexion. The latter is an important argument for *early* surgical correction before the joint deformity per se prevents full extension as a result of misshapen articular surfaces. Recurrence of the contracture is extremely frequent because of reconstitution of the calcaneo-ischial cord and popliteal scar formation and secondarily as a result of ankle equinus from the calcaneal insertion—the knee must flex to accommodate the persistent or recurrent equinus. The role of a weak quadriceps is obvious, although in practice its actual strength is difficult, if not impossible to test or document—the pretreatment strength of the muscle cannot be determined in an infant or toddler with a rigid flexion deformity that prevents extension. About all that can be determined is whether the muscle *contracts* when the leg is stimulated.

In arthrogryposis and similar conditions, obstacles to correction are mainly the periarticular fibrosis and underlying muscle paralysis. These joints are congenitally rigid because of lack of intrauterine movement, as evidenced by absence of flexion creases, for example. Periarticular tissue and joint capsules are contracted as a result. Early attempts to mobilize these joints with physical therapy are usually unrewarding because of lack of *active* movement, but an effort should always be made. At some point in a 12- to 24-month-old patient, a decision must be made about the prognosis for ambulation based on active movements of the lower extremities and, in particular, the presence of quadriceps function. In cases of total absence of quadriceps function, the decision to accept the flexed knee position and consequent nonambulatory status, and thus forego treatment of the knee flexion deformity, is completely justified.

Overall, the prognosis for obtaining and maintaining correction of congenital KFC of such causes—and thus useful ambulation—is guarded at best because of the often insurmountable problem of recurrence. Treatment must be commenced with the anticipation that recurrence is inevitable to some degree and that functional gains are elusive because of numerous possible complications, including nerve stretching and neuropathic pain, joint damage from extensive dissection producing avascular necrosis of the epiphysis and physis, incongruity and cartilage necrosis (Fig. 70–19), and inadequate muscle strength to allow nonsupported knee extension.

Treatment

ACUTE CORRECTION— PTERYGIUM/ARTHROGRYPOSIS

Correction by surgical release of the popliteal structures, combined with femoral and possibly tibial shortening, is

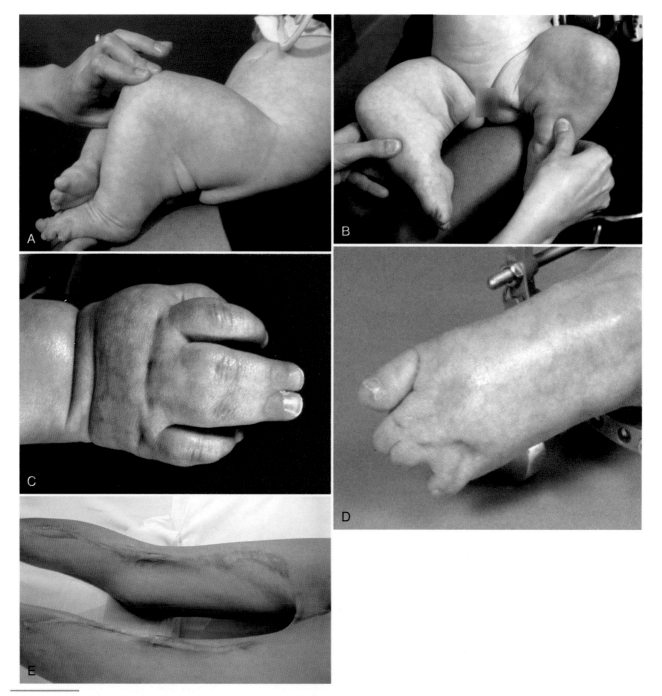

Figure 70–16. **A** and **B**, Clinical appearance of the lower extremities in an infant with popliteal pterygium syndrome (PPS). **C** and **D**, Syndactyly and toe deformities in PPS. **E**, Intercrural webbing affecting the perineal area (buttocks to the *right*).

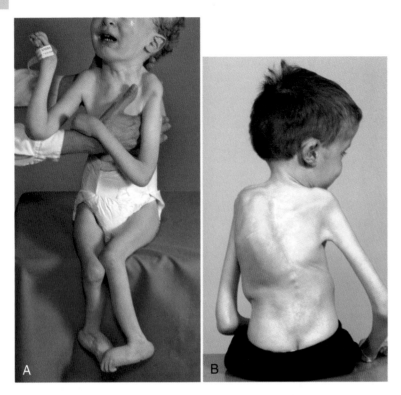

Figure   70–17.   **A,**   Congenital   contractural arachnodactyly (Beals' syndrome): elbow and knee flexion contractures in a 1-year-old. **B,** Spinal deformity in Beals' syndrome.

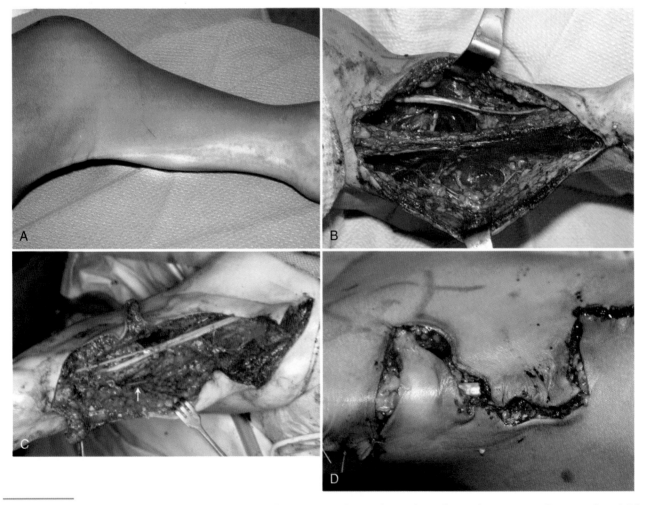

Figure 70–18. **A,** Superficial band with skin discoloration overlying khe ischiocalcaneal structure (foot to the *right*). **B,** Ischiocalcaneal muscle and band, with the sciatic nerve isolated. **C,** All popliteal soft-tissue structures have been released except the major nerve divisions and the vascular bundle *(arrow)*. **D,** After wound closure, the sciatic nerve is bowstrung directly under the skin.

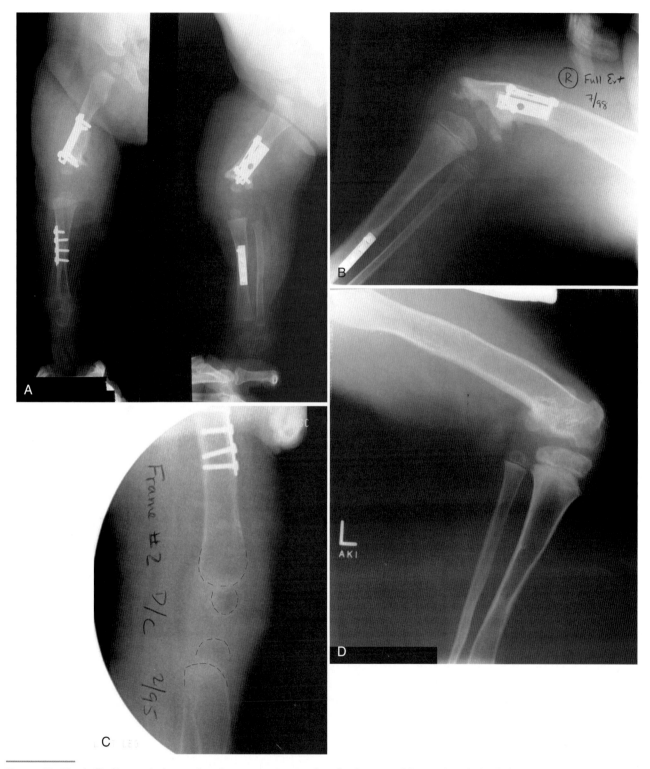

Figure 70–19. **A,** Radiograph 4 months after extensive popliteal release and femoral and tibial shortening were performed on the right lower extremity of the patient in Figure 70–16. **B,** Avascular necrosis of the distal femoral epiphysis and physis resulted. **C,** Left knee radiograph showing full extension of the same patient after a second attempt at distraction arthrodiastasis correction with the Ilizarov method (see also Figure 70–22). Soft-tissue release and femoral shortening followed the second frame correction. **D,** Result: recurrent deformity with severe degenerative changes 2 years later.

(Figure continues)

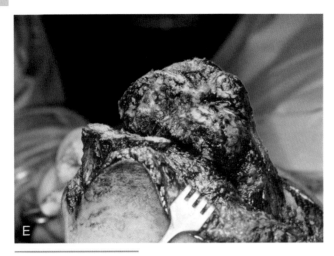

Figure 70–19, cont'd. **E,** Intraoperative view of the destroyed distal femur from **D.** The articular surface is covered with pannus, and cartilage cannot be identified. Knee fusion with rotationplasty was performed.

a first line of treatment for deformities of moderate severity, up to perhaps 60 degrees. The popliteal release may best be accomplished with the patient prone, although if hip mobility is normal and allows full internal and external rotation, the patient can be positioned supine, thus allowing access to both sides of the knee simultaneously. The latter is important because of the need to inspect the intercondylar notch and patellofemoral joint after posterior release since there is often a soft-tissue "pulvinar" in the notch blocking full extension that must be excised to complete the procedure and, in arthrogrypotic patients, the patellofemoral joint is often scarred or obliterated and the quadriceps mechanism must be freed from the femur and a suprapatellar pouch "created" (Fig. 70–20).

Regardless of patient position, the skin over the ischiocalcaneal band must be incised longitudinally with multiple Z-plasties and the actual cord exposed circumferentially from the ischial tuberosity to the calcaneal tuberosity. Exposure of the cord will reveal the sciatic nerve and its tibial, peroneal, and sural components, which should be completely dissected, mobilized, and protected (see Fig. 70–18). The ischiocalcaneal structure is then excised. The arcade of fascia enveloping the band can then be safely followed to the medial and lateral intermuscular septa and divided transversely just like a fasciotomy of the leg or plantar surface of the foot. This fascial division is best accomplished close to the joint, near the axis or rotation, but it can also be accomplished at points proximal and distal to the knee. Deeper structures in the popliteal fossa can then be dissected and released sharply, obviously protecting the deep midline vascular structures, which are in the normal anatomic location (see Fig. 70–18C). Beginning laterally, the biceps and IT band are released (Henry's approach), and posterior capsulotomy of the knee is the ultimate goal of the dissection. Medially, the hamstring tendons are released, leading to complete posteromedial capsulotomy. However, despite what appears to be a comprehensive, thorough

posterior knee release, the limiting factor—the sciatic nerve or its tibial component—usually prevents adequate extension and in fact bowstrings in the popliteal area so severely that skin closure over the nerve may be an issue (see Fig. 70–18D).

The femur should then be shortened,[46,52] as much as 3 to 4 cm if necessary, to achieve full or nearly full extension (see Figs. 70–19A and 70–20E and F). This shortening effectively "decompresses" the tissue around the knee, much like femoral shortening applied to reduction of a late-diagnosed congenital dislocation of the hip,[6] and allows extension without undue tension on the nerves. This can be accomplished in the distal diaphysis by plating the femur either laterally or posteriorly—the latter is theoretically preferable since the plate will then be on the tension side of the force at the osteotomy when the knee is extended with some force. An overly aggressive popliteal soft-tissue release combined with distal femoral shortening can result in avascular injury to the distal femoral physis (see Fig. 70–19B). The tibia can also be shortened to benefit ankle equinus, as well as decompress the popliteal structures further. Hyperextension osteotomy of the distal end of the femur has been used to correct KFC,[12] but in a young child provides only temporary improvement because of remodeling by distal physeal growth.

As suggested earlier, *anterior* arthrotomy must be considered for removal of the fibrofatty soft tissue that often fills the intercondylar notch and prevents the final 10 to 15 degrees of extension (see Fig. 70–20D). The patellofemoral joint may also need inspection as part of assessing whether full passive extension is possible. Finally, plication of the patellar tendon should be considered after femoral shortening in order to remove excessive redundancy, which will compromise eventual quadriceps strength. In children younger than 2 years, plication may not be necessary, but one will never be criticized for this final step in attempting to balance and augment the extension function in this deformity where such function is often lacking.

Once maximum extension has been achieved, the incisions are closed and a spica cast is applied to control the proximal part of the thigh because a long-leg cast has inadequate purchase on the thigh after femoral shortening. When the osteotomies have healed (5 to 6 weeks), the patient is actively mobilized, with concentration on active extension and unencumbered weightbearing. Bracing in full extension can be used if quadriceps weakness appears to be allowing excessive flexion. Long-term night bracing in full extension is often recommended, but its efficacy is unknown. As mentioned before, the tendency for recurrence is overwhelming, so attempts to delay it by long-term bracing are appropriate. Despite vigorous treatment of KFC in arthrogryposis, over half the patients lose ambulatory ability because of ineffective correction or recurrence and thus do not remain community ambulators.[42,55] Many patients with popliteal pterygium syndrome, depending on the initial severity, will remain community ambulators with repetitive surgery,[46,48] provided that the knees do not succumb to painful degenerative arthritis (see Fig. 70–19). Knee fusion or amputation may be resorted to in the latter situation.

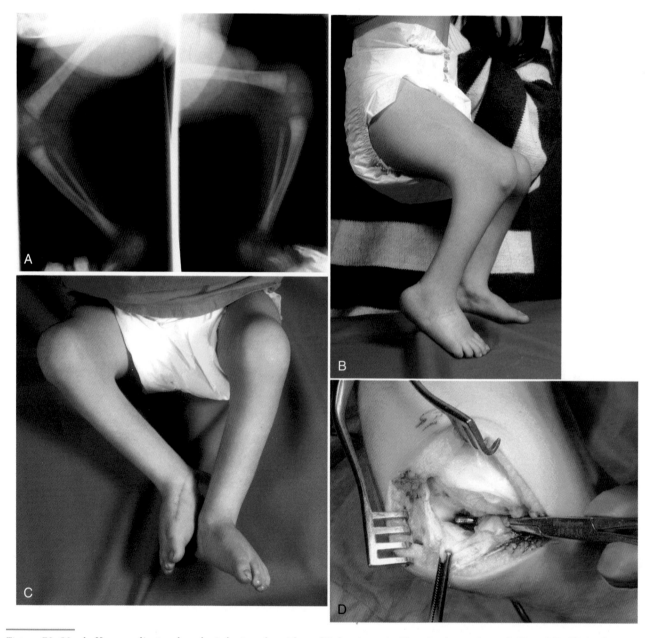

Figure 70–20. **A,** Knee radiographs of a infant male with multiple pterygia (Escobar's syndrome). **B** and **C,** Clinical appearance of the lower extremities. **D,** Anterior arthrotomy to excise fibrofatty soft tissue obstructing the intercondylar notch and blocking full extension.

(Figure continues)

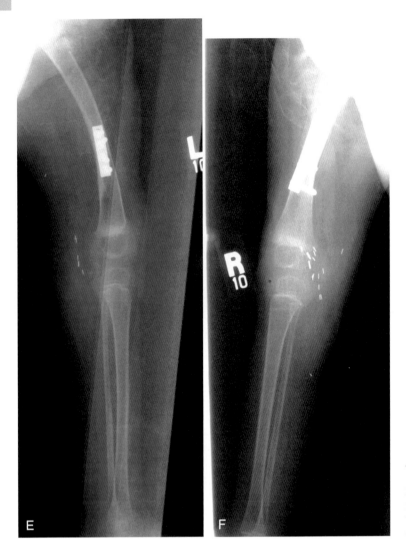

Figure 70–20, cont'd. **E** and **F,** Radiographs at $3\frac{1}{2}$ years of age after staged popliteal release, femoral shortening, and anterior arthrotomy, with latissimus dorsi free flaps for soft-tissue closure of the popliteal fossae.

Microvascular free tissue transfer has been used in place of Z-plasty in an attempt to further "decompress" the popliteal scarring that contributes to recurrence. Limited experience with latissimus dorsi free transfer (see Fig. 70–20) has shown that KFC recurrence can be delayed to some degree, but cannot be prevented simply by supplying noninvolved healthy tissue to cover the popliteal space. Because of the possible untoward effects of *bilateral* free latissimus flaps on the development of spinal deformity, this method may be appropriate only in patients nearing skeletal maturity, where the risk of progressive spinal deformity is minimal.

Full passive extension may not be achieved in spite of the comprehensive surgery just described, most commonly as a result of incomplete decompression of neurovascular structures, but also because of early joint incongruity. A form of *gradual* extension improvement can then be attempted postoperatively with either serial casts in progressively more extension or the use of an extension-desubluxation hinge cast (Quengel hinges, Fig. 70–21). The latter allows casting in flexion and then progressive gradual extension once early would healing has occurred, with the ability to translate the tibia anteriorly during correction to avoid knee subluxation. Care must be exercised to avoid pressure decubitus ulcers at the anterior distal aspect of the thigh, where careful padding and judicious cast trimming are crucial to prevent skin complications as progressive extension is achieved. A spica cast is recommended to avoid posterior proximal thigh skin pressure caused by the Quengel technique when a long-leg-only cast is placed.

GRADUAL CORRECTION— ILIZAROV TECHNIQUE

Gradual correction of joint contracture with an external fixator is an attractive option for severe congenital KFC. The amount of corrective force that can be applied to the bony skeleton is not limited by skin tolerance, and because the skeletal elements are controlled directly by the fixation wires or pins, joint subluxation can be avoided. The sciatic nerve and its branches—the structures directly limiting the amount of acute correction—tolerate slow stretching well. Both circular and monolateral devices using a hinge-distractor method have been reported.[7,11,18,25,41] Improvement in extension and alter-

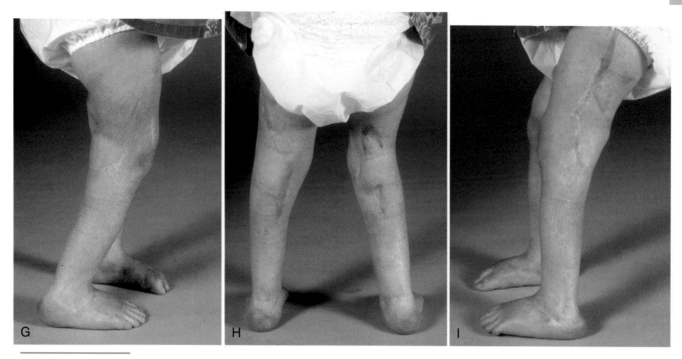

Figure 70–20, cont'd. **G-I,** Clinical appearance at 3½ years of age.

(Figure continues)

ation of the total arc range of motion to a more functional range can be achieved. The problem—as with acute correction—appears to be maintenance of correction, regardless of whether soft-tissue release has been performed simultaneously.[11,18,25]

Loss of correction with recurrence of both deformity and stiffness is common in our limited experience (Fig. 70–22; see also Fig. 70–19). Although gradual correction is very attractive, it still does not eliminate the problem of recurrences after Ilizarov correction of pterygia. The question arises whether a soft-tissue release *before* frame correction is advisable. The reasoning might be that the distraction arthrodiastasis actually *induces* increased fibrous tissue as the surgically treated popliteal structures are lengthened, in the same way that bone is created by distraction forces after osteotomy. Such "distraction histogenesis" invites recurrence by the stimulation of new popliteal fibrous tissue, which becomes apparent after frame removal. Thus, it is the author's opinion that Ilizarov correction of pterygia should *not* be preceded by soft-tissue release, but rather the deformity should be addressed by external fixation/arthrodiastasis alone and, at the first sign of recurrence (loss of extension) after healing of the pin tracts, be subjected to formal soft-tissue release and femoral shortening, as described earlier for acute correction.

The frame is constructed with double points of fixation on both the femur and tibia, usually with an arch proximal and a ring distal on the femur and two rings for the tibia (see Fig. 70–22A). The foot should be included in a static frame, fixed to the tibia in neutral position, whenever there is the potential for significant equinus during correction, which in practice means essentially every case

of KFC. An extra point of fixation to the distal femoral ring is a transverse wire through the femoral epiphysis to protect this physis from separation during correction,[11] although this is not mandatory—monolateral fixators have successfully corrected KFC,[41] obviously without such a protective wire for the distal femoral epiphysis. The hinge must be placed as a *distraction* hinge, with the axis of rotation being just distal to the anterior distal edge of the distal femoral condyle (see Fig. 70–22D). This is intended to prevent articular cartilage pressure damage, but in fact it is probably the least controllable complication of the procedure. The rate of angular correction can be calculated by using the triangulation formula or concentric radii,[25] but in practice it is generally tailored to the patient's tolerance and the appearance of any neuropraxia complications. Empirically, 4 mm of distraction per day on the motor rod seems to efficiently correct the deformity. Distal neuropathy, as evidenced by hyperesthesia or dysesthesia of the foot, warrants temporary slowing or a pause from correction and consideration of the use of gabapentin (Neurontin) if it does not resolve. Once full extension is achieved, it is generally recommended that the frame be maintained locked in full extension for 4 to 6 weeks.[25,41] Rapid flexion and extension through an arc of 30 degrees or more can be attempted during this period to "mobilize" the periarticular tissue once full extension is reached. The frame should then be removed and the knee placed in a cast for an additional 4 to 6 weeks to help maintain the correction and allow the pin tracts to heal in preparation for possible additional surgery, such as ischiocalcaneal cord excision and femoral shortening, to "decompress" the correction. Such surgery should be considered as soon as recurrence or loss of extension becomes apparent.

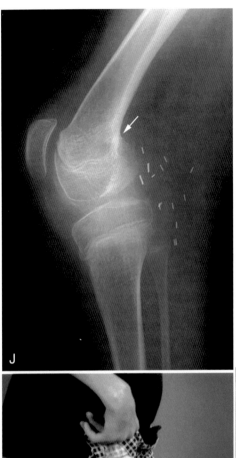

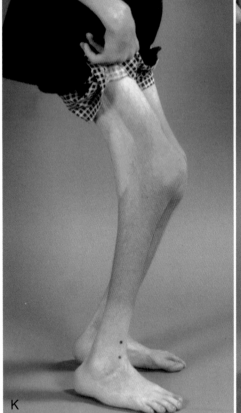

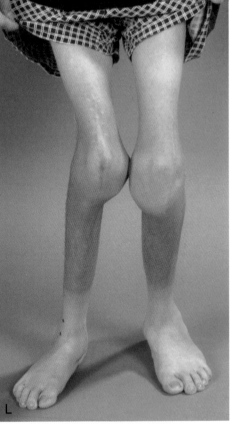

Figure 70–20, cont'd. **J,** Ten years postoperatively, a significant flexion deformity has recurred on the right. Premature growth arrest at the posterior physis is suspected *(arrow)*. Joint incongruity is also apparent. **K** and **L,** Clinical appearance at 14 years of age.

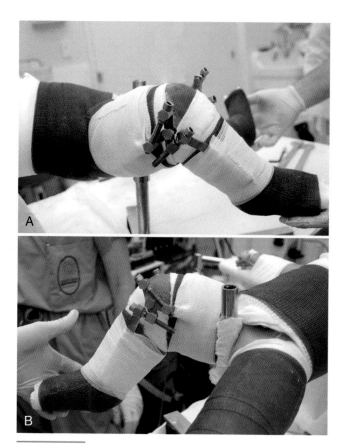

Figure 70–21. **A** and **B,** Extension-desubluxation hinge cast applied immediately after acute correction surgery. The proximal threaded screw extends the knee, whereas the distal one translates the tibia anteriorly to prevent posterior subluxation.

Although long-leg bracing is commonly recommended once the final cast is removed, in young children this is mechanically ineffective because of the limited control of the thigh, especially if the femur has been shortened. A nighttime extension orthosis may be the most practical for post-treatment splintage.

The results of Ilizarov correction of KFC are far more encouraging than those of acute correction, except for patients with popliteal pterygium syndrome, where recurrence is almost always expected;[11] 60% to 85% of knees gain significant correction and maintain it at up to 5 years' follow-up. Brunner et al[7] corrected 11 of 13 knees from 39 degrees of flexion to 17 degrees at follow-up without frame-related complications; Herzenberg et al[25] achieved good/excellent results in 9 of 14 knees, starting from an average 60 degrees of contracture corrected to 16 degrees at follow-up without complications; and Damsin and Ghanem[11] reported 13 corrections of greater than 90 degrees of contracture—by far the most severe contractures ever reported—to an average of 10 degrees at follow-up, excluding two cases with multiple pterygia syndrome that recurred and needed more treatment. Damsin and Ghanem encountered three fractures and one nerve palsy in their series, and 5 of 13 knees remained stiff after treatment, more a reflection of the severity of the joint pathology than a complication per se.

Perhaps the most discouraging aspect of severe KFC correction by the Ilizarov technique is the potential joint damage from cartilage pressure necrosis (see Fig. 70–19). There is no agreed upon method to avoid this complication, other than to proceed slowly and ensure that the joint is in fact distracted during the extension period. Recurrence of flexion deformity after correction to full extension may also be related to an inadequate quadriceps, which has not been addressed by patellar tendon plication, for example, in any series of Ilizarov corrections to date.

ANTERIOR FEMORAL STAPLING (HEMI-EPIPHYSEODESIS)

Mild (10 to 25 degrees) flexion deformities are amenable to nonoperative management, soft-tissue release with casting, or the more recently introduced anterior distal femoral hemi-epiphyseodesis.[33] The latter is a minimally invasive method to obtain correction via a hemi-epiphyseodesis effect with the use of traditional epiphyseal staples; it requires only that the distal femoral physis be functional and that greater than 2 years of growth remain. This technique is worth considering when an extensive surgical release or osteotomy is being considered for a less severe deformity.

AMPUTATION/ARTHRODESIS/ ROTATIONPLASTY

Failure to achieve a functional knee position, especially if accompanied by pain not amenable to bracing or medication and after perhaps two attempts to correct severe KFC, is an indication for either knee fusion or disarticulation. Any discussion of treatment of severe KFC must include a realization that especially if the failure is primarily unilateral, these alternatives are appropriate and useful. Since the majority of congenital KFC cases are *bilateral,* these salvage procedures are usually considered when one knee is considerably worse than the other. The decision to proceed with this type of salvage surgery must obviously be individualized.

Knee fusion with rotationplasty[1,19] should also be considered if the foot and ankle are functional despite the failed knee correction. The procedure simulates an internal knee amputation, with the limb being rotated 180 degrees externally after excising the distal femur and proximal tibia. This converts the ankle to a functional "knee," and with a below-knee prosthesis fitted to the foot, ankle plantar flexion becomes "knee" extension, with dorsiflexion becoming "knee" flexion. Since the rotated foot should be at the level of the contralateral knee, the use of this salvage method is generally limited to patients with one sound limb and one requiring knee ablation.

Summary/Commentary

Congenital KFC presents some of the most challenging treatment problems in orthopedics. In deformities greater

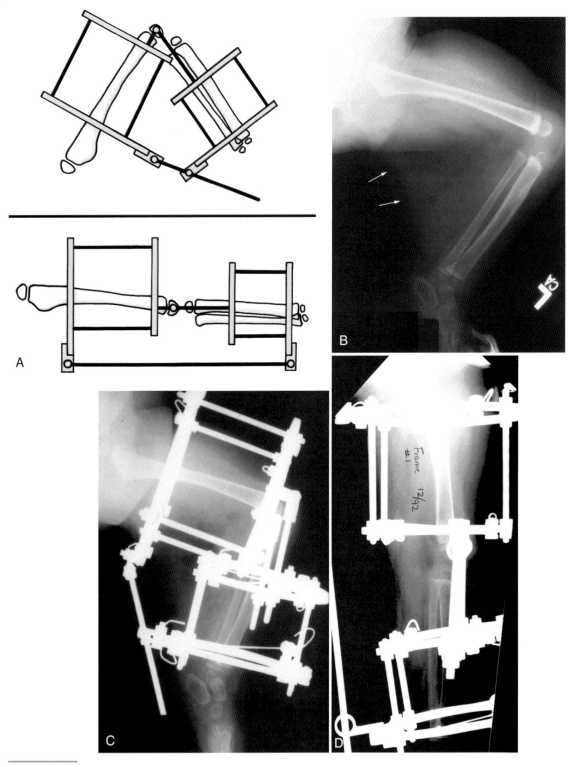

Figure 70–22. **A,** Diagram of a frame for correction of knee flexion contracture by the distraction hinge method. **B,** Radiograph of the left lower extremity (patient in Fig. 68-16) before frame application. The soft-tissue edge of the pterygium can be seen *(arrows)*. **C,** Radiograph of the initial position in the frame. **D,** Full extension achieved. Note the position of the knee hinge at the anterior edge of the distal end of the femur to accomplish joint distraction with extension.

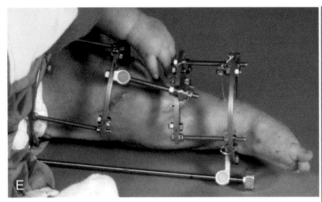

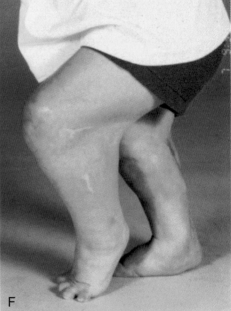

Figure 70–22, cont'd.   **E,** Clinical appearance with the knee extended. Failure to incorporate the foot allowed uncontrolled equinus and thereby contributed to recurrence. **F,** Recurrent deformity 1 year later. This extremity was treated a second time (see Fig. 70–19C), with a similar outcome.

than 45 degrees with a functional quadriceps, treatment to improve extension is indicated to avoid gait deterioration from quadriceps mechanical insufficiency. In young children, treatment may be important to achieve ambulation if the contracture is severe, and in patients with multiple syndromic deformities—arthrogryposis is the classic example—the decision to treat is difficult if the prognosis for functional ambulation is uncertain or poor.

Milder deformities are generally amenable to nonoperative management (bracing), soft-tissue release with casting (including extension-desubluxation hinges), or possibly stapling hemi-epiphyseodesis. In the more severe cases described in this chapter, extensive surgical approaches are indicated but unfortunately are fraught with recurrence as well as complications. Gradual correction by arthrodiastasis/extension (Ilizarov) methods, with or without soft-tissue release, is more effective and appears to be the treatment of choice for deformities greater than 60 degrees. Frame correction, however, is no panacea because the potential for complications is just as great as with acute correction and experience and attention to correction details are mandatory if there is to be a moderate chance of lasting success.

References

1. Alman BA, Krajbich JI, Hubbard S: Proximal femoral focal deficiency: Results of rotationplasty and Syme amputation. J Bone Joint Surg Am 77:1876, 1995.
2. Andrews M, Noyes FR, Barber-Westin SD: Anterior cruciate ligament allograft reconstruction in the skeletally immature athlete. Am J Sports Med 22:48, 1994.
3. Baker RH, Carroll NC, Dewar FP, et al: The semitendinosis tenodesis for recurrent dislocation of the patella. J Bone Joint Surg Br 54:103, 1972.
4. Bell MJ, Atkins RM, Sharrard WJW: Irreducible congenital dislocation of the knee: Aetiology and management. J Bone Joint Surg Br 69:403, 1987.
5. Bensahel H, Dal Monte A, Hjelmstedt A, et al: Congenital dislocation of the knee. J Pediatr Orthop 9:174, 1989.
6. Browne RS: The management of late diagnosed congenital dislocation and subluxation of the hip; with special reference to femoral shortening. J Bone Joint Surg Br 61:7, 1979.
7. Brunner R, Hefti F, Tgetgel JD: Arthrogrypotic joint contracture at the knee and the foot: Correction with a circular frame. J Pediatr Orthop B 6:192, 1997.
8. Charif P, Reichelderfer T: Genu recurvatum congenitum in the newborn: Its incidence, course, treatment, prognosis. Clin Pediatr (Phila) 4:587, 1965.
9. Conn H: A new method of operative reduction for congenital luxation of the patella. J Bone Joint Surg 7:370, 1925.
10. Curtis B, Fisher R: Congenital hyperextension with anterior subluxation of the knee; surgical treatment and long-term observations. J Bone Joint Surg Am 41:255, 1969.
11. Damsin J-P, Ghanem I: Treatment of severe flexion deformity of the knee in children and adolescents using the Ilizarov technique. J Bone Joint Surg Br 78:140, 1996.
12. Delbello DA, Watts HG: Distal femoral extension osteotomy in patients with arthrogryposis. J Pediatr Orthop 16:122, 1996.
13. Dugdale TW, Renshaw TS: Instability of the patellofemoral joint in Down syndrome. J Bone Joint Surg Am 68:405, 1986.
14. Eilert RE: Congenital dislocation of the patella. Clin Orthop 389:22, 2001.
15. Elchalal U, Ben Itzhak I, Ben-Meir G, et al: Antenatal diagnosis of congenital dislocation of the knee: A case report. Am J Perinatol 10:194, 1993.
16. Gao GX, Lee EH, Bose K: Surgical management of congenital and habitual dislocation of the patella. J Pediatr Orthop 10:255, 1990.
17. Ghanem I, Wattincourt L, Seringe R: Congenital dislocation of the patella. Part I: Pathologic anatomy; part II: Orthopedic management. J Pediatr Orthop 20:812, 2000.
18. Gillen JA, Walker JL, Burgess RC, Stevens DB: Use of Ilizarov external fixator to treat joint pterygia. J Pediatr Orthop 16:430, 1996.
19. Gillespie R, Torode IP: Classification and management of congenital abnormalities of the femur. J Bone Joint Surg Br 65:557, 1983.
20. Goldthwait JE: Slipping or recurrent dislocation of the patella. With the report of eleven cases. Boston Med Surg J 150:169, 1904.
21. Gordon JE, Schoenecker PL: Surgical treatment of congenital dislocation of the patella. J Pediatr Orthop 19:260, 1999.
22. Green JP, Waugh, W, Wood H: Congenital lateral dislocation of the patella. J Bone Joint Surg Br 50:285, 1968.
23. Guzzanti V, Falciglia F, Gigante A, et al: The effect of intra-articular ACL reconstruction on the growth plates of rabbits. J Bone Joint Surg Br 76:960, 1994.

24. Herold HZ, Shmueli G, Baruchin AM: Popliteal pterygium syndrome. Clin Orthop 209:194, 1986.

25. Herzenberg JE, Davis JR, Paley D, Bhave A: Mechanical distraction for treatment of severe flexion contractures. Clin Orthop 301:80, 1994.

26. Insall JA, Joseph DM, Aglietti P, et al: Bone-block iliotibial-band transfer for anterior cruciate insufficiency. J Bone Joint Surg Am 63:560, 1981.

27. Jacobsen K, Vopalecky F: Congenital dislocation of the knee. Acta Orthop Scand 56:1, 1985.

28. Johnson E, Audell R, Opeenheim WL: Congenital dislocation of the knee. J Pediatr Orthop 7:194, 1987.

29. Jones RDS, Fisher RL, Curtis BH: Congenital dislocation of the patella. Clin Orthop 19:177, 1976.

30. Judet R: Mobilisation of the stiff knee. J Bone Joint Surg Br 41:856, 1959.

31. Katz M, Grogono J, Soper K: The etiology and treatment of congenital dislocation of the knee. J Bone Joint Surg Br 49:112, 1967.

32. Ko J-K, Shih C-H, Wenger DR: Congenital dislocation of the knee. J Pediatr Orthop 19:252, 1999.

33. Kramer A, Stevens PM: Anterior femoral stapling. J Pediatr Orthop 21:804-807, 2001.

34. Langenskiold A, Ritsila V: Congenital dislocation of the patella and its operative treatment. J Pediatr Orthop 12:315, 1992.

35. Leveuf J, Pais C: Les dislocations congenitales du genou. Rev Chir Orthop 32:313, 1947.

36. Lo IK, Bell DM, Fowler PJ: Anterior cruciate ligament injuries in the skeletally immature patient. Instr Course Lect 47:35, 1998.

37. McCall RE, Lessenberry HB: Bilateral congenital dislocation of the patella. J Pediatr Orthop 7:100, 1987.

38. Mendez AA, Keret D, MacEwen GD: Treatment of patello-femoral instability in Down's syndrome. Clin Orthop 234:148, 1988.

39. Middleton D: The pathology of genu recurvatum. Br J Surg 22:696, 1935.

40. Miller RH 3rd : Knee injuries. In Canale ST (ed): Campbell's Operative Orthopaedics, 9th ed. St Louis, Mosby–Year Book, 1998, p 1218.

41. Mooney JF 3rd, Koman LA: Knee flexion contractures: Soft tissue correction with monolateral external fixation. J South Orthop Assoc 10:32, 2001.

42. Murray C, Fixsen JA: Management of knee deformity in classical arthrogryposis multiplex congenita (amyoplasia congenita). J Pediatr Orthop B 6:186, 1997.

43. Nakhostine M, Bollen SR, Cross MJ: Reconstruction of mid substance anterior cruciate rupture in adolescents with open physes. J Pediatr Orthop 15:286, 1995.

44. Niebauer JJ, King D: Congenital dislocation of the knee. J Bone Joint Surg Am 42:207, 1960.

45. Ooishi T, Sugioka Y, Matsumoto S, et al: Congenital dislocation of the knee: Its pathologic features and treatment. Clin Orthop 187: 287, 1993.

46. Oppenheim WL, Larson KR, McNabb MBB, et al: Popliteal pterygium syndrome: An orthopaedic perspective. J Pediatr Orthop 10:58, 1990.

47. Paletta GA Jr: Special considerations. Anterior cruciate ligament reconstruction in the skeletally immature. Orthop Clin North Am 34:65, 2003.

48. Parikh SN, Crawford AH, Do TT, et al: Popliteal pterygium syndrome: Implications for orthopaedic management. J Pediatr Orthop B 13:197, 2004.

49. Parker AW, Drez D Jr, Cooper J: Anterior cruciate ligament injuries in patients with open physes. Am J Sports Med 22:44, 1994.

50. Parsch K: Luxacion congenita de la rodilla. In de Pablos J (ed): La Rodilla Infantil. Majadahonda (Madrid), Ergon, 2003, pp 37-48.

51. Perry J, Antonelli D, Ford W: Analysis of knee joint forces during flexed knee stance. J Bone Joint Surg Am 57:961, 1975.

52. Saleh M, Gibson MF, Sharrard WJW: Femoral shortening in correction of congenital knee flexion deformity with popliteal webbing. J Pediatr Orthop 9:609, 1989.

53. Scott WN, Ferriter P, Marino M: Intra-articular transfer of the iliotibial tract. Two to seven-year follow-up results. J Bone Joint Surg Am 67:532, 1985.

54. Simonian PT, Staheli LT: Periarticular fractures after manipulation for knee contractures in children. J Pediatr Orthop 15:288, 1995.

55. Sodergard J, Ryoppy S: The knee in arthrogryposis multiplex congenita. J Pediatr Orthop 10:177, 1990.

56. Stadelmaier DM, Arnoczky SP, Dobbs J, et al: The effect of drilling and soft tissue grafting across open growth plates. A histologic study. Am J Sports Med 23:431, 1995.

57. Stanisavljevic S, Zemenick G, Miller D: Congenital, irreducible, permanent lateral dislocation of the patella. Clin Orthop 116:190, 1976.

58. Storen H: Congenital complete dislocation of patella causing serious disability in childhood: The operative treatment. Acta Orthop Scand 36:301, 1965.

59. Uhthoff HK, Ogata S: Early intrauterine presence of congenital dislocation of the knee. J Pediatr Orthop 14:254, 1994.

60. Windsor RE, Insall JN: Bone-block iliotibial band reconstruction for anterior cruciate insufficiency. Follow-up note and minimum five-year follow-up period. Clin Orthop 250:197, 1990.

CHAPTER 71

Meniscal Disorders

Mininder S. Kocher • Kevin Klingele

Meniscal injuries in pediatric athletes are being seen with increased frequency. Meniscal disorders include meniscal tears, discoid meniscus, and meniscal cysts. Unique considerations exist for the management of these conditions in children and adolescents. This chapter reviews the etiology, diagnosis, management, and prognosis of meniscal tears, discoid meniscus, and meniscal cysts in children.

MENISCUS

Historical Aspects

Understanding of the functional importance of the meniscus has evolved. In 1897, Bland-Sutton[9] characterized the menisci as "functionless remnants of intra-articular leg muscles." The sentiment was held onto through the 1970s, when menisci were routinely excised. In 1948, Fairbank[19] published the first long-term follow-up of patients after total meniscectomy.[19] His article warned that degenerative changes followed meniscectomy in a substantial proportion of patients. Reports since have established the deleterious consequences of total and even partial meniscectomy.[1,18,33,36,37,45,46,55,56,58,61] Nowhere are these consequences more important than in children and adolescents, in whom the long-term effects of meniscectomy are magnified by activity level and longevity.

Development

The menisci become clearly defined by 8 weeks of embryological development.[29] By week 14, they assume the normal mature anatomic relationships. At no point during their embryology are the menisci discoid in morphology.[29] The discoid meniscus represents an anatomic variant, not a vestigial remnant. Clark and Ogden[13] studied the developmental vasculature of the menisci. The blood supply arises from the periphery and supplies the entire meniscus. This vascular pattern persists through birth. During postpartum development, the vasculature begins to recede, and by the 9 months after birth, the central one-third is avascular. This decrease in vasculature continues until approximately age 10 years, when the menisci attain their adult vascular pattern. Injection dye studies by Arnoczky and Warren[6] have shown that only the peripheral 10% to 30% of the medial meniscus and 10% to 25% of the lateral meniscus receive vascular nourishment.

Anatomy

The medial meniscus is C shaped. The posterior horn is larger in anterior-posterior width than the anterior horn. The medial meniscus covers approximately 50% of the medial tibial plateau. The medial meniscus is attached firmly to the medial joint capsule through the meniscotibial or coronary ligaments. There is a discrete capsular thickening at its midportion, which constitutes the deep medial collateral ligament. The inferior surface is flat and the superior surface is concave so that the meniscus conforms to its respective tibial and femoral articulations. To maintain this conforming relationship, the medial meniscus translates 2.5 mm posteriorly on the tibia as the femoral condyle rolls backward during knee flexion.[22,23]

The lateral meniscus is more circular in shape and covers a larger portion, approximately 70%, of the lateral tibial plateau. The lateral meniscus is more loosely connected to the lateral joint capsule. There are no attachments in the area of the popliteal hiatus, and the fibular collateral ligament does not attach to the lateral meniscus. Accessory meniscofemoral ligaments exist in one-third of cases. These arise from the posterior meniscus. If this ligament inserts anterior to the posterior collateral ligament, it is called the *ligament of Humphrey,* and if it inserts posterior to the posterior collateral ligament, it is called the *ligament of Wrisberg.* Because of the lack of restraining forces, the lateral meniscus is able to translate 9 to 11 mm on the tibia with knee flexion. This ability may account for the lower incidence of lateral meniscal tears. Both menisci are attached anteriorly via the anterior transverse meniscal ligament.[22,23]

Meniscal blood supply arises from the superior and inferior and medial and lateral geniculate arteries. These vessels form a perimeniscal synovial plexus. There may be some contribution from the middle geniculate artery. King[30] published classic research in the 1930s indicating that the peripheral meniscus did communicate with the vascular supply and was capable of healing. It is believed that the inner two-thirds of the meniscus receives its nutrition through diffusion and mechanical pumping.

The menisci are composed primarily of type I collagen, 60% to 70% of its dry weight. Lesser amounts of types II, III, and VI collagen also are present. The collagen fibers are oriented primarily in a circumferential pattern, parallel with the long access of the meniscus.[22,23] There also are radial, oblique, and vertically oriented fibers. Proteoglycans and glycoproteins are present in smaller concentrations than in articular cartilage. The menisci also contain neural elements, including mechanoreceptors and type I and II sensory fibers. In a sensory mapping study, Dye and associates[17] showed that the probing of the peripheral meniscus led to pain, whereas stimulation of the central meniscus elicited little or no discomfort.

Function

It is now realized that the menisci have many functions. The menisci increase contact area and congruency of the femoral tibial articulation; this allows the menisci to participate in load sharing and reduces the contact stresses across the knee joint. It is estimated that the menisci transmit 50% to 70% of the load in extension and 85% of the load in 90 degrees of flexion.[2] Baratz and colleagues[7] showed that after total meniscectomy, contact area may decrease by 75% and contact stresses increase by 235%. They also documented the deleterious effects of partial meniscectomy, showing that the contact stresses increased in proportion to the amount of meniscus removed. Excision of small bucket-handle tears of the medial meniscus increased contact stress by 65%, and resecting 75% of the posterior horn increased contact stresses equivalent to that after total meniscectomy.[7] Repair of meniscal tears, by either arthroscopic or open techniques, reduced the contact stresses to normal. Multiple other studies have corroborated the mechanical importance of the meniscus.[22,23]

Meniscal tissue is about half as stiff as articular cartilage, allowing it to participate in shock absorption. Shock absorption capacity in the normal knee is 20% higher than in the meniscectomized knee.[35,57] The menisci also have a role in joint stability. In an anterior cruciate ligament (ACL)–deficient knee, the posterior horn of the medial meniscus plays a crucial passive stabilizing role. In an ACL-deficient knee, medial meniscectomy leads to a 58% increase in anterior translation at 90 degrees of flexion.[35,49] Given the presence of neural elements within their substance, it also is theorized that the menisci may have a role in proprioception.

MENISCAL TEARS

Epidemiology

The exact incidence of meniscal injuries in children and adolescents is unknown. Meniscal injuries in children younger than age 10 years are rare, unless associated with a discoid meniscus. The incidence of meniscal and other intra-articular disorders increases with age.[15] Younger children typically sustain physeal injuries and fractures, with a predominance of upper extremity injuries. With adolescence, increased size and speed and increased athletic demands result in higher energy injuries and an increase of intra-articular knee lesions.

Meniscal injury patterns differ in children. It is estimated that longitudinal tears constitute 50% to 90% of meniscal tears in children and adolescents.[33] Bucket-handle displaced tears are common (Fig. 71–1). Also in

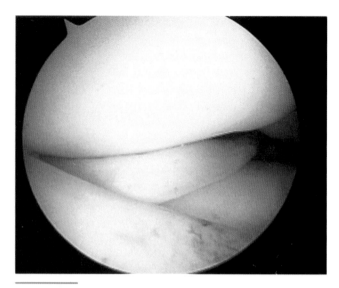

Figure 71–1. Bucket-handle displaced lateral meniscus tear in a 13-year-old female athlete.

these age groups, meniscal injuries commonly are associated with ACL injuries.[12,18,34,36] The incidence of medial meniscal tears is greater than lateral meniscal tears in the pediatric age group, especially in adolescents.[52] There seems to be a relatively increased incidence of lateral tears in the preadolescent age group, which may be due to the existence of lateral discoid menisci.[33]

Cannon and Vittori[12] estimated that repairable meniscal tears occur in 30% of all knees with acute ACL rupture and in 30% of patients younger than 20 years old. Approximately two-thirds of repairable meniscal tears are associated with ACL rupture, with most of these tears limited to the posterior horn.

Mechanism of Injury

Injury to the nondiscoid meniscus is virtually always traumatic in nature in children and adolescents. Multiple studies have shown that 80% to 90% of meniscal injuries in children and adolescents are sustained during sporting activities.[10,22,23,36,52] These numbers may be lower in the preadolescent age group. Meniscal tears most commonly occur with twisting motions, associated frequently with football, soccer, and basketball. Pain is the most common chief complaint. Other symptoms include effusion, snapping, giving way, and intermittent catching and locking.

Differential Diagnosis

The differential diagnosis of acute meniscal tear in a pediatric patient includes discoid meniscus, popliteal tendinitis, plica syndrome, osteochondritis dissecans, loose body, patellofemoral dysfunction, arthritis, tibial spine avulsion, and chondral or osteochondral injury.[33]

Physical Examination

The physical examination is the primary diagnostic tool for intra-articular and meniscal injuries. The most common findings, similar to adults, are joint line tenderness and effusion.[5,37] Because of the diversity of pathology and the difficulty of examination of children, diagnostic accuracy of physical examination for meniscus tear is only 29% to 59%.[32,33] In children, anteromedial or anterolateral joint line pain also may be due to patellofemoral pain, extensor mechanism dysfunction, iliotibial band friction syndrome, osteochondritis dissecans, or other lesions. The sensitivity of the McMurray maneuvers and Apley test has been estimated to be 58%, with even lower specificity.[33] Two studies by examiners with pediatric sports medicine experience have shown the diagnostic accuracy of physical examination to be 86.3% and 93.5% overall.[32,51] When medial meniscus tears were looked at alone, the sensitivity and specificity of physical examination were 62.1% and 80.7%.[32] The sensitivity and specificity for lateral meniscal tears were 50% and 89.2%.[32]

Imaging

Plain films can rule out other pathological conditions that can mimic meniscal tears, such as osteochondritis dissecans and loose bodies. MRI is considered the most useful adjunctive study in the diagnosis of intra-articular knee disorders. Sensitivity and specificity of 83% and 95% have been shown in skeletally immature patients.[32,51] Kocher and coworkers[32] showed that for medial meniscal tears, the sensitivity and specificity for MRI diagnosis were 79% and 92%. For lateral meniscal tears, the sensitivity and specificity were 67% and 83%.[32] Only the specificity for medial meniscal tears was significantly higher with MRI compared with physical examination.[32] The sensitivity and specificity of MRI decrease in younger children compared with older adolescents.[32,51] In studies that compared the diagnostic accuracy of physical examination versus MRI, physical examination rates were equivalent or superior to MRI.[32,51] These authors recommended judicious use of MRI in evaluating intra-articular knee disorders.

Normal signal changes exist in the posterior horn of the medial and lateral meniscus in children and adolescents.[31,32,51,63] These signal changes do not extend to the superior or inferior articular surfaces of the meniscus and likely represent vascular developmental changes.[33] When interpreting MRI of the developing knee, care must be taken to identify a meniscal tear only when linear signal changes extend to the articular surface.

Treatment

Some small, nondisplaced meniscal tears in the outer vascular region of the meniscus may heal nonoperatively or may become asymptomatic.[22,23,34] Nonoperative treatment usually consists of rehabilitation of the injured knee with the avoidance of pivoting and sports for 12 weeks.

Most meniscal tears in pediatric patients are larger and require surgical treatment.[22,23,33] Arthroscopic management is standard, with either partial meniscectomy (Fig. 71–2) using motorized shavers and baskets or meniscal repairs using outside-in, all-inside (Fig. 71–3), or inside-out techniques (Fig. 71–4).[14,22,23] In children and adolescents, meniscal repair should be attempted, in our opinion, instead of partial meniscectomy for middle-third and outer-third meniscal tears because of greater healing potential in this age group, the long life span of these patients, the poor results of total and near-total meniscectomy, and the lack of longer term results of partial meniscectomy. Inside-out techniques can be useful for anterior horn medial or lateral meniscal tears (see Fig. 71–4). For body and posterior horn tears, the traditional technique of meniscal repair has been inside-out repair with vertical or horizontal sutures. Zone-specific cannulas are helpful to direct the flexible suture needles to the appropriate position to avoid neurovascular structures. In addition, we routinely make an incision posteromedially

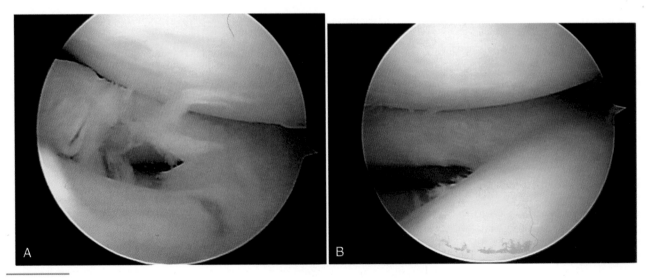

Figure 71–2. **A** and **B,** Partial meniscectomy of a complex medial meniscus tear in a 14-year-old male athlete.

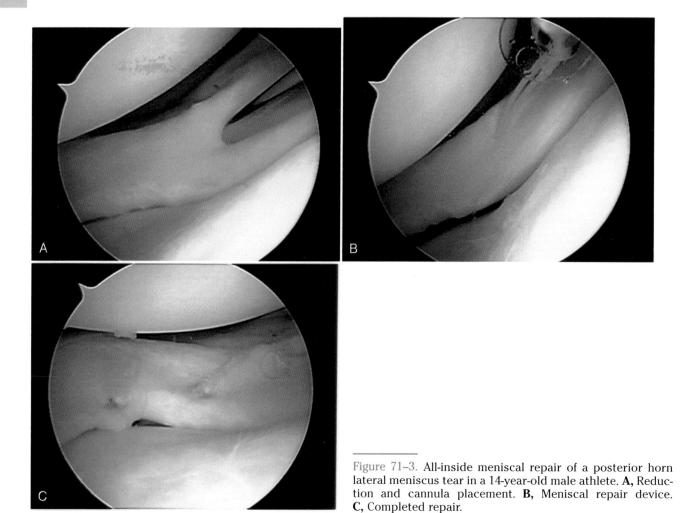

Figure 71–3. All-inside meniscal repair of a posterior horn lateral meniscus tear in a 14-year-old male athlete. **A,** Reduction and cannula placement. **B,** Meniscal repair device. **C,** Completed repair.

or posterolaterally to retrieve the suture needles and tie the sutures onto the joint capsule, protecting the saphenous nerve and vein medially and the peroneal nerve laterally. Newer, all-inside devices have eased the technique of meniscal repair (see Fig. 71–3). Reports of articular cartilage damage from the heads of bioabsorbable arrows and darts exist, however.[22,23]

Many of the available devices extend too far through the capsule in the small pediatric knee, with potential for neurovascular injury. We prefer newer, all-inside suture devices with a low profile in the joint. We tend to use these for posterior horn tears in adolescent knees. For smaller tears without substantial displacement, we use these alone. For larger tears with displacement, such as displaced bucket-handle tears, we use these devices in a hybrid manner with inside-out sutures (Fig. 71–5). Regardless of the instrumentation used for repair, certain surgical principles are important to obtain meniscal healing, including preparation of the repair site using abrasion or trephination, anatomic reduction of the meniscal tear, adequate strength and durability of repair, and protected mobilization.

The results of total or near-total meniscectomy in pediatric patients have been poor with early degenerative changes.[1,18,34,36,37,45,46,55,56,58,61] There have been relatively few studies on the long-term results of meniscal repair in children and adolescents. Mintzer and colleagues[38] reported on 29 patients younger than age 18 (25 had closed physes and 17 underwent concomitant ACL reconstruction). They reported 100% clinical healing at an average follow-up of 5 years. Noyes and Barber-Westin[41,48] looked at meniscal tears extending into the avascular zone in patients younger than 20 years old. Skeletal maturity had been reached in 88%. Their success rate in this group was 75%. This study showed a higher rate of healing with concomitant ACL reconstruction. Eggli[18] found an overall healing rate for repair of isolated meniscal tears of 88% in patients younger than age 30 compared with 67% in patients older than 30. Johnson and coworkers[26] showed a 76% healing rate at an average follow-up of greater than 10 years in a population that averaged 20 years old at the time of surgery. Factors that have been shown to correlate with increased healing of meniscal repairs include younger age, decreased rim width (peripheral tears), repairs of the lateral meniscus, concomitant ACL reconstruction, time from injury to surgery of less than 8 weeks, and tear length of less than 2.5 cm.[11,12,18,22,23,26,54]

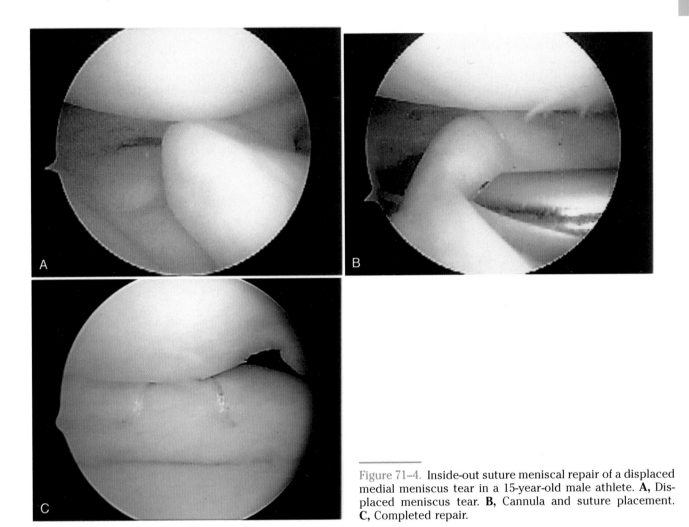

Figure 71–4. Inside-out suture meniscal repair of a displaced medial meniscus tear in a 15-year-old male athlete. **A,** Displaced meniscus tear. **B,** Cannula and suture placement. **C,** Completed repair.

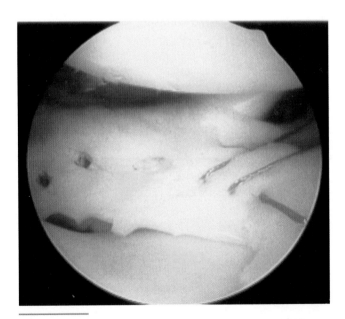

Figure 71–5. Hybrid meniscal repair using inside-out sutures and all-inside devices for a displaced lateral meniscus tear in an 11-year-old female athlete.

Rehabilitation

No unified consensus exists on rehabilitation after meniscal repair. Because most meniscal repairs are done in conjunction with ACL reconstruction, the rehabilitation plan must take this into account. For isolated meniscal repair, most surgeons prefer to restrict weightbearing and knee range of motion postoperatively. The goal is to decrease joint compressive and shearing forces that potentially could stress or disrupt the meniscal repair. This is followed by a protocol of progressive mobilization, range-of-motion exercises, strengthening exercises, sport-specific rehabilitation, and return to sports. Several studies have shown no deleterious effects of immediate limited motion and early protected weightbearing on healing with combined ACL reconstruction and meniscal repair.[11,22,23]

Our postoperative protocol for isolated meniscal repair involves touch-down weightbearing for 6 weeks postoperatively. Range of motion is restricted from 0 to 30 degrees for the first 2 weeks followed by 0 to 90 degrees for the next 6 weeks. Progressive mobilization, strengthening, and sport-specific therapy are performed under the direction of a physical therapy protocol. Return to sports is allowed at 3 months postoperatively, if there is full range of motion, adequate strength, no symptoms (pain, swelling, locking), and resolution of physical examination findings (joint line tenderness, McMurray maneuvers, terminal range joint line pain). Follow-up MRI is performed only in patients with persistent symptoms or physical examination findings. For meniscal repair in association with ACL reconstruction, return to sports is dictated by the ACL reconstruction, usually at 6 months postoperatively.

DISCOID MENISCUS

Since its first description in a cadaveric specimen by Young in 1889,[62] discoid lateral meniscus has become a well-documented meniscal abnormality seen in children. Although often synonymous with so-called snapping knee syndrome, discoid lateral menisci may manifest in a variety of ways. The true incidence of discoid lateral meniscus is unknown. Many children may remain asymptomatic, and few present with a true snapping knee. Nonetheless, the incidence is thought to be 3% to 5% in the general population.[16,27,28,33] The incidence is slightly higher in Asian populations.[16,27,28,33] Discoid morphology almost exclusively occurs within the lateral meniscus, but medial discoid menisci also have been reported.[16,27,28,33] In addition, the incidence of bilateral abnormality has been reported to be 20%.[3,8,44,50]

Etiology

Debate exists over the exact cause of a discoid lateral meniscus. Smillie[50] hypothesized that discoid morphology represented an arrest in embryological development, causing failure of central resorption within the meniscus. This theory has been disputed, however. During no stage of meniscal development is the meniscus found to be discoid in shape.[13,29] Further theories claim that increased mobility and subsequent repetitive microtrauma to the meniscus lead to its morphology and degenerative changes within its substance.[39] Early studies show that discoid menisci are more prone to mechanical stresses because of a thicker, less vascular structure, which often lacks periph-

eral attachments.[13] Other authors state that hypermobility does not explain the formation of the commonly seen, stable discoid meniscus with intact peripheral attachments.[60] Most authors now consider discoid meniscus as an anatomic variant, with a propensity for tearing owing to mechanical stresses and hypermobility as a result of meniscocapsular separation secondary to increased shear stress.[33,47,60] Reports of familial transmission and occurrence among identical twins support the congenital theory.[27]

Classification

The most widely documented classification system is that of Watanabe and associates,[59] who described three types of discoid lateral menisci, based on arthroscopic appearance (Fig. 71–6). Discoid menisci with intact peripheral attachments are either complete (type I), covering the entire tibial plateau, or incomplete (type II). Type III discoid lateral menisci, the so-called Wrisberg-ligament type, are complete or incomplete in morphology and lack posterior capsular attachments with the exception of the posterior meniscofemoral ligament (ligament of Wrisberg). This type of discoid meniscus is thought to produce the classic snapping knee syndrome.[16]

More recent reports have described variability not only in the size and shape of lateral menisci, but also in the peripheral rim stability and attachment.[27,28,40,60] As a result, newer classification systems have been proposed. Jordan and others[27,28] suggested a system based on peripheral stability, type of discoid meniscus (complete or incomplete), presence of associated meniscal tear, and presence or lack of clinical symptoms (Table 71–1).

The true incidence of the Wrisberg-type, or unstable, discoid meniscus is difficult to assess. Previous series have documented between 0 to 33% of symptomatic discoid menisci as unstable.[24,25,29,44,56] With variability in the morphology and the subjective nature of assessing hypermobility, reporting stability is problematic. In a review of 128 of our cases of discoid menisci, 28% were found to have peripheral rim instability, nearly 47% of which were detached along the anterior third peripheral attachment. We advocate a classification system based on type of discoid (complete or incomplete) and the presence of

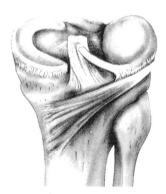
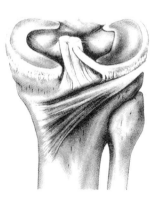
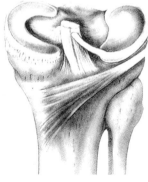

Type I   Type II   Type III

Figure 71–6. Watanabe classification of discoid lateral meniscus. Type I is complete variant, type II is partial variant, and type III is Wrisberg variant.

Table 71–1. Jordan Classification of Discoid Lateral Meniscus

CLASSIFICATION	CORRELATION	TEAR	SYMPTOMS
Stable	Complete/ incomplete	Yes/no	Yes/no
Unstable with discoid shape	Wrisberg type	Yes/no	Yes/no
Unstable with normal shape	Wrisberg variant	Yes/no	Yes/no

peripheral rim instability (stable or unstable) and associated meniscal tear.

Diagnosis

The clinical presentation of a discoid lateral meniscus varies. Symptoms often are related to the type of discoid present, peripheral stability of the meniscus, and the presence or absence of an associated meniscal tear.[4,16,20,27,40,47,60] Stable discoid menisci without associated tears often remain asymptomatic, identified only as incidental findings during MRI or arthroscopy. Unstable discoid menisci more commonly occur in younger children and often produce the so-called snapping knee syndrome. In such instances, a painless and palpable, audible or visible snap is produced with knee range of motion, especially near terminal extension. This snap is thought to be secondary to reduction of the subluxed, unstable meniscus as the joint space widens with knee extension. This is an uncommon presentation, however, because most discoid menisci are peripherally stable.

In children with stable discoid lateral menisci, symptoms often present when an associated tear is present. In contrast to acute meniscal tears, such symptoms may present insidiously without previous trauma. Signs and symptoms of a meniscal tear may exist, including pain, swelling, catching, locking, and limited motion. On physical examination, there may be joint line tenderness, popping, limited motion, effusion, terminal motion pain, and positive provocative tests (McMurray maneuvers, Apley test). Degenerative horizontal cleavage tears are the most common type of tear seen, reported in the largest series to occur in 58% to 98% of symptomatic discoid menisci.[3,8,44]

Imaging

Radiographic evaluation is often helpful to aid in diagnosis. Standard plain radiographs of both knees should be obtained, including anteroposterior, lateral, Merchant, and tunnel views. Characteristic findings on plain radiographs are often subtle, but include a widened lateral joint line, calcification of the lateral meniscus, squaring of the lateral condyle with concomitant cupping of the lateral tibial plateau, mild hypoplasia of the tibial spine, and an elevated fibular head.

On MRI, discoid meniscus is seen as three or more successive sagittal slices with continuity between the anterior and posterior meniscal horns or a transverse meniscal diameter of greater than 15 mm or greater than 20% of the tibial width on transverse images. In addition, MRI can detect the presence of an associated meniscal tear. MRI has a high positive predictive value for discoid meniscus.[32] That is, when MRI is positive, discoid meniscus is almost always present. MRI has low sensitivity for discoid meniscus, however.[32] That is, discoid meniscus still may be present despite negative MRI. When there is strong clinical suspicion for discoid meniscus despite negative MRI, the diagnosis still should be considered, and diagnostic arthroscopy may be necessary. Complete discoid menisci are detected more easily than partial discoid menisci. Normal morphology with detachment (Wrisberg type) can be difficult to detect on MRI. Techniques to improve the detection of discoid meniscus include newer meniscal sequences, finer cuts, and increased MRI and pediatric imaging experience.

Treatment

Several treatment options exist if the diagnosis of a discoid lateral meniscus is confirmed. For asymptomatic discoid lateral menisci, even if found incidentally on arthroscopy, conservative treatment is indicated. For stable, complete or incomplete discoid menisci, partial meniscectomy, "saucerization," is the treatment of choice. If meniscal instability with detachment also exists, meniscal repair also can be performed. Traditionally, complete meniscectomy via open or arthroscopic means was suggested for such lesions. The long-term results of complete meniscectomy and near-total meniscectomy in children are poor, however, with early degenerative changes.[1,18,34,36,37,45,46,55,56,58,61] Although there may be a rare instance where salvage of a discoid meniscus may seem unobtainable, better arthroscopic technology and techniques have made meniscal preservation the ideal treatment through saucerization and repair.

Arthroscopic saucerization should débride the discoid meniscus to a peripheral rim of 6 to 8 mm (Figs. 71–7 and 71–8).[21,24,25,34,42,43,53] Often an indentation on the lateral femoral condyle guides the depth of resection needed. If a meniscal tear is present, incorporation of its débridement into saucerization is most commonly performed. Most tears are of the horizontal cleavage variety, seen primarily in the posterior central area. Such tears can be débrided with adequate saucerization. If the tear extends into the peripheral vascular zone, repair should be attempted. Arthroscopic saucerization can be challenging to an inexperienced surgeon because visualization and performance within the lateral joint space can be limited by the thickened meniscus and the small size of the knee in pediatric patients. Saucerization is best begun with the knee in flexion by the aid of a straight biter, or scissor punch. Smaller baskets are available and are more appropriate for pediatric knees. A meniscal or cartilage knife can aid in contouring the abnormal meniscus. The knee can be placed in the figure-four position for further work. A

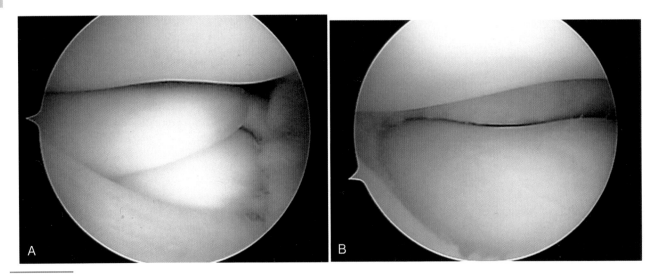

Figure 71–7. Saucerization of a partial discoid lateral meniscus. **A,** Presaucerization. **B,** Postsaucerization.

combination of small arthroscopic shavers and biters further facilitates saucerization. With horizontal cleavage tears, often the smaller of the present meniscal flaps is débrided, leaving an intact peripheral rim. Resection to widths greater than 8 mm is thought to increase the risk of recurrent tear.

A careful, methodical assessment of peripheral rim stability and attachment must be carried out after saucerization. The frequency of peripheral rim instability mandates a systematic probing of the remnant meniscus at all peripheral attachments. In contrast to the posteriorly unstable Wrisberg type of discoid meniscus, anterior peripheral detachment also can be seen. If peripheral instability is identified, meniscal repair is indicated. We prefer to perform meniscal repair using numerous inside-out sutures, using zone-specific cannulas and an open posterolateral incision to retrieve and tie the sutures, protecting the peroneal nerve. All-inside devices may be inappropriate for discoid lateral meniscus repair, given the extreme meniscal instability and the size of the implants.

Postoperatively, protected motion and weightbearing followed by progressive mobilization and rehabilitation is necessary. Younger children may be unable to ambulate effectively with crutches or comply with motion and weightbearing restrictions.

The results of arthroscopic saucerization with or without repair have not been established. Rosenberg and colleagues[47] presented a case report of arthroscopic attachment of a free posterior edge in a normal-shaped, Wrisberg-type lateral meniscus with good results at 1-year follow-up. Woods and Whelan[60] described four patients with unstable, discoid lateral menisci and lack of posterior attachment. All patients underwent repair; three

of four had good results at 37.5 months of follow-up. Similarly, Neuschwander and coworkers[40] identified six patients with lateral meniscal variants who underwent arthroscopic repair of posterior detachment, and four had an excellent result.

MENISCAL CYSTS

Popliteal cysts, or Baker's cysts, can occur in children. They usually present as a mass in the posteromedial aspect of the knee at the level of the popliteal crease. Usually, they are a painless, asymptomatic mass seen in children 4 to 8 years old.[33] Parents frequently are concerned about a tumor. Large cysts can cause pain in the back of the knee and a flexion contracture.

On physical examination, the cyst is more prominent with knee extension. In contrast to solid tumors, the cyst transilluminates. Radiographs usually are normal or show soft-tissue swelling. The diagnosis can be confirmed by ultrasound. MRI delineates the cyst and can identify any internal derangement.

The typical popliteal cyst arises from a plane between the medial head of gastrocnemius and semimembranosus. In contrast to popliteal cysts in adults, pediatric cases rarely are associated with intra-articular pathology.[32] The natural history of popliteal cysts is spontaneous resolution over 12 to 24 months in most pediatric popliteal cysts.[33] Treatment consists of reassurance and follow-up clinical examination. Surgical excision is reserved for large cysts that remain symptomatic. Cyst recurrence rates are relatively high, approximately 30% to 40%.[33]

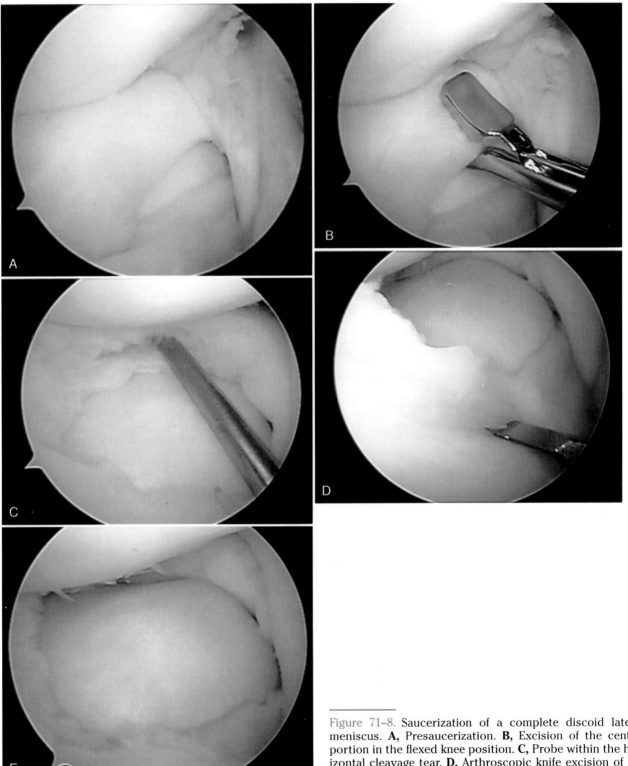

Figure 71–8. Saucerization of a complete discoid lateral meniscus. **A,** Presaucerization. **B,** Excision of the central portion in the flexed knee position. **C,** Probe within the horizontal cleavage tear. **D,** Arthroscopic knife excision of the excess anterior horn. **E,** Postsaucerization.

References

1. Aglietti P, Bertini FA, Buzzi R, et al: Arthroscopic meniscectomy for discoid lateral meniscus in children and adolescence: A ten year followup. Am J Knee Surg 12:83-87, 1999.
2. Ahmed AM, Burke DL: In-vitro measurement of static pressure distribution in synovial joints: Part I.Tibial surface of the knee. J Biomech Eng 105:216-225, 1983.
3. Aichroth PM, Patel DV, Marx CI: Congenital discoid lateral meniscus in children: A followup study and evaluation of management. J Bone Joint Surg Br 73:932-939, 1991.
4. Albertsson M, Gillquist S: Discoid lateral meniscus: A report of 29 cases. Arthroscopy 4:211-214, 1998.
5. Andrish JT: Meniscal injuries in children and adolescents: Diagnosis and management. J Am Acad Orthop Surg 4:231-237, 1996.
6. Arnoczky SP, Warren RF: Microvasculature of the human meniscus. Am J Sports Med 2:90-95, 1982.
7. Baratz ME, Fu FH, Mentago R: Meniscal tears: The effect of meniscectomy and of repair on intraarticular contact areas and stress in the human knee. Am J Sports Med 14:270-274, 1986.
8. Bellier G, Dupont JY, Larrain M, et al: Lateral discoid meniscus in children. Arthroscopy 5:52-56, 1989.
9. Bland-Sutton J (ed): Ligaments: Their Nature and Morphology, 2nd ed. London, JK Lewis, 1897.
10. Busch MT: Meniscal injuries in children and adolescents. Clin Sports Med 9:661-680, 1990.
11. Busek MS, Noyes FR: Arthroscopic evaluation of meniscal repairs after anterior cruciate ligament reconstruction and immediate motion. Am J Sports Med 19:489-494, 1991.
12. Cannon WD, Vittori JM: The incidence of healing in arthroscopic meniscal repairs in the anterior cruciate ligament-reconstructed knee versus stable knees. Am J Sports Med 20:176-181, 1992.
13. Clark CR, Ogden JA: Development of the menisci of the human knee joint: Morphological changes and their potential role in childhood meniscal injury. J Bone Joint Surg Am 65:538-547, 1983.
14. DeHaven KE, Arnoczky SP: Meniscus repair: Basic science, indications for repair, and open repair. Instr Course Lect 43:65-74, 1994.
15. DeHaven KE, Linter DM: Athletic injuries: Comparison by age, sport, gender. Am J Sports Med 14:218-224, 1986.
16. Dickhaut SC, DeLee JC: The discoid lateral meniscus syndrome. J Bone Joint Surg Am 64:1068-1073, 1982.
17. Dye SF, Vaupel GL, Dye CC: Conscious neurosensory mapping of the internal structures of the human knee without intraarticular anesthesia. Am J Sports Med 26:773-777, 1998.
18. Eggli S: Long-term results of arthroscopic meniscal repair: An analysis of isolated tears. Am J Sports Med 23:715-720, 1995.
19. Fairbank TJ: Knee joint changes after meniscectomy. J Bone Joint Surg Br 30:664-670, 1948.
20. Fleissner PR, Eilert RF: Discoid lateral meniscus. Am J Knee Surg 12:125-131, 1999.
21. Fujikawa K, Iseki F, Mikura Y: Partial resection of the discoid meniscus in the child's knee. J Bone Joint Surg Br 63:391-395, 1981.
22. Greis PE, Bardana DD, Holstrom MC, Burks RT: Meniscal injury: Basic science and evaluation. J Am Acad Orthop Surg 10:168-176, 2002.
23. Greis PE, Holstrom MC, Bardana DD, Burks RT: Meniscal injury: II. Management. J Am Acad Orthop Surg 10:177-187, 2002.
24. Hayashi LK, Yamaga H, Ida K, et al: Arthroscopic meniscectomy for discoid lateral meniscus in children. J Bone Joint Surg Am 70:1495-1500, 1988.
25. Ikeuchi H: Arthroscopic treatment of lateral discoid meniscus: Technique and long term results. Clin Orthop 167:19-28, 1982.
26. Johnson MJ, Lucas GL, Dusek JK, Henning CE: Isolated arthroscopic meniscal repair: A long term outcome study (more than 10 years). Am J Sports Med 27:44-49, 1999.
27. Jordan M: Lateral meniscal variants: Evaluation and treatment. J Am Acad Orthop Surg 4:191-200, 1996.
28. Jordan M, Duncan J, Bertrand S: Discoid lateral meniscus: A review. South Orthop J 2:239-253, 1993.
29. Kaplan EB: Discoid lateral meniscus of the knee joint. Bull Hosp Joint Dis 16:111-124, 1955.
30. King D: The healing of semilunar cartilage. J Bone Joint Surg 18:333-342, 1936.
31. King SL, Carty HML, Brady O: Magnetic resonance imaging of knee injuries in children. Pediatr Radiol 26:287-290, 1996.
32. Kocher MS, DiCanzio J, Zurakowski D, Micheli LJ: Diagnostic performance of clinical examination and selective magnetic resonance imaging in the evaluation of intraarticular knee disorders in children and adolescents. Am J Sports Med 29:292-296, 2001.
33. Kocher MS, Micheli LJ: The pediatric knee: Evaluation and treatment. In Insall JN, Scott WN (eds): Surgery of the Knee, 3rd ed. New York, Churchill-Livingstone, 2001, pp 1356-1397.
34. Kocher MS, Micheli LJ, Gerbino PG, Hresko MT: Tibial eminence fractures in children: Prevalence of meniscal entrapment. Am J Sports Med 31:404-407, 2003.
35. Levy IM, Torzilli PA, Warren RF: The effect of medial meniscectomy on anterior-posterior motion of the knee. J Bone Joint Surg Am 64:883-888, 1982.
36. Manzione M, Pizzutillo PD, Peoples AB, Schweizer PA: Meniscectomy in children: A long-term follow-up study. Am J Sports Med 11:111-115, 1983.
37. Medlar RC, Manidberg JJ, Lyne ED: Meniscectomies in children—report of long term results. Am J Sports Med 8:87-92, 1980.
38. Mintzer CM, Richmond JC, Taylor J: Meniscal repair in the young athlete. Am J Sports Med 26:630-633, 1998.
39. Nathan PA, Cole SC: Discoid meniscus: A clinical and pathological study. Clin Orthop 64:107-113, 1969.
40. Neuschwander DC, Drez D, Finney TP: Lateral meniscal variant with absence of posterior coronary ligament. J Bone Joint Surg Am 74:1186-1190, 1992.
41. Noyes FR, Barber-Westin SD: Arthroscopic repair of meniscal tears extending into the avascular zone in patients younger than twenty years of age. Am J Sports Med 30:589-600, 2002.
42. Ogata K: Arthroscopic technique: Two piece excision of discoid meniscus. Arthroscopy 13:666-670, 1997.
43. Patel D, Dimakopoulos P, Penoncourt P: Bucket handle tear of a discoid meniscus: Arthroscopic diagnosis and partial excision. Orthopaedics 9:607-608, 1986.
44. Pellacci F, Montanari G, Prosperi P, et al: Lateral discoid meniscus: Treatment and results. Arthroscopy 8:526-530, 1992.
45. Raber DA, Friederich NF, Buzzi R, et al: Discoid lateral meniscus in children: Long term followup after total meniscectomy. J Bone Joint Surg Am 8:1579-1586, 1998.
46. Rangger C, Klesti T, Gloetzer W, et al: Osteoarthritis after arthroscopic partial meniscectomy. Am J Sports Med 23:230-244, 1995.
47. Rosenberg TD, Paulos LE, Parker RD, et al: Discoid lateral meniscus: Case report of arthroscopic attachment of a symptomatic Wrisberg-ligament type. Arthroscopy 3:277-282, 1987.
48. Rubman MH, Noyes FR, Barber-Westin SD: Arthroscopic repair of meniscal tears that extend into the avascular zone: A review of 198 single and complex tears. Am J Sports Med 26:87-95, 1998.
49. Shoemaker SC, Markolf KL: The role of the meniscus in the anterior-posterior stability of the loaded cruciate deficient knee: Effect of partial versus total excision. J Bone Joint Surg Am 68:71-79, 1988.
50. Smillie I: The congenital discoid meniscus. J Bone Joint Surg Br 30:671-682, 1948.
51. Stanitski CL: Correlation of arthroscopic and clinical examinations with magnetic resonance imaging findings of injured knees in children and adolescents. Am J Sports Med 26:2-6, 1998.
52. Stanitski CL, Harvell JC, Fu F: Observations on acute knee hemarthrosis in children and adolescents. J Pediatr Orthop 13:506-510, 1993.
53. Stilli S, DiGennaro GL, Marchiodi L, et al: Arthroscopic surgery of the discoid meniscus during childhood. Chir Degli Org Mov 82:335-339, 1997.
54. Tenuta JJ, Arciero RA: Arthroscopic evaluation of meniscal repairs: Factors that affect healing. Am J Sports Med 22:797-802, 1994.
55. Vahvanen V, Aolto K: Meniscectomy in children. Acta Orthop Scand 50:791-795, 1979.
56. Vandermeer R, Cunningham F: Arthroscopic treatment of the discoid lateral meniscus: Results of long term followup. Arthroscopy 5:101-109, 1989.
57. Voloshin AS, Wosk J: Shock absorption of the meniscectomized and painful knees: A comparative in vivo study. J Biomed Eng 5:157-161, 1983.

58. Washington ER, Root L, Lierner U, et al: Discoid lateral meniscus in children—long term followup after excision. J Bone Joint Surg Am 77:1357-1361, 1995.
59. Watanabe M, Takada S, Ikeuchi H: Atlas of Arthroscopy. Tokyo, Igaku-Shoin, 1969.
60. Woods GW, Whelan JM: Discoid meniscus. Clin Sports Med 9:695-706, 1990.
61. Wroble RR, Henderson RC, Campion ER, et al: Meniscectomy in children and adolescents: A long term follow-up study. Clin Orthop 279:180-189, 1992.
62. Young RB: The external semilunar cartilage as a complete disc. In Cleland J, Mackey JY, Young RB (eds): Memoirs and Memoranda in Anatomy. London, Williams & Norgate, 1889, p 179.
63. Zobel MS, Borrello JA, Siegel MJ, Stewart NR: Pediatric knee MR imaging: Pattern of injury in the immature skeleton. Radiology 190:397-401, 1994.

CHAPTER 72

Osteochondritis Dissecans

Theodore J. Ganley • John M. Flynn

Osteochondritis dissecans (OCD) is an acquired condition affecting subchondral bone that manifests as a pathologic spectrum. Initially, softening of the overlying articular cartilage is noted with an intact articular surface (Fig. 72–1); this can progress to early articular cartilage separation, partial detachment of an articular lesion, and eventually osteochondral separation with loose bodies.[3,11,15,27,32,38,53,66] OCD is a relatively common cause of knee pain and dysfunction in children and adolescents. The etiology of OCD is unknown; however, repetitive microtrauma is often implicated.[11,15,27,53] OCD of the knee is subcategorized into a juvenile form and an adult form, depending on the status of the distal femoral physis, and classified based on anatomic location, surgical appearance, scintigraphic findings, and age.[11,12,15,27,30,53] Juvenile OCD has a much better prognosis than adult OCD, with greater than 50% of cases showing healing within 6 to 18 months from nonoperative treatment.[13,28,30,60,64] Adult OCD frequently requires operative intervention for healing.[4,13] Adult OCD and juvenile OCD lesions that do not heal have the potential for later sequelae, including osteoarthritis.[43,63]

HISTORY AND ETIOLOGY

Several factors have been implicated in the etiology of OCD, including inflammation, genetics, ischemia, accessory centers of ossification, and repetitive trauma. In 1887, König[40] suggested an inflammatory etiology using the name "osteochondritis dissecans." Further study did not support inflammation as a primary cause of OCD. Ribbing ascribed OCD to an ossification abnormality of the distal femoral epiphysis in 1955.[47] Although abnormalities in ossification do not account for most cases of OCD, some incidentally found lateral femoral condyle lesions in younger children that resolve spontaneously may represent an ossification variant. Based on their anatomic and histological findings, Green and Banks[28] proposed that ischemia was implicated in OCD, although further studies have failed to find avascular necrosis of the OCD fragment or a relative ischemic watershed of the lateral aspect of the medial femoral condyle.[14,36,57,58] Some investigators have suggested a genetic predisposition to OCD. Petrie[55] found OCD in only 1 of 86 first-degree relatives, although Mubarak and Carroll[48] reported 12 instances of family members with OCD over the course of four generations. It is widely believed that the common form of OCD is not familial. Endocrinopathies, ligamentous laxity, malalignment, apophysitis, epiphyseal dysplasia, and other osteo-chondropathies have not been described in association with OCD.

In 1933, Fairbanks[21] suggested that OCD might be due to a "violent rotation inwards of the tibia, driving the tibial spine against the inner condyle." Although anterior tibial spine impingement may not be the etiology of lesions in the most common location of the posterolateral aspect of the medial femoral condyle, the frequent occurrence of OCD in patients who are involved in sports with repetitive impact supports a repetitive trauma etiology.[22] OCD may begin after repetitive trauma causes a stress reaction, which may progress further to a stress fracture of the underlying subchondral bone. Without a reduction in repetitive loading, the ability of the subchondral bone to heal is exceeded, necrosis of the fragment occurs, and eventually fragment dissection and separation develop.

OCD lesions may resemble acute osteochondral fractures, chondral injuries, and osteonecrosis. The estimated incidence of OCD ranges from 15 to 29 cases per 100,000.[31,42] The mean age of OCD seems to be decreasing, and more girls seem to be affected.[11] The widespread use of MRI and arthroscopy in pediatric patients has likely resulted in greater recognition of OCD lesions. Trends in youth sports, such as the loss of free play, early sport specialization, multiple leagues in a single sport, and intensive training, also may be contributing factors.

DIAGNOSIS

Clinical Presentation

The presenting complaints of most children and adolescents with OCD are nonspecific. Because most patients have a stable lesion, aching and activity-related knee pain localized to the anterior aspect of the knee are the most common complaints. Symptoms resemble those produced by chondromalacia patellae and subtle forms of patellofemoral malalignment. In patellofemoral pain and OCD, climbing hills or stairs may produce symptoms. Children with OCD do not usually complain of knee instability.

Physical examination findings are often subtle. Children and adolescents with stable OCD lesions may walk with a slight antalgic gait. With careful palpation through varying amounts of knee flexion, a point of maximal tenderness often can be located over the anterior medial aspect of the knee. The tender area corresponds to the lesion, usually on the lateral aspect of the distal medial femoral condyle.

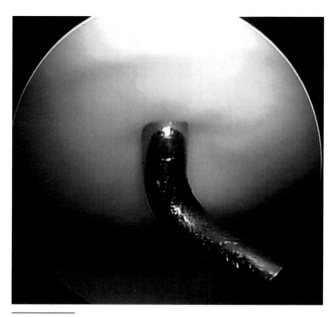

Figure 72–1. Probe showing softening of a femoral condyle osteochondritis dissecans lesion.

With stable lesions, knee effusion, crepitus, and extreme pain through a normal range of motion are rarely observed. Wilson's sign may be helpful, but is often not present.[16,67] Wilson's test is performed by starting with the knee flexed to 90 degrees. Then the tibia is internally rotated as the knee is extended from 90 degrees toward full extension. A positive Wilson's test elicits pain at about 30 degrees of knee flexion located over the anterior aspect of the medial femoral condyle. This pain is thought to result from contact of the medial tibial eminence with the OCD lesion. Ipsilateral quadriceps atrophy may be noted if the patient has been having pain for more than a few weeks.

The mechanical symptoms are more pronounced in the unusual circumstance in which the child or adolescent presents with an unstable lesion. An antalgic gait is common, and there is usually a knee effusion, possibly associated with crepitus, as the knee is taken through a range of motion. In stable and unstable presentations, both knees should be examined to determine whether or not the condition is bilateral.

Imaging Studies

Imaging protocols have received close attention in the literature as a result of the varied success of nonoperative treatment. The goals of imaging are to characterize the lesion, determine the prognosis of nonoperative management, and monitor the healing of the lesion (Fig. 72–2).

Imaging workup begins with plain radiographs including anteroposterior (Fig. 72–3A), lateral, and tunnel views. Tunnel view is particularly valuable because the typical OCD lesion is located on the lateral portion of the medial femoral condyle (Fig. 72–3B). If a patellar OCD is a possibility, a Merchant or skyline view should be added. Plain radiographs usually characterize and localize the

lesion and rule out other bony pathology of the knee region. In children 6 years old and younger, the distal femoral epiphyseal ossification center may exhibit irregularities that simulate the appearance of an OCD. In older children, the status of the physis (open, closing, or closed) should be assessed because this has major implications in the prognosis for healing. Cahill and Berg[12] developed a classification system based on lesion location and size, such that the type of lesion can be determined on the plain films.

MRI is most useful for determining the size of the lesion and the status of the cartilage in the subchondral bone.[37] The extent of bony edema, the presence of a high signal zone beneath the fragment (Fig. 72–4), and the presence of other loose bodies also are important findings on initial MRI (Table 72–1). Routine imaging studies during the course of nonoperative treatment in skeletally immature patients can help identify patients at risk for treatment failure. Evidence suggests that a high signal line on T2-weighted images, representing either healing vascular granulation tissue or articular fluid beneath the subchondral bone, is a predictor of instability.[9,19,50,56] A breach in the cartilage seen on T1-weighted MRI also may help predict treatment failure, particularly when seen in conjunction with a high signal line on T2-weighted images.[50] Investigations of the relationship between gadolinium enhancement and healing have been inconclusive.[9,41,65]

Technetium bone scans have been employed to provide information about the biological capacity of an OCD lesion to heal (Table 72–2).[12,44,52] Although some authors have found that serial bone scans indicate the extent of healing, this imaging technique has not been widely accepted, most likely owing to the length of the test, the need for intravenous access, and the perceived risk of the radiotracer injection.

NONOPERATIVE MANAGEMENT

Nonoperative management is the treatment of choice for skeletally immature children.[64] Because of the vague

Table 72–1. MRI Classification of Juvenile Osteochondritis Dissecans

STAGE	MRI FINDING
I	Small change of signal without clear margins of fragment
II	Osteochondral fragment with clear margins, but without fluid between fragment and underlying bone
III	Fluid is visible partially between fragment and underlying bone
IV	Fluid is completely surrounding the fragment, but the fragment is still in situ
V	Fragment is completely detached and displaced (loose body)

Data from Hefti F, Berguiristain J, Krauspe R, et al: Osteochondritis dissecans: A multicenter study of the European Pediatric Orthopedic Society. J Pediatr Orthop 8B:231-245, 1999.

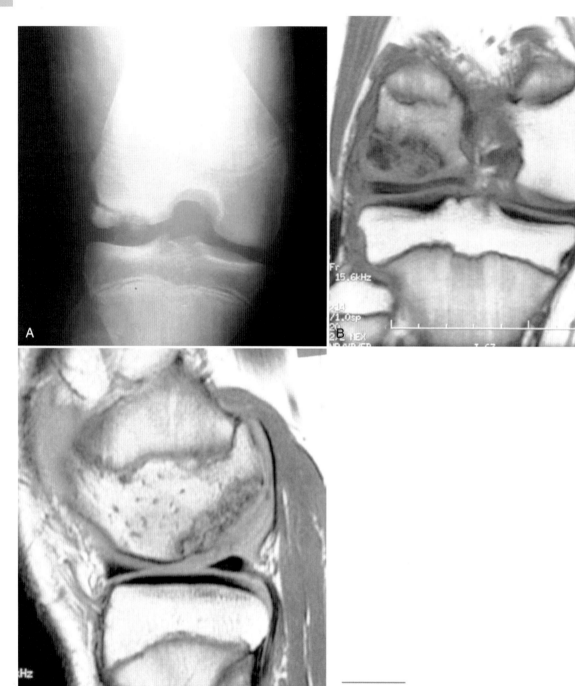

Figure 72–2. **A,** Anteroposterior x-ray of a large osteochondritis dissecans lesion of the lateral femoral condyle in an adolescent patient. **B** and **C,** Anteroposterior and lateral T1-weighted images of a large osteochondritis dissecans lesion in the posterolateral aspect of the lateral femoral condyle.

etiology of OCD, there has been a debate about whether immobilization is therapeutic or detrimental. If the goal is regeneration of injured subchondral bone, a cast or knee brace would provide immobilization, whereas continuous passive motion promotes cartilage health. Because the failure of the cartilage surface is most likely secondary to the failure of the underlying bone, it is widely accepted that rest, if not immobilization, is indicated.

The options for immobilization include casting, bracing, and standard knee immobilization. Partial weightbearing in slight flexion minimizes shear, while preserving a limited amount of compression across the lesion. Selecting an immobilization protocol can be difficult. Casts present children with the inconvenience of more restricted range of motion, but compliance with full-time immobilizer use in a young athlete can be a problem.

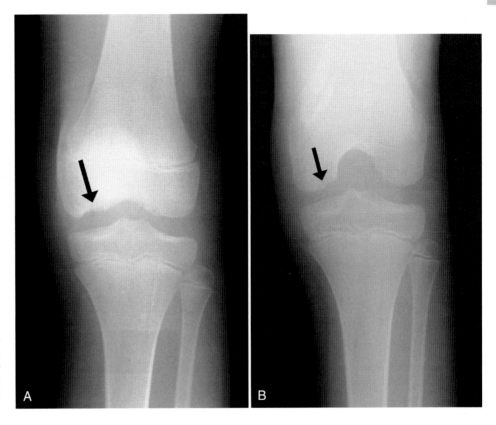

Figure 72–3. **A** and **B,** Anteroposterior and tunnel plain radiographs showing osteochondritis dissecans of lateral aspect of medial femoral condyle *(arrows).*

Table 72–2. Bone Scan Classification of Juvenile Osteochondritis Dissecans Lesions

STAGE	BONE SCAN FINDING
0	Normal radiographic and scintigraphic appearance
I	Lesion is visible on plain radiographs, but bone scan reveals normal findings
II	Bone scan reveals increased uptake in the area of the lesion
III	There is increased isotopic uptake in the entire femoral condyle
IV	There is uptake in the tibial plateau opposite the lesion

Data from Cahill BR: Osteochondritis dissecans of the knee: Treatment of juvenile and adult forms. J Am Acad Orthop Surg 3:237-247, 1995.

Hinged, unloader-type braces allow a greater range of motion than standard immobilization; however, the efficacy of bracing has yet to be proved in clinical studies.

We recommend a three-phase approach to the nonoperative management of OCD lesions. In phase I, knee immobilization with partial weightbearing is recommended. If the patient is pain-free, and radiographs show signs of healing after 6 weeks, he or she is allowed to begin weightbearing without immobilization and to begin a physical therapy protocol to improve knee range of motion and quadriceps and hamstring strength (phase II, weeks 6 to 12). Three months after diagnosis, a patient who has remained pain-free and shows radiographic evidence of healing begins phase III, in which running, jumping, and cutting sports are permitted under close observation. High-impact activities and activities that might involve shear stress to the knee should be restricted until the child has been pain-free for several months, and the radiographs show a healed lesion. Although children with juvenile OCD have a better prognosis for healing than adults with OCD, not all lesions in skeletally immature knees heal. Repeat immobilization can be considered if radiographs show progression of the lesion or if symptoms return.

Although immobilization is often successful in juvenile OCD, it may not be the ideal treatment option for a young athlete and his or her parents. Patients and their parents should be informed of the risks and benefits of nonoperative treatment relative to the risks and benefits of surgical management.

OPERATIVE MANAGEMENT

It is widely accepted that operative treatment should be considered for patients with unstable or detached lesions, in patients approaching skeletal maturity, and in patients whose lesions have not resolved with an appropriate period of nonoperative management.[4,11,20,29,32] The goals of operative treatment are to promote healing of subchondral bone, to maintain joint congruity, to fix rigidly unstable fragments, and to replace osteochondral defects with cells that can replace and grow cartilage.[26,60] Optimal surgical treatment provides a stable construct of subchondral bone, calcified tidemark, and repair cartilage with viability and biomechanical properties similar to native hyaline cartilage.

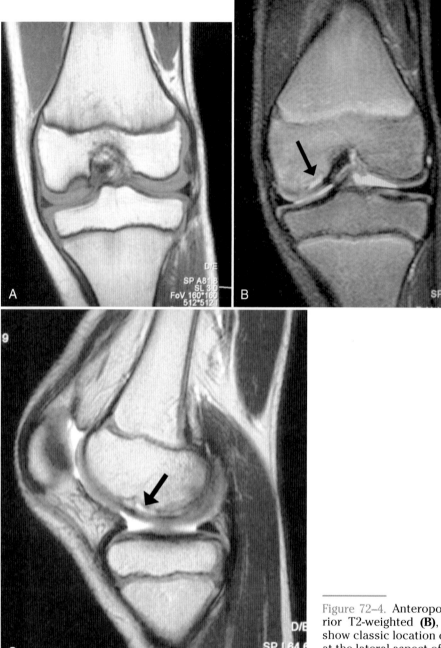

Figure 72–4. Anteroposterior T1-weighted **(A)**, anteroposterior T2-weighted **(B)**, and lateral T1-weighted **(C)** images show classic location of an osteochondritis dissecans lesion at the lateral aspect of the medial femoral condyle with fluid shown beneath the lesion *(arrows)*.

Arthroscopic drilling is indicated for stable lesions with an intact articular surface. Drilling creates channels to promote revascularization and healing (Fig. 72–5). Although more technically challenging, antegrade drilling (proximal to distal) precludes the disruption of the articular surface. Conversely, a transarticular technique is more straightforward from a surgical perspective, but creates articular cartilage channels that can heal with fibrocartilage.[6]

Arthroscopic transarticular drilling is effective in the treatment of OCD lesions in skeletally immature patients. Numerous authors have reported radiographic resolution and increases in Lysholm score throughout postoperative follow-up.[1,6,10] Treatment success is much better for chil-

dren with open physes compared with skeletally mature patients. Anderson and colleagues[6] noted healing in 18 of 20 lesions in a skeletally immature group, whereas only 2 of 4 healed at an average follow-up of 5 years in a skeletally mature group. Factors associated with inadequate healing after drilling include lesions in atypical locations, multiple lesions, and underlying medical conditions.[24] Younger age also has been shown to be a predictor of Lysholm score.[39]

The goal of operative treatment of flap lesions is the removal of the fibrous tissue found between the fragments and underlying bone without disrupting the underlying bone from the fragment or the subchondral bone at the base of the lesion. In patients with partially unstable

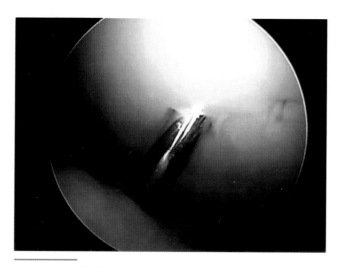

Figure 72–5. Drilling osteochondritis dissecans lesion with smooth Kirschner wire.

lesions or unstable lesions with adequate subchondral bone to match the defect and the fragment, open or arthroscopic fixation can be performed. For cases in which subchondral bone loss has occurred, autogenous bone graft can be packed into the crater before reduction and fixation. Rapid relief of discomfort on reduction has led some authors to theorize that pain is the result of increased pressure at the line of separation between the fragment and the epiphysis.[10,33,62]

The poor long-term results after excision of a loose OCD fragment in skeletally mature patients have led authors to recommend more aggressive attempts to preserve the articular cartilage and avoid excision of the fragments.[70] Cortical strips of bone from the metaphysis of the tibia also have been used.[26,49] Although Herbert screws and cannulated screws have been used successfully, second surgeries may be required for removal.[17,69] The use of a metal staple placed arthroscopically also has been described in the literature; however, broken staples were observed in more than one-third of the knees treated.[54] Despite the reported success of the operative fixation of OCD fragments, several complications associated with these techniques have been reported. The loosening and backing out of bioabsorbable screws can cause damage to adjacent articular surfaces, whereas unabsorbed screw heads and bone and osteochondral plugs have been found as intra-articular loose bodies.[18,23,34,59]

In a large unsalvageable fragment, the goal is to replace the defect with subchondral bone, calcified tidemark, and overlying cartilage. Drilling and abrasion arthroplasty or microfracturing with picks can be performed to recruit pluripotential cells from marrow that preferentially differentiate into fibrocartilage.[61] Although it is possible to resurface smaller lesions with these techniques, fibrocartilage does not respond to shear stress as effectively as native hyaline cartilage, and deterioration of the repaired site over time has been reported.[46] An alternative treatment option reported in the literature is the removal of the fragment and the débridement of the crater.[2] The results of long-term follow-up with weightbearing anteroposterior radiographs have shown the progression of Fairbanks

changes, however, and suggest a poor prognosis for lesions larger than 2 cm.[5]

A cartilaginous extracellular matrix can be generated in the defect with periosteum and transplant of the cambium layer. The results of studies with long-term follow-up suggest that this operative technique is not ideal because of the incidence of reoperation and persistent knee pain.[45,56] Concerns about the durability of reparative fibrocartilage have provided the impetus for the development of alternative techniques. Autologous osteochondral plugs obtained from non-weightbearing regions of the knee (e.g., the edge of the intercondylar notch or upper outer trochlea) also have been transplanted to replace defects.[7,8] Good results have been reported in more recent studies in patients with open growth plates and patients who have reached skeletal maturity.[51,68] Potential disadvantages of osteochondral grafts, such as donor site morbidity, including loose bodies originating from the donor site, are balanced by the advantages of biological internal fixation.[34] Successful secondary reconstruction with bone–articular surface allografts has been described in patients with significant surface defects in OCD, although no long-term results in skeletally immature patients are yet available.[25]

Autologous chondrocyte implantation also has been used in younger patients with no lower extremity malalignment to repair large, isolated femoral defects. Studies have reported high rates of successful repair, although information about long-term prognosis is not yet available.[7,54] King and associates[35] noted slightly better outcomes of autologous chondrocyte transplantation for large defects in articular cartilage of the distal femur in adolescent patients than previous reported results found in adult patients, probably owing to superior articular substance in the adjacent regions of the knee. Figure 72–6 is an algorithm for the treatment of OCD.

SUMMARY

The prevalence of OCD of the knee is increasing among children. Careful attention to presenting symptoms accompanied by successful imaging are an integral part of making the diagnosis. Timely recognition is essential because stable lesions with an intact articular surface usually can be treated successfully with a three-stage nonoperative management protocol. The fundamental principle of this protocol is the cessation of repetitive impact loading followed by the gradual return to normal activity, usually facilitated by some form of adjunctive immobilization. MRI may aid in the early prediction of a lesion's healing potential. For stable lesions that do not show signs of resolution after 6 to 9 months of following the nonoperative protocol, arthroscopic drilling should be considered to prevent progression to an unstable lesion. The excision of large lesions generally yields poor results, but chondral resurfacing techniques may decrease the risk of subsequent arthrosis. Unstable lesions and acute loose bodies require fixation and possible bone grafting and are associated with higher rates of complications. Most of these lesions heal, although the long-term prognosis is uncertain. Chronic loose bodies pose a greater challenge

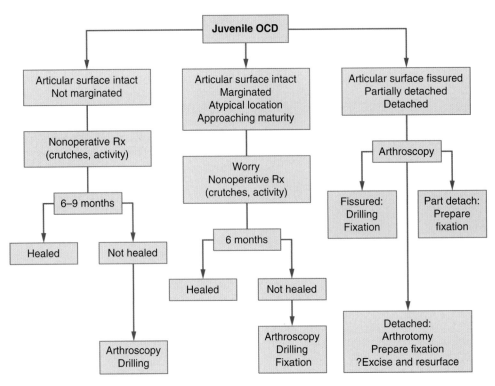

Figure 72–6. Algorithm for the treatment of osteochondritis dissecans (OCD) in a pediatric patient. (From Flynn JM, Kocher M, Ganley T: Osteochondritis dissecans of the knee. J Pediatr Orthop 24:434-443, 2004.)

for fixation and may have poor long-term healing potential.

References

1. Aglietti P, Buzzi R, Bassi PB et al: Arthroscopic drilling in juvenile osteochondritis dissecans of the medial femoral condyle. Arthroscopy 10:286-291, 1994.
2. Aglietti P, Ciardullo A, Giron F, et al: Results of arthroscopic excision of the fragment in the treatment of osteochondritis dissecans of the knee. Arthroscopy 17:741-746, 2001.
3. Aichroth P: Osteochondritis dissecans of the knee: A clinical survey. J Bone Joint Surg Br 53:440-447, 1971.
4. Anderson AF, Lipscomb AB, Coulam C: Antegrade curettement, bone grafting, and pinning of osteochondritis dissecans in the skeletally mature knee. Am J Sports Med 18:254-261, 1990.
5. Anderson AF, Pagnani MJ: Osteochondritis dissecans of the femoral condyles: Long-term results of excision of the fragment. Am J Sports Med 25:830-834, 1997.
6. Anderson AF, Richards DB, Pagnani MJ, et al: Antegrade drilling for osteochondritis dissecans of the knee. Arthroscopy 13:319-324, 1997.
7. Bentley G, Biant LC, Carrington RW, et al: A prospective, randomised comparison of autologous chondrocyte implantation versus mosaicplasty for osteochondral defects in the knee. J Bone Joint Surg Br 85:223-230, 2003.
8. Berlet GC, Mascia A, Miniaci A: Treatment of unstable osteochondritis dissecans lesions of the knee using autogenous osteochondral grafts mosaicplasty. Arthroscopy 15:312-316, 1999.
9. Bohndorf K: Osteochondritis (osteochondrosis) dissecans: A review and new MRI classification. Eur Radiol 8:103-112, 1998.
10. Bradley J, Dandy DJ: Results of drilling osteochondritis dissecans before skeletal maturity. J Bone Joint Surg Br 71:642-644, 1989.
11. Cahill BR: Osteochondritis dissecans of the knee: Treatment of juvenile and adult forms. J Am Acad Orthop Surg 3:237-247, 1995.
12. Cahill BR, Berg BC: 99m-Technetium phosphate compound joint scintigraphy in the management of juvenile osteochondritis dissecans of the femoral condyles. Am J Sports Med 11:329-335, 1983.
13. Cahill BR, Phillips MR, Navarro R: The results of conservative management of juvenile osteochondritis dissecans using joint scintigraphy: A prospective study. Am J Sports Med 17:601-606, 1989.
14. Chiroff RT, Cooke CP: Osteochondritis dissecans: A histologic and micro radiographic analysis of surgically excised lesions. J Trauma 15:689-696, 1975.
15. Clanton TO, DeLee JC: Osteochondritis dissecans: History, pathophysiology and current treatment concepts. Clin Orthop 167:50-64, 1982.
16. Conrad JM, Stanitski CL: Osteochondritis dissecans: Wilson's sign revisited. Am J Sports Med 31:777-778, 2003.
17. Cugat R, Garcia M, Cusco X, et al: Osteochondritis dissecans: A historical review and its treatment with cannulated screws. Arthroscopy 9:675-684, 1993.
18. Dervin GF, Keene GC, Chissell HR: Biodegradable rods in adult osteochondritis dissecans of the knee. Clin Orthop 356:213-221, 1998.
19. De Smet AA, Ilahi OA, Graf BK: Untreated osteochondritis dissecans of the femoral condyles: Prediction of patient outcome using radiographic and MR findings. Skeletal Radiol 26:463-467, 1997.
20. Ewing JW, Voto SJ: Arthroscopic surgical management of osteochondritis dissecans of the knee. Arthroscopy 4:37-40, 1988.
21. Fairbanks HAT: Osteochonritis dissecans. Br J Surg 21:67-82, 1933.
22. Flynn JM, Kocher MS, Ganley TJ: Osteochondritis dissecans of the knee. J Pediatr Orthop 24:434-443, 2004.
23. Friederichs MG, Greis PE, Burks RT: Pitfalls associated with fixation of osteochondritis dissecans fragments using bioabsorbable screws. Arthroscopy 17:542-545, 2001.
24. Ganley TJG, Amro RR, Gregg JR, Halpern KV: Antegrade drilling for osteochondritis dissecans of the knee. Presented at POSNA 2002 Annual Meeting, Salt Lake City, 2002.
25. Garrett JC: Osteochondritis dissecans. Clin Sports Med 10:569-593, 1991.
26. Gillespie HS, Day B: Bone peg fixation in the treatment of osteochondritis dissecans of the knee joint. Clin Orthop 143:125-130, 1979.

27. Glancy GL: Juvenile osteochondritis dissecans. Am J Knee Surg 12:120-124, 1999.

28. Green WT, Banks HH: Osteochondritis dissecans in children. J Bone Joint Surg Am 35:26-47, 1953.

29. Guhl JF: Arthroscopic treatment of osteochondritis dissecans. Clin Orthop 167:65-74, 1982.

30. Hefti F, Berguiristain J, Krauspe R, et al: Osteochondritis dissecans: A multicenter study of the European Pediatric Orthopedic Society. J Pediatr Orthop 8B:231-245, 1999.

31. Hughston JC, Hergenroeder PT, Courtenay BG: Osteochondritis dissecans of the femoral condyles. J Bone Joint Surg Am 66:1340-1348, 1984.

32. Iobst C, Kocher MS: Cartilage injury in the skeletally immature athlete. In Mirzayan R (ed): Cartilage Injury in the Athlete: Orthopaedic Management. New York: Thieme Medical Publishers, 2006.

33. Johnson LL, Uitvlugt G, Austin MD, et al: Osteochondritis dissecans of the knee: Arthroscopic compression screw fixation. Arthroscopy 6:179-189, 1990.

34. Kim SJ, Shin SJ: Loose bodies after arthroscopic osteochondral autograft in osteochondritis dissecans of the knee. Arthroscopy 16:E16, 2000.

35. King PJ, Ganley T, Lou JE, Gregg JR: Autologous chondrocyte transplantation for the treatment of large defects in the articular cartilage of the distal femur in adolescent patients. Presented at American Academy of Orthopaedic Surgeons Annual Meeting, New Orleans, 2003.

36. Koch S, Kampen WU, Laprell H: Cartilage and bone morphology in osteochondritis dissecans. Knee Surg Sports Traumatol Arthrosc 5:42-45, 1997.

37. Kocher MS, DiCanzio J, Zurakowski D, Micheli LJ: Diagnostic performance of clinical examination and selective magnetic resonance imaging in the evaluation of intra-articular knee disorders in children and adolescents. Am J Sports Med 29:292-296, 2001.

38. Kocher MS, Micheli LJ: The pediatric knee: Evaluation and treatment. In Insall JN, Scott WN (eds): Surgery of the Knee, 3rd ed. New York, Churchill Livingstone, 2001, pp 1356-1397.

39. Kocher MS, Micheli LJ, Yaniv M, et al: Functional and radiographic outcome of juvenile osteochondritis dissecans of the knee treated with transarticular arthroscopic drilling. Am J Sports Med 29:562-566, 2001.

40. König F: Ueber freie Körper in den Gelenken. Dtsch Z Chir 27:90-109, 1887.

41. Kramer J, Stiglbauer R, Engel A, et al: MR contrast arthrography (MRA) in osteochondrosis dissecans. J Comput Assist Tomogr 16:254-260, 1992.

42. Linden B: The incidence of osteochondritis dissecans in the condyles of the femur. Acta Orthop Scand 47:664-667, 1976.

43. Linden B: Osteochondritis dissecans of the femoral condyle. J Bone Joint Surg Am 59:769-776, 1977.

44. Litchman HM, McCullough RW, Gandsman EJ, et al: Computerized blood flow analysis for decision making in the treatment of osteochondritis dissecans. J Pediatr Orthop 8:208-212, 1988.

45. Madsen BL, Noer HH, Carstensen JP, et al: Long-term results of periosteal transplantation in osteochondritis dissecans of the knee. Orthopedics 23:223-226, 2000.

46. Mandelbaum BR, Browne JE, Fu F, et al: Articular cartilage lesions of the knee. Am J Sports Med 26:853-861, 1998.

47. Milgram JW: Radiological and pathological manifestations of osteochondritis dissecans of the distal femur: A study of 50 cases. Radiology 126:305-311, 1978.

48. Mubarak SJ, Carroll NC: Familial osteochondritis dissecans of the knee. Clin Orthop 140:131-136, 1979.

49. Navarro R, Cohen M, Filho MC, et al: The arthroscopic treatment of osteochondritis dissecans of the knee with autologous bone sticks. Arthroscopy 18:840-844, 2002.

50. O'Connor MA, Palaniappan M, Khan N, et al: Osteochondritis dissecans of the knee in children: A comparison of MRI and arthroscopic findings. J Bone Joint Surg Br 84:258-262, 2002.

51. Outerbridge HK, Outerbridge AR, Outerbridge RE: The use of a lateral patellar autologous graft for the repair of a large osteochondral defect in the knee. J Bone Joint Surg Am 77:65-72, 1995.

52. Paletta GA Jr, Bednarz PA, Stanitski CL, et al: The prognostic value of quantitative bone scan in knee osteochondritis dissecans: A preliminary experience. Am J Sports Med 26:7-14, 1998.

53. Pappas A: Osteochondritis dissecans. Clin Orthop 158:59-69, 1981.

54. Peterson L, Minas T, Brittberg M, et al: Treatment of osteochondritis dissecans of the knee with autologous chondrocyte transplantation: Results at two to ten years. J Bone Joint Surg Am 85(Suppl 2):17-24, 2003.

55. Petrie PW: Aetiology of osteochondritis dissecans: Failure to establish a familial background. J Bone Joint Surg Br 59:366-367, 1977.

56. Pill SG, Ganley TJ, Milam RA, et al: Role of magnetic resonance imaging and clinical criteria in predicting successful nonoperative treatment of osteochondritis dissecans in children. J Pediatr Orthop 23:102-108, 2003.

57. Reddy AS: Evaluation of the intraosseous and extraosseous blood supply to the distal femoral condyles. Am J Sports Med 26:415-419, 1998.

58. Rogers W, Gladstone H: Vascular foramina and arterial supply of the distal end of the femur. J Bone Joint Surg Am 32:867-874, 1950.

59. Scioscia TN, Giffin JR, Allen CR, et al: Potential complication of bioabsorbable screw fixation for osteochondritis dissecans of the knee. Arthroscopy 17:E7, 2001.

60. Smillie I: Treatment of osteochondritis dissecans. J Bone Joint Surg Br 39:248-260, 1957.

61. Steadman JR, Briggs KK, Rodrigo JJ, et al: Outcomes of microfracture for traumatic chondral defects of the knee: Average 11-year follow-up. Arthroscopy 19:477-484, 2003.

62. Thomson NL: Osteochondritis dissecans and osteochondral fragments managed by Herbert compression screw fixation. Clin Orthop 224:71-78, 1987.

63. Twyman R, Kailish D, Aichroth P: Osteochondritis of the knee: A long-term study. J Bone Joint Surg Br 73:461-464, 1991.

64. Van Demark RE: Osteochondritis dissecans with spontaneous healing. J Bone Joint Surg Am 35:143-148, 1952.

65. Vonstein D, Wall EJ, Nosir H, Laor T, Emery K: Juvenile osteochondritis dissecans of the knee: Healing prognosis based on x-ray and gadolinium enhanced MRI. Presented at POSNA, 2003 Annual Meeting, Amelia Island, FL, 2003.

66. Wall E, Von Stein D: Juvenile osteochondritis dissecans. Orthop Clin North Am 34:341-353, 2003.

67. Wilson JN: A diagnostic sign in osteochondritis dissecans of the knee. J Bone Joint Surg Am 49:477-480, 1967.

68. Yoshizumi Y, Sugita T, Kawamata T, et al: Cylindrical osteochondral graft for osteochondritis dissecans of the knee: A report of three cases. Am J Sports Med 30:441-445, 2002.

69. Rey Zuniga JJ, Sagastibelza J, Lopez Blasco JJ, Martinez Grande M: Arthroscopic use of Herbert screws in osteochondritis dissecans of the knee. Arthroscopy 9:668-670, 1993.

70. Wright RW, McLean M, Matava MJ, Shively RA: Osteochondritis dissecans of the knee: Long-term results of excision of the fragment. Clin Orthop 424:239-243, 2004.

CHAPTER 73

Anterior Cruciate Ligament Injuries/Posterior Cruciate Ligament Injuries and Acute Tibial Eminence Fractures in Skeletally Immature Patients

Carl L. Stanitski

ACUTE ANTERIOR CRUCIATE INJURY IN SKELETALLY IMMATURE PATIENTS

The anterior cruciate ligament (ACL) is a high-profile ligament secondary to the reporting by the media of ACL injuries in celebrity athletes and their usually successful return to play after reconstructive surgery. "ACL" has entered the lay lexicon, and patients and parents are aware of this structure and the grim athletic portents accompanying its injury. Over the past two decades, the ACL's role in normal knee function has been defined. The natural clinical history of skeletally mature patients with ACL-deficient knees who attempt to return to high-demand sports has been established, that is, progressive intra-articular compromise and onset of premature degenerative joint disease.[46] A subset of patients with ACL injury is now recognized—the skeletally immature athlete. In the past, ACL injuries in the truly immature patients were considered curiosities and data on ACL injuries in the almost mature adolescent were melded into adult series. The otherwise normal skeletally immature patient was simply considered to not suffer the meniscal and ACL injuries of the adult counterparts. The true prevalence and incidence of ACL injuries in the skeletally immature patient group are unknown, but it is certainly not an uncommon event given the significant number of children and youth participants in scholastic and community sports. The data suggest that ACL injury is especially common in female athletes. The precise cause of this gender difference, especially in soccer and basketball participants, is unknown. Theories of notch morphology variability,[29] lower-extremity mechanical alignment abnormalities, underlying conditioning deficits, and hormonal challenges have been proposed and are under scrutiny. A report by Hewitt and colleagues[22] suggests a loss of neuromuscular control with progressive physical maturation in girls resulting in abnormal landing patterns while jumping. In an interesting retrospective analysis, Kocher and coworkers[28] reviewed two groups of 25 skeletally immature patients, one with midsubstance tears and the other with type II or type III acute tibial eminence fractures. They compared the notch width index for each group and found no significant difference between the groups relative to age, gender, bone age, or skeletal maturity. Patients with midsubstance ACL tears did have narrower notch indices, but significant overlap was seen in the notch width indices between groups and a threshold value as an index for risk of ACL midsubstance injury could not be established. No normative data for notch width indices for age have been established. Awareness of an ACL tear in this age group has been heightened. Improvements in clinical acumen have been made, including the association of a "pop" and acute hemarthrosis, return to play limitation, and Lachman and pivot shift signs with quantitation of sagittal plane translation by arthrometry. Magnetic resonance imaging (MRI) techniques extend diagnostic capabilities when correlated with clinical findings. Arthroscopic findings remain the gold standard of diagnosis documentation.

Reports by Angel and Hall,[5] Lo and coworkers,[33] Stanitski and associates,[58] Guzzanti and colleagues,[17,18] and others[2,23,38,48,66] presented significant numbers of cases of arthroscopically documented ACL damage in truly skeletally immature patients, particularly ones with hemarthrosis, excluding those patients with tibial eminence fractures. Many previous studies of knee injuries in the immature patient suffered from major limitations, including study design, lack of diagnosis specificity and documentation, patient number, length of follow-up, activity modification, outcome quantitation, and imprecision in differentiating physiological from chronological maturity.[16,38,42,44]

The majority of growth in the lower extremity centers about the distal femoral and proximal tibial physes. Dimeglio[11] reports 5 cm of growth about the knee remains at the onset of puberty, which usually occurs at skeletal age 13 in girls and 15 in boys. In immature patients, the ACL attaches to the distal femoral and proximal tibial chondroepiphyses through a perichondral cuff that during adolescence transforms to a fibrocartilage-osseous interface at maturity. In the past it was assumed that the ACL was rarely injured in skeletally immature patients because of the relative vulnerability of the chondroepiphysis relative to ligament resistance. This attitude neglected to appreciate that junctional tissues involved responded differently to load rate, magnitude, and direction. Ligamentous injury, in general, is caused by lower magnitude forces at rapid load rates. Physeal damage occurs in response to high-energy forces at lower rates of loading.

The ACL's nutrition in children is via a perisynovial sheath and terminal osseous elements of the femur and tibia. Femoral intercondylar notch configuration and other intra-articular morphology are determined by the effects of use superimposed on a genetically determined template. Alterations in ACL morphology are often seen in congenital disorders of the lower extremities (e.g., congenital short femur, fibular hemimelia).

Natural History

Few retrospective and no prospective well-done natural history studies exist about isolated complete ACL tears in truly skeletally immature patients. Angel and Hall[5] used telephone and mail questionnaires to retrospectively review the outcome of 27 relatively mature children (mean age 14.5 years) with arthroscopically documented ACL tears[27] (67% partial) at an average of 51 months after injury. Physiological age of the cohort was not reported. Twenty-five patients were treated with physical therapy without immobilization, bracing, or sports limitation. At follow-up, half of the patients reported functional instability and pain, 11 had temporarily returned to full sports activity, and another 7 participated at a reduced level of play; 9 patients were unable to participate. Although the sports were not specified, this return to activity distribution is similar to that reported by Noyes and colleagues in their adult patients with ACL tears.[46] Mizuta and coworkers[44] reported the outcome of 18 girls (10 to 15 years old with an average age of 12.8 years) with ACL injuries observed for 36 to 51 months. No comment was made regarding physiological maturity, and no patient was placed at diminished athletic activity. One patient was able to return to full activity. Not surprisingly, most patients had poor Lysholm scores. Secondary meniscal tears were arthroscopically documented in 6 patients, and 3 others had clinical evidence of a meniscal tear. Pressman and colleagues[48] conducted a 12-year retrospective analysis of 42 patients with arthroscopically documented complete midsubstance ACL tears. Patients were from 5 to 17 years old at the time of injury with a follow-up evaluation at an average of 5.3 years done by telephone survey or clinical examination. Outcomes of 13 patients treated nonoperatively with derotation brace, physiotherapy, and initial casting showed significantly poorer functional knee scores than in a similar aged group treated by intra-articular surgical reconstruction. Brace and elimination of high-demand activities compliance were not addressed.

McCarroll and colleagues[38] observed 38 middle-school children (13 to 15 years old, average 13.5 years) with arthroscopically documented midsubstance ACL tears for an average of 4.2 years and a minimal follow-up of 2 years after injury. In this group of patients whose physiological age was not noted, 16 (42%) attempted to return to previous levels of athletic participation but all complained of "giving way," and 10 of these 16 patients developed documented meniscal tears; 2 of the 16 had chronic knee effusions. In the final report, of the 38 patients treated nonoperatively 37 had functional complaints of instability and 27 developed symptomatic meniscal tears after attempting to return to high-demand sports. In Graf and coworkers'[16] retrospective study of 12 patients with an average age of 14.5 years with arthroscopically proven ACL tears, eight meniscal tears (four medial, four lateral) were seen in 6 patients. Eight patients underwent rehabilitation and functional bracing, but all developed functional instability and multiple episodes of "giving way" while attempting to play at an average of 7 months from the injury to the first complaints of instability. This mirrors the 6-month period noted by Noyes and associates.[46] In Graf and colleagues' small series of 12 patients without documented physiological maturity, 7 patients developed additional meniscal damage at an average of 15 months after primary ACL injury despite brace use.[16]

Data are limited regarding partial ACL tears in truly skeletally immature patients. The amount of force from either a single episode or as a result of summated submaximal forces needed to convert a partial tear in an attenuated ligament to a complete tear is unknown. The percentage of injury to each of the ACL's bundles to indicate a partial tear has not been quantitated and classified. Kocher and coworkers[27] prospectively studied 45 skeletally mature and immature patients 17 years old or younger with acute hemarthroses, clinical findings of instability, and arthroscopically documented partial ACL tears treated with a structured rehabilitation program without ACL reconstruction. At a minimal follow-up of 2 years, only 31% of the patients required reconstruction. This surgical subgroup was primarily older patients with more than 50% tears and a high-grade pivot shift. Kocher and coworkers recommended nonreconstruction management for less than 50% partial ACL tears in children 14 years old or younger with low-grade Lachman and pivot shift tests.

Clinical Examination

Clinical evaluation in the hands of an experienced surgeon is an extremely accurate diagnostic method for ACL assessment, especially in the nonacute setting.[27,33,39,56] Immediately after the injury the patient is usually less than cooperative, owing to apprehension and pain during the various maneuvers to determine stability. I characterize the mechanism of injury as contact or noncontact and whether there is a component of deceleration and rotation.[65] It is uncommon to find an ACL tear in someone without elements of rotation and deceleration and knee hyperextension or flexion. The mechanism of injury seems to be similar to the one seen in adults, mainly, a noncontact stress combined with rapid directional change. A sensation of a "pop" in the knee is reported in about one-third of the patients with an acute ACL tear. Onset of effusion is rapid, and the patients are usually (~70%) unable to return to play. I group acute tears as ones seen less than 3 weeks after injury; subacute, at 3 to 12 weeks; and chronic, at more than 12 weeks after injury.[54] In addition to the usual characterization of historical points relative to the knee, additional data must be gathered about the patient's level of physiological maturity and projected remaining growth. Growth is a process of variable onset, rate, magnitude, and duration. Knowing parental and sibling heights as well as the growth status of the patient when combined with findings of maturity on clinical examination allows an educated approximation to be made of growth remaining. Onset of menarche should be determined because the peak height velocity growth phase occurs just before menarche. The apex of peak height velocity is reached at an average of 11.5 years in girls and 13.5 years in boys.[7] Determination of secondary sexual development as a physiological marker is necessary because physiological and not chronological age is required as a data point in the treatment algorithm.[13] Appearance of curly underarm hair is a clinical sign of maturity in boys, which equates in timing of maturation with menarche in girls.[59] Shoe size stability is a rough guide to impending skeletal maturity. Future sports participation plans, risks, and demands need to be addressed, including the high rate of repeat ACL injury with return to high-demand sports.

During clinical tests of knee stability, the opposite uninjured knee should serve as the control for tibial translation with assessment of the magnitude of translation and rotation and the endpoint quality. Many asymptomatic teenage girls have significant knee rotation and translation, including positive pivot shifts due to inherent, genetically determined, nonpathological ligamentous laxity. Tenderness to palpation should be sought around the patellar retinaculum, especially the patellofemoral and patellomeniscal ligaments, joint lines, and tibial and femoral physes. Joint line tenderness, particularly mid and posterior, commonly accompanies peripheral meniscal injury. Physeal tenderness may be misinterpreted as the site of collateral ligament injury in the skeletally immature patient. Effusion presence or absence as well as volume of effusion should be noted. An ACL tear of any consequence is always associated with an initial and persisting effusion. Arthrometric examination is usually difficult to perform shortly after injury because of patient guarding due to pain. Kocher and colleagues[30] suggest that the magnitude of a positive pivot shift in patients with ACL insufficiency may be a better measure of functional instability than Lachman or sagittal arthrometer testing.

Imaging

Initial imaging is via high-quality standard anteroposterior, lateral, notch, and patellar view radiographs. Other than in the case of a tibial eminence fracture, true avulsion of the ACL is a rare event, and the avulsed fragment in this circumstance is usually composed of mostly chondral tissue with only a fleck of bone. Osteochondral femoral and patellar fragments should be sought because the mechanism of injury of an ACL is similar to that causing acute patellar instability. Unsuspected osteochondritis dissecans lesions may also be seen. In addition to the just-mentioned potential findings, radiographs provide information about notch morphology, physeal injury, and physeal maturity. If an undisplaced physeal injury is suspected, stress views should not be done because they produce further damage to the physis and do

not add anything to the treatment plan for this undisplaced fracture. Follow-up radiographs in 10 to 14 days document the periosteal response expected in this type of injury.[57]

Magnetic resonance imaging (MRI) should be ordered by the treating surgeon for specific indications (e.g., when the diagnosis cannot be made by clinical examination). MRI should not be used as a screening test by nonsurgical physicians. Major errors occur in interpretations by radiologists of knee MR images in skeletally immature patients, as evidenced by reports of supposed meniscal tears in normal children. Several authors noted major discrepancies between clinical examination findings and radiology reports of knee MRI studies and between these reports and findings at arthroscopy.[27,39,56] In our study[56] there was a 75% presence of false-positive and false-negative results of MRI and only a 30% coincidence of MRI and arthroscopic findings. Clinical examination proved highly more accurate in this skeletally immature group of patients evaluated in a nonacute setting by a single surgeon. MRI studies provided no significant help in patient management. Acute ACL injury changes on MRI include increases in signal and change in morphology. Late changes are seen in the configuration of the posterior cruciate ligament (PCL) owing to the attachment of the fibrotic ACL stump. Transient subchondral changes, especially on the lateral femoral condyle, are common in the acute phase and reflect marrow edema. Clinical tenderness at these sites should not be confused with meniscal damage.

Treatment

All treatment plans are based on an accurate diagnosis achieved by clinical evaluation, imaging, and, if necessary, arthroscopic assessment. Treatment goals are a functional knee without progressive intra-articular damage and predisposition to premature osteoarthrosis. There are no well-documented follow-up studies of adequate length of truly skeletally immature patients with complete ACL tears without initial meniscal injury who have complied with nonoperative treatment with return to a non–high-demand sport program. In the emerging young athlete, a torn ACL is not a surgical emergency. One must take time to discuss treatment options and their impact on future sports involvement, vocational and avocational concerns, and the risks, complications, and outcomes of the various management programs, including re-rupture of the reconstructed ligament and/or tear of the contralateral ACL with return to high-demand sports. Data from adults suggest that despite short- and medium-term good clinical results, onset of degenerative arthrosis is not uniformly prevented after ACL reconstruction.[32,46] One aspect of this multifactorial problem is biomechanical. Sagittal plane laxity is eliminated, but normal rotatory femoral-tibial kinematics are not reestablished, especially in the lateral compartment.[35,36,60] Another part is biochemical, with prolonged changes in intra-articular concentrations of cytokines, proteases, and keratan sulfate after injury and reconstructive surgery. A third factor is activity level and intensity after reconstruction. Prospective, randomized, long-term clinical trials are needed to answer the impact of surgical intervention on development of arthrosis. The emerging athlete is often under significant pressure from peers, coaches, and often parents to return to play in replication of the professional athlete model. The orthopedic surgeon should assume the role of a knee counselor, especially to those patients whom he or she recognizes as "knee abusers" with high-risk activities.

Nonoperative treatment does not mean no treatment. The goal of the program must be defined from the outset. The plan may be a temporizing measure until the patient is mature enough to undergo an adult-type, complete transphyseal procedure or the nonoperative choice may be the definitive one for a patient willing to accept the athletic functional limitations consigned by not repairing the torn ACL.[66]

The nonoperative program I use for skeletally immature patients is in three phases.[12,55] Phase I begins shortly after injury, lasts 7 to 10 days, and includes progressive weightbearing with crutches, out-of-brace daily active knee flexion to comfort with passive knee extension, and use of a knee immobilizer for comfort. During this time, patient education regarding the consequences of imprudent high-level sports activity is reinforced.

Phase II lasts about 6 weeks. During that time, monitored and documented rehabilitation efforts are done to restore full range of motion and normalize the muscle balance of the lower extremity with focus on the quadriceps/hamstring complex. Active terminal knee extension is avoided, but full passive knee extension is emphasized. As the strength ratio is normalized, crutch use is diminished and then abandoned.

Phase III continues the rehabilitation and incorporates functional brace use; and when quadriceps and hamstring strength and endurance are equal to the opposite normal side by isokinetic testing at functional speeds (>260 degrees/s), return to low to moderated demand sports is allowed. Jogging and swimming are encouraged. The role of functional knee braces in children has not been defined, and issues of brace size, fit, and cost remain. Questions about the timing of brace use are also present (i.e., full time versus only during sports activities). The patient is seen monthly for the first 6 months to assess program compliance and to rule out further knee functional alterations.

Surgical management of an isolated ACL tear in the truly skeletally immature patient is controversial.[2-4,18,19,27,33,38,47,48,54,66] In patients with what I term an "ACL plus" knee injury,[55] that is, combined ACL and meniscal injury, consensus seems to exist for surgical reconstruction in this skeletally immature patient because of the poor prognosis for meniscal repair alone in the presence of cruciate compromise. Patients with isolated ACL tears who refuse to comply with a nonoperative program and attempt to return to high-demand sports are also candidates for surgical reconstruction.[2,16,18,19,33,43,44] Concerns exist about the consequences of physeal transgression by a variety of surgical methods and the restoration of ligamentous isometry in the growing skeleton. The percentage of femoral or tibial physeal invasion, even when central, that is safe and will not produce angular and lon-

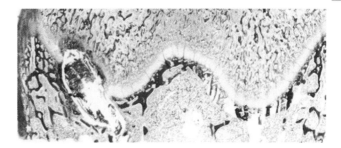

Figure 73–1. Histological section after ACl reconstruction in a lapin model. Note absence of femoral physeal arrest at graft tunnel that had been filled with a hamstring tendon.

gitudinal deformities in humans is unknown. Experimental laboratory models in various species have been used in an attempt to provide guidance.[14,17,25,53] Guzzanti and coworkers[17] used a lapin model with semitendinosus transfer through 2-mm tibial and femoral central transphyseal tunnels. Histological sections of the operative areas up to 6 months postoperatively showed no evidence of premature epiphyseodesis in the tunnels traversed by tendons (Fig. 73–1). Femoral physeal cross-sectional analysis showed 11% frontal and 3% sagittal plane involvements without alteration in length or axial deviation. Tibial cross-section analysis showed 12% frontal and 4% sagittal plane involvements. Two tibias developed valgus deformities, and one was shortened. Stadelmaier and colleagues[53] studied a small number of canines in whom a tensor fascial autograft was placed through tibial and femoral transphyseal drilled defects. In the control animal in which no fascia was placed through similar-sized defects, a transphyseal bone bridge was histologically apparent within 2 weeks after surgery. These authors also commented on the potential physeal-sparing effect of the biological material spacer in the tunnel. Janarv and colleagues[25] also used a lapin model in a pilot study to determine the true area of involvement of the drilled undulant femoral physis as well as the true area of the drill hole compared with a planar model of the physis. They found that use of the nonanatomic type of planar system underestimated the areas by 24% and 23%, respectively. In a second phase of the study, they determined that the relative size of a transphyseal drill injury required to cause a true growth disturbance was between 7% and 9%, comparable with data noted by previous investigators. They also found that free tendon grafts as well as grafts in continuity prevented bone bridge formation. However, all grafts were surrounded by a thin cylinder of bone. The remaining physeal growth may have been rapid enough to divide the cylinders and prevent bar formation. In a large graft, the authors question whether a firm cylinder of bone would cause permanent physeal effects. These authors also pointed out that in their studies as well as in other similar animal model studies, the remaining growth duration was quite brief until maturity in contrast to adolescent humans whose exposure to the effects of transphyseal surgery is more prolonged, especially in boys. Progression of physeal closure is not an acute event but rather one whose timing onset and rate are determined by multiple factors. One may consider the risk to invasion of the physis similar to a moving automobile's risk of collision. At high rates of speed, crash potential is significant. As the automobile's velocity decreases (e.g., when approaching a stop sign), the collision possibility likewise abates. Such is also true of the physis after its peak height velocity exposure. It must be pointed out that none of the animal series used transphyseal fixation techniques. Whether the effects of these quadruped models can be translated to the unique anatomy demanded by bipedal gait remains unanswered. The eventual outcome of any grafted tissue that provides the biological scaffolding for neoligament formation must be assessed in terms of the tissue's orientation, size, strength, growth, and isometric substitution potentials.

There are no data that specifically address timing of reconstruction of the acutely injured ACL in the skeletally immature patient. I like to wait 14 to 21 days to allow the initial inflammatory response to diminish and restore full passive extension. In the uncommon case of a patient with a blocked knee from a displaced meniscal tear, this delay is not possible. I use this interval to again emphasize the 6-month timeline required for recovery and return to sports, despite the contemporary accelerated rehabilitation programs, and to point out that the reinstitution of high-level sports participation after reconstruction is a function of biology and not arthroscopic technology.

ACL reconstruction requires consideration of the three Ts: tissues, tunnels, and techniques.[12,55] Autograft tissues include patellar or hamstring tendons, usually the semitendinosus with or without gracilis augmentation. Although allograft use for ACL reconstruction has been reported in adolescents,[3] concerns of potential viral transmission and sterilization effects on graft strength remain.[45] Synthetic replacement of the ACL either as an isolated structure or in combination as a ligament backup carries concerns about longevity, fixation, and foreign body synovitis from wear particles. Tunnels are technique dependent and may include grooves or drill holes in the tibial epiphysis, over-the-top femoral capsular placement,

femoral epiphyseal channels, or more vertical tibial transphyseal tunnel orientation in an attempt to improve isometry or may be via traditional tibial and femoral tunnels. In the skeletally immature patient, I consider tunnel choices as physeal sparing, partial transphyseal, or complete transphyseal.[54] Physeal-sparing techniques are used in the quite immature patient (Tanner stage 0 to I), usually one with an associated meniscal tear requiring treatment, or in the completely noncompliant patient. I use partial transphyseal procedures in the slightly more mature individual (i.e., Tanner stage II). Patients who are Tanner stage III (post peak height velocity growth, postmenarchal girls, boys with curly axillary and pubic hair) are treated by complete transphyseal techniques because their residual femoral and tibial physeal growth is very limited and any significant changes in height are due to spinal and not lower extremity growth.[7]

PHYSEAL-SPARING TECHNIQUES

These procedures attempt to provide a ligament restraint without transgressing the tibial or femoral physis. The major drawback with these methods is their inability to restore anatomic isometric placement of the neoligament. Either a distally based patellar tendon strip or medial hamstring graft in continuity is used (Fig. 73–2). Brief reported a technique using a hamstring tendon graft passed over the anterior tibia, under the meniscal coronary ligament, and affixed to the femur in an over-the-top position.[9] In his small series of patients, all who were older than age 14 years (skeletal maturity not defined) also had an extra-articular iliotibial band tenodesis. At a short follow-up period, the patients seemed to be doing well, but no functional, objective outcome data were reported. Parker and coworkers[47] described creating a groove in the proximal anterior tibial epiphysis, avoiding the physis, through which is passed a medial hamstring tendon graft that is attached to the femur in the over-the-top location

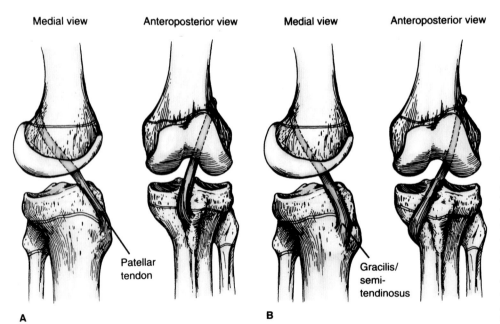

Medial view   Anteroposterior view   Medial view   Anteroposterior view

Patellar tendon

Gracilis/semi-tendinosus

A   **B**

Figure 73–2. Nontransphyseal ACL reconstruction with either (**A**) a patellar tendon segment or (**B**) a gracilis and/or semitendinosus autograft. (From Stanitski CL: ACL injury in the skeletally immature patient. J Am Acad Orthop Surg 3:153, 1995. Copyright 1995, American Academy of Orthopaedic Surgeons.)

(Fig. 73–3). The tibial groove's anterior/inferior to superior/posterior orientation was designed to place the transfer more centrally and improve its isometry (Fig. 73–4). Each of their six patients had associated meniscal tears and they were much younger than those reported by Brief.[9] In the Parker series,[47] outcomes were generally favorable at almost 2-year follow-up. Anderson[2] reported a physeal-sparing technique in 12 patients 11 to 15.9 years old (average, 13.3 years) who were observed for 2 to 8 years postoperatively (average, 4 years) (Fig. 73–5). Half the patients were Tanner III (i.e., significantly mature) at surgery. Outcomes were quite favorable by subjective and objective rating systems (Fig. 73–6). Guzzanti and coworkers[18] reported a novel physeal-sparing technique used in eight preadolescent patients with complete ACL tears (Fig. 73–7). All patients were Tanner I with a predicted average lower extremity growth of 10.8 cm. All were noncompliant with a nonoperative treatment protocol. All patients showed excellent postoperative functional scores with return to full sport activity. None had clinical or radiographic evidence of leg-length discrepancy or angular deformity (Fig. 73–8).

PARTIAL TRANSPHYSEAL TECHNIQUES

Patellar or medial hamstring tendon grafts in continuity are usually 6 to 8 mm in diameter and passed intra-articularly through a transphyseal tibial tunnel oriented more vertically than usual in an attempt to improve isometry of the reconstruction. Femoral fixation is at the over-the-top position. As with physeal-sparing techniques, the femoral attachment site must be chosen to not damage the

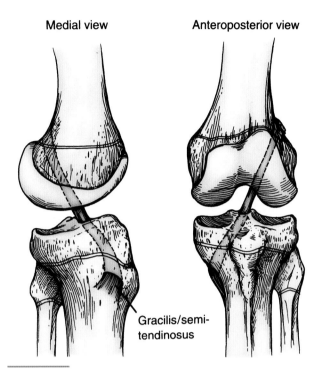

Medial view   Anteroposterior view

Gracilis/semi-tendinosus

Figure 73–3. Partial transphyseal ACL reconstruction using a hamstring (semitendinosus and/or gracilis) autograft through a transphyseal tibial tunnel with an over-the-top femoral position. A central patellar tendon autograft can be used as an alternative tissue. (From Stanitski CL: ACL injury in the skeletally immature patient. J Am Acad Orthop Surg 3:153, 1995. Copyright 1995, American Academy of Orthopaedic Surgeons.)

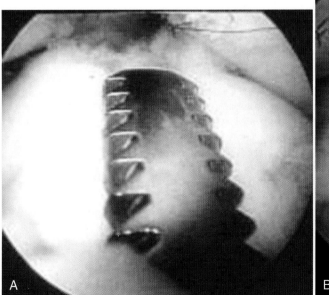
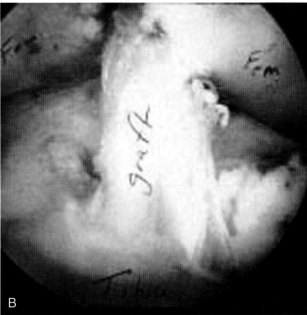

Figure 73–4. **A,** Rasp creating an anterior tibial epiphyseal groove under the transverse meniscal ligament. **B,** Transferred hamstring graft. (Courtesy of Dr. Scott Cameron, Marshfield Clinic, Marshfield, Wisconsin.)

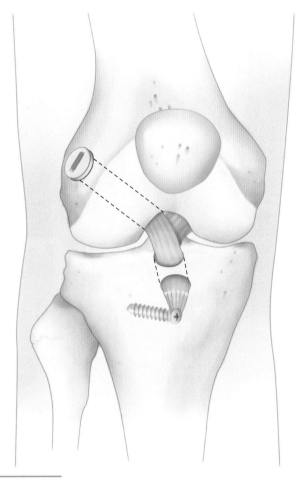

Figure 73–5. Physeal-sparing transepiphyseal ACL reconstruction. (From Anderson A: Transepiphyseal replacement of the anterior cruciate ligament in skeletally immature patients. J Bone Joint Surg Am 85:1260, 2003. Copyright of the artist, Delilah Cohn.)

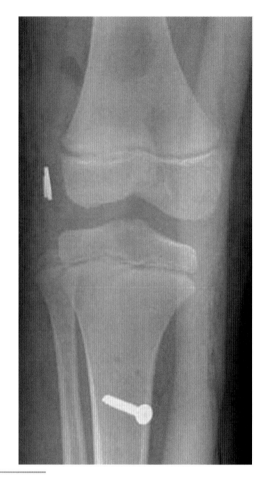

Figure 73–6. Anteroposterior radiograph of the knee of an 8-year-old boy after ACL reconstruction using the Anderson technique.

peripheral femoral physis, which is quite nearby, as shown by Behr and colleagues[6] (Fig. 73–9). Lo and associates[33] reported the largest series using this technique. Their 29 truly skeletally immature patients had excellent functional and objective measurement outcomes at follow-up that averaged more than 3 years. No clinical or radiographic evidence of limb deformity was seen. Guzzanti and coworkers[19] reported a partial transphyseal method using transepiphyseal tibial and transphyseal femoral tunnels for a 6-mm hamstring graft in 14 adolescents (Fig. 73–10). All were asymptomatic postoperatively and returned to full sport activities. The femoral tunnel represented less than 7% of the frontal plane and less than 1% of the transverse plane cross-sectional area of the femoral physis. No longitudinal or angular deformities were found at an average follow-up of 40 months, with a minimal 24-month follow-up (Fig. 73–11).

COMPLETE TRANSPHYSEAL TECHNIQUES

ACL reconstruction using complete transphyseal methods is the equivalent of adult-type procedures and is done in patients with advanced skeletal maturity (i.e., Tanner stage III or higher). McCarroll and coworkers[38] reported good results from complete transphyseal reconstructions in mature adolescents. In light of these outstanding results after reconstruction by this highly experienced group of knee surgeons, temporization on reconstruction in the immature patient was advocated by them until the patient was mature enough to undergo a complete transphyseal procedure. Compliance issues continue to plague all nonoperative program attempts.

Graft choice is surgeon dependent and may be a patellar bone/patellar tendon/tibial bone construct or a multistrand medial hamstring configuration.[64] Restitution of the normal anteromedial bundle to control sagittal translation and the posterolateral bundle for rotational balance is the goal of current four-strand hamstring reconstructions. Graft fixations are by intra-articular or extra-articular and intra-tunnel or extra-tunnel methods.

Postoperative Rehabilitation Program

The rehabilitation program is physiologically designed to minimize deleterious effects of immobilization, disuse, and misuse and to encourage maturation of the neoligament and its attachments through physiologically toler-

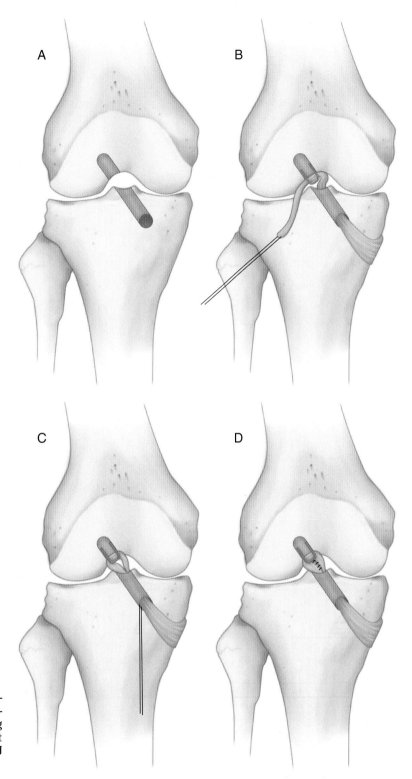

Figure 73–7. **A** to **D,** Guzzanti's physeal-sparing technique. (From Guzzanti V, Falciglia F, Stanitski CL: Physeal-sparing intraarticular anterior cruciate ligament reconstruction in preadolescents. Am J Sports Med 31:951, 2003.)

ated stresses. Progression to the next phase of the program occurs once objective criteria are achieved. The four-phase program I use[12,55] emphasizes restoration of range of motion and weightbearing; muscle strengthening; increases of speed, agility, power, and endurance; and sports readiness activities. Specific functional objectives must be met before returning to sports.

Phase I occurs immediately postoperative to 6 weeks. A knee immobilizer brace is set from −30 to 90 degrees and

worn during the day. The patient is encouraged to progressively increase weightbearing with crutch protection with the goal to be crutch free by 6 weeks. Modification of weightbearing and amount of knee flexion is done if concomitant meniscal reconstruction is performed. Active knee flexion is done within the brace's arc of motion. Out-of-brace passive knee extension is done four times daily, with emphasis on maintaining full extension. Closed-chain lower extremity–resisted exercises are incorporated

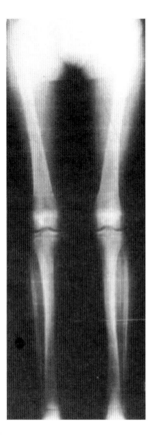

Figure 73–8. Postoperative teleoroentgenogram of the knee of a boy aged 11 years, 9 months at 2 years after Guzzanti reconstruction. Note incorporation of the staple into the lateral condyle. (From Guzzanti V, Falciglia F, Stanitski CL: Physeal-sparing intraarticular anterior cruciate ligament reconstruction in preadolescents. Am J Sports Med 31:952, 2003.)

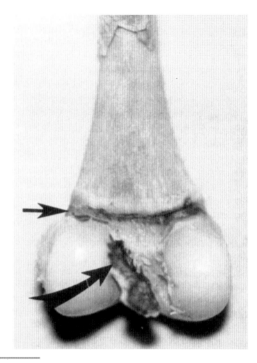

Figure 73–9. Note proximity of femoral lateral physis to proposed fixation point of ACL graft transfer. (*straight arrow* points to the lateral femoral epiphsis; *curved arrow* points to the origin of the ACL.) (From Behr CT, Potter GA, Paletta GA: The relationship of the femoral origin of the anterior cruciate ligament and the distal femoral physeal plate in the skeletally immature knee: An anatomical study. Am J Sports Med 29:782, 2001.)

for hip flexors and abductors and the gastrocnemius-soleus complex.

Phase II, at 6 to 12 weeks postoperatively, emphasizes restoring lower extremity muscle strength and endurance using a closed-chain, isokinetic program. At the end of this portion, quadriceps strength should be at least two-thirds of the opposite quadriceps by isokinetic testing at 120 degrees/s from −30 to 120 degrees of motion, and knee motion should be full.

In phase IIIA, at 12 to 18 weeks postoperatively, a functional brace is used and straight-line running is begun on level ground. As quadriceps/hamstring strength ratio is normalized, agility drills begin. Quadriceps strength should be 75% to 80% of normal at the end of this phase.

In phase IIIB, at 18 to 24 weeks postoperatively, advanced agility drills are added as lower extremity strength and endurance are normalized. In the final part of this phase, sports-specific tasks are introduced and are done at progressively higher speeds.

Phase IV occurs at 24 weeks and beyond. Return to full sport participation is permitted when full, painless motion is present and strength, endurance, stability, and agility are equal to that of the opposite normal side. Functional bracing is continued during sports for 6 months, usually at the athlete's request as a security measure.

The rehabilitation program is modified according to delays present in any phase. No specific complication management results have been presented in large numbers after ACL reconstruction of skeletally immature patients. Complications similar to ones seen in adults can be expected and include loss of motion, fibroarthrosis, and donor and insertion site problems. With introduction of current early motion and aggressive rehabilitation programs, problems of loss of motion are uncommon. The spectre of creating limb length, rotation, and angular deformities exists if imprudent decision making (inadequate assessment of physiological age, inappropriate surgical choice) or technical surgical errors (improper graft position, excessively large grafts, transphyseal bone or hardware) result in physeal compromise. Experimental and limited clinical data suggest that such growth complications are uncommon if appropriate indications and surgical approaches are observed.[2,18,19,33,47] General principles of management include the following: (1) bony avulsions should be anatomically reduced and fixed; (2) direct repair of intrasubstance lesions and extra-articular reconstructions are not successful; (3) excessive dissection for exposure for fixation should be avoided near physes, especially femoral; (4) transphyseal tunnels should be the smallest diameter and located centrally if possible with soft-tissue grafts placed in them without any transphyseal hardware or bone blocks; (5) assessment and definition of physiological age and growth remaining is essential for treatment planning; and (6) long-term follow-up to skele-

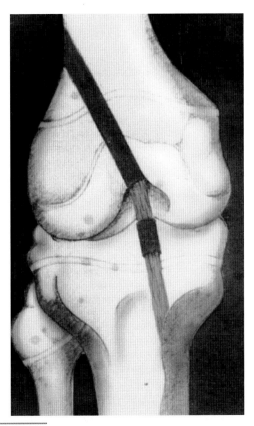

Figure 73–10. Partial transphyseal ACL reconstruction described by Guzzanti. (From Guzzanti V, Falciglia F, Stanitski CL: Preoperative evaluation and anterior cruciate ligament reconstruction technique for skeletally immature patients in Tanner stages 2 and 3. Am J Sports Med 31:944, 2003.)

tal maturity is required to be sure angular and/or length deformities do not occur.

In summary, skeletally immature patients do get ACL injuries and decisions regarding treatment must include the patient's physiological age and amount of growth remaining at the two major lower extremity physes. Non-operative treatment requires counseling about avoidance of high-demand sports that would lead to further intra-articular injury and premature joint senescence. If meniscal tears requiring surgical management occur, concomitant with a complete ACL tear, surgical reconstruction of both structures is recommended, tailoring the ACL technique appropriate for the patient's maturity. Three types of ACL reconstruction are considered: physeal sparing, partial transphyseal, and complete transphyseal. Each case must be assessed independently based on the patient's anatomic and physiological assets and liabilities.

TIBIAL EMINENCE AVULSION FRACTURES IN SKELETALLY IMMATURE PATIENTS

Avulsion fractures of the tibial intercondylar eminence occur because of the modulus mismatch present between the ACL and its insertion to the tibial proximal chondroepiphysis, especially in the 8- to 12-year age group.

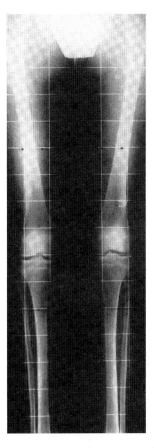

Figure 73–11. Postoperative radiograph of the legs of a 14-year-old boy at 30 months after partial transphyseal ACL reconstruction by the Guzzanti method. Note new staple position due to growth away from the femoral distal physis and no physeal deformity. (From Guzzanti V, Falciglia F, Stanitski CL: Preoperative evaluation and anterior cruciate ligament reconstruction technique for skeletally immature patients in Tanner stages 2 and 3. Am J Sports Med 31:946, 2003.)

This age spread reflects the progressive relative physiological skeletal maturity seen in this chronological span. The mechanism of injury is almost always knee hyperflexion, particularly associated with falls from a bicycle. Unfortunately, fractures of the tibial eminence have been dismissed as the "juvenile ACL injury" and true ACL tears are often misdiagnosed as commented on in the previous section. The natural history and outcome of the skeletally immature patient with a tibial eminence fracture are in marked counterdistinction from their counterpart with a complete ACL tear.

Patients with an acute tibial eminence avulsion fracture present with acute knee pain, limited knee motion from guarding due to pain, or true mechanical obstruction by the displaced fragment. Tenderness may be diffuse, but examination of the joint lines, collateral ligament areas, and femoral and tibial physes helps to identify other sites of associated injury. Because of the acuity of the injury and its attendant diminished patient cooperation with the clinical examination because of pain, muscle spasm, and guarding, associated sagittal laxity may not be appreciated at the initial assessment.

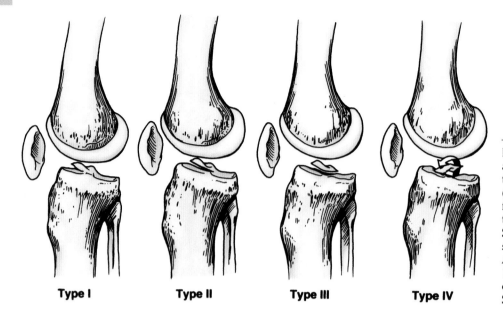

Figure 73–12. Tibial eminence avulsion fracture classification. Type III may be rotated (III+), and type IV represents fragment displacement, rotation, and comminution. (From Stanitski CL: ACL injury in the skeletally immature patient. J Am Acad Orthop Surg 3:151, 1995. Copyright 1995, American Academy of Orthopaedic Surgeons.)

Type I   Type II   Type III   Type IV

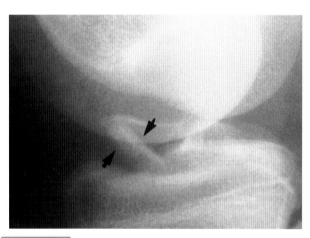

Figure 73–13. Lateral radiograph of a tibial eminence fracture in a 16-year-old boy. Note the well-defined cortical margins (*arrows*) of the fragment due to his maturity.

Standard four-view knee radiographs are the primary imaging studies, taking particular effort to ensure that a true lateral view is accomplished so classification of the injury can be done. It has been suggested that the tibial intercondylar eminence be considered as four distinct anatomic regions: medial and lateral "intercondylar tubercles or spines" and anterior and posterior "intercondylar areas or recesses."[1] The ACL footprint is situated between the lateral and medial meniscal anterior attachments in the anterior medial intercondylar recess. The anterior attachment of the lateral meniscus is posterior to the ACL insertion. Because of the often significant chondral segment of the fracture fragment, the injury may be dismissed as being only a small chip and the true extent of the damage underestimated. I find that the anteroposterior and tunnel views usually provide better data about fragment rotation and comminution than does the lateral radiograph. More sophisticated imaging methods (e.g., computed tomography [CT] and MRI) are usually not required and do not add a significant factor in the treatment decision. The initial radiographic classification of this injury dealt only with sagittal displacement of the fragment.[41] The classification was modified to encompass not only the amount of fragment sagittal displacement but also the fragment comminution and rotation to give a more accurate description of the lesion.[67] Fracture types indicate progressive increase in fragment sagittal displacement, with type I being the most benign and type IV representing significant displacement, rotation, and comminution (Fig. 73–12). Type I has minimal displacement (<3 mm); type II has an anterior flap elevation of one-third to one-half of the fragment; type III has sagittal and usually rotational displacement of the entire fragment; and type IV has comminution of the completely displaced fragment (Fig. 73–13). Cases with fracture metaphyseal extension may be seen (Fig. 73–14).

The outcome of tibial eminence avulsion fractures is usually quite good, with rapid healing and few functional complaints despite varying amounts of residual sagittal plane laxity and slight limitation of extension demonstrated on follow-up examination.[1,24,40,62,63,65,67] Even though patients were skeletally mature at follow-up in several series, they were still quite young and had not undergone the vocational and avocational stresses and demands of advancing age. With current enhanced techniques of diagnosis, associated injuries are being recognized with increasing frequency especially in type III and IV fractures. Medial collateral and meniscal (usually medial) damage has been reported in 4% to 20% of tibial eminence fracture cases[8,26,40,62] No data have been reported that specifically look at the outcome of patients with these associated injuries because these patients' outcomes were incorporated in the ones without associated injuries. Kocher and colleagues[26] retrospectively reviewed 80 immature patients with 57 type III and 23 type II surgically treated tibial eminence fractures, the latter nonreducible in extension. They found entrapment of the anterior horn of the medial (most common) or lateral meniscus or the intermeniscal ligament in 26% of type II and 65% of type III fractures.

Tibial eminence fractures represent a combination injury that includes ACL attenuation and chondroepiphy-

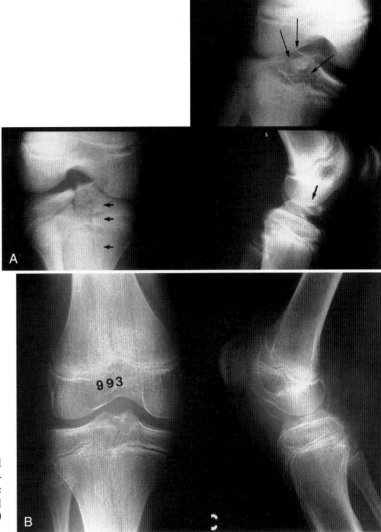

Figure 73–14. **A,** Radiographs of type III tibial eminence fracture with comminution and metaphyseal extension in an 8-year-old boy. (*Arrows* point to fracture line in epiphysis, physis, and metaphysis.) **B,** Radiographic appearance at 10 months after surgery.

seal fracture. Treatment of tibial eminence avulsion fractures depends on the fracture classification and associated injuries. In undisplaced, uncomplicated type I fractures, if the knee cannot be placed in full extension, local anesthetic is injected intra-articularly after hemarthrosis evacuation to allow full extension. Controversy exists as to the optimal knee casted position (i.e., full extension versus 30 degrees of flexion) to diminish ACL tension.[8,23,40,62,63,65] I use full extension and avoid hyperextension, which is painful and unnecessary. Placement in 30 degrees of knee flexion in a patient whose ACL is already attenuated does not seem to make physiological sense to me. The concept of knee extension for fracture reduction was advocated to allow fragment reduction by femoral condylar impingement on the fragment. This mechanism may be true for the uncommon case with fragments with large basilar extensions into the lateral and medial tibial compartments. In the majority of cases, fragments do not come into contact with the femoral condyles and reduction and maintenance of the reduction are effected by impingement of the fragment by the femoral intercondylar notch (Fig. 73–15). In type I cases, I immobilize the patient for 4 weeks in a cylinder cast with progressive weightbearing

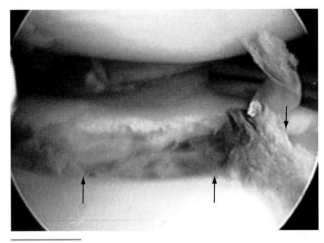

Figure 73–15. Medial compartment extension of a type II fracture. (*Arrows* indicate the articular and subchondral margins.)

with initial crutch-protected gait. Repeat lateral radiographs are done at weekly intervals for the first 2 weeks to ensure that the reduction is maintained. In type II fractures, reduction is done to prevent residual fragment deformity that may prevent full knee extension. After knee aspiration and intra-articular injection of local anesthetic, the knee is placed in extension and confirmation of reduction is done by a true lateral knee radiograph. A bolster is used at the ankle to provide knee extension and lateral

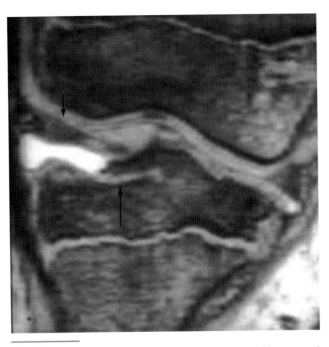

Figure 73–16. MR image of type II fracture with effusion and meniscus *(short arrow)* above the fracture site *(long arrow)*.

support at the knee and to prevent the tendency of the limb to externally rotate during the exposure. If anatomic fracture restoration within 2 mm is achieved, cylinder casting treatment is done for 6 weeks with progressive weightbearing with initial crutch protection. Repeat radiographs are done weekly for the first 2 weeks to document maintenance of fracture reduction. If anatomic reduction is not achieved, I recommend arthroscopic assessment of the fracture to ascertain the reason for fracture malreduction. At surgery, the meniscus (usually medial in my experience) is commonly found trapped in the fracture site (Figs. 73–16 and 73–17). A probe easily removes this obstruction to reduction. Meniscal stability and continuity need to be addressed as well. Knee extension is then achieved, and if the fragment is well reduced and no other associated injuries are present intra-articularly, the limb is incorporated in a cylinder cast with the knee in extension and the post-cast fracture reduction confirmed by lateral radiograph. If significant comminution of the fragment is present or anatomic restoration of reduction cannot be achieved, arthroscopic reduction and fixation of the fracture is carried out by techniques used for type III and IV fractures.

In type III or IV tibial eminence fractures, fracture reduction and fixation can be done by traditional arthrotomy or by arthroscopic techniques.[1,8,31,62,67] Meniscal injuries are dealt with by established principles and techniques, taking into account the meniscal injury's site, size, and stability. Fragment reduction is done by probe manipulation after any obstructions are removed from the fracture site, and fragment reduction is maintained using an ACL guide. If the fragment is large enough (>1 × 1 cm) and without comminution, fixation can be done using a cannulated screw placed through a percutaneous proximal-medial approach, taking care to not violate the proximal tibial physis.[1,8,62] The head of the screw (usually

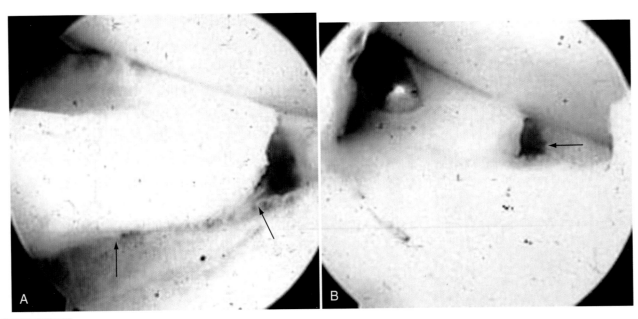

Figure 73–17. **A,** Arthroscopic view of medial meniscus trapped in the fracture site. **B,** Fracture reduction after elevation of meniscus.

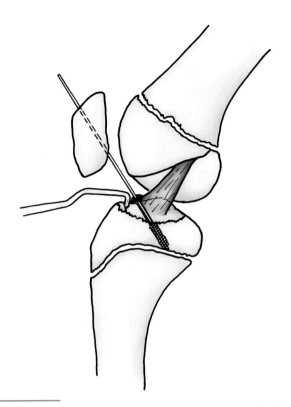

Figure 73–18. Percutaneous fixation of an acute tibial eminence avulsion fracture using a cannulated small fragment screw after arthroscopic fracture reduction. The guide pin is started medially at the upper pole of the patella. Note the prevention of physeal transgression of the fixation system. (From Wall EJ: Tibial eminence fractures in children. Op Tech Sp Med 6:209, 1998.)

< 20 mm) should be seated within the ACL base to avoid impingement in extension (Fig. 73–18). Countersinking the fragment into the epiphysis in an attempt to restore isometry to the attenuated ligament is not recommended. Type IV comminuted fractures do not lend themselves to screw fixation and are repaired using suture methods about the ACL bone "stump."[7,31,62] Once again, care is taken to avoid physeal damage with suture passage through the tibial epiphysis (Fig. 73–19). Postoperatively, patients with type III and IV fractures are immobilized in a cylinder cast with the knee in extension and crutch-protected weightbearing gait used initially. Lateral knee radiographs are done weekly for the first 2 weeks to document maintenance of fracture reduction. If the fracture fragment was large and noncomminuted and the fixation solid, immobilization is done for only 4 weeks, followed by use of controlled motion brace, similar to the ones used after ACL reconstruction. In cases with tenuous screw fixation, or in those requiring suture fixation because of fracture comminution, immobilization is continued for 6 weeks.

Complications after tibial eminence fracture are uncommon but include loss of extension, arthrofibrosis, fracture malunion, and nonunion with late re-avulsion. The period of immobilization should be as brief as is compatible with fracture healing and, in non–internally fixed fractures, is usually 6 weeks. Postimmobilization rehabilitation is similar to the type used after ACL reconstruction with emphasis on restoration of full extension. Arthrofibrosis with loss of flexion and extension may occur as a consequence of the inflammatory synovial response to the injury and associated hemarthrosis. If progressive gains in knee range of motion are not seen within the first month after immobilization with a stable fracture, arthroscopic lysis and débridement of adhesions should be done with postoperative caudal analgesia provided to allow aggressive rehabilitation. Knee manipulation should be avoided in these children because of the potential for femoral or tibial physeal fractures, especially in the post-immobilization period (Fig. 73–20). If symptomatic loss of knee extension occurs from eminence fracture malunion, notchplasty is done to eliminate impingement.

In summary, skeletally immature patients with tibial eminence fractures tend to do quite well. This injury should be suspected in 8- to 12-year-old patients with an acute knee injury from a fall from a bicycle. Minor loss of extension and sagittal plane laxity are often seen at follow-up but do not cause functional limitations, in general. In the relatively small percentage of patients with associated rotatory instability, the mechanism of injury (i.e., flexion/rotation) caused damage to the secondary restraints with resultant combined instability. This is in contrast to the direct flexion mechanism, which preserves the secondary capsular restraints. Associated meniscal and collateral ligament injuries should be sought, especially in older patients. Treatment is dependent on fracture type, with reduction and fixation needed for the more advanced types. Arthroscopic techniques of fracture reduction and fixation usually produce excellent outcomes. Because the fracture occurs through a chondroepiphysis, awareness of the potential for physeal injury with imprecise fixation methods must be kept in mind.

POSTERIOR CRUCIATE INJURY IN SKELETALLY IMMATURE PATIENTS

Disruption of the posterior cruciate ligament (PCL) is rare in adults, representing only 3% of all adult knee ligament injuries[21,51,61] and is so extremely rare in the skeletally immature patient as to warrant case reports.[10,13,34,37,50,52] In Ringer and Fay's 1990 literature review of PCL injury in children,[49] they accumulated 21 cases in patients younger than 16 years old and added 2 of their own cases in patients aged 5 and 12 years. Most cases were femoral avulsion injuries with attached bone fragments and not midsubstance tears. Follow-up in reported cases has been quite short, and almost all cases had limited objective functional outcome data. The prevalence and incidence of PCL injury in the immature patient is unknown, as is the natural history. Lateral and posterolateral corner ligament injuries commonly occur in conjunction with PCL injuries in adults and have been reported in maturing adolescents.[21,51,61] Minimal data are present regarding such injuries, either isolated or associated with a PCL injury, in truly skeletally immature patients. MacDonald and associates[37] report a 6-year-old boy with a midsubstance PCL tear treated nonoperatively who, after an asymptomatic

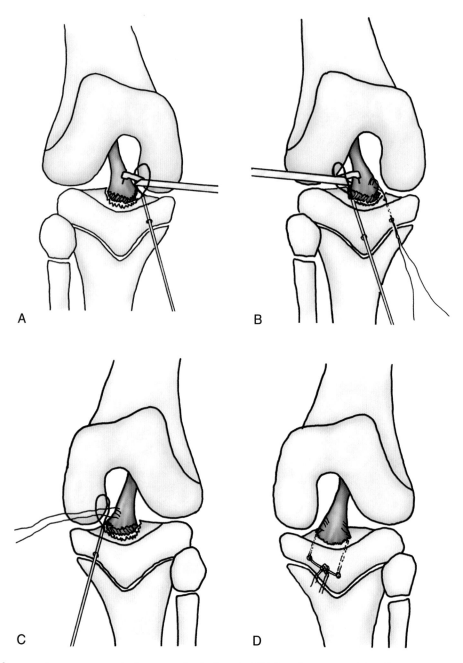

Figure 73–19. Arthroscopic management of a comminuted acute tibial eminence avulsion fracture not amenable to screw fixation. A ligament suture passer is placed through the epiphysis (**A** to **C**), sparing the physis; the sutures provide reduction and fixation when tied over the anterior tibial epiphysis (**D**). (From Wall EJ: Tibial eminence fractures in children. Op Tech Sp Med 6:209, 1998.)

interval, developed a feeling of "looseness" in his knee with a positive reverse pivot shift test, increased tibial external rotation, a small medial meniscal tear, and anterior knee pain 5 years later.

The mechanism of injury varies. Position of the knee at the time of injury dictates the type of tear. A significant amount of anatomic research about the PCL has been done by Harner and colleagues,[20,21] who defined components within the PCL based on the ligament's tensioning characteristics as a function of knee flexion and extension. The anterolateral bundle is the largest segment (twice the size of the posteromedial bundle), and its tension rises with increasing knee flexion. The smaller posteromedial bundle becomes taut in knee extension. The role of the third component, the meniscofemoral ligaments of Humphry (anterior) and Wrisberg (posterior)—one of which is found in about two-thirds of adults—in knee stability is still undefined despite this segment being stronger than the PCL's posterior medial bundle. It is uncommon for both meniscofemoral ligaments to be present. These three units blend to form the nonisometric PCL complex, which is the major restraint to posterior tibial displacement with a secondary function, along with the posterolateral ligament complex, of resisting tibial external rotation. A strong

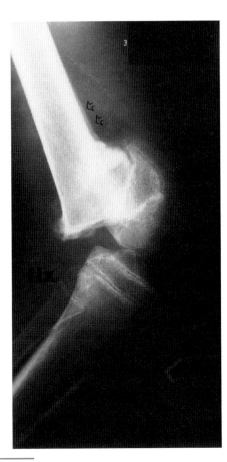

Figure 73–20. Distal femoral physeal displaced fracture after knee manipulation 8 weeks after reduction of a type II eminence fracture and 4 weeks after cast removal.

functional interaction occurs between the PCL and the posterolateral ligament complex as evaluated by the reverse pivot shift with the knee in 30 degrees of flexion. Hyperextension injury is often associated with playground merry-go-rounds where the foot is trapped, the knee extended, and rotation is continued, producing hyperextension. Hyperflexion injury is often caused by a fall with the ankle in plantarflexion and a direct blow to the anterior tibia. The anterolateral bundle's tension in flexion and its broad base on the femur commonly results in a PCL avulsion, usually with a bone or perichondral femoral fragment from knee hyperflexion. Posterior directed forces with the knee in extension are thought to cause midsubstance tears and not terminal avulsions.

Clinical Evaluation

Proper diagnosis is essential because the mechanism of injury of a PCL may be associated with a knee dislocation and not an isolated PCL tear. The patient usually complains of pain about the knee and will not bear weight on the affected limb nor will he or she actively move the knee through an arc of motion. Posterior midline tenderness is seen at the popliteal fossa. Lateral posterior tenderness may also be present with an associated posterolateral

corner injury. There is usually a minimal, delayed effusion with an isolated disruption of the PCL. A significant effusion may indicate a peripheral meniscal disruption or associated ACL tear. Distal neural, motor, and vascular status must be repeatedly documented to rule out compromise. The classic posterior drawer sign may be elicited along with the posterior sag or "ski-slope" sign with the knee flexed to 90 degrees and the tibia directed posteriorly, with its lack of posterior stability resulting in a concavity at the patellar tendon and proximal tibia. One must be sure to not be misled while performing the anterior drawer test and mistakenly interpret the tibial sagittal translation from posterior to the midline caused by a deficient PCL as an ACL tear with tibial anterior translation, the so-called false anterior drawer test. As with other clinical ligament stability tests, the quality of the endpoint must be evaluated in addition to any abnormal translation. Rubenstein and colleagues[51] reviewed 39 adults with varying grades of chronic PCL injury and found 96% accuracy, 90% sensitivity, and 99% specificity of diagnosis with clinical evaluation. Accuracy was highest for more advanced grades of injury. This group found the posterior drawer test to be the most sensitive and specific test, especially when the drop-off between the femur and tibia was palpated during the test. The quadriceps "active" drawer test is done with the affected knee and hip at 90 degrees and the foot stabilized by the examiner. The patient attempts to slide the foot distally by contracting the quadriceps. In a PCL-compromised knee, the quadriceps contraction causes anterior tibial translation to the neutral position, which is visible to the examiner. Physical examination should also assess other possible intra-articular injuries, such as meniscal tears, which are uncommon with an isolated PCL lesion. Integrity of the posterolateral corner ligamentous complex is assessed by the reverse pivot shift test and other standard maneuvers.

Imaging

Routine radiographs must be of high quality with emphasis on correct positioning of the lateral view to detect an avulsion fragment from the femur or tibia. Sagittal radiographic stress views may aid in diagnosis (Fig. 73–21). In young patients with significant chondral segments of their distal femoral and proximal tibial epiphyses, MR images can be useful to localize the site of injury. More mature patients usually have intrasubstance tears, also identifiable by MRI (Fig. 73–22).

Treatment

Treatment is based on precise diagnosis of the locus of injury. If an isolated avulsion injury occurs with a bone or cartilage fragment sufficient to allow anatomic restitution and fixation, surgical repair is done, taking care not to violate the respective femoral or tibial physis. For midsubstance tears, nonoperative treatment is preferred, as long as the diagnosis is not complicated with intra-

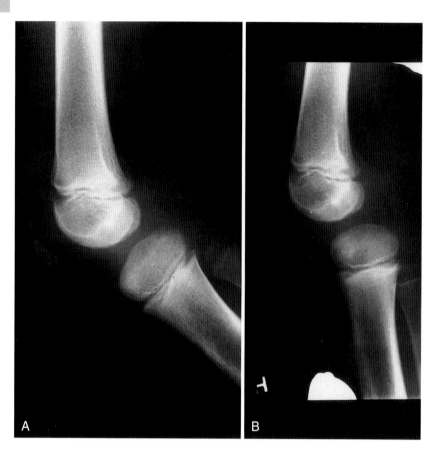

Figure 73–21. Radiographs of the knee of a 6-year old boy in flexion (**A**) and extension (**B**) with posterior drawer stress demonstrating posterior tibial translation due to femoral chondral avulsion of the PCL.

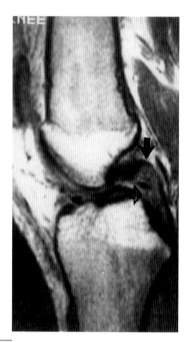

Figure 73–22. MR image of a 16-year-old boy's intrasubstance tear (*arrows*) of his PCL, which occurred from a posteriorly directed force with his knee in extension.

articular injury. Patients with midsubstance isolated PCL injuries are treated with cast immobilization in extension (avoiding hyperextension) for 3 weeks and then fitted with a controlled arc of motion brace that limits flexion to less than 70 degrees for an additional 3 weeks. Cast changes during this initial phase are dictated by changes in leg volume and must accommodate the knee to maintain extension and disallow posterior tibial sag. Partial protected weightbearing is allowed during these initial 6 weeks. Progressive restoration of knee motion and lower extremity muscle strength is done, but high-resistance open-chain hamstring and quadriceps exercises are avoided for 3 months.[61]

OUTCOMES

The data on the natural outcome of the PCL-compromised knee in adults are short term and quite varied. There are no long-term follow-up studies in skeletally immature patients, probably because of the rarity of the injury. Lobenhoffer and associates[34] reported a PCL reconstruction in a 3-year old with chronic femoral chondral PCL and meniscofemoral ligament avulsion injuries with 10 mm of posterior tibial displacement. Transepiphyseal tibial and femoral tunnels were used for a 2.2-mm graft. At 2-year follow-up, the patient was asymptomatic and the tunnels remained radiographically evident. No data were given regarding preoperative symptoms, function, and indications for surgery, nor were postoperative objective functional measures mentioned. The small tunnel and graft size may preclude later physeal growth abnormality, but a significant growth exposure time remains. Frank and Strother[13] reported a symptomatic 8-year-old boy with a chronic PCL injury associated with an avulsed femoral fragment. Treatment was by fragment excision. Instability remained 1 year after injury with a positive posterior drawer, active quadriceps PCL, and posterior sag tests. At follow up 2.5 years later, at age 10.5 years, the patient was asymptomatic and actively participated in karate and soccer. His clinical examination was normal except for a positive posterior sag sign. Nonstress knee radiographs were normal. Sanders and colleagues[52] reported two patients, 6 and 8 years old, with PCL injuries associated with a playground merry-go-round producing a hyperextension injury. In both cases, avulsion of the PCL occurred from the femur with varying amounts of bone and cartilage. In the older child, a tear of the meniscotibial ligament produced a peripheral medial meniscal tear. After direct fragment fixation in both cases and, in one case, meniscotibial ligament repair, the knees were fixed with crossed pins for stabilization. In the younger child's case, at 2 years follow up, he was essentially asymptomatic at normal activity but had a 5-degree loss of extension and lacked 15 degrees of full flexion. The older child had no follow-up data reported. MacDonald and coworkers[37] report a midsubstance PCL complete tear in a 6-year-old boy after a fall from a trampoline. The exact mechanism of injury could not be ascertained. He was treated without a formal rehabilitation program, immobilization, or sports limitation. Three months after injury he was asymptomatic but had persistence of posterior sag and false-positive anterior drawer signs. At evaluation 5 years after injury, at age 11 years, he complained of recent-onset anterior knee pain and a feeling of occasional knee laxity. In addition to persistence of positive posterior sag and false anterior drawer signs, increased external tibial rotation and a positive reversed pivot shift sign had developed. Repeat MRI showed the chronic PCL tear with evidence of a new, small, partial radial tear of the medial meniscus. Development of posterolateral laxity with anterior knee pain and a medial meniscal tear in the interim is cause of concern for early progressive asymmetric intra-articular loading, possibly leading to premature joint senescence.

The primary complication of an acute PCL tear is misdiagnosis. The injury may be missed completely or incorrectly diagnosed as an ACL injury, as noted in the previous section on clinical evaluation. Cases of PCL tibial avulsion fractures associated with femoral shaft fractures have been reported in 10- and 12-year-old boys[15] and remind us that evaluation of knee stability is paramount after stabilization of femoral and tibial fractures. A more ominous error occurs when a traumatic knee dislocation, although admittedly extremely rare in children, is not recognized because of spontaneous reduction and neural and vascular compromise ensues.

References

1. Accousti WK, Willis RB: Tibial eminence fractures. Orthop Clin North Am 34:365-375, 2003.

2. Anderson AF: Transepiphyseal replacement of the anterior cruciate ligament in skeletally immature patients: A preliminary report. J Bone Joint Surg Am 85:1255-1263, 2003.

3. Andrews M, Noyes FR, Barber-Westin SD: Anterior cruciate ligament allograft reconstruction in the skeletally immature athlete. Am J Sports Med 22:48-54, 1994.

4. Andrish JT: Anterior cruciate ligament injuries in the skeletally immature patient. Am J Orthop 30:103-110, 2001.

5. Angel KR, Hall DJ: Anterior cruciate ligament injury in children and adolescents. Arthroscopy 5:197-200, 1989.

6. Behr CT, Potter HG, Paletta GA Jr: The relationship of the femoral origin of the anterior cruciate ligament and the distal femoral physeal plate in the skeletally immature knee: An anatomic study. Am J Sports Med 29:781-787, 2001.

7. Berg EE: Comminuted tibial eminence anterior cruciate ligament avulsion fractures: Failure of arthroscopic treatment. Arthroscopy 9:446-450, 1993.

8. Berg EE: Pediatric tibial eminence fractures: Arthroscopic cannulated screw fixation. Arthroscopy 11:328-331, 1995.

9. Brief LP: Anterior cruciate ligament reconstruction without drill holes. Arthroscopy 7:350-357, 1991.

10. Clanton TO, DeLee JC, Snaders B, Neidre A: Knee ligament injuries in children. J Bone Joint Surg Am 61:1195-1201, 1979.

11. Dimeglio A: Growth in pediatric orthopaedics. J Pediatr Orthop 21:549-555, 2001.

12. Dorizas JA, Stanitski CL: Anterior cruciate ligament injury in the skeletally immature. Orthop Clin North Am 34:355-363, 2003.

13. Frank C, Strother R: Isolated posterior cruciate ligament injury in a child: Literature review and a case report. Can J Surg 32:373-374, 1989.

14. Garces GL, Mugica-Garay I, Lopez-Conzalez Coviella N, Guerado E: Growth-plate modifications after drilling. J Pediatr Orthop 14:225-228, 1994.

15. Goodrich A, Ballard A: Posterior cruciate ligament avulsion associated with ipsilateral femur fracture in a 10-year-old child. J Trauma 28:1393-1396, 1988.

16. Graf BK, Lange RH, Fujisaki CK, et al: Anterior cruciate ligament tears in skeletally immature patients. Meniscal pathology at presentation and after attempted conservative treatment. Arthroscopy 8:229-233, 1992.

17. Guzzanti V, Falciglia F, Gigante A, Fabbriciani C: The effect of intraarticular ACL reconstruction on the growth plates of rabbits. J Bone Joint Surg Br 76:960-963, 1994.

18. Guzzanti V, Falciglia F, Stanitski CL: Physeal-sparing intraarticular anterior cruciate ligament reconstruction in preadolescents. Am J Sports Med 31:949-953, 2003.

19. Guzzanti V, Falciglia F, Stanitski CL: Preoperative evaluation and anterior cruciate ligament reconstruction technique for skeletally immature patients in Tanner stages 2 and 3. Am J Sports Med 31:941-948, 2003.

20. Harner CD, Xerogeanes JW, Livesay GA, et al: The human posterior cruciate ligament complex: An interdisciplinary study: Ligament morphology and biomechanical evaluation. Am J Sports Med 23:736-745, 1995.

21. Harner CD, Hoher J: Evaluation and treatment of posterior cruciate ligament injuries. Am J Sports Med 26:471-482, 1998.

22. Hewett TE, Myer GD, Ford KR: Decrease in neuromuscular control about the knee with maturation in female athletes. J Bone Joint Surg Am 86:1601-1608, 2004.

23. Janarv PM: Anterior cruciate ligament injuries in skeletally immature patients. J Pediatr Orthop 16:673-677, 1996.

24. Janarv PM, Westblad P, Johannsson C, Hirsch G: Long-term follow-up of anterior tibial spine fractures in children. J Pediatr Orthop 15:63-68, 1995.

25. Janarv PM, Wikstrom B, Hirsch G: The influence of transphyseal drilling and tendon grafting on bone growth: An experimental study in the rabbit. J Pediatr Orthop 18:149-154, 1998.

26. Kocher MS, Micheli LS, Gerbino P, Hresko MT: Tibial eminence fractures in children. Prevalence of meniscal entrapment. Am J Sports Med 31:404-407, 2003.

27. Kocher MS, Micheli LJ, Zurakowski D, Luke A: Partial tears of the anterior cruciate ligament in children and adolescents. Am J Sports Med 30:697-703, 2002.

28. Kocher MS, Saxon HS, Hovis WD, Hawkins RJ: Management and complications of ACL injuries in skeletally immature patients:

Survey of the Herodicus Society and the ACL study group. J Pediatr Orthop 22:452-457, 2002.

29. Kocher MS, Saxon HS, Hovis WD, Hawkins RJ: Anterior cruciate ligament injury versus tibial spine fracture in the skeletally immature knee: A comparison of skeletal maturation and notch width index. J Pediatr Orthop 24:185-188, 2004.

30. Kocher MS, Steadman JR, Briggs KK, et al: Relationships between objective assessment of ligament stability and subjective assessment of symptoms and function after anterior cruciate ligament reconstruction. Am J Sports Med 32:629-634, 2004.

31. Kogan MG, Marks P, Amendola A: Technique for arthroscopic suture fixation of displaced tibial intercondylar eminence fractures. Arthroscopy 13:301-306, 1997.

32. Larson MD, Ulmer T: Ligament injuries in children. AAOS Instruct Course Lect 52:677-681, 2003.

33. Lo IK, Kirkley A, Fowler PJ, Miniaci A: The outcome of operatively treated anterior cruciate ligament disruptions in the skeletally immature child. Arthroscopy 13:627-634, 1997.

34. Lobenhoffer P, Wunsch L, Bosch U, Krettek C: Arthroscopic repair of the posterior cruciate ligament in a 3-year-old child. Arthroscopy 13:248-253, 1997.

35. Logan MC, Williams A, Lavelle J, et al: Tibiofemoral kinematics following successful anterior cruciate ligament reconstruction using dynamic multiple resonance imaging. Am J Sports Med 32:984-992, 2004.

36. Logan MC, Williams A, Lavelle J, et al: What really happens during the Lachman test? A dynamic MRI analysis of tibiofemoral motion. Am J Sports Med 32:369-375, 2004.

37. MacDonald PB, Black B, Old J, et al: Posterior cruciate ligament injury and posterolateral instability in a 6-year-old child: A case report. Am J Sports Med 31:135-136, 2003.

38. McCarroll JR, Shelbourne KD, Porter DA, et al: Patellar tendon graft reconstruction for midsubstance anterior cruciate ligament rupture in junior high school athletes: An algorithm for management. Am J Sports Med 22:478-484, 1994.

39. McDermott MJ, Bathgate B, Gillingham BL, Hennrikus WL: Correlation of MRI and arthroscopic diagnosis of knee pathology in children and adolescents. J Pediatr Orthop 18:675-678, 1998.

40. McLennan JG: Lessons learned after second-look arthroscopy in type III fractures of the tibial spine. J Pediatr Orthop 15:59-62, 1995.

41. Meyers MH, McKeever FM: Fracture of the intercondylar eminence of the tibia. J Bone Joint Surg Am 52:1677-1684, 1970.

42. Micheli LJ, Rask B, Gerberg L: Anterior cruciate ligament reconstruction in patients who are prepubescent. Clin Orthop Relat Res 364:40-47, 1999.

43. Mintzer CM, Richmond JC, Taylor J: Meniscal repair in the young athlete. Am J Sports Med 26:630-633, 1998.

44. Mizuta H, Kubota K, Shiraishi M, et al: The conservative treatment of complete tears of the anterior cruciate ligament in skeletally immature patients. J Bone Joint Surg Br 77:890-894, 1995.

45. Nemzek JA, Arnoczky SP, Swenson CL: Retroviral transmission by the transplantation of connective-tissue allografts: An experimental study. J Bone Joint Surg Am 76:1036-1041, 1994.

46. Noyes FR, Matthews DS, Mooar PA, Grood ES: The symptomatic anterior cruciate-deficient knee: I. The long-term functional disability in athletically active individuals. J Bone Joint Surg Am 65:154-162, 1983.

47. Parker AW, Drez D Jr, Cooper JL: Anterior cruciate ligament injuries in patients with open physes. Am J Sports Med 22:44-47, 1994.

48. Pressman AE, Letts RM, Jarvis JG: Anterior cruciate ligament tears in children: An analysis of operative versus nonoperative treatment. J Pediatr Orthop 17:505-511, 1997.

49. Ringer J, Fay M: Acute posterior cruciate ligament in sufficiency in children. Am J Knee Surg 3:192-203, 1990.

50. Ross AC, Chesterman PJ: Isolated avulsion of the tibial attachment of the posterior cruciate ligament in childhood. J Bone Joint Surg Br 68:747, 1986.

51. Rubinstein RA Jr, Shelbourne KD, McCarroll JR, et al: The accuracy of the clinical examination in the setting of posterior cruciate ligament injuries. Am J Sports Med 22:550-7, 1994.

52. Sanders JO: Anterior cruciate ligament reconstruction in the skeletally immature high performance athlete. Arthroscopy 16:392-393, 2000.

53. Stadelmaier DM, Arnoczky SP, Dodds J, Ross H: The effect of drilling and soft tissue grafting across open growth plates: A histologic study. Am J Sports Med 23:431-435, 1995.

54. Stanitski CL: Anterior cruciate ligament injury in the skeletally immature patient: Diagnosis and treatment. J Am Acad Orthop Surg 3:146-158, 1995.

55. Stanitski CL: Anterior cruciate injuries in the skeletally immature athlete. Oper Tech Sports Med 6:228-233, 1998.

56. Stanitski CL: Correlation of arthroscopic and clinical examinations with magnetic resonance imaging findings of injured knees in children and adolescents. Am J Sports Med 26:2-6, 1998.

57. Stanitski CL: Stress view radiographs of the skeletally immature knee: Different view. J Pediatr Orthop 24:342, 2004.

58. Stanitski CL, Harvell JC, Fu F: Observations on acute knee hemarthrosis in children and adolescents. J Pediatr Orthop 13:506-510, 1993.

59. Tanner JM, Davies PS: Clinical longitudinal standards for height and height velocity for North American children. J Pediatr 107:317-329, 1985.

60. Tashman S, Collon D, Anderson K, et al: Abnormal rotational knee motion during running after anterior cruciate ligament reconstruction. Am J Sports Med 32:975-983, 2004.

61. Veltri DM, Warren RF: Isolated and combined posterior cruciate ligament injuries. J Am Acad Orthop Surg 1:67-75, 1993.

62. Wall EJ: Tibial eminence fractures in children. Oper Tech Sports Med 6:206, 1998.

63. Wiley JJ, Baxter MP: Tibial spine fractures in children. Clin Orthop Relat Res 255:54-60, 1990.

64. Williams RJ 3rd, Hyman J, Petrigliano F, et al: Anterior cruciate ligament reconstruction with a four-strand hamstring tendon autograft. J Bone Joint Surg Am 86:225-232, 2004.

65. Willis RB, Blokker C, Stoll TM, et al: Long-term follow-up of anterior tibial eminence fractures. J Pediatr Orthop 13:361-364, 1993.

66. Woods GW, O'Connor DP: Delayed anterior cruciate ligament reconstruction in adolescents with open physes. Am J Sports Med 32:201-2, 2004.

67. Zaricznyj B: Avulsion fracture of the tibial eminence: Treatment by open reduction and pinning. J Bone Joint Surg Am 59:1111-1114, 1997.

CHAPTER 74

Physeal Injuries About the Knee

Carl L. Stanitski

The knee is a common site of injury. Three physes and three epiphyses (femur, tibia, and fibula) are present along with three traction sites of tendon/ligament insertions on immature cartilage—patella, tibial tubercle, and tibial eminence. Physeal fractures represent 15% to 20% of long bone fractures with a 2:1 ratio of boys to girls and upper to lower extremities.[2,25,26] Physeal fractures about the knee are uncommon, with an incidence of only about 2% of physeal injuries. Physeal fractures about the knee account, however, for a striking 50% of all post–physeal fracture growth abnormalities requiring later surgical intervention.[25] Peak injury ages are about 11 years in girls and 13 years in boys, a reflection of exposure to sports and vehicular trauma at those ages and physiological changes in physeal strength associated with onset of adolescence. Distal femoral physeal fractures also may be seen in infants from birth or nonaccidental trauma (Fig. 74–1).

ANATOMY

Distal femoral and proximal tibal physes contribute the major amounts of growth to the lower extremity. The femoral distal physis is the largest and most rapidly growing physis in the body, producing 70% of total femoral growth and 37% of lower limb growth with an average growth rate of 1 cm annually. The distal femoral epiphyseal secondary center of ossification is radiographically apparent and centered at the femoral diaphysis in coronal and sagittal planes at birth in term infants. Physiological complete closure of the distal femoral physis shows marked variability but usually is seen around 12 to 14 years in girls and 14 to 16 years in boys. The proximal tibial physis contributes approximately 55% of tibial total length and 25% of lower extremity total length with a growth rate averaging 0.6 cm/yr. The proximal tibial secondary ossification center is seen radiologically in about 60% of newborns and in 100% of infants by 2 months of age in normal, term infants and is centered in both planes relative to the tibial diaphysis. Proximal tibial physeal closure patterns and timing resemble those of the distal femoral physis.

Distal femoral and proximal tibial epiphyses are sites of major ligament and muscle origins and insertions. The femur is the site of lateral and medial collateral and anterior and posterior cruciate ligament origins and lateral and medial gastrocnemius muscle origins. The proximal tibial epiphysis serves as the insertion site for anterior and posterior cruciate and the deep layer medial collateral ligaments.

Distal femoral and proximal tibial physes have unique geometries to allow resistance to shear, especially the femur. The physeal/metaphyseal femoral undulations present in coronal and sagittal planes represent intersecting femoral metaphyseal grooves with four mammillary-like processes that provide resistance to shear and torsion. This pattern is more exaggerated in quadrupeds and evolved in humans' adaptation to bipedal gait. The proximal tibial physis is more transverse and has less defined mammillary interdigitations than the distal femoral physis. Peripheral femoral and tibial physeal latitudinal growth and resistance to hoop and shear stresses are provided by the zone of Ranvier and ring of Lacroix. The cleavage zone seen in physeal fractures is predominantly through the hypertrophic layer, but fracture geometry is proportional to many factors, including patient physiological age and growth remaining and fracture vector load, rate, and direction.

Physeal failure resistance has been thought to be only about one-third of the force required to cause ligament failure. This observation does not take into account, however, the physiological status of physeal maturity and load characteristics. Ligament failure generally follows high rates of loading with relatively low magnitude forces. In contrast, chondroepiphyseal failure is seen with low load rates and high forces. Sites of ligament and tendon insertions must be considered junctional tissues with transitional mechanical characteristics proportional to physiological maturity.

CLINICAL EVALUATION

A high level of suspicion is needed to diagnose physeal injuries about the knee. The primary clinical finding is tenderness to palpation at the involved physis. Distal neural and vascular integrity must be established, with special caution with displaced fractures, especially proximal tibial physeal ones. A thorough check of knee stability is mandatory after femoral shaft fracture stabilization to rule out physeal injury or knee ligamentous injury or both. Associated injuries about the knee can occur with physeal fractures (e.g., ligament tears and avulsions), especially in the physiological never-never land of adolescence.

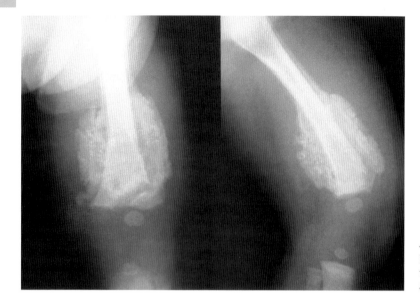

Figure 74–1. Florid periosteal healing after a type II distal femoral physeal fracture secondary to nonaccidental trauma in a 4-month-old.

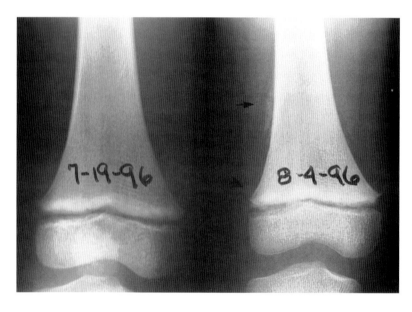

Figure 74–2. **A,** Original injury radiograph shows increased physeal width in a distal femoral physeal undisplaced fracture. **B,** Extended periosteal healing *(arrows)* in fracture 2 weeks after injury.

IMAGING

The fractures are usually readily apparent. The normal distal femoral and proximal physes are 3 to 5 mm thick, depending on their maturity. If a question of increased physeal width occurs, a comparison radiograph of the opposite knee in the same view is helpful. The past practice of coronal plane stress views of the knee in suspected physeal fractures is a relic of an era when differentiation between fracture and collateral ligament injury was required because operative treatment was done for collateral ligament complete tears. Because isolated collateral injuries are now managed nonoperatively, there is no indication to add additional trauma to an already compromised physis by demanding a stress view. Undisplaced physeal fractures require immobilization alone, and obser-

vation of callus formation on follow-up radiographs confirms the diagnosis (Fig. 74–2). Stress images may cause fracture displacement and do not change the treatment of an undisplaced fracture, and so these images should be eliminated as a diagnostic measure.[27]

Poland[19] did much of the original classification of physeal injuries about the knee in 1898 with findings based on anatomic, postmortem dissections. More recent classification systems are based on physeal, epiphyseal, and metaphyseal fragment geometry noted on radiographs. The most commonly used current classification of physeal fractures is the Salter and Harris[23] classification, which attempts to correlate diagnosis and prognosis based on radiographic pathoanatomy of fracture types I through V (Fig. 74–3). Rang added a type VI to reflect perichondrial ring injury, especially femoral, commonly seen with propeller injuries (Fig. 74–4).

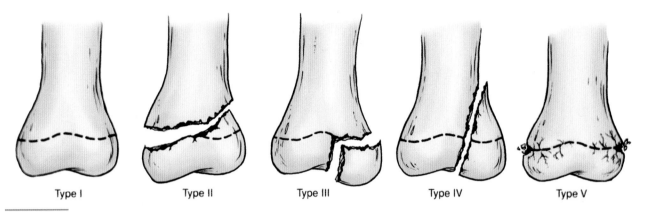

Type I   Type II   Type III   Type IV   Type V

Figure 74–3. Salter-Harris fracture classification of physeal fractures. In type I fractures, the fracture line traverses the physis, staying entirely within it. In type II fractures, the fracture line traverses the growth plate for a variable length, then exits obliquely through the metaphysis. Type III fractures also begin in the physis, but exit throughout the epiphysis toward the joint. Type IV fractures involve a vertical split of the epiphysis, physis, and metaphysis. Type V fractures are crush injuries to the physeal plate.

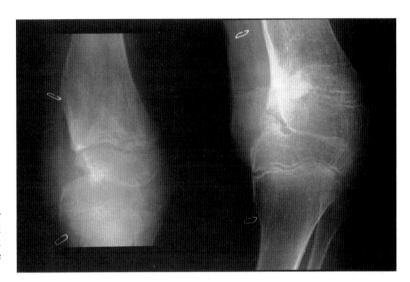

Figure 74–4. Radiographs of an 8-year-old boy 1 year after a lawnmower injury to the medial knee with progressive deformity. (From Stanitski CL: Epiphyseal fractures about the knee. Op Tech Sports Med 6:234-242, 1998.)

PROGNOSIS

Eventual outcome reflects multiple factors, including anatomic location, fracture pattern, closed versus open fracture, injury energy magnitude, and growth remaining at the physis. The initial radiograph reflects the resting position of the fracture at the time of the image and is a static picture of what had been a dynamic event. The position of the fracture fragments may not be representative of the initial magnitude of displacement. The abundant periosteal new bone formation after an innocuous-appearing, minimally displaced fracture is testimony of the fragment's excursion (Fig. 74–5). Avulsion injuries through a chondroepiphyseal zone or immature tendon junction may produce only a small fragment of bone, which may be misinterpreted radiographically as a small "chip" fracture when it represents only a small ossified portion of a much larger cartilaginous fragment. Clinical and radiographic follow-up is needed to ensure growth

arrest and potential deformity are recognized early and appropriate intervention is instituted. Evaluation and management of sequelae of physeal injuries are beyond the scope of this chapter. Tibial eminence fractures are reviewed elsewhere in this text.

DISTAL FEMORAL PHYSEAL FRACTURES

Distal femoral physeal/epiphyseal fractures represent about 10% of all long bone physeal injuries. Salter-Harris type II fractures predominate, followed closely by type I fractures. A bimodal age distribution is related to etiology, with vehicular trauma dominating the 6- to 12-year-old group and sports trauma dominating the 12- to 18-year-old group.[2,25,26] Accurate descriptions of this injury were presented by Poland[19] in 1898. He reviewed the anatomic findings in 114 patients, 24 of whom had their legs caught in wheel spokes as they tried to hitch a ride on a moving

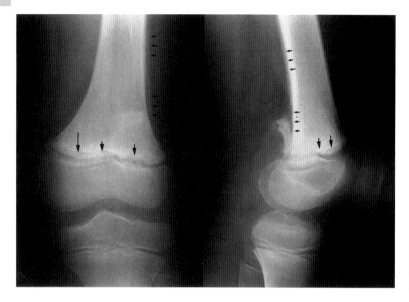

Figure 74–5. Periosteal new bone formation *(arrows)* after an "undisplaced" distal femoral physeal fracture.

carriage. A hyperextension injury often resulted in an open fracture and vascular compromise leading to death or amputation. In the 1950s, Aitken and Magill[1] first emphasized sports trauma as an etiologic factor in this fracture in their report of 15 distal femoral fractures in 13- to 17-year-old patients, 10 of whom were injured playing football. These authors suggested that, "The horse and wagon has been replaced by the football field as the source of this type injury."[1] In contrast to Poland's cases, only one of Aitken and Magill's patients had sagittal plane displacement. The remainder had closed, valgus injuries causing coronal displacement without neurovascular compromise, but significant potential for deformity owing to asymmetric growth. Coronal plane displacement continues to be the most common type of injury from vehicular or sports trauma. Valgus forces from football blocking or tackling or slide tackles in soccer are the main sources of sports trauma producing this injury. The initiating fracture site generates a tensile force across the physis, which propagates (Fig. 74–6). With fracture displacement, opposite side shear and compression forces are generated. The magnitude and direction of these forces define the fracture pattern produced. Type II injuries create a metaphyseal fragment, the radiographic Thurston-Holland sign, of varying size, depending on the force and mechanism of injury. The physis beneath this fragment is spared and, with growth, deformation occurs if the physis on the other side is damaged. Postinjury deformity may be due to malunion or asymmetric growth, or both, related to damage of the physis because of its unique, undulating geometry. The convolutions are sheared and heal as "spot welds" within the physis, causing focal growth arrests. In some cases, deformity is caused by accelerated symmetric or asymmetric physeal growth probably caused by fracture healing–induced hyperemia.

Treatment varies according to fracture type and the amount of fragment displacement. Infants with fractures from birth or nonaccidental trauma have a tremendous capacity for remodeling of the fracture; 20 degrees of posterior angulation and 10 to 15 degrees of coronal deformity spontaneously correct with growth.[25] Rotational

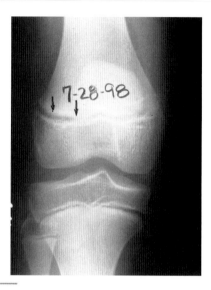

Figure 74–6. Distal femoral physeal type I fracture with lateral widening *(arrows)* after a varus load injury, an uncommon pattern.

deformities are not always well resolved, despite the prolonged growth remaining.

Undisplaced fractures are managed by cast immobilization with weekly radiographic follow-up initially to assess any change in fracture position. Immobilization is relatively brief, about 4 to 6 weeks, depending on the patient's age.

In older children, anatomic reduction of displaced fractures provides the best opportunity for optimal outcome and is mandatory for type III and IV fractures to restore articular and physeal congruity. Displaced type I fractures usually are reduced easily under general anesthesia. Placing the patient prone facilitates the reduction and allows easy targeting for pin fixation. Smooth crossed pin fixation is done across the epiphysis, physis, and metaphysis, ensuring the pins cross in the metaphysis, away from the fracture site (Fig. 74–7). Immobilization is with a long-leg cast with crutch-protected touch-down

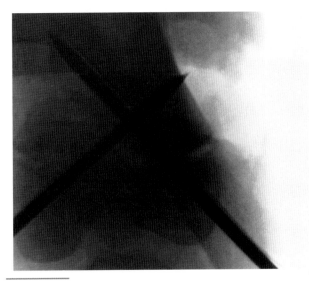

Figure 74–7. Intraoperative radiograph after closed reduction and fixation of a displaced type I fracture. Note pins crossing above the physeal fracture.

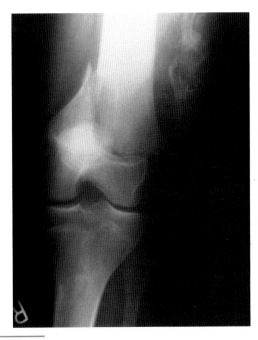

Figure 74–8. Salter-Harris type II fracture with a large metaphyseal fragment, the so-called Thurston-Holland sign. The size of the fragment allows a minimally invasive fracture fixation using a percutaneously placed cannulated screw postreduction.

gait allowed for 4 to 6 weeks post fixation. Pins are removed as soon as the fracture is healed. Early pin removal is believed to help prevent physeal bar formation at the fixation sites by rapid longitudinal physeal growth. No specific data in a controlled series have been presented to document this belief. Type II fractures also are treated with closed reduction. If the metaphyseal fragment is large enough, fixation of the fragment to the metaphysis using cannulated screws provides excellent stability (Fig. 74–8). If the fragment is not large enough to accommodate cannulated fixation, smooth pin stabilization of the metaphyseal fragment with an additional smooth pin from the main metaphyseal area into the epiphysis provides stability. One should not persist in attempting closed reductions in the uncommon event that anatomic reduction is not easily obtained. Rarely, soft-tissue interposition, usually periosteum, prevents reduction. Continued attempts at closed manipulation add injury to an already compromised physis. Type III and type IV displaced fractures require open reduction to ensure physeal and articular anatomic reduction. Fixation is done using smooth pins in the metaphyseal and epiphyseal segments (Fig. 74–9). Torg and associates[29] reported six cases in adolescent boys of type III fractures of the medial femoral condyle from sports trauma. Most of the fractures were occult. Treatment of these minimally displaced fractures was by cast immobilization in that era. Current percutaneous cannulated screw fixation methods are employed to ensure fracture stability.[26] Screw placement must avoid crossing the femoral notch (Fig. 74–10).

Associated injuries with distal femoral physeal fractures should be looked for and addressed, including collateral and anterior cruciate ligament injuries. In the 1980s, Bertin and Goble[3] reported a high rate of associated ligament injuries with various types of distal femoral and proximal tibial physeal fractures in patients with a wide age range (3 months to 17 years) at injury. They found 48% of fractures had an associated ligament injury: 38%

anterior cruciate, 17% medial collateral, and 7% combined medial collateral and anterior cruciate. Of the original study group, 40% were not seen at follow-up, which ranged from 10 to 180 months. Only 2 of the 16 patients with abnormal sagittal plane translation on examination complained of any functional instability. Thirteen patients with proximal tibial physeal fractures were reviewed. Of the five patients with positive anterior drawer signs and Lachman tests, none complained of functional instability. More recent reports of larger series of patients have not substantiated this high rate of associated ligament damage. Ligament injury is possible despite relative skeletal immaturity, especially in early adolescence (Fig. 74–11). Although uncommon, neural and vascular compromise can occur, especially with sagittal plane fracture displacement from hyperextension injuries, and requires emergent fracture reduction and fixation.

Prognosis for distal femoral physeal fractures is guarded, even with minimally displaced type I and II fractures, in contradiction to the prognosis afforded these injuries in the Salter-Harris classification. These fractures must be considered as "bad actors" and given respect for significant potential for late complications requiring surgical intervention (Figs. 74–12 and 74–13). Lombardo and Harvey[12] suggested that fractures that displaced greater than half of the femoral metaphyseal diameter were at greater risk for growth arrest and deformity development. It seems intuitive that increased displacement indicates higher-energy injury to the physis with subsequent growth consequences. Included in their series were 12 cases of varying types of displaced physeal fractures (8 type II, 3 type III, and 1 type IV) that were not reduced. The con-

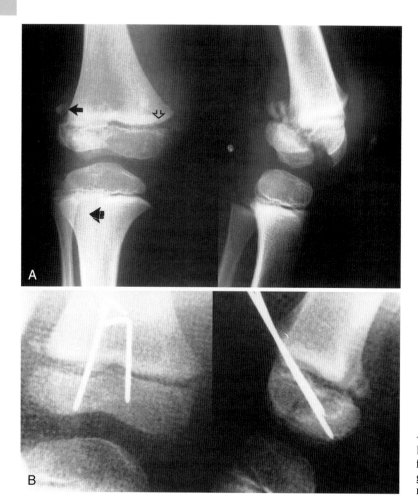

Figure 74–9. **A,** Type IV displaced epiphyseal fracture with physeal and articular incongruities *(arrows).* **B,** After open anatomic reduction and pin fixation.

clusion of Lombardo and Harvey[12] that development of deformity seemed to be related to the degree of initial fracture displacement, exactness of reduction, and type of fracture is put into question by the high number of unreduced cases, the outcome of which may have been more favorable if anatomic reduction were done, despite the amount of initial fracture displacement. Riseborough and coworkers[21] reported outcomes of femoral distal physeal fractures in a retrospective review of patients at Boston Children's Hospital that included patients initially treated at that institution and patients referred for treatment of deformity after fracture healing. They also noted the lack of prognostic correlation of fracture type and outcomes, especially with type I and type II injuries. Riseborough and coworkers[21] suggested that final results would be improved by anatomic reduction and greater use of internal fixation in type II through type IV fractures, a concept emerging in European centers at that time. A high potential for loss of fracture reduction exists after closed reduction without fixation. Thomson and colleagues[28] showed the best results in their series of displaced distal femoral physeal fractures after closed fracture reduction and pin fixation under general anesthesia. No loss of reduction was seen in this group in contrast to the 43% loss of reduction in patients undergoing similar reductions but only cast immobilization.

Angular deformity and limb-length discrepancies are the most common physeal growth compromise complications. Angular deformity was seen in an average of 24% (60 of 248), and significant longitudinal discrepancy (overgrowth or undergrowth) was documented in an average of 32% (79 of 248) of cases in a review of seven large series.[2,25,26] Sequelae of growth alterations usually are apparent by the first year after injury and commonly by 6 months. Longitudinal follow-up is required until lack of growth abnormalities are clinically and radiologically a certainty. Duration of follow-up is determined by the skeletal maturity of the patient at the time of injury.

PROXIMAL TIBIAL PHYSEAL FRACTURES

Fractures of the proximal tibial physis are rare, constituting fewer than 1% of physeal injuries. The proximal tibial physis is stabilized medially by the superficial portion of the medial collateral ligament's metaphyseal insertion, laterally by the fibular head buttress, anteriorly by the tibial tubercle projection, and posteromedially by the semimembranosus, which spans the physis. In view of this array of stabilizing factors, major trauma is needed to produce a fracture of this physis, especially a displaced

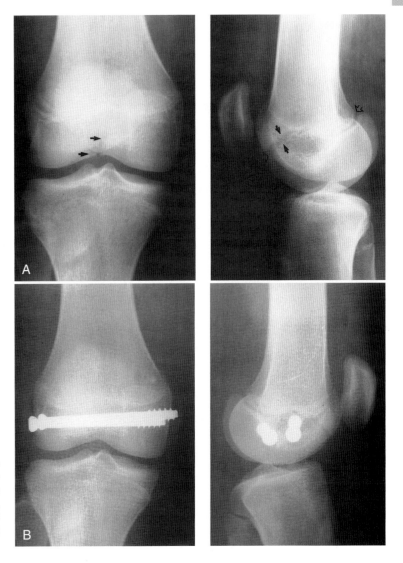

Figure 74–10. **A,** Type III distal femoral displaced epiphyseal fracture (*arrows*). **B,** Postoperative fixation using a percutaneous transepiphyseal cannulated screw technique, avoiding the femoral notch. (From Stanitski CL: Epiphyseal fractures about the knee. Op Tech Sports Med 6:234-242, 1998.)

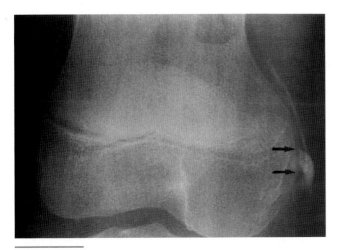

Figure 74–11. Radiograph of a 15-year-old boy 2 years after a distal femoral physeal fracture with an associated medial collateral ligament tear. Calcification is visible at the site of ligament injury *(arrows)*.

one. Most fractures are type I and type II; two-thirds of type II fractures are displaced after a valgus stress (Figs. 74–14 and 74–15).[2,20,24] A displaced type II fracture may have a concurrent proximal fibular fracture. The tibial injury occurs most commonly in 10- to 14-year-old boys. Poland,[19] using cadaveric material, showed that proximal tibial physeal separation was produced most easily in 8- to 13-year-olds (i.e., the ages most commonly seen clinically with such injuries). Sagittal posterior metaphyseal displacement occurs after a hyperextension force or a direct blow to the anterior tibia (e.g., after a fall). The transphyseal fracture displaces and produces vascular compromise at the vascular trifurcation. This type of proximal tibial physeal fracture should be considered the skeletally immature equivalent of an adult knee dislocation because of the high neural and vascular risks associated with it. Wozasek and coworkers[33] reported five patients with limb ischemia after this pattern of fracture. Four of the five cases had resolution of the vascular deficit after fracture reduction. In Shelton and Canale's series of 39 patients,[24] 2 had popliteal artery injuries with subsequent chronic vascular insufficiency. Type III physeal fractures

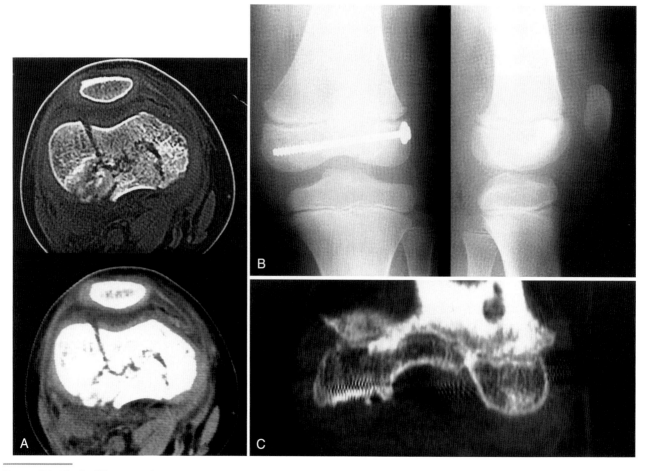

Figure 74–12. **A,** CT scans of a comminuted type III distal femoral epiphyseal fracture in a 10-year-old boy. **B,** Radiographs after open reduction and screw fixation. **C,** Follow-up CT scan 10 months later shows a large central physeal bar. (From Stanitski CL: Epiphyseal fractures about the knee. Op Tech Sports Med 6:234-242, 1998.)

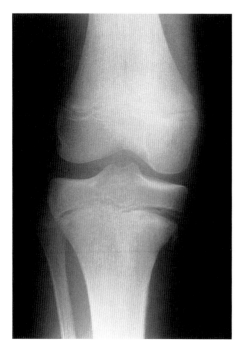

Figure 74–13. Undisplaced type I proximal tibial fracture with minimal medial physeal widening *(arrows)* after a valgus injury.

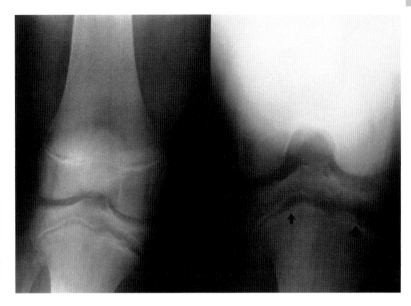

Figure 74–14. Anteroposterior and tunnel views of a 12-year-old boy with a type II minimally displaced proximal tibial physeal fracture with a small lateral metaphyseal fragment after valgus injury in soccer. Undulations within the tibial physeal/metaphyseal junction are visible *(arrows)*.

are uncommon. The injury follows a valgus load to the lateral knee and involves the lateral physis, often with an associated medial collateral ligament tear, which may be missed, resulting in late valgus instability and premature arthrosis. In older series, acute tibial tubercle avulsion fractures were included as type III or IV injuries. Currently, this avulsion injury is considered as a distinct entity. Type IV physeal fractures are rare and may involve medial or lateral sides. Propeller damage from lawnmowers or power boats often cause a peripheral slice injury and a Rang VI lesion.

Clinical findings reflect injury magnitude. Tenderness is present at the physis with deformity seen with displaced fractures. Fibular tenderness also should be looked for. Signs of intra-articular injury (effusion, joint line tenderness) and knee stability are identified, including medial collateral ligament tenderness. Initial assessment of all these factors may be difficult because of the patient's lack of cooperation owing to pain. Distal neural, vascular, and motor function and lower limb compartment turgor must be documented.

Anteroposterior and lateral view radiographs confirm the fracture in most cases. In undisplaced fractures, the physeal line may be widened on radiographs, and a comparison view may be helpful. As with suspected undisplaced distal femoral physeal fractures, stress views are contraindicated because they add trauma to an injured physis, and documentation of physeal instability to prove the presence of the fracture does not change the management of an undisplaced fracture.[27] Other imaging modalities usually are not needed. In cases of suspected vascular compromise, vascular contrast studies should be done without delay if vascular status is not normalized after emergent fracture reduction.

Treatment is dictated by fracture pattern and position. Undisplaced fractures are immobilized in a long-leg cast. Displaced type I or type II fractures usually can be treated with closed reduction. If difficulty is encountered with reduction, closed methods should be stopped to avoid additional damage to the already compromised physis. Open reduction is done to remove the obstacle to reduc-

tion, usually a flap of periosteum or a segment of the pes anserine.[32] After open or closed reduction, fixation with smooth pins is used to prevent fracture displacement in type I and type II injuries if any question of fracture stability is present (Fig. 74–16). Fixation of type III and type IV fractures can be done into the metaphyseal or epiphyseal segments of the fracture or both. Type III fractures can undergo closed reduction using a clamp with arthroscopic monitoring of the reduction to ensure joint surface congruity. Percutaneous screw fixation is placed across the epiphysis under fluoroscopic guidance, avoiding the physis (Fig. 74–17). Healing is rapid, occurring within 4 to 5 weeks. Careful observation after reduction and fixation is needed to ensure that distal neural or vascular compromise, which can be catastrophic, does not occur. Compartment syndrome is possible owing to bleeding into the anterior compartment. Knee coronal, rotatory, and sagittal stability should be determined after stabilization.

Prognosis for physeal fractures of the proximal tibia is quite good because the injury usually occurs near skeletal maturity with impending posterior to anterior closure of the transverse segment of the tibial physis (Fig. 74–18). Most complications (growth abnormalities, vascular impairment, peroneal nerve injury, and long-term knee instability with premature joint senescence) are associated with type III and type IV injuries. In Shelton and Canale's report,[24] 86% satisfactory outcomes were seen in 28 patients after skeletal maturity. A 10% incidence of growth consequence was seen in series by Sponseller[25] and Beatty and Kumar.[2] Clinical and radiographic assessment is continued until it is ensured that physeal injury growth sequelae are not present.

ACUTE PROXIMAL TIBIAL TUBERCLE AVULSION FRACTURES

Acute avulsion of the tibial tubercle is an uncommon fracture with reported incidence of fewer than 1% of all physeal injuries. The most vulnerable age for this fracture

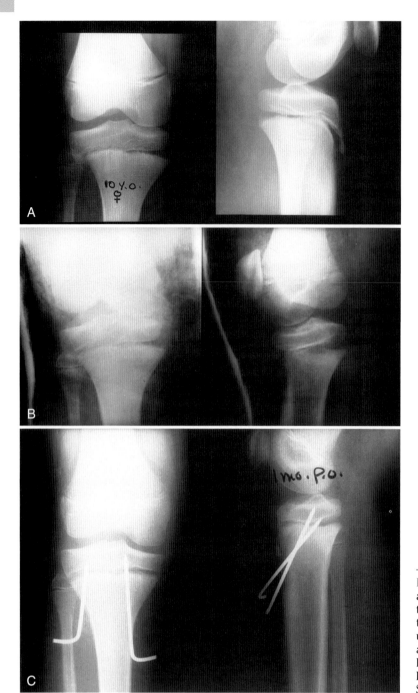

Figure 74–15. **A,** Initial injury radiographs of an 11-year-old girl's displaced type II proximal tibial physeal fracture. **B,** Post closed reduction radiographs show an unsatisfactory, unstable reduction. **C,** Radiographs 1 month after repeat closed reduction and fixation following pin stabilization. (From Stanitski CL: Epiphyseal fractures about the knee. Op Tech Sports Med 6:234-242, 1998.)

is 13 to 16 years, but there are reports of this injury in preadolescents.[4,5,13-15,17] The fracture is intimately related to tibial tubercle development and maturation. Ehrenborg and Engfeldt[6] divided tibial tubercle development into four stages: cartilaginous, apophyseal, epiphyseal, and bony. Ogden and associates[16] showed the existence of three histological zones in the tibial tubercle growth plate. There is progressive change from fibrocartilage to columnar cartilage proximal to distal, and the hypertrophic columnar cells, which predominate just before closure, have less resistance to tensile forces. Physiological physiodesis occurs in the same direction within the tubercle. This change predisposes to avulsion injury of the tibial tuberosity just before or during the later stages of physiological physiodesis. Watson-Jones[30] presented the first classification for acute fractures of the tibial tuberosity and defined three types. Ogden and colleagues[17] modified this classification to define the extent of injury and amount of displacement and comminution (Fig. 74–19). Ryu and Debenham[22] added a type IV, depicting an avulsion fracture of the entire proximal tibial physis. A type V has been reported[13] and constitutes a type IIIB tibial tubercle avulsion and an associated Salter-Harris type II fracture of the proximal tibia producing a Y-shaped configuration. Frankl and colleagues[8] suggested a type IC for fractures associated with patellar tendon avulsions.

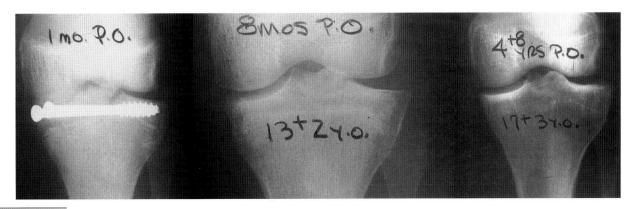

Figure 74–16. **A,** Status post reduction of a type III fracture in a boy 12 years, 6 months old with a reduction clamp and percutaneous cannulated screw fixation. Arthroscopy was used to document anatomic articular surface reduction. **B,** Sequential healing after hardware removal. **C,** Follow-up at skeletal maturity shows no deformity.

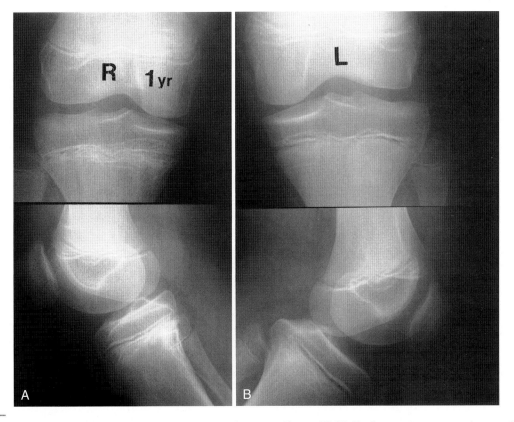

Figure 74–17. **A,** Follow-up radiographs of the patient shown in Figure 73-12. **B,** Comparison normal opposite side radiograph. Despite a small central bar, no deformity ensued.

Mechanisms of injury of acute tibial tuberosity avulsion fractures are related to sudden concentric or eccentric quadriceps loads producing a tensile force that exceeds the tubercle's apophyseal and surrounding perichondrial and periosteal strengths. One mechanism is by explosive quadriceps eccentric contraction during extension as in jumping. Another mode is acute passive flexion of the knee against a concentric quadriceps contraction, such as when landing from a jump or fall. Most reported injuries occur during athletic participation, particularly basketball.

Mosier and Stanitski[14] reported four preadolescent patients 9 to 12 years old who sustained acute tibial tubercle avulsion fractures. A boy 9 years, 4 months old who sustained a type IA fracture while jumping during a basketball game is the youngest reported patient with this injury to date. Most of these injuries in the younger group are type I and do not require surgery (Fig. 74–20). Because most type I acute tibial tubercle avulsion fractures are treated nonoperatively, they tend to be underrepresented in reports that deal only with surgical management of acute tibial tubercle avulsion fractures.

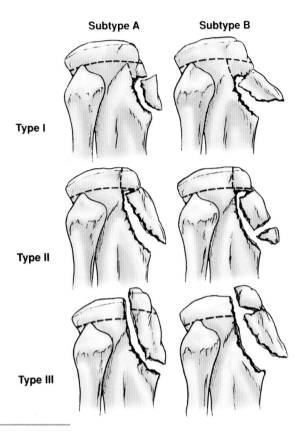

Figure 74–18. Ogden's modification of the Watson-Jones classification of tibial tubercle avulsion fractures. Type I is a distal fracture through the physis with breakout through the secondary ossification center. Type II is a more proximal fracture through the cartilage bridge between the ossification center of the tubercle and the proximal tibial physis. Type III propagates upward through the proximal tibial physis into the knee. Subtype A fractures are noncomminuted; subtype B fractures are comminuted.

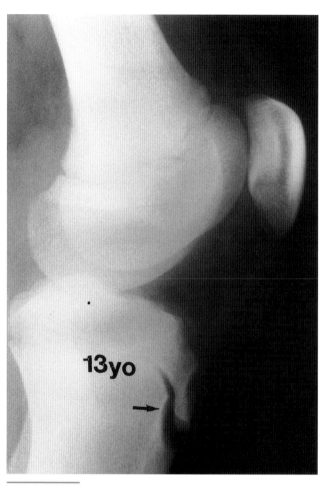

Figure 74–19. Type IA tibial tubercle avulsion fracture *(arrow)* in a 13-year-old boy high jumper.

Older series included acute tibial tubercle type III fractures as type III or type IV proximal tibial physeal injuries.

Avulsion fractures of the tibial tuberosity typically occur in strong, mature-appearing adolescent boys. Only six previous cases have been reported in girls.[4,5,14,17] The preponderance of male patients with fractures of the tibial tuberosity is thought to be secondary to the greater percentage of males participating in athletic jumping activities during adolescence. This increased exposure time during which adolescent boys undergo physiological physiodesis of the proximal tibial tubercle is suggested to contribute to this demographic pattern.

A possible relationship between Osgood-Schlatter disease and avulsion fractures of the tibial tuberosity has been suggested. No direct cause-and-effect relationship has been found, and the finding seems associative and not causative.

Clinical findings reflect the magnitude of the injury. Type I fractures have focal tenderness and swelling but no intra-articular signs or quadriceps insufficiency. With progressively more severe injuries, the fragment gap is palpable, patella alta is present, and hemarthrosis is evident,

reflecting the avulsion fracture with possible associated intra-articular injury. Evaluation of compartmental turgor and distal limb motor, sensory, and vascular integrity is mandatory.

Routine radiographs are confirmatory. The lateral view should be done with the tibia in slight internal rotation to obtain the best profile of the tubercle. Patella alta reflects a loss of continuity of the quadriceps mechanism.

Acute tibial tubercle avulsion fractures can have associated injuries, including tears of the medial collateral, lateral collateral, and anterior cruciate ligaments; medial and lateral menisci[7,11]; and compartment syndrome from bleeding into the anterior compartment.[18] Patellar tendon avulsion injuries may occur with the avulsion fracture. Mosier and Stanitski[14] reported a 10.5% rate of such avulsions (Fig. 74–21). They also presented a case of an acute quadriceps tendon tear, the only one associated with this type of fracture noted in the literature.

Goals of treatment of acute tibial tubercle avulsion fractures are anatomic fracture reduction, restoration of extensor mechanism alignment and isometry and maintenance of tibial articular surface congruency. Closed reduction and cylinder cast immobilization is used for fracture type IA, type IB, and type IIA. Type IIB fractures should undergo open reduction and internal fixation secondary

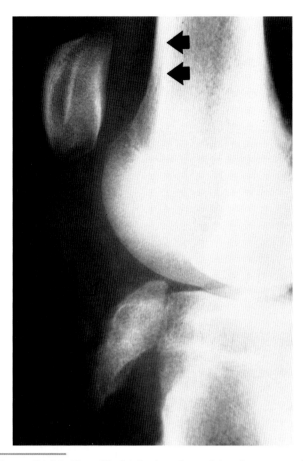

Figure 74–20. Type III tibial tubercle avulsion fracture with associated patellar tendon avulsion fracture *(open arrows)*. Note patella alta *(solid arrows)*.

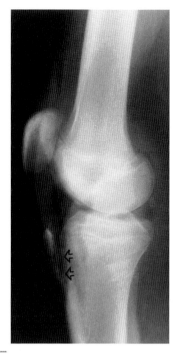

Figure 74–21. Late diagnosed type II tibial tubercle avulsion fracture *(arrows)* with healing and patella alta.

to the association of extensor mechanism disruption with these displaced and comminuted injuries. Type IIIA, type IIIB, and type IV tibial tubercle fractures (i.e., with intra-articular components) are treated by open reduction and internal fixation to ensure articular surface alignment, and other intra-articular injuries are addressed, including extensor mechanism disruption. A vertical midline incision is used with careful handling of the wound margins to minimize additional skin trauma to avoid wound necrosis. Anatomic fracture alignment is needed, and patella alta or infra is avoided. This alignment is particularly required in cases of late diagnosis with patella alta from quadriceps contracture (Fig. 74–22). Direct repair of the torn quadriceps expansion also is done. Various types of internal fixation have been used successfully (Figs. 74–23 and 74–24). Fixation devices should avoid the horizontal proximal tibial physis and central tibial tubercle in young patients. Suture fixation between the fracture and surrounding periosteum usually is adequate in such cases. An ambulatory long-leg cast is used for 3 to 4 weeks, and rehabilitation is begun. Quadriceps resistance exercises should be avoided until 6 weeks postinjury, but active knee range of motion is instituted on cast removal. Return to athletics is allowed in 6 to 8 weeks by patients with type I or minimally displaced type II fractures. Higher-grade injuries require 4 months of rehabilitation and healing

before returning to jumping sports. The patient must have a full range of motion with normal lower extremity muscle strength and endurance before return to athletics.

Complications from this fracture are rare. Only one case of genu recurvatum has been documented,[17] and no cases have been reported in otherwise normal patients. This fracture usually happens after proximal tibial horizontal physeal closure, and recurvatum is not an issue at this mature physis. Other reported complications include loss of flexion, nonunion, malunion, skin necrosis, patella infra, fracture through internal fixation, saphenous nerve neuroma, compartment syndrome, and deep venous thrombosis with pulmonary embolism.[4,5,17,18,31]

Acute avulsion fracture of the tibial tubercle is a relatively uncommon fracture. Treatment depends on fracture type. Overall, this injury has an excellent outcome, even with high grades of injury, and complications are rare.

PATELLAR AVULSION FRACTURES

The patella is the body's largest sesamoid bone and enhances knee extension mechanics. With a large amount of unossified cartilage relative to mineralized bone in young patients (Fig. 74–25), tensile forces at either pole may overcome this immature junction, resulting in an avulsion injury. Distal avulsion fractures are much more common than proximal ones and are seen in preadolescents (8 to 12 years old).[9,10]

Houghton and Ackroyd[10] raised awareness of distal patellar avulsion fractures when they coined the term *sleeve fracture* in their report of three patients, 8 to 12 years old, involved in sports. The sleeve reference was to the

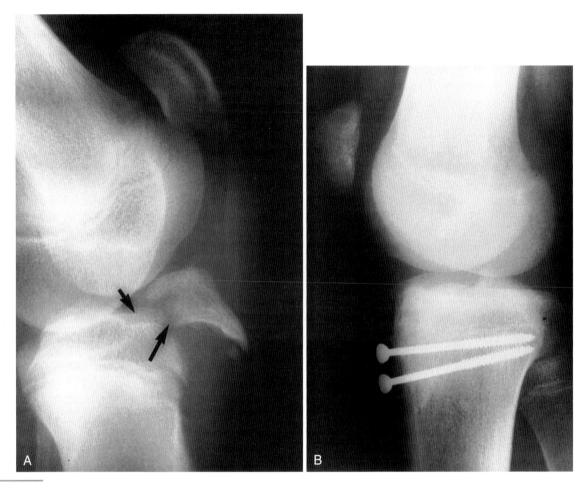

Figure 74–22. **A,** Type III fracture *(arrows)*. **B,** Six weeks after screw fixation and restoration of normal patellar alignment.

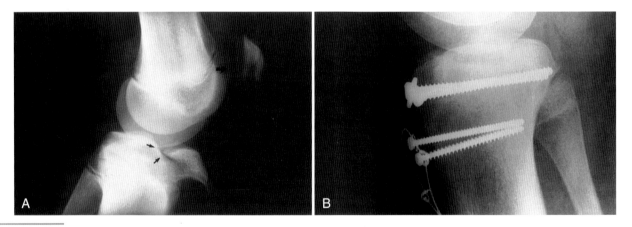

Figure 74–23. **A,** Type III fracture with distal comminution *(arrows)*. **B,** Status post fixation using a screw-wire construct.

large cuff of articular and unossified cartilage adherent to the smaller piece of bone. At the time of the injury, the avulsion injury involves the distal bone, articular cartilage, perichondrium, periosteum, and extensor retinaculum. Proximal avulsion injury is uncommon, and fracture displacement is less common. Similar anatomic components are involved with this injury as its distal counterpart.

Clinical findings reflect injury magnitude. The patient may be unable to walk and incapable of active knee extension. A palpable gap between fracture fragments is evident with displaced fractures. Patella alta is present.

Imaging findings belie the magnitude of injury because of the relatively small osseous fragment compared with the amount of cartilage involved. The injury often is dismissed

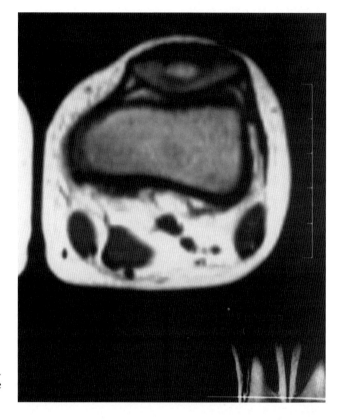

Figure 74–24. Axial view MRI of an 8-year-old boy's patella. Note the abundance of cartilage and limited amount of bone present at this age.

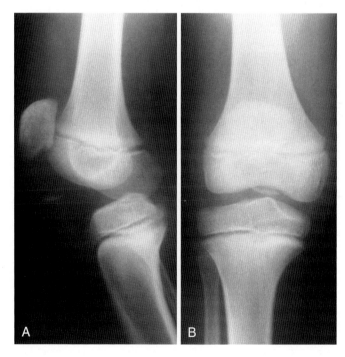

Figure 74–25. **A,** A sleeve fracture, which appears as a minor "chip" fracture. Note significant fragment displacement. **B,** Sleeve fracture fragment that could be misinterpreted as a tibial eminence fracture on this anteroposterior radiographic view.

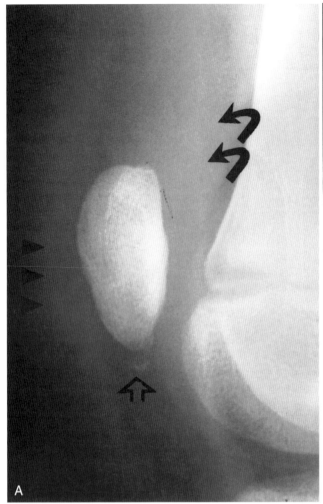

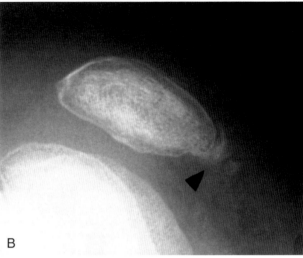

Figure 74–26. **A,** Preoperative radiograph of a displaced sleeve fracture with a large articular component *(open arrow)*. Note significant prepatellar swelling *(arrowheads)* and large effusion *(curved arrows)*. **B,** Follow-up radiograph after suture fixation. Note significant amount of new bone formation *(arrowhead)*.

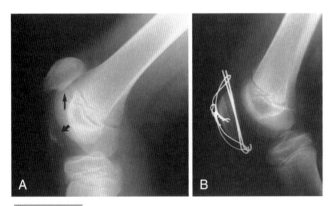

Figure 74–27. **A,** Radiograph of a 12-year-old girl with a significantly displaced sleeve fracture *(arrows)*. **B,** Post open reduction and fixation with smooth pins and figure-eight wire.

I bipartite patella. The last-mentioned usually has a smooth, transverse pattern.

Treatment reflects the amount of fragment displacement. Undisplaced or minimally displaced fractures are treated with ambulatory cast immobilization in knee extension for 3 to 4 weeks. Displaced fractures undergo open reduction with anatomic restoration of the patellar articular cartilage and fixation and repair of the associated extensor retinacular tear. Suture fixation may be used in fractures with small osseous fragments (Fig. 74–26). With larger bone segments, pin and wire constructs or screw fixation is recommended, followed by a 3-week period of casting (Fig. 74–27). In younger patients, radiographic evidence of healing may be slow because of the largely perichondrial response. Outcomes are generally good. The major problem with this fracture is lack of initial recognition of the pattern and extent of injury.

as a chip fracture of the patella, and proper diagnosis and treatment are delayed (see Fig. 74–25). A high index of suspicion is required for diagnosis. Differential diagnosis includes chronic changes at the inferior pole seen in Sinding-Larsen condition, Johannsen's condition, and type

References

1. Aitken AP, Magill HK: Fractures involving the distal femoral epiphyseal cartilage. J Bone Joint Surg Am 34:96-108, 1952.
2. Beaty JH, Kumar A: Fractures about the knee in children. J Bone Joint Surg Am 76:1870-1880, 1994.

3. Bertin KC, Goble EM: Ligament injuries associated with physeal fractures about the knee. Clin Orthop 177:188-195, 1983.
4. Bolesta MJ, Fitch RD: Tibial tubercle avulsions. J Pediatr Orthop 6:186-192, 1986.
5. Chow SP, Lam JJ, Leong JC: Fracture of the tibial tubercle in the adolescent. J Bone Joint Surg Br 72:231-234, 1990.
6. Ehrenborg G, Engfeldt B: The insertion of the ligamentum patellae on the tibial tuberosity: Some views in connection with the Osgood-Schlatter lesion. Acta Chir Scand 121:491-499, 1961.
7. Falster O, Hasselbalch H: Avulsion fracture of the tibial tuberosity with combined ligament and meniscal tear. Am J Sports Med 20:82-83, 1992.
8. Frankl U, Wasilewski SA, Healy WL: Avulsion fracture of the tibial tubercle with avulsion of the patellar ligament: Report of two cases. J Bone Joint Surg Am 72:1411-1413, 1990.
9. Grogan DP, et al: Avulsion fractures of the patella. J Pediatr Orthop 10:721-730, 1990.
10. Houghton GR, Ackroyd CE: Sleeve fractures of the patella in children: A report of three cases. J Bone Joint Surg Br 61:165-168, 1979.
11. Lipscomb AB, et al: Fracture of the tibial tuberosity with associated ligamentous and meniscal tears: A case report. J Bone Joint Surg Am 66:790-792, 1984.
12. Lombardo SJ, Harvey JP Jr: Fractures of the distal femoral epiphyses: Factors influencing prognosis: A review of thirty-four cases. J Bone Joint Surg Am 59:742-751, 1977.
13. McKoy BE, Stanitski CL: Acute tibial tubercle avulsion fractures. Orthop Clin North Am 34:397-403, 2003.
14. Mosier SM, Stanitski CL: Acute tibial tubercle avulsion fractures. J Pediatr Orthop 24:181-184, 2004.
15. Mosier SM, Stanitski CL, Levine RS: Simultaneous bilateral tibial tubercle avulsion fracture. Orthopedics 23:1106-1108, 2000.
16. Ogden JA, Hempton RJ, Southwick WO: Development of the tibial tuberosity. Anat Rec 182:431-445, 1975.
17. Ogden JA, Tross RB, Murphy MJ: Fractures of the tibial tuberosity in adolescents. J Bone Joint Surg Am 62:205-215, 1980.
18. Pape JM, Goulet JA, Hensinger RN: Compartment syndrome complicating tibial tubercle avulsion. Clin Orthop 295:201-204, 1993.
19. Poland J: Traumatic Separation of the Epiphyses. London, Smith, Elder, 1898.
20. Poulsen TD, Skak SV, Jensen TT: Epiphyseal fractures of the proximal tibia. Injury 20:111-113, 1989.
21. Riseborough EJ, Barrett IR, Shapiro F: Growth disturbances following distal femoral physeal fracture-separations. J Bone Joint Surg Am 65:885-893, 1983.
22. Ryu RK, Debenham JO: An unusual avulsion fracture of the proximal tibial epiphysis: Case report and proposed addition to the Watson-Jones classification. Clin Orthop 194:181-184, 1985.
23. Salter RB, Harris WR: Injuries involving the epiphyseal plate. J Bone Joint Surg Am 45:587-662, 1963.
24. Shelton WR, Canale ST: Fractures of the tibia through the proximal tibial epiphyseal cartilage. J Bone Joint Surg Am 61:167-173, 1979.
25. Sponseller PD: Fractures and dislocations about the knee. In Beatty JH, Kasser JR (eds): Rockwood and Wilkin's Fractures in Children, 5th ed. Philadelphia, Lippincott, Williams & Wilkins, 2001. Philadelphia, 1996.
26. Stanitski CL: Epiphyseal fractures about the knee. Op Tech Sports Med 6:234-242, 1998.
27. Stanitski CL: Stress view radiographs of the skeletally immature knee: A different view. J Pediatr Orthop 24:342, 2004.
28. Thomson JD, Stricker SJ, Williams MM: Fractures of the distal femoral epiphyseal plate. J Pediatr Orthop 15:474-478, 1995.
29. Torg JS, Pavlov H, Morris VB: Salter-Harris type-III fracture of the medial femoral condyle occurring in the adolescent athlete. J Bone Joint Surg Am 63:586-591, 1981.
30. Watson-Jones R: Fractures and Joint Injuries. Edinburgh, E & S Livingstone, 1955.
31. Wiss DA, Schilz JL, Zionts L: Type III fractures of the tibial tubercle in adolescents. J Orthop Trauma 5:475-479, 1991.
32. Wood KB, Bradley JP, Ward WT: Pes anserinus interposition in a proximal tibial physeal fracture: A case report. Clin Orthop 264:239-242, 1991.
33. Wozasek GE, et al: Trauma involving the proximal tibial epiphysis. Arch Orthop Trauma Surg 110:301-306, 1991.

CHAPTER 75

Patellar Instability in Childhood and Adolescence

Richard Y. Hinton • Krishn M. Sharma

Patellofemoral instability is a common cause of subjective complaints and activity impairment in the pediatric population. Conditions may vary from fixed, in utero dislocations to macrotraumatic injuries in previously asymptomatic, scholastic athletes. As discrepant as these scenarios may seem, they have in common a "relative" imbalance of the extensor mechanism of the knee. Effective evaluation plus treatment of patellofemoral instability is based on an understanding of the "normal envelope"[21] of extensor mechanism function and the multitude of factors that may disrupt its complex activity.

This chapter focuses primarily on patellofemoral instability in young, athletically active patients. We discuss the host, agent, and environmental risk factors that contribute to patellofemoral instability with a focus on age-specific information, a review of the pertinent literature, and a discussion of current treatment concepts. There is a cursory discussion of congenital, developmental, and habitual patella dislocation that includes detailed references for readers interested in the pathophysiology and surgical treatment of these conditions.

EMBRYOLOGY

The appendicular skeleton appears very early in embryological development. By the fourth week of gestation, the limb buds are easily identifiable, with maturation of the lower extremities trailing the upper ones by several days. The leg buds begin to bend anteriorly at the developing knee during the fifth week. By week 7, the distal end of the femur and the patella have undergone chondrification and the patellofemoral articulation is recognizable in its adult form. Initially, the lower limbs extend from the torso with the soles of the feet facing medially, toward one other. By the eighth week of gestation, the lower limbs complete a 90-degree, internal rotation, which brings them into their adult orientation.[23,57,68,75] It is thought that failure of the quadriceps myotome to complete this internal rotation is the most probable cause of in utero, congenital patellofemoral dislocation.[30,31,79] This failure of rotation leaves the extensor mechanism in a contracted, laterally dislocated position relative to the distal end of the femur.

Initial formation or malformation of the patellofemoral joint and other knee structures appears to be genetically driven without a dependence on function.[23,40] However, abnormal motion and stress across the articulation appear to play a role in progressive, developmental dysplasia. Individual abnormalities such as a shallow femoral sulcus, patellar hypoplasia, and patella alta tend to appear in relative amounts within a constellation of dysplastic changes. In cases of congenital, developmental, and habitual dislocation, early surgical restoration toward more normal extensor mechanism biomechanics may lead to partial normalization of patellofemoral architecture.[28,31,42]

ANATOMY AND BIOMECHANICS

The patella lies within the trochlea of the femur, bounded by the medial and lateral femoral condyles. Cartilaginous at birth, the patella begins ossification from multiple centers during early childhood. The relatively cartilaginous composition of the immature patella has diagnostic and clinical implications. The apparent lack of patellofemoral congruity and excessive shallowness of the femoral sulcus in the child's knee is in large part an illusion (Fig. 75–1). Nietosvaara[59] has shown that although the osseous patellofemoral sulcus angle is inversely proportional to age, ultrasound measurements of the cartilaginous sulcus are nearly constant throughout growth. A gradual thinning of the articular cartilage from the outer areas of the sulcus and retropatellar facets leads to an apparent deepening of the sulcus with age.[63] Even in a mature knee there is still a significant mismatch between the osseous outlines of the patellofemoral articulation and the geometry of the true articular cartilage surfaces (Fig. 75–2).[78] For these reasons, congenital and acquired patellofemoral dysplasia may be better represented on magnetic resonance imaging (MRI) than on plain radiographs.

Patella alta is one of the best substantiated radiographic risk factors for patella instability.[5,25,37,49,54,71] However, reliable measurement of this condition is limited by the cartilaginous nature of the patella and the tibial tubercle in the younger knee.[82] Alternatives to the traditional Isall-Salvatti method aim to minimize these effects. Koshino and Sugimoto's method[41] uses relationships of the midpatella to the midepiphyseal lines of the tibia and femur. This scheme may be most appropriate for younger children. The Blackburne-Peel[8] modification uses the relationship between posterior facet length and the distance to the tibial articular surface. This method is helpful

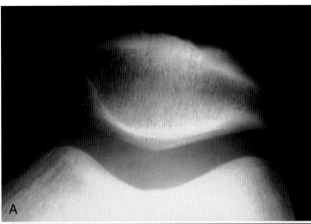

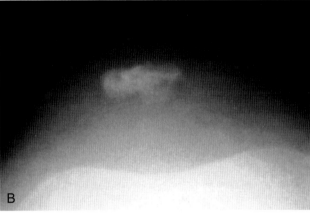

Figure 75–1. Sunrise view of the patellofemoral joint in an adult man (**A**) and an 8-year-old boy (**B**). (From Hinton RY, Sharma KM: Acute and recurrent patellar instability in the young athlete. Orthop Clin North Am 34:285-396, 2003.)

in adolescents in whom the inferior pole of the patella is not fully ossified or who have secondary tibial tubercle changes associated with Osgood-Schlatter disease.

The tibial tubercle also undergoes gradual ossification during childhood. Genu recurvatum is a potential complication with tubercle osteotomies and distal extensor realignment procedures. The appropriate age cutoff is not well described. However, older case series[35,47] report such complications in patients younger than but not older than 14.

The multilayer soft-tissue envelope about the patellofemoral joint has been described as having three layers on both the medial and lateral sides.[19,76,77,83] Medially, the superficial layer is the investing fascia over the sartorius muscle. The second layer includes the medial patellofemoral ligament (MPFL) and the parapatellar retinaculum. The superficial medial collateral ligament (MCL) is also in this second plane. The third medial layer contains the deep MCL and joint capsule. This arrangement places the MPFL in the same extracapsular environment as the MCL (Fig. 75–3). Such an environment is one that may promote ligamentous healing, as seen by the ability of the MCL to regain function and structure even after major injury. Laterally, there are fascial interconnections between the fibers of the iliotibial band, lateral hamstrings, lateral patellofemoral ligaments, and lateral quadriceps retinaculum that feed into the lateral aspect of the patella. Tightness in these structures may cause excessive posterior and lateral pull and thereby contribute to lateral patellar tilt and retropatellar pressure.

Muscle contraction may affect patellofemoral stability by "seating" the articulation as a result of increased joint reaction forces or by generating dynamic medial or lateral displacement forces.[77] The relative vectors of the individ-

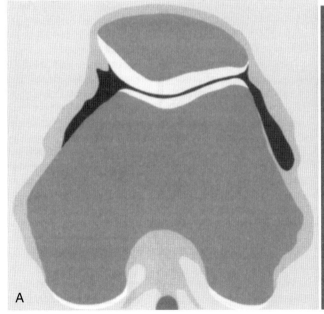

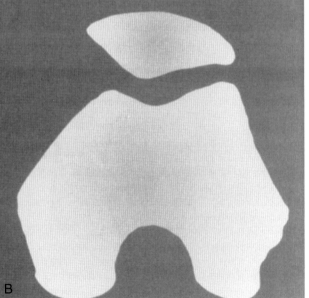

Figure 75–2. Diagram of a magnetic resonance arthrotomogram of the left knee in the axial plane showing articular cartilage congruence of the patellofemoral joint (**A**) and a diagram showing the osseous contour of same knee with "apparent" incongruence (**B**). (From Staeubli HU, Bosshard C, Porcellini P, Rauschning W: Magnetic resonance imaging for articular cartilage: Cartilage-bone mismatch. Clin Sports Med 21:417-433, viii-ix, 2002.)

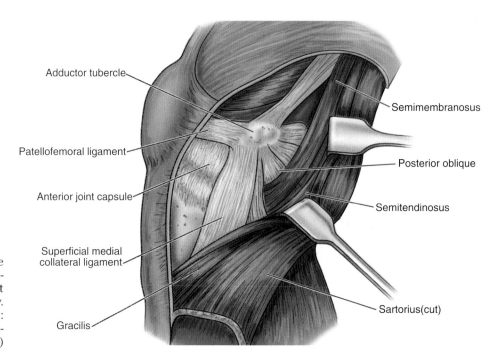

Figure 75–3. Diagram of the layer II medial-side knee structures. (From Clarke HD, Scott WN, Insall JN, et al: Anatomy. In Insall JN, Scott WN [eds]: Surgery of the Knee. Philadelphia, WB Saunders, 2001, p 52.)

ual quadriceps muscular components are determined by their level of attachment, angle of pull, and cross-sectional area. The vastus medialis obliquus (VMO) is a primary dynamic stabilizer. It is intimately associated with the MPFL and the adductor musculature. Though conceptually interesting, independent function, disuse, or rehabilitation of the VMO separate from the remaining quadriceps has not been proved.[43,64,67] Musculotendinous units are primarily dynamic actors, and advancement of the VMO to increase passive restraint to lateral patellar dislocation is unpredictable.[77]

The MPFL is an hourglass-shaped, ligamentous structure running transversely from the posterior part of the medial epicondyle, approximately 1 cm distal to the adductor tubercle, to the superomedial part of the patella. Though present as a distinct structure in 90% of specimens, the ligament can vary greatly in size and strength.[10,19,36] The femoral origin is intimately associated with the insertions of the adductor tendon and the superficial MCL (Fig. 75–4). Smirk and Morris[76] have investigated the isometricity of various origin and insertion positions for MPFL reconstruction. The best results were obtained by using the normal femoral and patellar attachments (Fig. 75–5). Superior displacement of the femoral attachment resulted in increased distance between insertion sites as the knee moved into greater flexion, which could lead to loss of knee flexion or disruption of the graft after MPFL reconstruction. Inferior displacement of the patellar insertion with a normal femoral attachment resulted in increasing graft laxity with knee flexion beyond 60 degrees. The MPFL has been shown to be the primary ligamentous restraint to excessive lateralization of the patella. A number of studies[10,19,29,36,62] comparing the roles of the MPFL, medial patellar retinaculum, patellotibial ligament, patellomeniscal ligament, and lateral retinaculum have found the MPFL to provide between 50%

and 80% of the soft-tissue restraint to lateral patellar displacement in functional positions of slight knee flexion.

Imaging and surgical exploration studies[50,72,73] have found the MPFL to be routinely injured at the time of patellar dislocation. Disruption appears to occur most often at the adductor tubercle, but it may take place along the length of the ligament or its patellar attachment. In patients with chronic dislocation, Nomura[62] reported the MPFL to be healed throughout its course with scar tissue, unhealed with femoral avulsion, or atrophied throughout its course. Laboratory studies and clinical reports[10,19,24,50,62,73] have found that repair or reconstruction of the MPFL is integral to reestablishing lateral patella stability.

The bony architecture of the patellofemoral joint also plays a role in stability. Trochlear dysplasia, altered convexity of the retropatellar surface, patella alta, and patellar hypoplasia have all been found to be risk factors for initial and recurrent patella instability.[25,37,40] The normal sulcus angle for young normal individuals has been reported to be 138 ± 3 degrees.[70,83] Mild trochlear dysplasia corresponds to a sulcus angle of 143 degrees, moderate dysplasia to an angle of 149 degrees, and severe dysplasia to a sulcus angle of 171 degrees.[16] Rünow[71] found the average sulcus angle in a large group of young patients with documented patellar dislocation to be increased to 146 ± 6 degrees. A very similar increase to 147 degrees has been reported by Aglietti et al[1] in symptomatic patella subluxers.

With the knee in full extension, the patella rests lateral and superior to the trochlea. Engagement occurs between 10 and 30 degrees of flexion. This is dependent on relative patella tendon length, and in individuals with patella alta, engagement will occur later in flexion. This condition leads to less stability in the early degrees of knee flexion in which most sporting activity occurs. For the

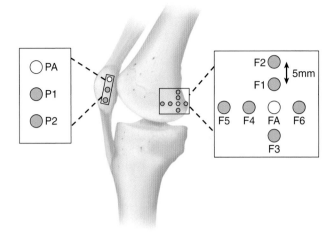

Figure 75–5. Potential graft attachment sites. FA, normal femoral attachment, 1 cm distal to the adductor tubercle. All femoral sites were 5 mm apart. PA, normal patellar attachment in the superior third of the patella. (Fom Smirk C, Morris H: The anatomy and reconstruction of the medial patellofemoral ligament. Knee 10:221-227, 2003.)

instability in many large group studies.[5,12,24,46] This may reflect the inability of a static measurement, usually made with the knee in a fully extended, non-weightbearing position, to capture a functional impairment.

RISK FACTORS

As with other musculoskeletal injuries, risk factors for patellofemoral instability are best viewed within the disease triad of *host* (patient characteristics), *agent* (macrotraumatic or repetitive microtraumatic energy exchange), and *environmental* (physical and social milieu of athletic participation) risk factors.[37,51] We classify young patients with patellofemoral instability into two large, somewhat overlapping groups (*TONES* and *LAACS*) based on "relative" risk factors, natural history, and characteristics (Box 75–1).

Host factors that may play an important role in patellar instability include age, gender, previous history of patellar instability, generalized ligamentous laxity, and patellofemoral dysplasia. Patellar dislocation rates are highest during the second decade of life,[5,25,71] probably because of higher athletic activity during this period and an underlying musculoskeletal predisposition in this age group. During a period of rapid growth, children and early adolescents are in the seemingly dichotomous situation of simultaneous musculotendinous tightness and relative ligamentous laxity. This is particularly apparent with the strap-like, two-joint musculotendinous units crossing the knee. Tightness in the iliotibial band, abductors, and lateral hamstrings may lead to increased valgus vector on the patella, which may be poorly balanced by lax medial ligamentous restraints and poorly developed quadriceps musculature. Age is also a significant risk factor for recurrence, with earlier initial dislocation being a positive pre-

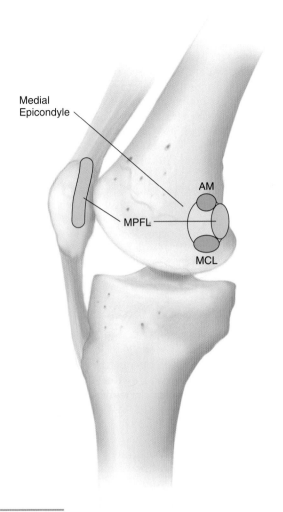

Figure 75–4. Schematic diagram showing the medial femoral epicondyle and its attachments for the adductor magnus tendon (AM), the medial patellofemoral ligament (MPFL), and the medial collateral ligament (MCL). (Fom Smirk C, Morris H: The anatomy and reconstruction of the medial patellofemoral ligament. Knee 10:221-227, 2003.)

adolescent and young adult population, the Insall ratio has been measured as 0.98 ± 0.13 for males and 1.08 ± 0.15 for females.[71] In a study of 104 patella dislocators, Rünow[71] found that the average Insall ratio was greater than 1.0 in all patients and that a ratio greater than 1.3 was significantly correlated with recurrent and bilateral dislocation. Several other studies have reported patella alta to be a significant risk factor for initial and recurrent patellar instability.[5,25,37,49,54,71]

The Q angle is subtended by a line drawn from the anterior superior iliac spine to the center of the patella or the trochlear groove and a second line drawn from the center of the tibial tubercle. An increased Q angle suggests a greater lateralizing vector on the patella. Unfortunately, there are no agreed-on standards for Q angle measurement with regard to the most appropriate degree of knee flexion, weightbearing status, and quadriceps activity. Though often discussed, an increased Q angle as a risk factor for instability has not been reliably associated with patella

Box 75-1. Classification of Patellofemoral Instability in Young Patients: TONES and LAACS

T: **T**raumatic, sports-related injury mechanisms
O: **O**lder at initial dislocation, **O**steochondral fractures more common
N: **N**ormal patellofemoral architecture and **N**ormal ligamentous function
E: **E**qual sex distribution
S: **S**ingle occurrence and **S**ingle-leg involvement

L: **L**axity, generalized and **Lower** age at onset
A: **A**traumatic in nature
A: **A**bnormal patellofemoral architecture and **A**bnormal ligamentous laxity
C: **C**hronic in nature, **C**ontralateral involvement, **C**omorbid conditions
S: **S**ex dependent, with greater number of females

dictor for higher recurrence rates.[11,25,26,54,55,71] Generalized ligamentous laxity is correlated with earlier onset, more recurrence, and dislocations that occur with lesser trauma.[71] However, patellar dislocation in a hyperlax patient carries a significantly lower risk of concurrent osteochondral fracture.[71,80] The patellofemoral dysplastic markers that have been most reliably linked to increased dislocation and recurrence risk are patella alta, increased sulcus angle, and lateral dominance of the retropatellar surface. These dysplastic changes usually occur as a constellation and are more often seen in younger, hyperlax female LAACS (see Box 75–1) type patients. However, there are often subtle abnormalities in these measurements among TONES (see Box 75–1) type patients as well. A key host characteristic for recurrent dislocation is a history of previous dislocation.[25]

Trauma, in varying degrees, is almost always associated with patellar dislocation. A large population-based study by Atkin et al[5] points to the "agent" of high sports participation as the major risk factor for first-time, acute patellofemoral dislocators. The most common mechanism of patella dislocation—noncontact external rotation of the lower part of the leg on a planted foot resulting in valgus overload of the extensor mechanism—is common in sports participation. In their group of TONES-type patients, they reported no predictive role for gender, family history, increased Q angle, or excessive hip rotation. Patella alta was the one traditional factor associated with higher risk in this patient group. In TONES patients, patella dislocation is a more traumatic event, with higher rates of MRI-documented disruption of the MPFL, VMO, and medial retinaculum. Fithian et al[25] suggested that increased soft-tissue trauma is a sign of macrotrauma to normal structures and that given adequate chance to heal, there will be a lower risk of recurrence than in cases in which the patella dislocates with less trauma. Osteochondral fracture rates are also significantly higher in TONES patients as a result of the greater stress required to dislocate the patellofemoral joint in patients with more normal

soft-tissue function. Interestingly, fractures tend to be either avulsion type or intra-articular osteochondral in nature, but the two rarely occur concurrently.[83] An initial avulsion may serve to decompress the patellofemoral joint and thus decrease stress between the retropatellar surface and the lateral femoral condyle. Sports, dance, and other high-demand activities are often the primary cause of injury in initial dislocators. Even in LAACS-type patients, most will report some level of trauma as precipitating a recurrent event. Only in the small group of "habitual" dislocators does the patella routinely dislocate with normal gait.

Today's young athletes are playing sports in an environment of relatively more game to practice time, consistently higher competitive levels, and early specialization in single sports. These factors combine to significantly increase injury exposure and risk. There is also increasing social pressure pushing the young athlete back to play before adequate postoperative or postinjury rehabilitation.

CLASSIFICATION

A myriad of classification systems have been devised for patellofemoral instability and maltracking. In his classic treatise on patellofemoral instability, Anders Rünow grouped initial dislocators into four groups. Group I had only minimal patella alta (Insall ratio of 1.0 to 1.3), minimal trochlear dysplasia, and no generalized hyperlaxity. Seventy-six percent of these patients experienced significant trauma causing the dislocation, they had an average age of 19 at initial onset and a low rate of recurrence, and osteochondral fractures occurred in 63%. Group II had generalized hyperlaxity and an Insall ratio of 1.0 to 1.3, whereas group III had normal soft-tissue function but an Insall ratio greater than 1.3. Group IV demonstrated both hyperlaxity and severe patella alta. For group IV patients the age at onset was 13, the recurrence rate was 74%, bilateral involvement occurred in 68%, significant trauma played a role in only 28%, and osteochondral fractures occurred in only 17% (Table 75–1). In a recent comprehensive population study, Fithian et al[25] classified acute dislocators into those with and without a history of previous dislocation. Those with a history of previous dislocation were more likely female and had a higher risk of future dislocation, a positive family history for patellar instability, higher rates of dysplastic hip disease, and increases in patella alta, patellar tilt, and patellar subluxation. As discussed earlier, we have found that grouping patients generally into the TONES and LAACS classifications is useful in assessing risk factors, discussing the natural history, and guiding treatment options.

In getting one's "clinical hands" around a patient with supposed patellofemoral instability the following questions are important to answer. (1) What is the personality of the injury? Is the situation one of a mechanically normal knee subjected to macrotrauma, or did the dislocation occur with minimal trauma in a patient with significant underlying mechanical risks factors? (2) Is this problem an aggravation or disability, as gauged by lost

Table 75–1. Classification of Patellar Instability

INSTABILITY GRADE	JOINT LAXITY	INSALL INDEX >1.3	PERCENT OF TOTAL GROUP	AGE AT ONSET (yr)	FREQUENT DISLOCATIONS (FRACTION)	BILATERAL DISLOCATIONS (FRACTION)	MODERATE TRAUMA (FRACTION)	FRACTURE(S) (FRACTION)	INSTABILITY SCORE
0	—	—	—	—	—	—	—	—	—
I	—	—	16	19	0.13	0.13	0.76	0.63	2.1
II	+	—	35	15	0.26	0.19	0.69	0.38	2.7
III	—	+	19	15	0.60	0.35	0.55	0.33	3.6
IV	+	+	30	13	0.74	0.68	0.26	0.17	5.0
Total/average			100	15	0.46	0.37	0.55	0.33	3.6

From Rünow A: The dislocating patella. Etiology and prognosis in relation to generalized joint laxity and anatomy of the patellar articulation. Acta Orthop Scand Suppl 201:1-53, 1983.

play/practice time, the presence of chronic quadriceps atrophy, or loss of explosive jumping ability? (3) Has there truly been adequate nonoperative care, and what was the response? (4) Are there signs or symptoms of concurrent knee injury, such as osteochondral fractures, other extensor mechanism overuse syndromes, or missed ligamentous injuries? (5) Is the instability truly first time, acute recurrent, or chronic? (6) Is the patella grossly unstable during clinical examination or daily activities? (7) What are the age, activity level, and athletic potential of the patient?

NATURAL HISTORY

Well-controlled, population-based studies have estimated the per capita risk for first-time dislocation in children and adolescents to be between 29 and 43 per 100,000.[5,25,60] The natural history of this fairly common major knee malady is not benign. A significant number of patients will experience recurrent instability and/or patellofemoral pain related to maltracking or osteochondral injury. For nonoperative patients, reported redislocation rates vary widely from 15% to 45%, and 30% to 50% may be expected to suffer anterior knee pain.[6,37] Less than perfect outcomes after nonoperative care suggest a need for early surgical intervention. However, the results of operative care have been mixed, appear to decline over time, and are less likely to succeed in the very LAACS-type patients who are apt to need surgery the most.[81] As discussed earlier, the natural history after an acute dislocation is dependent on host, agent, and environmental risk factors for the individual patient. Fithian et al[25] reported recurrent instability in 49% of patients with a previous history of instability and only a 17% recurrence rate in their group of first-time dislocators. Rünow[71] reported a redislocation rate of only 13% in his group I patients without laxity or patellofemoral dysplasia. However, the rate jumped to 74% in group IV patients with both generalized hypermobility and patellofemoral dysplasia. In their study of 100 young acute dislocators, Mäenpää et al[48] found a redislocation rate of 44%, patellofemoral pain in 19%, and no complaints after nonoperative treatment in only 37% of their patients. However, of the 14 patients who underwent surgical reconstruction, 47% continued to have a positive apprehension sign and 79% had significant retropatellar crepitance. In a randomized study of nonoperative and operative treatment, Nikku et al reported recurrent instability rates of 20% in their nonoperative and 18% in their operative group and overall better function in their nonoperative patients.[61] In a large group of male army conscripts with an average age of 20 who underwent surgery for acute or recurrent patellar dislocation, Mäenpää et al[48] found only 19% to have excellent results. Just 35% were able to finish their military service normally after surgical intervention.

INJURY HISTORY

The history of an acute patella dislocation is not always as straightforward as it may seem. The young athlete is able to recount a major injury, but rarely the details. The athlete has a painful, swollen, guarded knee, but rarely a fixed dislocation. Although injuries can occur from a direct fall onto the patella, the majority occur with the noncontact mechanism previously described. Children and younger adolescents can have a hard time differentiating this plant-twist mechanism from that leading to a noncontact anterior cruciate ligament (ACL) injury. Both result in sense of traumatic giving way, pain, hemarthrosis, and significant impairment. Both diagnoses must be considered and carefully ruled out in an acutely injured knee. A patient with recurrent, acute dislocation is usually able to relate an appropriate history and a feeling of "sameness" to the current dislocation episode. Symptomatic osteochondral fractures may result in complaints of mechanical locking and persistent effusion. Complaints associated with chronic subluxation are often vague. The child often complains of generalized anterior knee pain or burning and a sense of the knee giving way with quick stops, jumping, or change of direction. A history of multiple physician consultations and sporadic efforts at rehabilitation is often present.

PHYSICAL EXAMINATION

Fortunately, the patellofemoral articulation is very accessible to physical examination. Effort should be made to specifically correlate the underlying anatomic structures with superficial palpation. For example, injury to the MPFL can be inferred from tenderness at its origin at the adductor tubercle or a rent at its patellar attachment.

In the acute setting, arthrocentesis is both diagnostic and therapeutic. Hemarthrosis and fatty globules can be documented. Instillation of a local anesthetic and decompression of the joint may also improve the quality of examination. Pain is decreased and early range of motion and quadriceps activity are improved. A standard ligamentous examination of the knee should be performed to rule out concurrent injury. A sense of the overall tissue trauma should be established. Large palpable rents in the VMO, adductors, or MPFL and a grossly dislocatable patella are relative indicators for surgical intervention in a TONES-type patient. Generalized hypermobility is assessed, and an evaluation of mechanical and alignment risk factors can be made in the contralateral leg.

A LAACS patient with chronic patellar instability deserves an inclusive examination.[66] Overall alignment of the lower extremities should be determined in a weight-bearing position. This examination includes an assessment of generalized joint laxity, knee valgus, femoral/tibial rotation, and foot posture. Walking, jogging, jumping, and other sport-specific activity should be evaluated. An assessment of total lower extremity flexibility and strength should be made with a particular emphasis on the following: hip abductor/adductor strength balance, iliotibial band and hip flexor tightness, quadriceps atrophy, and painful arcs of resisted knee motion. The patient should be assessed for excessive guarding of the knee, hypersensitivity to light touch, or other signs of saphenous nerve irritation or early reflex sympathetic dystrophy.

More specific evaluation of the patellofemoral joint can then be carried out. Evaluation includes assessing the Q angle in full extension and 20 degrees of flexion. Patellar apprehension testing is then performed by attempting to displace the patella laterally over the lateral femoral condyle while observing the patient for signs of apprehension or discomfort. Medial and lateral patellar translation and endpoint compliance are assessed. The patella can normally be displaced both medially and laterally between 25% and 50% of the width of the patella. Patellar tilt should be evaluated. Lateral retinacular tightness may prevent the lateral facet from being tilted above the horizontal. Patella tracking is evaluated through a full range of motion with and without patellofemoral compression. Late engagement, patella alta or baja, lateralization, and painful arcs of motion are documented.

PATELLOFEMORAL IMAGING

With regard to patellofemoral instability, diagnostic imaging serves two broad functions. It provides information on extensor mechanism and concurrent knee injury, and it assesses architectural characteristics of the knee that may predispose to patellofemoral maltracking and instability. Unfortunately, most imaging studies are static and give little indication about the dynamic nature of the patellofemoral joint. As discussed earlier, the relative cartilaginous nature of a child's patellofemoral articulation also limits the usefulness of standard radiographs.

Radiographs should begin with standard anteroposterior, bent-knee weightbearing, true lateral at 20 to 30 degrees, and sunrise at 20 degrees. A true lateral radiograph can be helpful in assessing patella tilt, trochlea depth, dysplastic changes, and patella alta.[49] Some time should be devoted to assessment of patella alta because it is one of the radiographic risk factors most correlated with symptomatic instability.[5,44,54,71] There are many different methods and standard ratios. For young children we recommend the method of Koshino and Sugimoto[41] (Fig. 75–6A); for adolescents, the Blackburne-Peel method (Fig. 75–6B)[8]; and for a skeletally mature patient, the modified or standard Insall-Salvati method.[38] Walker et al[82] generated age-specific data for patella-to–patella tendon ratios with the Insall-Salvati method. We use the sunrise view at 20 degrees to determine a lateral patellofemoral angle by drawing a line across the top of the lateral and medial condyles and an intersecting line along the posterior face of the lateral facet. This angle should be open to the lateral side.[44] The degree of subluxation can also be assessed.

The Merchant view[56] is taken at 45 degrees of knee flexion and yields information on the patellofemoral relationship in a more seated position. The congruence angle defines the relationship of the patellar apex to the bisected femoral trochlea, and the sulcus angle defines the depth of the trochlear groove. A computed tomography scan can be used to evaluate tilt, translation, and congruence in varying degrees of knee flexion. Superimposed axial cuts may also be used to evaluate long-bone torsional deformities and to determine the rotational relationship between the tibial tubercle and the femoral sulcus in varying degrees of flexion.

Plain radiographs miss a high percentage of osteochondral fractures that occur at the time of patellofemoral dislocation. Dainer et al[15] found that 40% of arthroscopically documented lesions were missed on initial films. In a group of adolescent dislocators, Stanitski[80] found that only 34% of arthroscopically diagnosed osteochondral injuries were apparent on standard radiographs. The correlation of MRI with arthroscopic findings has also been questioned. However, newer articular cartilage imaging techniques promise better resolution and more accurate scans. Current and future techniques for patellofemoral imaging, including specific sequences, MR-arthrography, and dynamic MRI, can be found in recent review articles by Recht et al,[69] McCauley and Disler,[53] and Witonski.[84]

MRI also has an important role in determining the extent and location of injury to the MPFL.[50,72,77] The most common MRI findings associated with acute patellar dislocation are disruption of the MPFL and medial retinaculum and edema at the inferior border of the VMO. Though most commonly avulsed from its femoral attachment, the MPFL may be disrupted at any point along its course, and the disruption may be partial or complete. Hard-tissue abnormalities are also commonly seen. Medial patella avulsion fractures and osteochondral fractures from the retropatellar surface or lateral condyle are common. Rünow[71] found 46 fractures in his series of 140 dislocated

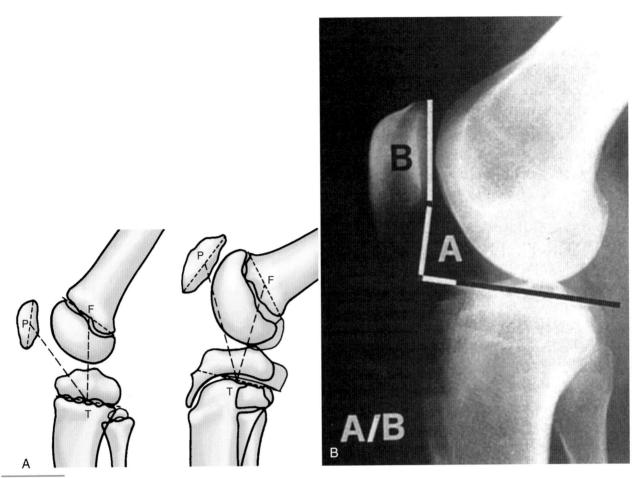

Figure 75–6. **A,** Epiphyseal line midpoint method of determining patella alta in skeletally immature patients **B,** Method of determining patella alta. (**A,** From Koshino T, Sigimoto K: New measurement of patellar height in the knees of children using the epiphyseal line midpoint. J Pediatr Orthop 9:216-218, 1989. **B,** from Blackburne JS, Peel TE: A new method of measuring patellar height. J Bone Joint Surg Br 59:241-242, 1977.)

knees. He and Stanitski[80] pointed out the significantly lower rate of osteochondral fractures in LAACS- versus TONES-type patients. Scheller and Martenson[74] and Rünow[71] have detailed the distribution of dislocation-related fractures and the infrequent occurrence of concurrent avulsion and osteochondral fractures.

TREATMENT

A number of factors must be considered when deciding on treatment of patellofemoral instability in a young patient, including the chronicity of the instability, the presence of predisposing mechanical risk factors, the degree of instability, the existence of concurrent injury, the age and activity level of the athlete, progression with nonoperative care, and desires of the athlete and family. The majority of patients with patellofemoral instability should be treated initially with a comprehensive, well-monitored nonoperative program. However, the indications for initial surgical intervention and earlier reconstruction are evolving.

Nonoperative Care

Most dislocations will spontaneously reduce on the field with terminal knee extension. If not, reduction should be done in a controlled setting with adequate sedation, full passive extension, and gentle pressure only as required. As discussed earlier, arthrocentesis is preformed for diagnostic and therapeutic benefit. Early immobilization in full extension is used for comfort and to let the injured soft tissues quiet down. However, quad sets, straight-leg raises, and single-plane motion are begun early and progressed as tolerated. Conceptually, the early nonoperative treatment is like that for initial MCL sprain. Early guarded motion and exercise are beneficial. It is unlikely that single-plane motion, particularly midflexion to full extension, will stretch the healing MPFL or cause recurrent instability. It is repetition of the injury mechanism or mechanically similar activities that must be avoided in the healing period. The MPFL is in the same layer II environment as the MCL. Although it is not known for certain, its healing potential may be similar.[77]

As strength and symptoms allow, patients progress out of their brace in the protected environment of physical therapy to single-plane walking, running, cutting, and finally sport-specific activity. Early modalities and exercise are aimed at decreasing pain and effusion while triggering quadriceps activity. It is much easier to maintain quadriceps function than to retrieve it after a period of complete immobilization and inactivity. Early motion also helps maintain articular cartilage health.

Rehabilitation involves optimizing the environment for quadriceps activity, restoring extensor mechanism balance, and improving lower extremity alignment. Long-term maintenance and preventive training programs are geared toward raising the level of extensor mechanism function to meet the demands of the sports environment without subsequent injury. Retropatellar irritation is a potential source of problems during extensor mechanism rehabilitation. Pain leads to significant quadriceps inhibition and may indicate increasing articular cartilage damage. Exercises should be done in a pain-free range and manner. In closed-chain exercises, patellofemoral stress increases as flexion increases. In open-chain exercises, the opposite is true. We have found that open-chain resistive exercises done in early to mid flexion are well tolerated. The patella is well seated, and areas of articular damage incurred at the time of dislocation in relatively more extension may not be weightbearing. Strengthening in more terminal extension is done with functional closed-chain exercises. Variable-arc isometrics is another way to avoid painful areas of patellofemoral compression. Despite traditional thought, selected VMO recruitment or strengthening has not been supported in the research.[43,64,67] It appears that the quadriceps both weaken and must be strengthened as a whole. However, quadriceps activity should be incorporated into functional patterns as soon as possible. Examples are working lateral pelvic tilts (hip abduction) or hip adduction (ball squeezes) with concurrent quadriceps contraction. Trampoline activities and multijoint exercises, such as short-arc squats, also require the quadriceps to work in a sport-specific manner. Patellar taping as described by Gilleard et al[32] has been shown to decrease pain, allow increased quadriceps activity, and improve weight acceptance in functional activities during the early rehabilitation period. The exact mechanism of the beneficial effects is unclear. It does not appear to be through a significant change in static patellar position. Potential reasons include changes in patellofemoral compressive forces possibly resulting from increasing rather than decreasing the area bearing weight and thereby decreasing force per unit area, proprioceptive feedback to improve recruitment of quadriceps activity, and subtle improvements in dynamic patella tracking. Patellar knee sleeves appear to serve a similar function on a more long-term basis.

Although quadriceps strengthening is paramount, selective stretching is required to achieve a balanced extensor mechanism. Stretching of the upper and lower iliotibial band, hamstrings, gastrocnemius, and hip flexors is preformed by the patient. Patellar mobilization can be done by the therapist to stretch a tight lateral retinaculum. Relative internal rotation of the lower extremity increases the lateralizing vector on the patella. Excessive or prolonged midfoot pronation may be a contributor, and semirigid orthotics are helpful in selected patients. Dynamic hip anteversion may also be improved with proximal strengthening.

Operative Care

Surgical interventions for patellofemoral instability are numerous. The phrase "over 100 procedures" has become synonymous with any discussion of surgery to address patellofemoral instability. Surgical care may involve acute repair or later reconstruction, bony or soft-tissue procedures, or proximal or distal realignment. Surgery may be aimed at anatomic restoration or compensatory realignment. Historically, many of the " nonanatomic" soft-tissue procedures have probably met with success because of the "healing" layer II environment of the medial aspect of the knee in which the MPFL is located. Lateral advancement of medial soft tissues containing a healed, but somewhat stretched MPFL may provide adequate restraint to patellar dislocation in some cases. However, there has been a recent trend toward anatomic restoration of the primary soft-tissue restraints to lateral patellar dislocation, specifically, the MPFL. This development reflects the trends in ACL reconstruction and shoulder instability surgery, which now incorporate anatomic restoration of the ACL or labrum rather than compensatory extra-articular, musculotendinous procedures.

There are several relative indications for operative intervention after patellar dislocation: (1) failure to progress with initial nonoperative care, (2) concurrent osteochondral injury that necessitates operative intervention, (3) continued gross patellar instability, (4) grossly palpable disruption of the MPFL-VMO-adductor mechanism, (5) high-level athletic demands coupled with mechanical risk factors and an initial mechanism not related to contact injury, and (6) recurrent dislocation and failure of a long-term nonoperative program. In general, TONES-type patients will get by with less surgery, most commonly repair or reconstruction of the MPFL. LAACS patients may often require combined proximal and distal realignment to address their chronic maltracking.

Osteochondral fractures must be suspected with all patellar dislocations. They may show up on diagnostic imaging or be manifested as mechanical symptoms and disproportionate pain during the early rehabilitation period. These fractures are rarely large or intact enough and do not have sufficient bony backing to warrant open reduction and fixation. Most are treated by loose-body removal, débridement of unstable shoulders, microfracture, and assessment for future chondral restoration procedures. Arthroscopic or open techniques may be used for the few fractures amenable to fixation.

SURGERY ADDRESSING THE MEDIAL PATELLOFEMORAL LIGAMENT

Surgery addressing the MPFL is appropriate when the primary deficiency is of medial soft tissue restraints. If significant malalignment and functionally increased Q angle are present, a distal realignment is required. In a combined deficiency, MPFL repair or reconstruction may be used in combination with a distal realignment. The safe age for tibial tubercle osteotomy is not well defined. However, a bone age of 14 to 15 years for boys and 12 to 13 years for girls should avoid any significant iatrogenic recurvatum.[35,47]

An injured MPFL may be addressed by acute repair, repair with augmentation, or reconstruction. A variety of graft options, fixation devices, and surgical techniques have been described, and the timing of surgery may vary, depending on a number of patient and clinical factors. In a patient with acute or early recurrent dislocation, the primary surgery is repair of the MPFL. Adjunctive reconstruction may be required if the native tissue is judged to be insufficient. With more chronic instability patterns, reconstruction of the MPFL is more routinely required. If preexisting lateral facet syndrome or significant lateral patellar tilt is present, concurrent lateral release may be performed. However, release is not routinely required. If distal realignment is required, posterior medialization or distal displacement of the tubercle should be avoided because of a significant risk for secondary retropatellar arthritis. Unfortunately, straight medialization and even anteromedialization may also increase medial retropatellar loading.[65] In a more immature patient with a significantly increased Q angle or patella alta, reconstruction of the MPFL may be augmented by using a limb of the hamstring graft to reconstruct the patellotibial ligament or by performing a patellar tendon split and turn under.

Medial Patellofemoral Ligament Repair/Reconstruction

Repair may be done acutely or after a period of initial healing. Acute repairs may be performed with suture to periosteum or by using suture anchors on the patellar or femoral sides. Acute repair must be accomplished at the site of MPFL disruption, most commonly at its femoral attachment, but it may also be accomplished at the superior medial patellar attachment or within its interstitial substance. MRI is useful in localizing the areas of MPFL damage. If the area of injury is uncertain or if initial repair at a particular site does not result in adequate tensioning, the ligament should be directly evaluated throughout its length. Ahmad et al[3] emphasized the importance of concurrently assessing the femoral attachment of the VMO, which may be ruptured. Repair of the VMO insertion back to the adductor tendon restores its normal biomechanics. Specific repair techniques and the necessary anatomic dissection have been described by previous authors.[3,29,77] The repair must be appropriately tensioned. There should be some laxity in the repaired MPFL in terminal knee extension. A normal patella can be translated 25% to 50% at full extension. The operative knee may be matched to an asymptomatic, contralateral knee with regard to medial/lateral translation and tilt. Others have suggested that 5 lb of lateralizing force on the repair or reconstruction at 30 degrees of flexion should result in no greater than 10 mm or no less than 5 mm of displacement.[14] With lateralization of the patella, there should be a firm endpoint to the repair. Although the graft should be placed in a relatively isometric position, it will tend to tighten as the knee moves to full flexion. Full range of motion should be possible without undue force or tension on the repair. If the native tissue is judged to be insufficient or inherently lax, the repair may be supplemented with a partial turndown of the adductor magnus tendon to increase the bulk of repaired tissue.

In patients with recurrent instability, deficient bony stabilizers, native soft-tissue laxity, and more pronounced dislocation, formal reconstruction of the MPFL may be required. A number of tissues, including the local adductor tendon, free hamstring autograft, iliotibial band, and synthetic materials, have been described.[17] The MPFL may be reconstructed alone or in combination with the medial patellotibial ligament. Fixation on the patellar side can be achieved with the use of bone tunnels, suturing, or suture anchors. On the femoral side, direct suturing, a post with a washer, a staple, and sling fabrication from the MCL have all been described for fixation. In a skeletally immature patient, hardware must be kept out of the femoral growth plate and excessive dissection about the peripheral growth plate avoided. Drez et al[20] describe a technique in which the MPFL and the medial patellotibial ligaments are reconstructed. A medial incision is made halfway between the medial patellar border and the adductor tubercle. Dissection is carried through subcutaneous tissue, and the patellar retinaculum and VMO are identified. A transverse incision is then made in the retinaculum beginning at the adductor tubercle and extending to the superomedial patellar border. The capsule of the joint is not violated. A semitendinosus and gracilis graft is then harvested and folded in half, and the center portion is sutured to the superomedial border of the patella with No. 2 nonabsorbable suture. The upper limb of the graft is then sutured to the femoral origin of the MPFL with the knee in full extension and slight medial pressure on the patella. The lower limb of the graft is sutured to the tibial periosteum, 1.5 cm distal to the joint line, to replicate the medial patellotibial ligament. The medial retinaculum is reapproximated to the medial border of the patella, and the transverse retinacular incision is closed (Fig. 75–7). Muneta et al[58] described the use of two smaller incisions: one at the medial border of the patella and the other centered over the medial epicondyle of the femur. The graft is tunneled in layer II between these two incisions. A double-stranded soft-tissue graft is fixed with a spiked washer at the femoral attachment site. Patellar fixation is accomplished through a 4.5-mm tunnel drilled from the center of the midportion of the articular surface of the patella at its medial edge to the center of the patella. A 3.2-mm hole is drilled from the anterior patellar surface to intersect the transverse hole. The graft is passed into the tunnel and fixed with a button or sewn back onto itself if graft length allows (Fig. 75–8). Deie et al[18] recently reported on MPFL reconstruction in a small group of patellar dislocators with an average age of 8.5 years. They used a semitendinosus graft taken with an open tendon stripper and left attached distally. Through a separate 2-cm incision over the femoral medial epicondyle a 1-cm slit was made in the posterior third of the MCL to act as a pulley. A curved incision was made over the patella and the graft transferred through the MCL pulley and tunneled in layer II to the medial aspect of the patella, where it was

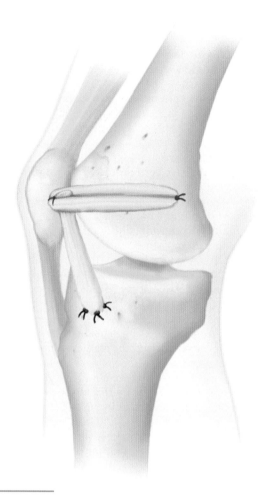

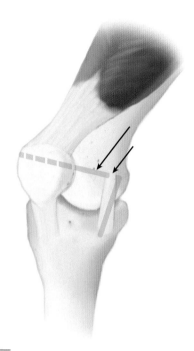

Figure 75–9. Reconstruction of the medial patellofemoral ligament. The semitendinosus tendon (*large arrow*) is transferred to the patella with a pulley in the posterior third of the proximal aspect of the medial collateral ligament (*small arrow*). (From Deie M, Ochi M, Sumen Y, et al: Reconstruction of the medial patellofemoral ligament for the treatment of habitual or recurrent dislocation of the patella in children. J Bone Joint Surg Br 85:887-890, 2003.)

Figure 75–7. Reconstructed medial patellofemoral ligament and medial patellotibial ligament. (From Drez D Jr, Edwards TB, Williams CS: Results of medial patellofemoral ligament reconstruction in the treatment of patellar dislocation. Arthroscopy 17:298-306, 2001.)

sutured to the anteromedial surface of the patella with moderate medial force on the patella and the knee in 30 degrees of flexion (Fig. 75–9).

For MPFL reconstruction we currently use three small incisions: one over the superomedial border of the patella, one over the medial epicondyle, and one for hamstring graft harvest. For acute repairs we use a single larger vertical incision midway between the origin and insertion of the MPFL. This technique allows full inspection of the origin, insertion, and intraligament substance. Our graft of choice is a doubled semitendinosus autograft, which provides adequate length and bulk. We bluntly dissect a tunnel in layer II of the medial part of the knee to pass the graft between the superomedial aspect of the patella and the epicondylar attachment of the MPFL. At the patella a shallow trough is burred in the upper two-thirds of the medial border, and two or three 3.5-mm suture anchors are used for fixation. On the femoral side we use a screw and soft-tissue washer for fixation. The folded end of the graft is initially fixed on the patella, with the two tails of the graft to be fixed left on the femur. This affords easy assessment and adjustment of graft tension around the post screw as the knee is taken through a range of motion and translation applied to the patella. We have not routinely reconstructed the medial tibiopatellar ligament. We usually fix the graft at approximately 20 degrees of flexion and allow 25% to 50% lateral translation and a crisp endpoint. We also use the mobility of the asymptomatic patella as a template (Fig. 75–10).

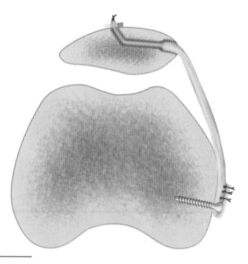

Figure 75–8. Drawing of patellofemoral fixation with a graft passing into the tunnel and fixed with a button. (From Muneta T, Sekiya I, Tsuchiya M, Shinomiya K: A technique for reconstruction of the medial patellofemoral ligament. Clin Orthop 359:151-155, 1999.)

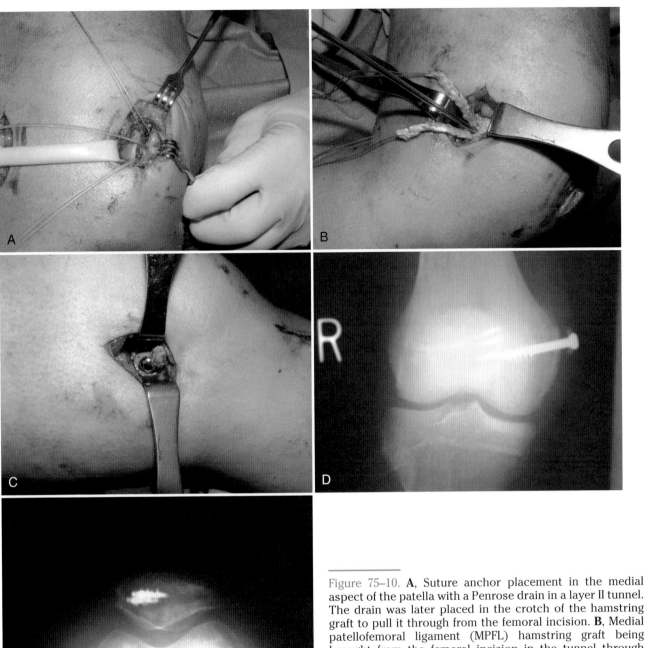

Figure 75–10. **A**, Suture anchor placement in the medial aspect of the patella with a Penrose drain in a layer II tunnel. The drain was later placed in the crotch of the hamstring graft to pull it through from the femoral incision. **B**, Medial patellofemoral ligament (MPFL) hamstring graft being brought from the femoral incision in the tunnel through layer II to the medial aspect of the patella. **C**, Screw and soft-tissue washer fixation at the MPFL femoral origin. **D**, Anteroposterior radiographic view of the suture anchors and screw/washer status after MPFL reconstruction. **E**, Sunrise radiographic view of the suture anchors and screw/washer status after MPFL reconstruction.

Postoperatively, extended immobilization must be avoided. After a week to allow the soft tissues to quiet down, progressive range of motion is begun. Maintaining quadriceps function is key to success, and an adjustable hinged brace is used to prevent extremes of flexion and significant valgus stress on the knee. Postoperative rehabilitation follows the nonoperative program as outlined earlier. Return to sporting activity can be anticipated in 6 months after reconstruction. Studies have reported a wide range of success with MPFL repair and reconstruction.[3,17,18,20,29,58,61,72] This variability may be related to selec-tion bias, definition of injury, concurrent osteochondral injuries, and the varied use of simultaneous procedures such as lateral release and/or distal realignment. In general, poor and fair results appear to be more related to retropatellar pain than to recurrent instability.

Non–Medial Patellofemoral Ligament Reconstruction in Younger Patients

Historically, the same type of nonanatomic procedures applied to patellofemoral instability in adult patients have been used in children, but with some modification to accommodate the immature tibial tubercle. These procedures are aimed at realigning or advancing the medial extensor mechanism and/or the distal patella tendon attachment to reduce lateralizing forces on the patella. McCall and Ratts[52] reported the successful use of extensive proximal and distal soft-tissue advancement coupled with lateral release in a large group of young patents with patellofemoral instability. Though effective in controlling instability, this procedure requires extensive dissection and may increase retropatellar contact force. Letts et al[45] reported on the use of semitendinosus tenodesis as first described by Galeazzi.[27] A semitendinosus graft left attached distally is placed through an obliquely drilled tunnel in the patella and sewn back on itself. This technique may be combined with medial reefing and/or lateral release. Good to excellent results in a skeletally immature population have been achieved in 62% to 82%. However, the routing of the graft does not duplicate that of the native MPFL. Dislocation recurrence rates may be as high as 10%, and the results may be compromised by persistent patellofemoral pain or chondromalacia.[45] In the Roux-Goldthwait procedure,[13] distal realignment is attempted by detaching the lateral half of the patella and transferring it medially under the remaining attached tendon. This may result in initial weakening of the patellar tendon and increased patellar tilt. The transferred tendon often atrophies and becomes of little biomechanical importance over time.

A number of arthroscopic soft-tissue balancing techniques for lateral patellar instability have been reported. They are essentially medial advancements coupled with an arthroscopic lateral release.[2,9,34] They have the advantages of being minimally invasive, seemingly as effective as similar open surgeries, and not burning any treatment bridges for young patients. Ahmad and Lee[2] described making an incision in the medial retinaculum, which is then repaired in a pants-over-vest fashion. The distance that sutures are passed from the edge of the incision will determine the degree of imbrication. Halbrecht[34] reported the use of suturing to bunch and tighten the medial retinaculum without incising it. Both authors combined medial reefing with arthroscopic lateral release. These procedures may be best in patients with more subtle instability, good soft-tissue quality, and relatively normal patellofemoral bony architecture. These procedures may also be used as an adjunct to distal realignment.

CONGENITAL, DEVELOPMENTAL, AND HABITUAL DISLOCATION

There has been significant confusion concerning the terminology of the early-onset, more involved forms of patellofemoral instability. After a thorough review of the pertinent literature, we suggest the following guidelines to be helpful.

Congenital dislocation: Persistent or fixed lateral dislocation of the patella detected at or near birth. It is manifested as knee flexion contracture with the patella tethered lateral to the femoral condyles. The probable cause is failure of normal embryological rotation of the quadriceps myotome during lower extremity development.

Developmental dislocation: Significant maltracking or dislocation resulting from abnormal growth and development and stress across the extensor mechanism. It is often associated with systemic or generalized syndromes.

Habitual dislocation: Dislocation with spontaneous reduction that occurs with every flexion-extension cycle. It is atraumatic and occurs with normal activities of daily living. Habitual dislocation is usually associated with significant patellofemoral dysplasia and tightness of the extensor mechanism.

Ghanem et al[30,31] pointed out that true congenital, in utero fixed dislocation of the patella is rare. It may occur as a result of arthrogryposis, skeletal dysplasia, and other related abnormalities. However, it should be differentiated from developmental dislocation in which the extensor mechanism is located normally at birth but progressively moves toward a fixed dislocation later in childhood. The probable cause of congenital dislocation is failure of normal medial rotation of the quadriceps myotome during in utero development.[30,79] In contrast, the patella dislocation often associated with Down's syndrome, nail-patella syndrome, acquired quadriceps fibrosis, and various neuromuscular conditions is related to abnormal biomechanical forces on an initially normally located patella. Although congenital dislocation is usually associated with more severe deformity, developmental dislocation can progress to a similar phenotypic manifestation of fixed lateral patellar dislocation, severe quadriceps contracture, and functional disability. It appears that early, comprehensive surgical realignment affords the best chance to normalize lower extremity function.[22,31,33,39] Such realignment involves aggressive mobilization of the entire patella/quadriceps mechanism, division of the lateral soft tissues, imbrication of the medial soft tissues, and possibly transfer of the insertion of the patellar ligament.

Habitual dislocators present a significantly different picture. Their problem involves spontaneous dislocation and reduction of the patella with every flexion-extension cycle of the knee. This condition does not significantly delay the age or ability of early ambulation. Consequently, it is usually diagnosed later at 5 to 10 years of age. It is relatively painless and not voluntary in nature. In contrast, recurrent dislocation is typically episodic, is often a result of minor trauma, is painful, and can lead to swelling. There is usually some degree of extensor mechanism contracture, so full range of motion is possible once the patella dislocates; however, with the patella held in place, flexion is limited. Several authors describe the underlying pathology as being quadriceps muscle contracture, often thought to be the result of local trauma.[4,7] In contrast to the more common recurrent dislocator, treatment of habitual dislocation would routinely require quadriceps lengthening and lateral release.

SUMMARY

Many reports on patellofemoral instability suffer the same flaws of inappropriate patient selection, poor definition of injury, and insufficient assessment of activity as found in other areas of the orthopaedic literature. A number of "truths" concerning risk factors and treatment interventions have seemingly been recycled through the literature without adequate substantiation. There appear to be two large groups of young patellar dislocators, which we have defined as TONES and LAACS based on their risk factors and natural history. Traditionally, patellar instability has been treated with variable periods of immobilization and sporadic rehabilitation, with full return to sports activity expected. The reality is that many young athletes suffer long-term retropatellar pain and sport-limiting extensor mechanism impairment. Although most athletes still benefit from an initial nonoperative program, this care must be aggressive, comprehensive, and responsive to early treatment outcomes. Concurrent osteochondral injuries are common and a major contributor to adverse outcomes. Diagnostically, MRI is improving in its ability to detail osteochondral injury and also plays an important role in determining the location and extent of MPFL injury. The primary stabilizing role of the MPFL and its injury as the essential lesion in patellar instability are just now being appreciated. There is growing interest in replacing the myriad of nonanatomic extensor mechanism reconstructions with more anatomically based MPFL-based surgeries.

References

1. Aglietti P, Insall JN, Cerulli G: Patellar pain and incongruence. I: Measurements of incongruence. Clin Orthop 176:217-224, 1983.
2. Ahmad CS, Lee FY: An all-arthroscopic soft-tissue balancing technique for lateral patellar instability. Arthroscopy 17:555-557, 2001.
3. Ahmad CS, Stein BE, Matuz D, Henry JH: Immediate surgical repair of the medial patellar stabilizers for acute patellar dislocation. A review of eight cases. Am J Sports Med 28:804-810, 2000.
4. Alvarez EV, Munters M, Lavine LS, et al: Quadriceps myofibrosis. A complication of intramuscular injections. J Bone Joint Surg Am 62:58-60, 1980.
5. Atkin DM, Fithian DC, Marangi KS, et al: Characteristics of patients with primary acute lateral patellar dislocation and their recovery within the first 6 months of injury. Am J Sports Med 28:472-479, 2000.
6. Beasley LS, Vidal AF: Traumatic patellar dislocation in children and adolescents: Treatment update and literature review. Curr Opin Pediatr 16:29-36, 2004.
7. Bergman NR, Williams PF: Habitual dislocation of the patella in flexion. J Bone Joint Surg Br 70:415-419, 1988.
8. Blackburne JS, Peel TE: A new method of measuring patellar height. J Bone Joint Surg Br 59:241-242, 1977.
9. Brief LP: Lateral patellar instability: Treatment with a combined open-arthroscopic approach. Arthroscopy 9:617-623, 1993.
10. Burks RT, Desio SM, Bachus KN, et al: Biomechanical evaluation of lateral patellar dislocations. Am J Knee Surg 11:24-31, 1998.
11. Cash JD, Hughston JC: Treatment of acute patellar dislocation. Am J Sports Med 16:244-249, 1988.
12. Caylor D, Fites R, Worrell TW: The relationship between quadriceps angle and anterior knee pain syndrome. J Orthop Sports Phys Ther 17:11-16, 1993.
13. Chrisman OD, Snook GA, Wilson TC: A long-term prospective study of the Hauser and Roux-Goldthwait procedures for recurrent patellar dislocation. Clin Orthop 144:27-30, 1979.
14. Conlan T, Garth WP Jr, Lemons JE: Evaluation of the medial soft-tissue restraints of the extensor mechanism of the knee. J Bone Joint Surg Am 75:682-693, 1993.
15. Dainer RD, Barrack RL, Buckley SL, Alexander AH: Arthroscopic treatment of acute patella dislocation. Arthroscopy 4:267-271, 1988.
16. Davies AP, Costa ML, Shepstone L, et al: The sulcus angle and malalignment of the extensor mechanism of the knee. J Bone Joint Surg Br 82:1162-1166, 2000.
17. Davis DK, Fithian DC: Techniques of medial retinacular repair and reconstruction. Clin Orthop 402:38-52, 2002.
18. Deie M, Ochi M, Sumen Y, et al: Reconstruction of the medial patellofemoral ligament for the treatment of habitual or recurrent dislocation of the patella in children. J Bone Joint Surg Br 85:887-890, 2003.
19. Desio SM, Burks RT, Bachus KN: Soft tissue restraints to lateral patellar translation in the human knee. Am J Sports Med 26:59-65, 1998.
20. Drez D Jr, Edwards TB, Williams CS: Results of medial patellofemoral ligament reconstruction in the treatment of patellar dislocation. Arthroscopy 17:298-306, 2001.
21. Dye SF: The knee as a biologic transmission with an envelope of function: A theory. Clin Orthop 325:10-18, 1996.
22. Eilert RE: Congenital dislocation of the patella. Clin Orthop 389:22-29, 2001.
23. Ellison AE, Berg EE: Embryology, anatomy, and function of the anterior cruciate ligament. Orthop Clin North Am 16:3-14, 1985.
24. Fairbank JC, Pynsent PB, van Poortvliet JA, Phillips H: Mechanical factors in the incidence of knee pain in adolescents and young adults. J Bone Joint Surg Br 66:685-693, 1984.
25. Fithian DC, Paxton EW, Stone ML, et al: Epidemiology and natural history of acute patellar dislocation. Am J Sports Med 32:1114-1121, 2004.
26. Fulkerson JP, Kalenak A, Rosenberg TD, Cox JS: Patellofemoral pain. Instr Course Lect 41:57-71, 1992.
27. Galeazzi R: Nuove applicazioni del trapianto muscolare e tendineo. Arch Ortop 38:19-22, 1921.
28. Gao GX, Lee EH, Bose K: Surgical management of congenital and habitual dislocation of the patella. J Pediatr Orthop 10:255-260, 1990.
29. Garth WP Jr, DiChristina DG, Holt G: Delayed proximal repair and distal realignment after patellar dislocation. Clin Orthop 377:132-144, 2000.
30. Ghanem I, Wattincourt L, Seringe R: Congenital dislocation of the patella. Part I: Pathologic anatomy. J Pediatr Orthop 20:812-816, 2000.
31. Ghanem I, Wattincourt L, Seringe R: Congenital dislocation of the patella. Part II: Orthopaedic management. J Pediatr Orthop 20:817-822, 2000.
32. Gilleard W, McConnell J, Parsons D: The effect of patellar taping on the onset of vastus medialis obliquus and vastus lateralis muscle activity in persons with patellofemoral pain. Phys Ther 78:25-32, 1998.
33. Gordon JE, Schoenecker PL: Surgical treatment of congenital dislocation of the patella. J Pediatr Orthop 19:260-264, 1999.
34. Halbrecht JL: Arthroscopic patella realignment: An all-inside technique. Arthroscopy 17:940-945, 2001.
35. Harrison MHM: The results of a realignment operation for recurrent dislocation of the patella. J Bone Joint Surg Br 37:559-567, 1955.
36. Hautamaa PV, Fithian DC, Kaufman KR, et al: Medial soft tissue restraints in lateral patellar instability and repair. Clin Orthop 349:174-182, 1998.
37. Hinton RY, Sharma KM: Acute and recurrent patellar instability in the young athlete. Orthop Clin North Am 34:385-396, 2003.
38. Insall J, Salvati E: Patella position in the normal knee joint. Radiology 101:101-104, 1971.
39. Jones RD, Fisher RL, Curtis BH: Congenital dislocation of the patella. Clin Orthop 119:177-183, 1976.
40. Katz MP, Grogono BJ, Soper KC: The etiology and treatment of congenital dislocation of the knee. J Bone Joint Surg Br 49:112-120, 1967.
41. Koshino T, Sugimoto K: New measurement of patellar height in the knees of children using the epiphyseal line midpoint. J Pediatr Orthop 9:216-218, 1989.
42. Langenskiold A, Ritsila V: Congenital dislocation of the patella and its operative treatment. J Pediatr Orthop 12:315-323, 1992.
43. Laprade J, Culham E, Brouwer B: Comparison of five isometric exercises in the recruitment of the vastus medialis oblique in persons with and without patellofemoral pain syndrome. J Orthop Sports Phys Ther 27:197-204, 1998.
44. Laurin CA, Dussault R, Levesque HP: The tangential x-ray investigation of the patellofemoral joint: X-ray technique, diagnostic criteria and their interpretation. Clin Orthop 144:16-26, 1979.

45. Letts RM, Davidson D, Beaule P: Semitendinosus tenodesis for repair of recurrent dislocation of the patella in children. J Pediatr Orthop 19:742-747, 1999.

46. Livingston LA, Mandigo JL: Bilateral Q angle asymmetry and anterior knee pain syndrome. Clin Biomech 14:7-13, 1999.

47. Macnab I: Recurrent dislocation of the patella. J Bone Joint Surg Am 34:957-967, 1952.

48. Mäenpää H, Huhtala H, Lehto MU: Recurrence after patellar dislocation. Redislocation in 37/75 patients followed for 6-24 years. Acta Orthop Scand 68:424-426, 1997.

49. Maldague B, Malghem J: [Significance of the radiograph of the knee profile in the detection of patellar instability. Preliminary report.] Apport du cliche de profil du genou dans le depistage des instabilites rotuliennes. Rapport preliminaire. Rev Chir Orthop Reparatrice Appar Mot 71(Suppl 2):5-13, 1985.

50. Marangi KS, White LM, Brossmann J, et al: Magnetic resonance imaging of the knee following acute lateral patella dislocation. Presented at the 63rd Annual Meeting of the American Association of Orthopaedic Surgeons, February 22-26, 1996, Atlanta.

51. Matthews LS, Hinton RY, Burke N: Lacrosse. In Fu FH, Stone DA (eds): Sports Injuries: Mechanism, Prevention, Treatment, 2nd ed. Philadelphia, Lippincott Williams & Wilkins, 2001, pp 568-582.

52. McCall RE, Ratts V: Soft-tissue realignment for adolescent patellar instability. J Pediatr Orthop 19:549-552, 1999.

53. McCauley TR, Disler DG: MR imaging of articular cartilage. Radiology 209:629-640, 1998.

54. McManus F, Rang M, Heslin DJ: Acute dislocation of the patella in children. The natural history. Clin Orthop 139:88-91, 1979.

55. Merchant AC: Classification of patellofemoral disorders. Arthroscopy 4:235-240, 1988.

56. Merchant AC, Mercer RL, Jacobsen RH, Cool CR: Roentgenographic analysis of patellofemoral congruence. J Bone Joint Surg Am 56:1391-1396, 1974.

57. Merida-Velasco JA, Sanchez-Montesinos I, Espin-Ferra J, et al: Development of the human knee joint ligaments. Anat Rec 248:259-268, 1997.

58. Muneta T, Sekiya I, Tsuchiya M, Shinomiya K: A technique for reconstruction of the medial patellofemoral ligament. Clin Orthop 359:151-155, 1999.

59. Nietosvaara Y: The femoral sulcus in children. An ultrasonographic study. J Bone Joint Surg Br 76:807-809, 1994.

60. Nietosvaara Y, Aalto K, Kallio PE: Acute patellar dislocation in children. Incidence and associated osteochondral fractures. J Pediatr Orthop 14:513-515, 1994.

61. Nikku R, Nietosvaara Y, Kallio PE, et al: Operative versus closed treatment of primary dislocation of the patella. Similar 2-year results in 125 randomized patients. Acta Orthop Scand 68:419-423, 1997.

62. Nomura E: Classification of lesions of the medial patello-femoral ligament in patellar dislocation. Int Orthop 23:260-263, 1999.

63. Ogden JA: Radiology of postnatal skeletal development. X. Patella and tibial tuberosity. Skeletal Radiol 11:246-257, 1984.

64. Philadelphia Panel evidence-based clinical practice guidelines on selected rehabilitation interventions for knee pain. Phys Ther 81:1675-1700, 2001.

65. Pidoriano AJ, Weinstein RN, Buuck DA, Fulkerson JP: Correlation of patellar articular lesions with results from anteromedial tibial tubercle transfer. Am J Sports Med 25:533-537, 1997.

66. Post WR: Clinical evaluation of patients with patellofemoral disorders. Arthroscopy 15:841-851, 1999.

67. Powers CM: Rehabilitation of patellofemoral joint disorders: A critical review. J Orthop Sports Phys Ther 28:345-354, 1998.

68. Ratajczak W: Early development of the cruciate ligaments in staged human embryos. Folia Morphol (Warsz) 59:285-290, 2000.

69. Recht M, Bobic V, Burstein D, et al: Magnetic resonance imaging of articular cartilage. Clin Orthop 391(Suppl):S379-S396, 2001.

70. Reider B, Marshall JL, Koslin B, et al: The anterior aspect of the knee joint. J Bone Joint Surg Am 63:351-356, 1981.

71. Rūnow A: The dislocating patella. Etiology and prognosis in relation to generalized joint laxity and anatomy of the patellar articulation. Acta Orthop Scand Suppl 201:1-53, 1983.

72. Sallay PI, Poggi J, Speer KP, Garrett WE: Acute dislocation of the patella. A correlative pathoanatomic study. Am J Sports Med 24:52-60, 1996.

73. Sandmeier RH, Burks RT, Bachus KN, Billings A: The effect of reconstruction of the medial patellofemoral ligament on patellar tracking. Am J Sports Med 28:345-349, 2000.

74. Scheller S, Martenson L: Traumatic dislocation of the patella. A radiographic investigation. Acta Radiol Suppl 336:1-160, 1974.

75. Sledge CB: Some morphologic and experimental aspects of limb development. Clin Orthop 44:241-264, 1966.

76. Smirk C, Morris H: The anatomy and reconstruction of the medial patellofemoral ligament. Knee 10:221-227, 2003.

77. Spritzer CE: "Slip sliding away": Patellofemoral dislocation and tracking. Magn Reson Imaging Clin N Am 8:299-320, 2000.

78. Staeubli HU, Bosshard C, Porcellini P, Rauschning W: Magnetic resonance imaging for articular cartilage: Cartilage-bone mismatch. Clin Sports Med 21:417-433, viii-ix, 2002.

79. Stanisavljevic S, Zemenick G, Miller D: Congenital, irreducible, permanent lateral dislocation of the patella. Clin Orthop 116:190-199, 1976.

80. Stanitski CL: Articular hypermobility and chondral injury in patients with acute patellar dislocation. Am J Sports Med 23:146-150, 1995.

81. Visuri T, Mäenpää H: Patellar dislocation in army conscripts. Mil Med 167:537-540, 2002.

82. Walker P, Harris I, Leicester A: Patellar tendon–to–patella ratio in children. J Pediatr Orthop 18:129-131, 1998.

83. Warren LF, Marshall JL: The supporting structures and layers on the medial side of the knee: An anatomical analysis. J Bone Joint Surg Am 61:56-62, 1979.

84. Witonski D: Dynamic magnetic resonance imaging. Clin Sports Med 21:403-415, 2002.

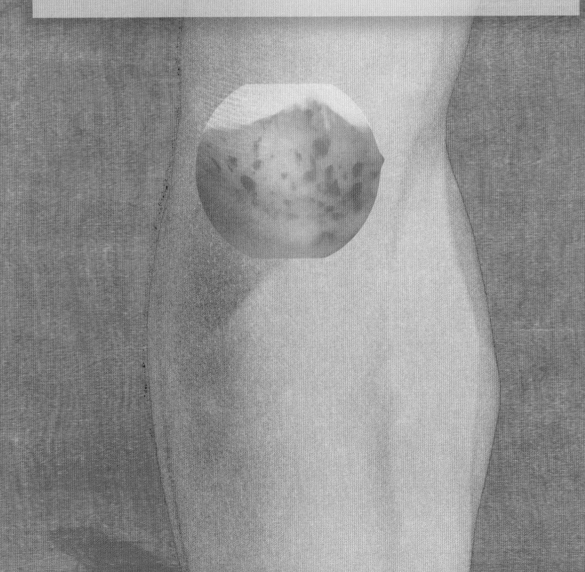

Joint Replacement and Its Alternatives

CHAPTER 76

Scoring Systems and Their Validation for the Arthritic Knee

Kevin J. Mulhall • Todd C. Battaglia • Thomas E. Brown Khaled J. Saleh

Total knee arthroplasty (TKA) is widely acknowledged to be one of the most successful and cost-effective procedures in orthopedic practice from the perspective of both patients and third-party payers.[30] Numerous long-term studies attest to the significant improvement in quality of life after TKA procedures, and further improvements have been achieved by recent technological advancements in prosthetic design, instrumentation, surgical techniques, and rehabilitation.[30] These results, when combined with an aging population, explain the dramatic rise in the number of TKA procedures performed in the United States and internationally.[24,25]

Unfortunately, most arthroplasty studies are reported retrospectively on small numbers of subjects with varying severity of disease and short follow-up periods. Furthermore, TKA results are reported in nonstandardized fashion and frequently use nonvalidated outcome measures. This situation creates difficulty in formulating predictive models that would enhance patient selection, rationalize geographic variation, or allow researchers to arrive at universally accepted treatment guidelines. These observations are not new, and various commentaries within the field have called for actions to address these shortcomings.[30]

To address these issues, considerable work has focused on deriving reliable and valid methods of assessing or scoring the outcomes of these procedures. The ultimate goal is to allow for continued rational improvement in patient care based on objective information from patient cohorts. These issues have also been addressed by the orthopedic community internationally through the establishment of large-scale data collection projects, with varying degrees of success. Accurate databases/data registries can be used to characterize practice patterns, identify and investigate prosthesis failure, establish benchmarks, develop guidelines, and quantify present and future health care resource utilization. Such data should inevitably lead to improvement in patient outcomes and should be based on valid, reliable outcomes measures, as well as provide study samples representative of the universal population and establish mechanisms to ensure high data integrity and accurate patient tracking. The focus of the current chapter, however, is to describe the specific outcomes scores that are currently in use for the assessment of TKA.

BACKGROUND TO HEALTH-RELATED QUALITY-OF-LIFE MEASUREMENT

Outcomes measures in general are a component of the broad area of quality-of-life measurement. This has become an increasingly important medical activity as people live longer and incur more chronic illnesses. Specific measurement of health-related quality of life (HRQL) is important both in patient care and in clinical research because it can help determine such issues as prognosis, compensation, placement, estimation of care requirements, and the nature, timing, and results of any medical or surgical interventions performed.

Health can be defined as "a state of complete physical, mental, and social well-being."[9] Health, however, is only one aspect of quality of life. Other factors such as income, freedom, and quality of the environment are also determinants of quality of life. It was because of this that the term "health-related quality of life" has been recommended as being more specific and applicable.[11]

Some HRQL measures consist of a single question, such as "how is your quality of life?" More commonly, HRQL instruments are questionnaires made up of a number of items or questions. These items are added up in a number of dimensions or domains that refer to the outcome of interest that is being measured. Domains include parameters such as mobility, self-care, and well-being.

Administration of HRQL questionnaires can be carried out by trained interviewers or can be self-administered. Response rates are typically maximized when an interviewer administers the HRQL instrument by limiting missing items and ensuring patient comprehension of each item on the questionnaire. However, this is an extremely costly and time-consuming type of administration, both because of the need to train the interviewer and because of the time spent performing interviews.

Self-administered HRQL measures are more cost efficient but may have a greater likelihood of a lower response rate, missing items, or misinterpreted questions. One compromise between the two approaches is to have an instrument completed by the subject under supervision.[6] Cost-effective supervision, in our experience, can be best achieved electronically in the form of software that will not allow the subject to move to the next question without appropriately completing the preceding question.

The goals of an HRQL questionnaire may be either

1. The ability to differentiate those who have a higher measure of HRQL from those who have a worse measure. This type of instrument is defined as a *discriminative instrument.*

2. The ability to measure how much HRQL changes over time after an intervention. This type is termed an *evaluative instrument.*

For either a discriminative or evaluative type of instrument, two fundamental properties are required. The first is *reproducibility,* or the ability of a test to reproduce the same results when repeated under the same conditions; the second is *accuracy,* which translates into whether the instrument is really measuring what it is intended to measure. Reproducibility in discriminative instruments is termed reliability, and for evaluative instruments it is termed responsiveness.[11]

Like all psychometric instruments, HRQL measures must meet two general standards:

1. *Reliability*—or the ability of the instrument to consistently discriminate between patients who have a great deal or a little of the characteristic of interest. In other words, a reliable instrument is one in which patients score consistently high or low across different observers (inter-rater), different situations (test-retest), and other factors.

2. *Validity*—or the demonstration that an instrument is actually assessing the characteristic of interest.

Validity may be further said to depend on whether a gold standard exists. Although no gold standards exist for HRQL, scenarios may arise when a specific target for an HRQL measure exists that can be treated as a *criterion.* In these circumstances an instrument is determined to be measuring what it is intended to if its results correspond to those of the criterion standards. Alternatively, when no gold or criterion standard exists, clinical research relies on techniques used by experimental psychologists to deal with this problem (such as face/content, concurrent and construct validity). The most reported type of validity is construct validity, which involves comparisons between measures. This method of instrument validation examines whether correlations exist—and to what degree—between the new instrument and a more established and perhaps better understood instrument. Such an example would be evaluation of a new arthroplasty instrument against the Short-Form-36 (SF-36) (Table 76–1).

A key property of an HRQL questionnaire is ease of interpretability. For discriminative instruments, ease of interpretability can be defined as whether an instrument score signifies the degree to which that state exists. For example, the degree of impairment experienced with osteoarthritis or rheumatoid arthritis can be classified into mild, moderate, or severe. Interpretability of an evaluative instrument refers to differences within patients during a specified period and can be signified as trivial, small, moderate, or large. It has also been stated that practicability is another critical facet of any HRQL instrument.[6] The essence of this belief is that even in the best context, greater effort should be made to facilitate the ease of application of HRQL instruments into medical decision making.

Table 76–1. Types of Validity

Face and content validity	A judgment by a criterion group of experts, patients, or caregivers that the questions asked appear to tap into the relevant domain and cover all the important content areas
Concurrent validity	The instrument correlates with other measures of the same underlying characteristic
Construct validity	The absence of a "gold standard" of the characteristic, construct validity amounts to the demonstration that the instrument changes in the anticipated direction when administered to groups who differ in other characteristics thought to be related to the characteristic of interest. The construct is the hypothesis relating the two characteristics

OUTCOMES MEASURES IN TOTAL KNEE ARTHROPLASTY

The ideal knee arthroplasty outcome system should be applicable to all patients so that genuine comparisons can be made for an individual at different time points or between different individuals after medical or surgical interventions. Unfortunately, such a system does not currently exist despite the desirability of a universal tool for assessing outcome after joint replacement surgery being identified as long ago as 1975.[16] Although a number of systems have been proposed to quantify the outcomes of different medical and surgical interventions, the validity of many of these instruments has not been established.

In a systematic review of rating scales for TKA, 34 different rating systems were identified in the published literature between 1972 and 1992.[7] The review highlighted the wide variations in characteristics recorded and the emphasis placed on each by the differing scoring systems. It has also been found that patients report that their most bothersome symptoms are not covered by most outcome questionnaires.[5] The challenge for any rating system of TKA is to objectively assess the function of the knee, independent of the overall function of the patient, which may be limited by something entirely different. The problem becomes more complex as one applies instruments designed for primary procedures to revision procedures where domains such as bone loss, ligament attenuation, component removal, extensor mechanism integrity, and other factors need to be considered in the assessment.

SPECIFIC AND GENERIC MEASURES OF HEALTH STATUS

The two basic methods of quality-of-life measurement that are used in arthroplasty analysis consist of generic and specific instruments. The strength of generic instruments, such as the Nottingham and the SF-36, is that these are single instruments that can detect differential effects on different aspects of health status. Generic instruments have the ability to compare various interventions for various conditions at various times and discriminate well among individuals with varying levels of self-reported general health status and comorbid conditions. However, the biggest weakness of generic instruments is that they can lack responsiveness as a result of not adequately focusing on the area of interest or study. Specific instruments, such as the Western Ontario and McMaster University osteoarthritis index (WOMAC), the Knee Society score, the Oxford questionnaire, and the Hospital for Special Surgery score, are disease-specific or population-specific instruments. Although specific instruments are more responsive than generic instruments, comparability across differing conditions may be difficult.

Generic Measures of Health Status

The SF-36 general health survey is a generic measure of health status and is probably one of the most widely used tools globally.[31,32] It comprises eight subscales with 35 items between them. One additional item is not used in the scores. The developers of the SF-36 proposed two summary scores, the physical component score (PCS—more heavily weighted toward dimensions of pain and physical function) and the mental component score (MCS—more weight given to mental health, vitality). Although the PCS more closely correlates with the status of the hip and knee patient, the MCS has also been shown to improve with joint replacement.

For example, the SF-36 has been shown to demonstrate highly significant improvement in physical function, social function, physical role function, emotional role function, mental health, energy, and pain 2 years after TKA. However, regression analysis failed to indicate a predictive relationship between preoperative and postoperative scores for any scale. So we can show with the SF-36 that TKA dramatically improves the quality of life and function of patients afflicted with arthritis, but because of the poor ability of the SF-36 to predict postoperative improvement on an individual basis, it cannot be used alone to determine treatment selection. It is findings such as these that support the inclusion of both a generic and a disease-specific HRQL measure to fully assess patient outcomes.

Specific Measures of Health Status

The most common specific instruments used in assessing TKA are the WOMAC,[2,3] the Knee Society score,[12] and the Hospital for Special Surgery scale.[13,15,30] Newer, even more directed developments in this field include the development and validation of a Knee Society Index of Severity for failed TKA.[28] A number of the many published instruments are outlined in Table 76–2, some of historical interest. It is striking how relatively few instruments have been fully validated for their intended use.

The WOMAC is a self-administered health questionnaire specifically designed for patients with osteoarthritis

Table 76–2. Summary of Common Scoring Systems for Assessment of Total Knee Arthroplasty

SYSTEM	YEAR	NUMBER OF PATIENTS	TOTAL SCORE	VALIDITY
HSS[13]	1973-92	10,394	100	Yes
HSS1[15]	1990	42	100	Yes
KS1[27]	1991-92	214	100	Yes
KS2[12]	1990-92	2170	*	Yes
Bristol[23]	1986-88	170	50	No
Oxford[6]	1998	117	60	Yes
Brigh	1982-92	840	100	No
Freeman et al	1973-89	228	100	No
FreeM	1977-92	523	110	No
Harr	1981-88	809	104	No
Hofm	1991	259	100	No
Hung	1982-88	136	100	No
Hung1	1988	37	100	No
Hung2	1985-92	1078	100	No
Hung3	1990	20	100	No
Laskin	1976	89	100	No
Lotke	1977-87	214	100	No
MayoM	1980-86	159	100	No
MtSi	1992	20	100	No
NewJ	1989-91	366	100	No
NTY[4]	1979-89	484	100	No
Potter et al	1972-85	220	0/37	No
Sloc	1973-84	105	100	No
Uclev	1988-89	200	100	No
Wang	1984	154	32	No
Weinfeld	1979-85	288	0/33	No
Wilson	1973-84	177	100	No

Brigh, Brigham and Women's Hospital; FreeM, Freeman Modified; Harr, Harris Hip Modified; Hofm, Hofmann et al; HSS, Hospital for Special Surgery; Hung, Hungerford et al (1, 2, 3 = modifications); KS1, Knee Society 1; KS2, Knee Society 2; Lotke, Lotke and Ecker; Mayo, Mayo Modified; MtSi, Mount Sinai; NewJ, New Jersey; NTY, Niwa, Terayama, and Yamamoto; Oxford, Oxford Knee Score; Sloc, Slocum and Larson; UClev, Hospital of Cleveland.

of the hip or knee and is one of the most widely used instruments for reporting outcomes after total joint arthroplasty. It consists of 24 multiple-choice items grouped into three categories: pain, stiffness, and physical function. The questions are ranked on a 5-point Likert scale (1 point, best result; 5 points, worst result), and the scores are summed for each category.

A major component of joint-specific scoring systems is range of motion (ROM). This measure is widely used because it is an easily understood, direct measure of the joint's condition. Despite the intuitive connection between joint flexibility and operative success, it remains to be shown how ROM influences the most important outcome: a patient's ability to use the prosthetic joint in activities of daily living.

In a study of knee ROM and outcome of TKA, only modest correlations were found between knee ROM and WOMAC function.[21] At 12 months, significantly worse WOMAC function scores were found in patients with less than 95-degree flexion than in patients with greater than 95-degree flexion. In linear regression models, WOMAC pain and function scores at 12 months were both correlates of patient satisfaction and perceived improvement in quality of life, but knee flexion was not. The conclusion here was that knee ROM is difficult to predict from self-administered surveys of a patient's functional status. In addition, use of the WOMAC questionnaire rather than collecting ROM data by self-administration was recommended.

The choice of the ideal outcome measure to assess TKA remains a complex issue. The authors believe that, pending future developments, the most appropriate method is a combination of acceptable knee scoring systems: a generic instrument (SF-36) plus a specific instrument (WOMAC). Both physician-oriented and patient-oriented methodologies should be used routinely.

FACTORS AFFECTING OUTCOMES

Domain Variability

In an assessment of 34 knee rating systems it was noted that considerable variability exists among the instruments with regard to key domains such as pain and function.[7] More specifically, the contribution of pain to the overall global score has a broad range with weights ranging from as little as 7% to as high as 60%. Functional assessment includes multiple factors that are not covered in a consistent fashion from one instrument to the next. Important attributes are not consistently reported in all instruments, such as the ability to ascend or descend stairs, walk, transfer, rise from a chair, squat or kneel, and sit for a specific period; extremity weakness; spinal pathology; and other comorbid conditions as they affect the knee.

Instrument Psychometric Properties

There is a paucity of psychometric testing (validation and reliability testing) in the literature of the various rating systems. For example, poor correlation has been found among the items in the Knee Society Clinical Rating System.[18] This poor correlation may signify that the instrument is not focused on the outcome of interest. A review of six assessment tools in knee arthroplasty subjects that included the Knee Society Clinical Rating System, WOMAC, SF-36, 6-minute walk, 30-second stair climb, and quality of life/time tradeoff demonstrated that each of the outcome measures offered a slightly different perspective.[17] However, the WOMAC and Knee Society scales were the most responsive outcome measures. A further comparison of the reliability and validity among three scoring systems (the American Knee Society score, the British Orthopaedic Association score, and the Oxford 12-item questionnaire) demonstrated that the Oxford 12-item questionnaire was the most reliable because of the elimination of interobserver variation.[19] This finding indicated that patient self-assessment was more reliable

and reproducible than the objective components of the other two investigator-dependent instruments.

Patient (and Physician) Expectations

Patients' expectations have been shown to strongly influence the postoperative outcome of TKA. Moreover, because these procedures are performed for pain relief and restoration of joint function, the goals of individual patients differ with respect to postoperative function and activity. Nonetheless, to a considerable extent, these goals determine whether TKA is successful and whether the patient believes that significant disability is still present.

In terms of functional outcomes, poor correlation has been found between objective physician-assessed knee scores and subjective patient-assessed visual analog scale scores. It has been demonstrated that surgeons usually focus on ROM, alignment, and stability whereas patients focus on functionality of the knee as a whole. Several studies have also demonstrated that surgeons tend to expect better symptomatic relief than do patients undergoing TKA.[22] Evaluations tend to be similar when patients have little or no pain and are satisfied with the result, but they diverge when patients' ratings for pain increase. This discrepancy increases when the patient is not satisfied with the outcome. These findings indicate that the use of self-administered patient questionnaires in conjunction with physician-generated assessment may provide a more complete evaluation of the results of TKA. Because it has also been shown that patient expectations are important independent predictors of improved functional outcome and satisfaction after TKA and are not correlated with preoperative functional health status, we need greater comprehension of exactly how expectations affect outcomes and whether it is possible to modify these factors.[20]

Range of Motion

Of the many factors that influence the outcome of TKA, preoperative ROM has been found to be an important factor affecting postoperative outcomes. In one study it was demonstrated that TKA patients with high ROM preoperatively will lose motion whereas those with poor preoperative motion will gain motion and those in the midrange stay in the midrange.[1] The statistical model was able to predict 50% to 60% of the postoperative change by simply looking at the preoperative scores. ROM therefore seems to be a reasonably predictable outcome that should be discussed with the patient beforehand, thus helping avoid the "unrealistic" goals or expectations of some patients.

Age

Whether patient age and the number and type of comorbid conditions have an effect on the outcome of TKA remains controversial. In a community-based cohort of primary TKA patients, preoperative and postoperative

WOMAC- and SF-36–based assessments showed no age-related differences in joint pain, function, or quality-of-life measures.[14] Although subjects in the older and younger groups had comparable numbers of comorbid conditions and complications, those in the older group were more likely to be transferred to a rehabilitation facility postoperatively.

Preoperative Functional Status

Over the last decade, the importance of functional assessment after TKA has been well recognized and has led to the creation of standard instruments to assess the outcome of these operations. The association of preoperative functional status with the outcome of TKA has been analyzed. SF-36 and WOMAC-based investigations have shown that patients with lower preoperative physical function and pain do not improve after TKA to the level achieved by those with higher preoperative function.[10] This finding indicates that surgery performed later in the natural history of functional decline secondary to osteoarthritis of the knee results in worse postoperative functional status. However, others have demonstrated that those with the poorest HRQL preoperatively gained most from the operation. Furthermore, it has also been found that patient satisfaction correlates significantly with general health and disease-specific outcome measures; the highest correlation occurred with the domains relating to pain and function, and patients operated on later were more satisfied with their outcomes.[26]

Activity

Activity measurements have also been used to assess arthroplasty patients. Indeed, these patients have been shown to be reliable in their self-evaluation of activity levels, with studies confirming the accuracy of self-administered questionnaires in assessing the frequency and level of activity by means of, for example, pedometry. Because activity may ultimately influence the relative longevity of given implants or an implant in different patient populations, it may prove to be an important indicator of survivorship outcomes.

The authors have also recently developed a new patient-administered activity scale for lower limb arthritis patients, the Lower Extremity Activity Scale.[29] It represents a simple and easily applied measure and also serves as an example of many of the principles espoused earlier, in terms of the development and validation of a new instrument. This scale has proven accurate in measuring actual patient activity and, for example, has clearly demonstrated that patients experience significant improvement in activity following TKA revision.

Radiographic Parameters

Several studies have analyzed the relationship between preoperative and postoperative radiographs and clinical outcomes. Uniform reporting of the radiographic results of TKA has enabled investigators to compare different implants. Domains assessed in this manner have included component position, extremity and knee alignment, and the prosthesis-bone interface as assessed on anteroposterior, lateral, and patella skyline or Merchant view radiographs. One group has measured the width of radiolucent lines in all zones around each of the three components in millimeters.[8] The sum of these measurements for each component results in a numerical score, with a high value or the presence of radiolucency in 10 or more zones signifying possible or impending failure.

FUTURE DIRECTIONS

It is widely accepted now that effective outcomes analysis is critical to the future development of quality care in knee arthroplasty. Nonetheless, the systems and instruments currently available either lack validity or fail to fully address patient variability and factors that influence outcomes. The current authors have recently reported a new method that addresses the multidimensional nature of patient improvement based on factor analysis of existing scales.[23] This method has indicated that new, more accurate and comprehensive, yet easily applied instruments will be possible in the future. Such developments will hopefully enable more widespread application of outcomes analysis and facilitate the use of such methods by all clinicians.

Surgeons need to remain at the forefront of outcomes analysis development and application in their role as patient advocates in order to ensure that appropriate systems are established according to the many principles outlined in this chapter. Leadership in this effort by clinicians is also important so that we can direct the development of arthroplasty in a clinically appropriate and progressive fashion. This will be possible only through the successful establishment of comprehensive, valid, and universally accepted TKA outcomes assessment.

References

1. Anuchi YS, McShane M, Kelly F, et al: Range of motion in total knee replacement. Clin Orthop 331:87-92, 1996.
2. Bellamy N: Pain assessment in osteoarthritis: Experience with the WOMAC osteoarthritis index. Semin Arthritis Rheum 18(4 Suppl 2):14-17, 1989.
3. Bellamy N, Buchanan WW, Goldsmith CH, et al: Validation study of WOMAC: A health status instrument for measuring clinically important patient relevant outcomes to antirheumatic drug therapy in patients with osteoarthritis of the hip or knee. J Rheumatol 15:1833-1840, 1988.
4. Callahan CM, Drake BG, Heck DA, Dittus RS: Patient outcomes following tricompartmental total knee replacement. A meta-analysis. JAMA 271:1349-1357, 1994.
5. Davies AP: Rating systems for total knee replacement. Knee 9:261-266, 2002.
6. Dawson J, Fitzpatrick R, Murray D, et al: Questionnaire on the perceptions of patients about total knee replacement. J Bone Joint Surg Br 80:63-69, 1998.
7. Drake BG, Callahan CM, Dittus RS, et al: Global rating systems used in assessing knee arthroplasty outcomes. J Arthroplasty 9:409-417, 1994.

8. Ewald FC: On behalf of the Knee Society: The Knee Society total knee arthroplasty roentgenographic evaluation and scoring system. Clin Orthop 248:9-12, 1989.

9. Feinstein AR: Clinical Epidemiology. The Architecture of Clinical Research. Philadelphia, WB Saunders, 1985, pp 170-190.

10. Fortin PR, Clarke AE, Joseph L, et al: Outcomes of total hip and knee replacement: Preoperative functional status predicts outcomes at six months after surgery. Arthritis Rheum 42:1722-1728, 1999.

11. Guyatt GH, Feeney DH, Patrick DL: Measuring health-related quality of life. Ann Intern Med 118:622-629, 1993.

12. Insall JN, Dorr LD, Scott RD, Scott WN: Rationale of the Knee Society clinical rating system. Clin Orthop 248:13-14, 1989.

13. Insall JN, Ranawat CS, Agiletti P, et al: A comparison of four models of total knee replacement prosthesis. J Bone Joint Surg Am 58:754-765, 1974.

14. Jones CA, Voaklander DC, Johnston DW, et al: The effect of age on pain, function, and quality of life after total hip and knee arthroplasty. Arch Intern Med 161:454-460, 2001.

15. Joseph J, Kaufmann EE: Preliminary results of Miller-Galante uncemented total knee arthroplasty. Orthopedics 13:511-516, 1990.

16. Kettelkamp DB, Thompson C: Development of a knee scoring scale. Clin Orthop 107:93-99, 1975.

17. Kreibich DN, Vaz M, Bourne RB, et al: What is the best way of assessing outcome after total knee replacement? Clin Orthop 331:221-225, 1996.

18. Lingard EA, Katz JN, Wright RJ, et al: Validity and responsiveness of the Knee Society Clinical Rating System in comparison with the SF-36 and WOMAC. J Bone Joint Surg Am 83:1856-1864, 2001.

19. Liow RYL, Walker K, Wajid MA, et al: Functional rating for knee arthroplasty: Comparison of three scoring systems. Orthopedics 26:143-149, 2003.

20. Mahomed NN, Liang MH, Cook EF, et al: The importance of patient expectations in predicting functional outcomes after total joint arthroplasty. J Rheumatol 29:1273-1279, 2002.

21. Miner AL, Lingard EA, Wright EA, et al: Knee range of motion after total knee arthroplasty: How important is this as an outcome measure? J Arthroplasty 18:286-294, 2003.

22. Moran M, Khan A, Sochart DH, et al: Expect the best, prepare for the worst: Surgeon and patient expectation of the outcome of primary total hip and knee replacement. Ann R Coll Surg Engl 85:204-206, 2003.

23. Mulhall KJ, Saleh KJ, North American Knee Arthroplasty Revision Study Group: Measuring improvement following total knee arthroplasty revision: A new perspective and findings in a multicenter prospective cohort study. Presented at the Fifth Combined Meeting of the Orthopaedic Research Societies of Canada, USA, Japan, and Europe, October 2004, Banff, Canada.

24. Orthopedic Network News: 2002 hip and knee implant review. CMS MedPar. Available at www.OrthopedicNetworkNews.com. Accessed 9/8/03.

25. Peyron JG: Osteoarthritis. The epidemiologic viewpoint. Clin Orthop 213:13-19, 1986.

26. Robertsson O, Dunbar MJ: Patient satisfaction compared with general health and disease-specific questionnaires in knee arthroplasty patients. J Arthroplasty 16:476-482, 2001.

27. Rougraff BT, Heck DA, Gibson AE: A comparison of tricompartmental and unicompartmental arthroplasty for the treatment of gonarthrosis. Clin Orthop 273:157-164, 1991.

28. Saleh KJ, Macaulay A, Radosevich DM, et al: The Knee Society Index of Severity for failed total knee arthroplasty: Development and validation. Clin Orthop 392:153-165, 2001.

29. Saleh KJ, Mulhall KJ, Bershadsky B, et al: Development and validation of a lower extremity activity scale with application in total knee arthroplasty revision patients. J Bone Joint Surg Am, in press.

30. Total Knee Replacement. Summary, Evidence Report/TechNlogy Assessment: Number 86. AHRQ Publication Number 04-E006-1, December 2003. Agency for Healthcare Research and Quality, Rockville, MD. http://www.ahrq.gov/clinic/epcsums/ kneesum.htm.

31. Ware JE Jr: Conceptualizing and measuring generic health outcomes. Cancer 67:774-779, 1991.

32. Ware JE Jr, Snow KK, Kosinski M, et al: SF-36 Health Survey Manual and Interpretation Guide. Boston, The Health Institute, 1993.

CHAPTER 77

Osteotomy about the Knee: American Perspective

James M. Leone • Arlen D. Hanssen

The basis of realignment osteotomy about an arthritic knee is to transfer weightbearing forces from the arthritic portion of the knee to a healthier location in the knee joint.[21] This redistribution of mechanical force to increase the life span of the knee joint distinguishes osteotomy from other treatment modalities of arthritic knees.[37] The prevalence of realignment osteotomy has steadily declined because of the success of total knee replacement (TKR) and the recent resurgence of enthusiasm for unicompartmental knee replacement.[13,67,97] Despite this rather significant decline, osteotomy about the knee remains a viable treatment option in carefully selected patients with knee arthritis.[6,40,83,84] The use of osteotomy has increased in patients who are undergoing other surgical procedures such as cartilage or meniscal transplantation or ligamentous reconstruction.[12,17,62,94] Over the past decade there has been an explosion of interest in developing modifications of the surgical technique,[7,49,52] new surgical instrumentation,[16,31] and new fixation devices,[93,95] as well as increasing interest in the use of external fixation devices[1,85,104] and computed tomography–free navigation systems aimed at improving the accuracy, reliability, and safety of realignment osteotomy.[47]

The goals of osteotomy include pain relief, functional improvement, and the capacity to maintain heavy functional demands otherwise precluded by prosthetic replacement. Alternative procedures should be compared with current standards of osteotomy and not historical controls because current patients undergoing osteotomy are generally considered worst-case scenarios for a successful long-term outcome with prosthetic replacement. The key to success after osteotomy is careful patient selection combined with skillful surgical technique.

PATIENT SELECTION PROCESS

The process of patient selection is possibly the single most important factor determining a successful result after osteotomy. A thorough synthesis of multiple variables is required to formulate the decision to proceed with osteotomy (Table 77–1). The primary indications for osteotomy include pain relief for degenerative arthritis associated with malalignment or a desired mechanical axis correction in conjunction with ligamentous reconstruction or transplantation of cartilage or meniscal allografts. It is often helpful to start by focusing on the relative and

absolute contraindications to corrective osteotomy during the patient selection process (Table 77–2).

Historical Variables

The ideal candidate for osteotomy is a thin, active individual in the fifth or sixth decade of life with localized, activity-related unicompartmental knee pain, no patellofemoral symptoms, a stable knee, and full knee extension with flexion of at least 90 degrees.[37,72] Although many patients do not meet all these ideal guidelines, a careful selection process will optimize clinical outcomes.

Emphasis on the location and character of pain, desired activity level, and appropriate patient expectations is particularly important when considering osteotomy. Diffuse and nonspecific knee pain reduces the chance of a successful outcome after osteotomy. Although it was previously believed that symptoms related to knee instability precluded osteotomy, the practice of treating malalignment in conjunction with concomitant ligamentous reconstruction is becoming increasingly common. Interested readers are referred elsewhere in this textbook for more information on the treatment of young active patients with malalignment and instability. An elderly patient with degenerative arthritis and instability would be optimally treated by TKR rather than osteotomy.[42]

Patients with osteoarthritis fare better than those with rheumatoid arthritis, and realignment osteotomy for inflammatory disorders is not recommended.[23] In the presence of secondary degenerative arthritis from a previous fracture, osteochondritis dissecans, or a prior medial meniscectomy, the results of osteotomy do not seem to be adversely affected, whereas patients who have undergone combined medial and lateral meniscectomy have disappointing outcomes.[68,87]

Degenerative arthritis of the patellofemoral joint has long been cited as a cause of failure after corrective osteotomy.[42] Conversely, long-term studies have shown a low incidence of unsatisfactory results attributed to the patellofemoral joint, and it is possible that realignment of the extremity may favorably alter patellofemoral mechanics inasmuch as it has been demonstrated that patellofemoral pain can improve after upper tibial osteotomy.[27,35] Significant retropatellar pain should be a cautionary factor during patient selection, but mild retropatellar pain should not preclude osteotomy if the

Table 77–1. Selection Factors for Realignment Osteotomy

HISTORICAL		Deformities away from the joint
Age		Joint line obliquity
Chronological		**EXAMINATION**
Physiological		
Patient's desired activity level		Malalignment
Pain		Magnitude
Location		Direction
Character		Previous incisions
Patellofemoral?		Body habitus
Rheumatological status		Range of motion
Previous meniscectomy		Total arc
Infection history		Flexion contracture
		Ligamentous deficiencies
RADIOLOGICAL		Patellofemoral mechanics
Anatomic axis		Adductor thrust
Mechanical axis		**MISCELLANEOUS**
Severity of arthrosis		Patient expectations
Magnitude of deformity		Surgeon capabilities
Tibiofemoral subluxation		Dynamic gait factors
Status of other compartments		Soft-tissue tension
		Upper body shift
Joint space opening		Potential complications
Amount of articular cartilage loss		Postoperative recovery
		Immobilization time
Calcium pyrophosphate deposition		Durability of the procedure
Osseous defects		Ease of revision to total knee arthroplasty

Table 77–2. Contraindications to Corrective Osteotomy

Absolute
Diffuse, nonspecific knee pain
Primary complaint of patellofemoral pain
Meniscectomy in the compartment intended for weightbearing
Arthrosis in the compartment intended for weightbearing
Underlying diagnosis of inflammatory disease
Unrealistic patient expectations

Relative
Age older than 60 years
Range-of-motion arc less than 90 degrees
Obesity (1.3 × ideal body weight)
Severe arthrosis
Tibiofemoral subluxation
Moderate or severe ligamentous instability

primary indication for osteotomy is unicompartmental tibiofemoral pain.[35]

Age assessment requires consideration of physiological status and lifestyle requirements. Many younger and sedentary patients may be better served by arthroplasty, whereas some elderly and active patients may be better suited for osteotomy. Arthroplasty provides more complete pain relief and shorter rehabilitation and is more reliable than osteotomy in most individuals older than 60 years.[42] Recently, it has been proposed that unicompartmental knee replacement is an ideal temporizing procedure for middle-aged patients in preference to osteotomy.[78,97] Others believe that unicompartmental knee replacement remains a prosthetic arthroplasty option that should not be considered a direct alternative to osteotomy and are concerned about increased complications in young active patients with prosthetic implants.[37,82,84,100]

Examination

Ipsilateral hip function should always be assessed, and if hip surgery is required, it should be completed before realignment osteotomy. Limb inspection should confirm the presence of axial malalignment and assess for the presence of lateral thrust because it is a potential risk factor for a poor clinical outcome.[77] In patients with high adduction moments, if sufficient correction of alignment is achieved at surgery, these moments of the knee do not seem to correlate with the clinical outcome.[102]

Previous skin incisions, which may affect the intended surgical exposure, should be noted. Knee motion should reveal a flexion arc of at least 90 degrees with less than 10 to 20 degrees of flexion contracture; however, these criteria have been established only by clinical convention. Patellofemoral symptoms or significant meniscal pathology should not be the primary cause of the patient's complaints, and every effort must be pursued to differentiate the potential sources of pain. It is imperative that the neurovascular status of the intended surgical limb be accurately assessed preoperatively and documented accordingly.

It cannot be overemphasized that osteotomy is technically more difficult in obese patients, particularly those with peripheral dystrophic weight distribution. Obesity has been associated with lower success rates after high tibial osteotomy (HTO) because the surgical technique and postoperative immobilization are more difficult in these individuals.[27] The long-term clinical results are also worse in individuals who exceed their ideal body weight by 1.32 times.[27] The activity level of these patients should be carefully assessed because sedentary, overweight individuals of any age may be better served by prosthetic replacement. It should be stressed that significant weight loss may also provide enough symptomatic relief to defer any operative intervention.

Counseling

The surgeon needs to discuss all treatment alternatives and convey that neither osteotomy nor arthroplasty provides a "normal joint." The long-term results, rehabilitation, pain relief, and durability of realignment osteotomy and arthroplasty should be differentiated for the patient.

A longer postoperative recovery period with less pain relief after rehabilitation is expected after osteotomy. These disadvantages need to be balanced against the possible catastrophic complications of infection or prosthetic failure with arthroplasty in a young and active patient.[6,90,100]

Specifically, realignment osteotomy is based on the concept that certain high-impact and excessive loading activities are not sanctioned with prosthetic arthroplasty.[37] Functional analysis of young patients after osteotomy reveals that many are able to participate in running and jumping activities that would probably lead to damage of a knee prosthesis.[6,69,75] Many patients also value the real potential for technological advances in arthroplasty over the expected survival period of an osteotomy and recognize that "buying time" with an osteotomy is a viable concept.

The expected results of TKR after osteotomy also need to be considered and discussed with the patient. Potential technical obstacles encountered include difficulty with exposure,[106] bony deficiencies necessitating grafts or wedges, difficulty in attaining ligament balance,[73] prolonged operative times,[36] and increased blood loss.[44,45,53] Other authors have noted that there are no significant differences in the technical difficulty or outcome of TKR after HTO.[64,79,91] The poorer long-term radiographic results of TKR after HTO occur in a specific subset of patients.[76] These patients are younger, heavier, and more active males who are also at risk for early wear of prosthetic components. A well-performed osteotomy in these patients seems reasonable if the goal is to postpone prosthetic replacement to a later stage in their lives when their activity level and age favor a decrease in the likelihood that they will require multiple revision surgeries. The literature detailing poor results of arthroplasty after osteotomy clearly indicates that technical difficulties or complications associated with osteotomy produce worse results with the subsequent arthroplasty.[15,106] Surgeons with only occasional experience performing corrective osteotomy should consider referral because a suboptimal surgical technique that may compromise subsequent procedures should not be the sole criterion used to abandon osteotomy.

Other important variables in this patient population also portend a poor result. Factors that prognosticated a worse outcome in HTO patients ($p < 0.01$) included (1) worker's compensation claim, (2) history of reflex sympathetic dystrophy after HTO, (3) early onset (less than 1 year) or no period of relief of pain after HTO, (4) multiple surgeries before HTO, and (5) occupation as a laborer.[66]

Radiographic Evaluation

The location and severity of the arthritis are determined with standing anteroposterior, lateral, intercondylar notch, and skyline patellar views. One should carefully inspect the contralateral tibiofemoral compartment for marginal osteophytes, which indicates the presence of diffuse arthritis. Tibiofemoral subluxation, excessive bony

erosion, and diffuse arthritic involvement are associated with poorer outcomes. A full-length, 51 × 14-inch weight-bearing radiograph is necessary to determine the mechanical axis.[89] Although there is generally high correlation between the anatomic and mechanical axes, long films are also helpful to determine whether deformities of the tibia or femur exist and the effect that these deformities have on overall mechanical alignment.

Preoperative Planning

The principal considerations in osteotomy planning include the location, direction, and magnitude of malalignment (Table 77–3). These variables need to be weighed concurrently during the planning phase to achieve appropriate angular correction. One of the reasons for premature failure after osteotomy is undercorrection or overcorrection of the deformity, which may be due to deficiencies in either the preoperative planning process or the surgical technique.[27,80,89] Clearly, philosophy, training, and experience heavily bias preference for a specific osteotomy technique. The rationale for choosing between one of these options is delineated in the discussion of these various techniques (Table 77–4). In recent times, varus deformities have been corrected by HTO, whereas most valgus deformities are corrected by distal femoral osteotomy. Previously, the most pragmatic approach for the majority of surgeons was a closing wedge osteotomy; however, opening wedge techniques are becoming increasingly more popular.[28,38,49,55]

Intra-articular deficiencies require special consideration when calculating the degree of desired angular correction. Slack collateral ligamentous restraint causes angular deformity, and each millimeter of tibiofemoral separation requires subtraction of roughly 1 degree per millimeter to avoid overcorrection (the correction factor will change depending on the actual proximal tibia width).[29] It is

Table 77–3. Components of Malalignment

Location
Extra-articular
　Femur
　Tibia

Intra-articular
　Joint line obliquity
　Ligamentous laxity
　Articular cartilage deficiency
　Osseous deficiencies

Direction
Sagittal
　Flexion
　Extension

Coronal
　Varus
　Valgus

Rotational

Magnitude
Mild (<10 degrees)
Moderate (10 to 20 degrees)
Severe (>20 degrees)

Table 77–4. Corrective Osteotomy Techniques

Tibial
Lateral closing wedge
Medial closing wedge
Medial opening wedge
Graft
Staple
Distraction histogenesis
Barrel vault (dome) osteotomy
Oblique metaphyseal wedge
Femoral
Medial closing wedge
Medial fixation
Lateral fixation
Oblique metaphyseal wedge
Lateral opening wedge
Lateral closing wedge

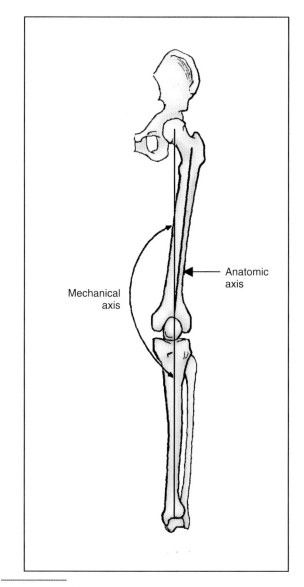

Figure 77–1. The mechanical axis, based on a line connecting the centers of the femoral head and the tibiotalar joint, averages 1.2 degrees of varus, whereas the femoral-tibial (anatomic) angle normally averages 5 degrees of valgus.

important to remember that ligamentous laxity will not be detected on standing radiographs when the laxity exists in the same compartment being overloaded. For example, lateral ligament laxity in a valgus knee or medial collateral ligament (MCL) laxity in a varus knee, not observed on radiographs, may cause overcorrection of alignment after realignment osteotomy once the load has been shifted toward the opposite compartment of the knee.

Some patients with proximal tibial varus deformity have excessive valgus angulation of the distal femoral articular surface. This obliquity of the distal femoral surface affects the magnitude of alignment correction and requires special consideration during preoperative planning because patients with femoral shaft–transcondylar angles of less than 9 degrees have an increased incidence of undercorrection.[81] Increased valgus orientation of the distal end of the femur can also result in deleterious overcorrection after HTO.[80] Extra-articular deformities distant from the knee joint may need to be addressed at the apex of the deformity rather than by periarticular correction.

The magnitude of coronal plane malalignment may dictate the location of the osteotomy or suggest the use of a particular technique. For example, excessive malalignment may contraindicate HTO if the tibial articular surface will be adversely tilted, and for malalignment exceeding 12 to 15 degrees, a supracondylar femoral osteotomy is recommended.[26] Alternatively, a dome or barrel vault osteotomy allows greater correction with less effect on the resultant joint line obliquity and should potentially be considered for varus deformities exceeding 20 degrees.[9] For severe deformities, a dual (double) osteotomy of both the distal femur and proximal tibia may also be deemed necessary.[11] Sagittal plane deformities can also be corrected with proper planning and appropriate adjustment of the osteotomy technique. As HTO techniques are being refined, more attention is being directed at the sagittal plane of correction in an attempt to better offload areas with significant cartilage damage.[4,59]

Historically, axial limb alignment was determined by measuring the femoral-tibial (anatomic) angle from standing radiographs and then judging the amount of correc-

tion required to restore this angle to normal, which typically averages 5 degrees of valgus (Fig. 77–1). The height of a tibial osteotomy wedge was then estimated by the rule of thumb that each millimeter provided roughly 1 degree of angular correction. This method of calculation is accurate only when the actual width of the tibial flare is 56 mm, and it is significantly altered by differences in tibial width or distortion as a result of radiographic magnification.[22] Use of this method without considering the actual tibial width invariably leads to undercorrection because the mean tibial width is 80 mm in men and 70 mm in women (Fig. 77–2). The mechanical axis averages 1.2 degrees of varus and is based on a line connecting the centers of the femoral head and the tibiotalar joint (see Fig. 77–1). This axis is more accurate than the anatomic axis when defining the load transmission forces

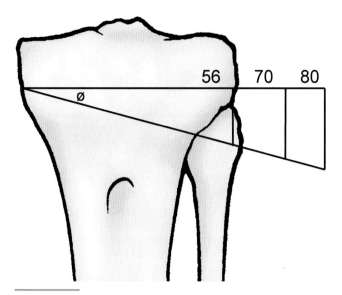

Figure 77–2. Given the same desired angle of correction (ø), the wedge height measurement progressively increases with increasing tibial width. The rule of thumb that 1 mm of wedge height equals 1 degree of angular correction results in undercorrection for tibial widths exceeding 56 mm.

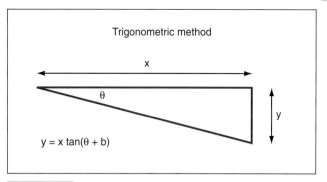

Figure 77–3. The trigonometric method of determining actual wedge height (y) is calculated with a trigonometric formula using known values of the desired angle of correction (ø) and actual tibial width (x). A direct measurement of tibial width at a point 2.0 to 2.5 cm distal to the joint line, on radiographs incorporating radiographic markers, is normalized by the amount of magnification present to obtain the actual tibial wedge height (x).

across the knee joint, particularly when femoral or tibial deformities are contributing to the malalignment.

One measurement method for HTO uses the mechanical axis on a full-length standing radiograph with radiographic markers to adjust for magnification. By using trigonometric principles and adjusting for radiographic magnification, the intended wedge height is determined by ascertaining the amount of angular correction required to place the mechanical axis at the desired location within the knee joint. The formula for these calculations is shown in Figure 77–3. A similar method, the weightbearing line method, divides the tibial plateau from 0% to 100% (medial to lateral) to determine the appropriate coordinate for the mechanical axis to intersect the knee joint (Fig. 77–4).[29] Lines to the center of the femoral head and the talar dome connect this coordinate, and the angle formed by these lines is the angle of desired correction. This angle is accordingly adjusted for distraction of the tibiofemoral joint surfaces allowed by ligamentous laxity and articular cartilage deficiency. The height of the wedge is then calculated by tracing the wedge on the radiograph and normalizing the measured height of the wedge by the amount of radiographic magnification. Both these measurement methods account for the actual width of the tibial plateau.

The use of a full-length radiograph for measurement of mechanical alignment is a static measurement only. Soft-tissue tension, joint line obliquity, and upper body gravity shift also affect tibiofemoral plateau pressure distribution during dynamic gait. Software programs are emerging to help with preoperative assessment of these factors and to assist the surgeon's final determination of the location, magnitude, and type of knee osteotomy.[31,47] The data printout generated by these programs details various osteotomy options and seems most useful for several

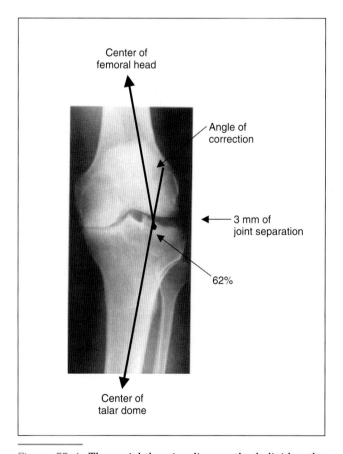

Figure 77–4. The weightbearing line method divides the tibial plateau from 0% to 100% (medial to lateral) to determine the desired intersection coordinate of the mechanical axis through the knee joint. The angle formed by lines drawn from this coordinate to the center of the femoral head and talar dome is corrected for tibiofemoral joint surface distraction allowed by ligamentous laxity to establish the desired angle of correction. Wedge height is calculated by tracing the wedge on the radiograph with the desired angle of correction. The wedge height measurement on the radiograph is then normalized by the radiographic magnification present.

specific circumstances: (1) to decide whether to perform a periarticular osteotomy or an osteotomy at the apex of the deformity away from the knee joint or (2) to determine whether joint line obliquity may be adversely affected after correction of severe malalignment with a particular technique and thereby suggest the need for a combined dual osteotomy of the tibia and femur. Currently, there are no data to suggest the upper limit of acceptance for resultant joint line obliquity, and we often accept up to 10 degrees of joint line obliquity before proceeding with a dual osteotomy (Figs. 77–5 to 77–9).

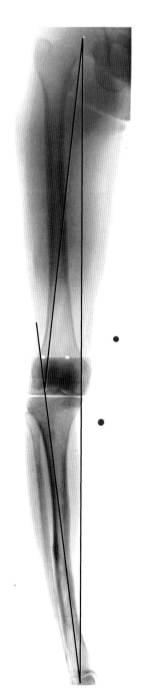

Figure 77–5. Standing full-length radiograph of an active 46-year-old woman with localized medial compartment knee pain. Note the tibial distal malunion.

For patients with mild or moderate deformity, the static measurement planning methods seem sufficient. Although these preoperative planning schemes provide objective criteria to guide surgery, even the most detailed plans rely on the ability of the surgeon to carry out the procedure accurately.

SURGICAL TECHNIQUES

The inherent principles of these techniques include appropriate placement of skin incisions, careful handling of soft tissues, respect for neurovascular structures, accurate execution of the osteotomy, and adequate skeletal fixation. The options for fixation and a discussion of complications associated with osteotomy are presented later in this chapter. Preparation for a skin incision should include forethought for an eventual TKR, and longitudinal incisions on the lateral or medial side of the knee should provide large bridges of skin to accommodate for any future midline or parapatellar approach. Carelessly placed incisions for the osteotomy may lead to catastrophic complications of wound healing and infection at a later arthroplasty.

The accuracy of the osteotomy based on preoperative planning and intraoperative technique cannot be overemphasized. With closing wedge techniques, apposition of bone surfaces facilitates prompt healing, whereas proper orientation and resection of bone ultimately determine final mechanical alignment. Opening wedge techniques provide more versatility intraoperatively, with the surgeon being able to manipulate the osteotomy site after the initial bone cut, although this technique also requires special attention to detail and must be carried out meticulously. The use of jig systems to assist in achieving correct placement and orientation of the osteotomy appears to be particularly useful for many surgeons who have limited experience performing these osteotomies.[16,41] The use of intraoperative radiographs and fluoroscopy to document that appropriate alignment has been achieved is recommended.

Historically, loss of patellar height was often seen with closing wedge osteotomy techniques because the knee was subsequently immobilized in a postoperative cast with resultant contracture of the patellar ligament. This complication has become less common as surgeons are now using more rigid fixation methods that allow for earlier knee mobilization during the immediate postoperative period.[2,16,105] Although loss of patellar height has also been seen with opening wedge techniques, the cause of this phenomenon differs in that the opening wedge technique causes an elevation of the joint line that results in patellar migration distally relative to the femoral trochlea rather than patellar ligament contracture.[108] The clinical implications of patella infra associated with HTO remain poorly understood.

Varus Deformity

For varus malalignment about the knee, many surgeons continue to prefer a lateral closing wedge osteotomy of the

X-ray magnification : 103%	Preop	Option 1	Option 2
FTA (degrees) :	189.57	176.38	176.69
Joint Obliquity (degrees) :	-1.67	4.35	0.22
Medial Load (%) :	100	41.73	40
Mechanical Deformity (degrees) :	9.57 varus	-3.62 valgus	-3.31 valgus
Peak Pressure (Mpa) :	3.69	0.61	0.59
Ligamentous Tension (N) :	190.92	0.00	0.00
Leg Length (cm) :	77.28	76.70	76.74
Tibial Closed Angle (degrees) :		14.00 valgus	9.00 valgus
Tibial Elevation (mm) :		20.00	20.00
Tibial Wedge Length (mm) :		16.61	11.20
Femoral Closed Angle (degrees) :			5.00 valgus
Femoral Elevation (mm) :			50.00
Femoral Wedge Length (mm) :			4.19

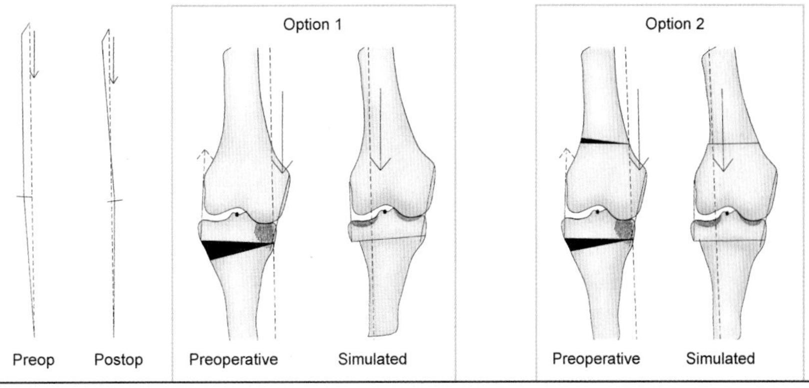

Figure 77–6. An OASIS data printout obtained from the full-length radiograph in Figure 77–5 details the several corrective osteotomy options. Option 1, with a proximal tibial wedge resection of 16.61 mm, is calculated to leave 4.35 degrees of resultant joint line obliquity. Option 2 describes a dual osteotomy designed to minimize resultant joint line obliquity. FTA, femorotibial angle.

proximal tibia.[16,20,37,51,56,72] Because of its perceived simplicity, medial opening wedge osteotomy is becoming more popular.[7,28,38,49,55,71] Both techniques are used to address varus malalignment with medial compartment arthritis, and each technique has inherent advantages and disadvantages. The decision to use one over the other must be based on the surgeon's philosophy and clinical experience (Table 77–5). Though less commonly performed, dome osteotomies and double osteotomies are also viable treatment options in selected individuals.[11,48,54]

LATERAL CLOSING TIBIAL WEDGE OSTEOTOMY

The following description, modified from the original report, is currently the preferred technique for a closing wedge osteotomy at our institution and is relatively straightforward when compared with some other techniques.[21] The primary modification of this technique is partial resection of the fibular head rather than total fibular head resection combined with advancement of the lateral ligamentous structures.

TABLE 77–5. Comparison Between High Tibial Osteotomy Techniques

HTO TYPE	FIXATION	ADVANTAGES	DISADVANTAGES
Opening wedge	Plate system External fixator or spatial frame (larger corrections) Bone graft (alone)	Potentially simpler Avoids the proximal tibiofibular joint Avoids the peroneal nerve More control of multiplanar correction (sagittal/coronal) Avoids the anterior compartment No bone loss	Less aggressive weightbearing/rehabilitation Often requires a graft with potential implications of healing/union May overlengthen the extremity May alter patella height
Closing wedge	Plate system Staples	More aggressive weightbearing/ rehabilitation Does not require a graft	More difficult to control tibial slope (often inadvertently decreased) Intraoperative adjustments more difficult Proximal tibiofibular joint violated Increased risk to the peroneal nerve Alters the shape of the upper part of the tibia with implications for joint reconstruction Bone loss/shortening May alter patella height

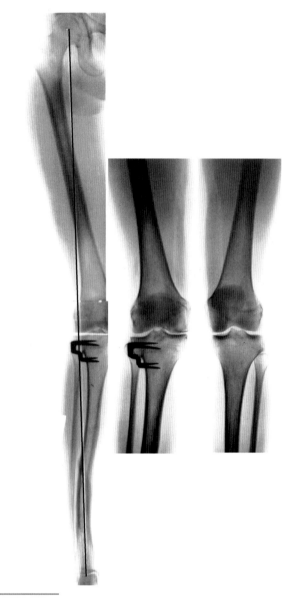

Figure 77–7. Postoperative full-length radiograph of a patient after a 16-mm lateral wedge resection osteotomy of the proximal end of the tibia demonstrating that the mechanical axis now intersects the lateral tibial compartment at the 75% coordinate. The inset standing radiograph demonstrates symmetry of the lower extremities.

The patient is positioned supine with a sandbag beneath the ipsilateral trochanteric region to place the extremity in neutral rotation. The extremity is exsanguinated and under tourniquet control, and the procedure is typically performed with the knee flexed to 90 degrees, although such flexure does not protect the popliteal artery from injury when compared with the fully extended position.[109] Though originally described as a long curvilinear incision, a short oblique incision coursing from fibular head toward the tibial tubercle is currently preferred. The iliotibial band is split longitudinally just anterior and parallel to the fibular collateral ligament, and the peroneal nerve is located by palpation only. The anterior tibial musculature

is then elevated subperiosteally from the proximal end of the tibia.

Removal of the inner third of the fibular head and cartilage is then accomplished with an osteotome. The posterior portion of the tibia is subperiosteally exposed to allow insertion of a broad malleable retractor to protect the neurovascular structures. An anterior retractor is placed between the patellar ligament and tibia just proximal to the tibial tubercle. The location of the joint line can be established with either a small arthrotomy or placement of medial and lateral Kirchner wires. At a point 2.0 to 2.5 cm below the joint line, a guide wire is inserted in a lateral-to-medial direction parallel to the tibial articular surface (Fig. 77–10A). The second pin is inserted at a point measured distally from pin No. 1 based on preoperative calculation of tibial wedge height. This pin is advanced obliquely to intersect with the first pin at the medial tibial cortex. Pin placement should be confirmed radiographically.

The osteotomy is performed parallel to the posterior slope of the tibial articular surface in the sagittal plane with a broad osteotome or an oscillating saw. The tibia is transected on the undersurface of pin No. 1 and the upper surface of pin No. 2. The width of the wedge can be adjusted to correct for flexion or extension deformity by altering the height of the wedge in the anteroposterior plane. Initially, the osteotomy traverses approximately 50% to 75% of the tibial width so that the outer wedge of bone can be removed to facilitate completion of the osteotomy with small osteotomes (Fig. 77–10B). It is important that the medial cortex not be transected, but rather be perforated four to five times with a long drill bit or small osteotome to maintain an intact periosteal hinge. The bone from the inner wedge is removed with small curets while taking great care to ensure removal of all cortical bone, especially in the posteromedial tibial corner.

Osteoclasis is then achieved by applying valgus stress to the extremity with the knee in full extension. The fibular head is inspected to verify that it is not preventing complete closure of the osteotomy. Mechanical alignment is verified by fluoroscopy with a rod extending from the femoral head to the talar dome. Fixation is then accomplished by inserting two stepped staples, the first staple positioned just anterior to the fibular head and the second staple yet more anterior (Fig. 77–10C). During staple insertion it is helpful to start advancing the proximal tine into the tibial plateau until the distal tine rests against the tibial cortex. Using a 3.2-mm drill bit, a starter hole is made just distal to the tine to facilitate compression at the osteotomy site and avoid propagation of a fracture through the thick tibial cortex.

Counterpressure against the medial portion of the tibia by a surgical assistant during final staple insertion helps prevent tibial translation and disruption of the medial periosteum. In overweight individuals, it is often difficult to provide adequate medial tibia counterpressure because of the thickness of the subcutaneous tissue. A large provisional pin inserted obliquely across the osteotomy site helps stabilize the tibia during staple insertion in these patients. The accuracy of apposition and the integrity of the medial periosteal hinge are then assessed dynamically with fluoroscopy. Bone graft from the removed wedge of

X-ray magnification : 105 %	Preop	Option 1	Option 2	Option 3
FTA (degrees) :	159.14	180.89	183.56	181.50
Joint Obliquity (degrees) :	-3.02	7.90	-15.73	-0.29
Medial Load (%) :	3.95	76.66	62.47	75.81
Mechanical Deformity (degrees) :	-20.86 valgus	-0.89 varus	3.56 varus	1.50 varus
Peak Pressure (Mpa) :	12.72	1.62	10.85	2.54
Ligamentous Tension (N) :	403.40	2.02	153.03	9.77
Leg Length (cm) :	74.18	74.22	73.89	74.25
Tibial Closed Angle (degrees) :			-25.00 varus	-9.00 varus
Tibial Elevation (mm) :			20.00	20.00
Tibial Wedge Length (mm) :			26.53	9.80
Femoral Closed Angle (degrees) :		-25.00 varus		-16.00 varus
Femoral Elevation (mm) :		50.00		50.00
Femoral Wedge Length (mm) :		16.74		11.21

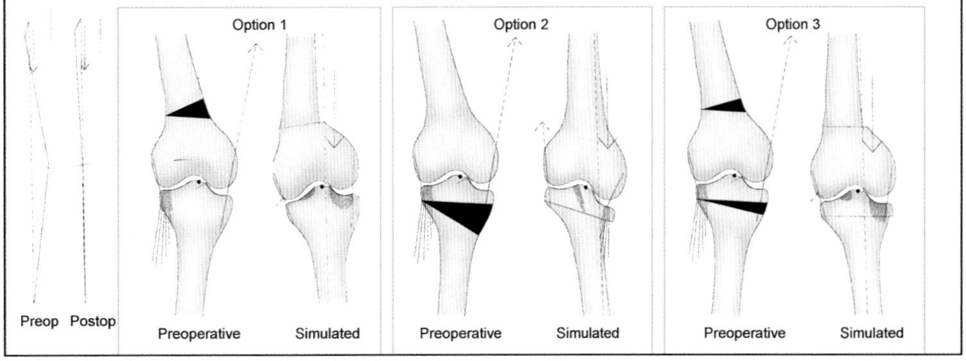

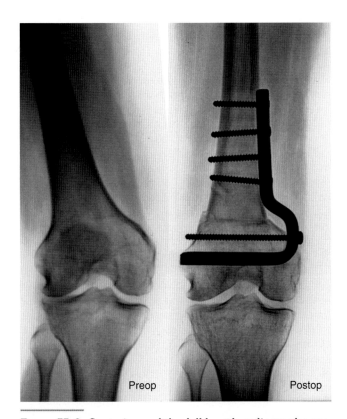

Figure 77–8. OASIS data printout obtained from a full-length standing radiograph of a 42-year-old active woman with painful genu valgum and osteoarthritis of the lateral compartment of her right knee. Option 2 demonstrates the anticipated resultant joint line obliquity created by a varus-producing osteotomy of the proximal end of the tibia. FTA, femorotibial angle.

Figure 77–9. Spot views of the full-length radiographs presented in Figure 77-8. Note the correction of the mechanical axis from the 95% coordinate in the preoperative radiograph to the 50% coordinate (neutral position) in the postoperative radiograph.

bone is placed adjacent to the staples. After tourniquet release, careful hemostasis is achieved, with particular attention paid to the region of the anterior tibial musculature. Deep drains are then inserted along the posterior aspect of the tibia and beneath the anterior compartment musculature. The wound is closed in layers and the extremity placed in a compressive dressing.

Postoperatively, the patient wears a hinged knee brace to allow early range of motion. Partial weightbearing is allowed for the initial 6 to 8 weeks, followed by progression to full weightbearing.

Because two-dimensional planning (based on preoperative and intraoperative radiographs or imaging) is being used to execute a three-dimensional procedure, the role of computer-assisted surgery has been explored with the hope of improving the placement and orientation of the osteotomy resection planes for closing wedge techniques.[31,47] The role of computer-aided surgery is presently evolving and may ultimately provide significant benefits in realignment surgery, particularly for surgeons with limited experience.

MEDIAL OPENING TIBIAL WEDGE OSTEOTOMY

Correction of malalignment with an opening medial wedge osteotomy has been reported to be successful (Fig. 77–11).[28,38,49,55] A number of technical improvements have contributed to both the safety and reproducibility of this technique.[52] Advantages of this technique include the requirement for only a single osteotomy with surgical dissection away from the peroneal nerve, no violation of the fibula and tibiofibular joint, and the capability of

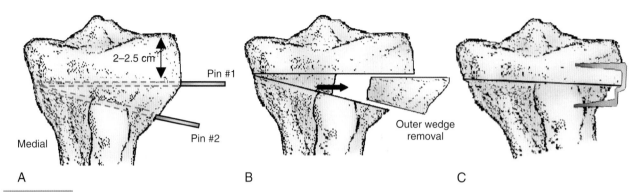

Figure 77–10. **A,** The first guide wire is inserted parallel to the tibial articular surface approximately 2.0 to 2.5 cm below the joint line. The second guide wire, inserted at a point distally based on the preoperative calculation of actual tibial wedge height, is advanced obliquely to intersect at the medial tibial cortex with the first guide wire. **B,** The outer 50% to 75% of the wedge is initially removed to allow completion of the inner portion of the wedge. **C,** The tibia is stabilized by the insertion of two stepped staples bridging the osteotomy site.

intraoperatively adjusting the correction. Inherent disadvantages include the potential need to procure an autogenous bone graft or the use of an alternative bone graft source such as an allograft or a synthetic bone graft substitute.[49] New fixation devices, such as the Puddhu plate[95] and the TomoFix,[93,95] have been specifically developed for medial opening wedge osteotomies.

The operative details of the procedure include positioning the patient supine with a sandbag beneath the ipsilateral trochanteric region to place the extremity in neutral rotation. A small vertical incision is made over the pes anserinus insertion halfway between the medial border of the patellar ligament and the posterior margin of the tibia to expose the sartorial fascia. This fascia is incised to expose the hamstring tendons. The osteotomy is often planned above the tibial tubercle. Retractors are carefully placed anterior and posterior to protect the patellar tendon and posterior neurovascular structures, along with the hamstring tendons and MCL. The superficial MCL inserts 5 to 7 cm distal to the joint and is usually retracted out of harm's way.

Under fluoroscopic imaging, a guide wire is drilled across the proximal tibia in a medial-to-lateral direction. The guide is positioned at the level of the superior aspect of the tibial tubercle and oriented obliquely to end approximately 1 cm below the joint line at the lateral tibial cortex. The tip of the fibular head can be used as a reference point. The starting point on the medial cortex is usually about 4 cm below the joint line. The guide pin should be repositioned until placement is optimal. The saw cut is then made on the underside of the pin and advanced to within 1 cm of the lateral edge of the tibia. Oftentimes, the cortical cut is made with a small sagittal saw, and flexible osteotomes are used to deepen the osteotomy. Continuous or frequent imaging should be performed to protect the lateral cortex. Once the osteotomy is completed (the anterior and posterior cortices are penetrated), the medial opening is created with an osteotomy wedge in a slow and careful fashion to the predetermined size. The anteroposterior slope can be matched or changed depending on the amount of deformity present and the preoperative goals. If replicating the native slope, it is

important to understand that the distraction anteriorly at the tubercle should be less than that at the posteromedial corner; otherwise, the slope will be increased. In cases in which the anterior opening is greater than 1 cm, a tibial tubercle osteotomy can be performed to advance the tubercle the same height as the osteotomy.[71]

Fluoroscopic imaging is used intraoperatively to evaluate the mechanical axis and ensure that it is appropriate. When the desired opening is achieved, the osteotomy is secured with a plate with the leg in extension (using two 6.5-mm cancellous screws proximally and two 4.5-mm cortical screws distally) and usually a bone graft or bone graft substitute. Before closing, the MCL can be fenestrated and allowed to slide if it is too taut. Fluoroscopy is also used at this stage to ensure that the graft is adequately seated. A drain is then inserted and the wound closed in layers. Postoperatively, the leg is placed in a hinged knee brace with toe-touch weightbearing for 6 to 8 weeks. Progression of weightbearing at that time is dependent on radiological evidence of bony union.

An alternative approach includes gradually opening the medial wedge with a variety of external fixation devices, including biplanar external fixators, semicircular external fixators, or small wire frames.[55,70,85] Advantages of these external fixation distraction histogenesis techniques include accurate correction of the desired mechanical axis at termination of distraction, ability to continuously adjust the correction over time, potentially less effect on patellar height, rapid mobilization of the patient, absence of limb length shortening, and maintenance of soft-tissue tension about the knee. In a matched-pair comparative analysis contrasting outcomes between a Coventry-type closing wedge valgus HTO and an HTO using an Ilizarov apparatus, there was a significantly greater decrease in pain and increase in function in the Ilizarov group at a mean follow-up of greater than 2 years.[1] Disadvantages of distraction histogenesis techniques include the use of an external fixation device, which can be cumbersome and poorly tolerated by patients. Pin site difficulties are the primary concern because many of these old pin tracts become colonized, with potential implications for deep infection if the knee is ultimately converted to a TKR.

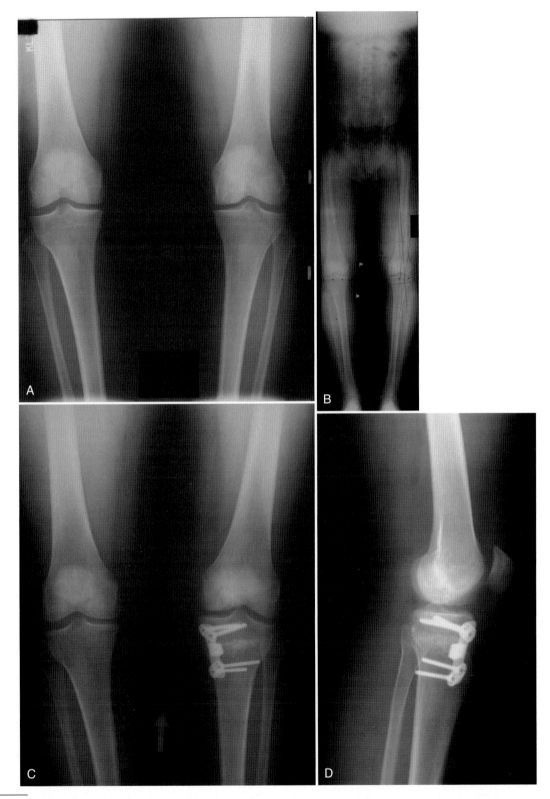

Figure 77–11. **A,** Patient with left knee medial compartment osteochondritis dissecans and post-traumatic medial compartment degenerative arthritis with varus malalignment. **B,** Preoperative templating for a planned left knee valgus-producing, medial tibial opening wedge osteotomy. Lines to the center of the femoral head and the talar dome connect at the 50% percent coordinate and 62.5% percent coordinate along the tibial plateau. The angle formed by the lines that connect at the 62% coordinate (lateral transection on the radiograph) outlines the desired correction to unload the medial compartment. **C,** Postoperative anteroposterior radiograph outlining the opening wedge osteotomy, which was fixed with an Arthrex opening wedge osteotomy locking plate. The osteotomy site was bone-grafted with cancellous allograft mixed with bone graft substitute. **D,** Postoperative lateral radiograph outlining the opening wedge osteotomy.

BARREL VAULT (DOME) TIBIAL OSTEOTOMY

A dome osteotomy involves the use of a curved osteotomy that allows rotation or translation of the distal end of the tibia on the proximal fragment.[9,57] A fundamental aspect of this procedure is that a portion of the fibula must be resected to allow correction of the malalignment.[57] Advantages of this method include avoidance of limb length alteration, potential for anterior displacement of the tibial tubercle to decrease patellofemoral joint reaction forces, and the capacity to address large corrections of malalignment without adversely affecting the resultant joint line obliquity. This procedure is technically demanding, yet with adequate experience proponents prefer this procedure because of the ability to adjust the mechanical axis exactly. Disadvantages of this technique include an increased incidence of complications, including pin tract infection, loss of correction after fixator removal, and peroneal palsy.[8]

DUAL (DOUBLE) OSTEOTOMY

A dual osteotomy is another alternative for patients with severe deformity in whom osteotomy would potentially and adversely alter the obliquity of the joint line. This procedure involves osteotomy of both the femur and tibia to correct malalignment.[11] Typically, the femoral wedge is performed as a lateral closing wedge when correcting varus malalignment and a medial closing wedge when correcting valgus malalignment. A recently published study of 29 double-level osteotomies has reported a 96% cumulative rate of survival at 100 months.[11] These authors attribute their high success to proper selection of patients, careful preoperative planning with biomechanical analysis that accounted for redistribution of the joint load, limited exposure of the knee joint, and modern techniques of internal fixation that allowed for early motion. Overall, the potential additional morbidity previously thought to be associated with double-osteotomy techniques should be considered and weighed against the disadvantages of slight joint line obliquity.

Valgus Deformity

Genu valgum is a much rarer entity than varus deformity of the knee. The biomechanical characteristics of varus and valgus knees are also different because most valgus knees have inherent superolateral obliquity of the joint line. Classically, distal femoral osteotomy has been recommended for valgus deformities exceeding 12 to 15 degrees or when the joint line obliquity would exceed 10 degrees after correction.[25] Although genu valgum may be corrected by a varus-producing proximal tibial osteotomy, the magnitude of the joint line obliquity is increased by the wedge resection and may be a cause of clinical failure. Excessive joint line obliquity produces ineffective weight transfer because some weight is applied as shear force against the intercondylar eminence when the femur subluxes on the tibia. In the current era, the use of a varus closing wedge osteotomy of the proximal tibia for correction of valgus malalignment is virtually obsolete. The reader is referred to Coventry's description of a closing wedge, varus-producing proximal tibial osteotomy.[25] Although dome osteotomy of the proximal tibia does not increase joint line obliquity, the superolateral obliquity of the distal femur associated with a valgus deformity is not corrected, and the persistent femoral valgus angulation continues to exert valgus force on the knee joint.

Osteotomy in the supracondylar region is the most effective method of addressing valgus deformity because the transcondylar line becomes perpendicular with the mechanical axis and MCL laxity is minimized.[60] For most surgeons today, valgus malalignment about the knee of any magnitude is best managed by femoral osteotomy, and a medial closing wedge osteotomy, with either lateral or medial fixation, seems to be the preferred technique.[3,18,30,32,58,92] Valgus deformity can also be corrected by an opening wedge osteotomy of the distal femur with insertion of tricortical autograft wedges supplemented by lateral plate fixation.[98]

Supracondylar femoral osteotomy is an "unforgiving" procedure for three specific reasons: difficulty cutting the wedge effectively, difficulty establishing effective stabilization of the closed osteotomy, and difficulty predicting the wedge size necessary to ensure proper correction of the limb. In many respects, it is clear that the biomechanics, preoperative planning, and operative technique of a supracondylar femoral osteotomy are quite different from that for a proximal tibial osteotomy. These three concerns are adequately addressed by the following surgical technique, which is characterized by a simple preoperative planning process and a straightforward surgical technique that minimizes wedge removal difficulties and reproducibly allows accurate extremity realignment.

MEDIAL CLOSING FEMORAL WEDGE OSTEOTOMY

This technique, which can be performed with either medial or lateral fixation, has been modified from the original description.[61] Essentially, this method uses the transcondylar line and a 90-degree AO blade plate to correct the mechanical axis to neutral. The patient is placed in the supine position; tourniquet control is optional. A 12- to 15-cm longitudinal incision extending from the joint line proximally can be placed anywhere from the midline to the medial side of the thigh. The vastus medialis obliquus is elevated from the medial septum and retracted anteriorly to expose the medial femoral condyle and femoral cortex. The joint line is located with a small arthrotomy or the use of a large needle.

With the knee flexed to 90 degrees, a guide wire is placed across the joint parallel with the articular surface of the distal end of the femur (Fig. 77–12). A second guide wire, inserted approximately 2.0 cm proximal and paral-

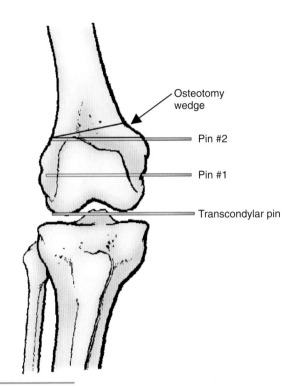

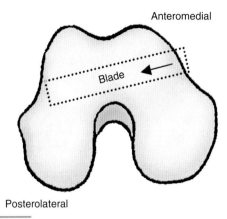

Figure 77–13. The blade plate should be inserted obliquely in an anteromedial-to-posterolateral direction to avoid penetration of the intercondylar notch or the anterior femoral articular surface.

Figure 77–12. Diagram depicting placement of the transcondylar pin, the location of pin No. 1 for entry of the blade plate, and the location of pin No. 2 used for the inferior portion of the osteotomy wedge. A truly parallel position of the transcondylar pin and blade plate entry is essential to obtain a neutral mechanical axis.

lel to the first pin, is directed in an anteromedial-to-posterolateral direction to aid insertion of the blade plate chisel at the correct angle (Fig. 77–13). It is imperative that radiographs be used to confirm a truly parallel position of these pins with the transcondylar line. The guide wire is inserted up to the lateral cortex of the femur to allow measurement of the proper blade plate length, which is usually 50 to 70 mm.

Three 4.5-mm holes are then drilled just above the second pin in the medial femoral condyle to prevent cortical comminution during chisel penetration. The chisel is impacted along the upper surface of pin No. 2 to the desired depth. The plate holder attached to the box chisel facilitates proper chisel entry and ensures correct apposition of the blade plate against the proximal end of the femur. Radiographs taken at this point document the proper chisel angle and ascertain that the chisel has not penetrated the intercondylar notch or the anterior femoral surface. Large malleable retractors are placed medially and posteriorly to protect the neurovascular structures.

Guide wires, placed in a medial-to-lateral direction and converging at the lateral cortex, are used to perform the osteotomy. The inferior guide wire is placed parallel with the transcondylar pin in the supracondylar region just proximal to the adductor tubercle (see Fig. 77–12). A longitudinal line extending above and below the site of the osteotomy is placed on the femur with a marking pencil

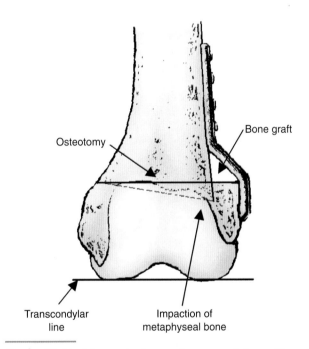

Figure 77–14. After osteotomy closure and impaction of the proximal fragment, the 90-degree AO osteotomy blade plate is secured to the proximal end of the femur, which is now perpendicular to the transcondylar line.

to ensure proper rotation of the limb at the time of osteotomy closure. The medial portion of the osteotomy is performed with an oscillating saw so that the outer 50% to 75% of the wedge can be removed before perforating the lateral cortex with several drill holes. Great care is taken to avoid transection of the lateral cortex and overlying periosteum with the saw. The height of the wedge can be a predetermined measurement, but preferably removal of only a 5- to 10-mm wedge allows impaction of the proximal fragment into the metaphysis of the distal fragment (Fig. 77–14). Such impaction promotes maximal bone apposition and improves stability of the osteotomy site.

The use of preoperative templates to determine the proper plate size is prudent. The proper 90-degree AO blade plate, selected by length of the blade and one of three sizes of offset, is then inserted into the femur. Osteoclasis is performed with a varus force applied to the extremity to close the osteotomy site, impact the proximal fragment, and enable application of the plate along the medial femoral cortex proximally. Multiple cortical screws are used to secure the plate to the femur via the dynamic compression technique; however, the AO outrigger compression device should be avoided because of the proximity of the vascular structures in the adductor canal. The medial femoral cortex and distal femoral articular surface should now be perpendicularly aligned, and the resultant mechanical axis should be approximately neutral (see Fig. 77–9). The removed bone wedge is then morselized and placed medially and posteriorly along the osteotomy site (see Fig. 77–14). The vastus medialis obliquus is reattached to the medial septum with several interrupted sutures over a drain placed at the osteotomy site. The wound is closed in layers and the limb placed in a compressive dressing.

Postoperatively, the patient should remain toe-touch weightbearing for 4 to 6 weeks. The patient then begins partial weightbearing in a hinged knee brace locked in extension for an additional 6 weeks. Weightbearing as tolerated is allowed at the 3-month follow-up if there is radiological evidence of bony union. Adequate fixation plus stability of the osteotomy site intraoperatively is a prerequisite for early active range of motion.

Because of concern regarding delayed union, nonunion, and hardware failure after supracondylar osteotomy with medially based fixation, a method of closing wedge osteotomy involving lateral fixation has been proposed.[65] This technique is based on the rationale that the lateral aspect of the femur becomes the tensile side of the knee after osteotomy and, under these circumstances, laterally based fixation is superior to fixation inserted medially. Indeed, these authors report a higher incidence of implant failure or nonunion with medial fixation than with lateral fixation. It is important to note that the technique described by these authors incorporates more than just fixation location because the osteotomy is performed obliquely and is stabilized with an interfragmentary screw. Undoubtedly, these technical aspects also contribute to the differences observed between the two techniques.

ARTHROSCOPY: DIAGNOSTIC VERSUS THERAPEUTIC

It is commonly believed that some patients might benefit from arthroscopic débridement in conjunction with corrective osteotomy. In one study, osteotomy patients undergoing simultaneous arthroscopic abrasion arthroplasty (group A) were compared with patients who underwent osteotomy alone (group B).[5] At 12-month follow-up, arthroscopic evaluation of group A knees revealed a significantly higher incidence of grade II cartilage repair; however, there was no difference in clinical outcome between the two groups at 2- to 9-year follow-up.

Another reason for considering arthroscopy might be to evaluate the stage of arthritis in the knee to predict the potential efficacy of osteotomy. Prognostic value has not been demonstrated when using arthroscopy to evaluate the joint before corrective osteotomy.[46] The observation of moderate or severe degenerative patellofemoral joint changes has not adversely affected the eventual clinical results.[46] Proliferation of fibrocartilage and regeneration of articular cartilage have been documented by comparing findings at second-look arthroscopy with those visualized preoperatively.[43,50,103] These data support the concept of mechanical realignment to facilitate the reparative capacity of the knee joint once unloaded, with one second-look study demonstrating a correlation between visible improvement of the articular surface, clinical outcome (functional score), and the degree of correction achieved.[43]

FIXATION

Skeletal fixation should be sufficiently rigid to allow early knee motion if desired and yet promote bone healing. Many options are available for fixation, and most are used in conjunction with a specific osteotomy technique. It is generally accepted that fixation of a distal femoral osteotomy requires a more rigid construct than does fixation of a proximal tibial osteotomy. Difficulties in fixation are more frequently reported with supracondylar osteotomy, and most authors agree that rigid internal fixation is required.

Various methods of fixation have been described for closing wedge techniques, including (1) cast immobilization without internal fixation, (2) external fixation devices, (3) staple fixation, (4) screw fixation, (5) buttress plates, (6) tension band plates, (7) "L"-plates, and (7) blade plate fixation.[33] Because of the difficulty associated with loss of correction, the use of internal or external fixation is preferable to cast immobilization without internal fixation. A cadaveric study comparing mechanical stability between blade plates, one-third tubular plates, bone staples, and an external fixator (Orthofix) after a closing wedge osteotomy showed higher stability with the use of external fixators or bone staples.[33] In our hands, although staple fixation has been inadequate for distal femoral osteotomy, it remains the preferred method of fixation for a closing wedge HTO. The benefits of using staple fixation include less soft-tissue dissection, less likelihood of hardware removal at subsequent TKR, and fewer problems with conformity in comparison to plate fixation. Fixation for opening wedge techniques can be accomplished successfully with specialized plates as discussed earlier in this chapter, but buttress plates and fixed-angled devices are also options. The blade plate remains a favorable option for fixation of distal femoral osteotomies, although other techniques have been described, such as fixation with a malleable plate.[92] Favorable rates of osteosynthesis were reported with this technique.[92]

One of the stated advantages of external fixation devices includes the absence of internal hardware. Though undoubtedly true, premature removal of external fixation is often dictated by pin site difficulties, and loss of correction may occur in these patients. Pin site difficulties are definitely more common when using external fixation techniques in the distal femur, and their use in this setting cannot be recommended.[30] The potential serious complications of septic arthritis of the knee joint or an infected total knee arthroplasty after previous pin site infection must be considered, especially in cases in which the treating surgeon does not have adequate experience with external fixation techniques. Although the incidence of this phenomenon is unknown, concern about the prognosis of these patients is warranted.

COMPLICATIONS

The technical difficulties and potential severity of complications associated with realignment osteotomy have undoubtedly biased the occasional surgeon to favor prosthetic treatment options. In general, complications can be categorized as major and minor (Table 77–6). Clearly, many complications arise from errors in selecting the appropriate patient, preoperative planning, surgical technique, and postoperative regimen. Patient selection factors and poor postoperative alignment, probably the most common complications of corrective osteotomy, are discussed in the section detailing results. Some of the other complications such as pin site infection, fixation problems, and adverse joint line obliquity have already been discussed.

Neurological injury after osteotomy ranks as one of the most adverse consequences of HTO. Causative factors include intraoperative injury (as a result of traction, compression, laceration, or penetration by an external fixation pin), tight postoperative dressings or casts, and progressive development of postoperative edema or hematoma. Some of these risks are technique specific because the incidence of neurological injury is lower with opening wedge techniques. Avoidance of dissection of the peroneal nerve,

careful placement of retractors, and maintenance of flexion of the knee during the operative procedure are useful adjuncts that help safeguard the nerve. Postoperative dressings should be well padded with the knee in a slightly flexed position.

The occurrence of a neurological deficit is clearly related to the performance and level of a concomitant fibular osteotomy.[107] A safe area for proximal fibular osteotomy is up to 20.5 mm distal to the tip of the fibular head.[88] When applicable, a distal fibular osteotomy should be performed at the junction of the middle and distal third of the fibula.[10] Injury to the posterior tibial nerve has also been described.[63] Vascular injury associated with HTO is fortunately rare, and most reported cases involve the popliteal artery.[109] As shown in 20 cadaveric dissections, flexion of the knee joint as compared with full knee extension does not protect the knee from popliteal artery injury.[109] The more extensive dissection required for plate and screw fixation with closing wedge techniques predisposes to anterior tibial artery compromise.[24]

Compartment syndrome is a rare, yet devastating complication after osteotomy. It has been demonstrated that suction drainage of the anterior compartment is helpful inasmuch as 8 of 10 patients with drains had postoperative compartment pressures of less than 30 mm Hg versus pressure elevation greater than 50 mm Hg in 7 of 10 patients without drains.[34] The importance of rapid diagnosis and the potential to avert an impending compartment syndrome before the onset of an established compartment syndrome must be emphasized to all members of the health care team when participating in the patient's care.

Deep infection is quite rare after corrective osteotomy, but the risk is higher when using external fixation devices. Thromboembolic disease occurs with lower frequency after osteotomy than after total knee arthroplasty, and the ideal method of prophylaxis is controversial. We prefer to use the same anticoagulation protocol for both osteotomy and arthroplasty.

Intra-articular fracture of the tibial plateau, which may occur during manipulation of the osteotomy, can be minimized by maintaining an adequate thickness of the proximal tibial fragment (usually 2 cm), removing the entire bone wedge (for a closing wedge technique) or extending the osteotomy bone cuts far enough laterally (for an opening wedge technique), allowing for plastic deformation of bone while slowly and carefully applying a directional force to the extremity, and carefully perforating the apical portion of the osteotomy when necessary. When using guide wires to direct a tibial osteotomy, one should cut on the undersurface of the most proximal wire. Evaluation of the osteotomy site by fluoroscopy before and intermittently during the manipulation will ensure that the osteotomy is adequately fashioned and appropriately responding to external realignment forces. The lateral tibial cortex (opening wedge) or medial tibial cortex (closing wedge) may also fracture through and destabilize the proximal osteotomy fragment during manipulation. If this complication occurs, the surgeon will need to apply supplemental fixation (usually staples) to address the resultant instability on that side. Fluoroscopy is also required to ensure that the hardware has not penetrated

Table 77–6. Complications Associated with Realignment Osteotomy

MAJOR	MINOR
Neurological injury	Superficial wound healing
Vascular injury	Pin site infections
Compartment syndrome	Skin numbness
Deep infection	Neuroma formation
Thromboembolic disease	Arthrofibrosis
Intra-articular fracture	Knee instability
Hardware failure	Adverse joint line obliquity
Nonunion	Patella infra
Malunion	Delayed union
Loss of correction	Inadequate pain relief
Undercorrection	Painful hardware
Overcorrection	Flare-up chondrocalcinosis
	Osteonecrosis of the tibial plateau

the joint itself. Excessive medial bone loss can cause an errant direction of the osteotome or saw and lead to direct osteotomy of the joint surface. Any plateau fracture should be reduced and adequately stabilized to maintain the proper position of the plateau for weight distribution and early range of motion. Osteonecrosis of the tibial plateau can also occur when the proximal tibial fragment is fashioned too thin.[24]

Joint stiffness has been rarely reported after HTO, whereas this phenomenon has been frequently reported after supracondylar osteotomy.[19,30,60] Rigid fixation and early range of motion minimize the prevalence of stiffness, but rapid healing of the osteotomy and maintenance of postoperative alignment should take priority. The stiffness associated with supracondylar osteotomy does make surgical exposure more difficult for subsequent knee arthroplasty in some patients.[15] Early range of motion also helps avoid quadriceps atrophy and may aid in the prevention of patellar ligament shortening after osteotomy.[105] It has been questioned whether patellar position is actually lowered after HTO.[101]

An acute postoperative flare-up of joint pain may be due to calcium pyrophosphate deposition and has been reported to occur in 4.6% of cases.[22] These flare-ups are generally documented by analysis of synovial fluid and radiographic evidence of crystalline deposition. Management with anti-inflammatory medications or intra-articular injection of corticosteroids is usually sufficient. It has previously been proposed that preoperative evidence of calcium pyrophosphate deposition, with the attendant generalized joint inflammation, should be a contraindication to corrective osteotomy.[22]

A cadaveric study suggests that conventional closing wedge HTO carried out without lateral collateral imbrication or advancement probably accounts for recurrence of varus deformity.[86] Recurrence of preoperative deformity over time has been correlated with clinical deterioration.[96] This study showed that a majority of patients have some recurrence of varus at a minimum of 5 years of follow-up but that only 18% had more than 5 degrees of recurrence.[96] In contrast, 83% had significant progression of lateral compartment arthritis.

Discussions regarding difficulty with successful union are ubiquitous in all reports of corrective osteotomy. Potential causes include the location of the osteotomy, the fixation method used, bone necrosis (secondary to heat generated by the power saw), fibular impingement against the proximal tibial fragment, and poorly performed osteotomy cuts. Tibial osteotomy below the tibial tubercle is associated with a fourfold increase in delayed union when compared with tibial osteotomy performed above the tibial tubercle.[99] The rate of nonunion after HTO performed above the tubercle ranges from 2% to 4% in the literature, which is distinctly less than the rates reported for supracondylar osteotomy (between 4.2% and 19%).[30,101] The opportunity to remove a section of bone and compress the opposing vascularized bone fragments in a closing wedge HTO has a clear advantage for establishing union versus an opening wedge technique, where an osteotomy is made and the wedge-shaped space created by distractive methods is commonly filled with nonvascularized bone graft or bone graft substitute.

RESULTS

High Tibial Osteotomy

It is clear that reported outcomes of HTO are quite variable. Factors that affect outcome, such as patient selection and surgical technique, have been clarified over the past 4 decades. The recent literature suggests that HTO provides durable and satisfactory long-term clinical results if the procedure is accurately performed in carefully selected patients, who are typically younger than 60 years and have less than a 12-degree angular deformity, pure unicompartmental disease, ligamentous stability, and a preoperative range-of-motion arc of at least 90 degrees.[14] The importance of patient selection is underscored by the results obtained in 39 osteotomies, many of which were performed without precise indications.[14] Among the 10 poor results, preoperative diagnoses included four cases of diffuse degenerative arthritis, two cases of inflammatory disease, one case of previous septic arthritis, and one case of post-traumatic arthritis with severe deformity. If these 10 patients were excluded from analysis, the percentage of overall satisfactory results would be 79% at 12 years' follow-up.

An equally important consideration for a successful clinical outcome includes the quality of the surgical technique. It is often difficult to ascertain the effects of patient selection and technical errors on the long-term outcome when evaluating many of these clinical series. Many HTO series reveal satisfactory results at 5 to 7 years of follow-up; the percentage of satisfactory clinical results then diminishes significantly (Table 77–7). A meta-analysis reviewing 19 previous HTO publications reported good or excellent results in 75.3% of patients at 60 months' follow-up and in 60.3% at 100 months' follow-up.[101] Several of these studies carefully analyzed subgroups of patients to further refine the prognostic factors associated with long-term success. The following quote requires careful consideration: "The passage of time seemed to influence the result only in knees that were undercorrected or overcorrected."[39] This quote can be appreciated in a series of 93 osteotomies, in which the overall 5-year survival rate was 90%, which then diminished to 45% at 10 years, thus hiding the results obtained in patients with good postoperative alignment. Favorable alignment was noted in 20 patients, with no failures observed at 11.5 years after the index surgery. This result sharply contrasts with the observed deterioration in 51 (75%) of 68 knees with postoperative undercorrection.

Excluding patient selection, the accuracy of postoperative alignment clearly appears to be a primary factor for success with the passage of time. The difficulty lies in determining the "appropriate postoperative alignment" because recommendations vary between reports. Some recommend 3 to 6 degrees of valgus,[39] others suggest 10 to 12 degrees,[19] and 6 to 14 degrees of anatomic valgus has even been advocated.[81] Coventry reported that for knees with 8 degrees or more of postoperative valgus, the survival rate was 94% at 5- and 10-year follow-up versus 63% survival at 5- and 10-year follow-up for knees corrected to 5 degrees or less of valgus angulation.[25]

Table 77–7. Survival Success of Selected Series of High Tibial Osteotomy

AUTHOR	YEAR	N	2 yr	5 yr	7 yr	10 yr	15 yr
Aglietti[2]	2003	102	—	96%	88%	78%	57%
Berman[14]	1991	39	87%	—	—	—	57%*
Billings[16]	2000	64	—	85%	—	53%	—
Cass[19]	1988	86	94%	87%	—	69%	—
Coventry[27]	1993	87	—	87% (96%)† (94%)‡	—	66% (91%)† (94%)‡	—
Hernigou[38]	2001	245	—	94%	—	85%	68%
Majima[56]	2000	48	91%§	—	—	61%	—
Naudie[72]	1999	85	—	95%	—	80%	60%
Ritter[79]	1988	78	95%	80%	58%	58%	58%*
Rudan[82]	1991	128	—	—	—	80%	70%
Sprenger[90]	2003	66	—	86%	—	74%	56%

*Twelve to 13 years.
†Body weight less than 1.17 times normal.
‡Postoperative alignment in 8 degrees or more of valgus.
§One year.

Finally, among 314 patients monitored for 10 to 19 years, in the 170 patients who had undercorrection, 54 subsequently required additional revision surgery for clinical deterioration, whereas in 144 patients with a normalized or overcorrected alignment, only 8 required surgical revision.[74] Based on this long-term experience, these surgeons suggest that a properly performed HTO rivals the longevity of current prosthetic replacements.

Distal Femoral Osteotomy

As with HTO, the reported success with distal femoral osteotomy has been variable (Table 77–8). Patient selection factors, good surgical technique, appropriate postoperative alignment, and the passage of time all affect the final clinical outcome. Many studies comment on the fact that some clinical failures were poor candidates for distal femoral osteotomy and report better success in patients meeting strict selection criteria.[30] In general, patients should be younger than 65 years and have good bone stock and isolated osteoarthritis of the lateral compartment, minimal ligamentous laxity, a range-of-motion arc of more than 90 degrees, and flexion contracture of less than 20 degrees.

Proper postoperative alignment appears to be an essential factor for a good long-term result, and again, the optimum range of alignment has not been determined. In one study the success rate was 77% if the alignment was corrected to neutral or varus, as opposed to 60% success in patients left in some degree of valgus.[30] We would agree with others that a tibiofemoral angle of approximately 0 degrees (neutral alignment) is the desired correction for a supracondylar osteotomy.[61]

Table 77–8. Results of Distal Femoral Osteotomy

AUTHOR	YEAR	N	SUCCESS (%)	FOLLOW-UP (yr)
Aglietti[3]	2000	18	77	9
Cameron[18]	1997	49	87	7*
Edgerton[30]	1993	24	71 (86)†	8.3 (5-11)
Finkelstein[32]	1996	21	64	11 (8-20)
Marin Morales[58]	2000	17	75	6.5
Mathews[60]	1998	21	57	3 (1-8)
McDermott[61]	1988	24	92	4 (2-11.5)
Miniaci[65]	1989	35	86 (100)†	5.4 (2-16.7)
Terry[98]	1992	35	60	5.4 (2-19)

*Endpoint of survival analysis.
†Isolated compartment disease.
‡Valgus deformity without arthrosis.

SUMMARY

Realignment osteotomy about the knee continues to meet many of the original expectations. Although the current indications are relatively narrow, the surgeon should be confident in choosing corrective osteotomy when appropriate criteria are met. The long-term results linked with careful patient selection, accurate surgical technique, and appropriate postoperative alignment portray a favorable outlook for these procedures, particularly since the population at large is more active and is expected to have increasing longevity.

References

1. Adili A, Bhandari M, Giffin R, et al: Valgus high tibial osteotomy. Comparison between an Ilizarov and a Coventry wedge technique for the treatment of medial compartment osteoarthritis of the knee. Knee Surg Sports Traumatol Arthrosc 10:169-176, 2002.
2. Aglietti P, Buzzi R, Vena LM, et al: High tibial valgus osteotomy for medial gonarthrosis: A 10- to 21-year study. J Knee Surg 16:21-26, 2003.
3. Aglietti P, Menchetti PP: Distal femoral varus osteotomy in the valgus osteoarthritic knee. Am J Knee Surg 13:89-95, 2000.
4. Agneskirchner JD, Hurschler C, Stukenborg-Colsman C, et al: Effect of high tibial flexion osteotomy on cartilage pressure and joint kinematics: A biomechanical study in human cadaveric knees. Winner of the AGA-DonJoy Award 2004. Arch Orthop Trauma Surg 124:575-584, 2004.
5. Akizuki S, Yasukawa Y, Takizawa T: Does arthroscopic abrasion arthroplasty promote cartilage regeneration in osteoarthritic knees with eburnation? A prospective study of high tibial osteotomy with abrasion arthroplasty versus high tibial osteotomy alone. Arthroscopy 13:9-17, 1997.
6. Amendola A: Unicompartmental osteoarthritis in the active patient: The role of high tibial osteotomy. Arthroscopy 19(Suppl 1):109-116, 2003.
7. Amendola A, Fowler PJ, Litchfield R, et al: Opening wedge high tibial osteotomy using a novel technique: Early results and complications. J Knee Surg 17:164-169, 2004.
8. Aydogdu S, Cullu E, Arac N, et al: Prolonged peroneal nerve dysfunction after high tibial osteotomy: Pre- and postoperative electrophysiological study. Knee Surg Sports Traumatol Arthrosc 8:305-308, 2000.
9. Aydogdu S, Sur H: [High tibial osteotomy for varus deformity of more than 20 degrees.] Rev Chir Orthop Reparatrice Appar Mot 84:439-446, 1997.
10. Aydogdu S, Yercan H, Saylam C, Sur H: Peroneal nerve dysfunction after high tibial osteotomy. An anatomical cadaver study. Acta Orthop Belg 62:156-160, 1996.
11. Babis GC, An KN, Chao EY, et al: Double level osteotomy of the knee: A method to retain joint-line obliquity. Clinical results. J Bone Joint Surg Am 84:1380-1388, 2002.
12. Badhe NP, Forster IW: High tibial osteotomy in knee instability: The rationale of treatment and early results. Knee Surg Sports Traumatol Arthrosc 10:38-43, 2002.
13. Berger RA, Meneghini RM, Sheinkop MB, et al: The progression of patellofemoral arthrosis after medial unicompartmental replacement: Results at 11 to 15 years. Clin Orthop 428:92-99, 2004.
14. Berman AT, Bosacco SJ, Kirshner S, Avolio A Jr: Factors influencing long-term results in high tibial osteotomy. Clin Orthop 272:192-198, 1991.
15. Beyer CA, Lewallen DG, Hanssen AD: Total knee arthroplasty following prior osteotomy of the distal femur. Am J Knee Surg 7:25-30, 1994.
16. Billings A, Scott DF, Camargo MP, Hofmann AA: High tibial osteotomy with a calibrated osteotomy guide, rigid internal fixation, and early motion. Long-term follow-up. J Bone Joint Surg Am 82:70-79, 2000.
17. Bonin N, Ait Si Selmi T, Donell ST, et al: Anterior cruciate reconstruction combined with valgus upper tibial osteotomy: 12 years follow-up. Knee 11:431-437, 2004.
18. Cameron HU, Botsford DJ, Park YS: Prognostic factors in the outcome of supracondylar femoral osteotomy for lateral compartment osteoarthritis of the knee. Can J Surg 40:114-118, 1997.
19. Cass JR, Bryan RS: High tibial osteotomy. Clin Orthop 230:196-199, 1988.
20. Choi HR, Hasegawa Y, Kondo S, et al: High tibial osteotomy for varus gonarthrosis: A 10- to 24-year follow-up study. J Orthop Sci 6:493-497, 2001.
21. Coventry MB: Osteotomy of the upper portion of the tibia for degenerative arthritis of the knee. A preliminary report. J Bone Joint Surg Am 47:984-990, 1965.
22. Coventry MB: Upper tibial osteotomy for gonarthrosis. The evolution of the operation in the last 18 years and long term results. Orthop Clin North Am 10:191-210, 1979.
23. Coventry MB: Upper tibial osteotomy. Clin Orthop 182:46-52, 1984.
24. Coventry MB: Upper tibial osteotomy for osteoarthritis. J Bone Joint Surg Am 67:1136-1140, 1985.
25. Coventry MB: Proximal tibial varus osteotomy for osteoarthritis of the lateral compartment of the knee. J Bone Joint Surg Am 69:32-38, 1987.
26. Coventry MB, Bowman PW: Long-term results of upper tibial osteotomy for degenerative arthritis of the knee. Acta Orthop Belg 48:139-156, 1982.
27. Coventry MB, Ilstrup DM, Wallrichs SL: Proximal tibial osteotomy. A critical long-term study of eighty-seven cases. J Bone Joint Surg Am 75:196-201, 1993.
28. Devgan A, Marya KM, Kundu ZS, et al: Medial opening wedge high tibial osteotomy for osteoarthritis of knee: Long-term results in 50 knees. Med J Malaysia 58:62-68, 2003.
29. Dugdale TW, Noyes FR, Styer D: Preoperative planning for high tibial osteotomy. The effect of lateral tibiofemoral separation and tibiofemoral length. Clin Orthop 274:248-264, 1992.
30. Edgerton BC, Mariani EM, Morrey BF: Distal femoral varus osteotomy for painful genu valgum. A five-to-11-year follow-up study. Clin Orthop 288:263-269, 1993.
31. Ellis RE, Tso CY, Rudan JF, Harrison MM: A surgical planning and guidance system for high tibial osteotomy. Comput Aided Surg 4:264-274, 1999.
32. Finkelstein JA, Gross AE, Davis A: Varus osteotomy of the distal part of the femur. A survivorship analysis. J Bone Joint Surg Am 78:1348-1352, 1996.
33. Flamme CH, Kohn D, Kirsch L, Hurschler C: Primary stability of different implants used in conjunction with high tibial osteotomy. Arch Orthop Trauma Surg 119:450-455, 1999.
34. Gibson MJ, Barnes MR, Allen MJ, Chan RN: Weakness of foot dorsiflexion and changes in compartment pressures after tibial osteotomy. J Bone Joint Surg Br 68:471-475, 1986.
35. Grelsamer R: High tibial osteotomy (HTO) is an effective procedure for medial and patellofemoral disease. Clin Orthop 260:310-311, 1990.
36. Haddad FS, Bentley G: Total knee arthroplasty after high tibial osteotomy: A medium-term review. J Arthroplasty 15:597-603, 2000.
37. Hanssen AD, Stuart MJ, Scott RD, Scuderi GR: Surgical options for the middle-aged patient with osteoarthritis of the knee joint. Instr Course Lect 50:499-511, 2001.
38. Hernigou P, Ma W: Open wedge tibial osteotomy with acrylic bone cement as bone substitute. Knee 8:103-110, 2001.
39. Hernigou P, Medevielle D, Debeyre J, Goutallier D: Proximal tibial osteotomy for osteoarthritis with varus deformity. A ten to thirteen-year follow-up study. J Bone Joint Surg Am 69:332-354, 1987.
40. Hofmann AA, Cook TM: High tibial osteotomy: Where did you go? Orthopedics 26:949-950, 2003.
41. Hofmann AA, Wyatt RW, Beck SW: High tibial osteotomy. Use of an osteotomy jig, rigid fixation, and early motion versus conventional surgical technique and cast immobilization. Clin Orthop 271:212-217, 1991.
42. Insall JN, Joseph DM, Msika C: High tibial osteotomy for varus gonarthrosis. A long-term follow-up study. J Bone Joint Surg Am 66:1040-1048, 1984.
43. Kanamiya T, Naito M, Hara M, Yoshimura I: The influences of biomechanical factors on cartilage regeneration after high tibial osteotomy for knees with medial compartment osteoarthritis: Clinical and arthroscopic observations. Arthroscopy 18:725-729, 2002.
44. Karabatsos B, Mahomed NN, Maistrelli GL: Functional outcome of total knee arthroplasty after high tibial osteotomy. Can J Surg 45:116-119, 2002.
45. Kawano T, Miura H, Nagamine R, et al: Alignment in total knee arthroplasty following failed high tibial osteotomy. J Knee Surg 16:168-172, 2003.
46. Keene JS, Dyreby JR Jr: High tibial osteotomy in the treatment of osteoarthritis of the knee. The role of preoperative arthroscopy. J Bone Joint Surg Am 65:36-42, 1983.
47. Keppler P, Gebhard F, Grutzner PA, et al: Computer aided high tibial open wedge osteotomy. Injury 35(Suppl 1):S-A68-S-A78, 2004.
48. Korn MW: A new approach to dome high tibial osteotomy. Am J Knee Surg 9:12-21, 1996.

49. Koshino T, Murase T, Saito T: Medial opening-wedge high tibial osteotomy with use of porous hydroxyapatite to treat medial compartment osteoarthritis of the knee. J Bone Joint Surg Am 85:78-85, 2003.

50. Koshino T, Wada S, Ara Y, Saito T: Regeneration of degenerated articular cartilage after high tibial valgus osteotomy for medial compartmental osteoarthritis of the knee. Knee 10:229-236, 2003.

51. Koshino T, Yoshida T, Ara Y, et al: Fifteen to twenty-eight years' follow-up results of high tibial valgus osteotomy for osteoarthritic knee. Knee 11:439-444, 2004.

52. Lobenhoffer P, Agneskirchner JD: Improvements in surgical technique of valgus high tibial osteotomy. Knee Surg Sports Traumatol Arthrosc 11:132-138, 2003.

53. Madan S, Ranjith RK, Fiddian NJ: Total knee replacement following high tibial osteotomy. Bull Hosp Jt Dis 61:5-10, 2002.

54. Madan S, Ranjith RK, Fiddian NJ: Intermediate follow-up of high tibial osteotomy: A comparison of two techniques. Bull Hosp Jt Dis 61:11-16, 2002.

55. Magyar G, Ahl TL, Vibe P, et al: Open-wedge osteotomy by hemicallotasis or the closed-wedge technique for osteoarthritis of the knee. A randomised study of 50 operations. J Bone Joint Surg Br 81:444-448, 1999.

56. Majima T, Yasuda K, Katsuragi R, Kaneda K: Progression of joint arthrosis 10 to 15 years after high tibial osteotomy. Clin Orthop 381:177-184, 2000.

57. Maquet P: Valgus osteotomy for osteoarthritis of the knee. Clin Orthop 120:143-148, 1976.

58. Marin Morales LA, Gomez Navalon LA, Zorilla RP: Treatment of osteoarthritis of the knee with valgus deformity by means of a varus osteotomy. Acta Orthop Belg 66:272-278, 2000.

59. Marti CB, Gautier E, Wachtl SW, Jakob RP: Accuracy of frontal and sagittal plane correction in open-wedge high tibial osteotomy. Arthroscopy 20:366-372, 2004.

60. Mathews J, Cobb AG, Richardson S, Bentley G: Distal femoral osteotomy for lateral compartment osteoarthritis of the knee. Orthopedics 21:437-440, 1998.

61. McDermott AG, Finklestein JA, Farine I, et al: Distal femoral varus osteotomy for valgus deformity of the knee. J Bone Joint Surg Am 70:110-116, 1988.

62. McGuire DA, Carter TR, Shelton WR: Complex knee reconstruction: Osteotomies, ligament reconstruction, transplants, and cartilage treatment options. Arthroscopy 18(9 Suppl 2):90-103, 2002.

63. McLaren CA, Wootton JR, Heath PD, Jones CH: Pes planus after tibial osteotomy. Foot Ankle 9:300-303, 1989.

64. Meding JB, Keating EM, Ritter MA, Faris PM: Total knee arthroplasty after high tibial osteotomy. A comparison study in patients who had bilateral total knee replacement. J Bone Joint Surg Am 82:1252-1259, 2000.

65. Miniaci A, Grossman SP, Jacob RP: Supracondylar femoral varus osteotomy in the treatment of valgus knee deformity. Am J Knee Surg 2:65-70, 1989.

66. Mont MA, Antonaides S, Krackow KA, Hungerford DS: Total knee arthroplasty after failed high tibial osteotomy. A comparison with a matched group. Clin Orthop 299:125-130, 1994.

67. Mont MA, Stuchin SA, Paley D, et al: Different surgical options for monocompartmental osteoarthritis of the knee: High tibial osteotomy versus unicompartmental knee arthroplasty versus total knee arthroplasty: Indications, techniques, results, and controversies. Instr Course Lect 53:265-283, 2004.

68. Morrey BF: Upper tibial osteotomy for secondary osteoarthritis of the knee. J Bone Joint Surg Br 71:554-559, 1989.

69. Nagel A, Insall JN, Scuderi GR: Proximal tibial osteotomy. A subjective outcome study. J Bone Joint Surg Am 78:1353-1358, 1996.

70. Nakamura E, Mizuta H, Kudo S, et al: Open-wedge osteotomy of the proximal tibia hemicallotasis. J Bone Joint Surg Br 83:1111-1115, 2001.

71. Naudie DD, Amendola A, Fowler PJ: Opening wedge high tibial osteotomy for symptomatic hyperextension-varus thrust. Am J Sports Med 32:60-70, 2004.

72. Naudie D, Bourne RB, Rorabeck CH, Bourne TJ: The Install Award. Survivorship of the high tibial valgus osteotomy. A 10- to 22-year followup study. Clin Orthop 367:18-27, 1999.

73. Noda T, Yasuda S, Nagano K, et al: Clinico-radiological study of total knee arthroplasty after high tibial osteotomy. J Orthop Sci 5:25-36, 2000.

74. Odenbring S, Egund N, Knutson K, et al: Revision after osteotomy for gonarthrosis. A 10- to 19-year follow-up of 314 cases. Acta Orthop Scand 61:128-130, 1990.

75. Odenbring S, Tjornstrand B, Egund N, et al: Function after tibial osteotomy for medial gonarthrosis below aged 50 years. Acta Orthop Scand 60:527-531, 1989.

76. Parvizi J, Hanssen AD, Spangehl MJ: Total knee arthroplasty following proximal tibial osteotomy: Risk factors for failure. J Bone Joint Surg Am 86:474-479, 2004.

77. Prodromos CC, Andriacchi TP, Galante JO: A relationship between gait and clinical changes following high tibial osteotomy. J Bone Joint Surg Am 67:1188-1194, 1985.

78. Repicci JA: Mini-invasive knee unicompartmental arthroplasty: Bone-sparing technique. Surg Technol Int 11:282-286, 2003.

79. Ritter MA, Fechtman RA: Proximal tibial osteotomy. A survivorship analysis. J Arthroplasty 3:309-311, 1988.

80. Rudan J, Harrison M, Simurda MA: Optimizing femorotibial alignment in high tibial osteotomy. Can J Surg 42:366-370, 1999.

81. Rudan JF, Simurda MA: High tibial osteotomy. A prospective clinical and roentgenographic review. Clin Orthop 255:251-256, 1990.

82. Rudan JF, Simurda MA: Valgus high tibial osteotomy. A long-term follow-up study. Clin Orthop 268:157-160, 1991.

83. Scott WN, Clarke HD: The role of osteotomy 2003: Defining the niche. Orthopedics 27:975-976, 2004.

84. Sculco TP: Orthopaedic crossfire—can we justify unicondylar arthroplasty as a temporizing procedure? In opposition. J Arthroplasty 17(4 Suppl 1):56-58, 2002.

85. Sen C, Kocaoglu M, Eralp L: The advantages of circular external fixation used in high tibial osteotomy (average 6 years follow-up). Knee Surg Sports Traumatol Arthrosc 11:139-144, 2003.

86. Shaw JA, Dungy DS, Arsht SS: Recurrent varus angulation after high tibial osteotomy: An anatomic analysis. Clin Orthop 420:205-212, 2004.

87. Slawski DP: High tibial osteotomy in the treatment of adult osteochondritis dissecans. Clin Orthop 341:155-161, 1997.

88. Soejima O, Ogata K, Ishinishi T, et al: Anatomic considerations of the peroneal nerve for division of the fibula during high tibial osteotomy. Orthop Rev 23:244-247, 1994.

89. Specogna AV, Birmingham TB, DaSilva JJ, et al: Reliability of lower limb frontal plane alignment measurements using plain radiographs and digitized images. J Knee Surg 17:203-210, 2004.

90. Sprenger TR, Doerzbacher JF: Tibial osteotomy for the treatment of varus gonarthrosis. Survival and failure analysis to twenty-two years. J Bone Joint Surg Am 85:469-474, 2003.

91. Staeheli JW, Cass JR, Morrey BF: Condylar total knee arthroplasty after failed proximal tibial osteotomy. J Bone Joint Surg Am 69:28-31, 1987.

92. Stahelin T, Hardegger F, Ward JC: Supracondylar osteotomy of the femur with use of compression. Osteosynthesis with a malleable implant. J Bone Joint Surg Am 82:712-722, 2000.

93. Staubli AE, De Simoni C, Babst R, Lobenhoffer P: TomoFix: A new LCP-concept for open wedge osteotomy of the medial proximal tibia—early results in 92 cases. Injury 34(Suppl 2):B55-B62, 2003.

94. Sterett WI, Steadman JR: Chondral resurfacing and high tibial osteotomy in the varus knee. Am J Sports Med 32:1243-1249, 2004.

95. Stoffel K, Stachowiak G, Kuster M: Open wedge high tibial osteotomy: Biomechanical investigation of the modified Arthrex Osteotomy Plate (Puddu Plate) and the TomoFix Plate. Clin Biomech (Bristol, Avon) 19:944-950, 2004.

96. Stuart MJ, Grace JN, Ilstrup DM, et al: Late recurrence of varus deformity after proximal tibial osteotomy. Clin Orthop 260:61-65, 1990.

97. Swienckowski JJ, Pennington DW: Unicompartmental knee arthroplasty in patients sixty years of age or younger. J Bone Joint Surg Am 86(Suppl 1):131-142, 2004.

98. Terry GC, Cimino PM: Distal femoral osteotomy for valgus deformity of the knee. Orthopedics 15:1283-1289, discussion 1289-1290, 1992.

99. Vainionpaa S, Laike E, Kirves P, Tiusanen P: Tibial osteotomy for osteoarthritis of the knee. A five to ten-year follow-up study. J Bone Joint Surg Am 63:938-946, 1981.

100. Vince KG, Cyran LT: Unicompartmental knee arthroplasty: New indications, more complications? J Arthroplasty 19(4 Suppl 1):9-16, 2004.

101. Virolainen P, Aro HT: High tibial osteotomy for the treatment of osteoarthritis of the knee: A review of the literature and a meta-analysis of follow-up studies. Arch Orthop Trauma Surg 124:258-261, 2004.

102. Wada M, Imura S, Nagatani K, et al: Relationship between gait and clinical results after high tibial osteotomy. Clin Orthop 354:180-188, 1998.

103. Wakabayashi S, Akizuki S, Takizawa T, Yasukawa Y: A comparison of the healing potential of fibrillated cartilage versus eburnated bone in osteoarthritic knees after high tibial osteotomy: An arthroscopic study with 1-year follow-up. Arthroscopy 18:272-278, 2002.

104. Weale AE, Lee AS, MacEachern AG: High tibial osteotomy using a dynamic axial external fixator. Clin Orthop 382:154-167, 2001.

105. Westrich GH, Peters LE, Haas SB, et al: Patella height after high tibial osteotomy with internal fixation and early motion. Clin Orthop 354:169-174, 1998.

106. Windsor RE, Insall JN, Vince KG: Technical considerations of total knee arthroplasty after proximal tibial osteotomy. J Bone Joint Surg Am 70:547-555, 1988.

107. Wootton JR, Ashworth MJ, MacLaren CA: Neurological complications of high tibial osteotomy—the fibular osteotomy as a causative factor: A clinical and anatomical study. Ann R Coll Surg Engl 77:31-34, 1995.

108. Wright JM, Heavrin B, Begg M, et al: Observations on patellar height following opening wedge proximal tibial osteotomy. Am J Knee Surg 14:163-173, 2001.

109. Zaidi SH, Cobb AG, Bentley G: Danger to the popliteal artery in high tibial osteotomy. J Bone Joint Surg Br 77:384-386, 1995.

CHAPTER 78

Osteotomy for the Arthritic Knee: A European Perspective

Pascal Poilvache

Do high tibial or low femoral osteotomies for the treatment of gonarthrosis belong in the past? Considering the improvement of the outcome of total[83,91,282] and unicompartmental[46,179,239,320] knee arthroplasties reported in recent years, the legitimate question arises whether osteotomies are still necessary. They seem likely to become an exception, similar to hip osteotomies in the case of coxarthritis. This trend clearly emerges—at least in the United States—when the number of osteotomies is compared with the number of prostheses.[360] Rather than becoming the exception, however, should not the indications for osteotomy be redefined? From the review of the literature that follows, it emerges that osteotomies should be aimed at young—at least physiologically—and active subjects, who present with a moderate deformation and arthrosis in its early stages.

By maintaining these criteria, are we not at risk of making osteotomies—which are not without complications—prophylactic operations only and possibly superfluous? The orthopedic literature is particularly lacking in longitudinal studies, assessing the long-term outcome of an early gonarthrosis arising from axial deviation. Two Swedish studies provide information on this subject, however. In a 10- to 17- year follow-up, Hernborg and Nilsson[122] reviewed 71 patients (94 knees) who had had gonarthrosis in the 1950s. More than half of the knees had deteriorated, particularly in the case of young patients and when axial deviation was present. Preexisting instability also worsened the prognosis. The femorotibial compartment that was intact at the time of the first radiographic examination remained so more often than not at the last examination.

Between 1972 and 1988, Odenbring and associates[258] monitored 189 knees with a medial arthrosis. After 14 years, tibial osteotomy had been performed in 85 knees, and arthroplasty had been done in another 33 knees. No major surgery had been undertaken in 71 knees. Of these 71 knees, 31 patients (40 knees) died, and most of the remaining 23 patients (31 knees) had unsatisfactory results; they managed only a low activity level. The authors concluded that the natural course of medial gonarthrosis had a poor prognosis because most patients with this condition eventually would have to undergo major knee surgery.

Bearing in mind this bad prognosis and the good long-term results of osteotomy when strict selection criteria are implemented and compliance with a rigorous technique is maintained, it seems that these procedures do have their place in the treatment of the early stages of gonarthrosis arising from axial deviation. This is all the more true now that multiple techniques for the early treatment of knee arthrosis have been developed, including administration of chondroprotective substances, reimplantation of cultured chondrocytes, meniscal grafts, cartilage transplantation, and ligament reconstruction in the presence of mild arthritis. These techniques aim at preventing the ultimate radical surgery of articular replacement. These techniques cannot be considered successful, however, unless the charges imposed on the damaged compartment are below the bearable threshold, and they often require an axial correction. Osteotomy of the knee has a long past,[34,61,75,96,152,215] dating back to the 19th century.[341] In a new millennium, a description of its merits is worthwhile.

HIGH TIBIAL OSTEOTOMY

Biomechanical Principles

Osteoarthrosis results from the loss of balance between the biological resistance of the joint and its mechanical stressing. The direct deleterious effect of excessive pressure on articular cartilage has been documented repeatedly in animal models.[260,277,285,363] McKellop and colleagues,[221,222] using pressure-sensitive films in cadaveric limbs, showed a relationship between the level and magnitude of the deformity and the contact pressure across the knee.

Treatment must reduce the articular stresses sufficiently to make them tolerable (Fig. 78–1). Maquet[203-205,207,208,210,211] proposed a biomechanical theory stating that the joint stability in a normal knee is the result of the equilibrium between two forces. The force P, eccentrically exerted by the part of the body supported by the knee, must be balanced by active muscular forces L and by passive ligamentous forces. Force R is the result or the vectorial sum of all of these forces. It creates compressive stresses and must act perpendicular to the weightbearing surfaces through their center of gravity (Fig. 78–2).[206,208]

According to Pauwels' law,[266] the quantity and the structure of osseous tissue depend on the magnitude of the stresses applied to it. The symmetric subchondral dense bone, of even thickness throughout, that underlies the tibial plateaus of a normal knee shows an even distribution of the articular compressive stresses. Akamatsu and associates,[10] in a series of 144 knees in which 23 were treated with high tibial osteotomy, measured by dual x-ray absorptiometry that the bone mineral density of the

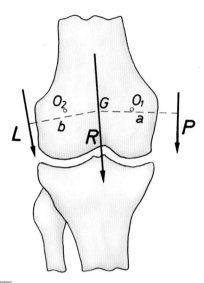

Figure 78–1. Loaded knee projected on the coronal plane. a, lever arm of P; b, lever arm of L; G, central point on the axis of flexion of the knee; L, lateral muscle stay; O1, center of curvature of the medial condyle; O2, center of curvature of the lateral condyle; P, force exerted by the part of the body supported by the knee; R, resultant of P and L. (From Maquet P: Osteotomy. In Freeman MAR [ed]: Arthritis of the Knee: Clinical Features and Surgical Management. Berlin, Springer-Verlag, 1980, p 148.)

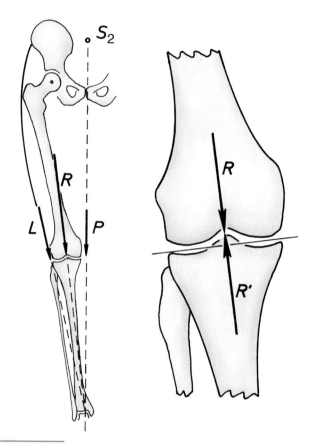

Figure 78–2. Normal knee. Force R acts perpendicular to the plane tangential to the tibial plateau. L, lateral muscle stay; P, force exerted by the part of the body supported by the knee; R, resultant of P and L; S_2, center of the second sacral vertebra. (From Maquet P: Osteotomy. In Freeman MAR [ed]: Arthritis of the Knee: Clinical Features and Surgical Management. Berlin, Springer-Verlag, 1980, p 148.)

medial femoral and tibial condyles was greater than the density of the lateral femoral and tibial condyles in all knees with medial compartmental osteoarthritis. The ratios of bone mineral density of the medial condyles to that of the lateral condyles were found to increase significantly with the progression of osteoarthritis and the increase of varus deformity. These ratios decreased sharply within 1 year after high tibial osteotomy. This finding was confirmed by Takahashi and colleagues,[321] and it is in concordance with the results of Koshino and Ranawat,[177] who studied remodeling of the femoral condyles before and after high tibial osteotomy using bone scintigraphy. They showed that the increased uptake of strontium-85 in the medial condyle before osteotomy decreased markedly at more than 1 year after osteotomy in knees with adequate correction of the varus deformity.

Force R can be displaced medially by a weakening of the muscles L, by an increase of the force P, by a varus deformity, or by a medial displacement of the center of gravity of the body (Fig. 78–3). This displacement alters the distribution and magnitude of the stresses in the joint and soon decreases its effective weightbearing surfaces.

Blaimont and coworkers[26,27] showed the role of the muscles in balancing the medially exerted gravity forces. Through radioscopic and electrophysiologic studies, they found that the tensor fasciae latae and the biceps femoris were the main stabilizers of the knee in the frontal plane. They act as a lateral shroud. Their moment of force is the product of their forces by their lever arm (Fig. 78–4). The investigators determined the maximum moment of force by measuring, under fluoroscopic control, the maximal load against which subjects were able actively to close the

lateral opening of their knee joints. The force of the biceps and the tensor was always diminished in medial arthritic knees. According to Blaimont and coworkers,[26,27] the aim of a valgus osteotomy should be to reduce the lever arm of the gravity force P to allow the weakened lateral muscles to stabilize the joint adequately and distribute the compressive stresses among the medial and lateral compartments of the knee.

If the role of the muscles is not taken into account, and accepting that the center of gravity of the body lies in S2,[92,281] one should see that, even in a perfectly aligned knee, in the midstance phase of gait, the medial compartment would be compressed, whereas the lateral compartment would be distracted, and that the knee would gap laterally at every step. In this case, the valgus deformity that should be created to unload the medial compartment effectively during gait would be unacceptable, as found by Shaw and Moulton[302] using a cadaveric osteotomy model. The action of the lateral muscles can explain why a normally aligned knee can develop medial osteoarthrosis, provided that the muscles are insufficient, and why some varus knees never wear with a good muscular activity.

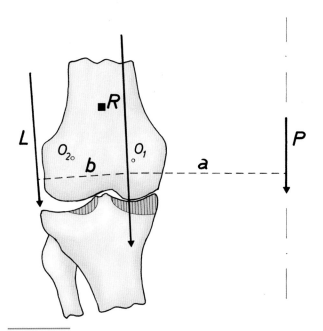

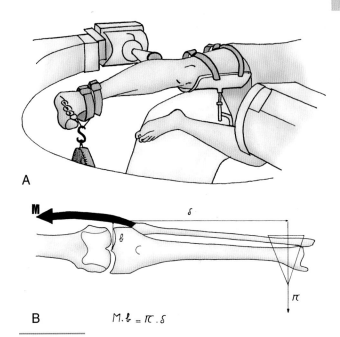

Figure 78–3. Increased stresses in the medial compartment of the knee resulting from a medial displacement of resultant R. a, lever arm of P; b, lever arm of L; L, lateral muscle stay; O1, center of curvature of the medial condyle; O2, center of curvature of the lateral condyle; P, force exerted by the part of the body supported by the knee; R, resultant of P and L. (From Maquet P: Osteotomy. In Freeman MAR [ed]: Arthritis of the Knee: Clinical Features and Surgical Management. Berlin, Springer-Verlag, 1980, p 148.)

Figure 78–4. **A** and **B,** Under fluoroscopic control, the maximal load against which the subject is able actively to close the lateral opening of the knee joint is measured. b, lever arm of M; d, lever arm of P; M, lateral muscular force; P, varus force applied on the ankle. (From Blaimont P, Burnotte J, Baillon JM, et al: Contribution biomécanique à l'étude des conditions d'équilibre dans le genou normal et pathologique: Application au traitement de l'arthrose varisante. Acta Orthop Belg 37:573, 1971.)

Blaimont and coworkers[27] also reported that a varus thrust, secondary to an insufficiency of the biceps and the tensor, was often observed in incipient medial gonarthrosis. They showed that, at this early stage of the disease, provided that the varus is minimal and that the subject is not overweight, reinforcing the lateral muscles can bring the knee back to equilibrium. Yasunaga[366] showed that the lateral thrust was significantly greater in medial compartmental osteoarthritic knees than in normal knees, and that a properly performed high tibial osteotomy was effective in restraining the lateral thrust.

Thomine and colleagues[326] further refined the concept of the adduction moment about the knee during gait. They divided the lever arm a of the gravity force P into two parts: an extrinsic one, which is independent of the axial alignment of the leg, and an intrinsic one, which reflects the axial alignment of the knee. Figure 78–5 schematizes this theory of the varus moment.

In a neutral knee (mechanical axis at 180 degrees), the distance between the line of force of gravity and the center of the knee is the extrinsic varus distance. In a varus knee, an intrinsic varus distance, consisting of the distance between a theoretical neutral mechanical axis and the center of the knee, is added to the extrinsic varus distance, forming the global varus distance. This concept clarifies the effect of the morphology of the patient on the adduction moment, independently of the axial alignment of the knee (Fig. 78–6): A broad pelvis, a coxa vara, a short femur, or a hip adduction increases the extrinsic varus distance. Conversely, a narrow pelvis, a coxa valga, a long femur, or a hip abduction decreases this extrinsic varus distance. The extrinsic varus distance plays a major role in the development of medial gonarthrosis. It explains why, in a varus arthritic knee, in which the lateral muscles are weakened,[26,27] some overcorrection is necessary to reestablish the balance between the varus gravity stresses and the valgus muscular stresses applied on the joint. The amount of overcorrection necessary is a function of the body weight, of the extrinsic varus distance, and of the force of the lateral muscles.

This static way of considering the adduction moment about the knee does not account for the dynamic variations that occur during gait. Studies of gait have shown that the distribution of joint loads within the knee during gait is highly dependent not only on the static angular deformity, but also on dynamic factors.[114,158,264,272,351] Prodromos and associates[272] and Wang and colleagues[351] have shown that the importance of the adduction moment, measured through gait analysis, plays a major role in the results of proximal tibial osteotomy. A patient who has a low adduction moment preoperatively has a higher probability of a good result for a longer time than one who has a high adduction moment.

Some patients with a varus knee seem to develop compensatory mechanisms that reduce the adduction moment. These mechanisms, which may continue postoperatively, include shortening of the stride and toeing-out (Fig. 78–7). Wada and coworkers[343] showed, provided

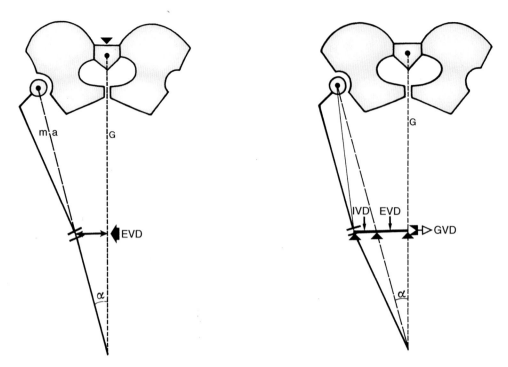

Figure 78–5. In a neutral knee, the mechanical axis passes through the center of the knee. The distance between the line of force of gravity and the center of the knee is the extrinsic varus distance (EVD). In a varus knee, an intrinsic varus distance (IVD), consisting of the distance between a theoretical neutral mechanical axis and the center of the knee, is added to the EVD, forming the global varus distance (GVD) ma, mechanical axis; G, line of force of gravity. (From Thomine JM, Boudjemaa A, Gibon Y, et al: Les écarts varisants dans la gonarthrose: Fondement théorique et essai d'évaluation pratique. Rev Chir Orthop 67:319, 1981. © Masson Editeur.)

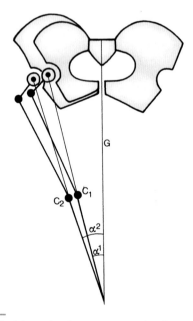

Figure 78–6. A broad pelvis increases the distance between the center of the knee (C) and the line of force of gravity (G), even if the mechanical axis is through the center of the knee. This increases the extrinsic varus distance. (From Thomine JM, Boudjemaa A, Gibon Y, et al: Les écarts varisants dans la gonarthrose: Fondement théorique et essai d'évaluation pratique. Rev Chir Orthop 67:319, 1981. © Masson Editeur.)

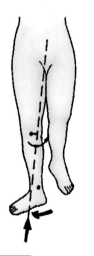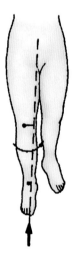

Figure 78–7. The toe-out of the foot is an adaptive mechanism that is used to lower the adduction moment during gait. (From Wang JW, Kuo KN, Andriacchi TP, et al: The influence of walking mechanics and time on the results of proximal tibial osteotomy. J Bone Joint Surg Am 72:905, 1990.)

that sufficient valgus alignment is achieved at surgery, that the preoperative peak adduction moment does not correlate with the clinical or radiographic outcome of high tibial osteotomy, whereas only alignment is associated significantly with long-term clinical results. This study supports the importance of overcorrection at surgery and the need for an accurate osteotomy technique.

Preoperative gait analysis should become a part of patient assessment when an osteotomy is considered. It could help to customize the amount of overcorrection needed for every individual knee, in a way similar to that of Blaimont previously, who measured the force of the lateral muscles.[27] Knees with a high adduction moment should be overcorrected to a greater extent than knees with a low adduction moment. A future perspective could be the development of rehabilitation techniques for reducing the adduction moment. This gait training could be combined with reinforcement of the lateral muscles—the biceps femoris and the tensor fasciae latae.

Another important factor in the pathogenensis of gonarthrosis is the rotational alignment of the lower limbs. Eckoff and colleagues[86,87] and Goutallier and associates[106] showed that rotational malalignment should be considered as a mechanical cause of arthrosis. Rotational malalignment can alter the pressure distribution in an otherwise normal joint. There is a positive correlation between decreased rotation in the femur and increased arthrosis of the medial femorotibial articulation[86,237] and between increased femoral anteversion and patellar arthrosis.[86,87,116,139] There is more version in the arthritic knee than in the normal knee.[86] The observation of a relationship between malrotation of the lower limbs and gonarthrosis is not new; in 1977, Blaimont and Schoon[28] reported two cases of medial compartmental arthrosis secondary to an abnormal internal tibial torsion and treated by a corrective osteotomy. The correlation of internal tibial torsion or decreased femoral external torsion with medial arthritic changes in the knee could aid in understanding why toeing-out is one of the compensatory mechanisms adopted by some patients to decrease the adduction moment during gait.

Patient Selection and Preoperative Evaluation

Patient selection is the most critical factor in planning and achieving a successful high tibial osteotomy. Selection criteria have become more restrictive in recent years, given the excellent alternatives offered by the advent of total[83,282,313] or unicompartmental[46,239,273,320,353,354] knee arthroplasties. Despite the increasing success of knee arthroplasty, tibial osteotomy still may be the more appropriate procedure for younger, active patients with unicompartmental arthritis because an arthroplasty implies limitations on postoperative physical activities and has a limited life expectancy.

There is no general agreement among surgeons concerning the choice between osteotomy and knee arthroplasty. This lack of consensus has been illustrated by a study of Wright and coworkers[361] comparing the rates of tibial osteotomies in Canada and the United States. Although there are national and even continental tendencies, this choice still remains in the hands of each individual surgeon and patient. Some broad criteria nevertheless can be presented. They concern not only the status of the knee, but also the general status of the patient.

AGE

Notwithstanding that the physiological rather than the chronological age should be considered, high tibial osteotomy is nowadays an operation reserved for reasonably young and active patients. There is no agreement yet about the meaning of "reasonably young." Langlais and Thomazeau[183] showed that even after 70 years, the failure rate of high tibial osteotomy is not higher, given a preoperative Ahlbäck's grade I or grade II osteoarthritis. Matthews,[219] Lootvoet,[194] Naudie,[244] and Odenbring[259] and their colleagues, analyzing the factors that influence the duration of satisfactory function after proximal tibial osteotomy, concluded that relative youth is a strong predictor of long function for an osteotomy-treated knee. This disagreement about the influence of age is secondary to the difficulty of separating age from other negative factors. Similar to other surgeons,[119] I reserve osteotomy for patients younger than 55 to 60 years, but exceptions are made to this rule.

LEVEL OF ACTIVITY

The preoperative activity level is probably more of a determinant than age in guiding the choice between osteotomy and arthroplasty, especially when the patient is between 50 and 60 years old. The preoperative level of activity is the best predictor for the postoperative level of activity.[242] Because a total or even a unicompartmental knee replacement can be a reasonable option in this age group, it is important to identify the patients whose activity level precludes an arthroplasty. A very high level of activity has potential adverse effects on the durability of the polyethylene articular surface of a knee arthroplasty and on the fixation of the implant. Nagel and associates,[242] in a retrospective study of the results of proximal tibial osteotomy in 34 men age 28 to 60 years, found that 17 engaged in manual labor to an extent that would have been of concern if they had had a total knee arthroplasty. Nineteen men continued to participate in sports involving running and jumping. Odenbring and coworkers[259] examined, after 7 to 18 years, 27 patients (28 knees), with a median age of 42 years, treated with a high tibial osteotomy for early medial gonarthrosis (Ahlbäck stage I). At follow-up, 22 knees were satisfactory; 9 patients managed high-activity sports or heavy work (Tegner score[323] 9 to 10); and 3 patients performed industrial work and walked in forested terrain (Tegner score 8).

PERSONALITY

As much as possible, the patient should take an active part in the decision-making process. The patient should be informed about the pros and cons of the possible options. The advantages and the disadvantages of these options might be perceived differently by each patient. If an osteotomy is planned, the patient should be aware that the pain relief could be incomplete and that it will not be permanent. The patient also should realize that the alignment of the limb would be modified. The patient's acceptance of these drawbacks is mandatory.

OTHER JOINTS

As a rule, the prerequisite to major knee surgery is a well-working ipsilateral hip. Weakness of the hip abductors, restricted hip mobility, and hip ankylosis have a detrimental effect on the knee[93,203,281,326] and should be corrected first when possible. An osteotomy requires a prolonged period of protected weightbearing. For this reason, the status of the contralateral lower limb and of the superior limbs should be assessed.

WEIGHT

Matthews and coworkers,[219] analyzing the factors that influence the duration of satisfactory function after proximal tibial osteotomy, stated that obesity had a negative impact on the outcome of this procedure. Coventry,[62] Brueckmann and Kettelkamp,[36] and Levigne and Bonnin[191] share the same opinion. Obese patients also are not ideal candidates for a knee arthroplasty[150,179]; it is difficult to make a decision based on this criterion. A multidisciplinary approach is advisable for these patients, and the problem of obesity should be considered at the same time as the gonarthrosis. An overweight woman older than 65 is not a valid candidate for an osteotomy.[299] I recommend a total knee replacement if a patient is older than 60 and if a patient is not willing to lose weight.

INFLAMMATORY DISEASES

Rheumatoid arthritis is a definite contraindication for osteotomy.[9,51,62,64] The efficacy of high tibial osteotomy has not been studied specifically in the other inflammatory diseases of the joints, but one should expect similarly poor results. Job and colleagues[157] compared the 5-year results of high tibial osteotomy in 146 osteoarthritic knees without chondrocalcinosis and in 94 osteoarthritic knees with chondrocalcinosis. There were 73% good clinical results in the first group and only 34% good results in the second group.

EXAMINATION OF THE KNEE

Clinical examination of the knee is decisive in the selection of the appropriate patient. During gait, the angular deformity, the torsional pattern of the limb, the position of the foot, a possible limp, a flexion deformity, and the presence or absence of a varus thrust[143,244] all should be assessed. In this chapter, the alignment is expressed as the hip-knee-ankle angle, the neutral alignment being arbitrarily numbered 0 for practical purposes.

There are limits of deformity that reliably can be corrected by a proximal tibial osteotomy. The results of prox-

imal tibial osteotomy are best when the varus deformity is 10 degrees or less[6,143,194] because the greater the deformity, the more severe the arthritic changes. High tibial osteotomy is best suited for knees with moderate arthritic changes, in which the deformity is secondary to proximal tibial bowing rather than to medial bone loss.[76,190,191,194,299] Varus deformity greater than 15 degrees generally is associated with increased medial bone loss,[194] bicompartmental deterioration, and lateral subluxation at the tibiofemoral joint.[11,143]

The torsional pattern of the limb and the position of the foot during gait influence the varus distances and the adduction moment, and they should be taken into account for planning the correction. A major limp, a flexion deformity, and a frank varus thrust generally reflect a more advanced stage of arthritis,[76,143,244] and the performance of a high tibial osteotomy should be considered cautiously. As stated by Andriacchi,[12] the varus thrust places all of the reaction force on the medial compartment and greatly increases the rate of degenerative changes associated with higher than normal medial compartment loads.

In the standing position, in addition to the static deformities, one should look for the presence of a popliteal cyst, varicose veins, and marked muscular atrophy. The clinical examination should continue in the sitting position. Inflammatory signs should be ruled out. Pain should be located predominantly on the medial side of the knee, and signs of patellofemoral arthritis should be sought. Possible arterial insufficiency should be looked for.

Knee stability also should be tested. Medial laxity is seldom important in medial arthritic knees and is often secondary to bone loss.[25,63] Because even after correction of the mechanical axis into valgus there remains an adduction moment about the knee during gait,[12,102,114,272,302,342,351] mild to moderate medial laxity should not contraindicate a valgus tibial osteotomy. In this situation, failure to take the laxity into account during surgery could lead to undercorrection, however, if the amount of correction is estimated visually by the intraoperative alignment of the limb.[27] A valgus stress manually applied to the knee could open the joint medially, which would not occur during gait because of the persistence of the adduction moment. For marked medial laxity associated with a varus knee, Cameron and Saha[45] recommend performing a combined opening and closing wedge osteotomy. Vielpeau[299] considers that medial laxity does not specifically indicate an opening wedge osteotomy because it would not re-tension the deep medial collateral ligament, and because attempts to tighten the superficial medial collateral ligament could lead to undercorrection.

The lateral collateral ligament may be stretched as the varus deformity develops. Active muscular contraction, primarily of the biceps[12,26,27] and of the tensor fasciae latae[26,27,204,208] and secondarily of the quadriceps,[12] produces dynamic stabilization against lateral joint opening, but at the expense of a greater joint contact force. Correction of the axis does not suppress the lateral laxity, but it restrains the lateral thrust of the knee,[366] reducing the high medial forces secondary not only to malalignment, but also to lateral joint opening. Lateral collateral ligament laxity cannot be considered as a contraindication for valgus tibial osteotomy, even if it usually reflects a more advanced stage of arthritis. Paley and coworkers[262] proposed a technique for tightening the lateral collateral ligament. Although I have no experience with this technique, I believe that tightening the lateral collateral ligament is usually unnecessary, provided that sufficient overcorrection has been achieved. The effect of lateral tibiofemoral separation should be taken into account for calculating of the desired amount of correction.[85,183]

The association of an old anterior cruciate ligament rupture with medial gonarthrosis may justify a valgus tibial osteotomy, especially when there is an added lateral laxity. The anterior cruciate ligament is a secondary restraint against lateral joint opening, and the conjunction of lateral and anterior laxity considerably increases the stresses on the medial compartment.[12] The relative indication of isolated osteotomy, isolated ligament reconstruction, and simultaneous or staged procedures is beyond the scope of this chapter.[15,78,141,184,189,250-252,358]

RADIOGRAPHIC EXAMINATION

Preoperative radiographs are necessary to select the appropriate patient and to plan the surgery. The radiological evaluation should include the following:

- Anteroposterior and lateral radiographs, on long films (18 × 43 cm), with the patient in the supine position, knees extended
- Skyline views
- "Shuss" posteroanterior radiographs (standing posteroanterior x-rays, knee flexed to 30 degrees)[278]
- Valgus and varus and stress anteroposterior radiographs, with the patient supine and the knee flexed to 20 degrees
- Hip-knee-ankle radiographs, with the patient standing on both legs

The first goal of the radiographic assessment is to confirm the indication for an osteotomy. The aim of knee osteotomy is to modify the axis of the limb, to shift compressive forces from a diseased compartment to a more normal compartmental joint space. The radiographs should show unicompartmental deterioration, associated with an abnormal lower extremity alignment and abnormal force transmission through the knee.

An increase of contact stresses in one compartment induces joint space narrowing, subchondral bone densification, and osteophyte formation. In the absence of these signs of overload, even in the case of axial malalignment, the origin of the knee pain should be investigated further. Bone scan, MRI, or arthrography should help to determine the cause of the symptoms and to plan the appropriate treatment.

If the opposite compartment is not intact, the indication for an osteotomy should be questioned. A metabolic or inflammatory disease should be suspected. As already mentioned, rheumatoid arthritis is a clear contraindication for knee osteotomy.[9,51,64,119] Chondrocalcinosis[157] also significantly affects the longevity of the osteotomy.

The patellofemoral joint also should be investigated. Although mild to moderate patellofemoral osteoarthrosis does not contraindicate an osteotomy,[84,123,127,143,145,148] the

patellar height and the patellar alignment could influence the technique of the osteotomy.[84,238,298,328]

Varus and valgus stress films are essential. They provide useful information about the condition of both compartments and of the ligaments. Joint space narrowing when stressing the presumably healthy compartment precludes osteotomy. A reliable preoperative recording of the knee alignment also is necessary to plan the osteotomy.

The full-length radiographs should determine the global alignment of the knee and evaluate the varus distances[326] to calculate the adductor moment. There are many different ways to obtain full-length radiographs.[109] Originally, full-length radiographs were obtained with the patient in the supine position. This position did not provide any information concerning the ligamentous laxity, however, and the amount of deformity could be underestimated in the case of bony defects or ligament overstretching. Unipodal standing full-length radiographs also have some disadvantages. Although walking is a succession of unipodal stances, a static unipodal station does not reproduce the dynamic aspect of the loading of the knee during the normal gait. When standing on one leg, the patient tilts the pelvis to bring the center of gravity of the body nearer to the hip of the weightbearing limb. This attitude decreases the extrinsic varizing distance and the adductor moment.[326] Another drawback of unipodal standing films is the difficulty of positioning elderly or disabled patients for them. Finally, ligament integrity is better evaluated with stress radiographs, performed with a constant and predetermined force instead of unipodal standing radiographs.[13,326] An acceptable compromise is the bipodal standing radiograph, which gives a correct estimation of the axial alignment of the lower limb and can be realized in almost every candidate for an osteotomy.

Errors in rotational positioning of the limb alter the reliability of the standing radiographs.[13,108,156,183,253,280,326,340] Several landmarks have been advocated to position the patient correctly. The most usual technique is to position the patient with the patella forward to obtain a true anteroposterior view of the knee. This technique is not valid in the case of marked femoropatellar dysplasia.

The most reproducible technique[13,183,253,280] is to define the frontal projection as perpendicular to a lateral view of the knee, which is monitored by superimposing the posterior aspects of the femoral condyles under fluoroscopic control (Fig. 78-8). Using a similar technique, Odenbring and associates[253] showed that the assessment of the hip-knee-ankle angle had a variability of 2 degrees at the most. A drawback of this technique is that the position imposed on the limb is not the same as when the patient is walking.

On a bipodal standing radiograph several landmarks are drawn:

- The center of the second sacral vertebra, which is a rough approximation of the center of gravity of the supported part of the body[26,92,281]
- The center of the hip
- The center of the ankle
- The mechanical axis of the femur, joining the center of the hip to the center of the intracondylar notch[92]

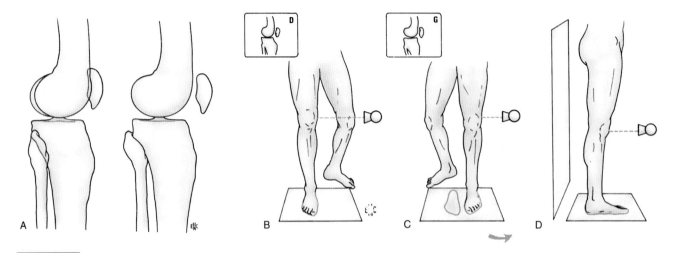

Figure 78–8. **A,** The superimposition of the posterior aspect of the condyles defines the reference profile. **B,** The patient stands on a cardboard sheet, his weight on one leg. The leg is turned under fluoroscopic control until a true profile is obtained. The outline of the foot is traced on the cardboard. **C,** The procedure is repeated for the other limb. If the patient stands on the two traced outlines, both knees are perfectly in profile. **D,** The cardboard is turned 90 degrees, and the camera is replaced by a large-size x-ray plate. The knees are x-rayed strictly full-face. (From Langlais F, Thomazeau H: Ostéotomies du genou. In Encyclopédie Médicochirugicale. Paris, Editions scientifiques et médicales Elsevier, 1989, p 1.)

- The mechanical axis of the tibia, joining the center of the proximal epiphysis to the center of the ankle[92]
- The mechanical axis of the lower extremity, joining the center of the hip to the center of the ankle[279]

The landmarks allow the measurement of the following (Fig. 78–9):
- The hip-knee-ankle angle, defined as the angle between the mechanical axis of the femur and the mechanical axis of the tibia[58,235]; the normal value is close to 0 degrees[58,235,280]
- The transcondylar angle, defined as the angle between the tangent line of the condyles and the mechanical axis of the femur[52,59,269,368]
- The tibial plateau–tibial shaft angle, defined as the angle between the tangent line of the tibial plateau and the mechanical axis of the tibia[52,58,269,368]
- The tibiofemoral separation, defined as the angle between a line tangent to the distal aspect of the femoral condyles and a line tangent to the tibial plateau[58,85]
- The varizing distances[326] (extrinsic, intrinsic, and global)

On the full-length radiographs or on long anteroposterior x-rays, the constitutional tibial varus also can be measured (Fig. 78–10). The constitutional tibial varus was described by Levigne[190] and Lootvoet and colleagues.[194] It represents the epiphyseal bony component of tibial varus. Its value is that of the angle formed by the mechanical axis of the tibia and the axis of the upper tibial epiphysis. In the absence of bone loss, the axis of the upper tibial epiphysis can be described as a line perpendicular to the tangent to the tibial plateaus. In the presence of bone wear, this epiphyseal axis can be estimated by drawing a line from the center of the tibial spines to the middle of the old physeal line. From the study of a group of 110 nonosteoarthritic patients, Levigne[190] showed that this way of determining the epiphyseal axis is reliable and is equivalent to drawing a line perpendicular to the tangent to the intact tibial plateaus.

The angle between the epiphyseal axis and the mechanical axis of the tibia allows one to distinguish the part of the deformity attributable to the tibial bone loss from that secondary to the bowing of the proximal tibia. This distinction is important to select correctly the candidates for a high tibial osteotomy because the result of a high tibial osteotomy is better when the varus deformity is mainly due to bowing than when the deformity is essentially due to wear.[30,76,191,194]

Another goal of the radiologic assessment is to select the site of the osteotomy. The normal upper tibia has a 3-degree varus slope.[59,119,162,234,235] In most varus knees, this varus slope is increased,[190,269] whereas it is decreased or even inverted in valgus knees.[190,269] In varus or neutral knees, the line tangent to the distal extent of the femoral condyles is perpendicular to the mechanical axis of the femur, but is inclined medially and distally in valgus knees.[59,62,183,269,304] Cooke and associates[60] described a subgroup of patients with varus arthritic knees showing excessive valgus angulation of the femoral joint surface together with proximal tibia vara. This pattern of deformity warrants special consideration because in some extreme cases it could require combined femoral and tibial osteotomies to restore the horizontality of the joint surfaces. The hip-knee-ankle angle is the sum of the angles between the mechanical axes of each bone and the corresponding articular surfaces and of the lateral or medial tibiofemoral separation, which is the angle between the articular surfaces of the femur and the tibia.

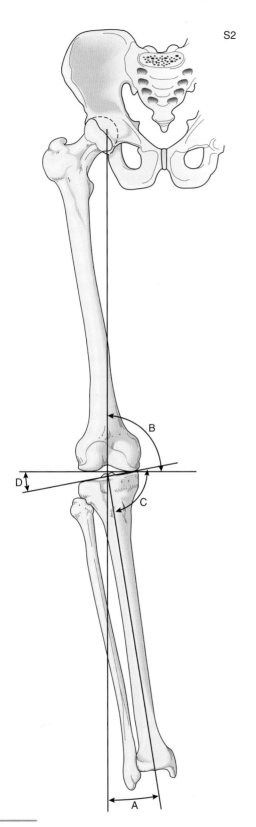

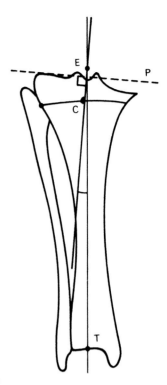

Figure 78–10. Constitutional tibial varus, after Levigne.[190] C, center of vestige of the epiphyseal growth plate; E, center of spines; P, line tangential to the tibial plateaus before medial wear; T, center of the ankle. EC, epiphyseal axis; EC-ET, constitutional tibial varus in degrees; ET, mechanical axis. (From Lootvoet L, Massinon A, Rossillon R, et al: [Upper tibial osteotomy for gonarthrosis in genu varum: Apropos of a series of 193 cases reviewed 6 to 10 years later]. Rev Chir Orthop Reparatrice Appar Mot 79:375, 1993. © Masson Editeur.)

In theory, the correction should be performed at the site of the maximal deformity to keep the joint line as perpendicular to the ground as possible. With a few exceptions, the osteotomy should be tibial in varus knees and femoral in valgus knees. Several authors[17,66,77,217] have reported good results when a tibial osteotomy is performed to correct a moderate valgus deformity. It seems reasonable to correct mixed tibial and femoral deformities on the tibial side, insofar as the resultant obliquity of the joint line would not exceed 10 degrees.

GAIT ANALYSIS

Peak adduction moments at the knee indicate the resultant loading in the medial compartment of the knee joint. Gait analysis can measure the distribution of load during walking.[12,102,158,264,272,351] Johnson and colleagues[158,159] showed that there is a lack of correlation between static analysis based on the mechanical axis and weightbearing in the knee calculated from gait analysis. Results from this study also showed a poor correlation between the mechanical axis and the peak adduction

Figure 78–9. Schematic drawing of a biopodal standing radiograph. **A,** Hip-knee-ankle angle. **B,** Transcondylar angle. **C,** Tibial plateau–tibial shaft angle. **D,** Tibiofemoral separation. S2, center of the second sacral vertebra.

moment about the knee. Several authors[12,102,114,158,272,351] postulated that an individual can adapt his or her gait and compensate dynamically for joint deformity. These compensatory mechanisms include slowing walking speed, shortening stride length, displacing the trunk toward the affected limb, and toeing-out.

Prodromos and coworkers[272] and Wang and coworkers[351] showed that the compensatory gait pattern that reduces the joint load may continue postoperatively, and that this reduction of the adduction moment is a key factor for the long-term clinical outcome. Wada and associates[342] suggested, on the basis of a prospective study of 32 patients with primary osteoarthritis of the medial compartment of the knee who underwent a high tibial osteotomy, that provided sufficient valgus alignment is obtained at surgery, the preoperative peak adduction moment of the knee does not correlate with clinical or radiographic outcomes of high tibial osteotomy. In this group, the average postoperative femorotibial angle was 167 to 169 degrees, which roughly corresponds to a 5-to7-degree mechanical axis, whereas in the study groups of Prodromos and coworkers[272] and Wang and coworkers[351] the average mechanical axis was 2 degrees valgus immediately after surgery and 1.2 degrees varus at follow-up. From these studies, one can infer that some overcorrection is necessary to provide good long-term results of high tibial osteotomy, and that the amount of overcorrection should be larger in knees with a high preoperative adduction moment.

A gait analysis probably should become a part of the preoperative assessment for all patients undergoing high tibial osteotomy to adapt the amount of overcorrection according to the importance of the adduction moment. Another field of investigation is the development of gait training techniques for reducing the adduction.

ARTHROSCOPY AND JOINT DÉBRIDEMENT

The usefulness of arthroscopy as a diagnostic tool before planning an osteotomy is limited. When the integrity of the supposed unaffected joint space is questionable, stress radiographs, arthrograms possibly combined with CT scans, or MRI should provide adequate information, obviating the need for more invasive investigations. The role of routine preosteotomy arthroscopy has been studied by Keene and associates.[167] They concluded that there was no correlation between preosteotomy arthroscopic findings and the clinical result of osteotomy. Hsu[138] also stated that preoperative arthroscopic grading, according to the criteria of Fujisawa and associates,[94] did not adequately predict the knee's functional outcome, but that postoperative arthroscopic grading was of some prognostic value.

Odenbring and colleagues[256] performed diagnostic arthroscopy at the time of high tibial osteotomy and 2 years after surgery in 16 patients. They found cartilage regeneration in eight medial tibial condyles and in nine medial femoral condyles. The main repair feature was proliferation of fibrocartilage that covered bone, covered areas of fibrillated cartilage, and filled clefts in hyaline cartilage. Cartilage regeneration was correlated to the degree of knee

alignment achieved after proximal tibial osteotomy. These findings have been confirmed by others.[161,178,349]

Débridement has been advocated as a complement to osteotomy.[197] In keeping with Johnson,[159] who reported that the combination of degeneration with varus deformity could be relieved by abrasion arthroplasty, Tippet[329] combined arthroscopic arthroplasty and dome osteotomy and reported satisfactory results in 90% of his cases. Korn[173] also combined the two procedures, with an interval of 4 to 6 weeks between the arthroscopy and the dome osteotomy, and claimed that prior arthroscopic abrasion arthroplasty provides early medial compartment resurfacing with fibrocartilage and that correction of varus deformity protects the developing fibrocartilage. In contrast, based on a large review of the literature, Goldman and coworkers[103] concluded that in degenerative knee arthritis, abrasion arthroplasty does not seem to offer any additional benefit to arthroscopic débridement alone.

Rand and Ritts,[283] based on a series of eight patients with persistent pain after upper tibial osteotomy subsequently treated with abrasion arthroplasty, concluded that this procedure was not a satisfactory salvage for a failed upper tibial osteotomy. Finally, whether arthroscopic débridement in conjunction with upper tibial osteotomy is more beneficial compared with osteotomy alone is not clearly determined. Arthroscopy in conjunction with osteotomy should be reserved for patients with mechanical symptoms suggesting meniscal abnormalities or loose bodies, in addition to unicompartmental osteoarthritis associated with deformity.[119]

Surgical Techniques

CLOSING WEDGE PROXIMAL TIBIAL VALGUS OSTEOTOMY WITH INTERNAL FIXATION BY BLADE-PLATE

My preferred technique for closing wedge proximal tibial valgus osteotomy is internal fixation by a "swan-neck" blade-plate, as described by Postel and Langlais,[270] Merle d'Aubigne,[226] and Langlais and Thomazeau[183] and in use at the Hospital Cochin in Paris since 1967. Large series[82,194,270,299] have shown the precision and the reliability of the procedure. Lootvoet and colleagues[194] analyzed the results of a series of 193 osteotomies performed with the same technique. In this series, the hip-knee-ankle angle was 7.7 ± 3.8 degrees of varus preoperatively, 2.7 ± 3.1 degrees of valgus at union, and 0.1 ± 5.1 degrees of valgus at review 6 to 10 years postoperatively.

This method not only provides a rigid internal fixation to allow early motion, but also offers an "automatic" correction, as opposed to other methods of fixation, such as the buttress plate.[135] The complication rate—which was feared to increase secondary to the larger surgical exposure required for plate fixation[65]—remains quite low. Lemaire[187] reported a series of 207 osteotomies fixed with an angled blade-plate, in which the complication rate was 7%. The most frequent complication was a transient partial peroneal nerve palsy (nine cases), with a full recovery in seven cases and a residual weakness of the great toe extensor in two cases. In this series, the fibula was osteotomized at the junction of its middle and upper thirds.

The principle of the "swan-neck" blade-plate is to use a special jig and a guide wire, over which the blade-plate is driven when the osteotomy is completed. The orientation of the guide wire sets the amount of correction. The correction depends on 2 angles: the angle of the jig and the angle of the blade-plate (Fig. 78–11).

A vertical incision usually is made beginning midway between the patella and the fibular head and extending distally for about 12 cm to the crest of the tibia. The incision is made closer to the midline to facilitate a possible revision. The upper tibia is exposed by making a fascial incision 5 mm away from the crest of the tibia, extending proximally into the iliotibial band, in line with its fibers. This incision creates a posteriorly hinged fasciomuscular flap to protect the peroneal nerve. This flap covers the blade-plate at the end of the procedure. The flap consists of the posterior part of the iliotibial band and of the tibialis anterior muscle. The fascial incision may be continued proximally through the patellar retinaculum as far as the vastus lateralis, if a lateral patellar release is needed. The tethering effect of the fibula is removed either by fibular shaft osteotomy or by separation of the superior tibiofibular joint.

The lateral joint line is identified with a needle. The guide wire is inserted in the upper tibia 10 to 15 mm distal to the joint line, using the special jig. The jig, which has the same profile as the blade-plate and which fits the lateral proximal tibia perfectly, is set for a predetermined amount of correction. This jig normally is set for use with a 90-degree blade-plate, but when greater correction is required, an alternative 100-degree blade-plate can be used.

The insertion point of the guide wire should be located midway between the posterior and the anterior aspect of the tibia, in the sagittal plane. The guide wire should be inserted strictly in the plane of flexion of the knee. It should be parallel to the joint line or slightly ascendant from medial to lateral in the frontal plane. The track for the blade-plate is started in the proximal fragment with a cannulated cutting tool, which is passed over the guide wire and aligned with the jig. Two guiding pins should be used to figure the wedge resection. The proximal limb of the osteotomy should be parallel with the guide wire and situated 15 to 20 mm distal to it. With the help of a template, a distal diaphyseal pin should be placed at an angle relative to the guide wire equal to the desired amount of resection. At the end of the procedure, these two pins should become parallel.

After wedge removal and completion of the osteotomy, the angular correction is performed by manually exerting a valgus force on the leg, with the knee in extension. The selected blade-plate is driven over the guide wire and fixed to the tibial cortex with three screws.

It is mandatory to obtain the correction without applying any constraint on the blade-plate because this would lead to a loss of correction either by sweeping of the blade into the cancellous bone or by bending the plate. When calculating the correction, one should take into account that the level of the osteotomy is distal relative to the joint line. The effect of the osteotomy on the hip-knee-ankle angle is smaller than if the same angular correction were performed at the level of the joint line. One should add approximately 2 degrees to the correction calculated on the basis of the hip-knee-ankle angle.[33,82]

Radiographic checks are made at two stages—the first after insertion of the guide wire and the second after insertion of the plate. The fascia is closed nonhermetically over a suction drain.

Continuous passive motion can be started in the recovery room. Active exercises begin on the first postoperative day. Walking is permitted with crutches. Weightbearing should be restricted to 15 kg until union of the osteotomy. This osteotomy technique permits more complex corrections, such as extension or internal rotation coupled to a valgus.

CLOSING WEDGE PROXIMAL TIBIAL VALGUS OSTEOTOMY WITH INTERNAL FIXATION BY PLATE

Hofmann and others[22,135] developed special instruments to resect the bone wedge with an improved precision. They recommended a standard lateral approach with division of the proximal tibiofibular capsule. Keith needles are used to identify the joint line, and a transverse osteotomy jig is fixed with 3.2-mm drill points. The transverse limb portion of the osteotomy is performed keeping the medial cortex intact (Fig. 78–12).

The desired correction is achieved using a slotted osteotomy jig with 2-degree increments to perform the oblique portion of the osteotomy (Fig. 78–13). An L buttress plate is applied to the proximal tibia with fully threaded cancellous screws, and an external compressor device is used to draw the osteotomy close before screws are placed in the plate distally. Postoperatively, patients are started on immediate continuous passive motion and allowed 50% weightbearing.

This technique is similar to the blade-plate technique. If the inner cortex of the tibia is disrupted, the risk of overcorrection is higher with a plate and a compressor than with a rigid blade-plate, and the stability of the fixation is lower (Fig. 78–14). Surer[318,319] developed a device to improve the stability of screw fixation. It uses a set screw to fix the screw to the plate (Fig. 78–15). Fixing the screw to the plate modifies the action of the screw, which then becomes directly involved in anchoring the implant. The stability of the fixation no longer depends on the simple application of the plate to the surface of the bone, but benefits from the hold of the screw in the bone. A series of plates using this principle has been designed and can be used for distal femoral osteotomies and for tibial opening or closing wedge osteotomies.

Several other fixation devices and guiding jigs are available,[160,167,174,227,238,240,261,327] but some of them do not combine the advantages of a rigid fixation and a precise and reliable correction. The other blade-plates available[174,238] are not guided by a wire as in the Postel Merle d'Aubigne technique, and the precision of the correction

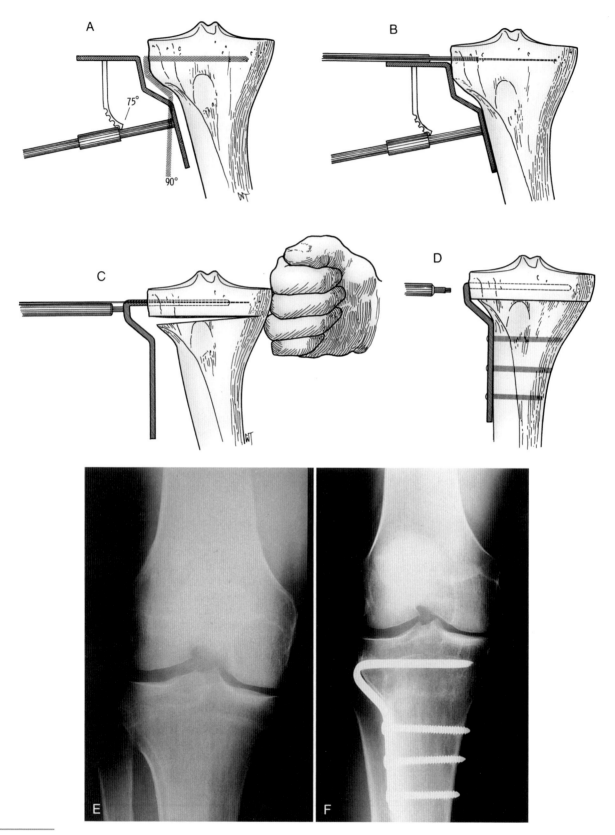

Figure 78–11. Blade-plate fixation. **A,** The guide instrument is set for the correction angle desired. **B,** A guide wire is drilled into the proximal tibia. **C,** After completion of the osteotomy, the blade-plate is driven into the proximal tibia over the guide wire. **D,** The blade is screwed to the tibia. **E** and **F,** Ten-year follow-up of a closing wedge osteotomy with blade-plate fixation. (**A-D** from Merle d' Aubigné R: Joint realignment in the management of osteoarthritis. In Straub LR, Wilson PD Jr [eds]: Clinical Trends in Orthopaedics. New York, Thieme-Stratton, 1982, p 246.)

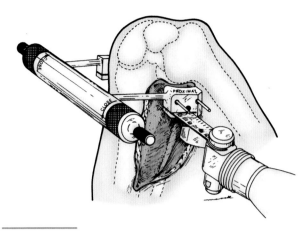

Figure 78–12. Transverse tibial osteotomy jig. (From Hofmann AA, Wyatt RW, Beck SW: High tibial osteotomy: Use of an osteotomy jig, rigid fixation, and early motion versus conventional surgical technique and cast immobilization. Clin Orthop 271:212, 1991.)

relies only on the exact measurement of the wedge and on the integrity of the medial tibial cortex.

Staple fixation, although advocated by several authors,[16,65,121,357,370] is not reliable enough to authorize early rehabilitation and often necessitates complementary cast immobilization. There is no advantage in using staples as a means of fixation because the plates and blade-plates now available are more stable[117] and do not carry additional risks of complication.

OPENING WEDGE OSTEOTOMY

Technique

Debeyre and colleagues[72,73,75] have employed a medial opening wedge osteotomy proximal to the tibial tubercule since 1951. Hernigou and coworkers[131] published the long-term results of this technique in 1987. The technique of the opening wedge osteotomy is straightforward. A longitudinal skin incision of approximately 8 cm is made over the anteromedial aspect of the tibia, along the anterior edge of the medial collateral ligament. The hamstring tendons are dissected, and the superficial medial collateral ligament is exposed and is separated from bone proximally as far as the level of the osteotomy, which should be started at least 3.5 cm distal to the medial joint line and directed laterally and proximally toward the tip of the fibula. A Steinmann pin can be inserted under fluoroscopic control to figure the osteotomy line. The fibula and tibiofibular joint do not need to be disturbed. The medial tibial cortex is cut with osteotomes, or the osteotomy can be initiated with an oscillating saw. The lateral tibial cortex should remain intact. The bone at the site of the osteotomy is forced open, and three bicortical wedges of appropriate size, obtained from the iliac crest, are inserted. Hernigou and coworkers[131] recommend fixation of the osteotomy with a T-plate and screws because the lateral part of the cortex may crack during the osteotomy or postoperatively. The wound is closed by repairing the divided tendons and

superficial medial collateral ligament, then approximating the subcutaneous tissue and skin.

Goutallier and coworkers[107] and Hernigou and Ma[130] reported their experience in substituting cement for full-thickness iliac crest wedges, combined with the use of a buttress plate fixation (Fig. 78–16). By reviewing 245 osteotomies performed with this technique, these investigators stated that using a cement wedge instead of an iliac bone graft does not expose the patient to any special complication and improves the accuracy of axial correction.

Puddu and colleagues[274] designed a special plate, which combines the roles of the buttress plate and the cement wedge (Fig. 78–17). This plate has two holes for one stainless steel 6.5-mm cancellous screw proximally and one 4.5-mm cortical screw distally. A plate with four holes can be used if the bone is soft. A set of five presized plates has been designed. The plates have metal blocks 4 mm deep and are of varying height (5 mm, 7.5 mm, 10 mm, 12.5 mm, and 15 mm). Plates with trapezoidal blocks, higher posteriorly than anteriorly, are currently available. The aim of these plates is to fix and stabilize the osteotomy. When the block is inserted into the osteotomy site, it prevents loss of correction. The opening osteotomy is facilitated by the use of a specially designed wedge-shaped instrument (Fig. 78–18). When the plate is fixed and the osteotomy is stabilized, a bone graft is obtained and inserted into the defect. Puddu advises taking the bone graft from the tibia itself if the osteotomy is 7.5 mm or less and from the iliac crest if the opening wedge is 1 cm or more. The distal part of the medial collateral ligament is left open and the wound is closed.

The knee is protected in a brace that permits a full range of motion. A suction drain is left in place for 24 hours postoperatively. Partial weightbearing is permitted after 40 days, and full weightbearing is allowed after 60 days if the x-rays show good healing at the operative site.

The AO group developed the Tomofix, a plate-fixator, based on the internal fixator principle (Fig. 78–19) and allowing secure fixation of locking head screws in the plate. Plates are adapted to the anatomy of the lateral femur and of the medial or lateral tibia. Lobenhoffer and colleagues[192,193] and Staubli and associates[312] reported the early results of opening wedge osteotomy stabilized with this medial plate. Stoffel and coworkers[314] showed the mechanical superiority of the Tomofix plate in opening wedge osteotomy after fracture of the lateral tibial cortex.

Calculation of Wedge Size for Opening Wedge Osteotomy

Hernigou and colleagues[124,132] analyzed mathematically the orientation of the superior tibial epiphysis in the frontal and sagittal planes. They determined mathematically the opening wedges and established tables expressing the height of the wedge's base as a function of the tibial width and the desired angular correction. The height of the wedge's base also can be determined graphically.[72] For a tibia 55 to 60 mm wide at the level of the osteotomy, 1 mm of opening roughly produces 1 degree of correction. Because the proximal tibia has a triangular cross-section,

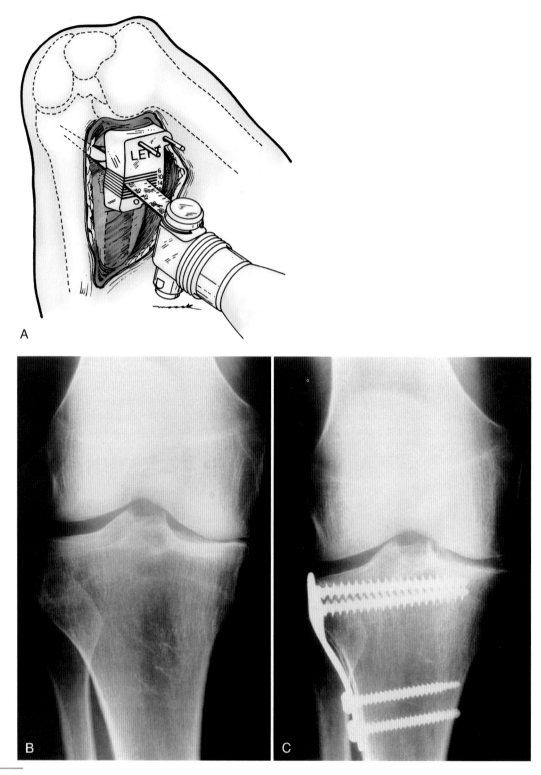

Figure 78–13. **A,** Oblique tibial osteotomy jig with 2-degree increments. **B,** Severe medial joint space narrowing in a 45-year-old woman secondary to a previous medial meniscectomy and a 5-degree varus deformity. **C,** Weightbearing antero-posterior radiograph of the same knee 5 years after closing wedge osteotomy with internal fixation by plate. (**A** from Hofmann AA, Wyatt RW, Beck SW: High tibial osteotomy: Use of an osteotomy jig, rigid fixation, and early motion versus conventional surgical technique and cast immobilization. Clin Orthop 271:212, 1991.)

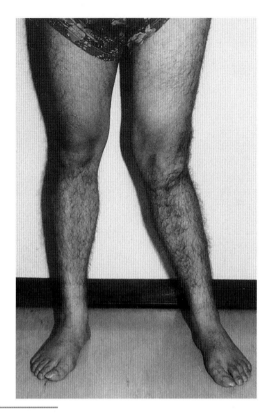

Figure 78–14. Severe overcorrection resulting in an unacceptable valgus malalignment. The closing wedge osteotomy had been performed with the help of a compresssion clamp that excessively crushed the lateral metaphyseal bone.

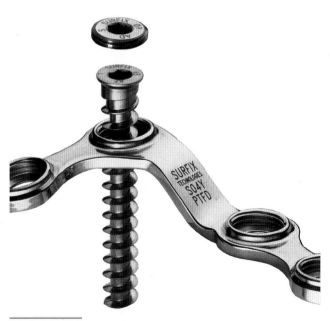

Figure 78–15. The fixation of the screw to the plate is achieved by the set screw, which is screwed into the plate. To be effective, the blockage requires two conditions: respecting coaxial alignment and cleaning all debris interposed between the plate, the screw, and the set screw. (From Surer P: Reliability of fixation with the Surfix plate: Analysis of the first 100 osteotomies. Eur J Orthop Surg Traumatol 7:47, 1997).

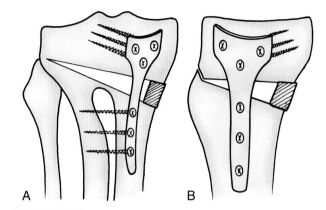

A   B

Figure 78–16. **A** and **B,** Opening wedge osteotomy with a cement wedge and a T-plate. The cement wedge should be posterior because the base of the opening wedge should be higher posteriorly than anteriorly to avoid a posterior tilt of the tibial plateaus. (From Goutallier D, Julieron A, Hernigou P: Cement wedge replacing iliac graft for medial opening wedge tibial osteotomy. Rev Chir Orthop 78:138, 1992. © Masson Editeur.)

the base of the wedge should be higher posteriorly than anteriorly to avoid a posterior tilt of the tibial plateaus.

Advantages and Disadvantages of Opening Wedge Tibial Osteotomy

The main advantage is leaving the fibula untouched. Another advantage is that this osteotomy can be combined with an anterior cruciate ligament reconstruction through the same incision.[274] The lengthening effect of an opening wedge osteotomy also should be considered.[129] The disadvantages are a longer uniting time and the necessity for bone grafting. Several bone substitutes have been used successfully instead of autologous bone graft, including tricalcium phosphate,[29] porous alumina ceramic,[35] and porous hydroxyapatite.[175,176]

I have used freeze-dried cancellous bone grafts[79,80] several times in opening wedge osteotomies stabilized by Puddu's plate. This seems a reasonable option, provided that the wedge's size is small. If the wedge height is superior to 7.5 mm, a bone graft should be taken from the iliac crest. In this situation, the other osteotomy techniques should be considered.

DOME-SHAPED PROXIMAL TIBIAL OSTEOTOMY

Technique

The dome or curviplane high tibial osteotomy was introduced by Blaimont[24,25] and popularized by Maquet.[207,211] This osteotomy is proximal to the tibial tubercle. It is semicylindrical, and its concavity is downward, circumscribing the tibial tuberosity (Fig. 78–20).

After oblique division of the fibula in its middle third, two Steinmann pins are inserted in the tibia, one proximal and the other distal to the osteotomy curve. The angle between the two pins should correspond to the planned

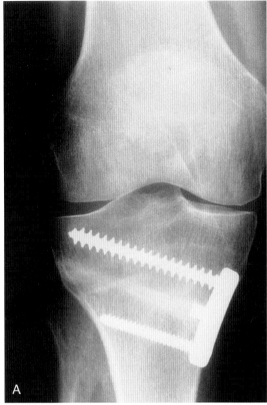

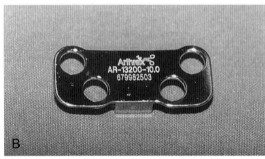

Figure 78–17. **A,** Medial opening wedge osteotomy combined with an anterior cruciate ligament reconstruction, using freeze-dried cancellous bone allograft and fixed with a two-hole Puddu plate. **B,** Alternatively a four-hole plate can be used.

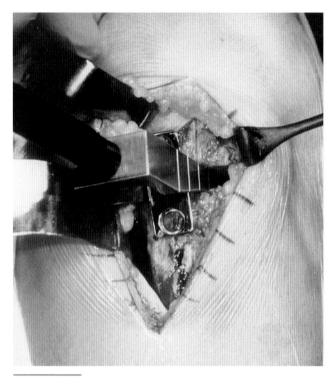

Figure 78–18. Graduated wedge-shaped instrument used to open the osteotomy. The plate is inserted between the two limbs of the instrument.

correction. This can be facilitated by the use of a special guide.[155,207,208,347] The barrel-vault tibial osteotomy is performed through a 5 cm longitudinal incision centered on the tibial tuberosity.

Special curved osteotomes (Fig. 78–21), which can glide easily behind the patellar tendon, can be used to initiate the osteotomy.[347] An alternative technique is to mark a curved line on the proximal tibia and to make holes along this line, either with Kirschner wires[207] or with 3-mm drills.[317,322] Korn[173] designed a curved double-bladed osteotomy guide, which directs the wires not only in the frontal plane, but also in the sagittal plane.

The osteotomy is completed with a thin osteotome, along the curved line formed by the Kirschner wire holes or the curved osteotome. The tibial fragments are rotated until both Steinmann pins are parallel. Two Charnley

clamps[207] or a Müller external fixator[347] linking the two pins fixes the fragments under compression. Unilateral external fixators placed on the lateral side of the tibia also have been used.[55,271]

Another method to assess intraoperatively that the appropriate correction has been obtained was described by Blaimont.[25] A long and straight metallic rod is aligned, under fluoroscopy, on the mechanical axis of the tibia. The position of the proximal end of the rod is checked: It should be medial to the femoral head and should project radiologically over the obturator hole. This position ensures that enough overcorrection has been obtained, provided that during this fluoroscopic control the possible medial collateral laxity has been annulled by maintaining the contact between the medial femoral condyle and the medial tibial plateau (Fig. 78–22). A suction drainage is left in place for 24 hours to reduce the risk of an anterior compartment syndrome,[211,347] and the tibial and fibular wounds are closed.

Postoperatively the knee is passively and actively flexed from the day after surgery. On the second day, the patient stands and walks with two crutches, putting some weight on the operated knee. After 8 weeks and x-ray evidence of healing, the Steinmann pins are removed. The crutches are discarded as soon as the patient feels stable on the operated leg.

Advantages and Disadvantages of the Dome Osteotomy

Maquet,[207,211] Blaimont,[24,25] and Lemaire[187] claimed that the dome osteotomy was more accurate than the other tech-

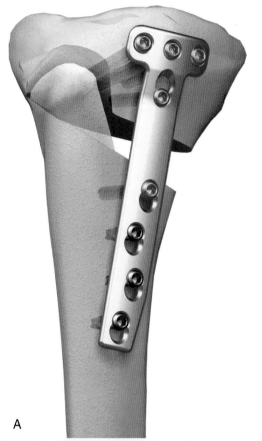

A

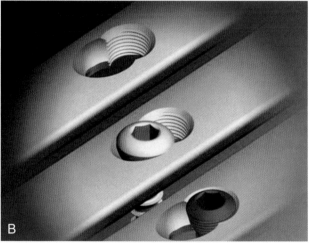

B

Figure 78–19. **A,** TomoFix medial high tibial plate. **B,** The locking compression plate hole consists of two parts: (1) a conical thread, allowing secure fixation of the locking head screw in the plate, and (2) a dynamic compression unit, allowing compression by eccentric insertion of a standard screw. (Courtesy of Synthes from the surgical technique "TomoFix Knee Osteotomy System." © 2003 Stratec Medical, Switzerland.)

niques. Maquet recommended combining an anterior displacement of the patellar tendon to the correction of the varus deformity. This procedure can be performed easily with a barrel vault osteotomy. Whether this association has any advantage is subject to debate, however.

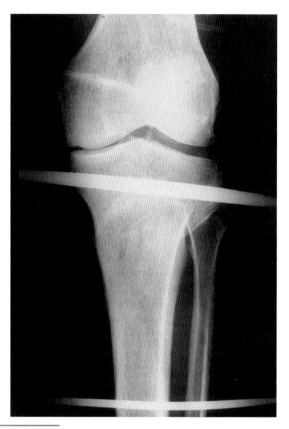

Figure 78–20. Dome high tibial osteotomy. The use of one proximal and one distal Steinmann pin is generally recommended, but two proximal and two distal pins can be used if extra stability is deemed necessary. Insertion of four Steinmann pins increases the risk of neurological complications.

The application of an external fixator allows postoperative correction of axial alignment, if necessary, and compression. The amount of correction using a dome osteotomy is theoretically unrestricted,[14,24,25,208,211] whereas it is limited by the amount of bone available when a closing wedge osteotomy is performed. The dome osteotomy tightens the medial collateral ligament, without affecting the position of the tibial tubercle relative to the joint line, as opposed to the opening wedge osteotomy.[25]

The main disadvantages are related to the use of the external fixator. The external fixator is cumbersome and is not easily accepted by some patients. The percutaneous Steinmann pins can damage the peroneal nerve or its branches[70,170,209] and can give rise to an infection[145,212] with a risk of late recurrence if the osteotomy has to be converted to a total knee replacement.

OPEN WEDGE TIBIAL OSTEOTOMY BY CALLUS DISTRACTION

Technique

In recent years, the technique of progressive opening wedge osteotomy by hemicallotasis has generated consid-

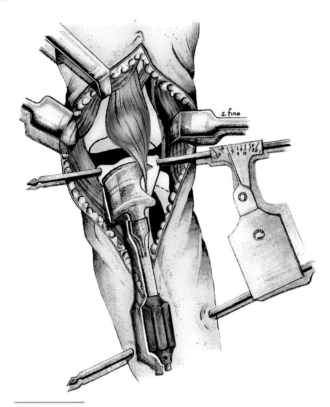

Figure 78–21. Tibial osteotomy using curved osteotomes and an angular guide. Under fluoroscopy, a Steinmann pin is inserted through the upper part of the tibial epiphysis, proximal to the osteotomy. The desired angle of correction is fixed on the guide. The guide, being slid on the first upper pin, gives the direction for the second Steinmann pin. After completion of the osteotomy, the exact correction is obtained by setting the Steinmann pins in parallel. (From Wagner J: Curvilinear osteotomy of the tibia. In Aichroth PM, Cannon WD Jr [eds]: Knee Surgery: Current Practice. London, Martin Dunitz, 1992, p 608.)

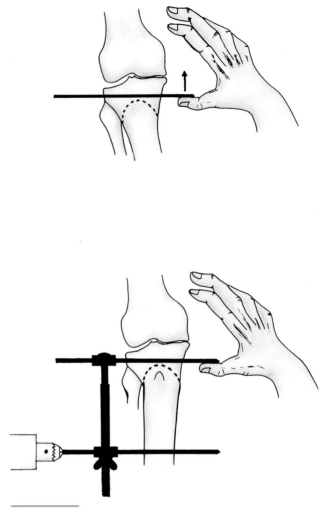

Figure 78–22. If the amount of correction is estimated visually by the intraoperative alignment of the limb, one should maintain manually the contact between the medial femoral condyle and the medial tibial plateau. In the presence of medial laxity, a valgus stress applied to the knee could open the joint medially, which would not occur during gait because of the persistence of the adduction moment. Failure to take the laxity into account during surgery could lead to undercorrection. (From Blaimont P: [Curviplane osteotomy in the treatment of gonarthrosis]. Acta Orthop Belg 48:97, 1982.)

erable interest.* The external fixator used in this technique can be either a ventral T-shaped fixator or a medial fixator (Fig. 78–23). These fixators have a lockable ball joint and a distraction device to make a progressive medial opening possible, keeping the lateral tibial cortex as a hinge. The use of an Ilizarov circular external fixator for progressive correction also has been described.[297] The osteotomy can be performed above the tibial tubercle[230,267,305] or at the distal part of it.[39,201,297] Some authors[267] advise performing a fibular osteotomy, but most[201,230,305] claim that fibular osteotomy is not required.

Partial weightbearing is allowed immediately. The distraction process starts 7 to 10 days after surgery. The gradual distraction is performed by the patient, usually at the speed of 1 mm per day (quarter turn four times a day). A greater distraction frequency, at a rate of 0.125 mm eight times a day, seems to provide better bone formation, resulting in a shorter external fixation period.[229] The dis-

traction phase lasts about 2 weeks, and a weekly radiological control is necessary during that period.

When the desired correction is achieved, the fixator is locked and left in place until union is obtained. The fixator usually is removed about 3 months after surgery. Low-intensity pulsed ultrasound applied during the consolidation phase of distraction osteogenesis could accelerate callus maturation and decrease the fixation time.[336] The pins are removed at the outpatient clinic.

Advantages and Disadvantages of Hemicallotasis

The supporters of this technique claim that it is relatively simple to perform; that it allows precise correction, early

*References 39, 71, 171, 172, 199, 201, 230, 231, 243, 267, 271, 297, 305, and 352.

colleagues[243] and Kitson and colleagues[171] showed that hemicallotasis did not cause patella infra. Another risk is the potential loss of correction because the mechanical properties of the newly formed bone are unknown at the time of the removal of the fixator.

Finally the follow-up periods in published studies are generally short (average follow-ups 18 months,[267] 16 months,[172] 14 months,[32] 5 to 36 months,[230] and 2 years[199,305]). Weale and associates[352] reported on the results of 76 osteotomies with a mean follow-up of 6 years and stated that hemicallotasis is a safe and reliable technique. Minor pin-tract sepsis was the most frequently occurring complication (28 of 76) in this series. One patient developed chronic osteomyelitis 2 years after surgery. The outcome was comparable with that of other techniques for osteotomy.

Other Techniques

Wagner and colleagues[344-346] described an oblique metaphyseal proximal tibial osteotomy just below the tibial tubercle. This technique is still popular in Germany.[268] It does not modify the patellar height. The main drawback of this technique is a longer healing time and a higher risk of nonunion.

Catagni and associates[48] developed a technique using the Ilizarov apparatus for correction and stabilization. Other groups have reported good results with this technique.[1,50,300] The osteotomy is distal to the tubercle and combines a valgus angulation and a small amount of translation. The time before removing the fixator averages 85 days. The drawbacks of this technique are the risk of pin-tract infection (10%), the bulkiness of the frame, and the required familiarity with the Ilizarov technique to avoid neurovascular complications.

FIBULAR OSTEOTOMY VERSUS DIVISION OF THE SUPERIOR TIBIOFIBULAR JOINT OR EXCISION OF THE FIBULAR HEAD

Opening wedge osteotomies, with immediate or gradual correction, usually leave the fibula untouched. Closing wedge osteotomies and dome osteotomies require relieving the tethering effect of the fibula, for which three methods can be used: fibular head excision, division of the superior tibiofibular joint, or osteotomy of the fibular shaft (Fig. 78–24).

In agreement with Maquet,[203,206,208] Blaimont and coworkers,[26,27] Andriacchi,[12] and others, I maintain that the lateral muscles—tensor fascia lata, biceps cruris—play a major role in counterbalancing the body mass, acting eccentrically on the knee during the stance phase of gait. In principle, division of the superior tibiofibular joint and excision of the fibular head are susceptible to further weakening dynamic stabilizers that already are insufficient in the varus arthritic knee[27] and affect the lateral collateral ligament.[238,301] This situation could contribute partly to some unpredictable results of high tibial osteotomy. Wagner and colleagues[348] showed the role of the fibula as a weightbearing bone together with the tibia. This role is even more important in the case of valgus or varus

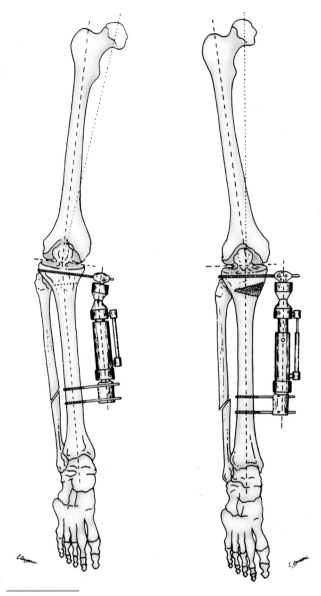

Figure 78–23. Medial external fixator used for progressive opening wedge osteotomy by hemicallotasis. (From Perusi M, Baietta D, Pizzoli A: [Surgical correction of osteoarthritic genu varum by the hemicallotasis technique]. Rev Chir Orthop Reparatrice Appar Mot 80:739, 1994. © Masson Editeur.)

mobilization, and weightbearing; and that it is a benign procedure performed through a short incision, not requiring a fibular osteotomy in most cases. The main drawback of hemicallotasis is the risk of pin-tract infection. Perusi and associates,[267] in a series of 58 osteotomies, reported 10 pin-tract infections treated by local antibiotics and 2 cases of septic arthritis. Magyar and coworkers[200] studied the complications after 308 open-wedge osteotomies by hemicallotasis performed in 17 hospitals. In 157 patients, pin-tract infections were recorded; most of these were minor and responded to wound toilet and antibiotic treatment. A second disadvantage, shared with the opening wedge osteotomy, is the lowering of the tibial tubercle relative to the joint line, although Nakamura and

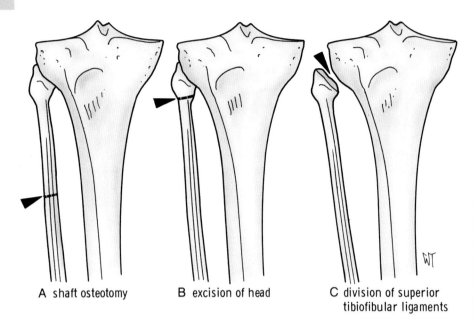

A shaft osteotomy   B excision of head   C division of superior tibiofibular ligaments

Figure 78–24. Methods of relieving the tethering effect of the fibula. **A,** Osteotomy of the fibular shaft. **B,** Excision of the fibular head. **C,** Division of the superior tibiofibular ligaments. (From Bauer GC, Insall J, Koshino T: Tibial osteotomy in gonarthrosis [osteoarthritis of the knee]. J Bone Joint Surg Am 51:1545, 1969.)

knee deformity. The fibular head excision[62,96] necessitates detaching the lateral ligament; the fabellofibular ligament, to which the popliteus tendon is attached; and the biceps tendon.

Although a repair of the lateral soft tissues is possible after the osteotomy, it seems doubtful that this repair could reproduce the complex anatomy and function of the posterolateral corner of the knee. Another disadvantage of fibular head excision is the risk of peroneal nerve injury. Coventry[62] did not have any peroneal palsy in his series, but Harris and Kostuik,[115] using a similar technique, reported 2 in 44 osteotomies.

Division of the superior tibiofibular joint implies proximal migration of the fibular head relative to the proximal tibial fragment after the osteotomy. This migration aggravates preexisting lateral collateral laxity or creates new laxity that did not exist previously.[301] It also destabilizes and proximalizes the point of action of the biceps. The increased lateral collateral laxity, together with the weakening of the biceps, impairs the improved load distribution achieved with the tibial osteotomy.[12,263,301] This is especially true if the secondary restraints to the lateral laxity (i.e., the anterior cruciate ligament, the posterior capsule, and the fascia lata) are damaged (Fig. 78–25).[12] The amount of proximal migration of the fibular head that is detrimental to the knee stability and to the action of the biceps has to be determined, but I believe that division of the tibiofibular joint should be restricted to the correction of small varus deformities (i.e., when the wedge height is ≤5 mm).

Fibular osteotomy avoids destruction of a normal joint, avoids proximal migration of the fibular head and loosening of the point of action of the biceps, and avoids increasing the laxity of the lateral collateral ligament.[238] The level of the osteotomy of the fibula influences the rate of peroneal nerve injuries.[70,170] High-risk regions can be located relative to the fibular head (Fig. 78–26).[170]

Curley and associates,[70] in a study of 16 patients assessed by electrophysiological recordings and intracompartmental pressure recording before and after high tibial osteotomy, observed that patients who had a proximal fibular osteotomy had greater electrical abnormalities postoperatively. Two of them developed common peroneal palsies. More commonly, an iatrogenic, isolated weakness or paralysis of the extensor hallucis longus muscle can occur in patients who have had a proximal tibial and fibular osteotomy. To investigate why this complication occurs, Kirgis and Albrecht[170] dissected the deep peroneal nerve and neighboring structures in 29 cadaveric specimens, paying special attention to the motor branches supplying the extensor hallucis longus. Of 46 motor nerves that were identified, 8 entered the muscle from the lateral side in an area 70 to 150 mm distal to the fibular head; all of them ran close to the fibular periosteum. Kirgis and Albrecht[170] suggested that, in some patients, the nerve supply to the extensor hallucis longus is at high risk of injury during a fibular osteotomy because of the proximity of the bone to the motor branches. Fibular osteotomy can be performed safely in the region between the middle and distal thirds of the fibula, about 160 mm distal to the fibular head.

INFLUENCE OF OSTEOTOMY ON THE TIBIAL SLOPE IN THE SAGITTAL PLANE

The normal upper tibia has a posterior slope.[149] Because the proximal tibia is triangular in section at the level of the osteotomy site, a wedge having the same height ventrally and dorsally would affect not only the alignment in the frontal plane, but also the tibial slope. In this case, an opening wedge would increase the posterior slope,[216] whereas a closing wedge would reduce the posterior slope.[299]

An excessive posterior slope is detrimental for the long-term result of the osteotomy.[128,299] It can provoke an anterior subluxation of the tibia,[99] particularly when the

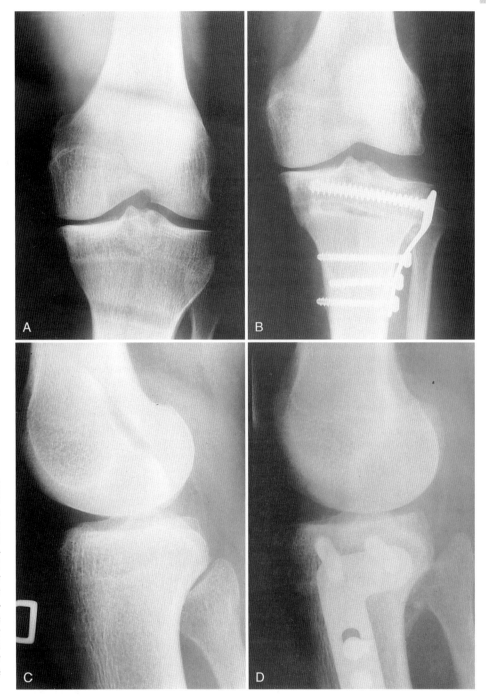

Figure 78–25. **A,** Medial gonarthrosis in a 33-year-old man, with an anterior cruciate ligament–deficient knee but without significant lateral laxity. **B,** Severe lateral collateral ligament laxity after lateral closing wedge osteotomy with division of the superior tibiofibular joint. **C,** Preoperative lateral x-ray of the same knee, showing the tibiofibular joint. **D,** Postoperative lateral x-ray showing the posterior and superior dislocation of the tibiofibular joint.

anterior cruciate ligament is deficient. For this reason, Hernigou and associates[131] advised that, when performing an opening wedge osteotomy, the posterior wedge should have a base that is exactly the height that is needed, whereas the base of the middle wedge should measure about 2 mm less, and the most anterior one should measure about 6 mm less. A closing wedge osteotomy tends to decrease the posterior tibial slope if the base of the wedge has the same height posteriorly and anteriorly. This decrease does not induce a posterior subluxation of the tibia except if the posterior cruciate ligament is damaged. These changes in the normal tibial slope com-

plicate the conversion of the osteotomy to a total knee replacement.

HIGH TIBIAL OSTEOTOMY AND THE PATELLOFEMORAL JOINT

Most authors agree that mild patellofemoral arthritis does not contraindicate a high tibial osteotomy and is of little prognostic significance.[68,72,119,145,148,169,208] Moderate to severe patellofemoral arthritis has a negative influence on

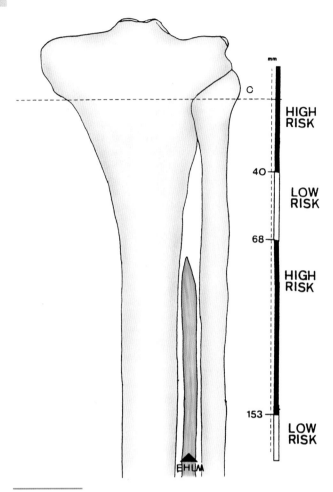

Figure 78–26. Frontal view showing a leg with a longitudinal scale. The scale illustrates regions that are at high and low risk for intraoperative injury relative to the presence of the motor branches from the truncus of the deep peroneal nerve. EHLM, extensor hallucis longus muscle. (From Kirgis A, Albrecht S: Palsy of the deep peroneal nerve after proximal tibial osteotomy: An anatomical study. J Bone Joint Surg Am 74:1180, 1992.)

prognosis, however.[127,275,291,299,331] As stated by Insall,[145] an osteotomy should be avoided in patients with marked patellofemoral arthritis, given the excellent alternative of total knee arthroplasty.

A high tibial osteotomy acts on the patella in different ways: It changes the patellar height, the Q angle, and the medial lateral position of the tibial tubercle. The change in the Q angle and in the medial lateral position of the tibial tubercle is minimal[105,127,299] whatever the osteotomy technique except for major angular corrections. The patellar height, in principle, is affected differently by the various osteotomy techniques.[328] A dome osteotomy or an osteotomy below the tibial tuberosity should not modify the proximal distal position of the tubercle, whereas an opening wedge should render it more distal, and a closing wedge should render it more proximal.[362] The length of the patellar tendon also can be altered after a high tibial osteotomy, as a consequence of scarring or immobilization.

Scuderi and coworkers[298] observed, in a study group of 66 patients who had had a proximal closing wedge tibial osteotomy, that 89% of the patellae as measured by the Insall-Salvati[142] index and 76.3% as measured by the Blackburne-Peel[23] index were lowered on the postoperative lateral radiograph. All knees were immobilized in a cylinder cast during healing of the osteotomy. More recently, Westrich and associates[356] showed, in a study group of 65 patients who underwent a high tibial osteotomy with a closing wedge osteotomy above the tibial tubercle, that 33 patients who underwent some type of internal fixation and received early range of motion postoperatively had less postoperative shortening of the patellar tendon, according to the Insall-Salvati index, than patients who were immobilized with a cast postoperatively. Dohin and colleagues,[84] in a group of 59 closing wedge osteotomies fixed by a blade-plate and immediately mobilized, showed that the patellar height was not modified, as measured by the Caton index.[49]

The aforementioned study results are a strong argument for using rigid internal fixation and early range of motion because this protocol should result in a better knee and facilitate any subsequent total knee arthroplasty.[56,171] It also is suggested that a closing wedge osteotomy should be preferred to an opening wedge osteotomy in the case of preoperative patella baja or patellofemoral arthritis.[328] Nevertheless, Hernigou and Goutallier,[127] studying the radiological changes in the patellofemoral joint 10 to 13 years after upper tibial valgus opening wedge osteotomy, found only minimal deteriorations that were not correlated with the functional results.

Whether advancement or medial transfer of the tibial tubercle in additon to high tibial osteotomy has any value in the presence of patellofemoral arthritis is doubtful. Although Maquet[211] recommended this combination, Nguyen and colleagues,[246] in a prospective study of similarly matched patients with medial and patellofemoral osteoarthritis, were unable to show any benefit from the addition of tubercle elevation to the osteotomy. Jackson and Waugh,[153] Hofmann and coworkers,[136] Goutallier and coworkers,[105] Hernigou and Goutallier,[127] and the members of the symposium of the Société Française de Chirurgie Orthopédique et Traumatologique, concerning the failures of high tibial osteotomies,[299] reached the same conclusion.

POSTOPERATIVE COMPLICATIONS

The complication rates of high tibial osteotomy vary considerably according to different series and include undercorrection, overcorrection, loss of correction, patella baja, restricted range of motion, intra-articular fractures, nonunion, infection, peroneal nerve dysfunction, compartment syndrome, vascular injury, and thromboembolic disease. Insall[145] analyzed the complications in 10 clinical series totaling 804 osteotomies. Of the 60 infections reported, 55 were superficial and 5 were deep; 37 of the infections occurred in association with transfixation pins and an external frame. Eight intra-articular fractures occurred, most of which were caused by a proximal tibial fragment that was too thin. There were 56 peroneal nerve palsies reported; 37 were associated with transfixation pins.

Hofmann and colleagues,[135] comparing 19 patients (group A) who underwent osteotomies with staple fixation or cast immobilization and 21 patients (group B) whose osteotomies were rigidly fixed by a buttress plate with immediate motion, found that 8 patients in group A had associated complications versus 1 patient in group B. The only complication in group B was a nondisplaced intra-articular fracture from overcompression of the buttress plate; in group A, there were two transient peroneal nerve palsies, one compartment syndrome, one nonunion, three delayed unions, one superficial infection, two nondisplaced intra-articular fractures and two losses of correction. The complication rate is technique dependent; cast immobilization, proximal fibular osteotomy or fibular head excision, and transfixation pins seem to increase the operative risk.

UNDERCORRECTION, OVERCORRECTION, AND LOSS OF CORRECTION

Undercorrection and overcorrection are secondary to incorrect preoperative planning or technical errors. Late recurrence of varus deformity was studied by Stuart and associates[315] in a series of 113 knees monitored for a minimum of 5 years. Varus recurred in 18%, lateral compartment arthritis progressed in 60%, and medial compartment arthritis progressed in 83% by 9 years after surgery. They concluded that the probability of arthritic progression is much higher than the probability of significant varus recurrence. In this report, the relationship between the postoperative hip-knee-ankle angle and the risk of recurrence of the deformity was not analyzed.

Hernigou and colleagues,[123] reviewing a series of 35 opening wedge osteotomies with a 20-year follow-up, stated that osteotomy rarely avoids the problem of recurrent deformity, which appears before 10 years when the initial correction is less than 3 degrees of valgus. Even correction between 3 and 6 degrees of valgus is not immune to recurrent varus deformity over the long-term (20 years); among knees between 3 and 6 degrees of valgus at the 1-year postoperative follow-up, most of them remained in this range of correction at 10 years, but half had lost some correction at 20 years. Hernigou and colleagues[123] also reported that a second valgus tibial osteotomy can be successful; 13 repeated tibial osteotomies produced a good result 20 years after the principal osteotomy.

In a large multicenter study,[299] it seemed that the deformity recurred in 14% of cases when the preoperative hip-knee-ankle angle was between 3 and 6 degrees valgus and in 38% of cases when this angle was between 0 and 2 degrees valgus. Overcorrection superior to 6 degrees valgus did not improve the result, was not well accepted by the patients, and should be avoided. Overcorrection superior to 10 degrees is not compatible with a normal gait and necessitates a revision of the osteotomy.[299]

PATELLA BAJA AND REDUCED RANGE OF MOTION

As already discussed, lowering of the patella can be minimized by early range of motion allowed by rigid internal or external fixation. In the case of preoperative patella infra, an opening wedge osteotomy should be avoided.

Odenbring and colleagues,[257] in a prospective study, randomized 32 knees in 32 patients to either a cylinder plaster cast or a hinged cast-brace after high tibial osteotomy for medial gonarthrosis. At 6 weeks, 3 months, and 1 year after surgery, the range of motion was better in the cast-brace group. Hofmann and associates,[135] comparing a group of 19 osteotomies with cast immobilization and a group of 21 osteotomies with rigid internal fixation and early motion, noted that three patients had less than 90 degrees flexion at 6 months in the first group, whereas all patients had gained 90 degrees flexion at 6 weeks in the second group. There are clear advantages in favor of early motion after high tibial osteotomy, and this should guide the choice for a strong fixation.

INTRA-ARTICULAR FRACTURES

Fracture of the tibial plateau usually can be avoided or corrected if recognized during surgery. The risk of fracture can be decreased if the proximal fragment is appropriately 2 cm or more thick,[67,168] if the osteotomy is continued to the opposite periosteum,[168] or if the opposite cortex is sufficiently weakened. The reported incidence is 2%.[119] This complication seems to be encountered more frequently in opening wedge osteotomies. Hernigou and colleagues[131] reported 10 undisplaced lateral plateau fractures in a series of 93 opening wedge osteotomies. There was no evidence that these undisplaced fractures had had any effect on the final results.

When using a blade-plate for fixation, care should be taken that the entry point of the blade is at least 10 to 15 mm distal to the joint line[183] and that its course is not too ascendant toward the sclerotic medial tibial plateau.[270] In this condition, Descamps and associates[81] did not observe any tibial plateau fracture in a series of 544 osteotomies with blade-plate fixation.

NONUNION

Delayed union or nonunion of the osteotomy is rare (Fig. 78-27). The reported rate of nonunion ranges from 0% to 3%.[47,144,241,330,331] Most authors report a 0.5% to 1% nonunion rate.[44,68,82,148,187,194] Jackson and Waugh[153] reported a threefold increase in the nonunion rate when the osteotomy was performed below the tuberosity rather than above it. Insall[145] believed that a thin proximal fragment is a risk factor for nonunion, perhaps because of avascular necrosis.

Mammi and colleagues[202] investigated the effect of electromagnetic field stimulation in a group of 40 consecutive patients treated with valgus tibial osteotomy, randomly receiving an active or a dummy stimulator post-

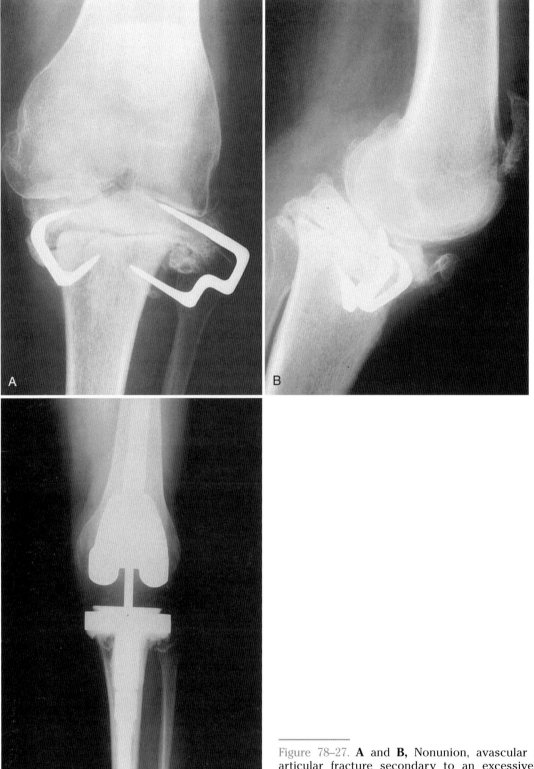

Figure 78–27. **A** and **B,** Nonunion, avascular necrosis, and intra-articular fracture secondary to an excessively proximal closing wedge osteotomy. **C,** Conversion to a total knee arthroplasty, requiring the use of a custom-constrained condylar implant.

operatively. They concluded that electromagnetic field stimulation had positive effects on the healing of tibial osteotomies. Coventry[65] reported that electrical stimulation has been effective in treating nonunion, if the position is acceptable.

Treatment of nonunion after osteotomy usually consists of bone grafting alone if rigid fixation is maintained or bone grafting and compression fixation in cases in which rigid fixation was not used initially.[119] This fixation may be internal, or an external fixator may be used.[65] Rozbruch and coworkers[288] proposed distraction osteogenesis for nonunion because this is a minimally invasive procedure that also allows correction of deformity and leg-length discrepancy. Cameron and associates[44] recommended a double T-plate technique when the proximal bone fragment is small, soft, or relatively avascular.

Infection

Deep infection is rare after high tibial osteotomy. Compiling the complications of 10 clinical series, for a total of 804 osteotomies, Insall[145] took a census of 5 deep and 55 superficial infections; 37 occurred when an external fixator was used. Maquet and colleagues,[212] in a series of 700 osteotomies, most of which were dome osteotomies, noted a 2.8% rate of skin necrosis and a 7.7% infection rate. The respective incidence of deep and superficial infections was not mentioned. Lortat-Jacob and associates[195] reported six cases of early reintervention for infection after high tibial osteotomy. In four cases, the internal fixation was left in place, with a good end result. One patient with gas gangrene required amputation, and another died from septic shock.

The hemicallotasis technique necessitates the use of an external fixator for a prolonged period. As already mentioned, Perusi and coworkers,[267] in a series of 58 osteotomies, reported 10 pin-tract infections treated by local antibiotics and 2 cases of septic arthritis. Septic complications related to the use of an external fixator should not be overestimated, however. Lemaire,[187] in a series of 201 dome osteotomies fixed by a compression frame, reported three infections; one was treated successfully by general antibiotics, and two were treated by curettage and antibiotic-impregnated polymethyl methacrylate beads left temporarily in the wound. The infection rate after high tibial osteotomy justifies routine antibiotic prophylaxis.[119]

Peroneal Nerve Dysfunction

Fibular osteotomy or resection of the fibular head can induce a common peroneal nerve palsy[70] or an isolated weakness of the extensor hallucis longus muscle.[170] Based on the already mentioned studies of Curley and associates[70] and Kirgis and Albrecht,[170] it seems that the fibular osteotomy should be performed distally, at the junction of the middle and distal thirds of the leg. Kirgis and Albrecht[170] defined two high-risk regions for an isolated injury of the motor branches to the extensor hallucis longus, the first one about 30 mm and the second one 68 to 153 mm distal to the fibular head. These authors stressed the danger related to the application of an external fixation device after a proximal tibial osteotomy. The nerve can be damaged directly by the pin or by the stab incision created for it. The distal Steinmann pin always should be placed in the safe region, 40 to 60 mm distal to the fibular tubercle, and it always should be inserted from the medial side.

In a large series of osteotomies, Maquet[209] recorded a 3.1% rate of motor deficits and a 4.1% rate of sensory deficits, of which 1.2% and 1.5% were definitive. Idusuyi and Morrey[140] documented 32 postoperative peroneal nerve palsies in a retrospective review of 10,361 consecutive total knee arthroplasties performed at the Mayo Clinic. They showed that epidural anesthesia for postoperative control of pain was significantly associated with peroneal nerve palsy. They postulated that the decrease in proprioception and sensation postoperatively allows the limb to rest in an unprotected state, making it susceptible to neurological ischemia from local compression. Although this association has not been documented in high tibial osteotomy, the neurological status of the patient should be monitored carefully if epidural anesthesia is used postoperatively. External rotation of the limb should be avoided to decrease the pressure on the nerve where it courses around the head of the fibula. The anesthesia should not produce prolonged sensory and motor blockade. The peroneus superficialis nerve also could be damaged when the fibular osteotomy is performed distally. The nerve should be avoided carefully at the time of the fascial incision.[183]

The technique of the tibial osteotomy itself also influences the rate of neurological complications. Flierl and associates[90] and Sabo and colleagues[294] retrospectively investigated 132 cases of closing wedge high tibial osteotomies using an external fixation device. When the osteotomy was performed through consecutive drill holes of increasing diameter followed by osteoclasis, persistent neurological deficits were encountered in 4.7% of cases, as opposed to 12.4% of cases when the osteotomy was performed with an oscillating saw. They concluded that the reduction of neurological complications was related to the less extensive approach of the drilling technique. I prefer using bone chisels instead of an oscillating saw for closing wedge osteotomies because the trajectory of the chisels is more easily controlled than the trajectory of a saw. Another advantage of using chisels is that they do not cause any thermal damage to bone.

Compartment Syndrome

The exact incidence of compartment syndrome after high tibial osteotomy is unknown.[98] Several technical precautions can help to decrease this risk. The tibialis anterior muscle should not be damaged during the approach and should not be crushed by the retractors. The proximal tibia should be accessed subperiosteally. The tourniquet should be released before closure, and careful hemostasis should be performed. The fascial incision should not be closed tightly.[183] A suction drain should be left in place,[98,183,211,347] and if a separate incision is made for the fibular osteotomy, it also should be drained. Tight dressings should be avoided. Epidural anesthesia can mask the signs of an impending ischemia. For that reason, I prefer to use patient-controlled analgesia rather than epidural in the postoperative phase of high tibial osteotomy. If epidural anesthesia is used, the amount of local anesthesic that is given should be sufficient to make the patient comfortable without producing prolonged sensory and motor blockade, and the status of the leg should be observed even more closely.

If in doubt, the tissue pressure should be monitored. Impending tissue ischemia must be considered when the tissue pressure reaches 30 to 10 mm Hg below the diastolic pressure. A higher pressure is a strong indication that fasciotomy should be performed.

Vascular Injury

Vascular injuries after osteotomy of the proximal tibia are rare. Three cases of false aneurysm of the popliteal artery after upper tibial osteotomy have been reported.[104,290] Sawant and Ireland[296] described a pseudoaneurysm of the anterior recurrent branch of the anterior tibial artery. Lang and coworkers[182] described a case of iatrogenic popliteal arteriovenous fistula after dome high tibial osteotomy. This complication was diagnosed after angiography, 8 weeks postoperatively, and was surgically treated.

Zaidi and associates[369] reported a case in which the popliteal artery was divided, although the osteotomy was performed with the knee at 90 degrees flexion. Using Doppler ultrasonography in 10 healthy volunteers to define the relationship of the popliteal artery to the back of the tibia and to assess the protection afforded by flexing the knee, these investigators showed that the distance between the popliteal artery and the posterior tibial cortex varied from 3.9 mm to 10.8 mm in normal knees in full extension. This distance became smaller with 90 degrees flexion in 12 knees and minimally larger in the other 8 knees. Zaidi and associates[369] also stressed that, although in most cases the artery is protected by the bulk of the popliteus muscle, in a few cases, high branching implies that the anterior tibial artery is closely applied to the tibia anterior to this muscle. Shetty and colleagues[303] performed an in vivo study of the popliteal artery in 100 knees, using color flow Doppler ultrasonography. The overall trend was for the popliteal artery to move away from the posterior tibial cortex when the knee was flexed to 90 degrees, but it moved closer to the posterior tibial surface in 25% and closer to the posterior tibia 1 to 1.5 cm below the joint line in 15%. There was a high branching anterior tibial artery in 6% of knees. Smith and colleagues[306] reached similar conclusions using MRI.

Haddad and coworkers[112] treated an arteriovenous fistula of the peroneal artery acquired after a dome osteotomy with midshaft fibular osteotomy. This fistula was undetected at first and presented as a recurrent hemarthrosis after a total knee replacement. It was treated by percutaneous embolization. To avoid this complication, Haddad and coworkers[112] recommended that fibular osteotomy should be carried out as distally and in the least traumatic manner as possible.

Thromboembolic Disease

In a review of the English literature, Heatley and coworkers[120] found 19 cases of pulmonary embolism, 5 of them fatal, among 1647 upper tibial osteotomies—an incidence of emboli of 1.2% and a mortality of 0.3%. The reported incidence of deep vein thrombosis was 2.8%, which is low in relation to the number of emboli. This low incidence can be explained by the sparse use of ultrasonography or venography in the reviewed series. Matthews and colleagues[219] reported an incidence of clinical thrombosis of 6%.

Turner and associates[337] performed postoperative venography on 84 consecutive patients who had undergone upper tibial osteotomy and showed deep vein thrombosis in 41%. Only 15% of the cases were diagnosed clinically, all in the calf veins, whereas 3 proximal thromboses and 12 mixed vein thromboses were revealed only by venography. One nonfatal pulmonary embolism also occurred in this series, in which prophylaxis with heparin, 5000 IU twice daily given subcutaneously, was delayed until the second postoperative day.

Leclerc and colleagues[186] randomly assigned a consecutive cohort of 129 patients undergoing knee arthroplasty or tibial osteotomy into two groups. In the first group, 30 mg of enoxaparin was administered subcutaneously every 12 hours, generally starting on the morning of the first postoperative day; the patients in the second group received an identical-looking placebo. Deep vein thrombosis was detected by either venography or noninvasive tests in 58% of patients in the placebo group and in 17% of patients in the enoxaparin group. Proximal vein thrombosis was found in 19% of the placebo patients and in none of the enoxaparin patients. There were no differences in bleeding complications or the amount of blood loss. One patient in the placebo group developed nonfatal pulmonary embolism.

In the aftercare of patients undergoing major surgery of the lower limbs, routine prophylaxis with low-molecular-weight heparin, starting 12 hours before surgery, has been my standard postoperative regimen since the 1980s. I have not detected increased bleeding secondary to this protocol. I strongly recommend the use of some form of thromboembolic prophylaxis after osteotomy.

Revision Surgery for Late Failure of High Tibial Osteotomy

Numerous reports deal with revision of failed high tibial osteotomy. Most describe the results and the technical pitfalls of revision using a total knee arthroplasty,* but some reports also consider the possibility of repeated osteotomy[123,299,335] and of revision with a unicompartmental knee arthroplasty.[284,299] Based on the existing literature, I suggest some answers to the following questions: What are the indications for the different revision procedures available? What technical mistakes at the time of osteotomy would make the revision difficult? What tips at the time of repeated surgery can ease the revision? What results can be expected from the revision of a valgus tibial osteotomy?

---

*References 11, 18, 31, 38, 100, 111, 125, 134, 163, 164, 180, 188, 198, 213, 223, 224, 232, 233, 245, 248, 249, 265, 289, 299, 309, 332, 333, 338, 350, 359, and 367.

The largest series of repeated surgery after failed high tibial osteotomy, including 225 knees, was reported at the 1991 annual meeting of the Société Française de Chirurgie Orthopédique et Traumatologique.[299] This series included 48 repeated osteotomies, 25 unicompartmental knee arthroplasties, 11 bicompartmental arthroplasties, and 141 total knee arthroplasties. The authors confirmed the good results of repeated high tibial osteotomy also reported by Hernigou and colleagues.[123] The condition for a successful repeated proximal tibia valgus osteotomy is that the failure of the initial osteotomy was exclusively secondary to undercorrection or loss of correction. Other causes of failure, such as inflammatory joint disease, chondrocalcinosis, painful femoropatellar arthritis, and lateral compartment degradation, should be ruled out. Repeat osteotomy also is indicated in cases of severe hypercorrection (Fig. 78–28). In this situation, the second osteotomy should be performed early to prevent the advent of degenerative changes in the lateral compartment. This approach is less difficult if the first osteotomy was an opening wedge. In this case, a medial closing wedge is the right solution. When the hypercorrection was secondary to a closing wedge osteotomy, correction with a lateral opening wedge increases the risk of peroneal nerve palsy, whereas a medial closing wedge increases the proximal tibial bone loss. A dome osteotomy could be an appropriate compromise for solving this difficult problem.

Revision with a unicompartmental knee arthroplasty gave good or excellent results in 24 of the 25 cases reported in this series. The prerequisites are approximately the same as for repeated valgus osteotomy, with the added condition of a normal anterior cruciate ligament. In contrast, Rees and colleagues[284] reported a high frequency of revision of the Oxford medial unicompartmental arthroplasty in knees previously treated by high tibial osteotomy, and they recommended that this implant should not be used in knees that previously have undergone a high tibial osteotomy. From the group of total or bicompartmental arthroplasties in this series, no clear conclusions can be drawn concerning the choice of the implant except that a hinged prosthesis definitely should be abandoned. From the other series of condylar total knee arthroplasties after failed high tibial osteotomy available, it is not possible to affirm the superiority of cruciate-retaining or cruciate-substituting designs for revision of high tibial osteotomy.

Several factors can make revision of a tibial osteotomy a difficult procedure. Most can be avoided by a proper realization of the osteotomy. These factors include previous incisions, flexion contracture, decreased range of motion, patella infra, epiphyseal malrotation or translation, hypercorrection, severe alteration of the normal posterior tibial slope, nonunion, avascular necrosis, sepsis, peroneal nerve palsy, collateral ligament laxity, and hardware removal.

The incision for a tibial osteotomy should be performed in such a manner that it would not complicate a future total knee arthroplasty. A midline or close-to-midline longitudinal incision should be chosen to allow the same incision to be used at the time of revision. The fixation of the osteotomy should be stable to authorize immediate motion and to avoid secondary displacement. Indications for combined valgus and rotation osteotomies are exceptional in arthritic knees; when confronted with severe patellofemoral pain in a medial arthritic knee, a total knee arthroplasty should be performed directly.

The shape of the wedge should be calculated to keep the posterior tibial slope within the normal range. One should not attempt to correct a flexion deformity through an extension osteotomy. A flexion deformity exceeding 15 degrees contraindicates a tibial osteotomy. Resecting the anterior and intercondylar osteophytes usually resolves a minor flexion contracture.[299]

Nonunion and avascular necrosis are often due to a too-thin proximal tibial fragment,[145] and care should be taken to osteotomize the tibia at least 2 cm distal to the joint line. If the anatomy of the peroneal nerve and of its branches is taken into account, the rate of neurological complications can be significantly lowered, provided that there is adequate surgical technique and postoperative care. Hypercorrection is the main cause of collateral ligament instability at reoperation; this stresses the necessity of accurate preoperative planning and reliable operation.

Large fixation devices, such as blade-plates, generally need to be removed at the time of revision. If the skin incision was adequate at the time of the osteotomy, hardware removal and knee arthroplasty can be performed in one session; otherwise the removal and the arthroplasty should be staged. The infection rate is increased when using transfixation pins, and if this technique is used, a strict aftercare protocol is mandatory. When in doubt at the time of revision, torpid bone infection can be diagnosed by C-reactive protein determination, MRI,[334] or leukocyte scintigraphy.[181,286,293]

Technical difficulties can be faced when performing a total knee arthroplasty in a knee in which a previous suboptimal proximal tibial osteotomy has been done. A midline longitudinal incision should be used, regardless of whether the previous osteotomy was through a lateral, longitudinal, or short horizontal incision.[359] When the osteotomy scar is lateral longitudinal, close to the midline, it can be reopened to enter the joint medially, raising a short skin flap, or laterally through the approach described by Buechel.[37] Segal and associates[299] advise the use of this lateral approach, particularly when the reason for failure of the tibial osteotomy is hypercorrection, because it allows the removal of the hardware through the same incision, to correct the valgus deformity without creating excessive instability, to displace the patella medially if needed, and to close the joint with the fat pad if the lateral retinaculum is left open. Because of soft-tissue scarring, subperiosteal exposure of the proximal tibia is more difficult in the postosteotomy knee, and the dissection should be performed with a scalpel rather than with a periosteal elevator or an osteotome.[164,233,359] If a medial approach is used, care should be taken to extend the incision to the tibial periosteum 1 cm medial to the tibial tubercle to leave a cuff of tissue that helps prevent inadvertent avulsion of the patellar ligament.[359]

Eversion of the patella can be difficult in a knee that has had a previous osteotomy because of scarring or patella infra or, after a closing wedge osteotomy, because of the decreased distance from the tubercle to the joint line.[232,298]

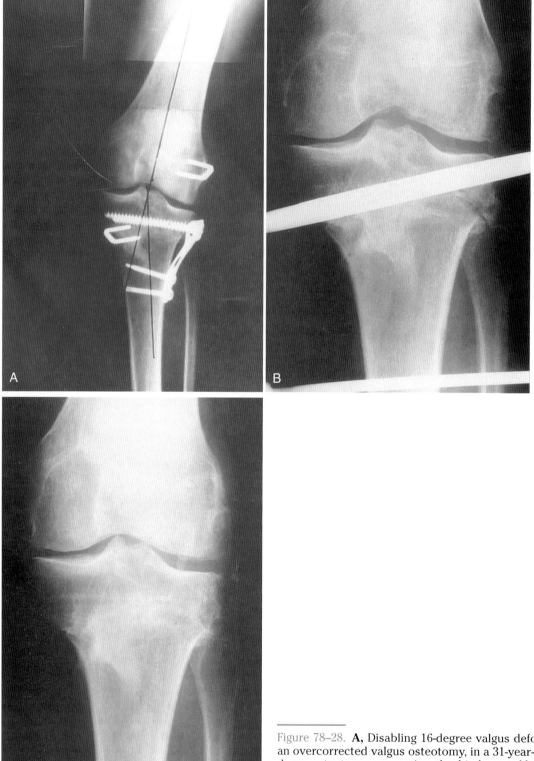

Figure 78–28. **A,** Disabling 16-degree valgus deformity, secondary to an overcorrected valgus osteotomy, in a 31-year-old laborer. **B,** Varus dome osteotomy, correcting the hip-knee-ankle angle to 3 degrees valgus. **C,** At 5 years after the varus osteotomy, the radiological and clinical outcome remains good.

A lateral retinacular release early in the operation may facilitate eversion.[232,245,359] In some instances, lateral retinacular release is insufficient, and a decision should be made from among three options: a quadriceps snip,[97,146,147] a quadriceps turndown,[100,232,233,359] or a tubercle osteotomy.[164,188,245,299] This choice seems to be mainly a matter of personal preference, although in the specific situation of a failed tibial osteotomy, tibial tubercle elevation seems more logical because it allows correction of the iatrogenic patella baja.

After a closing wedge osteotomy, the bone stock available from the proximal part of the tibia is reduced, and extra care should be taken to resect the least amount of bone from the tibial plateau that is necessary to obtain a satisfactory surface for fixation of the tibial component. Severe defects in the lateral plateau may require bone grafting[232,359] or metal wedges.[146] Angulation of the tibial plateau in the sagittal plane may have been significantly altered. In case of tibial recurvatum, even if care is taken not to over-resect the proximal tibia, the tibial insertion of the posterior cruciate ligament may be divided. This situation is best treated with a cruciate-substituting implant.[146,299]

In case of epiphyseal translation[188,245] or truncated metaphysis,[164,232] the use of prostheses that have a tibial component with a central peg may result in impingement of the tip of the peg on the lateral part of the tibial cortex. A custom-made tibial component[359] or an offset stem may be needed to accommodate the altered anatomy of the tibia. In severe cases, a second osteotomy to reverse the extra-articular deformity produced by the first osteotomy may be required.[43,232,299] This is the case when facing a hypercorrection of more than 10 degrees. Cameron and Welsh[43] advised performing a dome osteotomy to prevent further shortening of the extremity and an osteotomy of the fibula to permit adequate correction. A stemmed component should be used to bridge the osteotomy site[43,338] if the repeat osteotomy and the arthroplasty are done at the same time, although some authors[101] have advised, in the same operative session, to implant the prosthesis first, regardless of the deformity, and to correct the axis afterward, by a second osteotomy.

Ligament imbalance is especially prevalent in knees with overcorrected valgus. Krackow and Holtgrewe[180] have developed a complex ligament reconstruction for this subset of patients to allow simultaneous implantation of a minimally constrained total knee prosthesis. This reconstruction is associated with advancement of the medial collateral ligament and of the posterior cruciate ligament and posteromedial capsule. In a series of five patients, although the preoperative femorotibial alignment averaged 25 degrees valgus, the postoperative alignment and function were comparable to that with a standard primary total knee arthroplasty. The series available are too small to provide clear guidelines about when a lateral approach, a ligament reconstruction, or a second osteotomy should be performed.

Diverging conclusions have been presented concerning the outcome of total knee arthroplasty after high tibial osteotomy. Several authors[11,18,213,224,245,309] have reported that the results of total knee arthroplasty after high tibial osteotomy are comparable to the results of primary total knee arthroplasty. In contrast, other groups[125,164,233,359] have cited inferior results, with an increased incidence of complications and technical pitfalls. Parvizi and associates[265] evaluated the long-term clinical and radiographic outcome of 166 total knee arthroplasties after high tibial osteotomy and identified male gender, increased weight, young age, coronal laxity, and preoperative limb malalignment as risk factors for early failure.

Because high tibial osteotomy and unicompartmental arthroplasty are often in competition, Jackson and colleagues[154] and Gill and colleagues[100] compared the results of revision arthroplasty after these two procedures. The results of these two studies were conflicting. Jackson and colleagues[154] reported a higher complication rate in the post–tibial osteotomy group, mainly owing to wound healing problems. This result stresses again the importance of planning the osteotomy, including the skin incision, with a future total knee arthroplasty in mind. In contrast, Gill and colleagues[100] estimated that difficulty with exposure was not significantly greater in the osteotomy group and concluded that the functional level, complication rate, and technical results of revision total knee arthroplasty after unicompartmental knee arthroplasty for the initial treatment of unicompartmental arthritis approached, but did not equal, those obtained after high tibial osteotomy.

Although not formally established, I agree with the conclusions reached by Segal and colleagues,[299] who inferred from a review of 225 revisions for failed high tibial osteotomies that the results of revision are affected mainly when the initial osteotomy was performed incorrectly and, more specifically, when hypercorrection exceeded 10 degrees of mechanical valgus. Similar to Staeheli and coworkers,[309] my opinion is that a high tibial osteotomy, properly performed, does not "burn any bridges" insofar as a future arthroplasty is concerned (Fig. 78–29). The long-term fixation of the tibial component after failure of a tibial osteotomy should not be a concern because Toksvig-Larsen and coworkers,[332] using roentgen stereophotogrammetric analysis, showed that there was no difference in the prosthetic fixation for implants after primary total knee arthroplasty and for implants after total knee arthroplasty secondary to failed closing wedge osteotomy.

Results and Conclusions

The results of high tibial osteotomy have been studied and reported extensively since the 1960s. Insall[145] and Healy and Wilk[119] reviewed the experience of the 1960s through 1990s. The main conclusions that Insall[145] drew from his review were the following:

1. After a high tibial osteotomy, pain recurs in most knees, and most knees eventually require total knee arthroplasty.[219]
2. Younger patients with moderate varus deformities have the best results; obesity, undercorrection, and overcorrection[62,219] are adverse factors.
3. The ideal correction is a femorotibial angle between 170 degrees and 165 degrees
4. The overall preoperative state of the knee is the most important determinant of an eventual good result.[137]
5. Preoperative arthroscopic assessment of the knee is not useful.[167]
6. Previous medial meniscectomy[259] and anterior cruciate deficiency are not contraindications, but previous lateral meniscectomy may be.
7. The addition of tibial tubercle elevation to the osteotomy in the case of associated patellofemoral arthritis is unnecessary, and it increases the complication rate.[138,246]

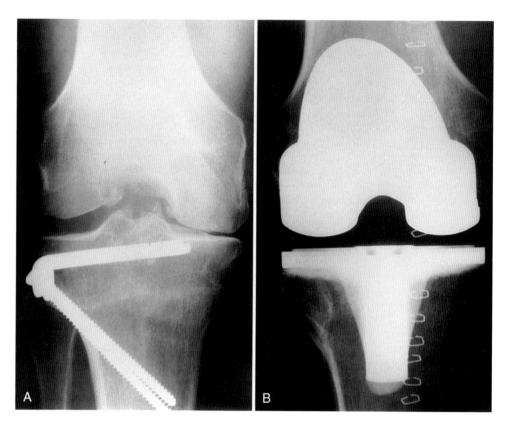

Figure 78–29. **A,** Late failure of a closing wedge high tibial osteotomy, internally fixed with a Giebel blade-plate. **B,** Uneventful one-step conversion to a total knee arthroplasty.

Taking into account the reports of the 1990s, my opinion remains similar to that of Insall, although some complementary information has been added, most of which has been discussed previously in this chapter.

The negative influence of the passage of time on the results of high tibial osteotomy has been confirmed repeatedly.* It is not clear, however, from the long-term follow-up studies available that a total knee arthroplasty would be the endpoint for most osteotomized knees, but rather that a conversion to total knee arthroplasty would be necessary in 5% to 15% of the osteotomized knees, although some authors report a relatively higher revision rate of about 20% to 25% at 10 years.[19,69] Holden and colleagues,[137] in a group of 51 proximal tibial valgus osteotomies reviewed with an average follow-up of 10 years, reported that 3 knees needed revision to a total arthroplasty. In a retrospective study of 128 osteoarthritic knees treated by valgus high tibial osteotomy, Rudan and Simurda[292] reported a relatively low revision rate of 10.9% over 15 years. Bouharras and colleagues[33] reported 4 conversions to total knee arthroplasties in a group of 118 high tibial osteotomies with an average follow-up of 8 years. Hernigou[123] reported 15 total knee arthroplasties after 93 osteotomies with a minimal follow-up of 20 years. Ivarsson and coworkers[151] reported 8 reoperations in a group of 65 knees reviewed at a mean of 11.9 years. Levigne and Bonnin,[191] in a study group of 217 osteotomies with an average follow-up of 9 years, reported 17 reoperations, including 5 repeat osteotomies, 1 unicompartmental knee arthroplasty, and 11 total knee arthroplasties. Lootvoet and colleagues[194] analyzed the results of a series of 193 upper tibial valgus osteotomies reviewed with an average follow-up of 8 years. Fourteen knees were operated on again because of a failure of the osteotomy; 3 repeat osteotomies, 1 unicompartmental arthroplasty, and 10 total knee arthroplasties were performed. Yasuda and colleagues[364,365] observed 56 osteotomies at a 10- to 15-year follow-up and reported 4 conversions to total knee arthroplasty. Odenbring and associates[255] reported on revision by repeat osteotomy or arthroplasty after tibial osteotomy in a consecutive series of 314 osteotomies at follow-up after 10 to 19 years; 52 knees had been revised by arthroplasty and 10 knees by repeat osteotomy.

The importance of precise postoperative alignment has been stressed in many reports.* There is no general agreement, however, about the optimal postoperative femorotibial alignment. If one tries to define a consensual ideal postoperative hip-knee-ankle angle, the obtained value approximates 3 to 6 degrees valgus, although Yasuda and colleagues[364,365] recommend a larger overcorrection, of up to 10 degrees valgus.

The influence of the preoperative grade of osteoarthritis on the long-term result of high tibial osteotomy also has been confirmed.[19,33,123,151,191,194,255,291,292] A preoperative Ahlbäck grade I or grade II is predictive of a good long-term result. Lootvoet and coworkers[194] reported an 84%

*References 4, 20, 22, 33, 54, 69, 123, 151, 194, 244, 255, 287, 315, 364, and 365.

*References 3, 19, 69, 123, 138, 151, 167, 191, 194, 244, 254, 255, 291, 292, 307, 308, 339, 364, and 365.

rate of good long-term results when the height of the preoperative medial joint space equaled or exceeded 50% of the normal height, whereas a narrowing greater than 50% reduced this rate to 60%. Excellent long-term results of high tibial osteotomy in young patients with Ahlbäck grade I medial gonarthrosis were reported by Odenbring and associates.[259] By measuring the constitutional tibial varus, Lootvoet and colleagues[194] and Levigne and Bonnin[190,191] also showed that when the cartilage lesion is secondary to bony deviation of the epiphysis in varus, a correction, even if incomplete, immediately brings mechanical relief. When there is a primary degeneration of cartilage, this "sick" cartilage does not tolerate any undercorrection.

The negative influence of age, obesity, hip disease, inflammatory diseases, preoperative deformity exceeding 10 degrees varus, femorotibial subluxation, and postoperative immobilization was discussed earlier. The mutual relationships between patellofemoral joint disorders and high tibial osteotomy and the advantages and disadvantages of the various osteotomy techniques and ways to deal with the fibula also have been analyzed.

From the numerous reported series of high tibial osteotomies, it is extremely difficult to make a precise estimate of the quality of the long-term results of this procedure. The selection criteria, surgical techniques, postoperative evaluation, and rating scales are extraordinarily disparate. Because most of the series are retrospective, few have reported the results of this procedure in a selected cohort of "ideal" candidates by the currently accepted standards. Because rigorous comparison between the series is impossible, I conclude this discussion by quoting the results and conclusions of two long-term follow-up studies conducted by Odenbring and colleagues.[255,259] The first study[259] describes the function after high tibial osteotomy for medial gonarthrosis in a group of 27 patients (28 knees) age 27 to 50 years. Of the 27 patients, 25, with an average follow-up of 11 years, had experienced improvement or great improvement, and 12 could participate in at least recreational exercise. Three-fifths of patients obtained a Lysholm[196] score of 84 points or more, and no revision to knee arthroplasty had been performed; sagittal instability or previous medial meniscectomy did not alter the results. This study shows that high tibial osteotomy is a beneficial procedure for young patients with gonarthrosis, including the increasing number of patients with gonarthrosis secondary to meniscal and ligamentous lesions, even if these patients maintain their active lifestyle.

The second study by Odenbring and colleagues[255] underlines the importance of surgical accuracy and appropriate correction of the angular deformity; in a group of 314 osteotomies at follow-up after 10 to 19 years, the revision rate was 54 of 170 in undercorrected knees and 8 of 144 in normocorrected or overcorrected knees. These knees were affected by early stages of gonarthrosis (Ahlbäck stages I through III).

High tibial osteotomy for medial gonarthrosis is a successful procedure in active, relatively young patients, with a good preoperative function and a low stage of arthritis. The results are better if the preoperative deformity is secondary to varus deviation of the epiphysis rather than to

medial wear of the joint. The axial correction should be accurate, and stable internal fixation with an early range of motion is advisable. The accuracy of the osteotomy and of its planning can be improved by a strict radiographic protocol, by the use of gait analysis,[166] by computer-aided analysis,[53,165] or by computer-assisted surgery.[225,276] The posterior tibial slope should not be altered by the osteotomy. Small corrections are performed easily with an opening wedge osteotomy. Closing wedge osteotomies are suitable for corrections of 10 to 15 degrees. In this case, a fibular shaft osteotomy seems biomechanically more logical than excision of the fibular head or division of the superior tibiofibular joint. The osteotomy of the fibula should be performed carefully at the junction of its middle and lower thirds. Given the risks related to transfixation pins, dome osteotomies should be set apart for the rare instances when a very large correction is necessary. Despite the remarkable results of knee arthroplasty, a place should remain for a surgical procedure aimed at maintaining the natural knee because this effort goes in the direction of the development of conservative treatment of arthritis, which is clearly the way of the future.

TREATMENT FOR VALGUS DEFORMITY

Principles

Valgus deformity of the knee usually is secondary to a valgus orientation of the distal part of the femur with regard to its long axis.[58,269,368] In this case, the line tangent to the distal extent of the femoral condyles is tilted medially and distally. To bring the joint line parallel to the floor through osteotomy, the deformity has to be corrected where it lies (i.e., in the distal femur).[58,119,145,304]

In some knees, the valgus deformity has a dual origin; the distal condyles are sloped medially, whereas the tibial plateau is sloped laterally.[190,269] In these knees, if the deformity is mild and the correction less than 10 degrees, a tibial osteotomy can be successful.[17,66,77,217] A tibial osteotomy should not be used for larger corrections, however, because the resultant tilt of the joint line in time would cause medial subluxation of the femur on the tibia,[113,145,304] whereas a tibial closing wedge osteotomy proximal to the tibial tubercle would create or increase laxity of the superficial medial ligament.[145]

Valgus deformities are tolerated better than varus deformities and develop arthritic changes later on.[183,204] This situation is explained by the adduction moment that places the gravity forces predominantly on the medial compartment during gait.[12,26,102,114,158,204,206,272,326,342] A severe valgus deformity is necessary to shift the gravity stresses toward the lateral compartment.[302] In the varus knee, the adduction moment is counteracted by the contraction of the lateral muscles[12,26,206,208]; this results in higher loading of the knee joint.[12] In contrast, in the valgus knee, the activity of the lateral muscles may decrease,[183,204] resulting in lower compressive forces across the joint.

A pathological ipsilateral hip joint can increase the stresses on the lateral compartment of the knee[93,145,183,281,326] by two main mechanisms. The gluteus major, the tensor fasciae latae, and the biceps act on the hip and the knee. If their activity is augmented to stabilize an abnormal hip, it increases the compressive forces on the lateral compartment of the knee at the same time.[204] If the hip is abducted during the stance phase of gait (i.e., if the pelvis tilts upward on the unaffected side), the center of gravity of the body is displaced laterally, also enhancing the stresses on the lateral compartment of the knee.[326] Whenever possible, a hip pathology should be treated before performing an osteotomy of the underlying knee.[145]

In varus knees, overcorrection is necessary because of the presence of an adduction moment during gait. In contrast, in valgus knees, there is no need for hypercorrection because it has been shown that in a neutrally aligned knee, most of the gravity forces are transmitted through the medial compartment.[12,206,208,302] The goal of a varus osteotomy should be to bring the hip-knee-ankle angle close to 0 degrees.

Patient Selection

The criteria of age and activity level should be even more restrictive for femoral supracondylar varus osteotomy than for proximal tibial valgus osteotomy because the time the bone takes to heal and the period of partial weight-bearing on crutches are longer. Because lateral compartmental arthrosis usually develops later in life than medial compartmental arthrosis, is often better tolerated, and has a lower incidence,[8,122] the indications for varus osteotomy of the knee are less frequent, and a total knee arthroplasty often is preferred. The procedure should be performed relatively early in the disease process before severe compromise of function has occurred,[88,214,218] and the arthrosis should be limited to the lateral compartment.[88,89,218]

Severe instability is a contraindication to osteotomy[145] because there are no dynamic restraints to medial laxity, which persists even if the alignment is correct. Extension loss of more than 15 degrees and flexion less than 90 degrees also are contraindications.[220,236] Hernigou and colleagues,[126] in a retrospective study of 96 valgus arthritic knees, noticed that femoral osteotomy or lateral unicompartmental arthroplasty led to poor results if undertaken in the presence of a preoperative recurvatum. Recurvatum seldom occurs as a consequence of valgus gonarthrosis and appears at a late stage of arthritic evolution. At this stage, a total knee arthroplasty is the appropriate option.

Stubbs[316] described a specific pattern of valgus knees, in which the degenerative changes are confined to the posterolateral portion of the knee. The symptoms often begin at a young age, the pain is posterolateral, and a history of trauma and a previous lateral meniscectomy frequently are noted. Bone-on-bone contact in the posterolateral corner of the knee can be seen with a posteroanterior flexion weightbearing view, but is not detected with standing radiographs in extension. Based on three failures in three osteotomized knees, Stubbs[316] considered that posterolateral arthritis of the knee may be a contraindication to valgus osteotomy because this offers an angular solution for a rotatory problem.

Surgical Techniques

Several techniques are available for the correction of a valgus deformity at the femur. The surgical procedure may be performed from a lateral approach employing an opening wedge osteotomy, or a medial wedge can be resected from a medial approach. A medial closing wedge osteotomy is the most common procedure (Fig. 78–30). Supracondylar dome osteotomies,[355] V osteotomies,[7] and intercondylar osteotomies[74] also have been described. Gugenheim and Brinker[110] reported favorable results of 14 supracondylar percutaneous dome osteotomies, using temporary external fixation and insertion of an intramedullary nail.

MEDIAL CLOSING WEDGE SUPRACONDYLAR OSTEOTOMY

The patient is placed in the supine position. A tourniquet generally is applied. A longitudinal medial or straight midline incision is made along the femur, beginning from just distal to the joint line and extending proximally for 15 cm. The fascia over the vastus medialis is incised, and the muscle is deflected forward and laterally. Dissection is carried distally to the joint capsule, but the joint is not entered. If the blade-plate that is to be used is cannulated and guided by a wire,[95,183,270] the technique is similar to that described for the closing wedge proximal tibial valgus osteotomy with internal fixation by blade-plate (Fig. 78–31). The guide wire is inserted using a special jig, set for a predetermined amount of correction. The track for the blade is initiated, then the desired wedge of bone is removed, the osteotomy is closed, and the blade-plate is driven over the guide wire and fixed to the femoral cortex with screws. The obtained angular correction is the complementary angle between the angle set on the guide and the 90-degree angle of the blade-plate. More often than not, the blade-plate that is used is not cannulated and is an AO-type, 90-degree offset, dynamic-compression blade-plate.[220] The correction relies in this case on the accurate positioning of pins under fluoroscopic control, but special jigs also have been designed to guide a 90-degree AO blade-plate.[185]

The first pin guides the osteotomy blade-plate. It is inserted across the distal femoral metaphysis, approximately 2.5 cm proximal to the femoral articular surfaces, using fluoroscopy. McDermott and colleagues[220] advised placing the blade parallel to the articular surfaces. This placement results in approximately 6 degrees of mechanical varus, which seems excessive, as already discussed. I believe the guiding pin should not be strictly parallel to the joint line, but slightly oblique distally and laterally, which is facilitated by using a guide. A second pin is placed proximally across the diaphysis, perpendicular to the long axis of the femur. These first two pins should become parallel at the end of the procedure. Then two pins are inserted, with the help of a goniometer or templates, to figure the wedge, which is removed. The proximal side of the wedge is perpendicular to the shaft of the femur. Care should be taken to keep a medial cortical bridge of

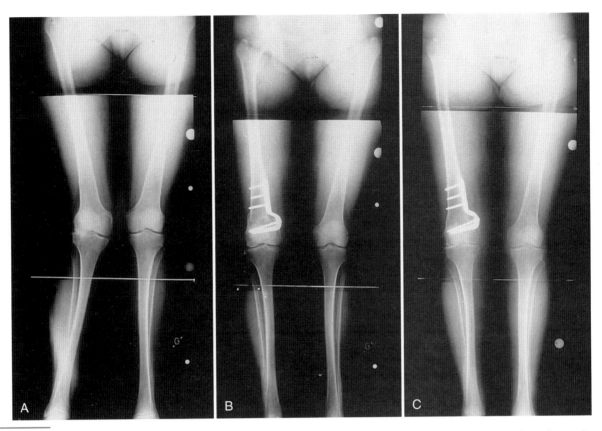

Figure 78–30. **A,** A 17-degree valgus deformity in a 55-year-old woman. **B,** Bipodal standing radiograph at 9 months after medial closing wedge supracondylar osteotomy. **C,** Satisfactory radiological and functional result at 10 years.

at least 2 cm between the osteotomy line and the blade. An oscillating saw is used to perform the osteotomy. The lateral cortex is weakened with a thin osteotome, but is not interrupted with the saw. As mentioned by Insall,[145] there is a tendency to overestimate the necessary wedge, which leads to overcorrection. It is wiser to start with a slightly thinner osteotomy than ultimately might be required.[236] If a greater correction is necessary, this usually can be obtained by crutching the distal femur in the softer metaphyseal bone rather than by taking additional bone from the distal segment. The blade-plate is driven across the distal metaphysis along the line of the initially placed pin, and the wedge is closed by manually exerting a varus force on the knee. Before an AO angled blade-plate can be inserted into bone, a channel must be drilled and precut with the U-profile chisel; this is performed more easily before completion of the osteotomy. Three to four screws secure the plate to the femur. The removed bone can serve as a graft. The tourniquet is released, careful hemostasis is performed, a suction drain is placed, and the wound is closed. Continuous passive motion is started immediately, and weightbearing is restricted until bony union is confirmed on radiographs.

Instead of a rigid blade-plate, Stahelin and colleagues[310,311] recommended the use of a malleable semi-tubular plate, bent to form an angled plate, and lag screws. Specific plates more recently have been designed for fixation of supracondylar closing wedge osteotomies. Similar to the plate designed for tibial closing wedge osteotomy, Surer[318,319] developed a distal femoral plate with set screws aimed at fixing the screws to the plate (Fig. 78–32).

LATERAL OPENING WEDGE SUPRACONDYLAR OSTEOTOMY

Lateral opening wedge supracondylar osteotomy has been described by Postel and Langlais.[183,270] It requires a lateral approach, and the use of a guided blade-plate angled at 95 degrees (Fig. 78–33). The patient is placed in the lateral position. The lateral side of the distal femur is exposed by a straight lateral approach, reflecting the vastus lateralis anteriorly. Using a jig, the guide wire is inserted in the epiphysis, 20 to 30 mm proximal to the joint line. Because the blade-plate has a 95-degree angle, the angle between the guide wire and the lateral femoral cortex should equal the sum of the desired correction plus 95 degrees. This wire should be parallel to the axis of flexion of the knee. Another wire figures the osteotomy line, which should leave a lateral cortical bridge of 25 mm proximal to the blade. The position of these two wires is checked under fluoroscopy. The osteotomy is performed with an oscillating saw, keeping the medial cortex temporarily intact. The blade-plate is inserted on the guide wire and partly driven into the epiphyseal bone, and the osteotomy

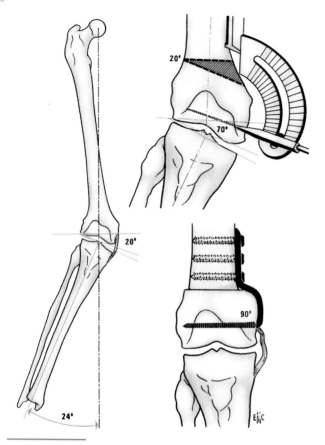

Figure 78–31. Medial closing wedge supracondylar osteotomy with the use of a cannulated blade-plate, guided by a wire. In this case, the 24-degree valgus deformity is secondary to a 20-degree distal femoral valgus deviation and to a 4-degree medial laxity. If the goal is to bring the hip-knee-ankle angle to 0 degrees, the correction and the resected wedge should be 20 degrees. The jig used to insert the guide wire should be set at 70 degrees because the blade-plate has a 90-degree angle. (From Langlais F, Thomazeau H: Ostéotomies du genou. In: Encyclopédie Médico-Chirurgicale: Techniques Chirurgicales, Orthopédie. Paris, Editions scientifiques et médicales Elsevier, 1989, p 1.)

is completed using thin chisels. The insertion of the blade-plate is achieved, opening the wedge laterally. Impaction can be realized manually by striking the flexed knee. The plate is fixed to the femur by three screws in the proximal fragment and one additional screw in the distal fragment. An AO 95-degree condylar blade-plate also can be used,[214] losing the advantage offered by the "automatic" correction. This opening wedge osteotomy does not require autologous bone grafting because medial impaction is created. It should not be used for corrections greater than 15 to 20 degrees, given the risk of stretching the peroneal nerve. Postoperative care is similar to that of closing wedge osteotomy.

Puddu and colleagues[274] designed plates with metal blocks of varying height, specifically devoted to lateral opening wedge supracondylar osteotomy (Fig. 78–34). Their use follows the same principles as for the block-plates designed for tibial opening wedge osteotomy. Specific locking plates (Tomofix, AO/Synthes) also have been developed for femoral opening wedge osteotomy (Fig. 78–35). With the Puddu plate and the Tomofix internal fixator, the medial femoral cortex acts as a hinge and should be kept intact. Impaction is not allowed, and the opening wedge should be filled in by a bone graft or a bone substitute.[247]

Complications

Supracondylar femoral osteotomy is technically demanding and is not performed frequently. It has a high rate of complications. Teinturier and colleagues,[324] in a series of 131 lateral supracondylar osteotomies, reported 4 infections treated by removal of the blade-plate, 1 nonunion successfully treated by iterative plating, and 5 deep vein thromboses. Weill and Jacquemin,[355] in a series of 39 dome supracondylar varus osteotomies internally fixed by a lateral blade-plate, reported 1 nonunion, 1 fracture secondary to a subsequent trauma, 1 hypocorrection with early reintervention, and 1 severe loss of motion. Aglietti and associates,[7] in a preliminary report of 14 V-shaped supracondylar osteotomies, followed by an immobilization period of 8 weeks, did not report any complications. Aglietti and Menchetti[5] reviewed the long-term results of 18 distal femoral varus osteotomies and reported no infection or nonunion. Edgerton and colleagues,[88,236] in a group of 24 knees treated by supracondylar osteotomies, usually fixed by staples, reported complications in 15 patients (63%), including a pin-tract infection in 1 patient treated with an external fixator, loss of correction and failure of fixation in 9 patients, and delayed union or nonunion in 7 patients. Of 24 medial closing wedge supracondylar osteotomies, McDermott and coworkers[220] reported 1 failure of fixation that required reoperation, 1 manipulation for stiffness at 6 months postoperatively, 1 superficial wound infection, and 1 nonfatal pulmonary embolism.

Learmonth[185] had no complications in 12 consecutive valgus knees corrected by a femoral closing wedge osteotomy performed with the help of a special jig. Cameron and colleagues,[41] reporting on 49 consecutive patients treated by supracondylar varus closing wedge osteotomy stabilized with a blade-plate, had 6 cases of delayed union, 1 case of loss of fixation, and 1 case of rotatory deformity. All delayed unions were treated successfully with lateral compression plating and occasionally with autogenous bone grafting from the iliac crest.[40] Healy and associates[118] evaluated the results of 23 distal femoral varus osteotomies and reported 2 cases of nonunion, 1 case of fracture, and 1 case of stiffness that necessitated a manipulation under anesthesia. Mathews and colleagues,[218] in a group of 21 supracondylar osteotomies, had a complication rate of 57%, including severe knee stiffness requiring manipulation under anesthesia (48%), nonunion/delayed union (19%), infection (10%), and fixation failure (5%). Five knees (19%) required total knee replacement within 5 years of surgery. Mironneau[228] analyzed the results of 28 supracondylar osteotomies, including 5 closing wedge osteotomies, 4 opening wedge

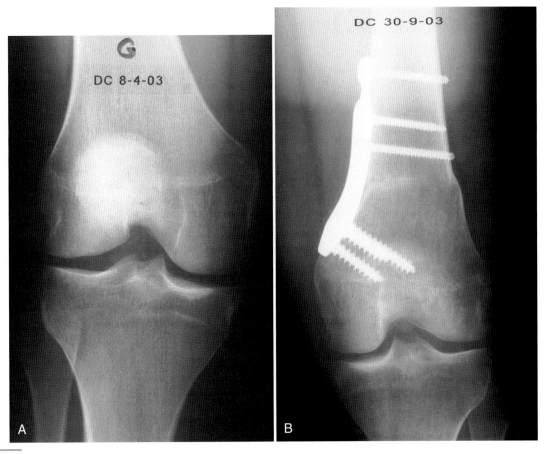

Figure 78–32. **A** and **B,** Closing wedge supracondylar osteotomy fixed by Surer's plate. The screws are locked to the plate by set screws. The osteotomy was performed to prevent progression of lateral unicompartmental arthritis secondary to lateral meniscectomy in a 19-year-old patient.

osteotomies, and 19 dome osteotomies, all fixed by a blade-plate. The morbidity was high, with three losses of fixation, one fracture, one nonunion, and one arthrofibrosis.

The reported complication rate varies and is technique dependent. As stated by Aglietti and associates,[7] avoiding to enter the knee joint should reduce the incidence of stiffness. A rigid internal fixation is mandatory, given the high rate of loss of fixation and nonunion when staples are used. It is uncertain whether the fixation provided by a medial blade-plate is sufficient, and one could look for better implants. The use of an oscillating saw could increase the risk of nonunion because of its thermal effect, and osteotomes or special saw blades with irrigation should be used. The lateral cortex should not be interrupted when performing a closing wedge osteotomy, and this could be eased by the use of a device for progressive closure of the osteotomy. McDermott and colleagues[220] feared that the use of the outrigger AO compression could endanger the femoral vessels in the Hunter canal, but a compression clamp similar to the ones designed for closing wedge high tibial osteotomy could be sufficient to close the resection site in a slow, controlled manner while

under compression. The use of the resected bone as a graft is recommended.

Results of Supracondylar Osteotomy

Few reports allow a clear estimation of the anticipated results of supracondylar osteotomy. The series are small, and the average follow-up time is short. The average follow-up in McDermott's series[220] was 4 years. Average follow-up was 2 years in Aglietti's preliminary series.[2] Average follow-up was 4 years for Healy and colleagues,[118] 3.5 years for Cameron and associates,[41] 41 months for Learmonth,[185] and 3 years for Teinturier and colleagues[324] and Mathews and coworkers.[218]

Some long-term results nevertheless have been published. They are generally good, despite a high complication rate. Mironneau[228] reported 8 excellent, 13 good, 4 fair, and 3 poor results in 28 patients with an average 7-year follow-up. He stated that the key factor was a precise axial correction and recommended bringing the mechanical axis to neutral except in the case of medial laxity. In

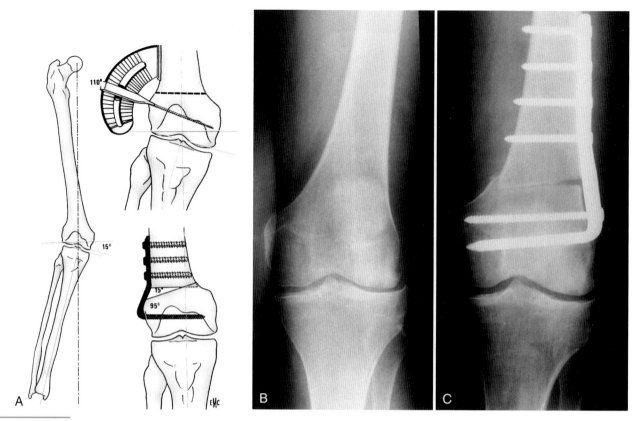

Figure 78–33. **A,** Lateral opening wedge osteotomy with the use of a cannulated blade-plate guided by a wire. In the absence of medial laxity, the correction should equal the preoperative valgus deformity. Because the blade-plate has a 95-degree angle, the jig should be set at 110 degrees to correct a 15-degree valgus deformity. **B,** A 9-degree valgus deformity in a 44-year-old woman. **C,** Immediate postoperative x-ray shows the medial impaction and the lateral opening created by the osteotomy. (**A** from Langlais F, Thomazeau H: Ostéotomies du genou. In: Encyclopédie Médico-Chirurgicale: Techniques Chirurgicales, Orthopédie. Paris, Editions scientifiques et médicales Elsevier, 1989, p 1.)

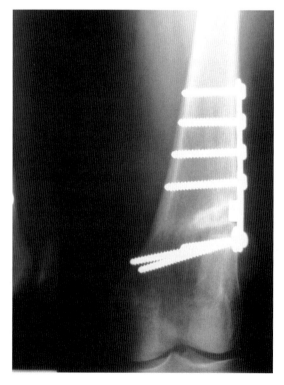

Figure 78–34. Puddu's lateral distal femoral plate, used for correction of a 15-degree valgus deformity secondary to asymmetric physeal closure.

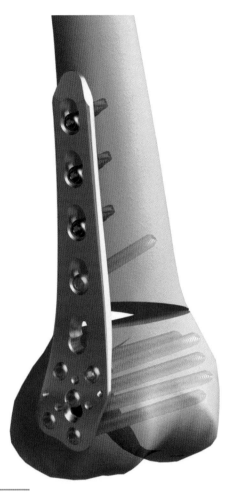

Figure 78–35. TomoFix lateral distal femoral plate. (Courtesy of Synthes from the surgical technique "TomoFix Knee Osteotomy System." © 2003 Stratec Medical, Switzerland.)

Using the Hospital for Special Surgery knee score in a group of 24 knees with an average follow-up of 8.3 years (range 5 to 11 years), Edgerton and colleagues[88] reported 71% good or excellent results. The severity of the disease was a statistically significant prognostic factor, as reflected by the preoperative and postoperative knee scores. The results were better when the disease was limited to the lateral compartment. This study did not document a tendency for a good result, when attained, to deteriorate with time, in contrast to the experience with proximal tibial osteotomy for varus deformity.

Aglietti and Menchetti[5] evaluated the results of 18 distal femoral varus osteotomies with an average 9-years follow-up. At follow-up, 77% of knees were rated as good or excellent by the Knee Society rating system. One knee required a subsequent total knee arthroplasty 5 years after osteotomy.

Finkelstein and coworkers[89] monitored 21 knees long-term or until failure. At an average follow-up of 11 years, 13 osteotomies were still successful, and 7 had failed; one patient had died. The probability of survival at 10 years was 64%. All the patients who had a failure subsequently underwent a total knee arthroplasty. The three early failures were attributed to poor selection of patients or failure of the fixation. The remaining four patients who had a failure were able to function for 72 to 98 months before they needed a conversion to a total knee arthroplasty. The authors did not find that a previous varus osteotomy of the distal part of the femur made a subsequent total knee arthroplasty more technically demanding, in contrast to Beyer and colleagues,[21] who reported increased technical difficulty when total joint arthroplasty was performed after supracondylar varus osteotomy. Cameron and Park[42] reviewed eight cases of total knee replacement after supracondylar varus femoral osteotomy and stated that, although in each case the distal femur was offset medially on the femoral diaphysis, it did not prove difficult to achieve correct mechanical alignment. Cameron and Park[42] advised hardware removal 6 months before total knee replacement. They stressed the importance of carefully templating the position of the femoral guidance system and of obtaining an intraoperative radiograph of the femoral guidance rod if there is any doubt about its accurate positioning. In these three series of conversion of supracondylar osteotomies to total knee arthroplasty, the ultimate result of arthroplasty was not compromised (Fig. 78–36).

From these reports, it seems that with proper selection of patients, exact correction of the femorotibial alignment, and stable fixation, varus osteotomy of the distal part of the femur is a reliable and effective procedure for the treatment of gonarthrosis of the lateral compartment in valgus knees. The ideal candidate is physiologically young and active, has an isolated grade I or grade II lateral compartmental arthrosis, and has a good preoperative function and range of motion. The candidate should not have recurvatum, posterolateral arthritis, marked medial laxity, or severe wear of the lateral tibial plateau. These criteria are stringent and are attained by a limited number of patients; most valgus arthritic knees are more suitable for a total knee replacement.

this situation, some hypercorrection is necessary. In the presence of medial laxity and severe wear of the lateral tibial plateau, an arthroplasty rather than an osteotomy should be performed.

Cognet and associates[57] reported the results of 75 closing wedge supracondylar osteotomies fixed by a guided blade-plate, with an average follow-up of 8.7 years (range 5 to 14 years). The mechanical axis at follow-up was 0.1 degree varus. Of all the patients, 77% were satisfied or very satisfied. The ideal candidate is active, has less than 15 degrees flexion contracture, and has an isolated lateral arthritis at an Ahlbäck[8] stage I or II.

Terry and Cimino[325] monitored a series of 36 knees for an average of 5.4 years, on which a medial closing wedge osteotomy (14 knees) or a lateral opening wedge osteotomy with bone grafting (22 knees) had been performed. Postoperative correction of the anatomic axis averaged 3.8 degrees valgus with a wide dispersion (range 8 degrees varus to 20 degrees valgus). Pain decreased or resolved in 21 of 35 knees (60 degrees), and activity level improved in 24 of 35 knees (69 degrees). One patient was unavailable for follow-up evaluation.

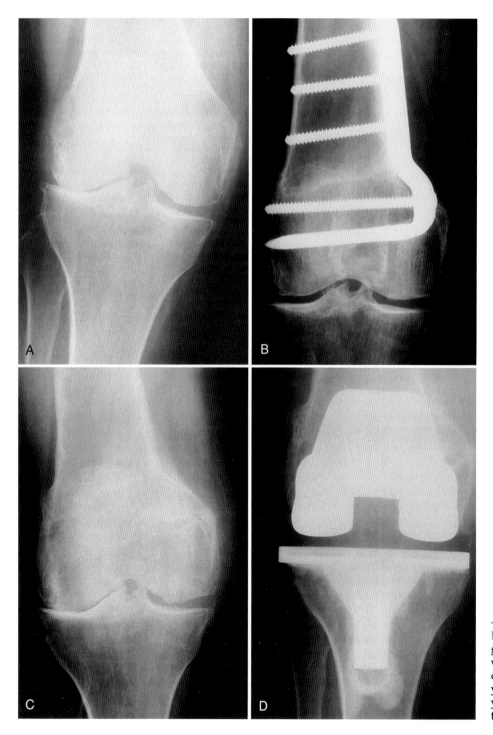

Figure 78–36. **A,** Severe lateral gonarthrosis in a 57-year-old woman. **B,** Result of a medial closing wedge osteotomy at 1 year. **C,** Deterioration at 11 years. **D,** Successful conversion to a total knee arthroplasty.

References

1. Adili A, Bhandari M, Giffin R, et al: Valgus high tibial osteotomy: Comparison between an Ilizarov and a Coventry wedge technique for the treatment of medial compartment osteoarthritis of the knee. Knee Surg Sports Traumatol Arthrosc 10:169-176, 2002.
2. Aglietti P, Buzzi R: Idiopathic osteonecrosis of the knee. Ital J Orthop Traumatol 10:217-226, 1984.
3. Aglietti P, Buzzi R, Gaudenzi A, et al: [Accuracy in high tibial osteotomy in varus gonarthrosis]. Arch Putti Chir Organi Mov 37:271-282, 1989.
4. Aglietti P, Buzzi R, Vena LM, et al: High tibial valgus osteotomy for medial gonarthrosis: A 10- to 21-year study. J Knee Surg 16:21-26, 2003.
5. Aglietti P, Menchetti PP: Distal femoral varus osteotomy in the valgus osteoarthritic knee. Am J Knee Surg 13:89-95, 2000.
6. Aglietti P, Rinonapoli E, Stringa G, et al: Tibial osteotomy for the varus osteoarthritic knee. Clin Orthop 176:239-251, 1983.
7. Aglietti P, Stringa G, Buzzi R, et al: Correction of valgus knee deformity with a supracondylar V osteotomy. Clin Orthop 217:214-220, 1987.
8. Ahlback S: Osteoarthrosis of the knee: A radiographic investigation. Acta Radiol (Stockh) 227(Suppl):1-72, 1968.
9. Ahlberg A, Scham S, Unander SL: Osteotomy in degenerative and rheumatoid arthritis of the knee joint. Acta Orthop Scand 39:379-388, 1968.
10. Akamatsu Y, Koshino T, Saito T, et al: Changes in osteosclerosis of the osteoarthritic knee after high tibial osteotomy. Clin Orthop 334:207-214, 1997.
11. Amendola A, Rorabeck CH, Bourne RB, et al: Total knee arthroplasty following high tibial osteotomy for osteoarthritis. J Arthroplasty 4(Suppl):S11-S17, 1989.
12. Andriacchi TP: Dynamics of knee malalignment. Orthop Clin North Am 25:395-403, 1994.
13. Augereau B: [Radiological assessment before femoral and tibial osteotomies]. Ann Radiol Paris 36:252-255, 1993.
14. Aydogdu S, Sur H: [High tibial osteotomy for varus deformity of more than 20 degrees]. Rev Chir Orthop Reparatrice Appar Mot 84:439-446, 1997.
15. Badhe NP, Forster IW: High tibial osteotomy in knee instability: The rationale of treatment and early results. Knee Surg Sports Traumatol Arthrosc 10:38-43, 2002.
16. Bae DK, Mun MS, Kwon OS: A newly designed miniplate staple for high tibial osteotomy. Bull Hosp Joint Dis 56:167-170, 1997.
17. Bauer GC, Insall J, Koshino T: Tibial osteotomy in gonarthrosis (osteo-arthritis of the knee). J Bone Joint Surg Am 51:1545-1563, 1969.
18. Bergenudd H, Sahlstrom A, Sanzen L: Total knee arthroplasty after failed proximal tibial valgus osteotomy. J Arthroplasty 12:635-638, 1997.
19. Berman AT, Bosacco SJ, Kirshner S, et al: Factors influencing long-term results in high tibial osteotomy. Clin Orthop 272:192-198, 1991.
20. Bettin D, Karbowski A, Schwering L, et al: Time-dependent clinical and roentgenographical results of Coventry high tibial valgisation osteotomy. Arch Orthop Trauma Surg 117: 53-57, 1998.
21. Beyer CA, Lewallen DG, Hanssen AD: Total knee arthroplasty following prior osteotomy of the distal femur. Am J Knee Surg 7:25-30, 1994.
22. Billings A, Scott DF, Camargo MP, et al: High tibial osteotomy with a calibrated osteotomy guide, rigid internal fixation, and early motion: Long-term follow-up. J Bone Joint Surg Am 82:70-79, 2000.
23. Blackburne JS, Peel TE: A new method of measuring patellar height. J Bone Joint Surg Br 59:241-242, 1977.
24. Blaimont P: The curviplane osteotomy in the treatment of the knee arthrosis. SICOT, 11th meeting, Mexico, October 10, 1969.
25. Blaimont P: [Curviplane osteotomy in the treatment of gonarthrosis]. Acta Orthop Belg 48:97-109, 1982.
26. Blaimont P, Burnotte J, Baillon JM, et al: Contribution biomécanique à l'étude des conditions d'équilibre dans le genou normal et pathologique: Application au traitement de l'arthrose varisante. Acta Orthop Belg 37:573-591, 1971.
27. Blaimont P, Burnotte J, Halleux P: La préarthrose du genou: Pathogénie biomécanique et traitement prophylactique. Acta Orthop Belg 41:177-200, 1975.
28. Blaimont P, Schoon R: A propos de 2 cas de gonarthrose associée à un vice de torsion interne du tibia. Acta Orthop Belg 43:476-481, 1977.
29. Bonnevialle P, Abid A, Mansat P, et al: [Tibial valgus osteotomy using a tricalcium phosphate medial wedge: A minimally invasive technique]. Rev Chir Orthop Reparatrice Appar Mot 88:486-492, 2002.
30. Bonnin M, Chambat P: [Current status of valgus angle, tibial head closing wedge osteotomy in media gonarthrosis]. Orthopade 33:135-142, 2004.
31. Booth REJ: TKA revision after osteotomy. Orthopedics 17:859-860, 1994.
32. Boss A, Stutz G, Oursin C, et al: Anterior cruciate ligament reconstruction combined with valgus tibial osteotomy (combined procedure). Knee Surg Sports Traumatol Arthrosc 3:187-191, 1995.
33. Bouharras M, Hoet F, Watillon M, et al: [Results of tibial valgus osteotomy for internal femoro-tibial arthritis with an average 8-year follow-up]. Acta Orthop Belg 60:163-169, 1994.
34. Bouillet R, Van Gaver PH: L'arthrose du genou: Étude pathogénique et traitement. Acta Orthop Belg 27:1-188, 1961.
35. Bove JC: [Utilization of a porous alumina ceramic spacer in tibial valgus open-wedge osteotomy: Fifty cases at 16 months mean follow-up]. Rev Chir Orthop Reparatrice Appar Mot 88:480-485, 2002.
36. Brueckmann FR, Kettelkamp DB: Proximal tibial osteotomy. Orthop Clin North Am 13:3-16, 1982.
37. Buechel FF: A sequential three-step lateral release for correcting fixed valgus knee deformities during total knee arthroplasty. Clin Orthop 260:170-175, 1990.
38. Burdin P, Bercovy M, Hernigou P, et al: [Total knee arthroplasty after tibial or femoral osteotomy: Round table of the French Society of Hip and Knee Surgery (SFGH) (78th Annual meeting of the SOFCOT). Abstracts]. Rev Chir Orthop Reparatrice Appar Mot 90:372-384, 2004.
39. Calista F, Pegreffi P: High tibial osteotomy: Osteotomy in minus or hemicallotasis with EAF? Chir Organi Mov 81:155-163, 1996.
40. Cameron HU: Repair of nonunion of supracondylar femoral osteotomy. Orthop Rev 21:349-350, 1992.
41. Cameron HU, Botsford DJ, Park YS: Prognostic factors in the outcome of supracondylar femoral osteotomy for lateral compartment osteoarthritis of the knee. Can J Surg 40:114-118, 1997.
42. Cameron HU, Park YS: Total knee replacement after supracondylar femoral osteotomy. Am J Knee Surg 10:70-71, 1997.
43. Cameron HU, Welsh RP: Potential complications of total knee replacement following tibial osteotomy. Orthop Rev 17:39-43, 1988.
44. Cameron HU, Welsh RP, Jung YB, et al: Repair of nonunion of tibial osteotomy. Clin Orthop 287:167-169, 1993.
45. Cameron JC, Saha S: Management of medial collateral ligament laxity. Orthop Clin North Am 25:527-532, 1994.
46. Carr A, Keyes G, Miller R, et al: Medial unicompartmental arthroplasty: A survival study of the Oxford meniscal knee. Clin Orthop 295:205-213, 1993.
47. Cass JR, Bryan RS: High tibial osteotomy. Clin Orthop 230:196-199, 1988.
48. Catagni MA, Guerreschi F, Ahmad TS, et al: Treatment of genu varum in medial compartment osteoarthritis of the knee using the Ilizarov method. Orthop Clin North Am 25:509-514, 1994.
49. Caton J, Deschamps G, Chambat P, et al: Les rotules basses: A propos de 128 observations. Rev Chir Orthop 68:317-325, 1982.
50. Causero A, Tcherkes-Zade T, Tcherkes-Zade D, et al: The Ilizarov technique in the treatment of osteoarthritic genu varum. Chir Organi Mov 87:235-240, 2002.
51. Chan RN, Pollard JP: High tibial osteotomy for rheumatoid arthritis of the knee: A one to six year follow-up study. Acta Orthop Scand 49:78-84, 1978.
52. Chao EY, Neluheni EVD, Hsu RW, et al: Biomechanics of malalignment. Orthop Clin North Am 25:379-386, 1994.
53. Chao EY, Sim FH: Computer-aided preoperative planning in knee osteotomy. Iowa Orthop J 15:4-18, 1995.

54. Choi HR, Hasegawa Y, Kondo S, et al: High tibial osteotomy for varus gonarthrosis: A 10- to 24-year follow-up study. J Orthop Sci 6:493-497, 1904.

55. Christodoulou N, Moussas T, Karaindros C, et al: [Osteosynthesis of tibial valgus osteotomies by goniometric CH-N external fixator]. Rev Chir Orthop Reparatrice Appar Mot 82:331-335, 1996.

56. Closkey RF, Windsor RE: Alterations in the patella after a high tibial or distal femoral osteotomy. Clin Orthop 389:51-56, 2001.

57. Cognet JM, Rouvillain JL, Mousselard HP, et al: Résultat des ostéotomies fémorales de varisation pour genu valgum: A propos de 75 cas revus à plus de cinq ans de recul. Rev Chir Orthop Reparatrice Appar Mot 84:46, 1998.

58. Cooke TD, Bryant JT, Scudamore RA: Biomechanical factors in alignment and arthritic disorders of the knee. In Fu FH, Harner CD, Vince KG (eds): Knee Surgery. Baltimore, Williams & Wilkins, 1994, pp 1061-1078.

59. Cooke TD, Li J, Scudamore RA: Radiographic assessment of bony contributions to knee deformity. Orthop Clin North Am 25:387-393, 1994.

60. Cooke TD, Pichora D, Siu D, et al: Surgical implications of varus deformity of the knee with obliquity of joint surfaces. J Bone Joint Surg Br 71:560-565, 1989.

61. Coventry MB: Osteotomy of the upper portion of the tibia for degenerative arthritis of the knee: A preliminary report. J Bone Joint Surg Am 47:984-990, 1965.

62. Coventry MB: Osteotomy about the knee for degenerative and rheumatoid arthritis. J Bone Joint Surg Am 55:23-48, 1973.

63. Coventry MB: Upper tibial osteotomy for gonarthrosis: The evolution of the operation in the last 18 years and long term results. Orthop Clin North Am 10:191-210, 1979.

64. Coventry MB: Upper tibial osteotomy. Clin Orthop 182:46-52, 1984.

65. Coventry MB: Upper tibial osteotomy for osteoarthritis. J Bone Joint Surg Am 67:1136-1140, 1985.

66. Coventry MB: Proximal tibial varus osteotomy for osteoarthritis of the lateral compartment of the knee. J Bone Joint Surg Am 69:32-38, 1987.

67. Coventry MB: Osteotomy of the upper portion of the tibia for degenerative arthritis of the knee: A preliminary report. 1965 [classical article]. Clin Orthop 248:4-8, 1989.

68. Coventry MB, Bowman PW: Long-term results of upper tibial osteotomy for degenerative arthritis of the knee. Acta Orthop Belg 48:139-156, 1982.

69. Coventry MB, Ilstrup DM, Wallrichs SL: Proximal tibial osteotomy: A critical long-term study of eighty-seven cases. J Bone Joint Surg Am 75:196-201, 1993.

70. Curley P, Eyres K, Brezinova V, et al: Common peroneal nerve dysfunction after high tibial osteotomy. J Bone Joint Surg Br 72:405-408, 1990.

71. de Pablos J, Gonzalez Herranz P, Barrios C: Progressive opening-wedge osteotomy for severe tibia vara in adults. Orthopedics 21:1253-1257, 1998.

72. Debeyre J, Artigou JM: [Long term results of 260 tibial osteotomies for frontal deviations of the knee]. Rev Chir Orthop Reparatrice Appar Mot 58:335-339, 1972.

73. Debeyre J, Artigou JM: [Indications and results of tibial osteotomy: Influence of laxity]. Rev Chir Orthop Reparatrice Appar Mot 59:641-656, 1973.

74. Debeyre J, Frain P: [An intercondylar femoral osteotomy technique in the management of knee deviations due to arthrosis]. Ann Chir 21:548-553, 1967.

75. Debeyre J, Patte D: Place des osteotomies de correction dans le traitement de la gonarthrose. Acta Orthop Belg 27:374-383, 1961.

76. Dejour H: Indications thérapeutiques dans l'arthrose fémoro-tibiale. In Dejour H, Neyret P (eds): Journées Lyonnaises de Chirurgie du Genou. Lyon, Hopital de Lyon Sud, 1991, pp 414-414.

77. Dejour H: L'ostéotomie tibiale de varisation: Résultats: À propos de 118 cas. In Dejour H, Neyret P (eds): Journées Lyonnaises de Chirurgie du Genou. Lyon, Hopital de Lyon Sud, 1991, pp 169-180.

78. Dejour H, Neyret P, Boileau P, et al: Anterior cruciate reconstruction combined with valgus tibial osteotomy. Clin Orthop 299:220-228, 1994.

79. Delloye Ch: Les implants osseux lyophilisés. Rev Chir Orthop 74:149-150, 1988.

80. Delloye Ch, Allington N, Munting E, et al: L'os de banque lyophilisé: Technique et résultats après trois années d'utilisation. Acta Orthop Belg 53:2-11, 1987.

81. Descamps L, Jarsaillon B, Schuster P, et al: [Angular synthesis in upper tibial valgus osteotomy in osteoarthritis: Apropos of a series of 544 cases]. Rev Chir Orthop 73:231-236, 1987.

82. Descamps L, Jarsaillon B, Schuster P, et al: [Angular synthesis in upper tibial valgus osteotomy in osteoarthritis: Apropos of a series of 544 cases]. Rev Chir Orthop 73:231-236, 1987.

83. Diduch D, Insall JN, Scott WN, et al: Total knee replacement in young, active patients: Long-term follow-up and functional outcome. J Bone Joint Surg Am 79:575-582, 1997.

84. Dohin B, Migaud H, Gougeon F, et al: [Effect of a valgization osteotomy with external wedge removal on patellar height and femoro-patellar arthritis]. Acta Orthop Belg 59:69-75, 1993.

85. Dugdale TW, Noyes FR, Styer D: Preoperative planning for high tibial osteotomy: The effect of lateral tibiofemoral separation and tibiofemoral length. Clin Orthop 274:248-264, 1992.

86. Eckhoff DG: Effect of limb malrotation on malalignment and osteoarthritis. Orthop Clin North Am 25:405-414, 1994.

87. Eckhoff DG, Montgomery WK, Kilcoyne RF, et al: Femoral morphometry and anterior knee pain. Clin Orthop 302:64-68, 1994.

88. Edgerton BC, Mariani EM, Morrey BF: Distal femoral varus osteotomy for painful genu valgum: A five-to-11-year follow-up study. Clin Orthop 288:263-269, 1993.

89. Finkelstein JA, Gross AE, Davis A: Varus osteotomy of the distal part of the femur: A survivorship analysis. J Bone Joint Surg Am 78:1348-1352, 1996.

90. Flierl S, Sabo D, Hornig K, et al: Open wedge high tibial osteotomy using fractioned drill osteotomy: A surgical modification that lowers the complication rate. Knee Surg Sports Traumatol Arthrosc 4:149-153, 1996.

91. Font-Rodriguez DE, Scuderi GR, Insall JN: Survivorship of cemented total knee arthroplasty. Clin Orthop 345:79-86, 1997.

92. Frain PH: Retentissement sur le genou des atteintes de la hanche: Bases théoriques. Rev Chir Orthop 53:713-714, 1967.

93. Frain PH, Mazas F, Kerboul M, et al: Retentissement sur le genou des atteintes de la hanche. Rev Chir Orthop 53:713-717, 1967.

94. Fujisawa Y, Masuhara K, Shiomi S: The effect of high tibial osteotomy on osteoarthritis of the knee: An arthroscopic study of 54 knee joints. Orthop Clin North Am 10:585-608, 1979.

95. Gardes JC: [Distal femoral osteotomy with internal closure for the correction of gonarthroses with genu valgum]. Rev Chir Orthop Reparatrice Appar Mot 69(Suppl 2):110-112, 1983.

96. Gariépy R: Genu varum treated by high tibial osteotomy. J Bone Joint Surg Br 46:783-784, 1964.

97. Garvin KL, Scuderi GR, Insall JN: Evolution of the quadriceps snip. Clin Orthop 321:131-137, 1995.

98. Gibson MJ, Barnes MR, Allen MJ, et al: Weakness of foot dorsiflexion and changes in compartment pressures after tibial osteotomy. J Bone Joint Surg Br 68:471-475, 1986.

99. Giffin JR, Vogrin TM, Zantop T, et al: Effects of increasing tibial slope on the biomechanics of the knee. Am J Sports Med 32:376-382, 2004.

100. Gill T, Schemitsch EH, Brick GW, et al: Revision total knee arthroplasty after failed unicompartmental knee arthroplasty or high tibial osteotomy. Clin Orthop 321:10-18, 1995.

101. Godeneche A, Besse JL, Moyen B, et al: Prothèse totale du genou et ostéotomie dans le même temps opératoire pour déviation axiale majeure (à propos de 11 cas). Rev Chir Orthop 84:42-43, 1998.

102. Goh JC, Bose K, Khoo BC: Gait analysis study on patients with varus osteoarthrosis of the knee. Clin Orthop 294:223-231, 1993.

103. Goldman RT, Scuderi GR, Kelly MA: Arthroscopic treatment of the degenerative knee in older athletes. Clin Sports Med 16:51-68, 1997.

104. Goubier JN, Laporte C, Saillant G: [False popliteal aneurysm after tibial osteotomy: A case report]. Rev Chir Orthop Reparatrice Appar Mot 86:621-624, 2000.

105. Goutallier D, Delepine G, Debeyre J: [The patello-femoral joint in osteoarthritis of the knee with genu varum (author's transl)]. Rev Chir Orthop Reparatrice Appar Mot 65:25-31, 1979.

106. Goutallier D, Garabedian JM, Allain J, et al: Influence of lower limb torsional deformities on the development of femoro-tibial degenerative arthritis. Rev Chir Orthop 83:613-621, 1997.

107. Goutallier D, Julieron A, Hernigou P: Cement wedge replacing iliac graft for medial opening wedge tibial osteotomy. Rev Chir Orthop 78:138-144, 1992.

108. Green SA, Green HD: The influence of radiographic projection on the appearance of deformities. Orthop Clin North Am 25:467-482, 1994.

109. Grelsamer RP: Unicompartmental osteoarthrosis of the knee. J Bone Joint Surg Am 77:278-292, 1995.

110. Gugenheim JJJ, Brinker MR: Bone realignment with use of temporary external fixation for distal femoral valgus and varus deformities. J Bone Joint Surg Am 85:1229-1237, 2003.

111. Haddad FS, Bentley G: Total knee arthroplasty after high tibial osteotomy: A medium-term review. J Arthroplasty 15:597-603, 2000.

112. Haddad FS, Prendergast CM, Dorrell JH, et al: Arteriovenous fistula after fibular osteotomy leading to recurrent haemarthroses in a total knee replacement. J Bone Joint Surg Br 78:458-460, 1996.

113. Harding ML: A fresh appraisal of tibial osteotomy for osteoarthritis of the knee. Clin Orthop 114:223-234, 1976.

114. Harrington IJ: Static and dynamic loading patterns in knee joints with deformities. J Bone Joint Surg Am 65:247-259, 1983.

115. Harris WR, Kostuik JP: High tibial osteotomy for osteo-arthritis of the knee. J Bone Joint Surg Am 52:330-336, 1970.

116. Harrison MM, Cooke TD, Fisher SB, et al: Patterns of knee arthrosis and patella subluxation. Clin Orthop 309:56-63, 1994.

117. Hartford JM, Hester P, Watt PM, et al: Biomechanical superiority of plate fixation for proximal tibial osteotomy. Clin Orthop 412:125-130, 2003.

118. Healy WL, Anglen JO, Wasilewski SA, et al: Distal femoral varus osteotomy. J Bone Joint Surg Am 70:102-109, 1988.

119. Healy WL, Wilk RM: Osteotomy in treatment of the arthritic knee. In Scott WN (ed): The Knee. St. Louis, Mosby, 1994, pp 1019-1043.

120. Heatley FW, Lea Thomas ML, Giddins GEB, et al: Deep vein thrombosis in barrel vault tibial osteotomy: A pilot study. J Bone Joint Surg Br 71:729, 1989.

121. Hee HT, Low CK, Seow KH, et al: Comparing staple fixation to buttress plate fixation in high tibial osteotomy. Ann Acad Med Singapore 25:233-235, 1996.

122. Hernborg JS, Nilsson BE: The natural course of untreated osteoarthritis of the knee. Clin Orthop 123:130-137, 1977.

123. Hernigou P: [A 20-year follow-up study of internal gonarthrosis after tibial valgus osteotomy: Single versus repeated osteotomy]. Rev Chir Orthop Reparatrice Appar Mot 82:241-250, 1996.

124. Hernigou P: Open wedge tibial osteotomy: Combined coronal and sagittal correction. Knee 9:15-20, 2002.

125. Hernigou P, Bassaine M: Prothèse totale de genou après ostéotomie tibiale d'addition et de soustraction. Rev Chir Orthop 84:43-43, 1998.

126. Hernigou P, Duparc F, de-Ladoucette A, et al: [Recurvatum in arthritic genu valgum. Contraindication for osteotomy and unicompartmental prosthesis]. Rev Chir Orthop Reparatrice Appar Mot 78:292-299, 1992.

127. Hernigou P, Goutallier D: [Outcome of the femoropatellar joint in osteoarthritic genu varum after tibial wedge osteotomy for angulation: 10 to 13 year regression]. Rev Chir Orthop 73:43-48, 1987.

128. Hernigou P, Goutallier D: Usure osseuse sous chondrale des plateaux tibiaux dans les gonarthroses fémoro-tibiales: Aspect radiologique sur l'incidence de profil: Corrélations anatomiques et conséquences. Rev Mal Osteoartic 57:67-72, 1990.

129. Hernigou P, Jaafar A, Hamdadou A: [Leg length changes after upper tibial osteotomy: Analysis of different preoperative planning methods]. Rev Chir Orthop Reparatrice Appar Mot 88:68-73, 2002.

130. Hernigou P, Ma W: Open wedge tibial osteotomy with acrylic bone cement as bone substitute. Knee 8:103-110, 2001.

131. Hernigou P, Medevielle D, Debeyre J, et al: Proximal tibial osteotomy for osteoarthritis with varus deformity: A ten to thirteen-year follow-up study. J Bone Joint Surg Am 69:332-354, 1987.

132. Hernigou P, Ovadia H, Goutallier D: Modelisation mathématique de l'ostéotomie tibiale d'ouverture et tables de correction. Rev Chir Orthop 78:258-263, 1992.

133. Herscovici DJ, Fredrick RW, Behrens F: Superior dislocation of the fibular head associated with a tibial shaft fracture. J Orthop Trauma 6:116-119, 1992.

134. Hofmann AA, Kane KR: Total knee arthroplasty after high tibial osteotomy. Orthopedics 17:887-890, 1994.

135. Hofmann AA, Wyatt RW, Beck SW: High tibial osteotomy: Use of an osteotomy jig, rigid fixation, and early motion versus conventional surgical technique and cast immobilization. Clin Orthop 271:212-217, 1991.

136. Hofmann AA, Wyatt RW, Jones RE: Combined Coventry-Maquet procedure for two-compartment degenerative arthritis. Clin Orthop 190:186-191, 1984.

137. Holden DL, James SL, Larson RL, et al: Proximal tibial osteotomy in patients who are fifty years old or less: A long-term follow-up study. J Bone Joint Surg Am 70:977-982, 1988.

138. Hsu RW: The study of Maquet dome high tibial osteotomy: Arthroscopic-assisted analysis. Clin Orthop 243:280-285, 1989.

139. Huberti HH, Hayes WC: Patellofemoral contact pressures: The influence of Q-angle and tendofemoral contact. J Bone Joint Surg Am 66:715-724, 1984.

140. Idusuyi OB, Morrey BF: Peroneal nerve palsy after total knee arthroplasty: Assessment of predisposing and prognostic factors. J Bone Joint Surg Am 78:177-184, 1996.

141. Imhoff AB, Linke RD, Agneskirchner J: [Corrective osteotomy in primary varus, double varus and triple varus knee instability with cruciate ligament replacement]. Orthopade 33:201-207, 2004.

142. Insall J, Salvati E: Patella position in the normal knee joint. Radiology 101:101-104, 1971.

143. Insall J, Shoji H, Mayer V: High tibial osteotomy: A five-year evaluation. J Bone Joint Surg Am 56:1397-1405, 1974.

144. Insall JN: High tibial osteotomy in the treatment of osteoarthritis of the knee. Surg Annu 7:347-359, 1975.

145. Insall JN: Osteotomy. In Insall JN, Windsor RE, Scott WN, et al (eds): Surgery of the Knee, 2nd ed. New York, Churchill Livingstone, 1993, pp 635-675.

146. Insall JN: Surgical techniques and instrumentation in total knee arthroplasty. In Insall JN, Windsor RE, Scott WN, et al (eds): Surgery of the Knee, 2nd ed. New York, Churchill Livingstone, 1993, pp 739-804.

147. Insall JN: Knee arthroplasty: Limits and other problems: Extensor mechanism complications. Orthopedics 19:809-811, 1996.

148. Insall JN, Joseph DM, Msika C: High tibial osteotomy for varus gonarthrosis: A long-term follow-up study. J Bone Joint Surg Am 66:1040-1048, 1984.

149. Insall JN, Kelly MA: Anatomy. In Insall JN, Windsor RE, Scott WN, et al (eds): Surgery of the Knee, 2nd ed. New York, Churchill Livingstone, 1993, pp 1-20.

150. Insall JN, Stern SH: Total knee arthroplasty in obese patients. J Bone Joint Surg Am 72:1400-1404, 1990.

151. Ivarsson I, Myrnerts R, Gillquist J: High tibial osteotomy for medial osteoarthritis of the knee: A 5 to 7 and 11 year follow-up. J Bone Joint Surg Br 72:238-244, 1990.

152. Jackson JP: Osteotomy for osteoarthritis of the knee. J Bone Joint Surg Br 40:826-826, 1958.

153. Jackson JP, Waugh W: The technique and complications of upper tibial osteotomy: A review of 226 operations. J Bone Joint Surg Br 56:236-245, 1974.

154. Jackson M, Sarangi PP, Newman JH: Revision total knee arthroplasty: Comparison of outcome following primary proximal tibial osteotomy or unicompartmental arthroplasty. J Arthroplasty 9:539-542, 1994.

155. Jiang CC, Hang YS, Liu TK: A new jig for proximal tibial osteotomy. Clin Orthop 226:118-123, 1986.

156. Jiang CC, Insall JN: Effect of rotation on the axial alignment of the femur: Pitfalls in the use of femoral intramedullary guides in total knee arthroplasty. Clin Orthop 248:50-56, 1989.

157. Job DC, Languepin A, Benvenuto M, et al: [Tibial valgization osteotomy in gonarthrosis with or without chondrocalcinosis: Results after 5 years]. Rev Rhum Mal Osteoartic 58:491-496, 1991.

158. Johnson F, Leitl S, Waugh W: The distribution of load across the knee: A comparison of static and dynamic measurements. J Bone Joint Surg Br 62:346-349, 1980.

159. Johnson LL: Arthroscopic arthroplasty historical and pathological perspectives: Present status. Arthroscopy 2:54-69, 1986.

160. Jokio PJ, Lindholm TS: The angle-measuring device, a practical resource in high tibial osteotomy. Ann Chir Gynaecol 80:54-58, 1991.

161. Kanamiya T, Naito M, Hara M, et al: The influences of biomechanical factors on cartilage regeneration after high tibial osteotomy for knees with medial compartment osteoarthritis: Clinical and arthroscopic observations. Arthroscopy 18:725-729, 2002.

162. Kapandji IA: The Physiology of the Joints, 2nd ed. New York, Churchill Livingstone, 1970, pp 74-75.
163. Karabatsos B, Mahomed NN, Maistrelli GL: Functional outcome of total knee arthroplasty after high tibial osteotomy. Can J Surg 45:116-119, 2002.
164. Katz MM, Hungerford DS, Krackow KA, et al: Results of total knee arthroplasty after failed proximal tibial osteotomy for osteoarthritis. J Bone Joint Surg Am 69:225-233, 1987.
165. Kawakami H, Sugano N, Yonenobu K, et al: Effects of rotation on measurement of lower limb alignment for knee osteotomy. J Orthop Res 22:1248-1253, 2004.
166. Kawakami H, Sugano N, Yonenobu K, et al: Gait analysis system for assessment of dynamic loading axis of the knee. Gait Posture 21:125-130, 2005.
167. Keene JS, Monson DK, Roberts JM, et al: Evaluation of patients for high tibial osteotomy. Clin Orthop 243:157-165, 1989.
168. Kettelkamp DB, Leach RE, Nasca R: Pitfalls of proximal tibial osteotomy. Clin Orthop 106:232-241, 1975.
169. Kettelkamp DB, Wenger DR, Chao EY, et al: Results of proximal tibial osteotomy: The effects of tibiofemoral angle, stance-phase flexion-extension, and medial-plateau force. J Bone Joint Surg Am 58:952-960, 1976.
170. Kirgis A, Albrecht S: Palsy of the deep peroneal nerve after proximal tibial osteotomy: An anatomical study. J Bone Joint Surg Am 74:1180-1185, 1992.
171. Kitson J, Weale AE, Lee AS, et al: Patellar tendon length following opening wedge high tibial osteotomy using an external fixator with particular reference to later total knee replacement. Injury 32(Suppl 4):SD-140-SD-143, 2001.
172. Klinger HM, Lorenz F, Harer T: Open wedge tibial osteotomy by hemicallotasis for medial compartment osteoarthritis. Arch Orthop Trauma Surg 121:245-247, 2001.
173. Korn MW: A new approach to dome high tibial osteotomy. Am J Knee Surg 9:12-21, 1996.
174. Koshino T, Morii T, Wada J, et al: High tibial osteotomy with fixation by a blade plate for medial compartment osteoarthritis of the knee. Orthop Clin North Am 20:227-243, 1989.
175. Koshino T, Murase T, Saito T: Medial opening-wedge high tibial osteotomy with use of porous hydroxyapatite to treat medial compartment osteoarthritis of the knee. J Bone Joint Surg Am 85:78-85, 2003.
176. Koshino T, Murase T, Takagi T, et al: New bone formation around porous hydroxyapatite wedge implanted in opening wedge high tibial osteotomy in patients with osteoarthritis. Biomaterials 22:1579-1582, 2001.
177. Koshino T, Ranawat NS: Healing process of osteoarthritis in the knee after high tibial osteotomy through observation of Strontium-85 scintimetry. Clin Orthop 82:149-156, 1972.
178. Koshino T, Wada S, Ara Y, et al: Regeneration of degenerated articular cartilage after high tibial valgus osteotomy for medial compartmental osteoarthritis of the knee. Knee 10:229-236, 2003.
179. Kozinn SC, Scott RD: Current concepts review: Unicondylar knee arthroplasty. J Bone Joint Surg Am 71:145-150, 1989.
180. Krackow KA, Holtgrewe JL: Experience with a new technique for managing severely overcorrected valgus high tibial osteotomy at total knee arthroplasty. Clin Orthop 258:213-224, 1990.
181. Krznaric E, Roo MD, Verbruggen A, et al: Chronic osteomyelitis: Diagnosis with technetium-99m-d, l-hexamethylpropylene amine oxime labelled leucocytes. Eur J Nucl Med 23:792-797, 1996.
182. Lang W, Ott R, Haas P, et al: Popliteal arteriovenous fistula after corrective upper tibial osteotomy. Arch Orthop Trauma Surg 112:99-100, 1993.
183. Langlais F, Thomazeau H: Ostéotomies du genou. In: Encyclopédie Médico-Chirurgicale: Techniques Chirurgicales, Orthopédie. Paris, Editions Scientifiques et Médicales Elsevier, 1989, pp 1-23.
184. Lattermann C, Jakob RP: High tibial osteotomy alone or combined with ligament reconstruction in anterior cruciate ligament-deficient knees. Knee Surg Sports Traumatol Arthrosc 4:32-38, 1996.
185. Learmonth ID: A simple technique for varus supracondylar osteotomy in genu valgum. J Bone Joint Surg Br 72:235-237, 1990.
186. Leclerc JR, Geerts WH, Desjardins L, et al: Prevention of deep vein thrombosis after major knee surgery—a randomized, double-blind trial comparing a low molecular weight heparin fragment (enoxaparin) to placebo. Thromb Haemost 67:417-423, 1992.
187. Lemaire R: [Comparative study of 2 series of tibial osteotomies with blade-plate fixation or with compression frame]. Acta Orthop Belg 48:157-171, 1982.
188. Lemaire R, Gillet P, Rondia J: [Semi-constrained prosthetic arthroplasty of the knee following tibial osteotomy]. Acta Orthop Belg 57(Suppl 2):130-137, 1991.
189. Lerat JL, Moyen B, Garin C, et al: [Anterior laxity and internal arthritis of the knee: Results of the reconstruction of the anterior cruciate ligament associated with tibial osteotomy]. Rev Chir Orthop Reparatrice Appar Mot 79:365-374, 1993.
190. Levigne CH: Interêt de l'axe épiphysaire dans l'arthrose. In Dejour H, Neyret P (eds): Journées Lyonnaises de Chirurgie du Genou. Lyon, Hopital de Lyon Sud, 1991, pp 127-141.
191. Levigne CH, Bonnin M: Ostéotomie tibiale de valgisation pour arthrose fémoro-tibiale interne: Résultats d'un échantillon de 217 ostéotomies revues avec un recul de 1 à 21 ans. In Dejour H, Neyret P (eds): Journées Lyonnaises de Chirurgie du Genou. Lyon, Hopital de Lyon Sud, 1991, pp 142-168.
192. Lobenhoffer P, Agneskirchner J, Zoch W: [Open valgus alignment osteotomy of the proximal tibia with fixation by medial plate fixator]. Orthopade 33:153-160, 2004.
193. Lobenhoffer P, Agneskirchner JD: Improvements in surgical technique of valgus high tibial osteotomy. Knee Surg Sports Traumatol Arthrosc 11:132-138, 2003.
194. Lootvoet L, Massinon A, Rossillon R, et al: [Upper tibial osteotomy for gonarthrosis in genu varum: Apropos of a series of 193 cases reviewed 6 to 10 years later]. Rev Chir Orthop Reparatrice Appar Mot 79:375-384, 1993.
195. Lortat JA, Hardy P, Benoit J: [Early reoperation for infection in orthopedic surgery of the leg (arthroplasties and hip surgical procedures excluded)]. Rev Chir Orthop Reparatrice Appar Mot 76:321-328, 1990.
196. Lysholm J, Gillquist J: Evaluation of knee ligament surgery results with special emphasis on use of a scoring scale. Am J Sports Med 10:150-154, 1982.
197. MacIntosh DL, Welsh RP: Joint debridement—a complement to high tibial osteotomy in the treatment of degenerative arthritis of the knee. J Bone Joint Surg Am 59:1094-1097, 1977.
198. Madan S, Ranjith RK, Fiddian NJ: Total knee replacement following high tibial osteotomy. Bull Hosp Joint Dis 61:5-10, 2002.
199. Magyar G, Ahl TL, Vibe P, et al: Open-wedge osteotomy by hemicallotasis or the closed-wedge technique for osteoarthritis of the knee: A randomised study of 50 operations. J Bone Joint Surg Br 81:444-448, 1999.
200. Magyar G, Toksvig-Larsen S, Lindstrand A: Hemicallotasis open-wedge osteotomy for osteoarthritis of the knee: Complications in 308 operations. J Bone Joint Surg Br 81:449-451, 1999.
201. Magyar G, Toksvig LS, Lindstrand A: Open wedge tibial osteotomy by callus distraction in gonarthrosis: Operative technique and early results in 36 patients. Acta Orthop Scand 69:147-151, 1998.
202. Mammi GI, Rocchi R, Cadossi R, et al: The electrical stimulation of tibial osteotomies: Double-blind study. Clin Orthop 288:246-253, 1993.
203. Maquet P: Biomécanique des membres inférieurs. Acta Orthop Belg 32:705-728, 1966.
204. Maquet P: Biomécanique du genou et gonarthrose. Rev Chir Orthop 53:111-138, 1967.
205. Maquet P: La sollicitation mécanique du genou durant la marche. Acta Orthop Belg 41:119-132, 1975.
206. Maquet P: Biomechanics of the Knee. New York, Springer, 1976.
207. Maquet P: Valgus osteotomy for osteoarthritis of the knee. Clin Orthop 120:143-148, 1976.
208. Maquet P: Osteotomy. In Freeman MAR (ed): Arthritis of the Knee: Clinical Features and Surgical Management. Berlin, Springer-Verlag, 1980, pp 148-183.
209. Maquet P: [Surgical treatment of femoro-tibial arthrosis]. Acta Orthop Belg 48:172-189, 1982.
210. Maquet P: Pathogénie de la gonarthrose. Acta Orthop Belg 48:45-56, 1982.
211. Maquet P: The treatment of choice in osteoarthritis of the knee. Clin Orthop 192:108-112, 1985.
212. Maquet P, Watillon M, Burny F, et al: [Conservative surgical treatment of arthrosis of the knee]. Acta Orthop Belg 48:204-261, 1982.

213. Marcacci M, Iacono F, Zaffagnini S, et al: Total knee arthroplasty after proximal tibial osteotomy. Chir Organi Mov 80:353-359, 1995.

214. Marin ML, Gomez NL, Zorrilla RP, et al: Treatment of osteoarthritis of the knee with valgus deformity by means of varus osteotomy. Acta Orthop Belg 66:272-278, 2000.

215. Marion J, Fischer L: [A case of bilateral deforming tibial osteochondrosis with tibia vara (Blount's disease)]. Lyon Chir 61:386-388, 1965.

216. Marti CB, Gautier E, Wachtl SW, et al: Accuracy of frontal and sagittal plane correction in open-wedge high tibial osteotomy. Arthroscopy 20:366-372, 2004.

217. Marti RK, Verhagen RA, Kerkhoffs GM, et al: Proximal tibial varus osteotomy: Indications, technique, and five to twenty-one-year results. J Bone Joint Surg Am 83:164-170, 2001.

218. Mathews J, Cobb AG, Richardson S, et al: Distal femoral osteotomy for lateral compartment osteoarthritis of the knee. Orthopedics 21:437-440, 1998.

219. Matthews LS, Goldstein SA, Malvitz TA, et al: Proximal tibial osteotomy: Factors that influence the duration of satisfactory function. Clin Orthop 229:193-200, 1988.

220. McDermott AG, Finklestein JA, Farine I, et al: Distal femoral varus osteotomy for valgus deformity of the knee. J Bone Joint Surg Am 70:110-116, 1988.

221. McKellop HA, Llinas A, Sarmiento A: Effects of tibial malalignment on the knee and ankle. Orthop Clin North Am 25:415-423, 1994.

222. McKellop HA, Sim FH, Redfern FC, et al: The effect of simulated fracture-angulations of the tibia on cartilage pressures in the knee joint. J Bone Joint Surg Am 73:1382-1391, 1991.

223. Meding JB, Keating EM, Ritter MA, et al: Total knee arthroplasty after high tibial osteotomy. Clin Orthop 375:175-184, 2000.

224. Meding JB, Keating EM, Ritter MA, et al: Total knee arthroplasty after high tibial osteotomy: A comparison study in patients who had bilateral total knee replacement. J Bone Joint Surg Am 82:1252-1259, 2000.

225. Menetrey J, Paul M: Possibilities of computer-assisted navigation in knee para-articular osteotomies. Orthopade 33:224-228, 2004.

226. Merle d'Aubigne R: Joint realignment in the management of osteoarthritis. In Straub LR, Wilson PD Jr (eds): Clinical Trends in Orthopaedics. New York, Thieme-Stratton, 1982, p 246.

227. Miniaci A, Ballmer FT, Ballmer PM, et al: Proximal tibial osteotomy: A new fixation device. Clin Orthop 246:250-259, 1989.

228. Mironneau A: L'osteotomie fémorale de varisation dans l'arthrose fémoro-tibiale externe essentielle. In Dejour H, Neyret P (eds): Journées Lyonnaises de Chirurgie du Genou. Lyon, Hopital de Lyon Sud, 1991, pp 181-190.

229. Mizuta H, Nakamura E, Kudo S, et al: Greater frequency of distraction accelerates bone formation in open-wedge proximal tibial osteotomy with hemicallotasis. Acta Orthop Scand 75:588-593, 2004.

230. Mollica Q, Leonardi W, Longo G, et al: Surgical treatment of arthritic varus knee by tibial corticotomy and angular distraction with an external fixator. Ital J Orthop Traumatol 18:17-23, 1992.

231. Mollica Q, Leonardi W, Travaglianti G: Correction of lower limb deformity using external fixation. Ital J Orthop Traumatol 18:297-302, 1992.

232. Mont MA, Alexander N, Krackow KA, et al: Total knee arthroplasty after failed high tibial osteotomy. Orthop Clin North Am 25:515-525, 1994.

233. Mont MA, Antonaides S, Krackow KA, et al: Total knee arthroplasty after failed high tibial osteotomy: A comparison with a matched group. Clin Orthop 299:125-130, 1994.

234. Moreland JR: Mechanisms of failure in total knee arthroplasty. Clin Orthop 226:49-64, 1988.

235. Moreland JR, Basset LW, Hanker GJ: Radiographic analysis of the axial alignment of the lower extremity. J Bone Joint Surg Am 69:745-749, 1987.

236. Morrey BF, Edgerton BC: Distal femoral osteotomy for lateral gonarthrosis. Instr Course Lect 41:77-85, 1992.

237. Moussa M: Rotational malalignment and femoral torsion in osteoarthritic knees with patellofemoral joint involvment. Clin Orthop 304:176-183, 1994.

238. Murphy SB: Tibial osteotomy for genu varum: Indications, preoperative planning, and technique. Orthop Clin North Am 25:477-482, 1994.

239. Murray DW, Goodfellow J, O'Connor J: The Oxford medial unicompartmental arthroplasty. J Bone Joint Surg Br 80:983-989, 1998.

240. Myrnerts R: The SAAB jig: An aid in high tibial osteotomy. Acta Orthop Scand 49:85-88, 1978.

241. Myrnerts R: High tibial osteotomy with overcorrection of varus malalignment in medial gonarthrosis. Acta Orthop Scand 51:557-560, 1980.

242. Nagel A, Insall JN, Scuderi GR: Proximal tibial osteotomy: A subjective outcome study. J Bone Joint Surg Am 78:1353-1358, 1996.

243. Nakamura E, Mizuta H, Kudo S, et al: Open-wedge osteotomy of the proximal tibia hemicallotasis. J Bone Joint Surg Br 83:1111-1115, 2001.

244. Naudie D, Bourne RB, Rorabeck CH, et al: The Insall Award: Survivorship of the high tibial valgus osteotomy: A 10- to -22-year followup study. Clin Orthop 367:18-27, 1999.

245. Neyret P, Deroche P, Deschamps G, et al: [Total knee replacement after valgus tibial osteotomy: Technical problems]. Rev Chir Orthop Reparatrice Appar Mot 78:438-448, 1992.

246. Nguyen C, Rudan J, Simurda MA, et al: High tibial osteotomy compared with high tibial and Maquet procedures in medial and patellofemoral compartment osteoarthritis. Clin Orthop 245:179-187, 1989.

247. Nicolaides AP, Papanikolaou A, Polyzoides AJ: Successful treatment of valgus deformity of the knee with an open supracondylar osteotomy using a coral wedge: A brief report of two cases. Knee 7:105-107, 2000.

248. Nizard RS, Cardinne L, Bizot P, et al: Total knee replacement after failed tibial osteotomy: Results of a matched-pair study. J Arthroplasty 13:847-853, 1998.

249. Noda T, Yasuda S, Nagano K, et al: Clinico-radiological study of total knee arthroplasty after high tibial osteotomy. J Orthop Sci 5:25-36, 2000.

250. Noyes FR, Barber-Westin SD, Hewett TE: High tibial osteotomy and ligament reconstruction for varus angulated anterior cruciate ligament-deficient knees. Am J Sports Med 28:282-296, 2000.

251. Noyes FR, Barber SD, Simon R: High tibial osteotomy and ligament reconstruction in varus angulated, anterior cruciate ligament-deficient knees: A two- to seven-year follow-up study. Am J Sports Med 21:2-12, 1993.

252. O'Neill DF, James SL: Valgus osteotomy with anterior cruciate ligament laxity. Clin Orthop 278:153-159, 1992.

253. Odenbring S, Berggren AM, Peil L: Roentgenographic assessment of the hip-knee-ankle axis in medial gonarthrosis: A study of reproducibility. Clin Orthop 289:195-196, 1993.

254. Odenbring S, Egund N, Hagstedt B, et al: Ten-year results of tibial osteotomy for medial gonarthrosis: The influence of overcorrection. Arch Orthop Trauma Surg 110:103-108, 1991.

255. Odenbring S, Egund N, Knutson K, et al: Revision after osteotomy for gonarthrosis: A 10-19-year follow-up of 314 cases. Acta Orthop Scand 61:128-130, 1990.

256. Odenbring S, Egund N, Lindstrand A, et al: Cartilage regeneration after proximal tibial osteotomy for medial gonarthrosis: An arthroscopic, roentgenographic, and histologic study. Clin Orthop 277:210-216, 1992.

257. Odenbring S, Lindstrand A, Egund N: Early knee mobilization after osteotomy for gonarthrosis. Acta Orthop Scand 60:699-702, 1989.

258. Odenbring S, Lindstrand A, Egund N, et al: Prognosis for patients with medial gonarthrosis: A 16-year follow-up study of 189 knees. Clin Orthop 266:152-155, 1991.

259. Odenbring S, Tjornstrand B, Egund N, et al: Function after tibial osteotomy for medial gonarthrosis below aged 50 years. Acta Orthop Scand 60:527-531, 1989.

260. Ogata K, Whiteside LA, Lester PA, et al: The effect of varus stress on the moving rabbit knee joint. Clin Orthop 129:313-318, 1977.

261. Ortlepp K, Siegling CW: [Results of follow-up studies following proximal corrective osteotomy of the tibia]. Beitr Orthop Traumatol 36:563-571, 1989.

262. Paley D, Bhatnagar J, Herzenberg JE, et al: New procedures for tightening knee collateral ligaments in conjunction with knee realignment osteotomy. Orthop Clin North Am 25:533-555, 1994.

263. Paley D, Maar DC, Herzenberg JE: New concepts in high tibial osteotomy for medial compartment osteoarthritis. Orthop Clin North Am 25:483-498, 1994.

264. Panula HE, Helminen HJ, Kiviranta I: Slowly progressive osteoarthritis after tibial valgus osteotomy in young beagle dogs. Clin Orthop 343:192-202, 1997.

265. Parvizi J, Hanssen AD, Spangehl MJ: Total knee arthroplasty following proximal tibial osteotomy: Risk factors for failure. J Bone Joint Surg Am 86:474-479, 2004.

266. Pauwels F: Biomécanique de l'Appareil Locomoteur: Contribution à l'Étude de l'Anatomie Fonctionnelle. Berlin, Springer-Verlag, 1979.

267. Perusi M, Baietta D, Pizzoli A: [Surgical correction of osteoarthritic genu varum by the hemicallotasis technique]. Rev Chir Orthop Reparatrice Appar Mot 80:739-743, 1994.

268. Pfeiffer M, Griss P: The valgisation osteotomy of the tibia: Results of a comparative follow-up study of the Coventry versus the Wagner technique. Z Orthop Ihre Grenzgeb 128:51-57, 1990.

269. Poilvache PL, Insall J, Scuderi GR, et al: Rotational landmarks and sizing of the distal femur in total knee arthroplasty. Clin Orthop 331:35-46, 1996.

270. Postel M, Langlais F: Osteotomies du genou pour gonarthrose. In: Encyclopédie Médico-Chirurgicale: Techniques Chirurgicales, Orthopédie. Paris, Editions Techniques, 1977, pp 1-17.

271. Price CT: Unilateral fixators and mechanical axis realignment. Orthop Clin North Am 25:499-508, 1994.

272. Prodromos CC, Andriacchi TP, Galante JO: A relationship between gait and clinical changes following high tibial osteotomy. J Bone Joint Surg Am 67:1188-1194, 1985.

273. Psychoyios V, Crawford RW, O'Connor J, et al: Wear of congruent meniscal bearings in unicompartpemtal knee arthropasty: A retrieval study of 16 specimens. J Bone Joint Surg Br 80:976-982, 1998.

274. Puddu G, Cerullo G, Cipolla M, et al: A plate for open wedge tibial osteotomy. Personal communication, 1997.

275. Putnam MD, Mears DC, Fu FH: Combined Maquet and proximal tibial valgus osteotomy. Clin Orthop 197:217-223, 1985.

276. Radermacher K, Portheine F, Anton M, et al: Computer assisted orthopaedic surgery with image based individual templates. Clin Orthop 354:28-38, 1998.

277. Radin EL, Paul IL, Rose RM: Role of mechanical factors in pathogenesis of primary osteoarthrits. Lancet 1:519, 1972.

278. Railhac JJ, Fournie A, Gay A, et al: Exploration radiologique du genou de face en légère flexion et en charge: Son intérêt dans le diagnostic de l'arthrose fémoro-tibiale. J Radiol 62:157-166, 1981.

279. Ramadier JO: Etude radiologique des déviations dans la gonarthrose. Rev Chir Orthop 53:139-147, 1967.

280. Ramadier JO, Buard JE, Lortat-Jacob A, et al: Mesure radiologique des déformations frontales du genou: Procédé du profil vrai radiologique. Rev Chir Orthop 68:75-78, 1982.

281. Ramadier JO, Merle DR: Genou: Gonarthroses avec déviations transversales du genou. In Merle dR, Postel M (eds): Chirurgie du Rhumatisme: Tome 2. Membre Inférieur. Paris, Masson, 1978, pp 232-253.

282. Rand JA, Ilstrup DM: Survivorship analysis of total knee arthroplasty: Cumulative rates of survival of 9200 total knee arthroplasties. J Bone Joint Surg Am 73:397-409, 1991.

283. Rand JA, Ritts GD: Abrasion arthroplasty as a salvage for failed upper tibial osteotomy. J Arthroplasty 4(Suppl):S45-S48, 1989.

284. Rees JL, Price AJ, Lynskey TG, et al: Medial unicompartmental arthroplasty after failed high tibial osteotomy. J Bone Joint Surg Br 83:1034-1036, 2001.

285. Reimann I: Experimental osteoarthritis of the knee in rabbits induced by alteration of the load-bearing. Acta Orthop Scand 44:496-504, 1973.

286. Reynolds JH, Graham D, Smith FW: Imaging inflammation with 99Tcm HMPAO labelled leucocytes. Clin Radiol 42:195-198, 1990.

287. Rinonapoli E, Mancini GB, Corvaglia A, et al: Tibial osteotomy for varus gonarthrosis: A 10- to 21-year followup study. Clin Orthop 353:185-193, 1998.

288. Rozbruch SR, Herzenberg JE, Tetsworth K, et al: Distraction osteogenesis for nonunion after high tibial osteotomy. Clin Orthop 394:227-235, 2002.

289. Rozbruch SR, Parvizi J, Hanssen AD, et al: Total knee arthroplasty following proximal tibial osteotomy: J Parvizi, AD Hanssen, and MJ Spangehl reply. J Bone Joint Surg Am 86:2571, 2004.

290. Rubens F, Wellington JL, Bouchard AG: Popliteal artery injury after tibial osteotomy: Report of two cases. Can J Surg 33:294-297, 1990.

291. Rudan JF, Simurda MA: High tibial osteotomy: A prospective clinical and roentgenographic review. Clin Orthop 255:251-256, 1990.

292. Rudan JF, Simurda MA: Valgus high tibial osteotomy: A long-term follow-up study. Clin Orthop 268:157-160, 1991.

293. Ruther W, Hotze A, Moller F, et al: Diagnosis of bone and joint infection by leucocyte scintigraphy: A comparative study with 99mTc-HMPAO-labelled leucocytes, 99mTc-labelled antigranulocyte antibodies and 99mTc-labelled nanocolloid. Arch Orthop Trauma Surg 110:26-32, 1990.

294. Sabo D, Flierl S, Thomsen M, et al: Fractioned drilling—a technique for wedge osteotomy of the knee. Int Orthop 19:352-354, 1995.

295. Sanfridsson J, Ryd L, Eklund K, et al: Angular configuration of the knee: Comparison of conventional measurements and the QUESTOR Precision Radiography system. Acta Radiol 37:633-638, 1996.

296. Sawant MR, Ireland J: Pseudo-aneurysm of the anterior tibial artery complicating high tibial osteotomy—a case report. Knee 8:247-248, 2001.

297. Schwartsman V: Circular external fixation in high tibial osteotomy. Instr Course Lect 44:469-474, 1995.

298. Scuderi GR, Windsor RE, Insall JN: Observations on patellar height after proximal tibial osteotomy. J Bone Joint Surg Am 71:245-248, 1989.

299. Segal P, Burdin PH, Cartier PH, et al: Les échecs des ostéotomies tibiales de valgisation pour gonarthrose et leurs reprises: Symposium. Rev Chir Orthop 78:85-128, 1992.

300. Sen C, Kocaoglu M, Eralp L: The advantages of circular external fixation used in high tibial osteotomy (average 6 years follow-up). Knee Surg Sports Traumatol Arthrosc 11:139-144, 2003.

301. Shaw JA, Dungy DS, Arsht SS: Recurrent varus angulation after high tibial osteotomy: An anatomic analysis. Clin Orthop 420:205-212, 2004.

302. Shaw JA, Moulton MJ: High tibial osteotomy: An operation based on a spurious mechanical concept: A theoretic treatise. Am J Orthop 25:429-436, 1996.

303. Shetty AA, Tindall AJ, Qureshi F, et al: The effect of knee flexion on the popliteal artery and its surgical significance. J Bone Joint Surg 85:218-222, 2003.

304. Shoji H, Insall J: High tibial osteotomy for osteoarthritis of the knee with valgus deformity. J Bone Joint Surg Am 55:963-973, 1973.

305. Siegrist O, Fritschy D, Manueddu C, Laurencet PA: Osteotomie de valgisation progressive du tibia proximal. 56° Congrès Annuel de la Société Suisse d'Orthopédie, [56th Annual Meeting of Swiss Orthopaedic Society], June 13, 1996.

306. Smith PN, Gelinas J, Kennedy K, et al: Popliteal vessels in knee surgery: A magnetic resonance imaging study. Clin Orthop 367:158-164, 1999.

307. Specchiulli F, Laforgia R, Solarino GB: Tibial osteotomy in the treatment of varus osteoarthritic knee. Ital J Orthop Traumatol 16:507-514, 1990.

308. Sprenger TR, Doerzbacher JF: Tibial osteotomy for the treatment of varus gonarthrosis: Survival and failure analysis to twenty-two years. J Bone Joint Surg Am 85:469-474, 2003.

309. Staeheli JW, Cass JR, Morrey BF: Condylar total knee arthroplasty after failed proximal tibial osteotomy. J Bone Joint Surg Am 69:28-31, 1987.

310. Stahelin T, Hardegger F: [Incomplete, supracondylar femur osteotomy: A minimally invasive compression osteosynthesis with soft implant]. Orthopade 33:178-184, 2004.

311. Stahelin T, Hardegger F, Ward JC: Supracondylar osteotomy of the femur with use of compression: Osteosynthesis with a malleable implant. J Bone Joint Surg Am 82:712-722, 2000.

312. Staubli AE, De Simoni C, Babst R, et al: TomoFix: A new LCP-concept for open wedge osteotomy of the medial proximal tibia—early results in 92 cases. Injury 34(Suppl 2):B55-B62, 2003.

313. Stern SH, Insall JN: Posterior stabilized prosthesis: Results after follow-up of nine to twelve years. J Bone Joint Surg Am 74:980-986, 1992.

314. Stoffel K, Stachowiak G, Kuster M: Open wedge high tibial osteotomy: Biomechanical investigation of the modified Arthrex Osteotomy Plate (Puddu Plate) and the TomoFix Plate. Clin Biomech (Bristol, Avon) 19:944-950, 2004.

315. Stuart MJ, Grace JN, Ilstrup DM, et al: Late recurrence of varus deformity after proximal tibial osteotomy. Clin Orthop 260:61-65, 1990.

316. Stubbs BT: Posterolateral arthritis of the knee. J Arthroplasty 10:427-432, 1995.

317. Sundaram NA, Hallett JP, Sullivan MF: Dome osteotomy of the tibia for osteoarthritis of the knee. J Bone Joint Surg Br 68:782-786, 1986.

318. Surer P: Un nouveau matériel d'ostéosynthèse: la plaque à ancrage "surfix": Son utilisation dans les ostéosynthèses métaphyso-épiphysaires du genou. Ann Orthop Ouest 27:127, 1995.

319. Surer P: Reliability of fixation with the Surfix plate: Analysis of the first 100 osteotomies. Eur J Orthop Surg Traumatol 7:47-49, 1997.

320. Tabor OB Jr, Tabor OB: Unicompartmental arthroplasty: A long-term follow-up study. J Arthroplasty 13:373-379, 1998.

321. Takahashi S, Tomihisa K, Saito T: Decrease of osteosclerosis in subchondral bone of medial compartmental osteoarthritic knee seven to nineteen years after high tibial valgus osteotomy. Bull Hosp Joint Dis 61:58-62, 2002.

322. Takahashi T, Wada Y, Tanaka M, et al: Dome-shaped proximal tibial osteotomy using percutaneous drilling for osteoarthritis of the knee. Arch Orthop Trauma Surg 120:32-37, 2000.

323. Tegner Y, Lysholm J: Rating systems in the evaluation of knee ligament injuries. Clin Orthop 198:43-49, 1985.

324. Teinturier P, Boulleret J, Terver S, et al: [Supracondylar osteotomy]. Rev Chir Orthop Reparatrice Appar Mot 61(Suppl 2):291-295, 1975.

325. Terry GC, Cimino PM: Distal femoral osteotomy for valgus deformity of the knee. Orthopedics 15:1283-1289, 1992.

326. Thomine JM, Boudjemaa A, Gibon Y, et al: Les écarts varisants dans la gonarthrose: Fondement théorique et essai d'évaluation pratique. Rev Chir Orthop 67:327, 1981.

327. Tigani D, Del Baldo A, Trentani P, et al: Closed-wedge tibial osteotomy: Conventional technique versus a new system of compression-dynamic fixation. Orthopedics 25:1265-1268, 2002.

328. Tigani D, Ferrari D, Trentani P, et al: Patellar height after high tibial osteotomy. Int Orthop 24:331-334, 2001.

329. Tippett JW: Articular cartilage drilling and osteotomy in osteoarthritis of the knee. In McGinty JB, Caspari RB, Jackson RW, et al (eds): Operative Arthroscopy, 2nd ed. Philadelphia, Lippincott-Raven, 1996, pp 411-426.

330. Tjornstrand B, Hagstedt B, Persson BM: Results of surgical treatment for non-union after high tibial osteotomy in osteoarthritis of the knee. J Bone Joint Surg Am 60:973-977, 1978.

331. Tjornstrand BA, Egund N, Hagstedt BV: High tibial osteotomy: A seven-year clinical and radiographic follow-up. Clin Orthop 160:124-136, 1981.

332. Toksvig-Larsen S, Magyar G, Onsten I, et al: Fixation of the tibial component of total knee arthroplasty after high tibial osteotomy: A matched radiostereometric study. J Bone Joint Surg Br 80:295-297, 1998.

333. Toksvig LS, Magyar G, Onsten I, et al: Fixation of the tibial component of total knee arthroplasty after high tibial osteotomy: A matched radiostereometric study. J Bone Joint Surg Br 80:295-297, 1998.

334. Totty WG: Radiographic evaluation of osteomyelitis using magnetic resonance imaging. Orthop Rev 18:587-592, 1989.

335. Tsuda E, Ishibashi Y, Sasaki K, et al: Opening-wedge osteotomy for revision of failed closing-wedge high tibial osteotomy: A case report. J Bone Joint Surg Am 86:2045-2049, 2004.

336. Tsumaki N, Kakiuchi M, Sasaki J, et al: Low-intensity pulsed ultrasound accelerates maturation of callus in patients treated with opening-wedge high tibial osteotomy by hemicallotasis. J Bone Joint Surg Am 86:2399-2405, 2004.

337. Turner RS, Griffiths H, Heatley FW: The incidence of deep-vein thrombosis after upper tibial osteotomy: A venographic study. J Bone Joint Surg Br 75:942-944, 1993.

338. Uchinou S, Yano H, Shimizu K, et al: A severely overcorrected high tibial osteotomy: Revision by osteotomy and a long stem component. Acta Orthop Scand 67:193-194, 1996.

339. Valenti JR, Calvo R, Lopez R, et al: Long term evaluation of high tibial valgus osteotomy. Int Orthop 14:347-349, 1990.

340. Van De Berg AJ, Collard Ph, Quiriny M: Gonarthrose et déviation angulaire du genou dans le plan frontal. Acta Orthop Belg 48:8-27, 1982.

341. Volkmann R: Ostetomy for knee joint deformity. Edinburgh Med J [transl from Berl Klin Wochenschr] 794, 1875.

342. Wada M, Imura S, Nagatani K, et al: Relationship between gait and clinical results after high tibial osteotomy. Clin Orthop 354:180-188, 1998.

343. Wada M, Imura S, Nagatani K, et al: Relationship between gait and clinical results after high tibial osteotomy. Clin Orthop 354:180-188, 1998.

344. Wagner H: Principles of corrective osteotomies in osteoarthrosis of the knee. Orthopade 6:145-177, 1977.

345. Wagner H: Principles of corrective osteotomy in osteoarthritis of the knee. Prog Orthop Surg 4:75-102, 1980.

346. Wagner H, Zeiler G, Baur W: [Indication, technic and results of supra- and infracondylar osteotomy in osteoarthrosis of the knee joint]. Orthopade 14:172-192, 1985.

347. Wagner J: Curvilinear osteotomy of the tibia. In Aichroth PM, Cannon WD Jr (eds): Knee Surgery: Current Practice. London, Martin Dunitz, 1992, pp 608-610.

348. Wagner J, Bourgois R, Hermanne A: Comportement mécanique du cadre tibio-péronier dans les genoux varum et valgum. Acta Orthop Belg 48:57-92, 1982.

349. Wakabayashi S, Akizuki S, Takizawa T, et al: A comparison of the healing potential of fibrillated cartilage versus eburnated bone in osteoarthritic knees after high tibial osteotomy: An arthroscopic study with 1-year follow-up. Arthroscopy 18:272-278, 2002.

350. Walther M, Konig A, Kirschner S, et al: Results of posterior cruciate-retaining unconstrained total knee arthroplasty after proximal tibial osteotomy for osteoarthritis: A prospective cohort study. Arch Orthop Trauma Surg 120:166-170, 2000.

351. Wang JW, Kuo KN, Andriacchi TP, et al: The influence of walking mechanics and time on the results of proximal tibial osteotomy. J Bone Joint Surg Am 72:905-909, 1990.

352. Weale AE, Lee AS, MacEachern AG: High tibial osteotomy using a dynamic axial external fixator. Clin Orthop 382:154-167, 2001.

353. Weale AE, Newman JH: Unicompartmental arthroplasty and high tibial osteotomy for osteoarthrosis of the knee: A comparative study with a 12- to 17-year follow-up period. Clin Orthop 302:134-137, 1994.

354. Weidenhielm L, Olsson E, Brostrom LA, et al: Improvement in gait one year after surgery for knee osteoarthrosis: A comparison between high tibial osteotomy and prosthetic replacement in a prospective randomized study. Scand J Rehabil Med 25:25-31, 1993.

355. Weill D, Jacquemin MC: [Cylindrical femoral supracondylar varisation osteotomy in the surgical treatment of gonarthrosis]. Acta Orthop Belg 48:110-130, 1982.

356. Westrich GH, Peters LE, Haas SB, et al: Patella height after high tibial osteotomy with internal fixation and early motion. Clin Orthop 354:169-174, 1998.

357. Wildner M, Peters A, Hellich J, et al: Complications of high tibial osteotomy and internal fixation with staples. Arch Orthop Trauma Surg 111:210-212, 1992.

358. Williams RJ, Kelly BT, Wickiewicz TL, et al: The short-term outcome of surgical treatment for painful varus arthritis in association with chronic ACL deficiency. J Knee Surg 16:9-16, 2003.

359. Windsor RE, Insall JN, Vince KG: Technical considerations of total knee arthroplasty after proximal tibial osteotomy. J Bone Joint Surg Am 70:547-555, 1988.

360. Wright J, Heck D, Hawker G, et al: Rates of tibial osteotomies in Canada and the United States. Clin Orthop 319:266-275, 1995.

361. Wright JG, Coyte P, Hawker G, et al: Variation in orthopedic surgeons' perceptions of the indications for and outcomes of knee replacement. Can Med Assoc J 152:687-697, 1995.

362. Wright JM, Heavrin B, Begg M, et al: Observations on patellar height following opening wedge proximal tibial osteotomy. Am J Knee Surg 14:163-173, 2001.

363. Wu DD, Burr DB, Boyd RD, et al: Bone and cartilage changes following experimental varus or valgus tibial angulation. J Orthop Res 8:572-585, 1990.

364. Yasuda K, Majima T, Tanabe Y, et al: Long-term evaluation of high tibial osteotomy for medial osteoarthritis of the knee. Bull Hosp Joint Dis Orthop Inst 51:236-248, 1991.

365. Yasuda K, Majima T, Tsuchida T, et al: A ten- to 15-year follow-up observation of high tibial osteotomy in medial compartment osteoarthrosis. Clin Orthop 282:186-195, 1992.

366. Yasunaga M: [The study of lateral thrust of the knee in normal and osteoarthritic knees—evaluation with an accelerometric technique]. Fukuoka Igaku Zasshi 87:242-252, 1996.

367. Yoshino N, Takai S, Watanabe Y, et al: Total knee arthroplasty with long stem for treatment of nonunion after high tibial osteotomy. J Arthroplasty 19:528-531, 2004.

368. Yoshioka Y, Siu D, Cooke TD: The anatomy and functional axes of the femur. J Bone Joint Surg Am 69:873-880, 1987.

369. Zaidi SH, Cobb AG, Bentley G: Danger to the popliteal artery in high tibial osteotomy. J Bone Joint Surg Br 77:384-386, 1995.

370. Zuegel NP, Braun WG, Kundel KP, et al: Stabilization of high tibial osteotomy with staples. Arch Orthop Trauma Surg 115:290-294, 1996.

CHAPTER 79

Historic Development, Classification, and Characteristics of Knee Prostheses

John N. Insall • *Henry D. Clarke*

The evolution of total knee replacement (TKR)—in its modern form approaching 40 years old—is not merely of historic interest. Surgeons with some years of experience will have noticed that fashion tends to repeat itself. For example, in the early years (1970 to 1974), a range of prostheses (unicondylar, bicondylar, and hinged) were used, depending on the preoperative condition and deformity. These prostheses fell into disrepute, and for a while tricondylar resurfacing prostheses were in vogue for virtually all procedures. In recent years, successful results have been obtained with unicondylar prostheses in selected patients, and both constrained and hinged prostheses have found a place in the surgical armamentarium for revision and complex primary surgery. In addition, interest in mobile-bearing prostheses has been rekindled as the limits of current fixed-bearing prostheses are defined. Yet another example of a trend that is re-emerging is the concept of uncemented fixation in TKR. After a decade of limited application of this form of fixation, new materials have prompted renewed interest. Whether this time such a development will provide a significant advantage remains to be seen. Indeed, since the last edition of this text was published, the proliferation of new materials, such as ceramics and cross-linked polyethylene, as well as prosthesis design changes to maximize flexion, minimize potential backside wear, optimize kinematics, and allow prosthesis insertion through minimally invasive approaches, has resulted in an ever-growing list of unanswered questions in the field of TKR. Therefore, at this important time in the field of TKR, as the original pioneers are succeeded by the next generation of surgeons, change should only be embraced once three criteria have been met: first, a problem that needs a solution should exist; second, the solution should be based on solid basic science research; and finally, the clinical results should be documented by the innovator and others. To help guide this pursuit of continuing improvement in total knee arthroplasty (TKA), we believe that it is useful to look at what has worked and what has not worked in the past.

EARLY PROSTHETIC MODELS

Interposition and Resurfacing Prostheses

The concept of improving knee joint function by modifying the articular surfaces has received attention since the 19th century. In 1860, Verneuil[252] suggested the interposition of soft tissues to reconstruct the articular surface of a joint. Subsequently, pig bladder, nylon, fascia lata, prepatellar bursa, and cellophane were some of the materials used for this purpose. The results were disappointing. In 1860, Ferguson[72] resected the entire knee joint, which resulted in mobility of the newly created subchondral surfaces (Fig. 79–1). When more bone was removed, the patients enjoyed good motion but lacked the necessary stability, whereas with less bone resection, spontaneous fusion often resulted. These early attempts were usually performed on knees damaged by tuberculosis or other infectious processes, along with concomitant ankylosis and deformity. The results of this procedure were sufficiently poor to discourage anything more than occasional attempts in severe cases.

Encouraged by the relative success of hip cup arthroplasty, Campbell[41] reported the successful use of a metallic interposition femoral mold in 1940. A similar type of arthroplasty was developed and used at Massachusetts General Hospital. The results, published by Speed and Trout[238] in 1949 and by Miller and Friedman[177] in 1952, were not very good, and this type of knee arthroplasty never achieved wide recognition.

In 1958, MacIntosh[162] described a different type of hemiarthroplasty that he had used in treating painful varus or valgus deformities of the knee. An acrylic tibial plateau prosthesis was inserted into the affected side to correct deformity, restore stability, and relieve pain. Later versions of this prosthesis[163] were made of metal (Fig. 79–2), and the somewhat similar McKeever prosthesis[65,175,213] showed considerably more success and was extensively used, particularly in patients with rheumatoid arthritis. Gunston[97] carried MacIntosh's ideas a step further and, instead of using a simple metal disk interposed within the joint, substituted metallic runners embedded in the femoral condyles that articulated against polyethylene troughs attached to the tibial plateau. To make a four-part system of this kind feasible, it was necessary to find a means of fixing the components rigidly to the bone. The solution was provided by acrylic cement.

Although the Gunston polycentric prosthesis[97] was the first cemented surface arthroplasty of the knee joint, the work of Freeman and colleagues[78,85] has had an even greater influence on the direction of both prosthetic design and surgical technique. The design objectives for a prosthesis (Fig. 79–3A and B) were outlined in 1973 by Freeman and colleagues.[85] The most important of these objectives are the following:

1. A salvage procedure should be readily available. Implantation of the prosthesis should require the removal of no more bone than for primary arthrodesis and should leave large, flat surfaces of cancellous bone.

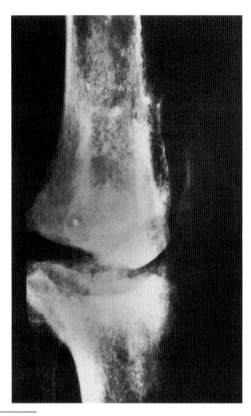

Figure 79–1. Resection arthroplasty creates a mobile, but usually unstable joint.

2. The chances of loosening should be minimized.
    a. The femoral and tibial components should be incompletely constrained relative to each other so that twisting, varus, or valgus moments cannot be transmitted to the bonds between the prosthesis and skeleton.
    b. The friction between components should be minimized.
    c. Any hyperextension-limiting arrangement should be progressive and not sudden in action.
    d. The prosthetic component should be fitted to the bone by means that spread the loads over the largest possible area of the bone-prosthesis interface.
3. The rate of production of wear debris should be minimized, and the debris produced should be as innocuous as possible. This objective leads to a preference for metal-on-plastic bearing surfaces, which should be as large as possible to keep the surface stress low.
4. The probability of infection should be minimized by having compact prosthetic components with few dead spaces.
5. The consequences of infection should be minimized by avoiding long intramedullary stems and intramedullary cement.
6. A standard insertion procedure should be available.
7. The prosthesis should give motion from 5 degrees of hyperextension to at least 90 degrees of flexion.
8. Some freedom of rotation should be resisted.
9. Excessive movements in any direction should be resisted by the soft tissues, particularly the collateral ligaments.

Most of these objectives remain valid today, although two additional points cited in the Freeman report remain issues for debate: (1) the place of the cruciate ligaments

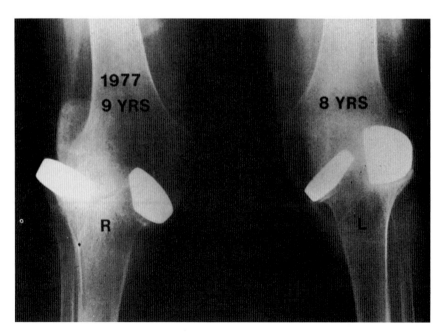

Figure 79–2. Use of the MacIntosh hemiarthroplasty in patients with rheumatoid arthritis often restores alignment and stability for a few years. However, as in this bilateral case, late dislocation and sinkage are common.

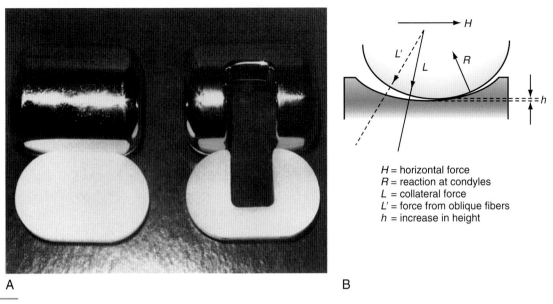

H = horizontal force
R = reaction at condyles
L = collateral force
L' = force from oblique fibers
h = increase in height

A   B

Figure 79–3. **A,** The original Freeman-Swanson prosthesis used two one-piece components. **B,** Stability is obtained by the roller-in-trough concept; dislocation can occur only if one component runs uphill on the other. Distraction is resisted by capsular and collateral ligament tension.

in TKA and (2) the need to replace the patellofemoral joint and the desirability of patellar resurfacing.

Other early examples of resurfacing prostheses (Figs. 79–4 and 79–5) were the Geometric,[51,52,250] Duocondylar,[195,232] UCI (University of California at Irvine),[263] and Marmor.[168-171]

Constrained Prostheses

A second line of development in knee arthroplasty occurred parallel to the concepts of interposition and, later, surface replacement. In 1951, Walldius[259] developed the hinged prosthesis that bears his name. The device was initially made of acrylic and later of metal.

Shortly thereafter, Shiers[224] described a similar device with even simpler mechanical characteristics (Fig. 79–6). A hinged prosthesis has considerable appeal. Technically, it is easy to use because the intramedullary stems make the prosthesis largely self-aligning, and all the ligaments and other soft-tissue constraints can be sacrificed because the prosthesis is self-stabilizing. The extent of damage to the knee is therefore of no consequence, and even the most extreme deformities can be corrected by dividing the soft tissues and resecting sufficient bone. Of course, the early hinged designs were uncemented, although later developments such as the GUEPAR (Fig. 79–7) were designed from the outset to be used with methylmethacrylate cement. Because of inherent limitations with a simple hinge, including limited range of motion and transmission of stress to the prosthesis-cement interface, the early hinged prostheses were supplanted by rotating-hinge devices that constrain the prosthesis in the coronal and sagittal planes, but allow rotation in the axial plane. Early designs included the Spherocentric (Fig 79–8) pros-

thesis, and current models include the Kinematic Rotating Hinge, the Rotating Hinge Knee, and the SROM prosthesis. In cases in which the maximal constraint offered by a linked hinge is not required, unlinked but constrained devices have been extensively used in revision and complex primary TKR. These devices include the TCP III (Total Condylar prosthesis)[58] (Fig. 79–9) and the Constrained Condylar Knee (CCK). The primary characteristic of these devices is a cam-and-post mechanism, similar to that found in a posterior-stabilized prosthesis, but thicker and taller, and it provides resistance not only to posterior translation but also to varus and valgus stress. At the present time, the use of cemented or uncemented stems with both hinged and constrained, but unlinked devices is based on surgeon preference.

EVOLUTION OF PROSTHETIC DESIGN

The prostheses discussed up to this point are now more or less obsolete. Although the early results were quite encouraging, further follow-up demonstrated various problems. The literature relevant to TKA includes many articles that report the clinical results of designs no longer in common use.* These published reports on results with early models are somewhat difficult to compare because different rating methods were used. A review conducted at the Hospital for Special Surgery (HSS) between 1971

*See references 5, 10-14, 16, 35, 37, 40, 43, 44, 47, 53, 54, 58, 60, 69-71, 75, 77, 79, 83, 84, 86, 87, 89, 94, 98, 105, 110, 112, 114, 115, 118, 121, 123-128, 132, 148, 150, 157-159, 166, 173, 174, 182, 183, 189, 190, 199, 201, 202, 204, 211, 222, 223, 225, 226, 228, 230, 231, 234, 244, 248, 251, 264, 265, 270, 272, 278.

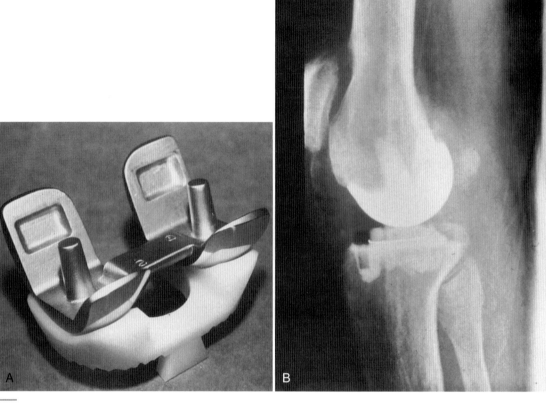

Figure 79–4. **A** and **B,** An early and widely used surface replacement was the Geometric prosthesis.

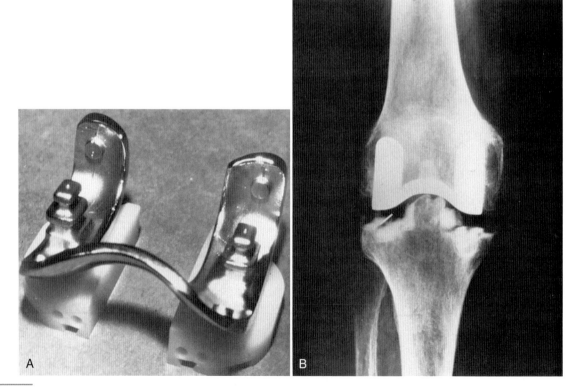

Figure 79–5. **A,** The Duocondylar prosthesis was anatomic in concept, retained both cruciate ligaments when present, but did not resurface the patellofemoral joint. Sinkage and loosening of the tibial components were an eventual problem with this design. **B,** Anteroposterior radiograph with the Duocondylar prosthesis inserted. Radiolucent lines around both tibial components are visible.

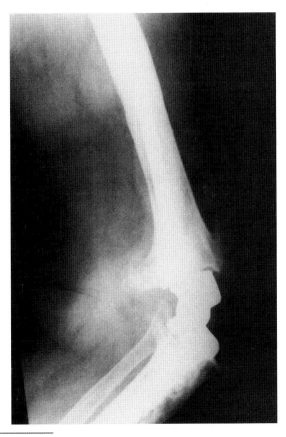

Figure 79–6. The Shiers prosthesis was a simple uniaxial metallic hinge.

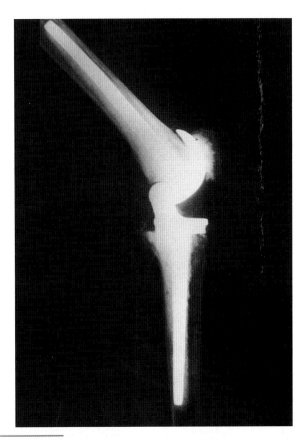

Figure 79–7. The GUEPAR hinge was like the Shiers uniaxial metallic hinge, but with the axis placed more posteriorly and femoral resurfacing for the patellar articulation.

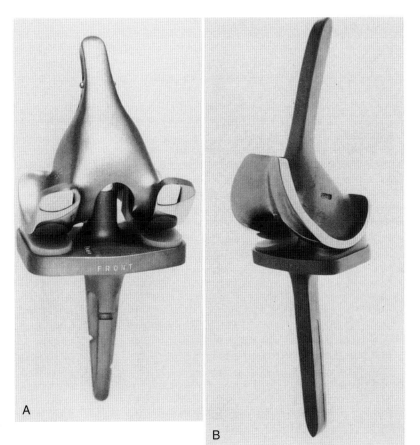

Figure 79–8. Spherocentric prosthesis. **A,** Standard version. **B,** Long-stemmed variant with a patellar flange. (Courtesy of Drs. Kauffer and Matthews.)

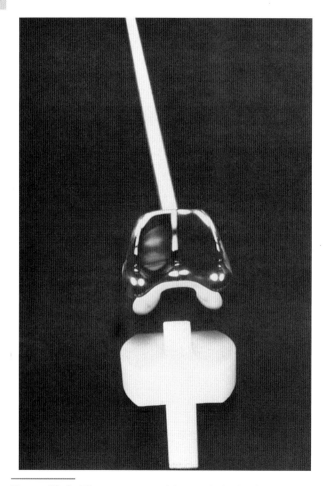

Figure 79–9. The constrained but unlinked TCP III. Varus and valgus constraint is provided by the rectangular central peg on the tibial component.

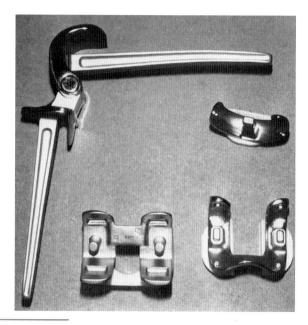

Figure 79–10. The graduated system concept selected the prosthesis according to the degree and extent of damage. The prostheses shown here in a clockwise direction are the unicondylar, Duocondylar, Geometric, and GUEPAR prostheses.

and 1973 is probably representative. This review[118] compared four different models (Fig. 79–10): the unicondylar (Fig. 79–11), Duocondylar, Geometric, and GUEPAR (see Fig. 79–7). The results were expressed by using the HSS 100-point knee-rating scale.

Postoperative knees were classified into four groups according to their scores on the HSS scale:

Excellent: 85+. These knees approached the normal and were obviously much improved in the opinion of both the patient and the examiner.

Good: 70 to 84. These knees showed obvious improvement after arthroplasty, but the result was not as good as in the excellent group.

Fair: 60 to 69. This group mostly consisted of knees in which the result of arthroplasty was deficient in some way (persistent pain, moderate instability, or unsatisfactory range of motion), but also included some in which the rating of the arthroplasty was downgraded by the patient's general condition (e.g., multiple-joint involvement in rheumatoid arthritis or systemic disease).

Failure: Less than 60. These knees were evidently unsatisfactory and below the rating achieved by knee fusion (which scores a 60 on the HSS knee-rating scale). This classification included knees

in which the prosthesis had been removed or replaced and knees in which the improvement, if any, did not seem to justify the risk of arthroplasty.

Considering the entire group of 178 arthroplasties studied in the four different models (23 unicondylar, 60 Duocondylar, 50 Geometric, and 45 GUEPAR), the results were considered excellent in 47 (26%), good in 66 (37%), fair in 37 (21%), and poor in 28 (16%) (Fig. 79–12). There was no statistically significant difference between the results obtained with each of the four prostheses studied. However, because it is easier to improve a bad knee than a relatively good one, the percentage of improvement was much greater with the GUEPAR than with the unicondylar (120% versus 45%).

Three specific problems were identified from this study: patellar pain, component loosening, and surgical technique. However, because the GUEPAR hinge was inserted into the worst knees originally, it gave the greatest percentage of improvement in the HSS knee-rating scale. At the time of the study, the conclusion reached was that the GUEPAR prosthesis appeared superior in a number of ways. It had been selected for use in the most severely involved knees and yet equaled any of the other prostheses in the quality of results both in rheumatoid arthritis and in osteoarthritis. It also gave the lowest proportion of failures and was the only model to improve range of motion postoperatively. However, the potential problems of loosening and mechanical failure with the GUEPAR prosthesis were noted. More than 100 GUEPAR prostheses were used at the HSS nearly 30 years ago, and these expected problems to a large extent materialized. Approximately 80% of the prostheses are loose both clinically and radiographically, although they are not necessarily symp-

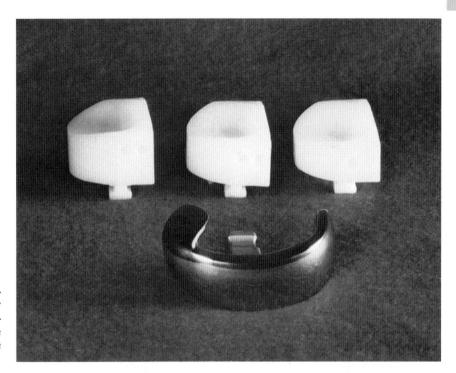

Figure 79–11. The unicondylar prosthesis was designed to resurface only the affected femorotibial compartment. The shape and curvature of the component were similar to that of the Duocondylar design.

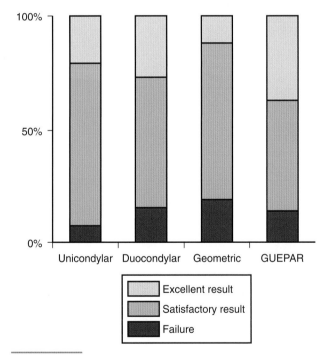

Figure 79–12. Graph showing the comparative results of four early prosthetic models.

tomatic (Fig. 79–13A). There have also been seven cases of stem breakage (four femoral and three tibial) (Fig. 79–13B), and as noted later, infection became a major problem. This study therefore reached some erroneous conclusions because of short follow-up—a point of great relevance today when many new prostheses are being used in patients with scanty clinical follow-up to support their merits.

Patellar Pain

None of the four early prosthetic models studied made any provision for patellofemoral function. Patellectomy did not seem to offer a solution to the problem of patellofemoral arthritis (Fig. 79–14). In our study, 38 patellectomies were performed in the group as a whole, 3 of which were done at a later date than the arthroplasty because of persistent patellar pain. A complaint of pain after patellectomy was as frequent as in patients in whom patellectomy had not been performed. In addition, patients who underwent patellectomy suffered from inadequacy of the extensor mechanism. In the GUEPAR group of 45 knees, pain on patellar compression was found in 22 on follow-up, and patellar erosion was observed in 5 patients. Patellar subluxation frequently occurred with the GUEPAR prosthesis despite wide lateral release of the patellar retinaculum at the time of arthroplasty (Fig. 79–15). Nonetheless, the subluxation was often not apparent to the patient and may be considered an incidental finding. Subluxation of the patella did not necessarily correlate with complaints of postoperative pain. However, with the Geometric prosthesis, 29 of 50 knees had pain on patellofemoral compression. Patellar subluxation was found in nine knees, and all were painful.

Loosening

A radiolucent line surrounding the prosthetic components was seen with great frequency. With the condylar replacements, the radiolucency was usually observed around the tibial component. It was present in 70% of knees with the unicondylar, 50% with the Duocondylar, and 80% with the Geometric prosthesis. A radiolucent line was observed

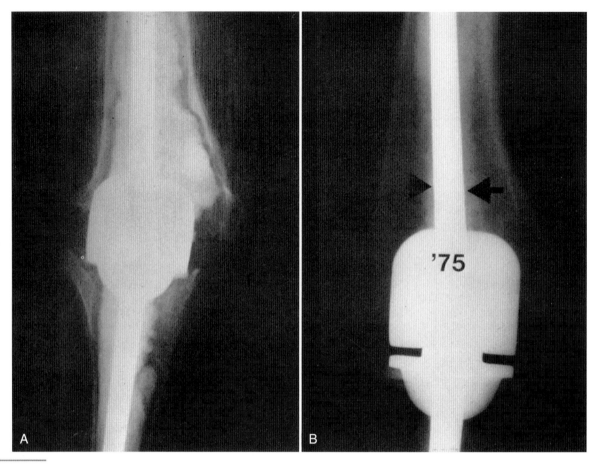

Figure 79–13. **A,** Radiograph of a grossly loose GUEPAR prosthesis 5 years after initial insertion. **B,** Stem breakage occurred with the GUEPAR prosthesis, usually at the site shown here in the radiograph, 5 cm proximal to the joint.

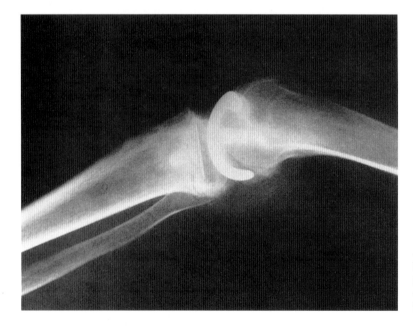

Figure 79–14. Patellectomy is not a satisfactory solution to patellofemoral pain. Patellectomy was performed in conjunction with implantation of a unicondylar prosthesis.

around the femoral component in 45% of the patients with a GUEPAR prosthesis. The radiolucent line was slightly more frequent in patients with osteoarthritis than in those with rheumatoid arthritis, and it was observed in all knees with osteoarthritis in which the Geometric prosthesis was used. Radiolucent lines are by no means always symptomatic, but when complete, progressive, and associated with pain on weightbearing, they generally indicate failure of fixation. Our subsequent experience has shown that the incidence of partial radiolucencies for a particular pros-

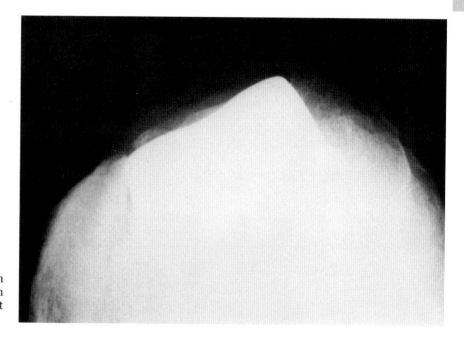

Figure 79–15. Patellar subluxation and dislocation often occurred with the GUEPAR prosthesis. It was not always symptomatic.

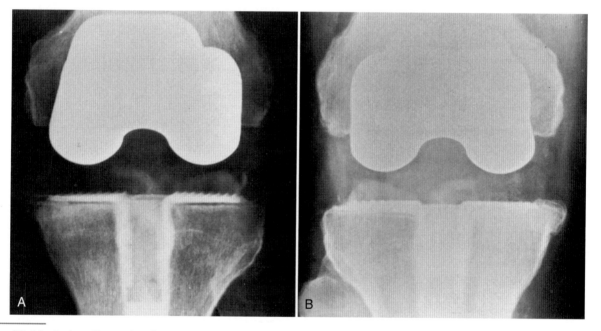

Figure 79–16. **A,** A radiograph taken 1 year after implantation shows a pronounced radiolucent line beneath the medial and lateral tibial plateaus. **B,** A radiograph of the same knee taken at 5 years shows a barely visible radiolucency.

thesis does not correlate with the eventual amount of component loosening. On the strength of a 10- to 12-year follow-up on one particular cemented prosthesis (the Total Condylar), we concluded that a detailed study of partial radiolucent lines about cemented knee replacements was worthless and a poor predictor of future failure (Fig. 79–16).

On the basis of early analysis of these data, it was clear that tibial loosening represented a failure in prosthetic design. The flat, cancellous surface of the upper part of the tibia is not a suitable bed for a flat prosthetic component because of poor resistance to shear stress. Moreover, this bone is not of sufficient strength to resist subsidence

of the tibial component, even if excavations are made to accommodate fixation fins or lugs on the bottom of the tibial prosthesis (Figs. 79–17 and 79–18). It was concluded that some form of cortical fixation would be essential for a successful TKA series.

Prosthesis Selection and Surgical Technique

Like many others, we initially believed in the concept of a graduated system in which selection of a prosthesis

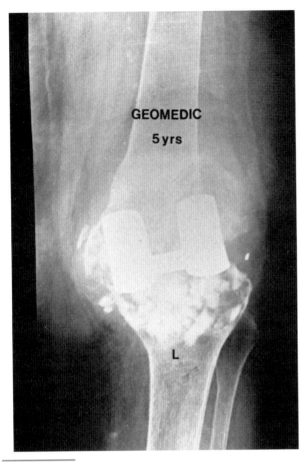

Figure 79–17. Failure of tibial fixation was a frequent problem with many early prosthetic designs. The problem was primarily attributable to collapse of the cancellous bone of the upper part of the tibia together with sinkage of the component.

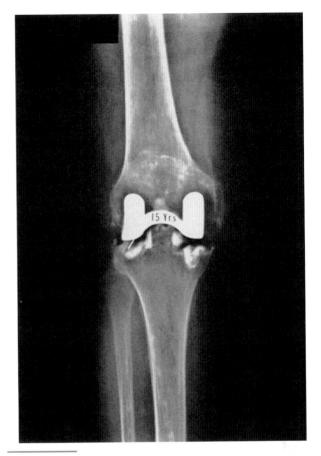

Figure 79–18. Radiograph of a 15-year follow-up of a Duo-condylar prosthesis that had two separate tibial components. There is the appearance of osteopenia around the femoral component runners. The knee continued to function well.

depended on the severity of damage found in the arthritic knee (see Fig. 79–10). For example, knees with cartilage erosion restricted to one femorotibial compartment were replaced with a unicondylar prosthesis, whereas in the most severely damaged and deformed knees, a hinged prosthesis was used. The bicondylar prosthesis occupied an intermediate position with respect to the severity of arthritis. Although the use of a hinged prosthesis is not technically demanding, the early condylar designs were difficult to insert and align, and there was very little margin for error. Obviously, the advantage of even the most sophisticated prosthetic design is lost if surgical placement is incorrect. Furthermore, an inherent draw-back in a graduated system of prostheses is that a model may be used for degrees of deformity exceeding the limits for which the prosthesis was intended. This error can itself be a cause of failure (e.g., dislocation) (Fig. 79–19). Clearly, there is no purpose in selecting one prosthetic design over another unless some advantage can be shown. For example, in our comparative study we did not find that the unicondylar prosthesis offered any advantage over bicondylar models. The merits of graduated knee systems remain a source of debate today.

Infection

Although deep periprosthetic infection was not a frequent cause of failure for the condylar designs, it has subsequently proved to be a major problem with the GUEPAR prosthesis. With further follow-up, 15 of 108 prostheses became infected (4 early and 8 late). This incidence of 14% is likely to rise because late infection occurs even many years after the arthroplasty. An example was an 85-year-old woman who had a GUEPAR prosthesis inserted in 1972. She did very well for 8 years until the onset of acute deep sepsis. There was no obvious focus elsewhere to suggest a metastatic infection. Because of her age and the extreme toxicity caused by virulent infection, a midthigh amputation had to be performed. More recently, a second amputation was performed for late-onset sepsis: the extreme devitalization of the tissues caused by metallic debris made any thought of salvage impossible. There have been reports of similar occurrences in the literature.[11]

At the HSS, dissatisfaction with the early prostheses led to design of the Total Condylar and Duopatellar prostheses, which were based on different philosophies about how

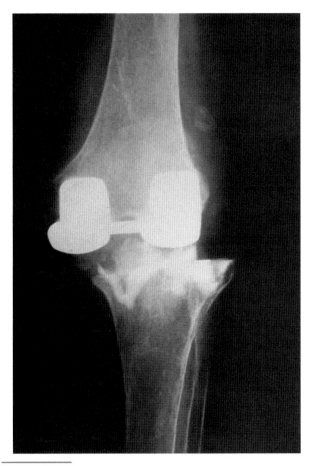

Figure 79–19. This Geometric prosthesis translocated and dislocated. This was the condition of the knee before the prosthesis was inserted and represents an error in prosthesis selection.

to manage the posterior collateral ligament (PCL). During the 1980s, prosthetic characteristics diverged further and were generally linked to whether the prosthesis was designed to substitute for or preserve the PCL. However, during the 1990s, a convergence of prosthetic designs has occurred, particularly in the United States.

TYPES OF PROSTHESES

Most simply, a prosthesis can be a surface replacement or a constrained design. These two categories may be further subdivided. Surface replacements comprise unicondylar and bicondylar designs. Unicondylar prostheses are discussed elsewhere in this text.* Bicondylar prostheses can be cruciate retaining, cruciate excising, or cruciate substituting. Constrained prostheses can be hinged or unlinked. The majority of hinged devices are now designed to allow rotation in the axial plane while eliminating motion in the coronal plane. Although in original designs the load was

transmitted solely through a metal axle that linked the femoral and tibial components, many newer designs allow for load sharing between the axle and a metal-on-polyethylene bearing, as found in surface replacement designs. As discussed earlier, the primary characteristic of unlinked designs, such as the CCK or TCP III, is a cam-and-post mechanism, similar to that found in a posterior-stabilized prosthesis, but thicker and taller. This mechanism provides resistance not only to posterior translation but also to varus and valgus stress and rotation. Although these devices offer less constraint in the coronal plane than a hinged prosthesis does, they are more constrained in the axial plane. To date, there is little information about which type of constrained device will prove superior in the long term.

Early Surface Replacement Designs

In the following sections we discuss early surface replacement designs.[255] Supplemental information about the individual innovators and the tremendous advances in TKA during the early years of the modern era can be found in the historical review by Robinson.[206] Much of the early debate about both prosthesis design and the techniques used to implant the components, including how to address the cruciate ligaments, arose from philosophic differences among the pioneers about whether it was better to design a knee prosthesis from an anatomic or a functional perspective.[206] It is interesting to note that the current generation of prostheses have converged in many ways, with most designs incorporating characteristics from each category that seem to have optimized long-term outcomes, for example, side-specific femoral components with optimized trochlear geometries from the anatomic approach and the moderately conforming coronal and sagittal geometry that was more associated with the functional approach.

Total Condylar Prosthesis

Although coined as the name of a specific prosthesis, the term *total condylar prosthesis* has more recently been used generically to describe a whole range of surface prostheses that share general characteristics with the original (Fig. 79–20).* Some of these later models differ in design details that may prove important in the long run.

The Total Condylar prosthesis, designed in 1973, was a true total replacement of the knee in that the patellofemoral joint was replaced as well as the femorotibial compartment. Designed from a functional perspective, the inherent geometry of the prosthesis was intended to substitute for the anatomic function of the cruciate ligaments, native articular geometry, and menisci. The salient features of the design are discussed in the following sections.[206]

*See references 15, 42, 101, 142, 143, 147, 149, 167, 172, 179, 180, 214, 217.

*See references 4, 7, 67, 73, 88, 104, 108, 109, 115, 116, 119, 120, 122, 131, 135, 139, 153, 194, 212, 221, 253, 254.

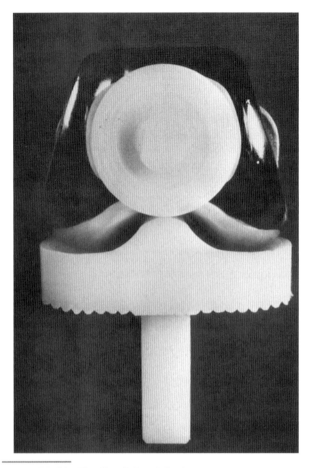

Figure 79–20. The Total Condylar Prosthesis.

Femoral Component. Made of cobalt chromium alloy, the femoral component contained a symmetrically grooved anterior flange that separated posteriorly into two symmetric condyles, each of decreasing radius posteriorly with a symmetric convex curvature in the coronal plane.

Tibial Component. The tibial component was made of high-density polyethylene in one piece with two separate biconcave tibial plateaus that mated (articulated) precisely with the femoral condyles in extension, thus permitting no rotation in this position. In flexion the fit ceased to be exact and rotation and gliding motions were possible. The symmetric tibial plateaus were separated by an intercondylar eminence designed to prevent translocation or sideways sliding movements. The peripheral margin of the articular concavities was of an even height both anteriorly and posteriorly. The undersurface of the component had a central fixation peg 35 mm in length and 12.5 mm in width. The anterior margin of the peg was vertical, but the posterior margin was oblique, thereby conforming with the posterior cortex of the tibia.

Patellar Component. Made of high-density polyethylene, the patellar component was dome shaped on its articular surface, closely conforming to the curvature of the femoral flange. A dome was selected because this shape did not require rotary alignment as an anatomic prosthe-

sis would. The bony surface of the prosthesis had a central, rectangular fixation peg.

Duopatellar Prosthesis

The Total Condylar Prosthesis was designed for cruciate excision. In contrast, the Duopatellar prosthesis,[71] a sibling prosthesis designed from an anatomic perspective at the HSS as a replacement for the Duocondylar model, was intended to preserve existing cruciate ligaments, particularly the PCL.[206] The general shape of the tibial runners was anatomic in the sagittal plane. Coronally, the condyles were flat with a median curvature.

The anterior connecting bar of the Duocondylar prosthesis was extended into a femoral flange. The initial version of the Duopatellar model had two separate tibial plateaus identical to the Duocondylar design: flat in the sagittal plane, but with a median curvature coronally to prevent translocation. The deep surface was dovetailed for cement fixation. Later, the two components were joined, and a central fixation peg similar to that of the total condylar prosthesis was added. A PCL cutout was provided. The patellar component of the Duopatellar prosthesis was identical to that of the Total Condylar Prosthesis.

Cruciate Excision, Retention, and Substitution

The Total Condylar and Duopatellar prostheses were designed for cruciate excision and retention, respectively.[7,9,59,80,84] Subsequent modifications to the Total Condylar prosthesis incorporated a cam on the femoral component and a central post on the tibial polyethylene (Fig. 79–21). This cam-and-post mechanism was designed to act as a functional substitute for the PCL and produce femoral rollback during flexion. With the development of this so-called Posterior-Stabilized prosthesis it was apparent that cruciate excision alone was not optimal. However, the relative merits of PCL retention versus PCL substitution have been debated vigorously within the orthopedic community for many years. The development of total knee prostheses has occurred along two distinct evolutionary paths based on these quite different principles.[206] In the following sections the anatomic function of the cruciate ligaments, the relative advantages and disadvantages of cruciate excision, and the subject of PCL retention versus PCL substitution will be reviewed. It has also become clear that if the PCL is retained, the function of the ligament must be optimized through a balancing technique. Difficulties with balancing the PCL, as well as late PCL rupture leading to flexion instability, have led to development of the so-called deep-dish polyethylene inserts that are currently offered as part of many cruciate-retaining prosthesis systems. These inserts have moderately conforming articular surfaces in the coronal and sagittal planes, together with an anterior lip that limits paradoxic anterior translation of the femur on the tibia. This is one example

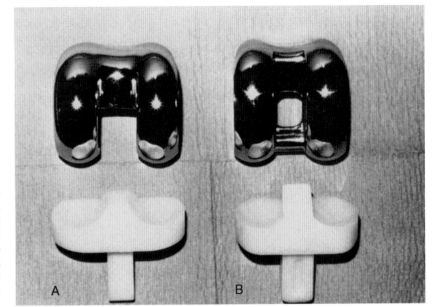

Figure 79–21. **A,** Total Condylar prosthesis. **B,** Posterior-Stabilized Condylar Knee, a newer derivative providing posterior cruciate substitution by means of a central cam mechanism. (From Insall JN, Lachiewicz PF, Burstein AH: The posterior stabilized condylar prosthesis: A modification of the total condylar design: Two to four year clinical experience. J Bone Joint Surg Am 64:1317, 1982.)

of how prosthesis design has converged in the past decade, thus making it more difficult to trace the origins of any particular design.

ANATOMIC FUNCTIONS OF THE CRUCIATE LIGAMENTS

One function of the cruciate ligaments, in addition to providing static anterior and posterior stability, is to impose certain movements on the joint surfaces relative to one another. The anterior cruciate ligament (ACL) is often absent in arthritic knees and has not been thought to be of much consequence in TKA. The importance of the ACL may have been underestimated inasmuch as unconstrained prostheses have increased sagittal plane laxity and fail more often when the ACL is absent.[266] Although the PCL is often attenuated in arthritic knees, it is usually present. It has been considered the collateral ligament for the medial compartment of the knee.[64] The PCL causes the femoral condyles to glide and roll back on the tibial plateau as the knee is flexed.[130] In a normal knee the shape of the plateau does not restrain this motion, and the laxity of the meniscal attachments allows the menisci to move posteriorly with the femur. This femoral rollback is crucial in prosthetic design. If the cruciates are excised, a more conforming tibial polyethylene component can be used to provide some degree of anterior and posterior stability. However, without the function of the PCL, femoral rollback will not occur, which theoretically limits the ultimate flexion that can be obtained. If the PCL is retained, the tibial surface must be flat or even posteriorly sloped[266] (Fig. 79–22). If a more conforming component is used in these circumstances, posterior impingement will occur (Fig. 79–23). Substitution of the PCL with a cam-and-post mechanism not only re-creates femoral rollback but also allows a conforming articulation to be used without risk

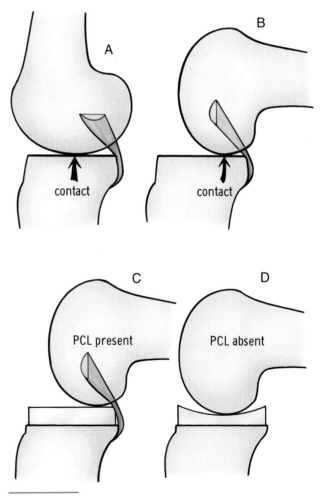

Figure 79–22. Effect of posterior cruciate ligament (PCL) retention on prosthetic design. **A** and **B,** Because of the rollback enforced by the PCL, the prosthetic tibial surface must be flat to allow this movement. **C** and **D,** When the PCL is absent, a dished tibial plateau is used.

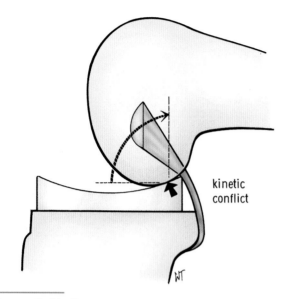

Figure 79–23. Kinematic conflict occurs if concepts are mismatched. In this case, the posterior cruciate ligament is preserved with the use of a dished tibial component. Impingement occurs posteriorly with flexion.

of posterior impingement. These considerations were reflected in the design of the total condylar, duopatellar, posterior-stabilized, and various PCL-retaining prostheses.

ARGUMENTS FOR CRUCIATE EXCISION

Correction of Deformity

Removal of the cruciate ligaments is an important element in the soft-tissue release of fixed varus or valgus deformities. Correction of these deformities is therefore facilitated by cruciate excision. In addition, clearance of the intercondylar notch provides clear visualization of the posterior capsule, which facilitates release and osteophyte removal during correction of flexion deformities.

Simpler Technique

Release of the cruciate ligaments facilitates surgical exposure, especially in tight knees, which makes the procedure less demanding. It is also technically easier to cut straight across the tibia than around the cruciate insertions. These factors make it easier to make the correct bone cuts and achieve accurate placement of the prosthesis.

Wear

Cruciate excision allows the use of a more conforming articulation, which increases the contact area and reduces contact stress.

ARGUMENTS AGAINST CRUCIATE EXCISION

Range of Motion

Without a functional PCL or PCL-substituting mechanism, rollback of the femoral component does not occur. This theoretically limits the ultimate flexion obtainable and, indeed, was noted as a clinical limitation with the original cruciate-sacrificing prosthesis, the Total Condylar prosthesis.

Instability

Failure to achieve flexion and extension balance can result in anterior-posterior laxity that may exceed the stability imparted by the moderately conforming articular surfaces. Such laxity may lead to symptomatic instability.

Loosening

The increased conformity of the articular surfaces used in the total condylar prosthesis theoretically results in increased stress at the bone-cement-prosthesis interface, which provoked concern that it would ultimately cause loosening. However, as discussed later in the section on PCL substitution, these concerns have not become clinically significant.

PCL RETENTION VERSUS SUBSTITUTION

Kinematics

Retention of the PCL was initially believed to allow preservation of normal knee kinematics after TKR. In particular, preservation of the normal femoral rollback caused by tightening of the PCL, which acts to move the tibiofemoral contact point posteriorly during flexion, thereby increasing quadriceps efficiency and range of motion, was thought to be critical in activities such as stair climbing. The natural PCL was initially perceived to be better in performing this kinematic function than the cam-and-post mechanism used in posterior-stabilized knee prostheses. However, fluoroscopic studies by Stiehl and coauthors[243] and Dennis and colleagues[55] have demonstrated that PCL-retaining prostheses do not replicate the kinematics of the normal knee. Instead, in many cases a paradoxic roll-forward of the femur with anterior translation of the tibiofemoral contact area occurs. This motion, which is the direct opposite of normal knee kinematics, may result from improper tension of the PCL (Fig. 79–24). Adverse consequences may include decreased flexion, reduced quadriceps efficiency, and posterior tibial polyethylene wear. In addition, Dennis and coauthors demonstrated that although posterior-stabilized prostheses did not completely reproduce normal knee kinematics, reliable roll-back did occur. Surgeons who advocate the use of PCL-retaining prostheses have emphasized the importance of balancing the PCL with techniques such as PCL release and recession.[205,215] However, the success of using these techniques to restore normal knee kinematics has not yet been proved. Based on current knowledge, it seems that PCL substitution more reliably results in desirable kinematics after TKR.

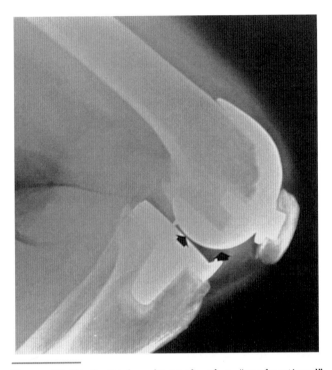

Figure 79–24. Sagittal radiograph of a "nonfunctional" posterior cruciate ligament. There has been "roll-forward" rather than "rollback" with knee flexion. The anterior margin of the femoral component abuts the anterior margin of the tibial component, as it does in a total condylar–type design.

Range of Motion

Early experience with use of the cruciate-sacrificing Total Condylar prosthesis produced flexion of about 90 to 95 degrees, which is near the theoretic limit for this type of prosthesis. Improved flexion with both posterior-stabilized and PCL-retaining prostheses has been reported. Pooled data from numerous studies demonstrate mean flexion of approximately 100 to 115 degrees with both types of prostheses.[21,187] Again, the importance of PCL recession and balancing in helping to allow optimal results with PCL-retaining prostheses has been advocated.[205,215] With careful surgical technique, reliable flexion of 110 to 115 degrees should be obtainable with either type of prosthesis. However, because of the experience and attention that seem to be required to correctly tension the PCL, we believe that the posterior-stabilized prosthesis is less technically challenging and produces more consistent results. The consequences of inadequately tensioning the PCL have been reported. Arthroscopic release of a tight PCL seems to be successful in improving flexion in select patients with PCL-retaining prostheses.[271]

Modifications to the latest generation of posterior-stabilized prostheses, the Legacy PS (Fig. 79–25), which included redesign of the trochlea to accommodate the natural patella, necessitated posterior translation of the cam-and-post mechanism. As a result of this change, the cam engages the post at approximately 70 degrees and then rides down the post, before eventually moving up the post with extreme flexion. This change has effectively increased the "jump distance," thereby allowing greater flexion before dislocation. In conjunction with modification of the posterior condyles to optimize the contact area in high flexion, as well as anterior scalloping of the polyethylene to reduce impingement on the extensor mechanism anteriorly, these changes have resulted in a new type of prosthesis that is intended for use in patients with good preoperative motion in whom high postoperative flexion is anticipated. Such a device is the Legacy PS Flex (Fig. 79–26), which can trace its heritage directly back to the original Insall-Burstein (IB) Posterior-Stabilized knee.

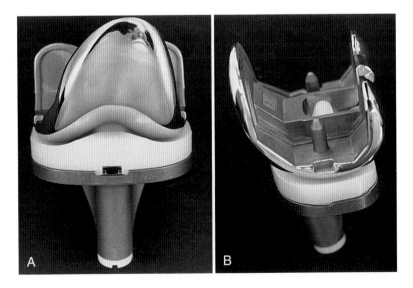

Figure 79–25. The Legacy PS prosthesis. **A,** Front view. **B,** Oblique view.

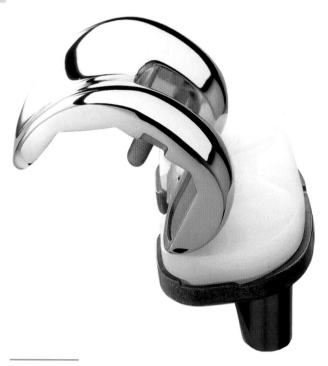

Figure 79–26. The LPS Flex prosthesis has been optimized for use in patients with good preoperative motion to allow safer flexion.

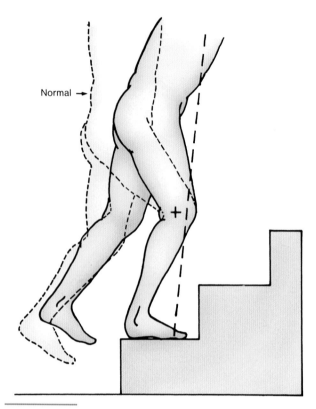

Figure 79–27. According to some gait analysis studies, there is a difference in stair climbing between cruciate-retaining and cruciate-sacrificing knee prostheses. It is reported that patients with the latter climb stairs with less knee flexion and a compensatory forward lean of the trunk. (From Andriacchi TP, Galante JO, Draganich LF: Relationship between knee extensor mechanics and function following total knee replacement. In Dorr LD [ed]: The Knee: Papers of the First Scientific Meeting of the Knee Society. Baltimore, University Park Press, 1985, p 83.)

Improvements in surgical technique, such as restoration of the posterior condylar offset and resection of posterior osteophytes, have also been emphasized in these cases to maximize postoperative motion. Similar design modifications have additionally been made to other posterior-stabilized knee prostheses, such as the Scorpio PS, as well as to cruciate-retaining prostheses, such as the Nex Gen CR Flex. Obviously, with a cruciate-retaining knee, the PCL must be adequately balanced for the prosthesis to function as intended.

Proprioception

Both cruciate ligaments contain mechanoreceptors, and therefore advocates of PCL retention have proposed that preserving the natural ligament would lead to superior proprioception after TKR. However, the current literature has not demonstrated a clear advantage. Simmons and coauthors were unable to identify any advantage in proprioception in patients who had a PCL-retaining prosthesis versus those with a PCL-substituting prosthesis.[229] Warren and coworkers found slightly different results.[261] After TKR all patients experienced improved proprioception regardless of whether a PCL-retaining or a PCL-substituting prosthesis had been used. However, the improvement was greater in patients with a PCL-retaining prosthesis. The improved proprioception in both groups was speculated to be due to elimination of pain, restoration of articular congruity, and retensioning of the collateral ligaments and soft tissues. These inconclusive results may be due to the inherent qualities of the PCL in patients

with arthritic knees. Kleinbart and coauthors have observed significant degenerative changes in the PCLs of patients with arthritic knees that exceed those in age-matched controls.[140] Therefore, a PCL that is preserved in a patient with a PCL-retaining prosthesis is likely to be abnormal and should not be expected to function normally either biomechanically or proprioceptively. The effects of PCL recession on the proprioceptive function of the ligament are not known.

Gait Analysis

Initial studies suggested that the mechanics of walking and stair climbing, in particular, is different in patients with PCL-retaining and PCL-substituting prostheses.[6,135] Andriacchi and Galante have described a characteristic forward lean of the trunk with less knee flexion in patients with PCL-substituting prostheses during stair climbing when compared with patients with PCL-retaining prostheses (Fig. 79–27).[6,8] This observation was suggested to represent a compensatory mechanism for the absence of the PCL. However, recent gait analysis by Wilson and coauthors and by Bolanos and coworkers dispute these findings. Bolanos and coauthors were unable to identify any significant differences in spatiotemporal gait parameters or knee range of motion during level walking or stair climbing in patients with PCL-retaining or PCL-substituting prostheses.[30] Wilson and colleagues also did not identify any differences in these parameters during stair climbing between patients with PCL-substituting prostheses and normal age-matched controls.[273] However, differences between patients after TKR and controls were identified during level walking and descending stairs. This evidence suggests that although gait patterns after TKR are different from those in normal controls, there is no clear effect of prosthesis type.

Correction of Deformity

Patients with significant preoperative fixed varus, valgus, or flexion deformities can be successfully managed with the use of PCL-retaining prostheses. However, because the PCL is one deforming factor in these cases, careful balancing with PCL release or recession may be required to achieve flexion and extension space symmetry.[96,205,215] Balancing of the PCL may be difficult and is experience dependent. The development of deep-dished polyethylene inserts for use in cruciate-retaining prostheses when the PCL is impossible to accurately tension reflects the difficulties in accomplishing this task. Laskin has reported inferior results in patients with fixed varus deformities exceeding 15 degrees in whom PCL-retaining rather than PCL-substituting designs were used.[154] In most circumstances, we believe that use of a posterior-stabilized prosthesis is technically less challenging and allows more reliable correction of the preoperative deformity. Failure to appropriately tension the PCL may lead to either reduced flexion or flexion instability.[188,262,271]

Stability

The more conforming tibial insert and cam-and-post mechanism of posterior-stabilized prostheses do not provide any constraint in the medial/lateral directions (Fig. 79-28). Neither the PCL-retaining nor the PCL-substituting prostheses are designed to compensate for instability in this plane and therefore require intact collateral ligaments. In the anterior and posterior directions, the inherent characteristics of the designs are different, and different problems are encountered if flexion-extension balance is not achieved. As previously discussed, a less conforming tibial polyethylene insert should be used in PCL-retaining prostheses because of the kinematic conflict that results during femoral rollback in flexion if a more conforming insert is used. If the PCL is functionally incompetent or stretches, posterior instability may occur because the minimally conforming or flat insert does little to prevent posterior translation of the femur. The phenomenon of symptomatic flexion instability in patients with PCL-retaining prostheses as a result of an incompe-

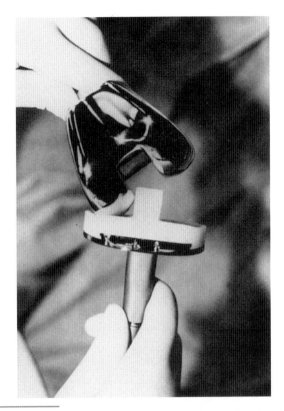

Figure 79-28. Posterior-stabilized prosthesis showing that the post-and-cam mechanism offers no restraint to varus or valgus stability.

tent PCL has recently gained more widespread recognition.[188,262] The consequences of overtensioning of the PCL have previously been discussed. Recent biomechanical studies have suggested that it is difficult to obtain the appropriate tension in the PCL.[111,164] However, the results of techniques used to balance the PCL have not been directly evaluated.

Although posterior-stabilized prostheses eliminate the PCL as a factor in preventing adequate flexion-extension balancing, anterior and posterior instability can still occur. In some patients with significant flexion instability, the jump distance of the cam-and-post mechanism may be exceeded during extreme flexion and acute dislocation results (Fig. 79-29). In previous series, a dislocation rate of 2% to 3% has been reported.[56,196] In one series, changes in design of the cam-and-post mechanism eliminated subsequent dislocations over a 2-year period.[196] Because of the uncertainties in achieving optimal tension in the PCL, we believe that PCL-substituting prostheses produce more reliable long-term anterior-posterior stability.

Polyethylene Wear

Polyethylene wear in current posterior-stabilized designs that have moderately conforming articular surfaces has not been a major clinical problem in older, less active patients.[48,196] In contrast, the higher contact stress encountered in the unconstrained flat-on-flat articulations, in

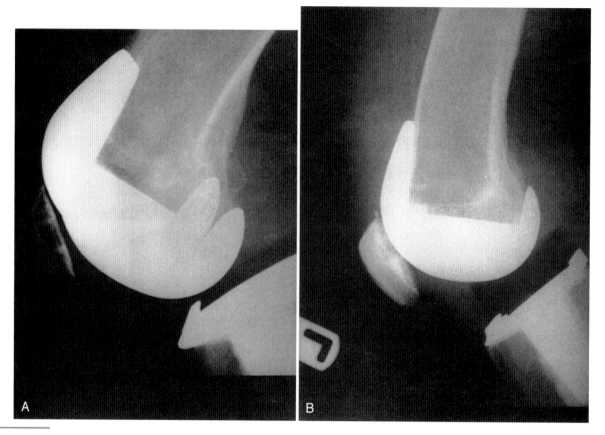

Figure 79–29. **A,** Radiograph of a dislocated posterior-stabilized prosthesis. The post of the tibial component has displaced posteriorly behind the cam of the femoral component. **B,** Radiograph after reduction.

conjunction with the heat-pressed, thin polyethylene inserts used in PCL-retaining prostheses during the 1980s, has led to documented rapid wear.[28,66,137,249] Failure to balance the PCL may also result in severe posteromedial polyethylene wear. Based on these results, the more conforming surfaces of posterior-stabilized implants seem better suited to optimizing long-term wear (Fig. 79–30).

Loosening

The increased constraint imposed by the moderately conforming articular surfaces of posterior-stabilized prostheses was initially considered to be detrimental to long-term fixation at the cement-bone-prosthesis interface because of increased stress transmission versus the relatively less conforming PCL-retaining prostheses. However, by proper design this shear stress can be altered to forces that are compressive (Fig. 79–31).

A theoretic seesaw motion may occur in PCL-retaining prostheses (Fig. 79–32). The rolling motion of the femur changes the metal-plastic contact point from anterior in extension to posterior in flexion. Thus, in extension the anterior portion of the tibia is compressed and in flexion the situation is reversed. This alternating compression-distraction may theoretically affect long-term fixation.

Long-term follow-up studies have failed to identify a significant clinical problem caused by these theoretic con-

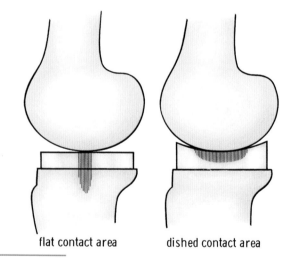

flat contact area   dished contact area

Figure 79–30. A dished component permits greater conformity, hence a larger contact area. The smaller contact area with a flat tibial component increases stress on the polyethylene.

cerns, with only rare cases of aseptic loosening with both types of prosthesis. In the senior author's experience with posterior-stabilized prostheses, no cases of aseptic loosening of the tibial component and only 2 cases of femoral component loosening occurred in 165 primary TKRs at a mean of 10 years' follow-up.[48] These results are similar to

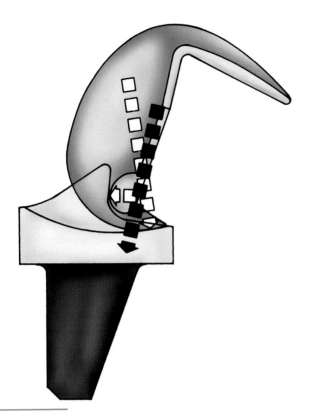

Figure 79–31. The cam mechanism of a posterior-stabilized knee simulates the function of the posterior cruciate ligament and causes rollback of the femur on the tibia with flexion. The resulting vector of forces passes distally through the fixation peg. (From Insall JN, Lachiewicz PF, Burstein AH: The posterior stabilized condylar prosthesis: A modification of the total condylar design: Two to four year clinical experience. J Bone Joint Surg Am 64:1317, 1982.)

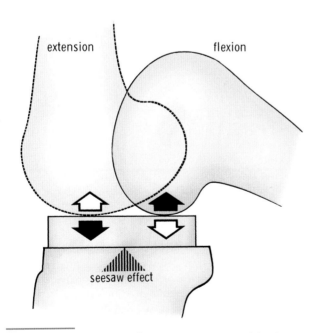

Figure 79–32. The seesaw effect. The back-and-forth movement on the tibial component caused by posterior cruciate ligament retention creates a rocking motion that may cause loosening.

those obtained with PCL-retaining designs. Malkani and coauthors from the Mayo Clinic have reported a 96% survival rate at 10 years' follow-up.[165] In summary, at 10- to 15-year follow-up there is little evidence to suggest that posterior-stabilized prostheses have an increased risk of aseptic loosening.

Current Surface Replacement Designs

The prostheses described in the preceding section have given rise to derivatives (Fig. 79–33). The Total Condylar prosthesis led to a series of posterior-stabilized prostheses initially developed by Insall and Burstein, including the IB Posterior-Stabilized prosthesis, modular IB II, NexGen Legacy PS (LPS), and the LPS Flex (see Figs. 79–25, 79–26, 79–28, and 79–34 to 79–36).* In addition, the Press Fit Condylar (PFC) PS and its successor, the PFC Sigma PS prosthesis (Fig. 79–37), were developed from the same foundation, as were the Optetrak PS and Advance PS prostheses.[206] The posterior cruciate duopatellar prosthesis evolved into the Kinematic I and II and the PFC CR prosthesis (Fig. 79–38).[206,274]

CEMENTLESS DESIGNS

Concerns about the long-term durability of cement fixation prompted the development of a variety of knee prostheses designed for cementless use during the 1980s. Because of theoretic concern about the increased stress transferred to the prosthesis-bone interfaces in posterior-stabilized designs that could potentially limit successful bone ingrowth, these uncemented devices were all designed to retain the PCL. The first design, developed by David Hungerford, was the Porous Coated Anatomic (PCA) (Fig. 79–39).† Other examples included the Porous Coated Anatomic II, Miller-Galante (Fig. 79–40),[144,145,208] Miller-Galante II, Tricon M,[151,185] Genesis (Fig. 79–41), and Ortholoc.[267] The Freeman-Swanson prosthesis[84,86] was modified into the Freeman-Samuelson prosthesis[81,210] (Fig. 79–42), which still used serrated polyethylene pegs for cementless fixation but offered a metal baseplate with intramedullary rods for the tibia and an intramedullary rod on the femoral component.

Unfortunately, the initial enthusiasm in some circles for these devices was not supported by the long-term results. Aseptic loosening and failure to achieve initial fixation, coupled with incidental problems related to the materials selected, as well as confounding problems caused by the flat-on-flat geometries that were used in most of these designs, led to higher failure rates than noted with comparable cemented prostheses during the first decade.[61,200] Consequently, these devices did not achieve widespread acceptance. More recently, the development of new bone ingrowth materials, especially those based on tantalum, have prompted renewed interest in this area, including

---

*See references 2, 3, 74, 95, 100, 117, 206, 219, 220, 240-242, 268.
†See references 22, 45, 50, 57, 76, 106, 107, 141, 181, 207, 209, 237.

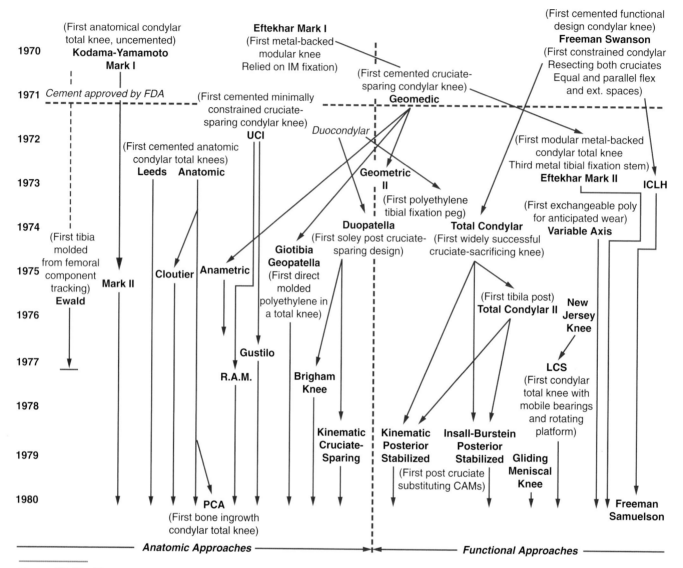

Figure 79–33. The evolution of the condylar total knee from 1970 to 1980. (Adapted from Robinson RP: The early innovators of today's resurfacing condylar knees. J Arthroplasty 20[Suppl 1]:2, 2005.)

the development of uncemented posterior-stabilized tibial components. However, the long-term results of this next generation of uncemented implants are not yet available.

Meniscal-Bearing Prostheses

Conventional fixed-bearing knee prostheses have proved clinically successful with very favorable results at 10 to 15 years.[48] However, with only a few exceptions, these results were obtained in older, less active patient populations.[56,62] Concern exists regarding the long-term durability of current prostheses in younger, more demanding patients, especially regarding problems related to polyethylene wear and osteolysis. Polyethylene wear may be reduced by radical improvements in the inherent qualities of the material itself, which have not yet been realized, or by decreasing the contact stress at the articular surfaces. Reduction in contact stress could be accomplished by increasing the conformity of the femoral component and polyethylene insert. However, because of the inherent trade-off between conformity and freedom of motion that exists in fixed-bearing prostheses, significant improvements in contact stress are not feasible. Therefore, at the present time a mobile-bearing prosthesis seems to represent the most plausible solution to this problem.[113] A mobile bearing eliminates the relationship between articular conformity and freedom of rotation that exists in fixed-bearing prostheses because rotation occurs at the interface between the tibial baseplate and the undersurface of the polyethylene insert and articular conformity is a property of the shape of the femoral component and superior surface of the polyethylene insert. Articular conformity can be maximized in a mobile-bearing prosthesis,

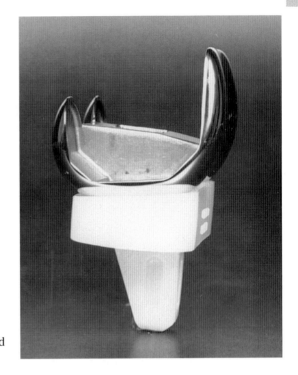

Figure 79–34. The original Insall-Burstein Posterior-Stabilized prosthesis.

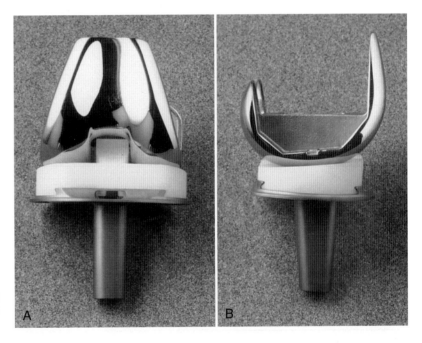

Figure 79–35. The modular Insall-Burstein II Posterior-Stabilized prosthesis. **A,** Front view. **B,** Side view.

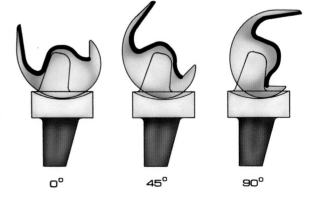

Figure 79–36. The TCP II was a precursor of the posterior-stabilized knee that provided a passive stop against posterior displacement in flexion, as well as a hyperextension stop in extension. (From Insall JN, Tria AJ, Scott WN: The total condylar knee prosthesis: The first five years. Clin Orthop 145:68, 1979.)

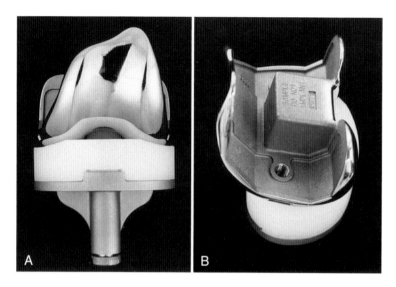

Figure 79–37. The PFC Sigma prosthesis. **A,** Front view. **B,** Oblique view.

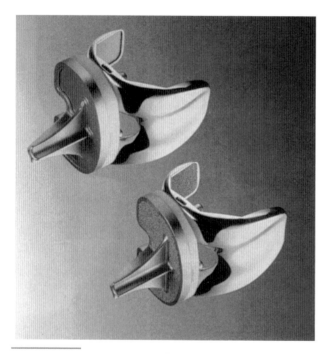

Figure 79–38. Press-Fit Condylar prosthesis. (Courtesy of Johnson & Johnson.)

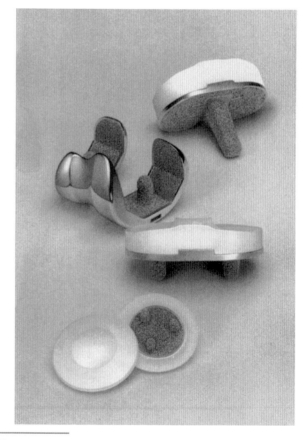

Figure 79–39. Porous Coated Anatomic prosthesis. (Courtesy of Howmedica.)

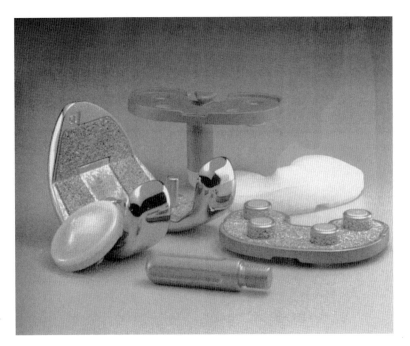

Figure 79–40. Miller-Galante prosthesis. (Courtesy of Zimmer.)

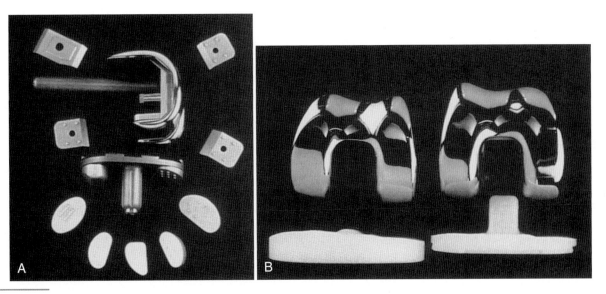

Figure 79–41. **A** and **B,** Genesis prosthesis. (Courtesy of Richards.)

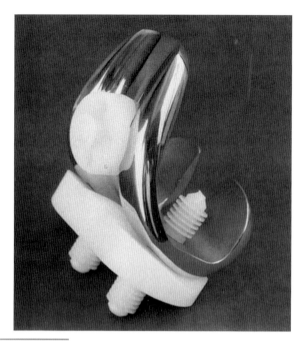

Figure 79–42. The Freeman-Samuelson prosthesis. (Courtesy of M.A.R. Freeman.)

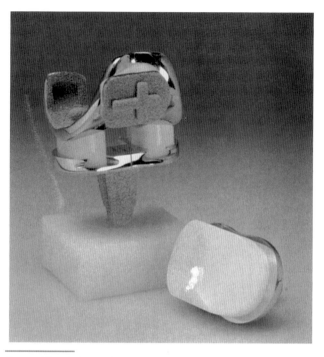

Figure 79–43. Low–Contact Stress prosthesis. (Courtesy of DePuy.)

thereby reducing contact stress and wear on the superior surface of the polyethylene while freedom of rotation is maintained.

The many nuances of mobile-bearing prosthesis design and our interest in the development of these prostheses will be reviewed more thoroughly in a subsequent chapter. Briefly, the concepts behind these prostheses are not new, as borne out by the Oxford prostheses.[18,31,33,90-93,247,269]

In 1976 Goodfellow and O'Connor introduced a bicondylar knee that attempted to solve the potential problem of polyethylene wear by providing a meniscal bearing, that is, a polyethylene tibial component that is fully congruent with the femoral component but free to move on a metallic tibial base tray. This concept hopes to provide the best possible wear characteristics with complete lack of constraint. The designers of the Oxford knee now recommend that this prosthesis be used only as a unicompartmental prosthesis when both the ACL and PCL are present and can be preserved. An absent ACL is now considered a contraindication to the Oxford knee. Buechel and associates have developed the meniscal-bearing concept into a series of prostheses known as the Low–Contact Stress (LCS) knee prostheses[23,38,39] (Fig. 79–43). These devices possess a femoral component similar to the total condylar prosthesis that is mated to meniscal-bearing tibial components that resemble those of the Oxford knee or, alternatively, a rotating platform for use when cruciate excision is indicated. There is also a metal-backed patellar component with a swiveling polyethylene surface of anatomic design.

Unlike the Oxford knee, the LCS model has a femoral component of decreasing radius posteriorly; congruency is reduced when the knee is flexed, so the contact area decreases in flexion, thereby losing a potential advantage of the original design.

A puzzle created by meniscal designs, particularly the Oxford model, is in deciding the position of the actual joint axis. Flexion takes place between the femur and the superior surface of the polyethylene bearing, whereas anteroposterior sliding and rotation occur at the inferior surface (a position 8 to 10 mm distal to the true joint line). Whether this curious anomaly has clinical significance has not been studied much.

Meniscal-bearing designs have the disadvantage of increased complexity, with movement occurring both proximal and distal to the polyethylene bearing and the potential for wear at both surfaces. Dislocation of the bearings has also been reported.[23] In Europe, a large number of mobile-bearing knees have been in widespread clinical use for nearly a decade, and long-term data that will identify designs and characteristics that are associated with improved outcomes will be forthcoming. In the United States, the LCS prosthesis was the only available mobile-bearing knee until the merger of DePuy and Johnson & Johnson. This merger allowed the development of mobile-bearing variants of both the PFC Sigma CR and PS prostheses. Except for these notable exceptions, the complexity of gaining Food and Drug Administration approval for new devices has restricted widespread introduction of other designs of mobile-bearing knees.

Constrained Prostheses

CONSTRAINED CONDYLAR KNEE

A derivative of the TCP III[25,46,58,103,133,138] design, the CCK has itself evolved into the Legacy Constrained Condylar Knee (LCCK) prosthesis (Fig. 79–44). These devices provide both posterior stability and medial-lateral stability by means of an enlarged post articulating closely with a femoral cam (Fig. 79–45). In its TCP III form, Donaldson and coworkers[58] found no loosening in 15 primary cases monitored for more than 2 years; all stems were cemented. The TCP III has evolved into the CCK for use with modular, press-fit stems. The CCK was initially used primarily for revision cases, but based on the good experience with the TCP III in primary knees, the CCK has proved very successful in managing difficult valgus knees in elderly low-demand patients.[63] Avoidance of extensive release procedures and possible peroneal nerve complications has hastened recovery and lessened morbidity.

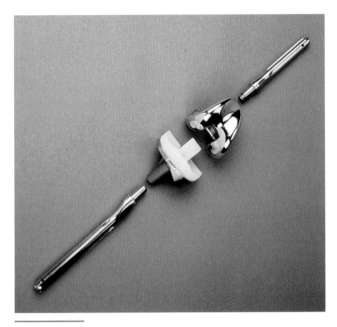

Figure 79–44. The LCCK prosthesis.

The LCCK metal components can be used with either its own constrained polyethylene tibial insert or a standard posterior-stabilized insert. Thus, during a difficult knee arthroplasty, an intraoperative decision can be made concerning the degree of constraint needed; for example, in severe valgus knees, we use the LCCK metal components, but when possible, we use a posterior-stabilized rather than a constrained tibial insert.

KINEMATIC ROTATING HINGE

Rand and colleagues[198] reported the results on 50 Kinematic Rotating-Hinge TKAs performed at the Mayo Clinic. The indications were either ligamentous instability, loss of bone, or both. The follow-up was 50 months (range, 29 to 79 months). There were 14 excellent, 12 good, 5 fair, and 5 poor results. Progression of radiolucent lines was observed in 13 knees, and 5 knees probably had radiographic loosening. The rate of sepsis was 16%, patellar instability developed in 22%, and breakage of the implant occurred in 6%. In these patients, 74% of the operations were revisions: a first revision in 17, a second revision in 16, a third revision in 3, and a fourth revision in 1. In a more recent report from the Mayo Clinic involving 69 Kinematic Rotating-Hinge knees at a mean of 75 months' follow-up, the results were similar, with an overall complication rate of 32%, an infection rate of 14.5%, and component breakage in 10%.[239] The results from these series were similar to previous experience with the GUEPAR prosthesis at the Mayo Clinic, although in this series the high percentage of revisions probably contributed to the poor results, especially the high rate of sepsis. Rand and coworkers combined the incidence of complications reported for several series with a total of 2099 hinged implants. In these combined series, loosening was reported in 27% of knees, sepsis in 7%, and wound-

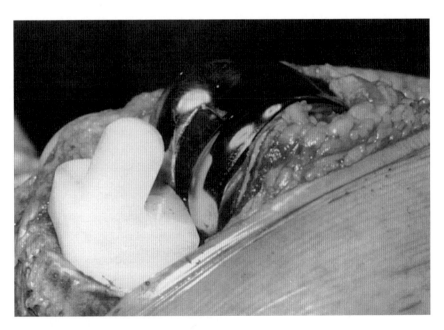

Figure 79–45. Articulation of the TCP III, a constrained condylar knee. A rectangular tibial post fits within a central femoral box or cavity, thereby providing varus-valgus stability as well as posterior restraint.

healing problems in 5.5%. The authors concluded that the Kinematic Rotating-Hinge prosthesis, though possessing theoretic advantages, gave no better results than the older nonrotating hinges. Mechanical failures have also been reported.[135]

GENERAL PROSTHETIC FEATURES

Interchangeability of Sizes

The natural variation that occurs between individual knee joints means that prosthetic components based on average dimensions do not always fit the femur and tibia of a particular joint equally well. Interchangeability of sizes, such that the femoral, tibial, and patellar components can be selected independently of each other according to the fit on their respective bones, becomes an attractive feature. Although it has long been possible to match patellar components with various femoral sizes, similar adaptability between the femoral and tibial components is a relatively new feature. As with other aspects of knee arthroplasty, some compromises are involved. Matching a smaller femur with a larger tibia (the usual combination) requires that the intercondylar distance or, more correctly, the bearing spacing between the femoral runners be constant for all sizes and that the tibial surface be almost flat. As we have seen, articulating a curved femur against a flat tibia produces a small contact patch with the attendant disadvantage of high localized stress on the polyethylene. The contact patch can be enlarged by also flattening the femoral surfaces (Fig. 79–46). However, malalignment or any situation that leads to asymmetric loading, even those occurring during the normal gait cycle, shifts the loading area to the periphery. This type of "edge" loading has been shown experimentally[19,255,257] to produce the greatest stress at the prosthesis-bone interface, perhaps

offsetting any benefits obtained from more complete tibial coverage.

Articular Geometry

Conforming joint surfaces should have the best wear resistance, particularly when the polyethylene is relatively thick.[19] However, conforming articulations are not fully interchangeable, may conflict with PCL kinematics, and can theoretically cause greater fixation stress.

Thatcher and colleagues,[245] discussing inherent laxity in knee prostheses, state that laxity is a function of joint conformity. They believe that the implanted prosthesis should compensate for soft-tissue structures that are deficient or removed. They think that the optimal laxity profile has not yet been determined but suggest that the articular geometry should possess partial conformity and comment on the classic inherent design compromise. The greater the conformity, the larger the contact area and the less the intrinsic stress and wear. However, conforming prostheses will create greater fixation stress, which may lead to loosening.

Wear is an increasing problem in TKA. Several factors have been implicated, including the quality of the polyethylene, the manufacturing process, the thickness of the tibial components, and the articular geometry.[236] It is also true that in the best of circumstances, polyethylene is not an ideal bearing material,[276] but attempts to improve its performance have not been successful.[275]

Many cases of severe wear and delamination of tibial components have been reported,[66,137] mainly involving thinner polyethylene components. The manufacturing process (which involved heat-pressing[28] the polyethylene to give a smoother surface) has been implicated, particularly in causing the most severe phenomenon of delamination, although design factors leading to high-contact stress are probably equally important inasmuch as other

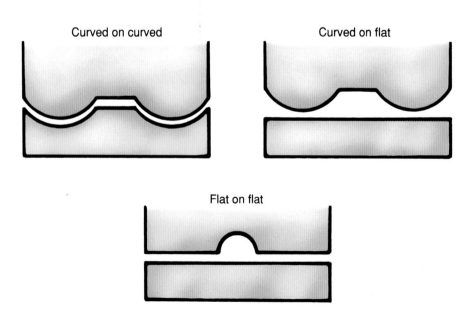

Figure 79–46. The more conforming the articulation, the larger the contact area and the less the stress on the polyethylene. In the frontal plane, curved-on-curved geometries are the best. Curved-on-flat geometry is the worst. Flat-on-flat surfaces can give a good area of contact but are sensitive to edge loading whenever the prosthesis is loaded unevenly, such as in leaning or pivoting movements.

models from the same manufacturer using similar poly-ethylene treatment have not shown the same degree of damage.

Design and Fixation of the Tibial Component

An important difference between prostheses is the method of tibial fixation.[160] The Total Condylar, Posterior-Stabilized Condylar, and Kinematic prostheses use a central peg. The PFC has a central tri-fin post. These prostheses are primarily designed for cement fixation. Others that can be inserted with or without cement have two to four short studs, augmented in most cases by screws. Long-term studies using central peg fixation and cement show tibial component loosening to be rare (Fig. 79–47).

There is good evidence from early experience with knee arthroplasty that separate tibial components are susceptible to fixation failure. Neither an anterior bar nor the use of fixation studs is helpful. Walker and coworkers[256] tested a variety of tibial components by applying compressive load with anteroposterior force, rotational torque, or varus-valgus moment (Fig. 79–48). The relative deflections, both compressive and distractive, were measured between the component and the bone. The fewest deflections occurred with one-piece metal components. Whether a central peg or two lateral studs were used did not seem to make much difference. Thick plastic components behaved much like metal-backed ones, except when a cruciate cutout was made. Metal backing seems particularly desirable for cruciate-retaining implants.

Railton and coworkers[193] found metal backing of the polyethylene without a central stem to be of little value in enhancing fixation. They did not address the question of optimal stem length or the use of cement. Yamamoto and coworkers,[277] discussing the results of the Kodama-Yamamoto Mark II prosthesis, which has an all-polyethylene tibial component with four small studs and is inserted without cement, express the opinion that a stem is unnecessary. They report a 4.4% incidence of femoral loosening accompanied by tibial sinkage in some. Cases with only tibial sinkage were not observed.

Lewis and colleagues[160] tested the fixation of six tibial component configurations by finite element analysis and concluded that metal-backed, single-post designs provided the lowest system stress overall when cement was used.

Clinical data on implants using metal tray and small stud fixation are mostly applicable to cementless fixation. Computer simulations of bone remodeling around porous-coated implants[186] demonstrate stress concentrations around small tibial pegs; this resulted in denser bone, with a decrease in density in more peripheral locations. This finding agrees with the clinical observation that bone ingrowth occurs most predictably around fixation pegs.

Walker and colleagues,[257] in a comparative study of uncemented tibial component designs, found that central stemmed and bladed designs performed better than short pegs placed near the periphery.

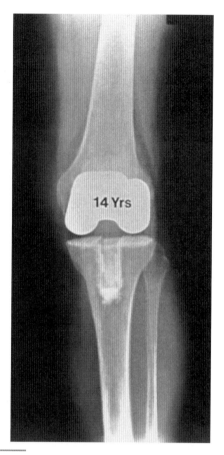

Figure 79–47. A radiograph of a Total Condylar prosthesis 14 years postoperatively. Note the thin cement mantle clearly showing ridges in the cement caused by the design of the tibial polyethylene. There is no evidence of cracking or fragmentation of the cement. This type of appearance was seen frequently in the more than 10-year follow-up of this prosthesis and indicates that a thick cement mantle is unnecessary.

Support of the plastic by means of a metal tray or endoskeleton is certainly desirable when the bone of the upper part of the tibia is deficient (severe erosive arthritis or revision operations), but when the bone is of good quality, metal backing may not offer an advantage. One-piece plastic components with a central peg have a low rate of loosening, but in 30% to 40% of cases a partial radiolucency develops. For the most part, these radiolucencies appear within the first year, are nonprogressive, and are of dubious clinical significance. The addition of a metal tray reduces the incidence of radiolucency, and it also seems to reduce the incidence of late tibial loosening (Fig. 79–49).

Modularity

Modularity, in the sense under discussion, refers to the ability to add stems, augments, and wedges to standard components so that, to a degree, the surgeon is able to make a custom prosthesis intraoperatively (Fig. 79–50). Most manufacturers now offer a complete knee prosthesis

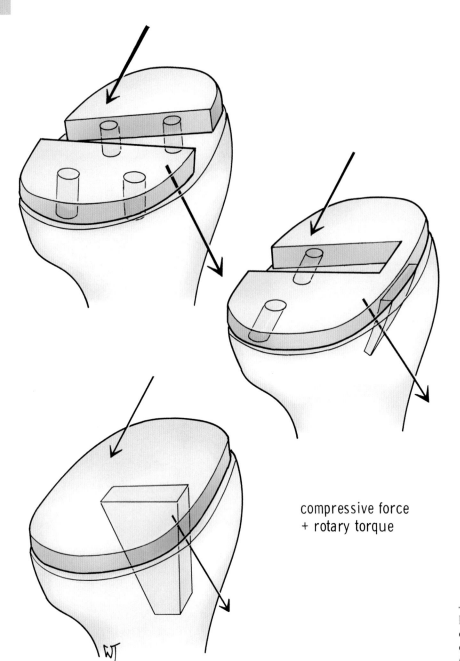

compressive force
+ rotary torque

Figure 79–48. Deflections at the bone-cement interface showing different configurations of the tibial component. (Courtesy of Dr. Peter Walker.)

system, such as the TCP III or LCCK, that offers all these modular components. Modularity is particularly useful for revision surgery when the bone deficiencies cannot be completely anticipated. It is also of value for primary knee replacement, for dealing with bone defects, and when prosthetic stability cannot be obtained. Modularity does not necessarily imply interchangeability, although both features may be present in a particular design.

Component Augmentation for Bone Defects

Cement,[161] cement and screws,[203] or bone grafts can be used to compensate for small bone defects.[36,152]

The senior author's experience indicates that onlay bone grafts should not be used on the femoral condyles or for revision defects. Cancellous grafting for contained defects is of course applicable in these circumstances. The advantage of bone grafting lies in the potential improvement of bone stock.

Another method is to use metal wedges (Fig. 79–51) and augments that can be adapted to fit existing defects without the need to remove sclerotic areas to expose bleeding cancellous surfaces. In this sense one can view them as more conservative. If they fail, the bone deficiency is not made worse. The metal pieces are either screwed or cemented to their components. Screw fixation, though mechanically satisfying, creates the possibility of metallic debris formation by micromotion (fretting). Cement may also not be the ideal bonding material

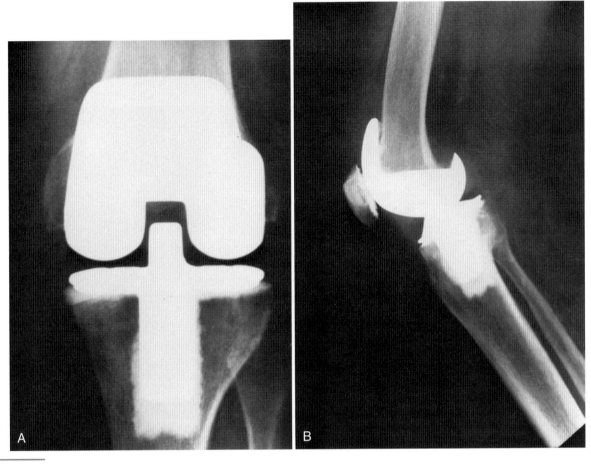

Figure 79–49. **A** and **B,** Anteroposterior and lateral radiographs of a tibial component with an endoskeleton. Metal backing of this type reduces tibial loosening at long-term follow-up.

between metal surfaces. At present, one or the other method must be used.

Prosthetic Stems

Prosthetic stems about the knee have a stigma that is related to their use with hinges and other constrained models, especially when the stems are cemented. However, Blauth and Hassenpflug and Bohm and Holy report continuing good results with the hinged-knee prosthesis that bears Blauth's name.[27,29] Reporting on the Stanmore hinge replacement, Lettin and colleagues[158,159] found 83% survivorship at 6 years (survivorship defined as prosthesis in situ), and Kaufer and Matthews[132] found an infection rate of 5% and revision rate of 15% for the spherocentric prosthesis monitored for an average of 8 years. Nonetheless, these reports appeared to be exceptions. In our experience, 15 of 108 GUEPAR prostheses became infected. All but four of them were late infections, and uncontrollable sepsis led to two above-the-knee amputations. Young[278] found that in a series of hinged prostheses all had failed by the end of 10 years. Hui and Fitzgerald[105] reported an 11.7% infection rate in 77 GUEPAR arthroplasties monitored for 2 or more years. They comment on

the difficulty of obtaining arthrodesis if the prosthesis has to be removed. Deburge[54] had a failure rate of 34% with the GUEPAR prosthesis that was attributable to major complications. Grimer and colleagues[94] recommend against routine use of the Stanmore prosthesis as a primary arthroplasty. Of 103 Stanmore knee replacements, they had 7 cases of infection and 4 of fracture around the prosthesis that contributed to major complications. Eight knees were revised for aseptic loosening and a further 14 were found to have radiological signs of loosening. There were two cases of amputation for fracture and sepsis. Only Wilson and colleagues[272] have reported favorable results over a long period with an uncemented Walldius prosthesis. The overall infection rate was 3.2%, and clinical evidence of loosening occurred infrequently. The 20 knees monitored for an average of 10 years showed little evidence of progressive deterioration. They attribute this result to the absence of cement. Walldius[260] himself has written on 27 years' experience with his prosthesis and states that good results are obtained in 80% of patients with a high degree of preoperative disability. No details are given.

In assessing these results, it must be pointed out that all relate to constrained prostheses with cemented stems (except the Walldius) and the worst results were obtained with metal-on-metal bearing surfaces, which generate

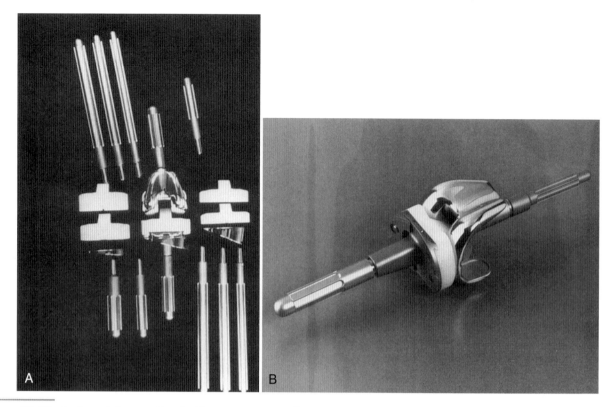

Figure 79–50. **A,** A modular prosthesis. The components offer stems, augments, and wedges, which are fixed with screws. There is also a choice of polyethylene components for posterior stabilization or for varus and valgus constraint. **B,** A revision-type, Constrained Condylar modular prosthesis assembled in the operating room. (Courtesy of Zimmer.)

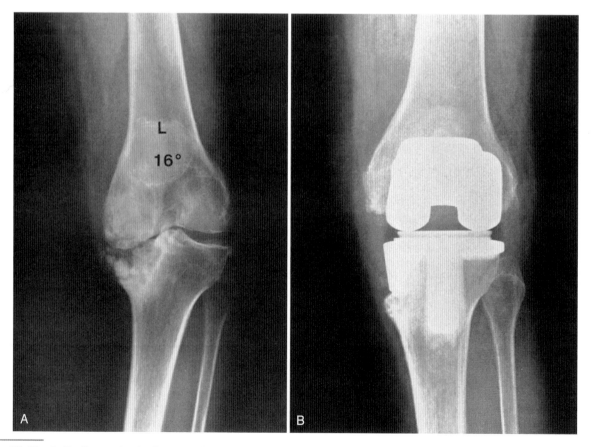

Figure 79–51. **A,** Radiograph of a knee with osteonecrosis of the medial aspect of the tibia and a massive tibial defect. **B,** Replacement of the knee with a custom prosthesis with a medial wedge.

large volumes of metallic debris.[191] Complete constraint of the degree provided by a hinge is rarely needed in knee arthroplasty, and lesser degrees of constraint such as provided by the TCP III or CCK do not seem to have particular disadvantages.[58] Murray and coauthors, from the Mayo Clinic, have reported 5-year results with the use of cemented stems in conjunction with the Kinematic Stabilizer prosthesis in 40 revision TKRs.[184] The incidence of radiolucent lines was 13% about the femoral stems and 32% about the tibial stems. However, the majority were incomplete, nonprogressive, and less than 1 mm. Only one femoral component and one tibial component were radiographically loose. Theoretic concerns regarding stress shielding were not noted in these cases. Therefore, it appears that in this time frame, cemented stems function adequately without significant complications. However, concern regarding bone loss and increased surgical difficulty at revision still remains. If the intention is merely to provide additional component support, in the case of deficient bone, stems need not be associated with constraint and do not need to be cemented.[178] The senior author used uncemented stems from 1977 onward with

both custom and modular components, and Bertin and colleagues have reported on Freeman's experience with uncemented stems in revision surgery.[24,99] In neither report was there any increase in the infection rate. Freeman used a stem of fixed diameter and did not attempt to obtain a press-fit (the so-called dangle stem) (Fig. 79–52). Bertin and colleagues noted the development of radiopaque lines adjacent to the stem in 88% of cases. In our study, similar lines were observed about 67% of femoral rods and 69% of tibial rods. A sclerotic halo about the tip of the prosthesis has also been noted in some cases (Fig. 79–53).[24] The importance of these findings is not fully understood but may be interpreted as evidence of the stem's function in resisting moments and load sharing. Although the stems need not have rigid fixation in the shaft, the medial tilting and slight displacement noticed in one case suggest that press-fitting the stems is desirable, especially in patients with more extensive bone loss (Fig. 79–54). In revision and reimplant surgery we now routinely use hand reamers to select a stem that makes contact with the cortices but do not attempt to expand the canal. With the flexibility of the current modular systems and the development of offset stems, this can routinely be accomplished without major difficulty.

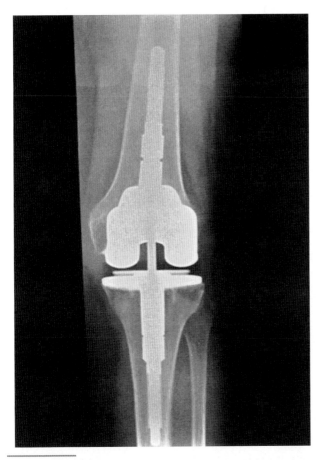

Figure 79–52. Radiograph of a knee prosthesis showing so-called dangle stems. These uncemented stems rest in the intramedullary canal and do not make contact with the cortices. Even so, roentgen stereophotogrammetric analysis data have shown on the tibial side that uncemented stems of this type have the lowest rates of migration and inducible displacement.

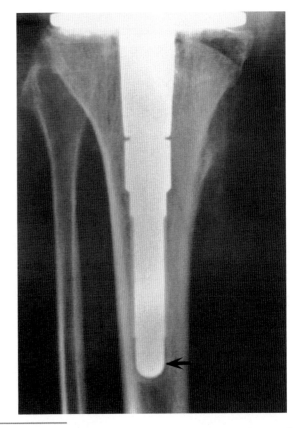

Figure 79–53. Radiograph showing sclerosis at the tip of an uncemented stem (arrow). The interpretation of this finding, which is fairly constant, is arguable. In part, it is probably due to bending of the more flexible bone, but it may also be indicative of the stem's role in resisting tilting movements.

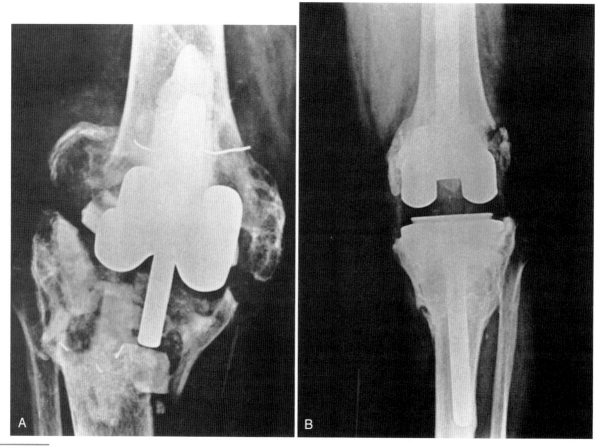

Figure 79–54. **A,** Failed Attenborough prosthesis with great loss of bone and fragmentation of the upper part of the tibia. **B,** Reconstruction with a custom prosthesis and a femoral head allograft in the tibia. The intramedullary rod was passed through a hole in the femoral head. Morselized cancellous graft was used to fill in remaining defects. The custom rod was undersized and has migrated into slight varus and stabilized in this position. Some cortical reaction is seen. This indicates the need for precise sizing of the intramedullary rods for this type of revision case, an advantage of modular systems. However, this knee functioned well until the patient's death 8 years postoperatively.

Custom Prostheses

Modular components have greatly reduced the need for custom prostheses in primary and revision surgery. However, custom devices are occasionally needed, most frequently in our experience for cases in which a previous high tibial osteotomy has been performed. The problem in these knees occurs when the osteotomy has produced an offset in the diaphysis and a tibial stem is desired (Fig. 79–55). The development of offset stems as part of current modular prosthesis systems has significantly reduced the number of custom components required in our experience.

Patellar Prostheses

RESURFACING

In rheumatoid arthritis the patella should always be replaced to remove all articular cartilage from the joint.

Some surgeons recommend selective resurfacing of the patella for patients with osteoarthritis.[216,227,233] Others think that the result is more predictable with routine patellar resurfacing (Fig. 79–56).[68,197,218,235] Undoubtedly, patellar resurfacing has its share of iatrogenic complications such as fracture[246] and soft-tissue overgrowth with impingement.[102] Fixation holes in the patella weaken its structure, central holes probably more so than peripheral ones (Fig. 79–57).

CONFIGURATION

Until recently, most patellar components were dome shaped. This configuration is not ideal because the convex contour might be expected to wear poorly on the basis of engineering experience (in an articulation the softer material should be concave). A component that is anatomic (e.g., PCA and LCS) has a more desirable configuration in this respect but requires careful rotary alignment to prevent binding against the femur (Fig. 79–58). In addition, correct static alignment, even if achieved at surgery,

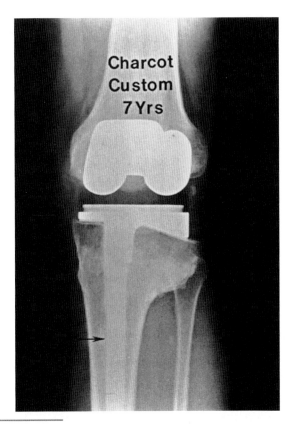

Figure 79–55. Radiograph of a custom prosthesis with a lateral wedge and offset stem. The prosthesis was designed for a patient with a neuropathic joint who had previously undergone high tibial osteotomy. The knee migrated into excessive valgus, leaving a lateral defect and an offset of the tibial diaphysis. A standard modular prosthesis would not have fit in this case.

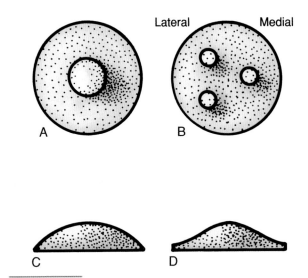

Figure 79–57. Patella shapes and methods of fixation. **A** and **C,** A dome patella with a central fixation lug. **B** and **D,** A sombrero patella with three fixation pegs.

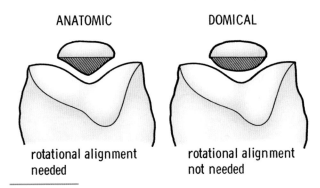

Figure 79–58. Rotational alignment is needed with a patellar replacement of anatomic shape.

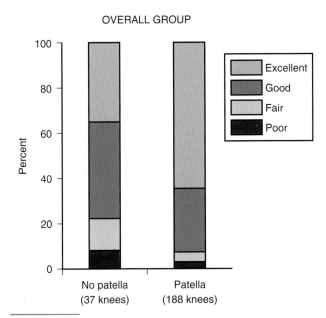

Figure 79–56. The clinical results are slightly better when a patellar component is used.

may not predict the functional pull of the quadriceps in active use, and the more desirable wear characteristics can be offset by increased torque on the component caused by malalignment. The LCS patellar design attempts to solve this problem by having an anatomic polyethylene articulation swivel on a metal baseplate. This design has been in use for more than 10 years and is apparently very successful. The tendency of the universal patellar dome to deform has led to the use of oval and sombrero shapes.[34] An oval patella provides greater coverage of the patellar bone, and a sombrero shape theoretically has more attractive wear characteristics. Other workers advocate inlaying the prosthesis into the central portion of the patellar bone[155] (Fig. 79–59), stating that the peripheral bony rim in contact with the femoral condyles does not cause symptoms. If this is so, the inlay patella is attractive, but the concept does not appear to be entirely rational. In any event, wear with a dome-shaped patellar component has not been seen as a problem in long-term clinical studies, but retrieval analysis raises some cause for concern (Fig. 79–60).

METAL-BACKED PATELLAR COMPONENT

Metal backing of the polyethylene has become a serious clinical problem (polyethylene dissociation and wear-through) (Fig. 79–61) whose full dimension has not yet been realized. It is apparent that many patellae were designed with inadequate polyethylene thickness.

Metal backing of the patellar component was inspired in part by the good experience with tibial component design and in part by the wish to obtain bone ingrowth.[76] This feature of design introduced very serious complications in the form of polyethylene wear-through or dissociation from the metal baseplate. It is impossible to design an onset patellar component with the necessary thickness of polyethylene to avoid wear-through without producing an unacceptably bulky component. This design difficulty has caused a widespread return to all-polyethylene patellar components generally used with cement, although press-fit inlaid components are used without cement.[26] The optimal patellar design remains uncertain.[49] However, Laskin and Bucknell[155] and others believe that metal-backed failures are due to a design problem that can be solved by increasing the thickness of the polyethylene and countersinking the base within the patellar bone. The LCS design continues to use a rotating platform with a metal base.

PROSTHETIC PATELLAR PROBLEMS

However the patella is treated, patellofemoral symptoms on stair climbing and other flexed-knee activities remain

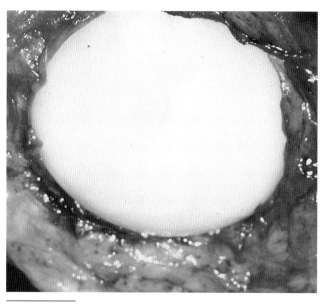

Figure 79–60. A patella showing considerable lateral polyethylene wear. This amount of polyethylene damage is unusual and was caused by lateral subluxation of the patella. Normally, only slighter flattening and deformation of dome-type patellae are noted.

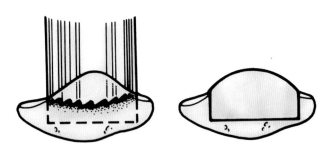

Figure 79–59. Insetting the patella allows greater thickness of polyethylene and the use of metal backing. There is a rim of peripheral exposed bone that can impinge against the femur.

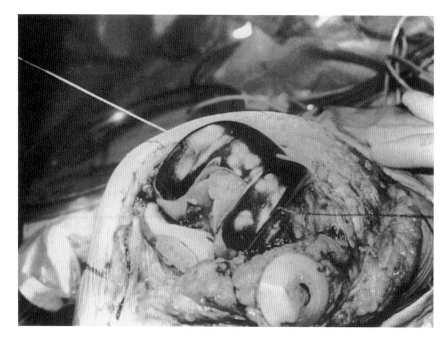

Figure 79–61. A Kinematic prosthesis showing central wear-through of a metal-backed patellar component.

a troublesome problem not yet fully resolved. Avoidance of a "high shoulder" profile of the femoral component in the junctional area between the flange and condylar runners in favor of a smooth, uniformly curved patellar sulcus reduces patellofemoral strain.[176] Technical factors, such as the orientation of the patellar osteotomy and the thickness of the patellar prosthesis composite, are important, as is avoidance of patella infra as a result of proximal alteration of the prosthetic joint line.

SHOULD THE PATELLA BE RESURFACED?

Some of the patellar problems can be avoided if the patellar prosthesis is omitted altogether (Fig. 79–62). Abraham and coworkers studied 100 knees, 47 of which underwent patellar resurfacing.[1] The prosthesis used was the Variable-Axis prosthesis. The two groups were similar in diagnosis, age, and sex. They were unable to find significant differences between the two groups with regard to walking distance, ability to climb stairs, ability to rise from a chair, motion, extensor lag, and quadriceps strength. One patient in the resurfacing group required a reoperation for subluxation, and two in the unresurfaced group required subsequent resurfacing. A number of more recent studies have noted similar findings. Keblish and colleagues reported on patients who had undergone bilateral TKR with patellar resurfacing on one side and retention of the natural patella on the other.[134] The patients expressed no preference between the two sides, and there were no differences in stair climbing or the incidence of anterior knee

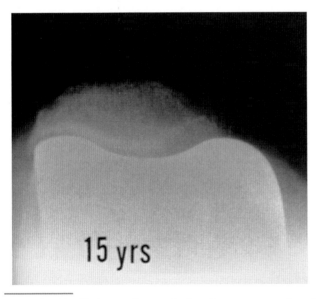

Figure 79–62. Skyline radiograph showing an unresurfaced patella 15 years postoperatively. In this case the patella has remodeled to fit the femoral groove. The knee is functioning satisfactorily, has good function on stairs, and is painfree. Unfortunately, this is not always the result with patellae that are left unresurfaced.

pain. Barrack and coauthors have also reported the results of a prospective, randomized study on patellar resurfacing involving 87 patients.[17] They were unable to detect a difference in the overall Knee Society score, function score, or patient satisfaction. Thirty-two patients had undergone bilateral TKR with resurfacing of the patella on one side and retention of the natural patella on the other. This subgroup of patients expressed no clear preference. Although the results were not significantly different between the two groups, a clear difference in complications was noted. A significantly higher rate of anterior knee pain was detected in the group in which the natural patella was retained (13% versus 7%), with a 10% prevalence of subsequent patellar resurfacing in this group. Boyd and coworkers also reported that in early to midterm follow-up, increased complications occur in patients with a retained natural patella.[32] At a mean of 3 years, the overall complication rate in the group with patellar resurfacing was 4% versus 12% in the unresurfaced group. Among patients with rheumatoid arthritis who had undergone patellar resurfacing, loosening of the patellar prosthesis occurred in 1%, whereas a 13% reoperation rate for subsequent resurfacing occurred in the group who initially had been left with the natural patella. Kajino and colleagues have reported superior pain relief in patients with rheumatoid arthritis after patellar resurfacing.[129] In this prospective, randomized study of patients who underwent bilateral TKR, only one knee was selected for patellar resurfacing. Although knee scores were not significantly different, patients experienced pain only on standing or during stair climbing on the side with a retained natural patella.

Enis and coauthors[68] have also reported a slight preference among 25 patients with bilateral arthroplasties in whom the patella was resurfaced, with the Townley prosthesis implanted on one side but not the other. The majority of patients expressed a preference for the resurfaced side, which they found to be relatively pain-free and stronger during flexed-knee activities, such as stair climbing. However, the difference was not very great. Our experience agrees with these results, which suggest slightly better results after patellar resurfacing, particularly in patients with inflammatory arthritis. However, in certain circumstances it may be preferable to leave the natural patella intact. It may be advisable to omit patellar resurfacing in the following situations:

1. The patellar articular surface is nearly normal.
2. The patient is obese. Stern and Insall have shown that with resurfacing, pain and complications are more frequent in obese patients.[240]
3. The patella is too small or eroded to accept a prosthesis.
4. The patient is young and active, which theoretically increases the risk of loosening and wear.

To allow the option to omit patellar resurfacing, it seems wise to design the femoral component to be compatible with the natural patella. The latest generation of posterior-stabilized prosthesis that we use is side specific with an extended trochlea that has a more gradual transition with the distal condyles to accommodate the natural patella. To facilitate these changes it was necessary to move the cam posteriorly.

EFFECT OF PATELLECTOMY ON TOTAL KNEE ARTHROPLASTY

Lennox and colleagues[156] described 11 patients who underwent TKA after a previous patellectomy. Good to excellent results were obtained in 5 of the 11 knees as compared with 11 of 11 in a control group with intact patellae. They did not find that presence or absence of the PCL was of importance. Two patients later underwent arthrodesis for continued complaints of pain. These authors found that a patient who preoperatively had more than three previous operations with minimal or moderate tibiofemoral arthritic changes and with severely compromised quadriceps function was unlikely to achieve an acceptable result from TKA.

Other investigators have reported similar results in their studies of knee arthroplasty after patellectomy.[146,192]

The senior author's experience has been that when extensor mechanism function was good before knee arthroplasty, the result was also functionally satisfactory. However, postoperative pain from the patellar tendon area could not be accurately predicted.

References

1. Abraham W, Buchanan JR, Daubert H, et al: Should the patella be resurfaced in total knee arthroplasty? Efficacy of patellar resurfacing. Clin Orthop 236:128, 1988.
2. Aglietti P, Buzzi R: Posteriorly stabilised total-condylar knee replacement: Three to eight years' follow-up of 85 knees. J Bone Joint Surg Br 70:211, 1988.
3. Aglietti P, Buzzi R, Gaudenzi A: Patellofemoral functional results and complications with the posterior stabilized total condylar knee prosthesis. J Arthroplasty 3:17, 1988.
4. Aglietti P, Rinonapoli E: Total condylar knee arthroplasty: A five-year follow-up study of 33 knees. Clin Orthop 186:104, 1984.
5. Andersen JL: Knee arthroplasty in rheumatoid arthritis: An analysis of 240 cases of hemi-, hinge and resurfacing arthroplasties. Acta Orthop Scand Suppl 180:1, 1979.
6. Andriacchi TP, Galante JO: Influence of total knee replacement design on walking and stair climbing. J Bone Joint Surg Am 64:1328, 1982.
7. Andriacchi TP, Galante JO: Retention of the posterior cruciate in total knee arthroplasty. J Arthroplasty 3(Suppl):S13, 1988.
8. Andriacchi TP, Galante JO, Draganich LF: Relationship between knee extensor mechanics and function following total knee replacement. In Dorr LD (ed): The Knee: Papers of the First Scientific Meeting of the Knee Society. Baltimore, University Park Press, 1985, p 83.
9. Andriacchi TP, Stanwyck TS, Galante JO: Knee biomechanics and total knee replacement. J Arthroplasty 1:211, 1986.
10. Arciero RA, Toomey HE: Patellofemoral arthroplasty: A three- to nine-year follow-up study. Clin Orthop 236:60, 1988.
11. Arden GP: Total replacement of the knee. J Bone Joint Surg Br 57:119, 1975.
12. Attenborough CG: Total knee replacement using the stabilized gliding prosthesis. Ann R Coll Surg Engl 58:4, 1976.
13. Attenborough CG: The Attenborough total knee replacement. J Bone Joint Surg Br 60:320, 1978.
14. Bain AM: Replacement of the knee joint with the Walldius prosthesis using cement fixation. Clin Orthop 94:65, 1973.
15. Barck AL: 10-year evaluation of compartmental knee arthroplasty. J Arthroplasty 4(Suppl):S49, 1989.
16. Bargar WL, Cracchiolo A III, Amstutz HC: Results with the constrained total knee prosthesis in treating severely disabled patients and patients with failed total knee replacements. J Bone Joint Surg Am 62:504, 1980.
17. Barrack RL, Wolfe MW, Waldman DA, et al: Resurfacing of the patella in total knee arthroplasty: A prospective, randomized, double-blind study. J Bone Joint Surg Am 79:1121, 1997.
18. Barrett DS, Biswas SP, MacKenney RP: The Oxford knee replacement: A review from an independent centre. J Bone Joint Surg Br 72:775, 1990.
19. Bartel DL, Bicknell VL, Wright TM: The effect of conformity, thickness, and material on stresses in ultra-high molecular weight components for total joint replacement. J Bone Joint Surg Am 68:1041, 1986.
20. Bartel DL, Burstein AH, Santavicca EA, et al: Performance of the tibial component in total knee replacement: Conventional and revision designs. J Bone Joint Surg Am 64:1026, 1982.
21. Becker MW, Insall JN, Farris PM: Bilateral total knee arthroplasty: One cruciate retaining and one cruciate substituting. Clin Orthop 271:122, 1991.
22. Bernasek TL, Rand JA, Bryan RS: Unicompartmental porous-coated anatomic total knee arthroplasty. Clin Orthop 236:52, 1988.
23. Bert JM: Dislocation/subluxation of meniscal bearing elements after New Jersey low-contact stress total knee arthroplasty. Clin Orthop 254:211, 1990.
24. Bertin KC, Freeman MAR, Samuelson KM, et al: Stemmed revision arthroplasty for aseptic loosening of total knee replacement. J Bone Joint Surg Br 67:242, 1985.
25. Bisla RS, Inglis AE, Lewis RJ: Fat embolism following bilateral total knee replacement with the GUEPAR prosthesis: A case report. Clin Orthop 115:195, 1976.
26. Blaha JD, Insler HP, Freeman MAR, et al: The fixation of a proximal tibial polyethylene prosthesis without cement. J Bone Joint Surg Br 64:326, 1982.
27. Blauth W, Hassenpflug J: Are unconstrained components essential in total knee arthroplasty? Long-term results of the Blauth knee prosthesis. Clin Orthop 258:86, 1990.
28. Bloebaum RD, Nelson K, Dorr LD, et al: Investigation of early surface delamination observed in retrieved heat-pressed tibial inserts. Clin Orthop 269:120, 1991.
29. Bohm P, Holy T: Is there a future for hinged prostheses in primary total knee arthroplasty? A 20 year survivorship analysis of the Blauth prosthesis. J Bone Joint Surg Br 80:302, 1998.
30. Bolanos AA, Colizza WA, McCann PD, et al: A comparison of isokinetic strength testing and gait analysis in patients with posterior cruciate–retaining and substituting knee arthroplasties. J Arthroplasty 13:906, 1998.
31. Bourne RB, Rorabeck CH, Finlay JB, et al: Kinematic I and Oxford knee arthroplasty: A 5-8-year follow-up study. J Arthroplasty 2:285, 1987.
32. Boyd AD, Ewald FC, Thomas WH, et al: Long term complications after total knee arthroplasty with or without resurfacing of the patella. J Bone Joint Surg Am 75:674, 1993.
33. Bradley J, Goodfellow JW, O'Connor JJ: A radiographic study of bearing movement in unicompartmental Oxford knee replacements. J Bone Joint Surg Br 69:598, 1987.
34. Brick GW, Scott RD: The patellofemoral component of total knee arthroplasty. Clin Orthop 231:163, 1988.
35. Brodersen MP, Fitzgerald RH Jr, Peterson LFA, et al: Arthrodesis of the knee following failed total knee arthroplasty. J Bone Joint Surg Am 61:181, 1979.
36. Brooks PJ, Walker PS, Scott RD: Tibial component fixation in deficient tibial bone stock. Clin Orthop 184:302, 1984.
37. Bryan RS, Peterson LFA: Polycentric total knee arthroplasty: A prognostic assessment. Clin Orthop 145:23, 1979.
38. Buechel FF, Pappas MJ: Long-term survivorship analysis of cruciate-sparing versus cruciate-sacrificing knee prostheses using meniscal bearings. Clin Orthop 260:162, 1990.
39. Buechel FF, Pappas MJ, Makris G: Evaluation of contact stress in metal-backed patellar replacements: A predictor of survivorship. Clin Orthop 273:190, 1991.
40. Callihan SM, Halley DK: Prospective analysis of Sheehan total knee arthroplasty. Clin Orthop 192:124, 1985.
41. Campbell WC: Interposition of Vitallium plates in arthroplasties of the knee: Preliminary report. Am J Surg 47:639, 1940.
42. Cartier P, Cheaib S: Unicondylar knee arthroplasty: 2-10 years of follow-up evaluation. J Arthroplasty 2:157, 1987.
43. Cartier P, Sanouiller J-L, Grelsamer R: Patellofemoral arthroplasty: 2-12-year follow-up study. J Arthroplasty 5:49, 1990.

44. Cavendish ME, Wright JTM: The Liverpool Mark II knee prosthesis: A preliminary report. J Bone Joint Surg Br 60:315, 1978.

45. Cheng CL, Gross AE: Loosening of the porous coating in total knee replacement. J Bone Joint Surg Br 70:377, 1988.

46. Chotivichit AL, Cracchiolo A III, Chow GH, et al: Total knee arthroplasty using the total condylar III knee prosthesis. J Arthroplasty 6:341, 1991.

47. Cloutier JM, Gauthier F, Rizkallah R: Arthroplasty of the knee using the Marmor prosthesis. J Bone Joint Surg Br 58:142, 1976.

48. Colizza WA, Insall JN, Scuderi GR: The posterior stabilized total knee prosthesis: Assessment of polyethylene damage and osteolysis after a ten-year-minimum follow-up. J Bone Joint Surg Am 77:1713, 1995.

49. Collier JP, McNamara JL, Surprenant VA, et al: All-polyethylene patellar components are not the answer. Clin Orthop 273:198, 1991.

50. Cooke TDV, Collins A, Wevers HW: Failure of a knee prosthesis accelerated by shedding of beads from the porous metal surface. Clin Orthop 258:204, 1990.

51. Coventry MB, Finerman GAM, Riley LH, et al: A new geometric knee for total knee arthroplasty. Clin Orthop 83:157, 1972.

52. Coventry MB, Upshaw JE, Riley LH, et at: Geometric total knee arthroplasty. II. Patient data and complications. Clin Orthop 94:177, 1973.

53. Deane G: The evolution and clinical use of the Deane intercondylar knee. J Bone Joint Surg Br 63:476, 1981.

54. Deburge A, GUEPAR: GUEPAR hinge prosthesis: Complications and results with two years' follow-up. Clin Orthop 120:47, 1976.

55. Dennis DA, Komistek RD, Hoff WA, et al: In vivo knee kinematics derived using an inverse perspective technique. Clin Orthop 331:107, 1996.

56. Diduch DR, Insall JN, Scott WN, et al: Total knee replacement in young active patients: Long-term follow-up and functional outcome. J Bone Joint Surg Am 79:575, 1997.

57. Dodd CAF, Hungerford DS, Krackow KA: Total knee arthroplasty fixation: Comparison of the early results of paired cemented versus uncemented porous coated anatomic knee prostheses. Clin Orthop 260:66, 1990.

58. Donaldson WF III, Sculco TP, Insall JN, et al: Total condylar III knee prosthesis: Long-term follow-up study. Clin Orthop 226:21, 1988.

59. Dorr LD, Ochsner JL, Gronley J, et al: Functional comparison of posterior cruciate–retained versus cruciate-sacrificed total knee arthroplasty. Clin Orthop 236:36, 1988.

60. Ducheyne P, Kagan A II, Lacey JA: Failure of total knee arthroplasty due to loosening and deformation of the tibial component. J Bone Joint Surg Am 60:384, 1978.

61. Duffy GP, Berry DJ, Rand JA: Cement versus cementless fixation in total knee arthroplasty. Clin Orthop 356:66, 1998.

62. Duffy GP, Trousdale RT, Stuart MJ: Total knee arthroplasty in patients 55 years old or younger: 10 to 17 year results. Clin Orthop 356:22, 1998.

63. Easley ME, Insall JN, Scuderi GR, Bullek DD: Primary constrained condylar knee arthroplasty for the arthritic valgus knee. Clin Orthop 380:58, 2000.

64. Elias SG, Freeman MAR, Gokcay EI: A correlative study of the geometry and anatomy of the distal femur. Clin Orthop 260:98, 1990.

65. Emerson RH Jr, Potter T: The use of the McKeever metallic hemi-arthroplasty for unicompartmental arthritis. J Bone Joint Surg Am 67:208, 1985.

66. Engh GA: Failure of the polyethylene bearing surface of a total knee replacement within four years: A case report. J Bone Joint Surg Am 70:1093, 1988.

67. England SP, Stern SH, Insall JN, et al: Total knee arthroplasty in diabetes mellitus. Clin Orthop 260:130, 1990.

68. Enis JE, Gardner R, Robledo MA, et al: Comparison of patellar resurfacing versus nonresurfacing in bilateral total knee arthroplasty. Clin Orthop 260:38, 1990.

69. Evanski PM, Waugh TR, Orofino CF, et al: UCI knee replacement. Clin Orthop 120:33, 1976.

70. Ewald FC, Jacobs MA, Miegel RE, at al: Kinematic total knee replacement. J Bone Joint Surg Am 66:1032, 1984.

71. Ewald FC, Thomas WH, Poss R, et al: Duo-patella total knee arthroplasty in rheumatoid arthritis. Orthop Trans 2:202, 1978.

72. Ferguson W: Excision of the knee joint: Recovery with a false joint and a useful limb. Med Times Gaz 1:601, 1861.

73. Figgie HE III, Davy DT, Heiple KG, et al: Load-bearing capacity of the tibial component of the total condylar knee prosthesis: An in vitro study. Orthop Clin 183:288, 1984.

74. Figgie HE III, Goldberg VM, Heiple KG, et al: The influence of tibial-patellofemoral location on function of the knee in patients with the posterior stabilized condylar knee prosthesis. J Bone Joint Surg Am 68:1035, 1986.

75. Finerman GAM, Coventry MB, Riley LH, et al: Anametric total knee arthroplasty. Clin Orthop 145:85, 1979.

76. Firestone TP, Teeny SM, Krackow KA, et al: The clinical and roentgenographic results of cementless porous-coated patellar fixation. Clin Orthop 273:184, 1991.

77. Freeman MAR, Insall JN: Tibio-femoral replacement using two unlinked components and cruciate resection (the ICLH and total condylar prostheses). In Freeman, MAR (ed): Arthritis of the Knee: Clinical Features and Surgical Management. New York, Springer-Verlag, 1980, p 254.

78. Freeman MAR, Insall JN, Besser W, et al: Excision of the cruciate ligaments in total knee replacement. Clin Orthop 126:209, 1977.

79. Freeman MAR, Levack B: British contribution to knee arthroplasty. Clin Orthop 210:69, 1986.

80. Freeman MAR, Railton GT: Should the posterior cruciate ligament be retained or resected in condylar nonmeniscal knee arthroplasty? The case for resection. J Arthroplasty 3(Suppl):S3, 1988.

81. Freeman MAR, Samuelson KM, Bertin KC: Freeman-Samuelson total arthroplasty of the knee. Clin Orthop 192:46, 1985.

82. Freeman MAR, Samuelson KM, Elias SG, et al: The patellofemoral joint in total knee prostheses: Design considerations. J Arthroplasty 4(Suppl):S69, 1989.

83. Freeman MAR, Samuelson KM, Levack B, et al: Knee arthroplasty at the London Hospital: 1975-1984. Clin Orthop 205:12, 1986.

84. Freeman MAR, Sculco T, Todd RC: Replacement of the severely damaged arthritic knee by the ICLH (Freeman-Swanson) arthroplasty. J Bone Joint Surg Br 59:64, 1977.

85. Freeman MAR, Swanson SAV, Todd RC: Total replacement of the knee using the Freeman-Swanson knee prosthesis. Clin Orthop 94:153, 1973.

86. Freeman MAR, Todd RC, Bamert P, et al: ICLH arthroplasty of the knee: 1968-1977. J Bone Joint Surg Br 60:339, 1978.

87. Gibbs AN, Green GA, Taylor JG: A comparison of the Freeman-Swanson (ICLH) and Walldius prostheses in total knee replacement. J Bone Joint Surg Br 61:358, 1979.

88. Goldberg VM, Figgie MP, Figgie HE III, et al: Use of a total condylar knee prosthesis for treatment of osteoarthritis and rheumatoid arthritis: Long-term results. J Bone Joint Surg Am 70:802, 1988.

89. Goldberg VM, Henderson BT: The Freeman-Swanson ICLH total knee arthroplasty: Complications and problems. J Bone Joint Surg Am 62:1338, 1980.

90. Goodfellow JW, Kershaw CJ, D'A Benson MK, et al: The Oxford knee for unicompartmental osteoarthritis: The first 103 cases. J Bone Joint Surg Br 70:692, 1988.

91. Goodfellow J, O'Connor J: Kinematics of the knee and the prosthetic design. J Bone Joint Surg Br 59:119, 1977.

92. Goodfellow JW, O'Connor J: Clinical results of the Oxford knee: Surface arthroplasty of the tibiofemoral joint with a meniscal bearing prosthesis. Clin Orthop 205:21, 1986.

93. Goodfellow JW, Tibrewal SB, Sherman KP, et al: Unicompartmental Oxford meniscal knee arthroplasty. J Arthroplasty 2:1, 1987.

94. Grimer RJ, Karpinski MRK, Edwards AN: The long-term results of Stanmore total knee replacements. J Bone Joint Surg Br 66:55, 1984.

95. Groh GI, Parker J, Elliott J, et al: Results of total knee arthroplasty using the posterior stabilized condylar prosthesis: A report of 137 consecutive cases. Clin Orthop 269:58, 1991.

96. Firestone TP, Krackow KA, Davis JD IV, et al: The management of fixed flexion contractures during total knee arthroplasty. Clin Orthop 284:221, 1992.

97. Gunston FH: Polycentric knee arthroplasty: Prosthetic simulation of normal knee movement. J Bone Joint Surg Br 53:272, 1971.

98. Gunston FH, MacKenzie RI: Complications of polycentric knee arthroplasty. Clin Orthop 120:11, 1976.

99. Haas SB, Insall JN, Montgomery W III, et al: Revision total knee arthroplasty with use of modular components with stems inserted without cement. J Bone Joint Surg Am 77:1700, 1995.

100. Hanssen AD, Rand JA: A comparison of primary and revision total knee arthroplasty using the kinematic stabilizer prosthesis. J Bone Joint Surg Am 70:491, 1988.

101. Hernigou PH, Goutallier D: GUEPAR unicompartmental lotus prosthesis for single-compartment femorotibial arthrosis: A five- to nine-year follow-up study. Clin Orthop 230:186, 1988.

102. Hirsh DM, Sallis JG: Pain after total knee arthroplasty caused by soft tissue impingement. J Bone Joint Surg Am 71:591, 1989.

103. Hohl WM, Crawfurd E, Zelicof SB, et al: The total condylar III prosthesis in complex knee reconstruction. Clin Orthop 273:91, 1991.

104. Hood RW, Vanni M, Insall JN: The correction of knee alignment in 225 consecutive total condylar knee replacements. Clin Orthop 160:94, 1981.

105. Hui FC, Fitzgerald RH Jr: Hinged total knee arthroplasty. J Bone Joint Surg Am 62:513, 1980.

106. Hungerford DS, Kenna RV, Krackow KA: The porous-coated anatomic total knee. Orthop Clin North Am 13:103, 1982.

107. Hungerford DS, Krackow KA: Total joint arthroplasty of the knee. Clin Orthop 192:23, 1985.

108. Hvid I, Kjaersgaard-Andersen P, Wethelund J-O, et al: Knee arthroplasty in rheumatoid arthritis: Four- to six-year follow-up study. J Arthroplasty 2:233, 1987.

109. Hvid I, Nielsen S: Total condylar knee arthroplasty: Prosthetic component positioning and radiolucent lines. Acta Orthop Scand 55:160, 1984.

110. Ilstrup DM, Coventry MB, Skolnick MD: A statistical evaluation of geometric total knee arthroplasties. Clin Orthop 120:27, 1976.

111. Incavo SJ, Johnson CC, Beynnon BD, et al: Posterior cruciate ligament strain biomechanics in total knee arthroplasty. Clin Orthop 309:88, 1994.

112. Insall JN: Reconstructive surgery and rehabilitation of the knee. In Kelley WN, Harris ED Jr, Ruddy S, et al (eds): Textbook of Rheumatology. Philadelphia, WB Saunders, 1980, p 1980.

113. Insall JN: Adventures in mobile-bearing knee design: A mid life crisis. Orthopedics 21:1021, 1998.

114. Insall JN, Aglietti P: A five- to seven-year follow-up of unicondylar arthroplasty. J Bone Joint Surg Am 62:1329, 1980.

115. Insall JN, Freeman MAR, Matthews LS, et al: Present status of total knee replacement. [Symposium]. Contemp Orthop 2:592, 1980.

116. Insall JN, Kelly M: The total condylar prosthesis. Clin Orthop 205:43, 1986.

117. Insall JN, Lachiewicz PF, Burstein AH: The posterior stabilized condylar prosthesis: A modification of the total condylar design: Two to four year clinical experience. J Bone Joint Surg Am 64:1317, 1982.

118. Insall JN, Ranawat CS, Aglietti P, et al: A comparison of four models of total knee replacement prostheses. J Bone Joint Surg Am 58:754, 1976.

119. Insall JN, Ranawat CS, Scott WN, et al: Total condylar knee replacement: Preliminary report. Clin Orthop 120:149, 1976.

120. Insall JN, Scott WN, Ranawat CS: The total condylar knee prosthesis: A report of two hundred and twenty cases. J Bone Joint Surg Am 61:173, 1979.

121. Insall JN, Tria AJ: The total condylar prosthesis type II. Orthop Trans 3:300, 1979.

122. Insall JN, Tria AJ, Scott WN: The total condylar knee prosthesis: The first five years. Clin Orthop 145:68, 1979.

123. Insall JN, Walker P: Unicondylar knee replacement. Clin Orthop 120:83, 1976.

124. Jones EC, Insall JN, Inglis AE, et al: GUEPAR knee arthroplasty results and late complications. Clin Orthop 140:145, 1979.

125. Jones GB: Arthroplasty of the knee by the Walldius prosthesis. J Bone Joint Surg Br 50:505, 1968.

126. Jones GB: Walldius arthroplasty of the knee. J Bone Joint Surg Br 52:390, 1970.

127. Jones WT, Bryan RS, Peterson LFA, et al: Unicompartmental knee arthroplasty using polycentric and geometric hemicomponents. J Bone Joint Surg Am 63:946, 1981.

128. Jonsson B, Astrom J: Alignment and long-term clinical results of a semiconstrained knee prosthesis. Clin Orthop 226:124, 1988.

129. Kajino A, Yoshino S, Kameyama S, et al: Comparison of the results of bilateral total knee arthroplasty with and without patellar replacement for rheumatoid arthritis: A follow-up note. J Bone Joint Surg Am 79:570, 1997.

130. Kapandji IA: The Physiology of the Joints, vol. 2, The Lower Limb. London, Churchill Livingstone, 1970, p 120.

131. Katz MM, Hungerford DS, Krackow KA, et al: Results of total knee arthroplasty after failed proximal tibial osteotomy for osteoarthritis. J Bone Joint Surg Am 69:225, 1987.

132. Kaufer H, Matthews LS: Spherocentric arthroplasty of the knee. J Bone Joint Surg Am 63:545, 1981.

133. Kavolus CH, Faris PM, Ritter MA, et al: The total condylar III knee prosthesis in elderly patients. J Arthroplasty 6:39, 1991.

134. Keblish PA, Varma AK, Greenwald AS: Patellar resurfacing or retention in total knee arthroplasty. J Bone Joint Surg Br 76:930, 1994.

135. Kelman GJ, Biden EN, Wyatt MP, et al: Gait laboratory analysis of a posterior cruciate–sparing total knee arthroplasty in stair ascent and descent. Clin Orthop 248:21, 1989.

136. Kester MA, Cook SD, Harding AF, et al: An evaluation of the mechanical failure modalities of a rotating hinge knee prosthesis. Clin Orthop 228:156, 1988.

137. Kilgus DJ, Moreland JR, Finerman GAM, et al: Catastrophic wear of tibial polyethylene inserts. Clin Orthop 273:223, 1991.

138. Kim Y-H: Salvage of failed hinge knee arthroplasty with a total condylar III type prosthesis. Clin Orthop 221:272, 1987.

139. Kjaersgaard-Andersen P, Hvid I, Wethelund J-O, et al: Total condylar knee arthroplasty in osteoarthritis: A four- to six-year follow-up evaluation of 103 cases. Clin Orthop 238:167, 1989.

140. Kleinbart FA, Bryk E, Evangelista J, et al: Histologic comparison of posterior cruciate ligaments from arthritic and age-matched knee specimens. J Arthroplasty 11:726, 1996.

141. Knahr K, Salzer M, Schmidt W: A radiological analysis of uncemented PCA tibial implants with a follow-up period of 4-7 years. J Arthroplasty 5:131, 1990.

142. Kozinn SC, Marx C, Scott RD: Unicompartmental knee arthroplasty: A 4.5-6-year follow-up study with a metal-backed tibial component. J Arthroplasty 4(Suppl):S1, 1989.

143. Kozinn SC, Scott R: Unicondylar knee arthroplasty. J Bone Joint Surg Am 71:145, 1989.

144. Kraay MJ, Meyers SA, Goldberg VM, et al: "Hybrid" total knee arthroplasty with the Miller-Galante prosthesis: A prospective clinical and roentgenographic evaluation. Clin Orthop 273:32, 1991.

145. Landon GC, Galante JO, Maley MM: Noncemented total knee arthroplasty. Clin Orthop 205:49, 1986.

146. Larson KR, Cracchiolo A III, Dorey FJ, et al: Total knee arthroplasty in patients after patellectomy. Clin Orthop 264:243, 1991.

147. Larsson S-E, Larsson S, Lundkvist S: Unicompartmental knee arthroplasty: A prospective consecutive series followed for six to 11 years. Clin Orthop 232:174, 1988.

148. Laskin RS: Modular total knee replacement arthroplasty: A review of eighty-nine patients. J Bone Joint Surg Am 58:766, 1976.

149. Laskin RS: Unicompartmental tibiofemoral resurfacing arthroplasty. J Bone Joint Surg Am 60:182, 1978.

150. Laskin RS: RMC total knee replacement: A review of 166 cases. J Arthroplasty, 1:11, 1986.

151. Laskin RS: Tricon-M uncemented total knee arthroplasty: A review of 96 knees followed for longer than 2 years. J Arthroplasty 3:27, 1988.

152. Laskin RS: Total knee arthroplasty in the presence of large bony defects of the tibia and marked knee instability. Clin Orthop 248:66, 1989.

153. Laskin RS: Total condylar knee replacement in patients who have rheumatoid arthritis: A ten-year follow-up study. J Bone Joint Surg Am 72:529, 1990.

154. Laskin RS: Total knee replacement with posterior cruciate ligament retention in patients with a fixed varus deformity. Clin Orthop 331:29, 1996.

155. Laskin RS, Bucknell A: The use of metal-backed patellar prostheses in total knee arthroplasty. Clin Orthop 260:52, 1990.

156. Lennox DW, Hungerford DS, Krackow KA: Total knee arthroplasty following patellectomy. Clin Orthop 223:220, 1987.

157. Lettin AWF, Deliss LJ, Blackburne JS, et al: The Stanmore hinged knee arthroplasty. J Bone Joint Surg Br 60:327, 1978.

158. Lettin AWF, Kavanagh TG, Craig D, et al: Assessment of the survival and the clinical results of Stanmore total knee replacements. J Bone Joint Surg Br 66:355, 1984.

159. Lettin AWF, Kavanagh TG, Scales JT: The long-term results of Stanmore total knee replacements. J Bone Joint Surg Br 66:349, 1984.

160. Lewis JL, Askew MJ, Jaycox DP: A comparative evaluation of tibial component designs of total knee prostheses. J Bone Joint Surg Am 64:129, 1982.

161. Lotke PA, Wong RY, Ecker ML: The use of methyl-methacrylate in primary total knee replacements with large tibial defects. Clin Orthop 270:288, 1991.

162. MacIntosh DL: Hemiarthroplasty of the knee using a space occupying prosthesis for painful varus and valgus deformities. J Bone Joint Surg Am 40:1431, 1958.

163. MacIntosh DL: Arthroplasty of the knee in rheumatoid arthritis. J Bone Joint Surg Br 48:179, 1966.

164. Mahoney OM, Noble PC, Rhoads DD, et al: Posterior cruciate function following total knee arthroplasty: A biomechanical study. J. Arthroplasty 9:569, 1994.

165. Malkani AL, Rand JA, Bryan RS, et al: Total knee arthroplasty with the Kinematic condylar prosthesis: A ten year follow-up study. J Bone Joint Surg Am 77:423, 1995.

166. Manchester Knee Arthroplasty [editorial]. J Bone Joint Surg Br 61:225, 1979.

167. Marks KE, Nelson CL, Lautenschlager EP: Antibiotic-impregnated acrylic bone cement. J Bone Joint Surg Am 58:358, 1976.

168. Marmor L: The modular (Marmor) knee: Case report with a minimum follow-up of two years. Clin Orthop 120:86, 1976.

169. Marmor L: Results of single compartment arthroplasty with acrylic cement fixation: A minimum follow-up of two years. Clin Orthop 122:181, 1977.

170. Marmor L: Marmor modular knee in unicompartmental disease: Minimum four-year follow-up. J Bone Joint Surg Am 61:347, 1979.

171. Marmor L: Unicompartmental knee arthroplasty: Ten- to 13-year follow-up study. Clin Orthop 226:14, 1988.

172. Marmor L: Total knee arthroplasty in a patient with congenital dislocation of the patella: Case report. Clin Orthop 226:129, 1988.

173. Matthews LS, Goldstein SA, Kolowich PA, et al: Spherocentric arthroplasty of the knee: A long-term and final follow-up evaluation. Clin Orthop 205:58, 1986.

174. Mazas FB: GUEPAR total knee prosthesis. Clin Orthop 94:211, 1973.

175. McKeever DC: Tibial plateau prosthesis. Clin Orthop 18:86, 1960.

176. McLain RF, Bargar WF: The effect of total knee design on patellar strain. J Arthroplasty 1:91, 1986.

177. Miller A, Friedman B: Fascial arthroplasty of the knee. J Bone Joint Surg Am 34:55, 1952.

178. Miura H, Whiteside LA, Easley JC, et al: Effects of screws and a sleeve on initial fixation in uncemented total knee tibial components. Clin Orthop 259:160, 1990.

179. Moller JT, Weeth RE, Keller JO: Unicompartmental arthroplasty of the knee: Cadaver study of tibial component placement. Acta Orthop Scand 56:115, 1985.

180. Moller JT, Weeth RE, Keller JO, et al: Unicompartmental arthroplasty of the knee: Cadaver study of the importance of the anterior cruciate ligament. Acta Orthop Scand 56:120, 1985.

181. Moran CG, Pinder IM, Lees TA, et al: Survivorship analysis of the uncemented porous-coated anatomic knee replacement. J Bone Joint Surg Am 73:848, 1991.

182. Moreland JR, Thomas RJ, Freeman MAR: ICLH replacement of the knee: 1977 and 1978. Clin Orthop 145:47, 1979.

183. Murray DG, Webster DA: The variable-axis knee prosthesis: Two-year follow-up study. J Bone Joint Surg Am 63:687, 1981.

184. Murray RB, Rand JA, Hanssen AD: Cemented long-stem revision total knee arthroplasty. Clin Orthop 309:116, 1994.

185. Nilsson KG, Karrholm J, Ekelund L: Knee motion in total knee arthroplasty: A roentgen stereophotogrammetric analysis of the kinematics of the Tricon-M knee prosthesis. Clin Orthop 256:147, 1990.

186. Orr TE, Beaupré GS, Carter DR, et al: Computer predictions of bone remodeling around porous-coated implants. J Arthroplasty 5:191, 1990.

187. Pagnano MW, Cushner FD, Scott WN: Role of the posterior cruciate ligament in total knee arthroplasty. J Am Acad Orthop Surg 6:176, 1998.

188. Pagnano MW, Hanssen AD, Lewallen DG, et al: Flexion instability after primary posterior cruciate retaining total knee arthroplasty. Clin Orthop 356:39, 1998.

189. Phillips H, Taylor JG: The Walldius hinge arthroplasty. J Bone Joint Surg Br 57:59, 1975.

190. Rackemann S, Mintzer CM, Walker PS, et al: Uncemented press-fit total knee arthroplasty. J Arthroplasty 5:307, 1990.

191. Rae T: A study on the effects of particulate metals of orthopaedic interest on murine macrophages in vitro. J Bone Joint Surg Br 57:444, 1975.

192. Railton GT, Levack B, Freeman MAR: Unconstrained knee arthroplasty after patellectomy. J Arthroplasty 5:255, 1990.

193. Railton GT, Waterfield A, Nunn D, et al: The effect of a metal-back without a stem upon the fixation of a tibial prosthesis. J Arthroplasty 5(Suppl):S67, 1990.

194. Ranawat CS, Boachie-Adjei O: Survivorship analysis and results of total condylar knee arthroplasty. Eight- to 11-year follow-up period. Clin Orthop 226:6, 1988.

195. Ranawat CS, Insall J, Shine J: Duo-condylar knee arthroplasty: Hospital for Special Surgery design. Clin Orthop 120:76, 1976.

196. Ranawat CS, Luessenhop CP, Rodriguez JS: The press-fit condylar modular total knee system: Four to six year results with a posterior-cruciate–substituting design. J Bone Joint Surg Am 79:342, 1997.

197. Rand JA: Patellar resurfacing in total knee arthroplasty. Clin Orthop 260:110, 1990.

198. Rand JA, Chao EYS, Stauffer RN: Kinematic rotating-hinge total knee arthroplasty. J Bone Joint Surg Am 69:489, 1987.

199. Rand JA, Coventry MB: Ten-year evaluation of geometric total knee arthroplasty. Clin Orthop 232:168, 1988.

200. Rand JA, Trousdale RT, Ilstrup DM, Harmsen WS: Factors affecting the durability of primary total knee prostheses. J Bone Joint Surg Am 85:259, 2003.

201. Riley D, Woodyard JE: Long-term results of Geomedic total knee replacement. J Bone Joint Surg Br 67:548, 1985.

202. Riley LH, Hungerford DS: Geometric total knee replacement for treatment of the rheumatoid knee. J Bone Joint Surg Am 60:523, 1978.

203. Ritter MA: Screw and cement fixation of large defects in total knee arthroplasty. J Arthroplasty 1:125, 1986.

204. Ritter MA, Campbell E, Faris PM, et al: Long-term survival analysis of the posterior cruciate condylar total knee arthroplasty: A 10-year evaluation. J Arthroplasty 4:293, 1989.

205. Ritter MA, Faris PM, Keating EM: Posterior cruciate ligament balancing during total knee arthroplasty. J Arthroplasty 3:323, 1988.

206. Robinson, RP: The early innovators of today's resurfacing condylar knees. J Arthroplasty 20(Suppl 1):2, 2005.

207. Rorabeck CH, Bourne RB, Nott L: The cemented kinematic-II and the non-cemented porous-coated anatomic prostheses for total knee replacement: A prospective evaluation. J Bone Joint Surg Am 70:483, 1988.

208. Rosenberg AG, Barden RM, Galante JO: Cemented and ingrowth fixation of the Miller-Galante prosthesis: Clinical and roentgenographic comparison after three- to six-year follow-up studies. Clin Orthop 260:71, 1990.

209. Rosenqvist R, Bylander B, Knutson K, et al: Loosening of the porous coating of bicompartmental prostheses in patients with rheumatoid arthritis. J Bone Joint Surg Am 68:538, 1986.

210. Samuelson KM: Bone grafting and noncemented revision arthroplasty of the knee. Clin Orthop 226:93, 1988.

211. Samuelson K, Nelson L: An all-polyethylene cementless tibial component: A five- to nine-year follow-up study. Clin Orthop 260:93, 1990.

212. Schurman DJ, Parker JN, Ornstein D: Total condylar knee replacement: A study of factors influencing range of motion as late as two years after arthroplasty. J Bone Joint Surg Am 67:1006, 1985.

213. Scott RD, Joyce MJ, Ewald FC, et al: McKeever metallic hemiarthroplasty of the knee in unicompartmental degenerative arthritis: Long-term clinical follow-up and current indications. J Bone Joint Surg Am 67:203, 1985.

214. Scott RD, Santore RF: Unicondylar unicompartmental replacement for osteoarthritis of the knee. J Bone Joint Surg Am 63:536, 1981.

215. Scott RD, Thornhill TS: Posterior cruciate supplementing total knee replacements using conforming inserts and cruciate recession: Effect on range of motion and radiolucent lines. Clin Orthop 309:146, 1994.

216. Scott RD, Volatile TB: Twelve years' experience with posterior cruciate–retaining total knee arthroplasty. Clin Orthop 205:100, 1986.

217. Scott RD, Welsh RP, Thomas WH: Unicompartment unicondylar total knee replacement in osteoarthritis of the knee. Orthop Trans 2:203, 1978.
218. Scott WN, Rozbruch JD, Otis JC, et al: Clinical and biomechanical evaluation of patella replacement in total knee arthroplasty. Orthop Trans 2:203, 1978.
219. Scott WN, Rubinstein M: Posterior stabilized knee arthroplasty. Six years' experience. Clin Orthop 205:138, 1986.
220. Scott WN, Rubinstein M, Scuderi G: Results after knee replacement with a posterior cruciate–substituting prosthesis. J Bone Joint Surg Am 70:1163, 1988.
221. Scott WN, Tria A, Insall JN: Total knee arthroplasty: Past present, future. Orthop Surv 3:135, 1979.
222. Shaw NE, Chatterjee RK: Manchester knee arthroplasty. J Bone Joint Surg Br 60:310, 1978.
223. Sheehan JM: Arthroplasty of the knee. J Bone Joint Surg Br 60:333, 1978.
224. Shiers LGP: Arthroplasty of the knee: Preliminary report of a new method. J Bone Joint Surg Br 36:553, 1954.
225. Shindell R, Neumann R, Connolly JF, et al: Evaluation of the Noiles hinged knee prosthesis: A five-year study of seventeen knees. J Bone Joint Surg Am 68:579, 1986.
226. Shoji H, D'Ambrosia RD, Lipscomb PR: Failed polycentric total knee prostheses. J Bone Joint Surg Am 58:773, 1976.
227. Shoji H, Yoshino S, Kajino A: Patellar replacement in bilateral total knee arthroplasty: A study of patients who had rheumatoid arthritis and no gross deformity of the patella. J Bone Joint Surg Am 71:853, 1989.
228. Simison AJM, Noble J, Hardinge K: Complications of the Attenborough knee replacement. J Bone Joint Surg Br 68:100, 1986.
229. Simmon S, Lephart S, Rubash H, et al: Proprioception after unicondylar knee arthroplasty versus total knee arthroplasty. Clin Orthop 331:179, 1996.
230. Skolnick MD, Bryan RS, Peterson LFA: Unicompartmental polycentric knee arthroplasty. Description and preliminary results. Clin Orthop 112:208, 1975.
231. Sledge CB, Ewald FC: Total knee arthroplasty experience at the Robert Breck Brigham Hospital. Clin Orthop 145:78, 1979.
232. Sledge CB, Stern P, Thomas WH, et al: Two-year follow-up of the duo-condylar total knee replacement. Orthop Trans 2:193, 1978.
233. Smith SR, Stuart P, Pinder IM: Nonresurfaced patella in total knee arthroplasty. J Arthroplasty 4(Suppl):S81, 1989.
234. Sonstegard DA, Kaufer H, Matthews LS: The spherocentric knee: Biomechanical testing and clinical trial. J Bone Joint Surg Am 59:602, 1977.
235. Soudry M, Walker PS, Reilly DT, et al: Effects of total knee replacement design on femoral-tibial contact conditions. J Arthroplasty 1:35, 1986.
236. Soudry M, Mestriner LA, Binazzi R, et al: Total knee arthroplasty without patellar resurfacing. Clin Orthop 205:166, 1986.
237. Spector M: Historical review of porous-coated implants. J Arthroplasty 2:163, 1987.
238. Speed JS, Trout PC: Arthroplasty of the knee: A follow-up study. J Bone Joint Surg Br 31:53, 1949.
239. Springer BD, Hanssen AD, Sim FH, Lewallen DG: The kinematic rotating hinge prosthesis for complex knee arthroplasty. Clin Orthop 392:283, 2001.
240. Stern SH, Bowen MK, Insall JN, et al: Cemented total knee arthroplasty for gonarthrosis in patients 55 years old or younger. Clin Orthop 260:124, 1990.
241. Stern SH, Insall JN: Total knee arthroplasty in obese patients. J Bone Joint Surg Am 72:1400, 1990.
242. Stern SH, Insall JN, Windsor RE, et al: Total knee arthroplasty in patients with psoriasis. Clin Orthop 248:108, 1989.
243. Stiehl JB, Komistek RD, Dennis DA, et al: Fluoroscopic analysis of kinematics after posterior-cruciate–retaining knee arthroplasty. J Bone Joint Surg Br 77:884, 1995.
244. Tew M, Waugh W, Forster IW: Comparing the results of different types of knee replacement: A method proposed and applied. J Bone Joint Surg Br 67:775, 1985.
245. Thatcher JC, Zhou X-M, Walker PS: Inherent laxity in total knee prostheses. J Arthroplasty 2:199, 1987.
246. Thompson FM, Hood RW, Insall JN: Patellar fractures in total knee arthroplasty. Orthop Trans 5:490, 1981.
247. Tibrewal SB, Grant KA, Goodfellow JW: The radiolucent line beneath the tibial components of the Oxford meniscal knee. J Bone Joint Surg Br 66:523, 1984.
248. Townley CO: The anatomic total knee resurfacing arthroplasty. Clin Orthop 192:82, 1985.
249. Tsao A, Mintz L, McRae CR, et al: Failure of the porous-coated anatomic prosthesis in total knee arthroplasty due to severe polyethylene wear. J Bone Joint Surg Am 75:19, 1993.
250. Turner RH, Matza R, Hamati YI: Geometric and anametric total knee replacements. In Savastano AA (ed): Total Knee Replacement. New York, Appleton-Century-Crofts, 1980, p 171.
251. Vanhegan JAD, Dabrowski W, Arden GP: A review of 100 Attenborough stabilised gliding knee prostheses. J Bone Joint Surg Br 61:445, 1979.
252. Verneuil A: De la création d'une fausse articulation par section ou résection partielle de l'os maxillaire inférieur, comme moyen de rémedier a l'ankylose vraie ou fausse de la machoire inférieure. Arch Gen Med 15(ser 5):174, 1860.
253. Vince KG, Insall JN, Bannerman CE: Total knee arthroplasty in the patient with Parkinson's disease. J Bone Joint Surg Br 71:51, 1989.
254. Vince KG, Insall JN, Kelly MA: The total condylar prosthesis: 10- to 12-year results of a cemented knee replacement. J Bone Joint Surg Br 71:793, 1989.
255. Walker PS: Human Joints and Their Artificial Replacements. Springfield, IL, Charles C Thomas, 1977.
256. Walker PS, Greene D, Reilly D, et al: Fixation of tibial components of knee prostheses. J Bone Joint Surg Am 63:258, 1981.
257. Walker PS, Hsu H-P, Zimmerman RA: A comparative study of uncemented tibial components. J Arthroplasty 5:245, 1990.
258. Walker PS, Ranawat C, Insall JN: Fixation of the tibial components of condylar replacement knee prostheses. J Biomech 9:269, 1976.
259. Walldius B: Arthroplasty of the knee joint using endoprosthesis. Acta Orthop Scand Suppl 24:19, 1957.
260. Walldius B: Arthroplasty of the knee—twenty-seven years' experience. In Savastano AA (ed): Total Knee Replacement. New York, Appleton-Century-Crofts, 1980, p 195.
261. Warren PJ, Olanlokun TK, Cobb AG, et al: Proprioception after total knee arthroplasty: The influence of prosthetic design. Clin Orthop 297:182, 1993.
262. Waslewski GL, Marson BM, Benjamin JB: Early, incapacitating instability of posterior cruciate ligament–retaining total knee arthroplasty. J Arthroplasty 13:763, 1998.
263. Waugh TR, Evanski PM: University of California, Irvine (UCI) knee replacement—design, operative technique, and results. In Savastano AA (ed): Total Knee Replacement. New York, Appleton-Century-Crofts, 1980, p 217.
264. Waugh W, Tew M: Total replacement of the knee [letter]. J Bone Joint Surg Br 61:225, 1979.
265. Webster DA, Murray DG: Complications of variable axis total knee arthroplasty. Clin Orthop 193:160, 1985.
266. White SH, O'Connor JJ, Goodfellow JW: Sagittal plane laxity following knee arthroplasty. J Bone Joint Surg Br 73:268, 1991.
267. Whiteside LA, Amador DD: The effect of posterior tibial slope on knee stability after Ortholoc total knee arthroplasty. J Arthroplasty 3(Suppl):S51, 1988.
268. Whiteside LA, Amador DD: Rotational stability of a posterior stabilized total knee arthroplasty. Clin Orthop 242:241, 1989.
269. Whittle MW, Jefferson RJ: Functional biomechanical assessment of the Oxford meniscal knee. J Arthroplasty 4:231, 1989.
270. Williams EA, Hargadon EJ, Davies DRA: Late failure of the Manchester prosthesis: Its relationship to the disease process. J Bone Joint Surg Br 61:451, 1979.
271. Williams RJ III, Westrich GH, Siegel J, et al: Arthroscopic release of the posterior cruciate ligament for stiff total knee arthroplasty. Clin Orthop 331:185, 1996.
272. Wilson FC, Fajgenbaum DM, Venters GC: Results of knee replacement with the Walldius and geometric prostheses: A comparative study. J Bone Joint Surg Am 62:497, 1980.
273. Wilson SA, McCann PD, Gotlin RS, et al: Comprehensive gait analysis in posterior-stabilized knee arthroplasty. J Arthroplasty 11:359, 1996.
274. Wright RJ, Lima J, Scott RD, et al: Two- to four-year results of posterior cruciate–sparing condylar total knee arthroplasty with an uncemented femoral component. Clin Orthop 260:80, 1990.

275. Wright TM, Astion DJ, Bansal M, et al: Failure of carbon fiber–reinforced polyethylene total knee–replacement components. J Bone Joint Surg Am 70:926, 1988.

276. Wright TM, Bartel DL: The problem of surface damage in polyethylene total knee components. Clin Orthop 205:67, 1986.

277. Yamamoto S, Nakata S, Kondoh Y: A follow-up study of an uncemented knee replacement: The results of 312 knees using the Kodama-Yamamoto prosthesis. J Bone Joint Surg Br 71:505, 1989.

278. Young HH: Use of a hinged Vitallium prosthesis (Young type) for arthroplasty of the knee. J Bone Joint Surg Am 53:1658, 1971.

CHAPTER 80

Unicompartmental Total Knee Arthroplasty

Wolfgang Fitz • Richard D. Scott

Despite more than 2 decades of controversy, the status of unicompartmental knee arthroplasty (UKA) remains uncertain. In the beginning of the 1970s several authors reported early discouraging results with unicondylar arthroplasty and questioned its role except perhaps for lateral compartmental disease.[18,26] During the next 10 years, more favorable results began appearing,[1,29,47] largely as a result of refined surgical technique and narrowing of patient selection to candidates better suited for the procedure.

The concept of unicompartmental total knee replacement is attractive as an alternative to tibial osteotomy or tricompartmental replacement in an osteoarthritic patient with unicompartmental disease confirmed at arthrotomy.[14,24,53] When compared with osteotomy, UKA has a higher initial success rate and fewer early complications.[19,47] Any internal derangement can be relieved at the time of arthrotomy. Intra-articular débridement can lead to improvement in range of motion. Patients with bilateral disease can have both knees operated on during the same anesthetic, with full recovery within 3 months of surgery. Osteotomies in the same patient are often spaced 3 to 6 months apart, and as much as a year may be required to achieve full recovery from the time of the initial procedure.

With the introduction of minimally invasive techniques by Repicci and Eberle,[39] UKA has experienced an enormous surge of interest in the last several years with clear advantages of this technique: less blood loss, less pain, and quicker recovery. Price et al,[36] for example, compared 40 minimally invasive with 20 traditional open UKA procedures and looked at clinical parameters to document the benefit of minimally invasive techniques. The mean number of days until patients were able to perform an active straight-leg raise after surgery was 1.2 for minimally invasive surgery versus 2.1 days for open UKA (range, 1 to 3 and 0 to 4). Patients were able to bend more than 70 degrees at 2.2 versus 4.4 days (range, 2 to 8 and 0 to 40), and independence on stairs was achieved at 4.2 versus 7.3 (range, 2 to 6 and 5 to 13) days. One concern with minimally invasive techniques is that improper exposure may compromise component positioning. The literature is somewhat controversial, and no prospective randomized studies are available. Whereas Price et al,[36] Keys, and Mueller et al[31] showed comparable radiographic component positioning, Fisher noted a significant tendency with minimally invasive techniques to put the tibial component in more varus. In 88 consecutive minimally invasive UKA procedures, the tibial component was an average of 5.4 degrees in varus, significantly greater than with the open technique, which had an average of 4.1 degrees. Computer-assisted surgery has been proved in a prospective study comparing 20 minimally invasive UKAs with the conventional minimally invasive technique to be superior as a result of navigation. Ninety-five percent of UKAs were within 4 degrees as compared with 70% in the traditional group. Surgery took an average of 19 minutes longer.[35]

In a flat-on-flat total knee replacement (TKR) design, peak stress increases beyond the yield strength of polyethylene in neutral alignment to 3 degrees of varus. Komistek and Dennis measured up to 38 MPa of stress in the same design, which should apply to stress in UKA and thus emphasizes the importance of component positioning.[22] The influence of component malpositioning is well documented in TKR survivorship.

Prospective randomized studies have documented the benefit of computer-assisted surgery in significantly improving component positioning in TKR. In one such study using computed tomography to assess component positioning, all seven measured positions were significantly better in the computer-guided group. The same applies for minimally invasive UKA.[35]

When compared with tricompartmental arthroplasty, unicompartmental replacement has the advantage of preserving both cruciate ligaments, thereby yielding a knee with nearly normal kinematics.[24,41,53] A study of 42 patients with a bicompartmental or tricompartmental arthroplasty on one side and a unicompartmental replacement on the other showed that more patients preferred the unicompartmental side because it felt more like a normal knee and had better function.[10,33]

Another potential advantage over tricompartmental replacement is preservation of bone stock in the patellofemoral joint and opposite compartment. Theoretically, this should make revision easier to perform should it become necessary.

This advantage, however, has not been supported by several studies of revision of unicompartmental replacements.[2,25,34] The results of revision were not superior to those after revision of bicompartmental or tricompartmental replacement, and the bone stock deficiency in the femoral condyle or tibial plateau often had to be augmented with bone graft or special components. These deficiencies are frequently the result of poor surgical technique or prostheses that invade the bone stock unnecessarily. More modern techniques using surface replacements on the femoral and tibial sides have made the procedure as conservative in practice as it is in theory. Today, there are more systems available in which the tibia is cut first with the use of extramedullary alignment guides. Femoral component positioning is then based on the tibial cut without intramedullary femoral guidance. The thromboembolic potential from intramedullary guidance is thus eliminated.

Survivorship analysis for tricompartmental replacement has indicated that with or without cruciate retention, survivorship can be above 90% after 10 years of follow-up.[37,38,43,48] Survivorship studies generated from early unicompartmental series show that survivorship is not as good at 10 years, with a decline into the 85% range.[5,16,29,45,51,52] These series were generated, however, at a time when patient selection was still evolving and surgical techniques were not yet perfected. Later reports may show better survivorship into the second decade.[8]

PATIENT SELECTION

Osteotomy remains the procedure of choice in a young, active male patient with unicompartmental osteoarthritis.

Pain during rest and poor range of motion are relative contraindications to osteotomy. Internal derangement is not a contraindication to osteotomy but should be relieved by an arthroscopic procedure before or after the osteotomy. Subluxation and extreme angular deformity are contraindications to both osteotomy and unicompartmental replacement. Metallic interpositional arthroplasty may occasionally be advisable when osteotomy is contraindicated and the patient is considered too young or too heavy to be a candidate for total knee arthroplasty (Fig. 80–1).[11,15,46] Until recently, the ideal candidate for unicompartmental replacement was an osteoarthritic patient with a physiological age older than 60 and a sedentary lifestyle.[24,50] With studies showing the survivorship of tricompartmental arthroplasty to be superior to that of unicompartmental arthroplasty after the first decade, the selection process must be reconsidered. Patients in their 60s and 70s would seem to have a greater chance of living out their life without a revision if they undergo a tricompartmental procedure. Unicompartmental replacement now might assume its role in two groups of patients. One group consists of middle-aged osteoarthritic patients (especially women undergoing a "first arthroplasty"). Advantages include a reliable initial result, anatomic

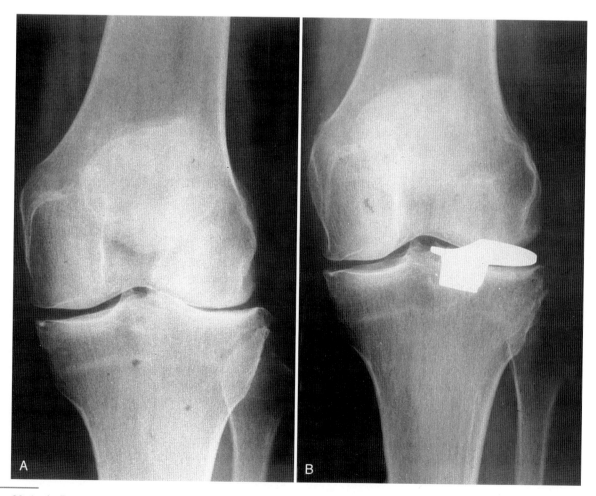

Figure 80–1. **A,** Preoperative anteroposterior (AP) radiograph of a 50-year-old ski instructor with advanced lateral compartmental osteoarthritis and early medial changes. **B,** AP radiograph 8 years after McKeever hemiarthroplasty. The patient returned to downhill skiing.

realignment (versus osteotomy with clinical valgus, which can be cosmetically objectionable), retention of both cruciate ligaments for higher performance, and easy salvage. A published report of early results in middle-aged patients supported this concept but recommended caution in heavy, active middle-aged men.[42]

Body weight remains a controversial issue and a relative contraindication. Studies published in recent years may suggest obesity to be less a contraindication than 15 years ago.[2,52] Using body mass index as a variable, Murray et al did not find any relationship between body mass index and the final result in their 10-year follow up.[32] Ridgeway et al[40] found no correlation between weight and outcome at a minimum 5-year follow-up. The second group of potential candidates consists osteoarthritic octogenarians undergoing their "first and last" arthroplasty. Advantages include faster surgery, faster recovery, less blood loss, less energy consumption, and a less expensive prosthesis. Modification of the surgical technique to avoid intramedullary guidance may further reduce perioperative morbidity and mortality. In a prospective study comparing computer-guided TKR with and without intramedullary guidance, a significant reduction in postoperative confusional state was observed in patients who underwent TKR without intramedullary guidance.[9] An unpublished series of 42 octogenarians from our clinic shows that at 5 to 10 years after surgery, the prostheses survived the patient in all but 1 case.

Once arthroplasty has been chosen over osteotomy, the final decision between unicompartmental replacement versus bicompartmental or tricompartmental replacement is made at arthrotomy.[24,47,53] Although the patient may be an ideal candidate for unicompartmental arthroplasty, as indicated by clinical examination and radiography, several contraindications to the procedure may be discovered at the time of arthrotomy. We consider an absent anterior cruciate ligament (ACL) to be a significant (though not absolute) contraindication to unicompartmental replacement because it is usually accompanied by ligamentous laxity, which can promote eventual lateral subluxation of the tibia on the femur and secondary opposite-compartment disease. Inspection of the opposite compartment and patellofemoral joint may show significant degenerative changes that make unicompartmental arthroplasty inadvisable.

In varus knees there are two typical findings. First, impingement of osteophytes anterior to the insertion of the ACL can cause erosion of the lateral condyle close to the notch, which is called a kissing lesion. Second, changes in the medial trochlea or medial patella facet are seen and can be accepted as long as it is not bare bone because correction of the varus deformity will unload this area.

Mild chondromalacia in the opposite compartment can be accepted, but areas of eburnated bone are definite contraindications. In a varus osteoarthritic knee with medial compartment arthritis, a secondary lesion appears on the medial aspect of the lateral femoral condyle with early lateral subluxation. This lesion is usually accompanied by intercondylar osteophyte formation (Fig. 80–2). If the subluxation is slight and the lesion small, it can be débrided and corrected by unicompartmental arthroplasty.

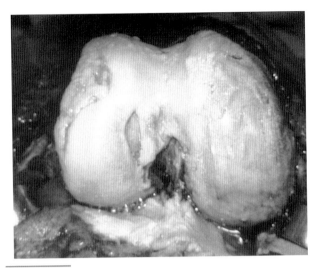

Figure 80–2. Erosion of the medial aspect of the lateral femoral condyle secondary to tibial spine impingement.

If the subluxation is great and the lesion large, bicompartmental or tricompartmental arthroplasty is advisable.

Eburnated bone in the patellofemoral compartment is also a contraindication to unicompartmental arthroplasty. Some surgeons, however, will accept patellofemoral degeneration, including areas of eburnated bone, and still proceed with unicompartmental arthroplasty. We will accept significant chondromalacia but not usually eburnated bone.

A third contraindication discovered at arthrotomy consists of a significant inflammatory component in the patient's disease. It may be in the form of a very strong synovial reaction or the discovery of diffuse crystal deposits from either gout or pseudogout. Inflammatory disease in any form substantially increases the risk for secondary degeneration of the opposite compartment in subsequent years. Crystal deposition as seen in pseudogout is considered a relative contraindication.[9]

IMPLANT DESIGN

Over the past 2 decades many lessons have been learned concerning the ideal design features of unicompartmental arthroplasty. Many early femoral components were narrow in their mediolateral dimension and suffered a high incidence of subsidence of the component into condylar bone.[44,47] The ideal component should be wide enough to maximally cap the resurfaced condyle and widely distribute the weightbearing force and, therefore, decrease the chance of subsidence and loosening. For this reason, multiple sizes should be available to accommodate both small and large patients. Revision studies have shown the inadvisability of deeply invading the condyle with fixation methods.[2,25,34] Relatively small fixation lugs appear to be sufficient as long as there are two lugs to gain rotational fixation to the bone or some sort of fin provided for this purpose. The posterior metallic condyle should fully cap the posterior condyle of the patient to allow physiological range of motion without impingement. The amount of

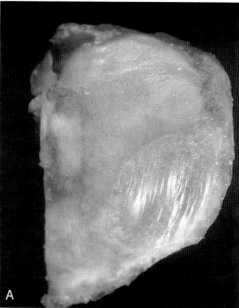
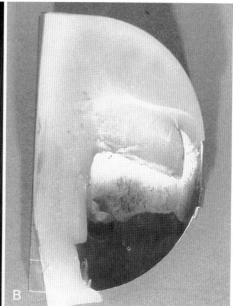

Figure 80–3. **A,** Typical anterior and peripheral wear pattern in medial osteoarthritis. **B,** Worn medial metal-backed tibial component showing an anterior and peripheral wear pattern.

bone resection required for insertion should be minimal. Preferably, the femoral component should be supported on top of the distal subchondral bone without any resection, but this requires sacrifice of more bone from the tibial side. The ideal compromise is to resect 4 to 6 mm of distal condyle while still preserving adequate distal femoral bone to allow easy conversion to a TKR. At the same time, such distal femoral resection preserves an equivalent amount of proximal tibial bone.

The coronal articulating topography of the prosthetic components also calls for a compromise. A flat surface on the femoral component articulating with a flat surface on the tibial component may potentially improve metal-to-plastic contact, but is difficult to technically line up precisely enough to avoid edge contact throughout the range of motion. An articulating surface with a small radius of curvature articulating on the tibial side with a flat surface creates too much point contact. A femoral surface with a small radius of curvature matched to a similarly small radius on the tibial side can create too much constraint. The ideal surfaces of both components are therefore probably those with a relatively large radius of curvature that allows adequate metal-to-plastic contact without excessive constraint.

In the sagittal plane, conformity might at first seem attractive to increase contact area and lower the stress that causes polyethylene wear. Worn unicompartmental tibial component retrievals have yielded important information regarding wear patterns and their implications on prosthetic design (Fig. 80–3). It appears that the polyethylene wear pattern tends to reproduce the preoperative wear pattern of the osteoarthritic knee.[30] As noted by White and associates,[54] the wear pattern tends to be anterior and peripheral on the medial tibial plateau in a varus knee. If a fixed-bearing unicompartmental knee is too conforming, a higher incidence of component loosening is reported.[17,42]

A mobile- or meniscal-bearing articulation is an attractive way to maximize contact area and decrease contact stress while avoiding excessive constraint.[12,13] This technique, however, usually requires slightly more tibial resection to accommodate the thinnest bearing and runs the slight additional risk of bearing subluxation.

The shape of the tibial component as it sits on the tibial plateau should probably be anatomic. Such shape will maximize contact between the prosthesis and bone and widely distribute the weightbearing force to resist subsidence and loosening. It will also provide maximum plastic for an anterior and peripheral wear pattern. This will necessitate an asymmetric shape with right and left components (Fig. 80–4). As is necessary on the femoral side, multiple sizes will be required on the tibial side to accommodate both small and large patients.

Metal backing of the tibial component is controversial. It was initiated in the early 1980s in order to distribute

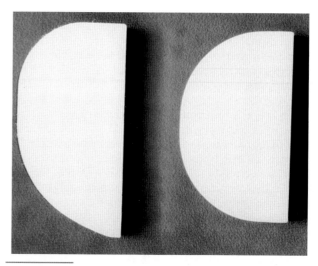

Figure 80–4. Comparison of anatomic symmetric and asymmetric tibial components.

the weightbearing force more uniformly on the cut surface of the plateau. Early results with metal-backed components were superior to those with all-polyethylene components, but possibly because of improved patient selection and operative technique rather than the use of metal backing.[23] When metal-backed components were monitored for more than 5 years, failures were seen in 6-mm components because of wear-through of the polyethylene to the metal backing. The wear-through resulted when there were areas of polyethylene less than 4 mm thick and design flaws in the method of fixation of the polyethylene to metal. These problems were similar to those seen with metal-backed patellar components.[3,28] Depending on the type of metal used (titanium versus chrome cobalt), the minimal composite thickness of a metal-backed tibial component must be 8 to 10 mm. This necessity makes metal backing less attractive than previously thought, and there appears to be a trend back to all-polyethylene tibial components.

A vertical skin incision starts at the top of the patella along the medial edge of the patellar tendon and ends distally just medial to the tibial tubercle and just below the joint line. A medial parapatellar capsulotomy is performed. After adequate exposure has been achieved, the three compartments of the knee are carefully inspected. When the ACL is sufficient, we typically see a wear pattern on the medial anterior and middle third of the tibia. If bare bone is exposed in the posterior third of the tibia, ACL insufficiency is suspected and the procedure changed to TKR. Unicompartmental arthroplasty is absolutely contraindicated if there is an inflammatory synovitis or relatively contraindicated if there are crystalline deposits of calcium pyrophosphate. The cartilage in the opposite compartment should appear to be healthy. Chondromalacia in the patellofemoral compartment is not a contraindication to unicompartmental arthroplasty, but eburnated bone on the patella or trochlea probably mandates tricompartmental replacement, especially eburnated bone on the contralateral side.

The knee is bent to 90 degrees of flexion and then a bent Hohman or Z-retractor is positioned lateral to the ACL and the patella pushed to the contralateral side. For a lateral UKA, the arthrotomy is accordingly performed along the lateral edge of the patellar tendon.

For medial compartmental arthroplasty, the coronary ligament is incised at the anterior horn of the medial meniscus, and a periosteal sleeve is elevated from the anteromedial aspect of the tibia with an osteotome (Fig. 80–5).

For lateral compartmental replacement, the coronary ligament is left intact medially while avoiding derangement of the anterior horn of the medial meniscus. The ligament is incised lateral to the midline, and a periosteal sleeve is elevated from the anterolateral aspect of the tibia as far as Gerdy's tubercle. Alternatively, some surgeons recommend a lateral parapatellar incision for a valgus deformity and lateral compartment arthroplasty.[20] This will provide excellent exposure of the lateral compartment but may make TKR more difficult if deemed necessary and the surgeon is not familiar with the lateral approach. Magnetic resonance imaging or arthroscopy is recommended preoperatively to detect possible meniscal pathology in the

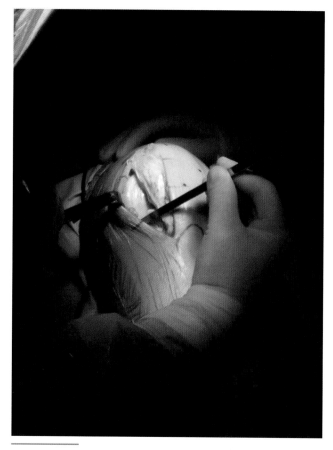

Figure 80–5. A periosteal sleeve is elevated from the anteromedial aspect of the tibia with a curved osteotome.

medial tibiofemoral joint because a minimally invasive lateral approach will not provide sufficient exposure of the medial aspect of the joint.

After adequate exposure has been achieved, the three compartments of the knee are carefully inspected and a decision made concerning the number of compartments that need replacement.

INTERCONDYLAR OSTEOPHYTES

As osteoarthritis of the medial compartment progresses, there is usually a tendency for lateral subluxation of the tibia on the femur during weightbearing. As a result, the lateral tibial spine impinges on the medial aspect of the lateral femoral condyle, and "kissing" osteophytes develop, accompanied by erosion of the medial aspect of the lateral femoral condyle (see Fig. 80–2). If these osteophytes are not removed, intercondylar impingement can persist after unicompartmental arthroplasty and result in pain while weightbearing. If the kissing lesion is large, tricompartmental arthroplasty may be necessary.

As lateral compartment osteoarthritis progresses, lateral subluxation of the tibia on the femur does usually not occur until the deformity is so severe that unicompartmental arthroplasty is not appropriate. The medial collateral ligament and medial capsule gradually elongate as the

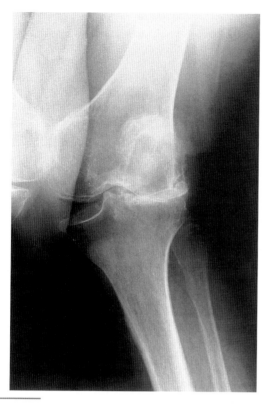

Figure 80–6. Lateral unicompartmental osteoarthritis with significant laxity of the medial collateral ligament.

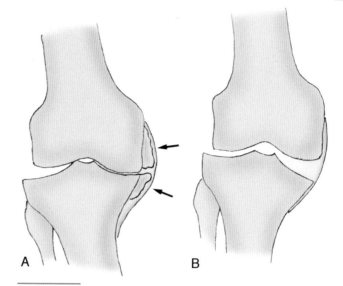

Figure 80–7. **A,** Diagram showing how medial osteophytes on the femur and tibia tent up the medial collateral ligament and capsule. **B,** After removal of the osteophytes, the varus deformity can be corrected.

valgus deformity progresses (Fig. 80–6). With significant medial laxity, the knee can no longer be stabilized by unicompartmental arthroplasty, and bicompartmental arthroplasty accompanied by lateral release is necessary.

PERIPHERAL OSTEOPHYTES

In an osteoarthritic knee with a varus deformity, peripheral osteophytes build up on the periphery of the medial femoral condyle and medial plateau of the tibia. The medial collateral ligament and capsule may be tented over these osteophytes, thereby resulting in relative shortening of these structures, which prevents passive correction of a varus deformity. When the osteophytes are removed, the resultant relative lengthening of the medial collateral ligament and capsule allows passive correction of the varus deformity (Fig. 80–7). A formal medial ligament release is rarely necessary because such a need would imply that there is a varus deformity too great for unicompartmental arthroplasty.

Balancing the Flexion Gap

The extramedullary tibial alignment guide is attached to the tibia with one proximal or two pins. The two pins are placed lateral to the sagittal cut to avoid stress risers, which have been reported to be a potential cause of stress

fractures.[7] A stylus is used to resect 2 to 4 mm off the deepest defect of the tibia. This provides a minimal resection of approximately 1 to 2 mm on the very medial edge of the tibia. The authors prefer minimal tibial resection to preserve as much bone as possible and use the thinnest tibial implant available. This all-polyethylene tibial component has a thickness of 7 mm. To avoid undermining the ACL insertion, the sagittal tibial cut is done first, with the saw blade left in situ just 1 mm below the cutting surface (Fig. 80–8). The blade should be about 2 mm lateral to the lateral edge of the medial condyle and exactly in the middle of the ascending portion of the medial spine. Most of the time the direction of the sagittal cut is determined by the condyle itself or by orienting the saw blade parallel to the wear pattern of the tibia. A Z-retractor is positioned medially along the joint line to protect the medial collateral ligament. The natural slope is restored, but a posterior slope greater than 7 degrees is not recommended. The cut is completed and the resected surface of the tibia removed and compared with tibial trial components for determination of size.

At this point, flexion gap balancing is performed by sliding a spacer block representing the thickness of the tibial component (e.g., 7 mm) between the tibial surface and the posterior condyle (Fig. 80–9). Alternatively, the extension gap can be balanced first (see the next section).

To balance the flexion gap, the weight of the thigh has to be taken out of the equation by lifting the thigh with one arm. The block should slide backward with mild resistance. In most cases the flexion gap is too tight. The authors do not recommend that the tibia be recut to increase the slope, but instead, as a first step cartilage should be removed from the posterior condyle with a pituitary. If this is not enough, a thin wafer can be taken off the posterior condyle with the saw until proper tensioning of the flexion gap is achieved.

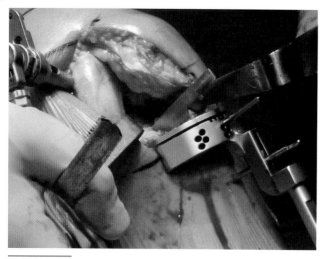

Figure 80–8. A bent Hohman retractor is placed lateral to the anterior cruciate ligament (ACL) to push the patella aside. The medial collateral ligament is protected with a Z-retractor. To avoid stress risers through drill holes underneath the tibial component, the alignment guide is pinned by placing both pins lateral to the sagittal tibial cut. Alternatively, only the proximal pin can be used. The reciprocating saw blade is left in situ 1 or 2 mm below the horizontal cutting level to protect the insertion of the ACL from the horizontal oscillating saw.

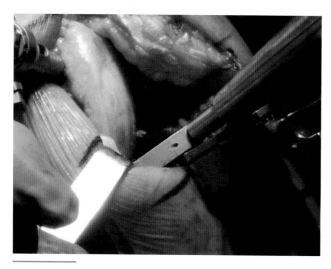

Figure 80–9. A spacer block representing the thickness of the tibial component is pushed underneath the posterior condyle until proper tensioning is achieved. For a tight flexion gap, the first step is to remove residual cartilage off the posterior condyle. Such removal enlarges the flexion gap by about 1 to 2 mm. If needed, a thin bone wafer can be taken off the posterior condyle. With conservative tibial bone resection, very rarely the flexion gap is too loose. If so, the thickness of the tibial component is increased until the flexion gap is balanced. Alternatively, the knee is first balanced in extension. If the spacer block is too loose, the distal femoral cut is distalized.

In rare instances the flexion gap is too loose. If this occurs, take the next thicker tibial spacer block (e.g., 9.5 mm) and repeat this step.

For a lateral UKA the same principles apply with some modifications. The most important principle is that there is more play in the lateral compartment. Conservative tibial resection is recommended. Balancing is similar to that for a medial UKA, but looser; play of 2 to 3 mm instead of 1 to 2 mm (medial UKA) is suggested.

Balancing the Extension Gap

With the tibial trial left in place, the knee is extended and valgus stress applied. An opening of 1 mm under stress is recommended. In most cases, the extension gap is too loose. By using shims in 1-mm increments between the distal end of the femur and the distal femoral cutting block, less distal femur is resected and the extension gap tightened. The second important step is rotation of the femoral component. The femoral prosthesis should be only slightly externally rotated. To assess the amount of external rotation, the knee is extended from 90 degrees in small increments and the center of the tibial trial is marked with a Bovie on the femoral condyle in different positions (90, 60, 30, 0 degrees) (Fig. 80–10). Then, with the knee in extension, the center of the tibial trial is marked anterior to the linea terminalis. This point represents the tip of the femoral component. External rotation of more than 5 degrees is not recommended so that the possibility of edge loading is minimized.

It is also important to calculate the amount of slope into the extension gap assessment to avoid hyperextension.

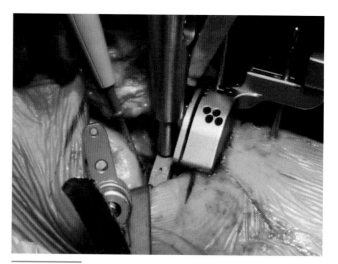

Figure 80–10. Alignment of the femoral and tibial components is achieved by placing the center of the femoral component in the center of the tibial tray. The center of the tibial tray (black line) is marked on the femoral condyle (electrocautery) in extension, the knee is slowly flexed, and every 30 to 40 degrees a Bowie mark is left on the condyle. This provides good assessment of femorotibial mismatch. If necessary, the tibial component can be rotated more externally or internally.

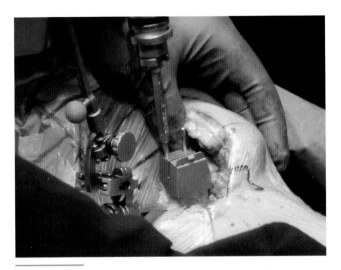

Figure 80–11. The tibial spacer block is used to balance the extension gap. In extension, the distal femoral cutting block is pinned with two short pins, after the gap is balanced. If the extension gap is too loose, shims in 1-mm increments can be placed on top of the cutting block to move the distal femoral cut more distally.

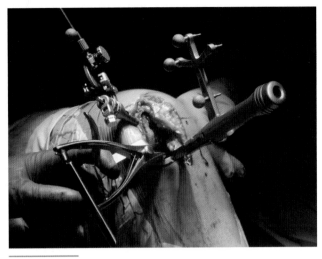

Figure 80–12. The tibial tray preparation is completed by using a laminar spreader for fixation to the tibial cutting surface instead of additional drill holes. The keel is prepared with a 4-mm drill or mill, with a 5-mm bone bridge preserved anterior to the posterior cortex.

For example, for a 5-degree slope the knee should be held in 5 degrees of flexion to fix the distal femoral cutting block. If the distal femoral cutting block is pinned in full extension, the knee will hyperextend 5 degrees, as determined by the tibial slope (Fig. 80–11).

The cutting block is also moved laterally with about 1 to 2 mm of uncovered bone left medially. In principle, for medial UKA the femoral component is shifted laterally. For lateral UKA the femoral component is not shifted medially, but the tibial component is translated medially with 2 to 3 mm of resected tibia laterally left uncovered.

Final Tibial Preparation

The tibial component should cover the tibial cutting surface without medial or posterior overhang. The authors prefer a laminar spreader to position the tibial template onto the tibial cutting surface instead of additional pin holes (Fig. 80–12) before preparing the tibial keel with a 4-mm bur or drill. It is recommended that a 5-mm bone bridge be preserved anterior to the posterior cortex.

FEMORAL COMPONENT

Placement

The femoral component should be placed in the center of the mediolateral dimension of the femoral condyle, measured after removal of peripheral and intercondylar osteophytes. If the femoral component is placed laterally in a medial compartmental arthroplasty (too close to the intercondylar notch), the procedure may fail. Failure mecha-

nisms include the absence of mediolateral constraint of the tibial component, which can lead to impingement of the femoral component on the medial tibial spine. If, however, a laterally placed femoral component is mated to a medial tibial component with intercondylar constraint, the tibia will move laterally on the femur when the components are seated and the lateral tibial spine will impinge on the lateral femoral condyle.

The femoral component should extend far enough anteriorly to cover the weightbearing surface that comes in contact with the tibia in full extension. The anterior extent of the weightbearing surface is usually well defined by the junction between the eburnated bone of the femoral condyle and the intact cartilage remaining in the trochlear groove. The leading edge of the femoral component must be countersunk into this junction to prevent patellar impingement during flexion of the knee.

The same principles apply to placement of a femoral component onto the lateral femoral condyle. On the lateral condyle the patella is more vulnerable to impingement on the leading edge of the femoral component. This problem can be avoided by undersizing the femoral component.

Size

The size of the femoral component should accurately reproduce the anteroposterior dimension of the femoral condyle. In borderline cases, the larger size should always be inserted first to conserve bone. The posterior condylar bone should be resected to at least the thickness of the metallic implant. It is better to resect slightly too much of the posterior condyle than too little to avoid making the components too tight in flexion.

TIBIAL COMPONENT

Placement

The tibial component should be positioned on the tibia so that with the knee correctly aligned, this component is directly under the femoral component in the mediolateral dimension and the articulating surfaces of the two components are rotationally congruent during weightbearing (Fig. 80–13). The congruency of components should be determined with the knee in full extension. It should not be judged while the knee is flexed and the patella is everted because in this position the displaced quadriceps mechanism artificially externally rotates and laterally subluxates the tibia on the femur. If there is a preoperative quadriceps contracture, the force of the displaced quadriceps is even greater. After placement of the tibial component, proper congruency in the frontal plane should be judged by observing tracking of the components as the knee is flexed and extended with the patella located in the trochlear groove. Viewed from the front, the line of resection of the tibial plateau should be within 4 degrees of a right angle to the longitudinal axis of the tibia. Computer guidance will facilitate alignment to within ±1 degree. Viewed from the side, the line of resection varies from 0 to 10 degrees of posterior slope, depending on the individual case; 3 to 5 degrees of posterior slope is usually appropriate, and a slope of more than 7 degrees should be avoided.

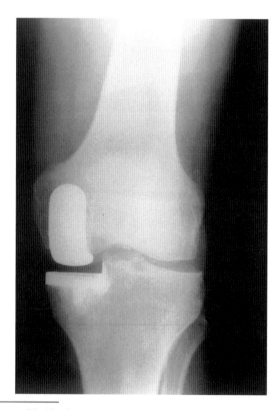

Figure 80–13. Anteroposterior radiograph showing well-positioned components after medial unicompartmental arthroplasty.

Size

Ideally, the proper thickness of the tibial component is the thickness necessary to restore the worn tibial plateau to its normal height after resection. In a varus knee, if the medial collateral ligament and capsule have been properly released by removal of medial osteophytes, correction of the deformity should be possible without resorting to thicker tibial components. If the articulated components are too tight, the tibia will subluxate toward the opposite compartment and produce excessive pressure there. After medial compartment replacement, the medial joint space should open up 1 or 2 mm when valgus stress is applied with the knee in full extension. The same principles apply to replacement of the lateral compartment.

The alignment goals for unicompartmental arthroplasty are different from those for osteotomy or tricompartmental replacement. The deformity should not be overcorrected as advocated for osteotomy.[21]

COMPUTER-GUIDED UNICOMPARTMENTAL KNEE ARTHROPLASTY

Optimal positioning of the tibial component in UKA is perpendicular to the mechanical axis of the tibia. Prospective randomized studies have shown that computer guidance improves component alignment in TKA and UKA.[9,35,49] The technique involves the fixation of two light-reflecting arrays. A two-pin array with two 2.3-mm Schanz screws is inserted into the distal third of the tibia (Fig. 80–14), and a 4.5-mm Schanz screw is positioned in the medial aspect of the femoral condyle; the femur and tibia are then registered. Varus or valgus malalignment can be documented preoperatively and the requested correction determined. At this point the authors prefer computer guidance for the tibial cut only. The traditional extramedullary alignment guide provides excellent ability

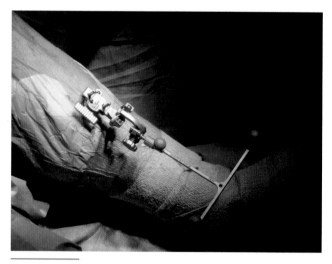

Figure 80–14. Two 2.3-mm Schanz screws are placed in the distal third of the tibia to attach the tibial array.

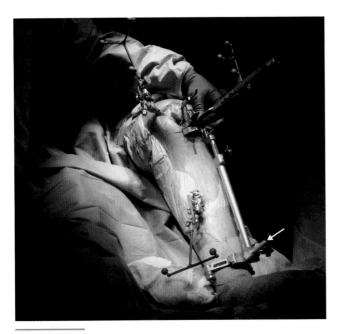

Figure 80–15. Computer-guided unicompartmental arthroplasty. After placing a two-pin array in the tibia and a 4.5-mm Schanz screw in the medial femoral condyle, registration is completed and computer assistance used for the tibial cut. The first pin is percutaneously introduced (*arrow*) about 2 mm lateral to the medial edge of the tibial tubercle. Then a stylus is used to take 2 to 4 mm off the deepest portion of the medial tibial plateau. After fine-tuning the tibial cutting block by moving it medially or laterally for varus/valgus adjustments or more anterior or posterior for a posterior slope between 3 and 7 degrees, a second pin is applied and the cut made.

to fine-tune for optimal varus and valgus alignment and posterior slope. Use of a stylus for a measured resection of the tibia helps fixate the tibial cutting block before insertion of the pins (Fig. 80–15). After the tibia is cut, the tibial cutting surface is verified, documented, and if necessary corrected (Fig. 80–16). Then the femur is prepared as described earlier. The instrumentation for the femoral condyle is slightly modified; Figures 80–16 to 80–18 show this modification. Figure 80–19 presents an example of kinematic analysis of the UKA intraoperatively with the computer. The picture shows the contact point of the round femoral condyle on the tibia. The contact point is supposed to be as close to the center in the medial lateral dimension as possible.

POSTOPERATIVE REHABILITATION

The postoperative regimen after unicompartmental arthroplasty is similar to that after bicompartmental or tricompartmental arthroplasty. It is often noted, however, that rehabilitation goals are met faster and patients suffer less postoperative pain, swelling, and blood loss[10] when minimally invasive techniques are used. After closure of the capsule, note is made of the patient's potential flexion against gravity since it is unreasonable to expect improvement in this function during the initial postoperative period. It can easily be documented with computer guidance. Our current postoperative protocol includes the use of low-dose warfarin (Coumadin) (started the night before surgery) combined with pulsatile compression stockings to minimize the chance of postoperative venous throm-

Figure 80–16. The tibial cut is documented with computer guidance. The authors recommend a deviation of not more than ±1 degree. The advantage of computer guidance is that the cut can be optimized if necessary.

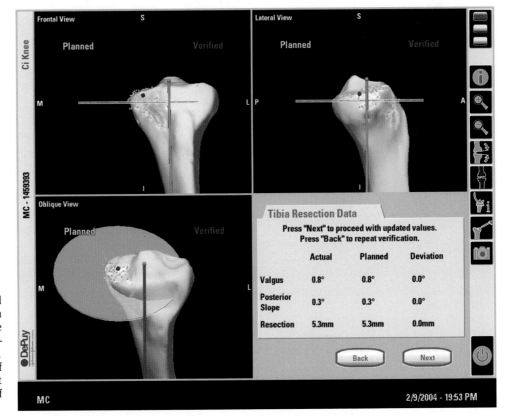

	Actual	Planned	Deviation
Valgus	0.8°	0.8°	0.0°
Posterior Slope	0.3°	0.3°	0.0°
Resection	5.3mm	5.3mm	0.0mm

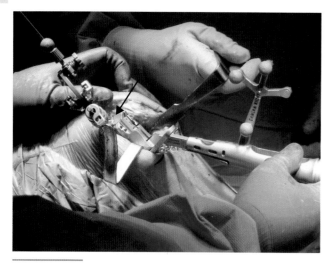

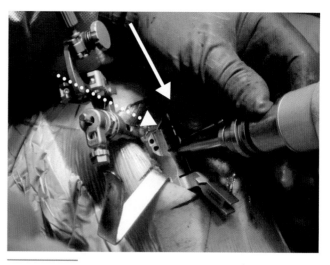

Figure 80–17. With the knee in 90 degrees of flexion the femoral cutting block is positioned on the distal femoral cutting surface by using the mark (*black arrow*) made earlier. It is translated laterally with a 1- to 2-mm uncovered rim of bone left medially, but simultaneously covering the width of the condyle. A 5-mm shim is used to push the base of the femoral cutting block against the posterior condyle.

Figure 80–18. The femoral cutting block is translated laterally until the cutting block is in line with the mark on the top of the femoral condyle (*arrow*). The waist of the cutting block determines the width of the femoral component and should be moved laterally to allow 1 to 2 mm of the medial femoral cutting surface not to be covered by the component (*dashed arrow*). All remaining preparations are completed with this one cutting block.

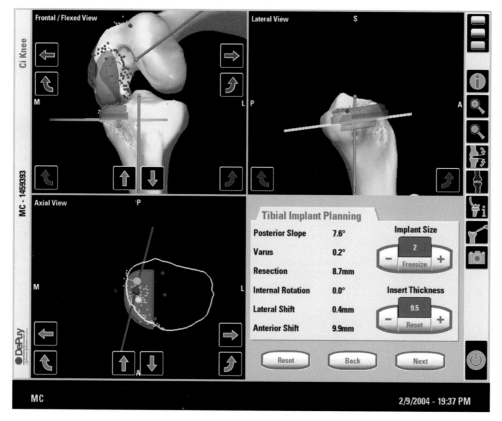

Figure 80–19. Second-generation computer guidance allows motion analysis of the trial implants: The *yellow point* represents the center of the tibial component and the *red point* the actual contact point of the femoral component in 90 degrees of flexion. We recommend that the contact point stay in the center of the tibial component.

bosis. In high-risk patients (age, obesity, cancer, family or personal history of deep venous thrombosis or pulmonary embolism, hormone replacement therapy, or birth control), low-molecular-weight heparin is initiated on postoperative day 1 and given until the international normalized ratio is therapeutic.

Continuous passive motion is begun immediately in the recovery room as tolerated. The motion machine is used during the day and a knee immobilizer may be applied at night to minimize the chance for development of a significant flexion contracture. The continuous passive motion machine is advanced as tolerated until 90 degrees is achieved and maintained. Quadriceps-setting exercises and attempts at straight-leg raising are initiated as tolerated and are achieved on postoperative day 1 or 2. The patient commences walking on the day of surgery with a walker or crutches, with weightbearing as tolerated. The patient may progress to a cane as tolerated. The limitation in progression to crutches or a cane is more a safety concern.

A knee immobilizer should be used during ambulation until the patient has a secure ability to perform straight-leg raises. Most patients walk within 1 week with a cane and discontinue the cane at 2 weeks though a cane is recommended for 2 to 4 weeks for safety.

CEMENTLESS UNICOMPARTMENTAL ARTHROPLASTY

The role of cementless unicompartmental arthroplasty is uncertain. In theory, it is appealing if it could be shown to be conservative in comparison to cemented unicompartmental arthroplasty. In practice, cementless unicompartmental arthroplasty is actually more radical than a cemented procedure. For most cementless components, more bone resection is required on the femoral side. Failure rates are reported to be higher in terms of loosening on both the femoral and tibial sides.[4] Metal-backed components are most likely required on the tibial side. Cementless unicompartmental arthroplasty must remain experimental until better methods and results are reported.

SUMMARY

Despite almost 3 decades of experience, the role of unicompartmental arthroplasty .remains controversial. It appears to offer an attractive alternative to osteotomy or tricompartmental arthroplasty in selected osteoarthritic patients. The procedure can be conservative with preservation of the cruciate ligaments along with bone stock in the opposite compartment and patellofemoral joint.

With appropriate patient selection, prosthetic design, and operative technique, a unicompartmental replacement can function as the initial conservative replacement in middle-aged osteoarthritic patients, especially women. It may also be appropriate in an elderly patient with a life expectancy of less than 10 years. Osteotomy should still be considered in young, active individuals, especially males.

References

1. Bae KK, Guhl JF, Keane SP: Unicompartmental knee arthroplasty for single compartment disease. Clin Orthop 176:235, 1983.
2. Barrett WH, Scott RD: Revision of failed unicondylar arthroplasty. J Bone Joint Surg Am 69:1328, 1987.
3. Bayley JC, Scott RD, Ewald FC, et al: Failure of the metal-backed patellar component after total knee replacement. J Bone Joint Surg Am 70:668, 1988.
4. Bernasek TL, Rand JA, Bryan RS: Unicompartmental porous coated anatomic total knee arthroplasty. Clin Orthop 236:52, 1988.
5. Bert JM: Ten year survivorship of metal-backed unicompartmental arthroplasty. J Arthroplasty 13:901, 1998.
6. Broughton NS, Newman JH, Bailey RA: Unicompartmental replacement osteoarthritis of the knee. J Bone Joint Surg Br 68:447, 1986.
7. Brumby SA, Carrington R, Zayontz S, et al: Tibial plateau stress fracture. A complication of unicompartmental knee arthroplasty using 4 guide pinholes. J Arthroplasty 18:809, 2003.
8. Cartier P, Sanouiller JL, Grelsamer RP: Unicompartmental knee arthroplasty surgery. J Arthroplasty 11:782, 1996.
9. Chauhan SK, Scott RG, Breidahl W, Beaver RJ: Computer-assisted knee arthroplasty versus a conventional jig-based technique. A randomised, prospective trial. J Bone Joint Surg Br 86:372, 2004.
10. Cobb AG, Kozinn SC, Scott RD: Unicondylar or total knee replacement: The patient's preference. J Bone Joint Surg Br 72:166, 1990.
11. Emerson RH, Potter T: The use of the metallic McKeever hemiarthroplasty for unicompartmental arthritis. J Bone Joint Surg Am 67:208, 1985.
12. Goodfellow JW, O'Connor JJ: Clinical results of the Oxford knee: Surface arthroplasty of the tibiofemoral joint with a meniscal-bearing prosthesis. Clin Orthop 205:21, 1986.
13. Goodfellow JW, Tribewal MB, Sherman KP, et al: Unicompartmental Oxford meniscal knee arthroplasty. J Arthroplasty 2:1, 1987.
14. Grelsamer RP: Unicompartmental osteoarthritis of the knee. J Bone Joint Surg Am 77:278, 1995.
15. Hallock RH, Fell BM: Unicompartmental tibial hemiarthroplasty: Early results of the UniSpacer knee. Clin Orthop 416:154, 2003.
16. Heck DA, Marmos L, Gibson A, et al: Unicompartmental knee evaluation. Clin Orthop 286:154, 1993.
17. Hodge WA, Chandler HP: Unicompartmental knee replacement: A comparison of constrained and unconstrained designs. J Bone Joint Surg Am 74:877, 1992.
18. Insall JN, Walker PS: Unicondylar knee replacement. Clin Orthop 120:83, 1976.
19. Jackson M, Sarongi PP, Newman JH: Revision total knee arthroplasty: Comparison of outcome following primary proximal tibial osteotomy or unicompartmental arthroplasty. J Arthroplasty 9:539, 1994.
20. Keblish PA: Valgus deformity in total knee replacement: The lateral retinacular approach. Orthop Trans 9:28, 1985.
21. Kennedy W, White R: Unicompartmental total knee arthroplasty of the knee: Postoperative alignment and its influence on overall results. Clin Orthop 321:278, 1997.
22. Komistek RD, Dennis DA: Contact stresses vs. implant conformity in TKA. Internal Report: Rocky Mountain Musculoskeletal Research Laboratory, Denver, 1996.
23. Kozinn SC, Marx C, Scott RD: Unicompartmental knee arthroplasty. J Arthroplasty 4:1, 1989.
24. Kozinn SC, Scott RD: Current concepts review: Unicompartmental total arthroplasty. J Bone Joint Surg Am 71:145, 1989.
25. Lai, Rand JA: Revision of failed unicompartmental total knee arthroplasty. Clin Orthop 287:193, 1993.
26. Laskin RS: Unicompartmental tibiofemoral resurfacing arthroplasty. J Bone Joint Surg Am 60:182, 1978.
27. Levine WN, Ozuna RM, Scott RD, et al: Conversion of failed modern unicompartmental arthroplasty to total knee arthroplasty. J Arthroplasty 11:797, 1996.
28. Lombardi AV Jr, Engh GA, Volz RG, et al: Fracture/dissociation of the polyethylene in metal-backed patellar components in total knee arthroplasty. J Bone Joint Surg Am 70:675, 1988.
29. Marmor L: Unicompartmental knee arthroplasty: Ten to thirteen year follow-up study. Clin Orthop 226:24, 1987.
30. McCallum JD, Scott RD: Duplication of medial erosion in unicompartmental knee arthroplasties. J Bone Joint Surg Br 77:726, 1995.
31. Muller PE, Pellengahr C, Witt M, et al: Influence of minimally invasive surgery on implant positioning and the functional outcome for medial unicompartmental knee arthroplasty. J Arthroplasty 19:296, 2004.
32. Murray DW, Goodfellow JW, O'Connor JJ: The Oxford medial unicompartmental arthroplasty: A ten-year survival study. J Bone Joint Surg Br 80:983, 1998.
33. Newman JH, Ackroyd CE, Shah NA: Unicompartmental or total knee replacement? Five-year results of a prospective randomized trial of 102 osteoarthritic knees with unicompartmental arthritis. J Bone Joint Surg Br 80:862, 1998.

34. Padgett DE, Stern SH, Insall JN: Revision total knee arthroplasty for failed unicompartmental replacement. J Bone Joint Surg Am 73:186, 1991.

35. Perlick L, Bathis H, Tingart M, et al: Minimally invasive unicompartmental knee replacement with a nonimage-based navigation system. Int Orthop 28:19, 2004.

36. Price AJ, Webb J, Topf H, et al: Rapid recovery after Oxford unicompartmental arthroplasty through a short incision. J Arthroplasty 16:970, 2001.

37. Ranawat CS, Oheneba BA: Survivorship analysis and results of total condylar knee arthroplasty. Clin Orthop 226:6, 1988.

38. Rand JA, Illstrup DM: Survivorship analysis of total knee arthroplasty: Cumulative rates of survival of 9200 total knee arthroplasties. J Bone Joint Surg Am 73:397, 1991.

39. Repicci JA, Eberle RW: Minimally invasive surgical technique for unicondylar knee arthroplasty. J South Orthop Assoc 8:20, 1999.

40. Ridgeway SR, McAuley JP, Ammeen DJ, Engh GA: The effect of alignment of the knee on the outcome of unicompartmental knee replacement. J Bone Joint Surg Br 84:351, 2002.

41. Rougraff BT, Heck DA, Gibson AE: A comparison of tricompartmental and unicompartmental arthroplasty for the treatment of gonarthrosis. Clin Orthop 273:157, 1991.

42. Schai PA, Suh JT, Thornhill TS, et al: Unicompartmental knee arthroplasty in middle-aged patients. J Arthroplasty 13:365, 1998.

43. Schai PA, Thornhill TS, Scott RD: Total knee arthroplasty with the PFC system. J Bone Joint Surg Br 80:850, 1998.

44. Scott RD: Robert Brigham unicondylar knee surgical techniques. Tech Orthop 5:15, 1990.

45. Scott RD, Cobb AG, McQueary FG, et al: Unicompartmental knee arthroplasty: Eight- to twelve-year follow-up with survivorship analysis. Clin Orthop 271:96, 1991.

46. Scott RD, Joyce MJ, Ewald PC, et al: McKeever metallic hemi-arthroplasty of the knee in unicompartmental degenerative arthritis. J Bone Joint Surg Am 67:203, 1985.

47. Scott RD, Santore R: Unicondylar unicompartmental replacement for osteoarthritis of the knee. J Bone Joint Surg Am 63:536, 1981.

48. Scuderi GR, Insall JN, Windsor RE, et al: Survivorship of cemented knee replacement. J Bone Joint Surg Br 71:798, 1989.

49. Sparmann M, Wolke B, Czupalla H, et al: Positioning of total knee arthroplasty with and without navigation support. A prospective, randomised study. J Bone Joint Surg Br 85:830, 2003.

50. Stern SH, Becker MW, Insall JN: Unicondylar knee arthroplasty: An evaluation of selection criteria. Clin Orthop 286:143, 1993.

51. Swant M, Stulberg SD, Jiganti J, et al: The natural history of unicompartmental arthroplasty: An eight-year follow-up study with survivorship analysis. Clin Orthop 286:130, 1993.

52. Tabor OB Jr, Tabor OB: Unicompartmental arthroplasty: A long-term follow-up study. J Arthroplasty 13:373, 1998.

53. Thornhill TS, Scott RD: Unicompartmental total knee arthroplasty. Orthop Clin 20:25, 1989.

54. White SH, Ludkowski PF, Goodfellow JW: Anteromedial osteoarthritis of the knee. J Bone Joint Surg Br 73:582, 1991.

CHAPTER 81

Unicompartmental Knee Arthroplasty: A European Perspective

Jean-Noël A. Argenson

Unicompartmental knee arthroplasty (UKA) is the logical treatment option for an isolated femorotibial lesion of the knee. When the other compartments of the knee are preserved and when the cruciate ligaments are present, there is no need to perform a total knee arthroplasty (TKA). When comparing the outcomes of UKA and TKA, several studies have shown that recovery is faster after UKA, and patient satisfaction is greater because the knee feels more natural.[13,28,31,40] UKA has a specific mode of failure, however, which is progression of disease in the unreplaced compartments (Fig. 81–1). This progression might be related to surgical technique, but the most critical issue is patient selection. Improper patient selection combined with limited instrumentation and suboptimal designs may explain the less than satisfactory results originally published for UKA and the subsequent decreased interest, especially in the United States.[23,29,33] Interest in UKA has been maintained in Europe since the first experience in the 1970s, and different new designs arrived in the 1980s. Since the early 1990s, new implant designs have been introduced with reliable instrumentation, which make the procedure as reliable as TKA. With proper patient selection and a more reliable surgical technique, the 10-year results of modern UKA are now available and show survivorship greater than 90% after 10 years of follow-up.[2,8,12,38,54,55] The other potential advantage over tricompartmental replacement is the preservation of bone stock in the patellofemoral joint and opposite compartment, making revision easier to perform should it become necessary. The initial results of revision of UKA were not encouraging, requiring the use of graft or wedges, but most of the time the failed UKA corresponded to a nonconservative surgical technique.[7,28,43] More recent surface replacement designs should utilize the original conservative procedure and make the revision comparable to a primary TKA.[24,32,36]

Modern UKA is a conservative resurfacing arthroplasty of the knee that preserves the two other compartments and the cruciate mechanism, acting as a four-bar linkage guiding the femorotibial movements.[41] In vivo kinematic studies performed in patients implanted with UKA showed that femorotibial contact patterns similar to those observed for the normal knee were observed after UKA.[4] A more recent development in UKA is the possibility to perform the arthroplasty using a minimally invasive surgery (MIS) technique. The goal of MIS is to reduce the hospital stay and to accelerate the return to normal activities with appropriate knee function. The initial concept was developed using surfacing-type replacement arthroplasties requiring limited instrumentation and adequate surgical skill.[48] The technique has been popularized by the development of dedicated instrumentation using either reproducible cutting jigs or milling tools.[1,37,46] The first results are encouraging in terms of patient recovery and radiographic positioning, but adequate visualization is mandatory to avoid poor component positioning as was described in the early days of UKA, in the 1970s. New worldwide interest in UKA is due to the possibilities of fast recovery and minimal surgical morbidity permitted by MIS and improvements in UKA design allowing greater and safer motion capabilities, especially for the active patients who are candidates for UKA.

UNICOMPARTMENTAL KNEE ARTHOPLASTY: THE EUROPEAN EXPERIENCE

After the initial experience of Marmor in the United States in 1972, many variations of the Marmor Modular Knee were introduced in Europe at that time. Marmor published his own experience later, in the mid-1980s,[34] but the concept of resurfacing the tibial and the femoral side of one femorotibial compartment gained great attention in several European countries. The principles of these resurfacing systems were to minimize saw cuts by adapting the femoral component to the condyle and to use an inlay polyethylene tibial component cemented in the subchondral tibial bone, while preserving the cortical rim. The St. Georg Sled, mostly used in Northern Europe, was based on the same concept. The second generation of Marmor-like designs introduced a metal backing of the tibia, to bring modularity to the procedure and to distribute the weightbearing forces more uniformly on the cut surface of the plateau. Although the initial results seemed satisfactory in terms of more friendly surgical technique,[27] wear failure of the tibial plateau was attributed mainly to the use of 6-mm thickness polyethylene. It is now recognized that the minimum thickness should be 8 mm for flat-bearing designs. Meanwhile the Unicondylar Knee prosthesis was used in the United States and Europe[23] as an alternative to the Polycentric Knee or the Duocondylar design, resurfacing both tibofemoral compartments of the knee. This initial attempt to resurface both femorotibial compartments of the knee while preserving the cruciate ligaments represented the first form of the Oxford mobile bearing system by Goodfellow and O'Connor in 1978.[18a]

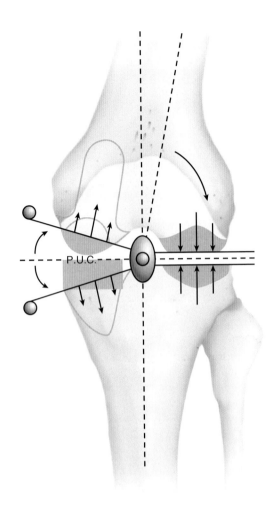

Figure 81–1. Diagram showing the mechanism of overcorrection leading to progression of osteoarthritis in the unreplaced tibiofemoral compartment after unicompartmental knee arthroplasty.

The concept was used for unicompartmental arthroplasty and is based on a fully congruent mobile articulating surface, which aims to increase the area of contact and then reduce polyethylene wear. Measurement of retrieved bearings has shown a mean linear wear rate of 0.03 mm/yr or less (0.01 mm/yr) after normal function of the knee.[1,47]

Cartier in France introduced instrumentation specifically dedicated to UKA, promoting the concept that UKA was not a half TKA, and that some type of persistent undercorrection of the deformity was suitable in opposition to the principle of TKA.[10a] The cutting jig systems brought the same type of instrumentation than that used for TKA with posterior and chamfer cuts of the femoral condyle based on intramedullary instruments. The advantage of this type of instrumentation was to provide a reproducible surgical technique, allowing the component to be placed perpendicular to the mechanical axis as previously determined on preoperative radiographs. Most of these designs have been used widely in Europe and the United States since the late 1980s, and long-term follow-

up of the Brigham, Duracon, PFC Uni, and Miller-Galante is now available through the Swedish Registry.[52] Independent publications also have reported survivorship comparable to that reported for TKA.[2,38,45] Most of this experience was realized using cemented components, which remain the standard nowadays for UKA in Europe. The first reported use of porous-coated designs was not encouraging,[9] but hydroxyapatite coating has gained some limited acceptance in some European centers.[15]

PATIENT SELECTION

The most frequent indication for UKA is osteoarthritis affecting mainly the medial femorotibial compartment. Avascular osteonecrosis is also a classic indication, despite some case of osteonecrosis progression reported in Marmor's series.[35] In my own experience, the results of UKA performed for a preoperative diagnosis of avascular osteonecrosis were satisfactory at a mean follow-up of 6 years.[2] Any type of inflammatory arthritis, such as rheumatoid arthritis, is recognized as a formal contraindication for UKA because this can be a cause of rapid degeneration of the unreplaced compartments. Mild chondrocalcinosis, which is mostly a radiographic finding, may be accepted as an indication to perform UKA, in contrast to the productive chondrocalcinosis often associated with cyclic effusion of the knee.

The clinical examination of the knee before choosing UKA as the treatment option needs to focus on range of motion, with a minimum preoperative flexion of 90 degrees required to implant the femoral component through a short incision. A femoral contracture may be improved by only a few degrees after UKA, and this should be recognized preoperatively. The clinical evaluation of the patellofemoral joint also is mandatory, to seek out any kind of anterior knee pain described by the patient during stair climbing and descending or during squatting. The stability of the joint must be evaluated carefully for the anterior cruciate ligament (ACL) by performing the anterior drawer test and for the state of the collateral ligaments. The unicompartmental implant fills the gap left by the worn cartilage, bringing the collateral ligament back to normal tension after the procedure. The clinical results of UKA using mobile meniscal or fixed bearings[14,18] and the in vivo kinematic evaluation of patients with flat fixed tibial bearings have highlighted the importance of a functional ACL for unicondylar knee replacement.[4] The clinical outcome for these sedentary patients with a probable secondary distention of the ACL confirmed that a correct clinical function of the knee may be achieved in these low-demand patients using fixed bearings, despite ACL deficiency. For these patients, I concur with the findings of Hernigou and Deschamps,[22] who studied the effect of posterior tibial slope on the outcome of UKA and recommended avoiding posterior slope superior to 7 degrees if the ACL is absent at the time of implantation. For younger patients, I have considered combined ACL/UKA surgery in a limited group of patients, with good results on stability and pain, but limited range of motion as compared with isolated UKA (Fig. 81–2).

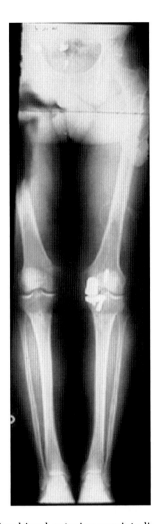

Figure 81–2. Combined anterior cruciate ligament/unicompartmental knee arthroplasty surgery performed in a 44-year-old woman working as a hospital nurse at 7 years of follow-up. The patient returned to mountain hiking.

Age and weight still represent debatable issues for the indication of UKA because the procedure often is presented as an alternative to either osteotomy or TKA.[19,57] My own experience showed that the best indication for osteotomy is a young, heavy, active man with limited unicompartmental osteoarthritis (no complete loss of joint space) and bony deformity. Compared with osteotomy, UKA has a higher initial success rate and fewer early complications.[24,59] Regarding age and based on the comparative results at 10 years of UKA and TKA, Scott and colleagues[55,56] considered that UKA now might assume a role in two groups of patients—middle-aged osteoarthritic patients (especially women undergoing a "first arthroplasty") and osteoarthritic octogenarians having their "first and last" arthroplasty. With survivorship studies of modern UKA comparable to TKA after the first decade, the selection process must be reconsidered, and patients in their 60s and 70s would seem to have a greater chance of living out their life with either a TKA or a UKA, which in any case would be easier to revise. In patients 60 years old or younger, the results of modern UKA reported by

Schai and coworkers[54] and Pennington and associates[44] are encouraging in this high-demand population. Early reports of UKA considered obesity as a relative contraindication for UKA.[7,20,27] I have not considered obesity as a contraindication, and I concur with more recent studies showing no correlation between weight and outcome.[49,58] UKA is at higher risk of failure in a heavy, active middle-aged man than in an obese, sedentary patient.

The radiographic evaluation is a critical step in patient selection for UKA. In all cases, I use a full weightbearing view of the limb in bipedal or single-leg stance. This view measures the global tibiofemoral angle and calculates the angle between femoral anatomic axis and limb mechanical axis to be reported at the time of the distal femoral cut. It also evaluates any extra-articular bony deformity that cannot be corrected by the unicompartmental implant and searches for any femoral hip stem that might require the use of a shorter intramedullary femoral rod. Kozinn and Scott[27] suggested that UKA should be limited to preoperative frontal deformity less than 15 degrees of varus/valgus, and this statement commonly has been accepted by various authors.[2,8,38,53,57,58] Most important deformities are more or less associated with ligament retraction requiring collateral ligament release, which must be avoided during UKA because of the risk of postoperative frontal femorotibial subluxation. In rare cases of deformity caused partly by extra-articular bone deviation, such as a metaphyseal varus deformity, I have considered combined or staged osteotomy/UKA surgery (Fig. 81–3).

The most important views are the stress views performed in varus (for a medial UKA) and used to confirm the indication of unicompartmental replacement with full loss of cartilage in the medial affected compartment. The stress view in valgus confirms the full thickness of cartilage in the unaffected lateral compartment and the entire correction of the deformity to neutral. In the case of absence of correction or overcorrection, this view indicates the necessity for collateral ligament balance and the use of TKA. The lateral view of the joint confirms the absence of anterior tibial translation greater than 10 mm referencing the posterior edge of the tibial plateau and shows that tibial erosion is limited to anterior and midportions of the tibial plateau.

The axial patellofemoral views confirm the appropriate cartilage thickness of the patellofemoral joint. The presence of peripatellar osteophytes may not be a contraindication for unicondylar replacement, and these osteophytes can be removed even by minimal incision. Although the status of the patellofemoral joint is not a criterion of suitability for some authors,[38,60] the full loss of patellofemoral cartilage is now, for me, a contraindication for performing unicondylar replacement.[2] The use of MRI, CT, or preoperative arthroscopy has little or no place in my practice for deciding to perform UKA. The final decision may be made in some cases at the time of surgery, however, after inspection of the opposite compartment and gentle traction on the ACL.

Laskin,[30] in analyzing 300 knees undergoing TKA and evaluating the selection criteria presented by Kozinn and Scott,[27] found that 15% of the knees were eligible for UKA at intraoperative inspection. This 15% rate of indication

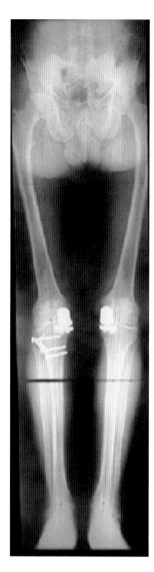

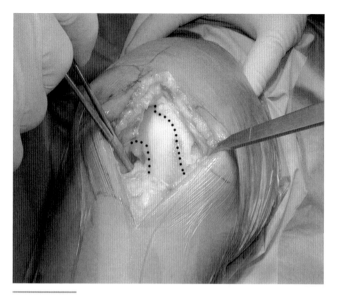

Figure 81–4. Operative view through a minimal incision shows the osteophytes to be removed and the anterior cruciate ligament with the knee at 45 degrees of flexion.

Figure 81–3. Staged opening wedge tibial osteotomy and unicompartmental knee arthroplasty performed in a 46-year-old man who had a preoperative 8-degree metaphyseal varus deformity and a global varus deformity of 16 degrees. The patient returned to horse riding competition.

for UKA corresponds to the figures currently reported in Europe, in contrast to the 6% rate of potential candidates for a UKA reported by Ritter and colleagues.[50]

SURGICAL TECHNIQUE

Approach

The MIS approach is now the technique of choice for UKA, as a result of advances in instrumentation based on a single compartment of the knee and allowing the procedure to be performed without patellar eversion and without incision in the quadriceps tendon.[1,37,46] The initial results of such a technique for UKA are promising not only

for patient recovery, but also for implant positioning.[16,37,53] The routine operating table is used with the knee flexed at 90 degrees for skin incision, the thigh tourniquet inflated, and the foot resting on the table. Frequent extension/flexion manipulations are necessary during the procedure, because some structures are preferentially visualized at either low or high degrees of flexion. The length of the skin incision varies from 6 to 8 cm, depending on skin elasticity and patient corpulence. The upper limit of the incision (for a medial UKA) is the medial pole of the patella, extending distally toward the medial side of the tibial tuberosity but ending 2 cm above the joint line previously located; this means that two-thirds of the incision should be proximal to the joint line. When the synovial cavity is opened, the part of the fat pad in the way of the condyle is excised, and a dedicated, curved, thin Homan retractor is placed on the medial side of the incision. Moving the retractors mediolaterally from one side to the other allows skin elasticity and avoids soft-tissue tension through a short incision. A medial UKA is performed through a medial parapatellar arthrotomy, and a lateral UKA is performed through a lateral capsular incision. The anterior and mid-portion of the meniscus are excised at that step; the posterior aspect is removed after the posterior femoral cut. The first step is to bring the knee at 45 degrees of flexion to evaluate the joint by checking the resistance of the ACL with an appropriate hook and evaluating the state of the other tibiofemoral joint and the patellofemoral joint. The osteophytes are removed on the peripheral side of the femoral condyle, in the intercondylar notch to avoid late impingement with the ACL, and finally around the patella and the tibial plateau (Fig. 81–4). After removing the peripheral osteophytes, there is relative lengthening of the medial collateral ligament and capsule, allowing passive correction of the deformity.

Tibial Component

In my practice, the tibial cut is always performed first for UKA and TKA, but, because the cuts are independent in the intramedullary technique, the surgeon can start with the femoral side as well. When using an extramedullary technique, the tibial cut and the distal femoral cut are linked to have them parallel to each other and perpendicular to the mechanical axis. In this technique, the deformity is corrected with the leg in extension.

The extramedullary tibial cutting guide is placed distally around the ankle with the axis of the guide lying slightly medial to the center of the ankle joint. The proximal part of the guide is translated on the anterior affected tibia (Fig. 81–5). The diaphyseal part of the guide is parallel to the anterior tibial crest, and the anteroposterior position of the guide is adjusted distally to reproduce the natural upper tibial slope, usually 5 degrees of posterior slope. The amount of resection is decided after using a palpator located on the lowest part of the medial affected

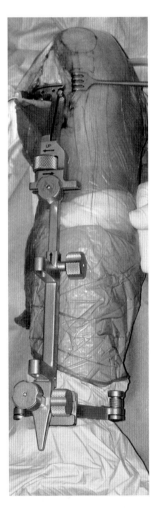

Figure 81–5. The tibial cut is realized with an extramedullary cutting guide aligned on the tibial crest in the frontal plane and with a 5-degree posterior slope in the sagittal plane. The cutting jig is fixed on the superomedial part of the tibia (for a medial unicompartmental knee arthroplasty).

plateau. The horizontal tibial resection should reproduce the height of the nonaffected lateral plateau.[11] The cut in the frontal plane is realized at a right angle to the tibial mechanical axis or within 5 degrees, according to epiphyseal deformity.[12,56] With an MIS approach, it is important to protect the medial collateral ligament while performing the horizontal tibial cut.

The sagittal tibial cut is realized most of the time as a freehand cut aligned close to the tibial spine's eminence without violating the ACL and using a reciprocating saw, the anterior starting point decided after checking the alignment of the lateral edge of the medial femoral condyle (for a medial UKA) on the tibial plateau when the knee is brought close to full extension. The ideal size for the tibial component is one that provides the best mediolateral coverage without overhang in the medial soft-tissue structures (for a medial UKA).

Femoral Component

Identically to the tibial cut, the femoral resection should be conservative, regardless of the resection technique chosen: resurfacing, distal reaming with posterior cutting, or cutting technique as in TKA with distal, posterior, and chamfer cuts. The last-mentioned technique reproduces the femoral anatomic/mechanical angle during the distal cut, allowing a resection perpendicular to the mechanical axis. The drilling of the femoral medullary canal through a short incision often requires bringing the knee to lower degrees of flexion; otherwise, in flexion the patella might induce wrong alignment of the intramedullary guide. It is also crucial to protect the skin at the proximal part of the incision while performing this cut to avoid any skin damage.

The placement of the femoral component (and, before that, of the cutting guide) is a critical issue in UKA, because it should be placed in the center of the mediolateral dimension of the femoral condyle and centered over the tibial component when the knee is extended. In the case of false mediolateral positioning, there is a risk either of impingement on the tibial spines or of edge loading on the tibial polyethylene. After the cuts have been made, the next step is to remove any posterior osteophytes using an osteotome, to increase the range of flexion and avoid any posterior impingement with the polyethylene in high flexion.

The ideal anteroposterior size of the femoral component should extend far enough anteriorly to cover the weight-bearing surface that comes in contact with the tibia in full extension and leave 1 to 2 mm of exposed bone on the cut surface at the junction with the trochlear groove. The leading edge of the femoral component must be countersunk into this junction to prevent patellar impingement during flexion of the knee.[56]

Alignment

It is possible before performing the final preparation of the tibia to use dedicated spacers to check the correspondence between flexion and extension space. In some designs, it is also possible, before drilling the final peg or keel holes, to use trial components to make flexion/extension tests looking for tilting. Having the patella not dislocated from the patellar groove in the MIS approach avoids the artificial external rotation of the tibia and allows for an appropriate tracking of component congruity. A persistent tilting of the tibial component may be due to any remaining posterior impingement or an inadequate tibial cut.[11]

A trial polyethylene liner is inserted at that step, which also is considered crucial because this provides the final alignment of the leg. A protective laxity checked close to full extension, with a joint space opening up 1 or 2 mm when valgus stress is applied, is necessary to avoid any overcorrection of the deformity leading to progression of osteoarthritis in the unreplaced tibiofemoral compartment. Important residual varus deformity also should be avoided for medial UKA, as more recently reported,[49] to minimize the risk of polyethylene wear when using flat polyethylene inserts. Hernigou and Deschamps[21] showed, at a minimum 10 years of follow-up, that severe undercorrection of the deformity in varus was associated with increased wear in the tibial component after medial UKA. The ideal correction as measured on the postoperative full-weightbearing view probably consists of a tibiofemoral axis crossing the knee between the tibial spines and the lateral third of the tibial plateau (Fig. 81–6).[26]

Lateral Unicompartmental Replacement

The skin incision, using a minimal approach of the lateral compartment, needs to be lateral, especially at the distal portion, owing to the frequent divergence of the lateral femoral condyle. When the lateral arthrotomy is performed, visualization of the joint is often easier than on the medial side because of the natural mobility of the lateral tibiofemoral joint. The tibial resection should stay minimal, because the disease is more often on the femoral side. In the case of femoral dysplasia, it is often necessary to use a "more proximal distal" femoral cut.

The alignment of the femoral anteroposterior cutting guide on the tibial cut is crucial because of the natural shape of the femoral condyle. It is often necessary to mark the correct alignment in extension rather than in flexion to avoid medial edge loading and impingement between the femoral implant and the tibial spines. The polyethylene insert is often thicker than for the medial side in the case of femoral dysplasia, but the principle of undercorrecting the deformity for all cases of lateral UKA remains the basis for successful long-term results.

Lateral replacement, in my practice, corresponds to 10% of the indications for UKA, and the long-term results confirm that lateral osteoarthritis can be treated successfully by unicondylar replacement.[2,6,42] The in vivo kinematic evaluation of patients implanted with lateral UKA found a greater posterior displacement of the femorotibial contact point during flexion as compared with patients implanted with medial UKA because it is in the nonimplanted knee.[4]

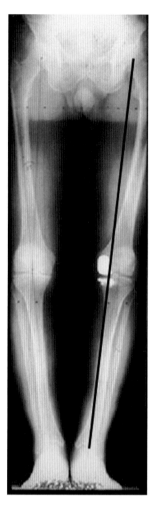

Figure 81–6. Full weightbearing view of the limbs shows a hip-knee-ankle axis crossing the knee joint just medial to the tibial spines, leaving an undercorrected 3-degree varus deformity after a medial unicompartmental knee arthroplasty.

Postoperative Recovery

Before closure of the capsule, a local anesthesic may be administered in the intraoperative tissue for pain management. I routinely use drains for UKA, removed at 48 hours postoperatively. Although same-day discharge is not yet common in Europe, I have noted significant changes in my own practice since the use of the MIS approach (Fig. 81–7), as previously reported.[16,37,53] These changes include immediate weightbearing at postoperative day 1 protected by crutches for 1 week, immediate quadriceps active exercises, and patient discharge after postoperative day 3.[3]

RESULTS OF UNICOMPARTMENTAL KNEE ARTHROPLASTY

Survivorship studies generated from early unicompartmental series show that survivorship rates at 10 years were decreasing into the 85% range.[10,20,23,56,58] With better

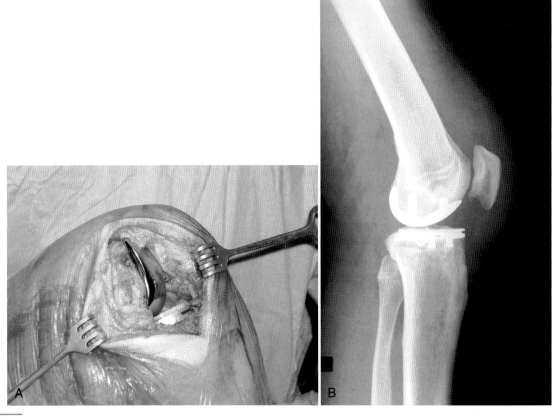

Figure 81–7. Intraoperative view **(A)** and postoperative sagittal radiograph **(B)** show a medial unicompartmental knee arthroplasty implanted through an 8-cm skin incision and without disruption of the extensor mechanism.

patient selection and reproducible instrumentation, more recent series show 10 year-survivorship regularly at 90% or greater.[2,8,11,38]

Using fixed bearings, Scott and Santore[56] documented 90% survivorship at 9 years in 64 knees implanted with the Brigham prosthesis. At 10 years, Berger and associates[8] projected a 98% rate of implant survival in 51 knees, and Argenson and colleagues,[2] using the same cemented metal-backed UKA, projected a 94% survivorship in 160 knees. More recently, using the same Miller-Galante UKA, Naudie and associates[39] reported a 90% 10-year survival rate in 113 knees with medial UKA. With mobile bearings, the Oxford group reported medial UKA survivorship of 97% at 10 years.[38] Robertsson and coworkers[52] analyzed the Swedish registry for the same implant and found a 4-year revision rate of 10% in a large multicenter study. Bearing exchange is a frequent reason for revision in mobile bearing designs, especially in the lateral compartment with an incidence of 10% for the Oxford UKA in the Swedish register.[52] Keblish and Briard,[25] studying the outcome of 177 LCS UKAs in a two-center study, reported a 82% survivorship at 11 years with 15 knees requiring bearing exchange alone. The analysis of a community-based implant registry by Gioe and coworkers,[17] studying 516 UKAs from nine designs and performed by 23 surgeons, showed 88.6% survivorship at 10 years compared with 94.8% for primary TKA. In most of the more recent studies, the specific mode of failure of UKA is pro-gression of osteoarthritis in the unreplaced compartments, which can be related either to inadequate patient selection or to surgical technique. Many authors now also support the view that revision of a modern UKA is a relatively common and simple procedure. Patients from the Swedish registry are more satisfied after revision of a failed UKA than after revision of TKA.[51]

SUMMARY

Unicondylar knee replacement should not be considered as a temporary procedure, and the 10-year survival can be as good as with TKA if patient selection and surgical principles are followed carefully. UKA is more conservative than TKA, and revision is easier. Although component loosening has become as rare as in TKA, progression of osteoarthritis in the unreplaced compartment is still a specific mode of failure, which can be decreased significantly by appropriate patient selection and adequate surgical technique. Polyethylene wear, associated with flat, metal-backed tibial components, may be a problem over the long-term, particularly in heavy and active patients, and continued follow-up is necessary.

These same criteria should be addressed for the MIS technique with correct implant positioning. The quicker recovery and the different evolutions in recent years in dedicated instrumentation and prosthetic design have made unicompartmental arthroplasty the standard of treatment for patients with severe osteoarthritis limited to one tibiofemoral compartment. The other femorotibial compartment and the patellofemoral joint should be intact. In the future, the use of computer-assisted surgery probably will increase the precision of the procedure performed with MIS technique.

References

1. Argenson JN: The mini incision: Routine approach. Orthopaedics 27:482, 2004.
2. Argenson JN, Chevrol-Benkeddache Y, Aubaniac JM: Modern unicompartmental knee arthroplasty with cement: A three to ten year follow-up study. J Bone Joint Surg Am 84:2235, 2002.
3. Argenson JN, Flecher X, Figuera A, Aubaniac JM: Unicompartmental knee arthroplasty by minimally invasive or conventional approach. Rev Chir Orthop 89(Suppl 6):3S120, 2003.
4. Argenson JN, Komistek RD, Aubaniac JM, et al: In vivo determination of knee kinematics for subjects implanted with a unicompartmental arthroplasty. J Arthroplasty 17:1049, 2002.
5. Argenson JN, O'Connor JJ: Polyethylene wear in meniscal knee replacement: A one to nine year retrieval analysis of the Oxford knee. J Bone Joint Surg Br 74:228, 1992.
6. Ashraf T, Newman JH, Evans RL, Ackroyd CE: Lateral unicompartmental knee replacement survivorship: An experience over 21 years. J Bone Joint Surg Br 84:1126, 2002.
7. Barrett WH, Scott RD: Revision of failed unicondylar arthroplasty. J Bone Joint Surg Am 69:1328, 1987.
8. Berger RA, Nedeff DD, Barden RM, et al: Unicompartmental knee arthroplasty: Clinical experience at 6 to 10-year follow-up. Clin Orthop 367:50, 1999.
9. Bernasek TL, Rand JA, Bryan RS: Unicompartmental porous coated anatomic total knee arthroplasty. Clin Orthop 236:52, 1988.
10. Bert JM: Ten year survivorship of metal-backed unicompartmental arthroplasty. J Arthroplasty 13:901, 1998.
10a. Cartier P, Cheaib S: Unicompartmental knee arthroplasty: A 2 to 10 years of follow-up evaluation. J Arthroplasty 2:157, 1987.
11. Cartier P, Deschamps G: Surgical principles of unicompartmental knee replacement. In Cartier P, Epinette JA, Deschamps G, Hernigou P (eds): Unicompartmental Knee Arthroplasty. Paris, Expansion Scientifique Française, 1996, pp 137-143.
12. Cartier P, Sanouiller JL, Grelsamer RP: Unicompartmental knee arthroplasty surgery: 10-year minimum follow-up period. J Arthroplasty 11:782, 1996.
13. Cobb AG, Kozinn SC, Scott RD: Unicondylar or total knee replacement: The patient's preference. J Bone Joint Surg Br 72:166, 1990.
14. Deschamps G, Lapeyre B: Rupture of the anterior cruciate ligament: A frequently unrecognized cause of failure of unicompartmental knee prostheses: A propos of a series of 79 Lotus prostheses with a follow-up of more than 5 years. Rev Chir Orthop Reparatrice Appar Mot 73:544, 1987.
15. Epinette JA, Edidin AA: Hydroxyapatite-coated unicompartmental knee replacement. In Cartier P, Epinette JA, Deschamps G, Hernigou P (eds): Unicompartmental Knee Arthroplasty. Paris, Expansion Scientifique Française, 1996, pp 243-259.
16. Fisher DA, Watts M, Davis KE: Implant positioning in knee surgery: A comparison of minimally invasive, open unicompartmental, and total knee arthroplasty. J Arthroplasty 18(7 Suppl 1):2, 2003.
17. Gioe TJ, Killeen KK, Hoeffel DP, et al: Analysis of unicompartmental knee arthroplasty in a commune based implant registry. Clin Orthop 416:111, 2003.
18. Goodfellow JW, O'Connor JJ: The anterior cruciate ligament in knee arthroplasty: A risk factor with unconstrained meniscal prostheses. Clin Orthop 276:245, 1992.
18a. Goodfellow J, O'Connor J: The mechanics of the knee and prosthesis design. J Bone Joint Surg 60B:358, 1978.
19. Grelsamer RP: Unicompartmental osteoarthritis of the knee. J Bone Joint Surg Am 77:278, 1995.
20. Heck DA, Marmor L, Gibson A, Rougraff BT: Unicompartmental knee arthroplasty: A multicenter investigation with long-term follow-up evaluation. Clin Orthop 286:154, 1993.
21. Hernigou P, Deschamps G: Alignment influences wear in the knee after medial unicompartmental arthroplasty. Clin Orthop 423:161, 2004.
22. Hernigou P, Deschamps G: Posterior slope of the tibial implant and the outcome of unicompartmental knee arthroplasty. J Bone Joint Surg Am 86:506, 2004.
23. Insall JN, Walker PS: Unicondylar knee replacement. Clin Orthop 120:83, 1976.
24. Jackson M, Sarangi PP, Newman JH: Revision total knee arthroplasty: Comparison of outcome following primary proximal tibial osteotomy or unicompartmental arthroplasty. J Arthroplasty 9:539, 1994.
25. Keblish PA, Briard JL: Mobile bearing unicompartmental knee arthroplasty: A 2-center study with an 11-year (mean) follow-up. J Arthroplasty 19(7 Suppl 2):87, 2004.
26. Kennedy W, White R: Unicompartmental total knee arthroplasty of the knee: Postoperative alignment and its influence on overall results. Clin Orthop 221:278, 1997.
27. Kozinn SC, Scott R: Unicondylar knee arthroplasty. J Bone Joint Surg 71:145-150, 1989.
28. Lai CH, Rand JA: Revision of failed unicompartmental total knee arthroplasty. Clin Orthop 287:193, 1993.
29. Laskin RS: Unicompartmental tibiofemoral resurfacing arthroplasty. J Bone Joint Surg Am 60:182, 1978.
30. Laskin RS: Unicompartmental knee replacement: Some unanswered questions. Clin Orthop 392:267, 2001.
31. Laurencin CT, Zelicof SB, Scott RD, Ewald FC: Unicompartmental versus total knee replacement in the same patient: A comparative study. Clin Orthop 273:151, 1991.
32. Levine WN, Ozuna RM, Scott RD, et al: Conversion of failed modern unicompartmental arthroplasty to total knee arthroplasty. J Arthroplasty 11:797, 1996.
33. Mallory TH, Danyi J: Unicompartmental total knee arthroplasty: A five to nine year follow-up study of 42 procedures. Clin Orthop 175:135, 1983.
34. Marmor L: Unicompartmental knee arthroplasty: Ten to thirteen year follow-up study. Clin Orthop 226:24, 1987.
35. Marmor L: Unicompartmental arthroplasty for osteonecrosis of the knee joint. Clin Orthop 294:247, 1993.
36. McAuley JP, Engh GA, Ammeen DJ: Revision of failed uni compartmental knee arthroplasty. Clin Orthop 392:279, 2001.
37. Muller PE, Pellenghar C, Witt M, et al: Influence of minimally invasive surgery on implant positioning and the functional outcome for medial unicompartmental knee arthroplasty. J Arthroplasty 19:296, 2004.
38. Murray DW, Goodfellow JW, O'Connor JJ: The Oxford medial unicompartmental arthroplasty: A 10 year survival study. J Bone Joint Surg Br 80:983, 1998.
39. Naudie D, Guerin J, Parker DA, et al: Medial unicompartmental knee arthroplasty with the Miller-Galante prosthesis. J Bone Joint Surg Am 86:1931, 2004.
40. Newman JH, Ackroyd CE, Shah NA: Unicompartmental or total knee replacement? Five-year results of a prospective randomised trial of 102 osteoarthritic knees with unicompartmental arthritis. J Bone Joint Surg Br 80:862, 1998.
41. O'Connor JJ, Shercliff TL, Biden E, Goodfellow JW: The geometry of the knee in the sagittal plane. Proceedings of the Institution of Mechanical Engineers, Part 17. J Eng Med 203:223, 1989.
42. Ohdera T, Tokunaga J, Kobayashi A: Unicompartmental knee arthroplasty for lateral gonarthrosis: Midterm results. J Arthroplasty 16:196, 2001.
43. Padgett DE, Stern SH, Insall JN: Revision total knee arthroplasty for failed unicompartmental replacement. J Bone Joint Surg Am 73:186, 1991.
44. Pennington DW, Swienckowski JJ, Lutes WB, Drake GN: Unicompartmental knee arthroplasty in patients sixty years of age or younger. J Bone Joint Surg Am 85:1968, 2003.
45. Perkins TR, Gunckle W: Unicompartmental knee arthroplasty: 3 to 10 year results in a community hospital setting. J Arthroplasty 3:293, 2002.
46. Price AJ, Webb J, Topf H, et al: Rapid recovery after Oxford unicompartmental arthroplasty through a short incision. J Arthroplasty 16:970, 2001.

47. Psychoyios V, Crawford RW, Murray DW, O'Connor JJ: Wear of congruent meniscal bearings in unicompartmental knee replacement. J Bone Joint Surg Br 80:976, 1998.
48. Repicci JA, Eberle RW: Minimally invasive surgical technique for unicondylar knee arthroplasty. J South Orthop Assoc 8:20, 1999.
49. Ridgeway SR, McAuley JP, Ammeen DJ, Engh GA: The effect of alignment of the knee on the outcome of unicompartmental knee replacement. J Bone Joint Surg Br 84:351, 2002.
50. Ritter MA, Faris PM, Thong AE, et al: Intra-operative findings in varus osteoarthritis of the knee: An analysis of pre-operative alignment in potential candidates for unicompartmental arthroplasty. J Bone Joint Surg Br 86:43-47, 2004.
51. Robertsson O, Dunbar M, Pehrsson T, et al: Patient satisfaction after knee arthroplasty: A report on 27,372 knees operated on between 1981 and 1995 in Sweden. Acta Orthop Scand 71:262, 2000.
52. Robertsson O, Knutson K, Lewold S, Lundgren L: The Swedish knee arthroplasty register: Outcome with special emphasis on 1988-1997. Scientific Exhibit AAOS, San Francisco, 2001.
53. Romanowski MR, Repicci JA: Minimally invasive unicondylar arthroplasty: Eight-year follow-up. J Knee Surg 15:17, 2002.
54. Schai PA, Suh JT, Thornhill TS, et al: Unicompartmental knee arthroplasty in middle-aged patients. J Arthroplasty 13:365, 1998.
55. Scott RD, Cobb AG, McQueary FG, et al: Unicompartmental knee arthroplasty: Eight- to twelve-year follow-up with survivorship analysis. Clin Orthop 271:96, 1991.
56. Scott RD, Santore R: Unicondylar unicompartmental replacement for osteoarthritis of the knee. J Bone Joint Surg Am 63:536, 1981.
57. Squire MW, Callaghan JJ, Goetz DD, et al: Unicompartmental knee replacement: A minimum 15 year follow-up study. Clin Orthop 367:61, 1999.
58. Tabor OB Jr, Tabor OB: Unicompartmental arthroplasty: A long term follow-up study. J Arthroplasty 13:373, 1998.
59. Thornhill TS, Scott RD: Unicompartmental total knee arthroplasty. Orthop Clin 20:25, 1989.
60. Weale AE, Murray DW, Crawford R, et al: Does arthritis progress in the retained compartments after "Oxford" medial unicompartmental arthroplasty? A clinical and radiological study with a minimum ten-year follow-up. J Bone Joint Surg Br 81:783, 1999.

CHAPTER 82

Minimally Invasive Surgery for Unicondylar Arthroplasty of the Knee

Giles R. Scuderi • Alfred J. Tria, Jr.

Minimally invasive surgery for knee arthroplasty began in the early 1990s with the work of Repicci for unicondylar knee arthroplasty (UKA).[16,18] Although there had been a long history of UKA dating back to the early 1970s,[7,10,11,13] the techniques and surgical approaches were modeled after total knee arthroplasty (TKA).[3,8,9,12,15,17,19,21] The results were not equal to TKA, and many surgeons abandoned the procedure. The minimally invasive surgical approach introduced a new method to perform the surgery and helped to improve the results by emphasizing the differences between TKA and UKA. Minimally invasive surgery forced the surgeon to consider UKA as a separate operation with its own techniques and its own principles. UKA now has a place in the armamentarium for surgery of the knee. Many of the prostheses are not new, but the surgical approach and the decision making are quite different and have led to much more successful results.

PREOPERATIVE PLANNING

The preoperative evaluation of the patient includes the history, physical examination, and radiograph. It is critical to choose the correct patient for the operation and to observe the limitations that it imposes. The patient should identify a single compartment of the knee as the primary source of the pain, and the physical examination should correlate with the history. Tenderness should be isolated to one tibiofemoral compartment, and the patellofemoral examination should be negative. The posterior cruciate and collateral ligaments should be intact and stable with distinct endpoints. The literature suggests that the anterior cruciate ligament (ACL) should be intact[6]; however, there are cases in which the ACL is absent and the knee is quite stable. In the latter setting, the ligament deficiency has no effect on the unicondylar replacement. The varus or valgus deformity does not have to be completely correctable to neutral, but the procedure is more difficult to perform with fixed axial deformity. The range of motion in flexion should be greater than 105 degrees.

The standing radiograph is the primary imaging study (Fig. 82–1). Although it is ideal to have a full view of the hip, knee, and ankle, it is not absolutely necessary. The 14 × 17-inch standard cassette allows measurement of the anatomic axes of the femur and the tibia, which will permit adequate preoperative planning for the surgical procedure. An anteroposterior flexed knee view (notch view) is helpful to rule out any involvement of the opposite condyle. The patellar view, such as a Merchant, will allow evaluation of the patellofemoral joint and will confirm that there is no significant malalignment. The lateral radiograph is used to further judge the patellofemoral joint and to measure the slope of the tibial plateau (Fig. 82–2). The tibial slope can vary from 0 to 15 degrees and can be changed during the surgery to adjust the flexion extension gap balancing.

The radiographs provide important guidelines for the surgery. The varus deformity should not exceed 10 degrees, the valgus should not exceed 15 degrees, and the flexion contracture should not exceed 10 degrees. Deformities outside these limits will require soft-tissue balancing that will make the UKA difficult to complete. There should be minimal translocation of the tibia beneath the femur (Fig. 82–3), and the opposite tibiofemoral compartment and the patellofemoral compartment should show minimal involvement. Translocation indicates that the opposite femoral condyle has degenerative changes, and this will certainly compromise the clinical result. Although Stern and Insall indicated that only 6% of all patients satisfy the requirements for the UKA,[20] we have found the incidence to be 10% to 15%. However, it is important to avoid broadening the indications outside the limitations noted to preserve a high success rate with good longevity.

Magnetic resonance imaging (MRI) is sometimes helpful for evaluation of avascular necrosis of the femoral condyle or to confirm the integrity of the meniscus in the opposite compartment when the patient complains of an element of instability. However, MRI is not necessary on a routine basis.

Scintigraphic studies are sometimes helpful to identify the extent of involvement of one compartment versus the other. But, once again, this is not a routine diagnostic test.

SURGICAL TECHNIQUE

The operation can be performed with epidural, spinal, or general anesthesia. Femoral nerve blocks have become more common, but they may on occasion have an associated motor block of the quadriceps muscle that will have an effect on the physical therapy on the day of surgery. It is important that the anesthesia team understands that the patients will be required to walk and begin physical therapy within 2 to 4 hours of the completion of the oper-

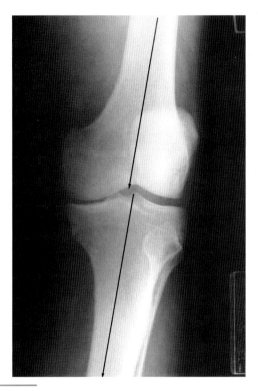

Figure 82–1. Anteroposterior standing radiograph of a left knee.

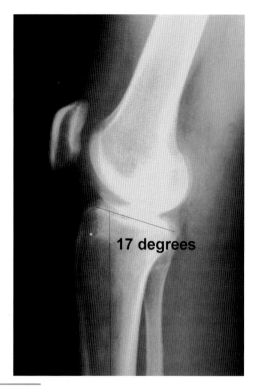

Figure 82–2. Lateral radiograph of the knee showing a 17-degree tibial slope.

ation and the anesthesia must be in harmony with this approach.

The surgery is usually performed with an arterial tourniquet; however, this is not mandatory. The limited minimally invasive surgical incision necessitates continuous repositioning of the knee. The surgeon should be prepared for this and either have adequate assistance or use a leg-holding device to facilitate exposure (Fig. 82–4).

The skin incision is made with the knee in flexion, on either the medial or lateral side of the patella (depending on the compartment to be replaced), and begins from the superior pole of the patella to 2 cm distal to the joint line. It is typically 7 to 10 cm long. The incision should not be centered on the joint line and biased toward the involved compartment, because this will limit the exposure to the femoral condyle. In the varus knee, a limited medial parapatellar arthrotomy is performed, extending from the lower border of the vastus medialis to a point just distal to the joint line along the proximal tibia. Occasionally, a short, transverse cut in the capsule 1 to 2 cm beneath the vastus medialis (Fig. 82–5) is helpful when the surgeon's experience is limited and when exposure is difficult in the "tight" knee. With greater experience, the transverse extension is not necessary. It is important to emphasize that this transverse cut is not a subvastus approach but merely an incision in the capsule of the knee midway between the vastus medialis and the tibial joint line. The deep medial collateral ligament is released on the tibial side to improve the exposure of the joint. The release is not performed for the purposes of alignment correction. This is the beginning of the divergence of UKA from the TKA surgery. The surgery is only performed on one side of the joint. The goal of the surgery is to replace one side

and to balance the forces so that the arthroplasty and the opposite compartment share the weightbearing equally. If the medial ligamentous complex is released, there is the potential for overloading the opposite side, with resultant pain and failure.

In the lateral UKA, the transverse extension is not necessary. The vertical incision is taken down to the tibial plateau, and the iliotibial band is sharply released from Gerdy's tubercle and elevated posteriorly (Fig. 82–6). The arthrotomy is closed in a vertical fashion, and the iliotibial band heals onto the tibial metaphysis.

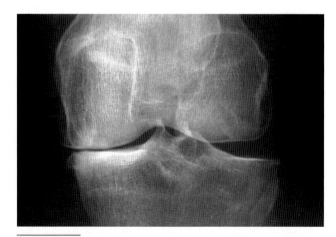

Figure 82–3. Translocation of the lateral tibial spine contacting the lateral femoral condyle on a standing anteroposterior radiograph of the knee. This is a relative contraindication to unicondylar knee arthroplasty.

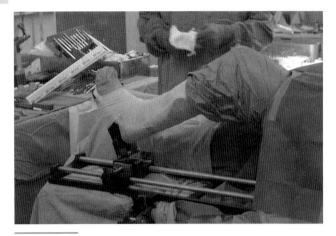

Figure 82–4. The leg holder (Innovative Medical Products, Inc., Plainville, CT) allows flexion and extension of the knee along with internal and external rotation.

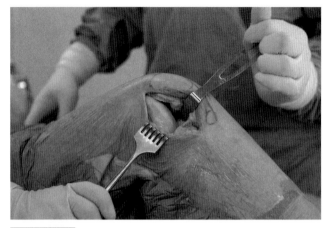

Figure 82–6. The lateral view of a right knee shows the anterior tibial joint line after the iliotibial band has been released and retracted posteriorly.

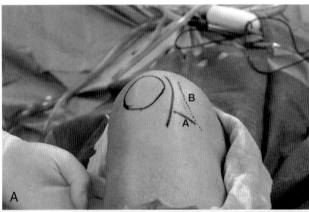

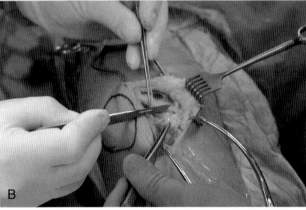

Figure 82–5. **A,** The medial incision extends from the top of the patella to just below the tibial joint line (A). B is the outline of the margin of the medial femoral condyle. **B,** The medial arthrotomy can include a T in the capsule (made with the tip of the knife blade).

With minimally invasive surgery, the patella is not everted in the procedure and the vastus medialis is not violated either by a dividing incision or a subvastus approach. The sparing of the surrounding soft-tissue structures and the preservation of the extensor mechanism in its entirety makes the procedure minimally invasive.

With the completion of the arthrotomy, the peripheral osteophytes should be removed from the femoral condyle and the tibial plateau. All compartments of the joint should be inspected. It is not unusual to see some limited arthritic involvement in the other areas. There should be no surprises at the time of the surgery, and the preoperative evaluation should be thorough enough to preclude a conversion to a TKA in the large majority of the cases. Diagnostic arthroscopy is not necessary but can sometimes be included to confirm the anatomy of the opposite side in an unusual case. After exposing the joint, the distal femoral cut can be completed using an intramedullary reference, an extramedullary guide, or a spacer block technique.

The Intramedullary Technique

The intramedullary technique is valuable for its accuracy and ease of use. An entrance hole is made on the distal femoral surface centered just above the roof of the intercondylar notch (Fig. 82–7). The intramedullary canal is suctioned free of its contents to discourage fat embolization, and the instrument is positioned. The depth of the distal femoral cut affects the extension gap and also the anatomic valgus of the distal femur (Fig. 82–8). The angle (or tilt) of the cut determines the perpendicularity of the component to the tibial plateau surface in full extension (Fig. 82–9). Flexion contractures of the knee can be corrected with the medial UKA but not with the lateral replacement. If there is a flexion contracture and the distal anatomic femoral valgus is 5 degrees or less in the varus knee, the standard amount of bone is removed to replace millimeter for millimeter with the prosthesis. If the distal femoral valgus is 6 degrees or more in the varus knee, 2 mm of additional bone is removed from the distal femur to decrease the excess valgus and to increase the space in full extension. Increasing the space in full extension helps to correct the flexion contracture and enables the surgeon to decrease the associated depth of the tibial cut. The deeper femoral cut saves 2 mm of bone on the tibial side[2]

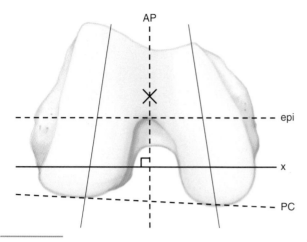

Figure 82–7. The intramedullary hole is located just above the roof of the intercondylar notch (marked with the letter X).

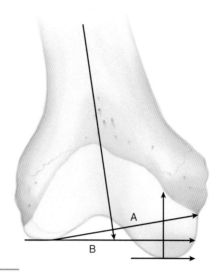

Figure 82–8. The two cuts on the medial femoral condyle show that the deeper resection (line A) results in less valgus than line B (3 degrees versus 5 degrees). This also allows for more space in full extension.

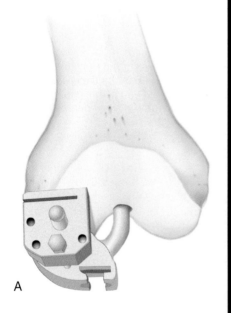

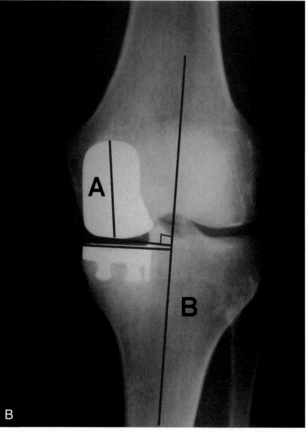

Figure 82–9. **A,** The intramedullary guide allows for a distal cut of 2, 4, 6, or 8 degrees. This setting adjusts the angle of the femoral component with relation to the tibial plateau cut surface. It does not adjust the overall varus or valgus of the knee because it is only cutting one condyle. **B,** The femoral component "tilt" is defined as the angle between the long axis of the component (line A) referenced to the axis of the tibial shaft (line B).

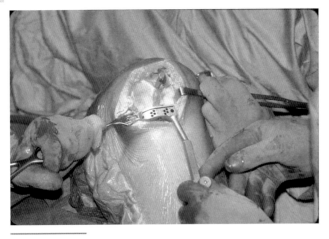

Figure 82–10. The tibial cut is completed with an extramedullary guide.

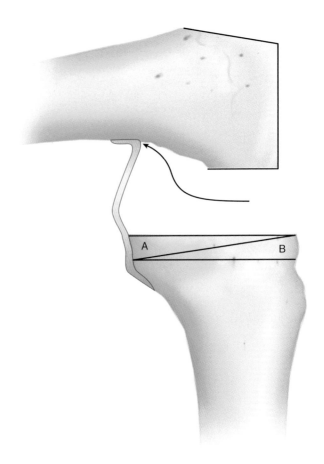

Figure 82–11. The slope of the tibial cut can be changed to correct flexion-extension imbalance. The flexion gap is often larger than the extension gap. The cut A can be lowered anteriorly and the slope decreased to line B, which will equalize the gaps.

and results in a total distal femoral resection of 8 mm. The resection does not elevate the femoral joint line as it would in a TKA. Most TKA femoral components remove a minimum of 9 mm for the prosthesis so that this change does not adversely affect revision to a TKA.

In the valgus knee, the maximal acceptable deformity is 15 degrees and the distal femur is cut millimeter for millimeter for replacement. The deformity will be slightly decreased with a standard resurfacing because the prosthesis and the cement mantle are slightly thicker than the bone that is removed. Because the lateral femoral condyle is less prominent than the medial condyle in full extension, flexion contractures cannot be corrected as easily on the lateral side. A deeper cut on the lateral femoral condyle will only increase the distal femoral valgus without changing the extension gap significantly.

After completing the distal femoral cut, it is easier to proceed to the tibial preparation because this in turn opens up the space in 90 degrees of flexion and makes positioning the femoral finishing guide much easier. The tibial cut is made with an extramedullary instrument (Fig. 82–10). The tibial cut can be angled from anterior to posterior. Most systems favor a 5- to 7-degree posterior slope similar to the preoperative alignment. The slope of the cut also affects the flexion-extension balancing. The flexion gap is usually larger than the extension gap because of the flexion contracture that is present in almost all arthritic knees. As the flexion contracture increases to 10 degrees, the extension gap becomes tighter. If the slope of the tibial cut is decreased from the anatomic slope of the preoperative tibial radiograph, the cut can be made deeper anteriorly to give greater space in extension while maintaining the same flexion gap posteriorly (Fig. 82–11).

With the completion of the tibial cut, the remainder of the femoral cuts can be completed with the appropriate blocks for guidance of the saws. If the intramedullary approach is used, an intramedullary retractor can be used to retract the patella (Fig. 82–12). The femoral runner should be a slight bit smaller than the original femoral condyle surface and should be perpendicular to the tibial plateau at 90 degrees of flexion and centered medial to lateral on the condyle. If the femoral condyle divergence is extreme in 90 degrees of flexion, the femoral compo-

nent should be positioned perpendicular to the tibial cut surface (parallel to the long axis of the tibia). This positioning may result in some overhang of the femoral runner into the intercondylar notch (Fig. 82–13).

The Extramedullary Technique

The extramedullary instruments avoid violating the intramedullary canal, ensure parallelism of the distal femoral and proximal tibial cuts, and sometimes allow a smaller incision. The extramedullary instrument system inserts a distractor into the affected compartment in full extension and adjusts the two linked cuts for the distal femur and the proximal tibia with extramedullary rods that reference the ankle and the femoral head (Fig. 82–14). It is important to remember not to overcorrect the deformity when using these techniques. The distal femoral cut is made in full extension; and, then, the proximal tibial cut can be made in flexion following the same principles as mentioned earlier. The femoral finishing guide is used in the extramedullary technique in the same manner as in the intramedullary approach.

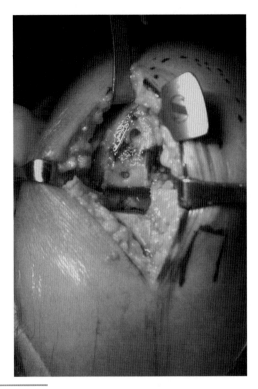

Figure 82–12. The intramedullary retractor is useful to visualize the joint (labeled with Z).

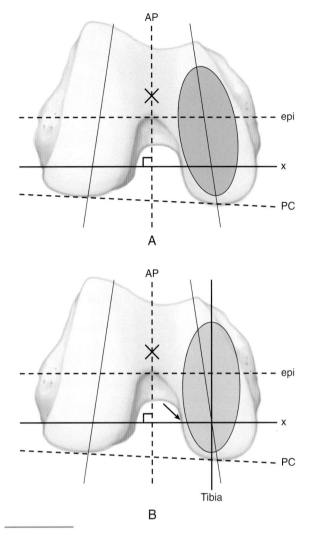

Figure 82–13. **A,** If the femoral component is aligned with the cut articular surface of the femur, the divergence of the condyles may be too great and the subsequent position may lead to edge loading on the polyethylene tibial insert. **B,** The femoral component should be perpendicular to the tibial insert even if this leads to a nonanatomic position on the femoral surface and slight overhang of the component into the intercondylar notch *(arrow).*

The Extramedullary Spacer Block Technique

The extramedullary spacer block technique performs the tibial resection first with the extramedullary instrument. The tibial resecting guide is set parallel to the tibial shaft, and the resection guide is secured to the proximal tibia. A depth gauge is used to determine the level of resection, which is usually 2 to 4 mm from the lowest point on the tibial plateau. Once the desired depth of resection is determined, a retractor is placed medially to protect the medial collateral ligament. With the knee flexed, the proximal tibia is resected. Caution must be taken not to undercut the attachment of the anterior cruciate ligament and the lateral tibial plateau. With a reciprocating saw, the sagittal cut is made in line with the medial wall of the intercondylar notch. The resected tibial bone is removed and the resultant gap is checked with a spacer block to ensure that the appropriate amount of bone has been resected and that the axial alignment is correct. If the gap is too tight, additional bone should be resected from the proximal tibia. If the gap is too loose, a thicker spacer block is placed.

After resection of the proximal tibia, the knee is brought into full extension and the appropriate spacer block is inserted into the joint space. With the knee in full extension, the distal femoral resection guide is secured to the spacer block (Fig. 82–15A). An alignment tower confirms positioning of the resection guide (see Fig. 82–15B). The distal femoral resection guide is secured to the distal femur and the distal femur is resected. The distal femoral cut can be completed in full extension, but caution must be taken not to overcut the femur and have the saw blade violate the popliteal area. If desired, the femoral cut can be started in extension and finished in flexion. Once the distal femur is resected, the extension gap is checked with a spacer block and alignment rod (see Fig. 82–15C). This technique is simple and guarantees parallel cuts.

Final Preparation and Implantation

On completion of the basic bone cuts, the femur and tibia are finished to accept the implants. The appropriate-sized femoral finishing guide is selected. There should be 1 to 2 mm of exposed bone along the anterior edge of the guide. If the finishing guide appears to be between sizes,

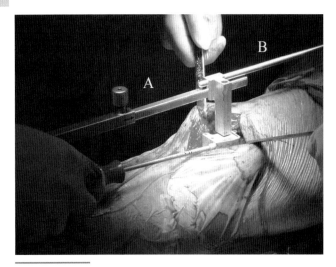

Figure 82–14. The extramedullary distractor (Zimmer, Warsaw, IN) is placed between the femur and the tibia on the medial side. The tibial rod (A) is aligned parallel to the tibial axis and the femoral rod (B) is aligned with reference to the proximal femoral head. Care must be taken to avoid overcorrection with this technique.

it is preferable to pick the smaller size. This guide should also be rotationally set so that the posterior surface is parallel to the resected tibia. Final preparation of the femur is then complete. On the tibial side, a template that covers the entire surface without overhang is chosen.

Once the femoral and tibial preparation is complete, the flexion-extension gap should be tested with the trial components in position. In the ideal case there should be 2 mm of laxity in both positions (Fig. 82–16). It is best not to overtighten the joint and to accept greater rather than less laxity. Excess tightness may lead to early polyethylene failure and also contributes to increase pressure transmission to the opposite side. Three separate items determine the overall varus or valgus of the knee: the depth of the tibial cut, the tibial polyethylene thickness, and the depth of the femoral cut. The tibia can be cut exactly perpendicular, and the distal femoral cut can be set in 4 degrees of valgus; but with the insertion of an excessively thick polyethylene, the knee can be shifted into 6 or more degrees of valgus and overcorrected despite properly aligned bone cuts. In the setting of TKA, changing the thickness of the tibial insert affects spacing in full extension and 90 degrees of flexion but it does not affect the varus of valgus of the knee, which remains the same.

If the UKA spacing is not symmetric, the tibial cut should be altered. Typically, the extension space will be smaller than the flexion space. This can be corrected by starting the tibial cut slightly deeper on the anterior surface and decreasing the slope angle. Once again, in TKA the extension space is easily increased by removing more bone from the distal femur. In UKA, deepening the femoral cut will change the distal femoral valgus and will also increase the size of the component because the anteroposterior surface will be widened. This may lead to poor bone contact with the new femoral component and possible early loosening. Thus, it is best to modify the spacing with changes on the tibial side. If the space in

extension is larger than the flexion space, this usually means that the slope of the tibial cut was made too shallow and the slope should just be increased. Figure 82–17 outlines the corrections that can be made if the spacing is not ideal.

After testing the components for stability, range of motion, and flexion-extension balance, the final components are cemented in place. There are cementless designs for UKA with somewhat encouraging results, but the authors have not embraced that technology. When the tibial component is a modular design, the metal tray can be cemented in place first and this allows excellent visualization of the posterior aspect of the joint and also allows more space for the femoral component cementing. The all-polyethylene insert does give more thickness to the prosthesis. However, the thicker polyethylene blocks visualization for the cementing; and, if full-thickness polyethylene failure occurs, the exchange will require invasion of the underlying tibial bone. The modular tibial tray allows polyethylene exchange without bone invasion and backside wear does not seem to be a problem in UKA surgery. The femoral runner is cemented after the tibial tray, and the polyethylene is inserted last.

The tourniquet is released before the closure and adequate hemostasis is established. The closure of the arthrotomy is performed in a routine fashion over a single drain. The patellar tracking should be checked before closing the subcutaneous tissues. At the time of closure, some surgeons inject the surrounding tissues with a local anesthetic to permit more comfortable activity immediately after the surgery. We have not found this to be particularly helpful, but it is certainly not contraindicated.

POSTOPERATIVE MANAGEMENT

Full weightbearing ambulation and range-of-motion exercises are begun as soon as the patient is alert, oriented, and able to stand. Fondaparinux (Arixtra, Sanofi-Synthelabo) or enoxaparin (Lovenox) is used for prophylaxis for deep venous thrombosis after surgery. At times a Doppler ultrasound study of both lower extremities is performed before discontinuation.[1,4] The patient is discharged on the first or second day after surgery to home. Physical therapy typically lasts 4 to 6 weeks after the operation, and most patients have full range of motion at that point.

RESULTS

At present there are few reports using the minimally invasive surgical approach. Berger's report[2] included a 10-year follow-up with 98% longevity using standard open arthrotomy techniques. The average age of the patients was 68, and the indications for the procedure were quite strict. Price reported early follow-up of an abbreviated incision for UKA with good results.[14] He compared 40 Oxford UKAs using a minimally invasive surgical type incision with 20 Oxford UKAs performed with a standard incision. The average rate of recovery of the minimally invasive

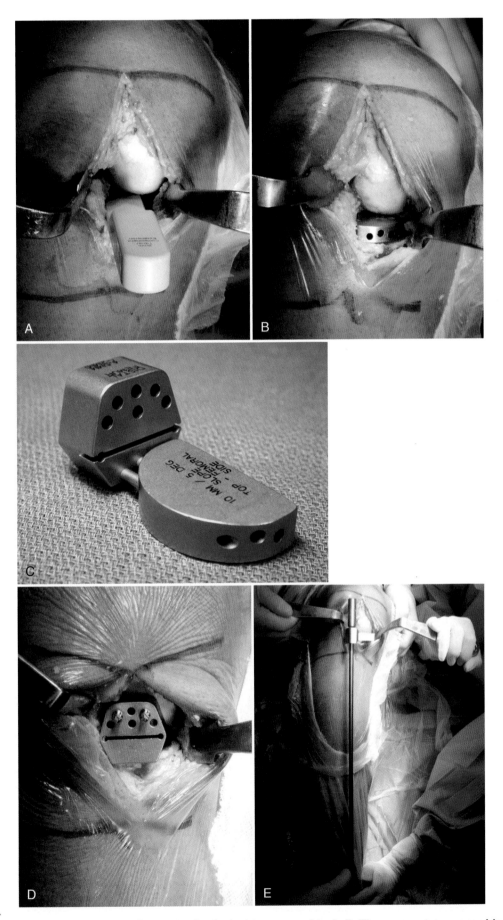

Figure 82–15. **A,** After tibial resection the gap is checked with a spacer block. **B,** The appropriate spacer block is inserted into the joint space. **C,** The spacer block and distal cutting guide assembly are shown. **D,** The distal cutting guide is secured to the distal femur. **E,** Alignment is confirmed with the appropriate block and rod.

UKAs was twice as fast. The accuracy of the implantation was evaluated using 11 variables on fluoroscopically centered postoperative radiographs and was found to be the same as that of the open UKAs. Price concluded that more rapid recovery was possible with less morbidity. The technique did not compromise the final result of the UKA. Repicci and Eberle reported on 136 knees with 8 years of follow-up using the minimally invasive surgical technique.[16] There were 10 revisions (7%): 3 for technical errors, 1 for poor pain relief, 5 for advancing disease, and 1 for fracture. The revisions for technical errors occurred from 6 to 25 months after surgery. The revisions for

advancing disease occurred from 37 to 90 months after surgery. Repicci and Eberle concluded that minimally invasive UKA is "an initial arthroplasty procedure (that) relieves pain, restores limb alignment, and improves function with minimal morbidity without interfering with future TKA."

One of us (AJT) has performed 325 UKAs using the Miller-Galante Unicondylar Knee Arthroplasty (Zimmer, Warsaw, IN). Forty-one patients underwent surgery in the year 2000 and now have more than 2 years of clinical follow-up. There were 24 women and 17 men, including six bilateral surgeries, four simultaneous and two staged 6 to 8 weeks apart. There were 47 knees: 45 varus and 2 valgus. The average age was 68 with a range from 42 to 93. Thirty percent of the patients were younger than the age of 60, and 20% were older than the age of 75. The average preoperative range of motion of the knee was 121 degrees, and the postoperative range of motion was 132 degrees. One knee was converted to a TKA because of patellar subluxation occurring 9 months after the surgery. The revision was performed at 14 months after the original TKA. One patient sustained an undisplaced tibial plateau fracture 2 weeks after surgery and this healed without intervention. There were no infections or component loosenings. The average preoperative Knee Society pain score was 45, and this improved to 80 after surgery. The Knee Society function score improved from 47 to 78.[5] Although these are very early results, most of the series with poor results started to see failures within the first 2 years after the procedure.

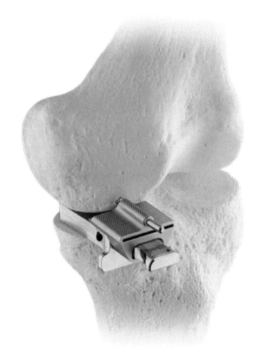

Figure 82–16. The tongue depressor is 2 mm thick and demonstrates the proper laxity in full extension of the knee and the matching proper laxity in 90 degrees of flexion.

CONCLUSION

The results of UKA have improved steadily through the late 1990s into the year 2000. The minimally invasive surgical technique has fostered better results and has helped to set UKA apart from TKA in the minds of the operating surgeons. As the prosthetic designs and surgical techniques continue to improve, minimally invasive surgical UKA should have results similar to those of TKA in the first 10 to 15 years and give patients a choice before TKA

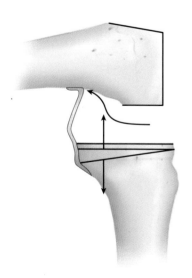

UKA Spacing

Flex/Ext →	0	1	2
↓ 0	Recut 2mm	↓ S	↓ S
1	↑ S	Recut 1mm	↓ S
2	↑ S	↑ S	Perfect!

S = Slope

Figure 82–17. The measurements of laxity of the knee in full extension and in 90 degrees of flexion with the appropriate changes that should be made in the slope of the tibial cut to equalize the gaps.

that will permit greater activity and improved quality of life without compromising the result of a later TKA.

References

1. Bauer KA, Eriksson BL, Lassen MR, Turpie AG: Fondaparinux compared with enoxaparin for the prevention of venous thromboembolism after elective major knee surgery. N Engl J Med 345:1305-1310, 2001.
2. Berger RA, Nedeff DD, Barden RN, et al: Unicompartmental knee arthroplasty. Clin Orthop Relat Res 367:50-60, 1999.
3. Colizza W, Insall J, Scuderi G: The posterior stabilized total knee prosthesis: Assessment of polyethylene damage and osteolysis after a ten year minimum follow-up. J Bone Joint Surg 77:1716-1720, 1995.
4. Eriksson BL, Bauer KA, Lassen MR, Turpie AG: Fondaparinux compared with enoxaparin for the prevention of venous thromboembolism after hip-fracture surgery. N Engl J Med 345:1298-1304, 2001.
5. Gesell MW, Tria AJ Jr: MIS unicondylar knee arthroplasty: Surgical approach and early results. Clin Orthop Relat Res 428:53-60, 2004.
6. Goodfellow JW, Kershaw CJ, Benson MK, O'Connor JJ: The Oxford knee for unicompartmental osteoarthritis: The first 103 cases. J Bone Joint Surg Br 70:692-701, 1988.
7. Goodfellow JW, O'Connor JJ: The mechanics of the knee and prosthesis design. J Bone Joint Surg Br 60:358-369, 1978.
8. Insall J, Ranawat C, Scott WN, Walker P: Total condylar knee replacement: Preliminary report. Clin Orthop Relat Res 120:149-154, 1976.
9. Insall J, Tria A, Scott W: The total condylar knee prosthesis: The first five years. Clin Orthop Relat Res 145:68-77, 1979.
10. Insall J, Walker P: Unicondylar knee replacement. Clin Orthop Relat Res 120:83-85, 1976.
11. Laskin RS: Unicompartment tibiofemoral resurfacing arthroplasty. J Bone Joint Surg Am 60:182-185, 1978.
12. Malkani A, Rand J, Bryan R, Wallrich S: Total knee arthroplasty with the kinematic condylar prosthesis: A ten year follow-up study. J Bone Joint Surg 77:423-431, 1995.
13. Marmor L: Marmor modular knee in unicompartmental disease: Minimum four-year follow-up. J Bone Joint Surg Am 61:347-353, 1979.
14. Price AJ, Webb J, Topf H, et al, and the Oxford Hip and Knee Group: Rapid recovery after Oxford unicompartmental arthroplasty through a short incision. J Arthroplasty 16:970-976, 2001.
15. Ranawat C, Flynn W, Saddler S, et al: Long-term results of the total condylar knee arthroplasty: A 15-year survivorship study. Clin Orthop Relat Res 286:96-102, 1993.
16. Repicci JA, Eberle RW: Minimally invasive surgical technique for unicondylar knee arthroplasty. J South Orthop Assoc 8:20-27, 1999.
17. Ritter MA, Herbst SA, Keating EM, et al: Long-term survivorship analysis of a posterior cruciate retaining total condylar total knee arthroplasty. Clin Orthop Relat Res 309:136-145, 1994.
18. Romanowski MR, Repicci JA: Minimally invasive unicondylar arthroplasty: Eight year follow-up. J Knee Surg 15:17-22, 2002.
19. Scott RD, Volatile TB: Twelve years experience with posterior cruciate retaining total knee arthroplasty. Clin Orthop Relat Res 205:100-107, 1986.
20. Stern SH, Becker MW, Insall J: Unicompartmental knee arthroplasty: An evaluation of selection criteria. Clin Orthop Relat Res 286:143-148, 1993.
21. Stern S, Insall J: Posterior stabilized prosthesis: Results after follow-up of nine to twelve years. J Bone Joint Surg Am 74:980-986, 1992.

CHAPTER 83

Patellofemoral Arthroplasty

Jess H. Lonner

Isolated patellofemoral arthritis can be the source of great pain and disability. Often, this clinical entity is treated effectively with nonsurgical interventions, such as weight reduction, physical therapy, and judicious use of injectable or oral medications. However, when the pain is refractory to these efforts, surgery may be considered. A number of surgical options have been used for patellofemoral arthritis, including arthroscopic débridement and lavage, patellar unloading procedures (such as tibial tubercle elevation or tibial tubercle anteromedialization), patellectomy, cartilage grafting techniques, patellar resurfacing, patellofemoral arthroplasty, and total knee arthroplasty. This chapter discusses the role of patellofemoral arthroplasty for isolated patellofemoral chondral degeneration. Results may be optimized by limiting the procedure to patients with arthritis strictly localized to the anterior compartment of the knee and without significant patellar malalignment, by accurately aligning the prosthesis and balancing the soft tissues to optimize patellar tracking, by using an implant that engages the patella within the trochlear groove but has limited constraint and a sagittal radius of curvature that mates well with the native distal femur, and by minimizing activities postoperatively that require repetitive loading in deep flexion.

Patellofemoral arthroplasty has never gained widespread use, particularly because earlier design flaws predisposed to a relatively high rate of failure as a result of patellar maltracking, catching, and anterior knee pain. However, newer and improving designs that have reduced the incidence of patellofemoral dysfunction, as well as interest in less invasive alternatives to standard total knee arthroplasty, have stimulated considerable enthusiasm for patellofemoral arthroplasty.

EPIDEMIOLOGY

Chondromalacia patellae has been observed in 40% to 60% of patients at autopsy and in 20% to 50% of patients at the time of arthrotomy for other diagnoses.[46] The prevalence of isolated patellofemoral arthritis is high; it occurred in as many as 11% of men and 24% of women older than 55 with symptomatic osteoarthritis of the knee in one study.[34] This gender predilection is undoubtedly related to the often subtle patellar malalignment and dysplasia that is common in women. The patellofemoral cartilage is also vulnerable to direct traumatic injury in view of its unprotected location in the body.

NONSURGICAL TREATMENT

Nonsurgical management is the mainstay of treatment of isolated patellofemoral arthritis; to be certain, it is the minority of patients who ultimately require an operation. A directed therapy program emphasizing short-arc quadriceps strengthening, stretching of the lateral retinacular structures, and preservation of motion is frequently successful in mitigating symptoms. There is some evidence to suggest that vastus medialis obliquus dysfunction may be associated with patellofemoral pain.[39] This serves to reinforce the importance of a directed strengthening program. When the anterior knee pain associated with patellofemoral arthrosis is refractory to months of nonoperative interventions, such as weight reduction, physical therapy, and judicious use of injectable or oral medications, surgery may be considered.

SURGICAL ALTERNATIVES

Arthroscopic Surgery

Arthroscopic options for patellofemoral chondromalacia and arthritis include lavage and débridement, with or without marrow stimulation. Arthroscopic débridement and lavage may be beneficial in patients who have recurrent effusions by decreasing the debris load, which may be a source of inflammation. Furthermore, removal of an unstable chondral flap lesion on the patella or trochlear groove can improve the mechanical symptoms. However, these interventions have varied results, and patients should be counseled regarding the likelihood of only partial and temporary symptomatic relief and the persistence of functional limitations. The poor intrinsic healing capabilities of articular cartilage limit the value of arthroscopic treatment of patellofemoral arthritis, particularly in the absence of mechanical symptoms.

Various technical modalities are available for débridement of chondromalacia, including mechanical shavers, thermal devices, and lasers. Lasers have produced limited short-term improvement in symptoms but have extremely worrisome potential complications, including extensive damage to cartilage and necrosis of subchondral bone. Thermal devices have had more predictable results. In one study comparing thermal and mechanical débridement, the short-term results of radiofrequency ablation were superior to those with a shaver. However, the long-term effects of thermal energy on articular cartilage have yet to be defined, and thus its use should be approached with prudence.

Federico and Reider analyzed a series of 36 patients who underwent arthroscopic chondroplasty for isolated chondromalacia patellae without patellar malalignment.[13] Patients with traumatic chondromalacia had 60% good or excellent results as compared with 41% good or excellent results in all others. Lateral retinacular release, after chondral degeneration has already occurred, is often ineffective in resolving anterior knee pain.[38] Schonholtz and Ling performed chondroplasty for varying degrees of chondromalacia of the patella to remove loose fibrillation, but not to penetrate through subchondral bone or to débride intact cartilage.[42] At a mean 40-month follow-up, the authors reported good to excellent results in 49% of patients and fair results in 44%. They noted that 78% of patients were satisfied and that the grade of chondromalacia did not correlate with the outcome. Marrow stimulation techniques, such as microfracture, have also fared relatively poorly in treating lesions of the patellofemoral articulation. The reparative fibrocartilage tissue, composed primarily of type I collagen, is incapable of withstanding the excessive shear stress common to the patellofemoral articulation.

Tibial Tubercle Unloading Procedures

Anteromedialization of the tibial tubercle is a time-tested and well-established procedure for the treatment of patellar maltracking associated with patellofemoral malalignment.[16-18] Whereas anteriorization of the tibial tubercle reduces patellofemoral joint reaction force by increasing the angle between the patellar tendon and quadriceps tendon and increases the lever arm for extensor mechanism function, medialization of the tibial tubercle improves the Q angle and thereby decreases the strong lateral vectors acting on the patella. Combining these two components can therefore both improve patellar tracking and relieve the pain associated with subchondral overload of the lateral patellar facet. The obliquity of the tibial tubercle osteotomy allows for adjustment in the extent of anteriorization, and bone grafting is not necessary. The angle can be adjusted to accommodate varying degrees of subluxation and articular cartilage damage. Although Fulkerson has reported excellent to good results in 89% of patients monitored for more than 5 years, no patients with substantial chondromalacia (Outerbridge grade III or IV) had excellent results and satisfaction was achieved in only 75%.[17]

Direct anteriorization of the tibial tubercle has also been advocated in patients with patellofemoral arthrosis when there is no patellar subluxation or malalignment.[33] Symptom improvement with the classic Maquet osteotomy has ranged from 30% to 90%.[15,21,33] Biomechanical studies have demonstrated reductions in contact pressure; however, contact areas may shift proximally, thereby paradoxically overloading the proximal portion of the patella in deep flexion.[9] The optimal patient to benefit from a Maquet osteotomy is one with post-traumatic arthrosis or chondromalacia involving the inferior half of the patella. Patients with proximal arthrosis or diffuse patellofemoral arthrosis and those with multiple previous patellofemoral surgeries will have compromised outcomes. Its limited indications, unpredictable results, and risk of complications such as wound necrosis and osteotomy nonunion restrict the practical application of this procedure.

Cartilage Grafting

Autologous chondrocyte implantation for isolated patellar cartilage lesions has produced satisfactory results in approximately 75% at 2- to 10-year follow-up.[8,36] Proponents advise that residual patellar malalignment is a common reason for failure of this technique and should therefore be addressed before or simultaneous with autologous chondrocyte implantation.[36] Autologous osteochondral transplantation has been advocated by its innovator for patellofemoral lesions.[19] Although the duration of follow-up is not clear, Hangody reported 79% satisfactory results in those with patellar and/or trochlear mosaicplasties.[19]

Patellectomy

Patellectomy has been shown experimentally to reduce extension power by 25% to 60%, with a concomitant requisite increase in quadriceps force of 15% to 30% to achieve adequate extension torque.[23] Tibiofemoral joint reaction force may increase as much as 250%, thus explaining the propensity for tibiofemoral arthrosis after patellectomy.[12] Variable pain relief, residual quadriceps weakness, and secondary instability, with a failure rate as high as 45%, truly relegate patellectomy to being a salvage procedure for the rare patient who does poorly with other more successful interventions.[22] Additionally, the results of total knee arthroplasty can be compromised after patellectomy.[39] Therefore, patellectomy is less desirable than patellofemoral arthroplasty or total knee arthroplasty for the treatment of isolated patellofemoral arthrosis.

Total Knee Arthroplasty

Total knee arthroplasty is generally effective for elderly patients with isolated patellofemoral arthritis and yields good and excellent results in 90% to 95% of patients at midterm follow-up, although anterior knee pain has been reported in as many as 7% to 19% of patients.[26,37,40] In a study comparing total knee arthroplasty for isolated patellofemoral arthrosis with that for tricompartmental arthrosis, Knee Society clinical scores, bipedal stair climbing capacity, and ability to rise from a seated position were all significantly better in the former group.[26] Given the predictably good results of total knee arthroplasty, it is preferable to patellofemoral arthroplasty in elderly patients with isolated patellofemoral arthrosis. However, in younger patients with isolated patellofemoral arthrosis, patellofemoral arthroplasty may be favorable.

PATELLOFEMORAL ARTHROPLASTY

Patellofemoral arthroplasty may be considered in the treatment algorithm for patients with localized patellofemoral arthrosis or severe recalcitrant chondromalacia (Fig. 83–1A-F). Early designs resurfaced only the patella, using a metal implant, and left the trochlea untouched. Although the patella is commonly more degenerated than the trochlea, results have been variable with this technique.[2,32] With the recognition that residual anterior knee pain may have been related to trochlear chondromalacia, first-generation patellofemoral resurfacing arthroplasties using a polyethylene patellar component and metallic trochlear component were developed.[6,32]

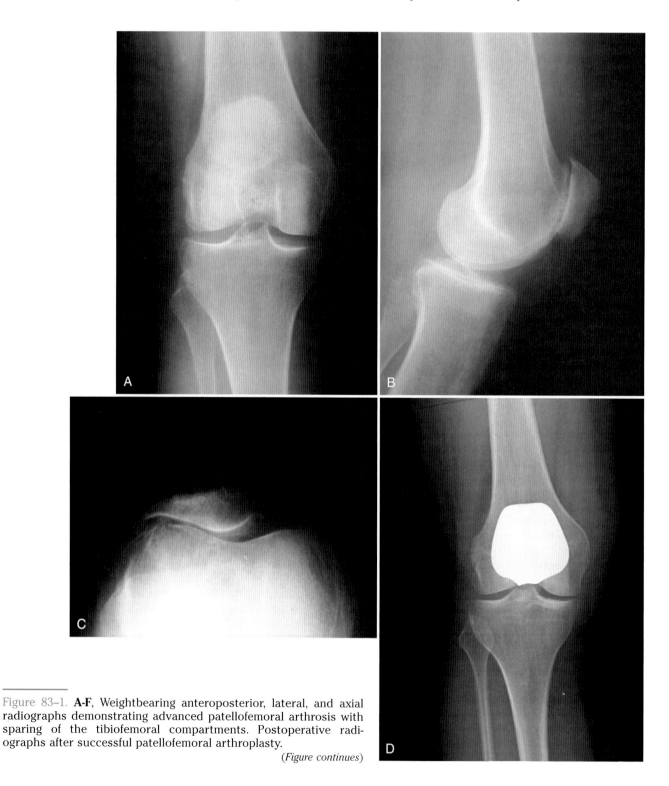

Figure 83–1. **A-F,** Weightbearing anteroposterior, lateral, and axial radiographs demonstrating advanced patellofemoral arthrosis with sparing of the tibiofemoral compartments. Postoperative radiographs after successful patellofemoral arthroplasty.

(Figure continues)

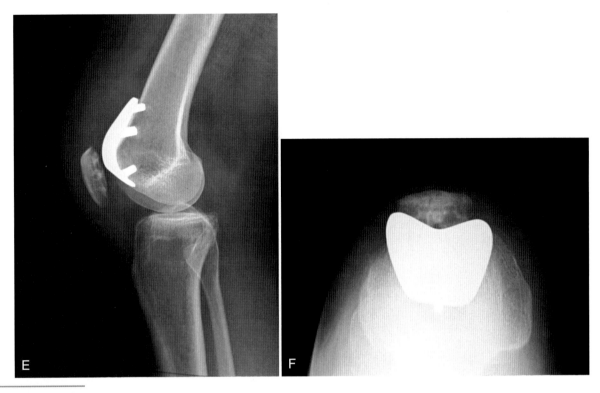

Figure 83–1, cont'd.

Patient Selection for Patellofemoral Arthroplasty

The outcome of patellofemoral arthroplasty can be optimized by limiting its application to patients with isolated patellofemoral osteoarthrosis, post-traumatic arthrosis, or severe chondrosis (Outerbridge grade IV), and then only after an extended supervised program of nonoperative measures. Additionally, this option is best reserved for patients with severe pain and functional limitations or those with considerable discomfort during activities such as stair or hill ambulation, squatting, or prolonged sitting. The procedure should not be performed in patients with inflammatory arthritis or chondrocalcinosis involving the menisci or tibiofemoral chondral surfaces, nor should it be offered to patients with inappropriate expectations.[27-29] Alternative causes of anterior knee pain should be excluded, such as patellar tendinitis, synovitis, patellar instability, sympathetic-mediated pain, or pain referred from the back or ipsilateral hip.

Although it can be most effective for treating patellofemoral dysplasia,[20] patellofemoral arthroplasty should be avoided in patients with considerable patellar maltracking or malalignment, unless these abnormalities are corrected preoperatively. This is not to say, however, that slight patellar tilt, observed on preoperative tangential radiographs or at the time of arthrotomy, or trochlear dysplasia should be considered contraindications to this procedure. In such cases, lateral retinacular release may be necessary at the time of arthrotomy.[27-29] Persistent patellar subluxation may cause pain and snapping and, potentially, polyethylene wear of the prosthesis. Patients with excessive Q angles should undergo successful tibial tubercle realignment before patellofemoral arthroplasty. Additionally, identification of tibiofemoral arthrosis during preceding arthroscopic procedures or arthrotomy for patellofemoral arthroplasty should prompt abandonment of this procedure. The presence of even focal grade III tibiofemoral chondromalacia can compromise the outcome after patellofemoral arthroplasty, although these patients will often acknowledge resolution of the most prominent component of pain.

As with other knee arthroplasty procedures, this treatment method should be restricted to patients willing to modify their activity levels to minimize stress overload and accelerated implant wear. Laborers and athletes who opt to continue their trade or aggressive recreational involvement are not ideal candidates for this procedure. Patients should be discouraged from activities that require excessive loading in deep flexion. Despite intuitive concerns, no data are available on whether obesity or cruciate ligament insufficiency places patellofemoral arthroplasty at risk for failure.

Although there are no hard and fast rules regarding age criteria for patellofemoral arthroplasty, it is an excellent alternative to total knee arthroplasty or patellectomy for patients younger than 55 with isolated anterior compartment arthrosis.[27-29,43] Elderly patients may be better suited to total knee arthroplasty because of its remarkable track record and proven survivorship and because some degree of tibiofemoral chondromalacia is ubiquitous in more elderly patients, but this contention is not universally supported[1,35] and the decision should be individualized for each patient.

Clinical Evaluation

Evaluation of a patient under consideration should be thorough to confirm that the pain is, in fact, localized to the anterior compartment of the knee and that it emanates from the patellofemoral chondral surfaces and not the soft tissues. This can usually be done by taking a detailed history of the problem and performing a meticulous physical examination.

The key elements of the history that should be elaborated include whether there was previous trauma to the knee, a history of patellar dislocation, or preceding patellofemoral "problems." A history of recurrent atraumatic patellar dislocation may suggest considerable malalignment and may need to be corrected before considering patellofemoral arthroplasty. A clear description of the location of the pain is important—discomfort anywhere but directly retropatellar or just lateral or medial to the patella will not be relieved by patellofemoral arthroplasty. Patellofemoral pain is often exacerbated by activities such as stair climbing and descent, ambulating on hills, standing from a seated position, sitting with the knee flexed, and squatting. Walking on level ground tends to not be as problematic. A description of anterior crepitus is common. After establishing the location and quality of pain, it is important to ascertain whether there were previous interventions, such as physical therapy, weight reduction, medications, injections, or surgery.

With respect to the physical examination, pain on patella inhibition testing, patellofemoral crepitus, and retropatellar knee pain with squatting are typical. Any associated medial or lateral tibiofemoral joint line tenderness should raise one's suspicion of more diffuse chondral disease (even in the presence of relatively normal radiographs) and may be a contraindication to patellofemoral arthroplasty. It is also essential to rule out other potential sources of anterior knee pain, such as pes anserinus bursitis, patellar tendinitis, prepatellar bursitis, instability, or pain referred from the ipsilateral hip or back. Careful assessment of patellar tracking and the Q angle is also important. As stated earlier, even subtle tracking abnormalities and malalignment can predispose to inferior outcomes, particularly with certain designs. In patients with high Q angles, therefore, a tibial tubercle realignment procedure (anteromedialization) should be performed before patellofemoral arthroplasty. Anterior or posterior cruciate ligament insufficiency is not a contraindication to this procedure; however, cruciate ligament reconstruction may be advisable to reduce the risk of anterior knee pain and instability and to potentially preserve the tibiofemoral articular cartilage.

Generally, weightbearing radiographs are ample imaging studies. Standing anteroposterior and midflexion posteroanterior radiographs are critical to determine the presence of tibiofemoral arthritis. Mild squaring off of the femoral condyles and even small marginal osteophytes may be accepted, provided that the patient is devoid of tibiofemoral pain during functional activities and physical examination and minimal chondral degeneration is observed at arthroscopy or arthrotomy. Lateral radiographs will occasionally demonstrate patellofemoral osteophytes, but they are generally more useful in identifying whether patella alta or baja is present. Axial radiographs will demonstrate the position of the patella within the trochlear groove and the extent of arthritis, although it is not uncommon to have apparent patellofemoral joint space preservation with minimal or no osteophytes despite significant cartilage loss. Often, subchondral sclerosis and facet "flattening" may be the only radiographic clues (see Fig. 83–1A-F). Computed tomography and magnetic resonance imaging are not necessary for evaluating patellofemoral arthrosis, although they can be useful for evaluating patellar instability. Photographs from previous arthroscopic treatment will provide valuable information regarding the extent of anterior compartment arthrosis and the status of the tibiofemoral articular cartilage and menisci.

Surgical Technique

During arthrotomy it is essential to avoid cutting normal articular cartilage or the menisci. Before proceeding with patellofemoral arthroplasty, carefully inspect the entire joint to make sure that the tibiofemoral compartments are free of disease.

The trochlear component should be externally rotated parallel to the epicondylar axis to enhance patellar tracking.[28,29] Osteophytes bordering the intercondylar notch should be removed. The trochlear component should maximize coverage of the trochlea without extending beyond the medial-lateral femoral margins anteriorly, encroaching on the weightbearing surfaces of the tibiofemoral articulations, or overhanging into the intercondylar notch. Preparation of the recipient trochlear bed should avoid excessive removal of subchondral bone, but the component edges should be flush with or recessed approximately 1 mm from the adjacent articular cartilage. The patella is resurfaced by the same principles observed in total knee arthroplasty: restoration of the original patella thickness and medialization of the component. The exposed cut surface of the lateral portion of the patella that is not covered by the patellar prosthesis should be beveled to avoid the potentially painful articulation on the trochlear prosthesis.

Assessment of patellar tracking is performed with the trial components in place. Attention is directed at identifying patellar tilt, subluxation, or catching of the components. Patellar tilt and mild subluxation can usually be addressed successfully by performing a lateral retinacular release. As stated earlier, more severe extensor mechanism malalignment (such as an excessive Q angle) should have been addressed preoperatively. With appropriate patient selection and surgical technique, proximal realignment at the time of surgery should be unnecessary in most cases, even when there is preoperative patellofemoral dysplasia and slight patellar tilt or subluxation.

Postoperative Management

Isometrics and range-of-motion exercises are started immediately. Use of a continuous passive motion machine during hospitalization (average, 2 or 3 days) may accelerate flexion recovery, but it is probably not necessary for all patients. Full weightbearing is permitted immediately, with support by crutches and a cane until adequate recovery of quadriceps strength is noted. In some circumstances, full recovery of quadriceps strength can take 6 months or longer because of the often severe preoperative quadriceps atrophy that is encountered in patients with patellofemoral arthritis. Thromboembolic prophylaxis is maintained for 4 to 6 weeks. Twenty-four hours of perioperative antibiotics is advisable, and appropriate precautions regarding antibiotic prophylaxis for dental procedures or other interventions should follow the standard recommendations of the American Academy of Orthopaedic Surgeons.[20]

Patellofemoral Scoring Systems

Relevant measures of the clinical outcome of interventions for patellofemoral arthritis are useful for communicating among practitioners, gauging the success of treatment, and comparing interventions. Although the Knee Society score and Hospital for Special Surgery score are useful for evaluation of knee arthritis treatments in general, patellofemoral-specific evaluation scales have great value when addressing patients with isolated patellofemoral disease and the treatments that are directed specifically at that underlying process. Several scales have been reported, including the Bristol score (Table 83–1), the Bartlett score (Table 83–2), the Fulkerson score (Table 83–3), and an additional scoring system that this author uses in his practice (Table 83–4). Each of these scales ascribes a certain amount of points that depend on the degree of pain, subjective and objective assessment of symptoms, and functional performance. An additional feature of the Bristol patella score is allocation of points based on physical findings observed during the physical examination.

Clinical Results

With a few exceptions, the clinical results of patellofemoral arthroplasty have been relatively constant despite differences in component design and variable indications for surgery over the past 2 or 3 decades. Most series have reported good and excellent results in roughly 85% of cases, although there have been some outliers (Table 83–5). However, in the series reviewed no uniform objective assessment measures or scoring systems were used, thus making accurate comparison of studies impossible. Additionally, several reports included patients treated with simultaneous patellofemoral and unicompartmental tibiofemoral arthroplasty, without distinguishing the clinical outcomes of those with isolated patellofemoral arthroplasty.[3,4,10] Patellar instability resulting from soft-tissue imbalance, component malposition, or malalignment of the extensor mechanism is the major source of failure in patellofemoral arthroplasty and a prominent source of residual anterior knee pain. The geometric features of some trochlear components may predispose to patellofemoral complications such as such as pain, snapping, and subluxation.[6,10,11,29,30,44,45] The radius of curvature, breadth, and degree of constraint of the trochlear component can affect patellar tracking and outcomes.[29] Although the ideal trochlear design is not yet understood, implant geometry should be such that it can be implanted flush with the anterior femoral cortex and the surrounding cartilage surfaces of the condyles. An

Table 83–1. Bristol Patella Score

SYMPTOMS

Anterior Knee Pain	
Severe	0
Moderate	1
None	2

Pain—Stairs	
Severe	0
Moderate	1
None	2

CLINICAL EXAMINATION

Patella Tenderness	
Severe	0
Moderate	1
None	2

Crepitus-Clicking-Catching	
Severe	0
Moderate	1
None	2

Malalignment	
Severe	0
Moderate	1
None	2
Total (maximum 10 points)	[ ]

From Bristol Patella Score. Bristol University, Bristol, England.

Table 83–2. Bartlett Patella Score

Anterior Knee Pain	
None	15
Mild	10
Moderate	5
Severe	0

Quadriceps Strength	
Good 5\5	5
Fair 4\5	3
Poor <4\5	1

Ability to Rise from Chair	
Able with ease (no arms)	5
Able with ease (with arms)	3
Able with difficulty	1
Unable	0

Stair Climbing	
One foot per stair—no support	5
One foot per stair—with support	4
Two feet per stair—no support	3
Two feet per stair—with support	2
Unable	0
Total (maximum 30 points)	[ ]

From Feller JA, Bartlett RJ, Lang DM: Patellar resurfacing versus retention in total knee arthroplasty. J Bone Joint Surg Br 78:226–228, 1996.

Table 83–3. Fulkerson Patellofemoral Joint Evaluation Score

CATEGORY	POINTS
Limp	
None	5
Slight or periodic	3
Severe and constant	0
Assistive Devices	
None	5
Cane or brace	3
Unable to bear weight	0
Stair Climbing	
No problem	20
Slight impairment	15
Very slowly	10
One step at a time	5
Unable	0
Crepitation	
None	5
Annoying	3
Limits activity	2
Severe	0
Instability (Giving Way)	
Never	20
Occasionally with vigorous activity	10
Frequently with vigorous activity	8
Occasionally with daily activities	5
Frequently with daily activities	2
Everyday	0
Swelling	
None	10
After vigorous activity only	5
After walking or mild activity	2
Constant	0
Pain	
None	35
Occasionally with vigorous activity	30
Marked with vigorous activity	20
Marked after walking 1 mile or mild to moderate rest pain	15
Marked with walking <1 mile	10
Constant and severe	0
Final Grading	
Excellent	91-100
Good	81-90
Fair	70-80
Poor	<69

From Fulkerson JP, Shea KP: Disorders of patellofemoral alignment. J Bone Joint Surg Am 72:1424-1429, 1990.

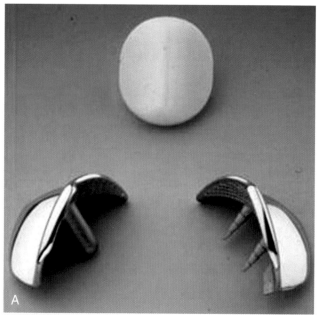
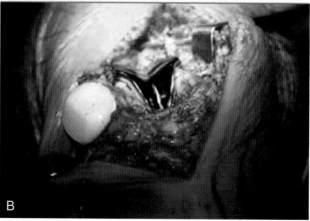

Figure 83–2. **A** and **B**, Richards II and III patellofemoral arthroplasties. The former has one central fixation lug; the latter has three fixation spikes. (Courtesy of Smith Nephew Richards, Memphis, TN.)

inadequate radius of curvature can cause patellar catching and maltracking, particularly when the implant is placed in a flexed orientation.[29] The trochlear component geometry should be relatively unconstrained and broad anteriorly to allow some freedom of tracking in extension. Narrow trochlear components can be unforgiving and predispose to catching and maltracking.[29] Improved designs have substantially reduced the incidence of patellofemoral complications, with tibiofemoral arthritis being the major source of failure.[29]

In the reported series, less than 1% of patellofemoral arthroplasties have failed because of loosening or wear of the implants, although follow-up in most series has averaged less than 7 years.* Provided that patellofemoral tracking is satisfactory, tibiofemoral degeneration may ultimately be the most common source of "failure" of contemporary patellofemoral arthroplasties. In one series with long-term follow-up, Kooijman reported that after a mean of 15.6 years (range, 10 to 21 years) after isolated patellofemoral arthroplasty, 25% of patients required secondary surgeries for progressive tibiofemoral arthritis, including 2 proximal tibial osteotomies and 10 total knee arthroplasties.[24] In other words, 75% of the implants studied were still functioning well into the second decade after implantation.

In a study by Blazina et al of 57 Richards I and II implants (Smith Nephew Richards, Memphis TN) (Fig. 83–2), nine patients had patellofemoral revisions because of implant malposition and one patient underwent

*References 1, 5, 6, 10, 11, 29, 30, 35, 44, 45.

Table 83–4. Lonner Patellofemoral Score

PATELLO FEMORAL PAIN ASSESSMENT		FUNCTIONAL ASSESSMENT	
Pain Walking on Level Ground		**Distance Able to Walk on Level Ground**	
None	10	Unlimited	5
Mild	8	More than 10 blocks	4
Moderate	3	Between 5 and 10 blocks	3
Severe	0	5 or fewer blocks	1
Pain Climbing Stairs		**Stair Climbing**	
None	10	Normally	10
Mild	8	Normally, with a railing	8
Moderate	3	One at a time with a railing	3
Severe	0	Unable to climb stairs	0
Pain Descending Stairs		**Stair Descent**	
None	10	Normally	10
Mild	8	Normally, with a railing	8
Moderate	3	One at a time with a railing	3
Severe	0	Unable to descend stairs	0
Pain Sitting in a Chair with Knee Bent		**Rising from a Chair**	
None	10	Normally, without pain	10
Mild	8	Normally, with pain	8
Moderate	3	Using hands for assistance	3
Severe	0	Unable	0
Pain Sitting with Knee Straight		**Ambulate**	
None	10	Without support	5
Mild	8	With 1 cane or crutch	3
Moderate	3	With 2 crutches	0
Severe	0	**Patella Catches/Gives Way**	
Night Pain		Never	5
No	5	With stairs or rising from chair	3
Yes	0	With any activity	0
Total pain score:	/55		
		Total functional score:	/45
		Total patellofemoral score:	/100

removal of the trochlear component and patellectomy at a mean follow-up of 2 years.[6] The authors advised that the procedure should be limited to patients with severe patellofemoral degeneration but without patellofemoral maltracking or malalignment. They also suggested that the geometry of the implants should have limited constraint and accommodate a certain degree of freedom so that subtle maltracking or technical errors would not cause catching of the implant on the trochlear edges.[6] A report by de Winter et al,[11] with a mean follow-up of 11 years, found that 7 of 26 Richards II patellofemoral arthroplasties required additional surgery as a result of patellar maltracking or implant malalignment. Two patients underwent patellar realignment, three underwent patellectomy, and two underwent total knee arthroplasty either for patellofemoral malalignment or for tibiofemoral arthritis. In a series by Krajca-Radcliffe and Coker,[25] 88% of patients with a Richards I or II patellofemoral arthroplasty had good or excellent results, but 70% had residual extensor lag, most quite subtle, at a 5.8-year mean follow-up. One patient had ongoing pain of unclear etiology and one had patellofemoral malalignment and patellar subluxation. In a series of 25 patellofemoral arthroplasties by Arciero and Toomey,[3] several failure mechanisms were reported, including persistent patellofemoral malalignment (1), component malposition (causing catching and subluxation with initiation of flexion) (2), and persistent anterior knee pain (1). Three patients in that series had

the presence or eventual development of tibiofemoral arthritis that required additional surgery at an average 5-year follow-up. An aggressive preoperative quadriceps-strengthening program should be performed, particularly in patients with considerable muscle atrophy. Cartier et al[10] reported on 72 patellofemoral Richards II and III arthroplasties with a multitude of concomitant surgical procedures, including unicompartmental arthroplasty and proximal tibial osteotomy, distal patellar realignment, or proximal patellar realignment. There were two patients with lateral patellar subluxation, one with patella baja resulting in "catching" of the patella on the trochlea, and four with progressive tibiofemoral degeneration. Kooijman et al reported an 86% long-term success rate in 45 patellofemoral arthroplasties.[24] However, secondary soft-tissue surgery was necessary in 18% of patients early on, and revision of the patellofemoral arthroplasty was necessary for catching, imbalance, or malposition in seven patients.[24]

Argenson et al reported on 66 Autocentric (DePuy, Warsaw, IN) (Fig. 83–3) patellofemoral arthroplasties with 14 concomitant procedures, including 9 tibiofemoral osteotomies and 5 distal realignments.[4] Fifteen percent were revised to total knee arthroplasty, although the precise reasons were not provided. The authors reported the best results after patellar fracture or patellar subluxation. Patients with primary degenerative arthritis of the patellofemoral articulation tended to fail at a higher rate

Table 83–5. Results of Patellofemoral Arthroplasty Series

SERIES	IMPLANT	NO. OF PFA's	AGE	DIAGNOSIS	DURATION OF FOLLOW-UP (YR)	GOOD/EXCELLENT RESULTS (%)
Blazina[6]	Richards types I & II	57	39 (range, 19-81)	NA	2 (range, 8-42 mo)	NA
Arciero[3]	Richards type II (14); CFS-Wright (11)	25	62 (range, 33-86)	OA (25); malalignment or instability (14)	5.3 (range, 3-9 yr)	85
Cartier[10]	Richards types II & III	72	65 (range, 23-89)	Dysplasia/grade IV chondromalacia (29); PTA (3); chondrocalcinosis (5)	4 (range, 2-12 yr)	85
Argenson[4]	Autocentric	66	57 (range, 19-82)	Dysplasia or dislocation (22); PTA (20); OA (24)	5.5 (range, 2-10 yr)	84
Krajca[25]	Richards types I & II	16	64 (range, 42-84)	Primary OA (10); PTA (2); recurrent dislocation (1)	5.8 (range, 2-18 yr)	88
Tauro[45]	Lubinus	62	66 (range, 50-87)	PTA (2); primary OA (74)	7.5 (range, 5-10 yr)	45
de Winter[11]	Richards type II	26	59 (range, 22-90)	Primary OA (17); malalignment (8); PTA (1)	11 (range, 1-20 yr)	76
Ackroyd[1]	Avon	95	NA	NA	2-5	83
Smith[44]	Lubinus	45	72 (range, 42-86)	Primary OA (44); PTA (1)	4 (range, 6 mo-7.5 yr)	69
Koojiman[24]	Richards type II	45	50 (range, 20-77)	OA (45)	17 (range, 15-21 yr)	86
Lonner[29]	Lubinus	30	38 (range, 34-51)	Primary OA (26); PTA (4); s/p tibial tubercle realignment (10)	4 (range, 2-6 yr)	84
Lonner[29]	Avon trochlea; Nexgen patella	25	44 (range, 28-59)	Primary OA (25); s/p realignment (2)	6 mo (range, 1 mo-1 yr)	96
Merchant[35]	LCS	15	49 (range, 30-81)	Chronic subluxation or recurrent dislocation with secondary DJD (13); chondrosis (2)	3.8 (range, 2.3-5.5 yr)	93

DJD, degenerative joint disease; LCS, Low Contact Stress Patellofemoral Joint; NA, not available; OA, osteoarthritis; PFA, patellofemoral arthroplasty; PTA, post-traumatic arthritis; s/p, status post.

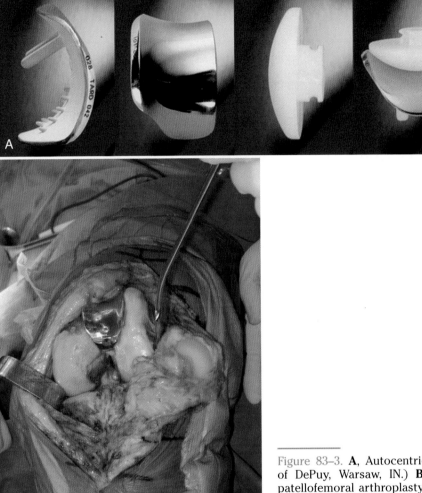

Figure 83–3. **A,** Autocentric patellofemoral arthroplasty. (Courtesy of DePuy, Warsaw, IN.) **B,** Operative appearance of autocentric patellofemoral arthroplasty 10 years after implantation. Revision to total knee arthroplasty was necessary for progressive tibiofemoral arthrosis.

than did those with underlying dysplasia or post-traumatic arthrosis, probably because of the subclinical presence of tibiofemoral degeneration at the time of arthroplasty or the subsequent development of tibiofemoral arthritis. The authors reported no cases of loosening in a cohort of cemented trochlear components, but in 4 of 24 uncemented implants, trochlear loosening occurred at a mean of 5.5 years after implantation. The authors concluded that trochlear components should be cemented. Merchant reported the short-term results of patellofemoral arthroplasty using the Low Contact Stress Patellofemoral Joint (LCS, DePuy Orthopaedics, Warsaw, IN) (Fig. 83–4) in 15 knees in 15 patients with an average age of 49 years (range, 30 to 81). At a mean follow-up of 3.8 years (range, 2.3 to 5.5 years), the authors had 93% excellent or good results. This design capitalizes on the success of the LCS total knee system (DePuy Orthopaedics, Warsaw, IN), which has an anatomically shaped mobile-bearing patella that has the potential to "self-align" within the trochlear component.[35] Although the authors cite the ability to retain the patellar component if revision to LCS total knee arthroplasty is necessary, the patellar implant will probably not safely articulate

against other tibiofemoral arthroplasties and may have to be revised during revision arthroplasty, unless the LCS total knee system is used. Additionally, even though the virtues of the low-stress concept of mobile-bearing components in total knee arthroplasty are sound, the sulcus angle of the trochlear component in this implant is 140 degrees, which despite the mobile bearing of the patellar component, may subject the implants to increased stress because of the retentive geometry, particularly if there is any degree of maltracking.

The results may be less predictable with some designs. Tauro et al[45] reported a 55% unsatisfactory rate after patellofemoral arthroplasty with the Lubinus implant (Fig. 83–5) that included the need for revision in 21 knees (28%) at a mean follow-up of 7.5 years. Fifteen knees were successfully revised for maltracking (5 to total knee arthroplasty and 10 to a patellofemoral arthroplasty with a different geometry), and 5 knees were revised to total knee arthroplasty for progressive tibiofemoral osteoarthritis. The authors reported patellar malalignment in 32% of cases, although it was not always symptomatic. There are potential design flaws with this particular implant, including an obtuse radius of curvature, a narrow anterior

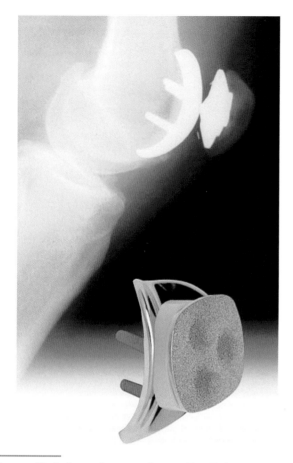

Figure 83–4. Low Contact Stress Patellofemoral Joint. (Courtesy of DePuy, Warsaw, IN.)

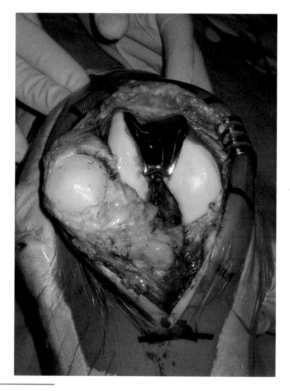

Figure 83–5. Lubinus patellofemoral arthroplasty.

trochlear surface, and limited proximal extension, all of which predispose to malposition of the trochlear component, patellar catching, and snapping in the first 30 degrees of flexion. Smith et al reviewed 45 Lubinus patellofemoral arthroplasties and found that results were worse when there was evidence of medial compartmental arthritis preoperatively.[44] In that series, five knees were converted to total knee arthroplasty—four for tibiofemoral arthritis and one for patellofemoral maltracking. Two additional patients were successfully converted to a patellofemoral arthroplasty from a different manufacturer, although the new implant was not identified.

One series reported a stratification of results, depending on which of two disparate knee designs were used. Thirty consecutive patellofemoral arthroplasties using the Lubinus implant (Link, Hamburg, Germany) were compared with 25 consecutive patellofemoral arthroplasties using the Avon (Stryker/Howmedica, Mahwah, NJ) (Fig. 83–6) trochlear component with the Nexgen (Zimmer, Warsaw, IN) all-polyethylene dome-shaped patellar component. The Nexgen patellar prosthesis has a central dome and is congruous with the Avon trochlear prosthesis. The Avon patellar component has a medialized offset dome. If future revision to a total knee arthroplasty is necessary, the central dome–shaped, all-polyethylene patellar prosthesis can be retained if not worn or loose, and it can be anticipated to articulate with most contemporary femoral implants.[31] Patients in each group had similar demographic characteristics, range of motion, and knee scores. Satisfactory results were noted in 84% of patellofemoral arthroplasties, including the Lubinus implant (30 cases) and the Avon implant (Howmedica, Stryker/Howmedica, Mahwah, NJ) (25 cases). The incidence of fair and poor results, patellofemoral dysfunction, subluxation, catching, and substantial pain was reduced from 17% with the first-generation design of the Lubinus prosthesis to less than 4% with the second-generation design of the Avon implant, although follow-up with the latter was short.[29] With the latter implant, patellar subluxation and catching have been markedly reduced; although there have been

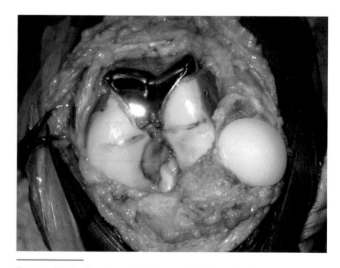

Figure 83–6. Avon patellofemoral arthroplasty.

several cases of mild anterior knee pain from soft-tissue crepitus or inflammation, the incidence is comparable to that observed after total knee arthroplasty.

Analysis of the design characteristics of disparate patellofemoral arthroplasties puts into perspective the reasons for some of the patellofemoral complications that have been associated to a greater extent with some but not other implants. The critical variables of trochlear component geometry include the sagittal radius of curvature, the proximal extension of the anterior flange, the medial-lateral breadth of the implant, and the level of constraint. Some first-generation designs had an obtuse radius of curvature, which commonly led to malposition of the trochlear prosthesis, with the implant flexed and offset proximally from the anterior surface of the femoral cortex (Fig. 83–7). This feature probably contributed to the high percentage of patellar snapping, clunking, and maltracking with those particular implants.[29,44,45] Trochlear components that have a radius of curvature that more approximates most distal femora, with nearly a 90-degree angle of curvature, have a lesser tendency to have these problems (Fig. 83–8). Another design feature to consider is the medial-lateral breadth of the anterior flange of the trochlear implants. Broader anterior surfaces (Fig. 83–9) allow a greater degree of freedom for patellar excursion and tracking than narrow implants do, which are much more confining and unforgiving of subtle tilt or subluxa-

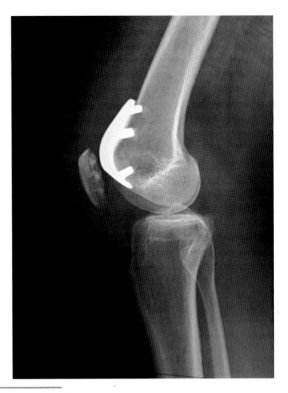

Figure 83–8. Postoperative lateral radiograph after patellofemoral arthroplasty with the Avon trochlear prosthesis radiograph showing the implant to be flush with the anterior femoral cortex. The radius of curvature is approximately 90 degrees. (From Lonner JH: Patellofemoral arthroplasty. Pros, cons, and design considerations. Clin Orthop 428:158-165, 2004.)

tion (Fig. 83–10). Finally, earlier implants with limited proximal extension on the anterior surface of the femur were vulnerable to snapping and catching of the patellar prosthesis at the point of transition from its initial articulation with the anterior femoral surface in full extension

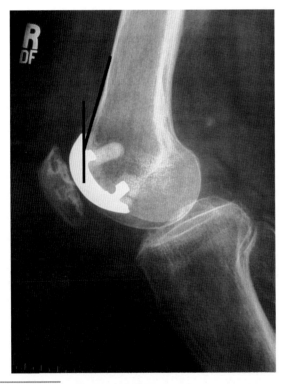

Figure 83–7. Lateral postoperative radiograph after patellofemoral arthroplasty with the Lubinus prosthesis illustrating one of the potential problems with this design, namely, that the trochlear implant must be flexed, which leaves it offset from the anterior femoral shaft and makes the patella prone to catching and subluxing. (From Lonner JH: Patellofemoral arthroplasty. Pros, cons, and design considerations. Clin Orthop 428:158-165, 2004.)

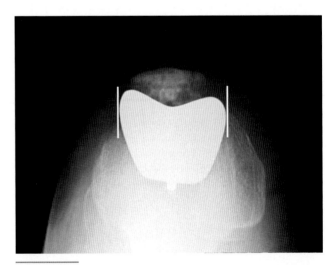

Figure 83–9. Broader anterior trochlear coverage, such as provided by the size "small" Avon prosthesis. (From Lonner JH: Patellofemoral arthroplasty. Pros, cons, and design considerations. Clin Orthop 428:158-165, 2004.)

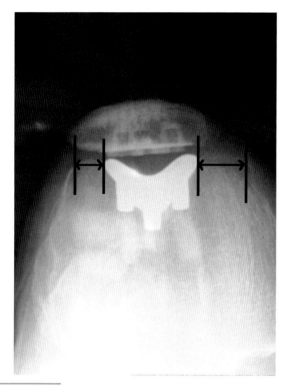

Figure 83–10. Axial radiograph of a "large" sized Lubinus trochlear component that is quite narrow. This increases the risk of subluxation with even small degrees of maltracking. There is little room for freedom of excursion. The *arrows* show the extent of uncapped cartilage anteriorly. (From Lonner JH: Patellofemoral arthroplasty. Pros, cons, and design considerations. Clin Orthop 428:158-165, 2004.)

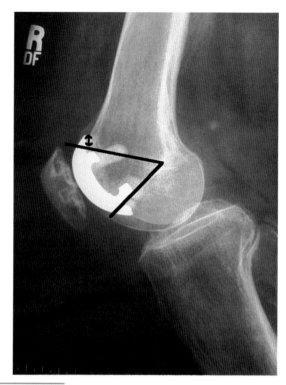

Figure 83–11. The limited proximal extension of the Lubinus femoral prosthesis above the physeal scar predisposes to catching and subluxing as the patella transitions from the native femur onto the prosthesis in the initial 30 degrees of flexion. (From Lonner JH: Patellofemoral arthroplasty. Pros, cons, and design considerations. Clin Orthop 428:158-165, 2004.)

onto the trochlear prosthesis at approximately 10 to 30 degrees of flexion, particularly if the trochlear component was flexed or offset anteriorly (Fig. 83–11). This is less likely with a trochlear prosthesis that extends further proximally because the patellar component articulates entirely with the trochlear component in extension (Fig. 83–12). The problem may be compounded by the degree of trochlear constraint in the axial plane. Trochlear components have different sulcus angles, which has an impact on patellar constraint. For instance, the trochlear angles (sulcus angles) of the Lubinus, Avon, and LCS are approximately 110, 125, and 140 degrees, respectively (Figs. 83–13 and 83–14). An increased degree of freedom within the trochlear groove is more forgiving in extension than in implants with lower sulcus angles.

Evolving designs can considerably reduce the incidence of ongoing patellofemoral dysfunction, which would leave progressive tibiofemoral arthritis or late loosening as the primary potential mechanism of failure of patellofemoral arthroplasty. If the early patellofemoral failures are excluded, the short-term failure rate is reduced. This is similar to the experience of Ackroyd et al, who reported that patellofemoral dysfunction as a result of maltracking occurred in 1% of patients with the Avon patellofemoral prosthesis at 2 to 5 years[1] versus 32% with the Lubinus patellofemoral prosthesis at 5 to 10 years.[45] The Avon prosthesis has a radius of curvature that mates better with

the femur and has a broader anterior surface that is more forgiving and captures the patella better than a narrow implant would (see Fig. 83–4A-D).

Wear of the adjacent articular cartilage from articulation of the patellar prosthesis on the uncapped femoral cartilage is a concern after patellofemoral arthroplasty. It is established that the patellofemoral joint reaction force increases in a normal knee from approximately 3.3 times body weight at 60 degrees of loaded flexion to 7.8 times body weight at 130 degrees of squatting.[41] Beyond 60 degrees, the edges of the patellar components or the cut, exposed lateral osseous patellar surface may begin to articulate, at least in part, with the adjacent femoral condyles as the trochlear components taper distally, and such articulation can predispose to wear of the exposed articular cartilage. Presently, there is no ideal bearing surface for the patella that can optimally articulate with both the femoral prosthesis and the surrounding articular cartilage.

Late failure as a result of component subsidence or loosening has not been reported with great frequency in published series. Even though the femoral component is implanted onto subchondral bone with minimal bone stock loss, long-term stress shielding of the distal femur may eventually develop, and if conversion to total knee arthroplasty is required, this bone stock deficiency may need to be addressed. However, in the short term, sub-

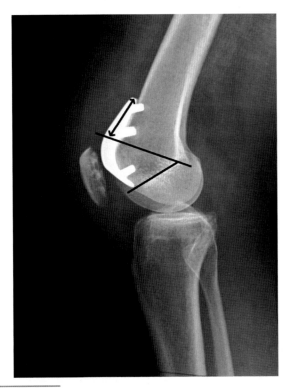

Figure 83–12. The greater proximal extension of the Avon trochlear implant above the physeal scar ensures that the patella articulates with the femoral prosthesis at all times in extension. (From Lonner JH: Patellofemoral arthroplasty. Pros, cons, and design considerations. Clin Orthop 428:158-165, 2004.)

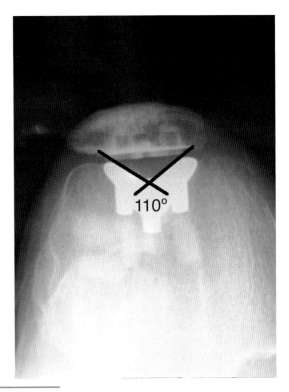

Figure 83–13. Axial radiograph showing the trochlear angle of the Lubinus implant to be approximately 110 degrees. (From Lonner JH: Patellofemoral arthroplasty. Pros, cons, and design considerations. Clin Orthop 428:158-165, 2004.)

stantial bone stock deficiency generally need not be anticipated.

The presence of pain with ambulation and need for conversion to total knee arthroplasty are obviously more likely in patients with some degree of underlying tibiofemoral arthrosis, once again underscoring the importance of careful patient selection and counseling. However, even in patients with absence of gross tibiofemoral cartilage wear at the time of arthroplasty, progressive painful tibiofemoral arthritis may develop. Arthrofibrosis is uncommon after patellofemoral arthroplasty. Although it has been reported with an incidence of 7.6% to 12% in two series, both included a number of patients who had undergone concomitant unicompartmental tibiofemoral arthroplasty but did not mention whether the tendency for arthrofibrosis was increased in those who underwent bicompartmental arthroplasty.[3,4]

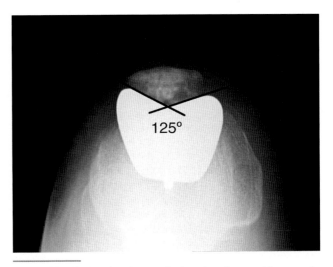

Figure 83–14. Axial radiograph showing the trochlear angle of the Avon implant to be approximately 125 degrees. (From Lonner JH: Patellofemoral arthroplasty. Pros, cons, and design considerations. Clin Orthop 428:158-165, 2004.)

Summary

Patellofemoral arthroplasty can be an effective treatment alternative for patellofemoral arthritis resulting from primary osteoarthrosis, dysplasia, or post-traumatic arthrosis in patients younger than 55 or 60 who have normal patellofemoral alignment without considerable maltracking or subluxation. Patients who have undergone previous distal realignment procedures such as tibial tubercle anteromedialization or direct anteriorization may be candidates for patellofemoral arthroplasty.

Patellofemoral arthroplasty may provide patients with substantial relief of pain from isolated patellofemoral arthrosis; however, the procedure is technically demanding and the results can be affected by the geometric features of the trochlear component. Residual instability may result in early failure, thus highlighting the importance of excluding patients with uncorrectable patellar instability or malalignment. Implant malposition, potentially hastened by particular designs, may also contribute to failures from maltracking and mechanical catching of the patella.[27,29,45] Sparing of the tibiofemoral compartments, menisci, and cruciate ligaments allows preservation of a more kinematically sound knee joint than total knee arthroplasty does. It is a particularly attractive option for young active patients with isolated patellofemoral arthrosis in whom neither total knee arthroplasty nor patellectomy is desirable, and it can be easily converted to total knee arthroplasty if necessary.

Though sparse, long-term data suggest that loosening of cemented trochlear and all-polyethylene patellar components is uncommon and that only approximately 25% of patients may need additional surgery for progressive tibiofemoral arthritis at a mean of 15 years after patellofemoral arthroplasty.[24] With emerging designs, the incidence of anterior knee pain after patellofemoral arthroplasty should be comparable to that after total knee replacement surgery, namely, approximately 4% to 7%.[26,37] Finally, even small amounts of tibiofemoral cartilage loss may compromise the results enough to warrant restricting this procedure to younger patients. The predictable success of total knee arthroplasty makes it the preferable choice in elderly patients with isolated patellofemoral arthritis.

References

1. Ackroyd CE, Newman JH, Webb JM, Eldridge JDJ: The Avon patellofemoral arthroplasty. Two to five year results. Presented at the Annual Meeting of the American Academy of Orthopaedic Surgeons, February 2003, New Orleans.
2. Aglietti P, Insall JN, Walker PS, Trent P: A new patella prosthesis. Design and application. Clin Orthop 107:175-187, 1975.
3. Arciero RA, Toomey HE: Patellofemoral arthroplasty. A three to nine year follow-up study. Clin Orthop 236:60-71, 1988.
4. Argenson JN, Guillaume JM, Aubaniac JM: Is there a place for patellofemoral arthroplasty? Clin Orthop 321:162-167, 1995.
5. Baker CL, Hughston JC: Miyakawa patellectomy. J Bone Joint Surg Am 70:1489-1494, 1988.
6. Blazina ME, Fox JM, Del Pizzo W, et al: Patellofemoral replacement. Clin Orthop 144:98-102, 1979.
7. Bristol Knee Score, Bristol University, Bristol, England.
8. Brittberg M, Tallheden T, Sjogren-Jansson E, et al: Autologous chondrocytes used for articular cartilage repair. An update. Clin Orthop 391(Suppl):S337-S348, 2001.
9. Burke DL, Ahmed AM: The effect of tibial tubercle elevation on patellofemoral loading. Trans Orthop 5:162, 1980.
10. Cartier P, Sanouiller JL, Grelsamer R: Patellofemoral arthroplasty. J Arthroplasty 5:49-55, 1990.
11. de Winter WE, Feith R, van Loon CJ: The Richards type II patellofemoral arthroplasty: 26 cases followed for 1-20 years. Acta Orthop Scand 72:487-490, 2001.
12. Dinham JM, French PR: Results of patellectomy for osteoarthritis. Postgrad Med J 48:590-593, 1972.
13. Federico DJ, Reider B: Results of isolated patellar debridement for patellofemoral pain in patients with normal patellar alignment. Am J Sports Med 25:663-669, 1997.
14. Feller JA, Bartlett RJ, Lang DM: Patellar resurfacing versus retention in total knee arthroplasty. J Bone Joint Surg Br 78:226-228, 1996.
15. Ferguson AB Jr: Elevation of the insertion of the patellar ligament for patellofemoral pain. J Bone Joint Surg Am 64:766-771, 1982.
16. Fulkerson JP: Anteromedialization of the tibial tuberosity for patellofemoral malalignment. Clin Orthop 177:176-181, 1983.
17. Fulkerson JP, Becker GJ, Meaney JA, et al: Anteromedial tibial tubercle transfer without bone graft. Am J Sports Med 18:490-497, 1990.
18. Fulkerson JP, Shea KP: Disorders of patellofemoral alignment. J Bone Joint Surg Am 72:1424-1429, 1990.
19. Hangody L, Fules P: Autologous osteochondral mosaicplasty for the treatment of full-thickness defects of weight-bearing joints. J Bone Joint Surg Am 85(Suppl 2):25-32, 2003.
20. Hanssen AD, Osmon DR, Nelson CL: Prevention of deep periprosthetic joint infection. J Bone Joint Surg Am 78:458-471, 1996.
21. Heatley FW, Allen PR, Patrick JH: Tibial tubercle advancement for anterior knee pain. A temporary or permanent solution. Clin Orthop 208:215-224, 1986.
22. Ivey FM, Blazina ME, Fox JM, Del Pizzo W: Reoperation following patellectomy for chondromalacia. Orthopedics 2:134, 1979.
23. Kaufer H: Mechanical function of the patella. J Bone Joint Surg Am 53:1151-1560, 1971.
24. Kooijman HJ, Driessen APPM, van Horn JR: Long-term results of patellofemoral arthroplasty. J Bone Joint Surg Br 85:836-840, 2003.
25. Krajca-Radcliffe JB, Coker TP: Patellofemoral arthroplasty. A 2 to 18 year follow up study. Clin Orthop 330:143-151, 1996.
26. Laskin RS, Van Steijn M: Total knee replacement for patients with patellofemoral arthritis. Clin Orthop 367:89-95, 1999.
27. Lonner JH: Patellofemoral arthroplasty. Semin Arthroplasty 11:234-240, 2000.
28. Lonner JH: Patellofemoral arthroplasty. Tech Knee Surg 2:144-152, 2003.
29. Lonner JH: Patellofemoral arthroplasty: Pros, cons, design considerations. Clin Orthop 428:158-165, 2004.
30. Lonner JH, Booth RE: Patellofemoral arthroplasty. J Am Acad Orthop Surg June 2005.
31. Lonner JH, Mont MA, Sharkey P, et al: Fate of the unrevised all-polyethylene patellar component in revision total knee arthroplasty. J Bone Joint Surg Am 85:56-59, 2003.
32. Lubinus HH: Patella glide bearing total replacement. Orthopedics 2:119, 1979.
33. Maquet P: Advancement of the tibial tuberosity. Clin Orthop 115:225-230, 1976.
34. McAlindon RE, Snow S, Cooper C, Dieppe PA: Radiographic patterns of osteoarthritis of the knee joint in the community: The importance of the patellofemoral joint. Ann Rheum Dis 51:844-849, 1992.
35. Merchant AC: Early results with a total patellofemoral joint replacement arthroplasty prosthesis. J Arthroplasty 19:829-836, 2004.
36. Minas T, Chiu R: Autologous chondrocyte implantation. Am J Knee Surg 13:41-50, 2000.
37. Mont MA, Haas S, Mullick T, Hungerford DS: Total knee arthroplasty for patellofemoral arthritis. J Bone Joint Surg Am 84:1977-1981, 2002.
38. Osborne AH, Fulord PC: Lateral release for chondromalacia patellae. J Bone Joint Surg Br 64:202-205, 1982.
39. Paletta G, Laskin RS: Total knee replacement in the patient who had undergone patellectomy. J Bone Joint Surg Am 77:1708-1712, 1995.
40. Parvizi J, Stuart MJ, Pagnano MW, Hanssen AD: Total knee arthroplasty in patients with isolated patellofemoral arthritis. Clin Orthop 392:147-152, 2001.
41. Reilly DT, Martens M: Experimental analysis of the quadriceps muscle force and patello-femoral joint reaction force for various activities. Acta Orthop Scand 43:126-137, 1972.
42. Schonholtz G, Ling B: Arthroscopic chondroplasty of the patella. Arthroscopy 1:92-96, 1985.
43. Sisto DJ: Patellofemoral degenerative joint disease. In Fu FH, Harner CD, Vince K (eds): Knee Surgery. Baltimore, Williams & Wilkins, pp 1203-1221.
44. Smith AM, Peckett WRC, Butler-Manuel PA, et al: Treatment of patellofemoral arthritis using the Lubinus patellofemoral arthroplasty. A retrospective review. Knee 9:27-30, 2002.
45. Tauro B, Ackroyd CE, Newman JH, Shah NA: The Lubinus patellofemoral arthroplasty. A five to ten year prospective study. J Bone Joint Surg Br 83:696-701, 2001.
46. Vuorinen O, Paakkala T, Tunturi T, et al: Chondromalacia patellae: Results of operative treatments. Arch Orthop Trauma Surg 104:175-181, 1985.
47. Witvrouw E, Cambier D, Danneels L, et al: The effect of exercise regimens on reflex response time of the vasti muscles in patients with anterior knee pain: A prospective randomized intervention study. Scand J Med Sci Sports 13:251-258, 2003.

CHAPTER 84

Surgical Techniques and Instrumentation in Total Knee Arthroplasty

Thomas Parker Vail • Jason E. Lang

Surgical techniques and instrumentation in total knee arthroplasty (TKA) are based on the pioneering innovation and careful thoughts of John Insall. In updating this chapter, every effort has been made to maintain the tone and emphasis on basic concepts relevant to successful knee arthroplasty so well written in the last iteration of this chapter by Insall and Easley. Changes in this chapter reflect new thought that has developed out of published reports and clinical experience in the intervening years.

RELEVANT KNEE ANATOMY AND ALIGNMENT

It is important to examine a patient's knee in three positions: weightless, standing, and when walking. The weightless examination, with the patient either seated or supine, allows careful assessment of ligament competence, range of motion, and passive patellar tracking. With the patient standing, one can assess overall axial alignment of the leg, the angle of the joint line in stance, and the static position of the patella. Evaluation of the patient while walking allows one to add a dynamic component to the examination, determine the presence of antalgic movement, and assess the contribution of soft-tissue impingement of the thighs and varus or valgus thrust during active stance. There is considerable variation in body habitus, and one must be cautious in describing what is "normal." However, the following description represents consensus.[73,106]

Static Alignment

The mechanical axis of the leg (Fig. 84–1) is formed by a line that passes from the center of the hip through the center of the knee into the center of the ankle joint. The offset is the distance between the femoral shaft and the center of rotation of the hip, which is determined by the length and angle of the femoral neck. There is a valgus angle of 7 degrees (variability in this angle has to do with the width of the pelvis in addition to the offset of the femoral neck) between the femoral and tibial shafts. The proximal-to-distal mechanical axis forms an angle of 3 degrees with the midline vertical axis of the body. The transverse axis of the knee joint is perpendicular to the midline vertical axis of the body and thus forms a 3-degree

angle with the axis of the tibial shaft and a 10-degree angle with the axis of the femoral shaft. Hungerford and Krackow[71] and Townley[172] have pointed out that the "normal" angle of varus is variable as a result of inherited and developmental anatomic factors such as pelvic width, femoral neck varus, femoral and tibial bowing, physeal growth, and femoral length. Because of this arrangement, the distribution of body weight when standing is more medial than lateral in each knee.[69,76,119,172]

Dynamic Alignment

During normal walking, the center of gravity of the body moves toward the supporting leg during each gait cycle. However, the distribution of contact force across the knee joint is not symmetric; it is estimated that between 60% and 75% of this force is carried by the medial compartment of the knee.[65,80,119]

Johnson et al[80] noted that during normal walking, a greater medial load than would be predicted is observed because of the laterally directed ground reaction force. The force does not rest on a perpendicular tibial plateau because the anatomic tibial plateau is sloped 2 to 10 degrees posteriorly and distally. However, when the menisci are taken into account, tibial plateaus are not posteriorly sloped; only the bony surfaces give the appearance of posterior slope. Furthermore, the medial tibial subchondral bone is concave ("dished") relative to the more convex lateral tibial subchondral surface. When combined with the 3-degree angle of the tibial anatomic axis relative to the transverse knee axis, a varus moment is imparted during normal gait. This lateral "thrust" is resisted by the lateral stabilizing force arising from the capsule, the lateral collateral ligament (LCL), the cruciate ligaments, the ligamentum patellae, and the iliotibial band (ITB).[106]

Abnormal patterns of gait can also affect loading of the knee joint. Muscle imbalance as a result of deconditioning or obesity can accentuate a varus thrust or cause the thighs to rub together during the swing phase of gait. Gait studies performed on obese patients have demonstrated locomotor adaptations, such as slower speed, shorter steps, increased double support time, and decreased range of motion of the knee.[111,113,161] Additionally, Sharma et al[156] reported on a correlation between body mass index and severity of osteoarthritis in knees with varus malalignment that was not seen in knees with valgus malalignment. Likewise, compensatory external rotation of the foot is a

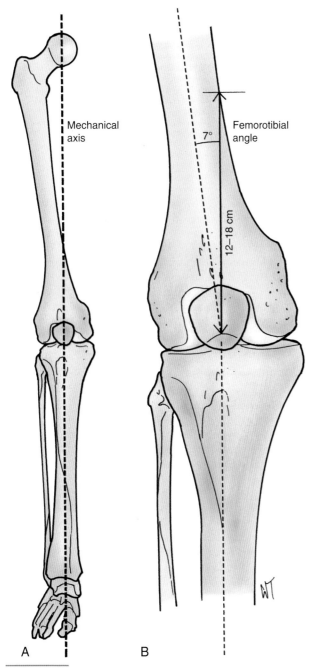

Figure 84–1. The mechanical axis (**A**) usually corresponds to a femorotibial angle (**B**) of about 7 degrees and intersects the medial femoral cortex 12 to 18 cm proximal to the knee.

mechanism of unloading a painful medial compartment during stance.

OBJECTIVES OF PROSTHETIC REPLACEMENT

The foregoing description applies to the normal condition, but it must be appreciated that many patients with

osteoarthritis of the knee have contributing anatomic variations such as habitual varus or valgus alignment. One must ask how closely prosthetic components should duplicate normal anatomy; for example, should the forces across a knee arthroplasty be borne predominantly by the medial compartment? How should the alignment of a prosthetic knee joint be changed to accommodate pathological alterations in gait that are not restored to normal even after prosthetic replacement?

It was Insall's opinion that the objective of prosthetic replacement is to distribute contact stress across the artificial joint as symmetrically as possible while avoiding overloading of one compartment. This philosophy can require altering an individual's prearthritic anatomy. For example, it is likely that many patients with medial compartment arthritis of the knee have been bowlegged since childhood; to restore prearthritic alignment, though "normal" for these people, would result in a component positioned in more varus than is generally considered acceptable after knee arthroplasty.

There are also practical considerations that affect proper implant alignment. Given the factor of human error, reproducibility is important. Instrumentation and careful technique can minimize the incidence of component malposition. Computer navigation of knee surgery may have a positive impact on the issue of reproducibility in the future by decreasing the number of "outliers."[24] For most surgeons, it is easier to make a right-angle bone cut than an oblique one, and it is easier (and thus more reproducible) to make a cut across the upper part of the tibia at right angles to the tibial shaft rather than make a cut that is inclined 3 degrees medially and 10 degrees posteriorly (Fig. 84–2). Moreover, if angle cuts are not appropriately adjusted from a rotational perspective, further inaccuracies result; for example, an intended 10-degree posterior slope may result in a combination of posterior and valgus slope if the cutting guide is internally rotated (Fig. 84–3). In addition, since referencing off the pathological bone surfaces is likely to result in errors in both angular and rotational alignment because of loss of bone and absence of the soft-tissue contribution to alignment, one might choose to not reproduce the original joint surfaces. In pathological states, which in themselves create secondary changes in the ligaments, this difficulty is obviously compounded.

Insall believed that restoration of "normal" anatomy was not often achieved and perhaps was not important to success. Evidence to support this assertion is that early models of knee prostheses were crude, often grossly mismatched in size, incompatible with ligamentous structures, and often inexpertly inserted. Many of these devices failed, but a surprising number not only worked well but continued to do so for many years, thus proving the human body's remarkable resilience (Fig. 84–4). As clinical experience increased, surgical expertise improved, and prosthetic design became more sophisticated, more durable, and more "natural." Today, in addition to painlessness, normality of feel, less invasive approaches, and a high level of function are expected. Furthermore, some individuals require special consideration, such as Middle Eastern and Asian patients, who need significant knee flexion during prayer.

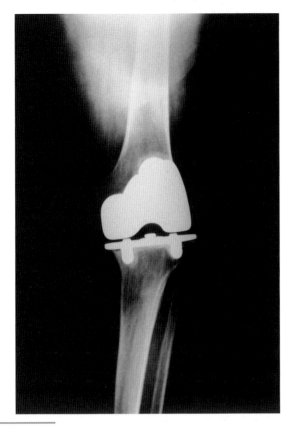

Figure 84–2. Radiograph of a prosthesis with a varus tibial cut. The instrument system designed for this prosthesis recommended a 3-degree tibial cut because this slope more closely duplicates normal anatomy. In practice, it often led to a greater and undesirable sloping cut in the tibia.

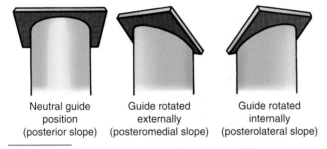

Neutral guide position (posterior slope) Guide rotated externally (posteromedial slope) Guide rotated internally (posterolateral slope)

Figure 84–3. Care must be taken when making a 10-degree posterior slope on the tibial cut. The guide must be placed in the neutral position. When it is externally rotated, a posteromedial slope (varus) will be produced. When the guide is internally rotated, a posterolateral slope (valgus) will result.

Polyethylene wear continues to be a major clinical issue. Designers of knee implants have two possible routes to minimize wear potential: decreasing contact stress or changing the mechanical properties of the bearing surface. Ideal "anatomic," highly conforming joint surfaces may conflict with the bioengineering requirements needed to reduce wear. In addition, modularity has introduced the potential for wear secondary to micromotion between the polyethylene insert and the tibial tray.[56,128,176,178] At least

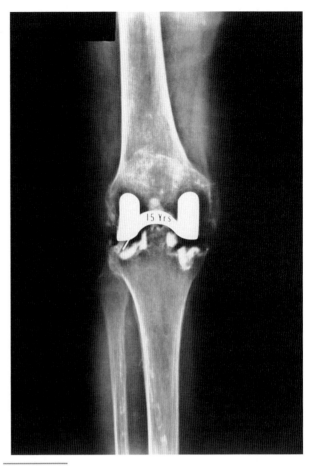

Figure 84–4. Radiograph at a 15-year follow-up of a duo-condylar prosthesis with two separate tibial components. There is the appearance of osteopenia around the femoral component runners. The knee continued to function well.

partial conformity between the components is considered necessary to reduce high polyethylene stress and provide acceptable durability. All current fixed-bearing designs are compromises between conformity and mobility. Increasing conformity at the bearing surface can be combined with mobility at the backside to reduce contact stress without restricting mobility. This combination of conformity and motion is the theory behind the mobile-bearing total knee concept. Cross-linking of polyethylene may have an impact on the generation of wear debris in knee arthroplasty, but the optimal balance between improvement in wear properties and reduction in mechanical properties remains to be defined.[27]

THEORIES OF SURGICAL TECHNIQUE

The development of implants and instruments led to two distinct surgical techniques during the early days of knee arthroplasty: the gap technique and the measured resection technique.[38] Over time, instrument systems have adopted aspects of both philosophies, thus blurring the distinctions. The gap technique was developed in conjunction with the design of cruciate-substituting prostheses. The measured resection technique was developed by surgeons and designers who favored cruciate retention and emphasized measured femoral and tibial resection as the primary consideration.

Gap Technique

The gap technique[55,73,75] is used in conjunction with cruciate-substituting prostheses and some cruciate-retaining devices (often accompanied by posterior cruciate release from the posterior tibial insertion). Ligament releases (see later) are performed to correct fixed deformity by bringing the limb into approximate alignment before the bone cuts are made (Fig. 84–5).

The gap technique was developed at a time when a limited number of anteroposterior femoral sizes were available, which frequently dictated that a relatively small femoral component be fitted onto a larger distal femur. This typically necessitated over-resection of the posterior femoral condyles. To appropriately balance the flexion gap and avoid flexion instability, less proximal tibial resection was performed at the risk of creating a tight extension gap. In fact, the largest available tibial polyethylene insert was approximately 15 mm. Leaving a substantial amount of proximal tibial bone was in accordance with the belief that the proximal tibial bone weakened significantly with resection greater than 5 mm. The gap technique is still used, but because most systems have a full complement of component sizes, posterior femoral over-resection is less likely, and the flexion gap may be balanced even with proximal tibial resection greater than 10 mm.

A particular sequence of steps in balancing the flexion gap was not deemed essential for the gap technique; the femur or tibia may be osteotomized first, the goal being to create a balanced flexion gap (Fig. 84–6). Insall would traditionally perform the tibial cut first but would often begin with contouring the femur when referencing instruments were adequately placed on the posterior femoral condyles. The proximal tibial osteotomy is performed 10 mm below the least compromised articular cartilage (Fig. 84–7). A perpendicular tibial cut establishes proper limb alignment with reference to the distal femoral cut. Harada et al[64] suggested that the proximal end of the tibia weakens below a depth of 5 mm, thus prompting many surgeons to resect as little bone as possible and requiring the use of thinner polyethylene inserts at the risk of stress-related wear.[192] Clinical experience plus later research on tibial bone strength[58] has supported a 10-mm cut below the joint line, thereby obviating the need to use excessively thin polyethylene components. When the gap theory is applied to cruciate-retaining designs, the posterior cruciate ligament (PCL) may be retained if it is appropriately balanced and the joint line position is restored with modular tibial inserts.

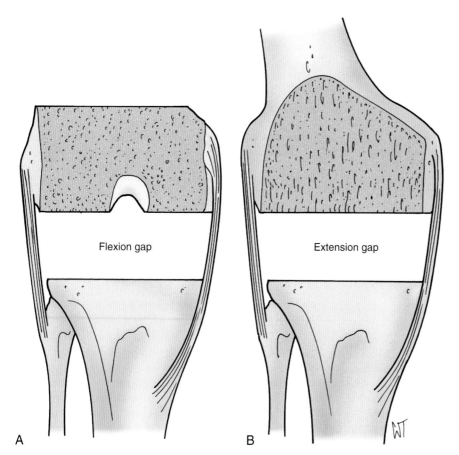

Flexion gap

Extension gap

A   B

Figure 84–5. The extension gap (**B**) must exactly equal the flexion gap (**A**).

ROTATIONAL ALIGNMENT OF THE FEMUR

Rotational alignment of the femoral component is determined by the distal femoral anatomy and is influenced to some degree by the condition of the medial soft tissues. When medial release is not required for axial alignment, some external rotation of the femoral anteroposterior cutting block is needed to compensate for the normal medial inclination of the tibial plateau and the flexion laxity of the lateral ligamentous structures (Fig. 84–8). Only by this external rotation can a rectangular "flexion gap" be produced (Figs. 84–9 and 84–10). However, when a medial soft-tissue release is performed, a rectangular flexion gap is created by the ligament release itself, and the femoral template can be positioned anatomically relative to the epicondylar axis of the distal end of the femur.

Proper femoral rotation is essential because inappropriate rotation of the femoral component may result in flexion imbalance and patellofemoral problems.[7,12,133] Although an arbitrary external rotation of 3 degrees is often satisfactory,[53,134] several methods have been developed in an effort to accurately determine appropriate femoral rotation (Fig. 84–11):

1. Medial and lateral epicondyles[14,130]
2. Posterior femoral condyles[63]
3. Anteroposterior femoral axis ("Whiteside's line")[8,185]
4. Tibial shaft axis[164]
5. Ligament tension

Femoral rotation is difficult to instrument precisely because of surface landmark inconsistencies and obscurities; accordingly, surgeons must form their own judgment and make sure to err on the side of external rotation, *never* internal rotation.[7,12,133] The posterior condylar axis is frequently used as the reference for femoral rotation; however, posterior condylar erosion as part of the arthritic process, particularly in a valgus knee, often distorts this reference angle, and thus it should probably not be relied on as the sole method of determining femoral rotation.[63,164] The anteroposterior axis of the femoral sulcus, described by Whiteside,[8,185] has also been shown to be an accurate reference point for determining femoral rotation, although it has been noted to be less reliable in cases of trochlear dysplasia and some valgus knees.[130] The tibial shaft axis has likewise been described as an effective reference axis for defining femoral rotation.[164] Using the anatomic axis of the tibia is particularly useful because it should facilitate balancing the flexion space when perpendicular proximal tibial cuts are made for TKA.

Insall preferred the epicondylar axis to most closely recreate the patient's natural femoral rotation.[14,130] The center of the medial epicondyle is located in the sulcus that lies between the proximal origin of the superficial medial collateral ligament (MCL) and the proximal origin of the deep MCL. The medial epicondylar ridge at the origin of the superficial MCL can be identified by isolating the condylar vessels that lie proximal and anterior to the medial epicondylar ridge. From these vessels the epicondylar ridge can readily be outlined; the center of this outline is the sulcus, which can typically be palpated

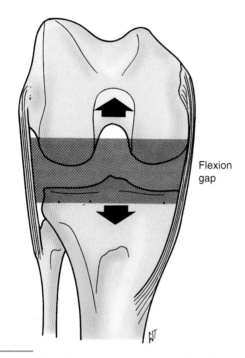

Figure 84–6. The flexion gap is created first by removing bone from the tibial plateaus and posterior femoral condyles.

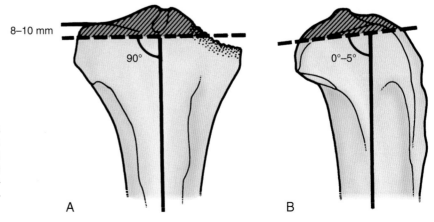

Figure 84–7. The correct cut on the tibia ignores defects and removes 10 mm from the less compromised side, cut at right angles to the long axis in the coronal plane (**A**) and sloped posteriorly no more than 5 degrees in the sagittal plane (**B**).

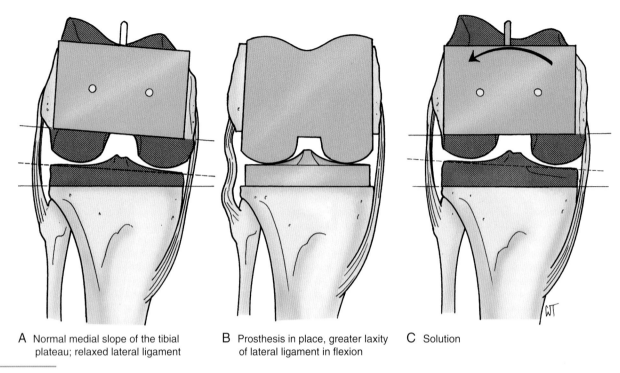

A Normal medial slope of the tibial
   plateau; relaxed lateral ligament

B Prosthesis in place, greater laxity
   of lateral ligament in flexion

C Solution

Figure 84–8. Imitating the normal anatomy results in lateral laxity in flexion.

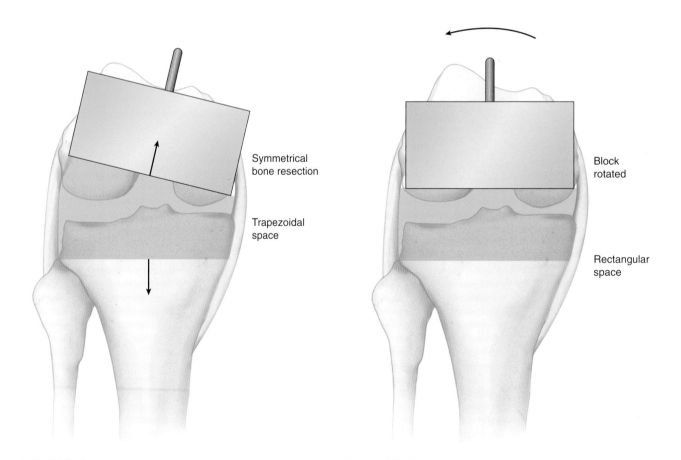

Symmetrical
bone resection

Trapezoidal
space

Block
rotated

Rectangular
space

Figure 84–9. In an osteoarthritic knee, lateral laxity is accentuated; when symmetric bone is excised from the posterior femoral condyles, the resulting space on distraction is trapezoidal.

Figure 84–10. By externally rotating the femoral component and removing an asymmetric amount of bone from the posterior femoral condyles, soft-tissue length is equalized and the resulting space is rectangular.

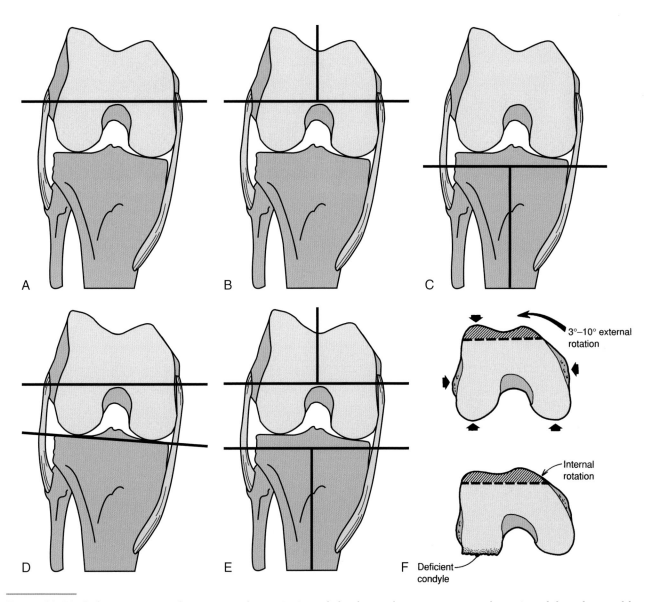

Figure 84–11. Reference points for rotational positioning of the femoral component are the epicondyles, the trochlear surface, the tibial shaft, and the posterior condyles. **A,** The transepicondylar axis. **B,** The anteroposterior trochlear sulcus ("Whiteside's line"). **C,** The tibial shaft axis. **D,** The posterior condylar angle. **E,** The transepicondylar axis is perpendicular to the anteroposterior sulcus line and the tibial shaft axis. **F,** When the posterior condyles are used for rotational reference, one must beware of erosion of the condyles. For example, in valgus knees, posterior erosion of the lateral femoral condyle is often present, which may result in internal rotation of the femoral component.

without dissection (Fig. 84–12). The lateral epicondyle is the most prominent point on the lateral aspect of the distal end of the femur. Here, too, following the leash of condylar vessels confirms the exact location of the lateral epicondyle, which lies immediately distal to the vessels (Fig. 84–13). The line across the distal end of the femur connecting the epicondyles is the epicondylar axis.

The benefit of having several different methods of assessing femoral rotation is that one or more can be used to confirm the surgeon's preferred method (Fig. 84–14). Several investigators have compared these various methods. Poilvache et al[130] correlated the transepicondylar, anteroposterior, and posterior condylar axes. Berger et al[14] and Griffin et al[62] described the relationship of the epicondylar axis to the posterior condylar axis. Whiteside[8,185]

defined the relationship of the anteroposterior and posterior condylar axes. Stiehl and Cherveny[164] demonstrated that referencing from the tibial shaft axis is more accurate than referencing from the posterior condylar axis. More recently, Katz et al[84] found that using the transepicondylar axis was less predictable and resulted in excessive external rotation when compared with the anteroposterior axis and the balanced tension line. Fehring[50] reported rotational errors of at least 3 degrees occurring in 45% of patients when rotation was determined by fixed bony landmarks as compared with the balanced tension line. Ultimately, determination of whether the rotation is "correct" will be made by proper tracking of the patella and unconstrained movement of the tibiofemoral articulation.

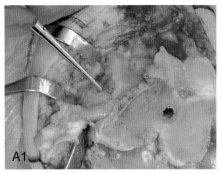
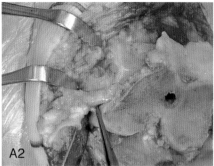
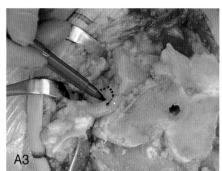

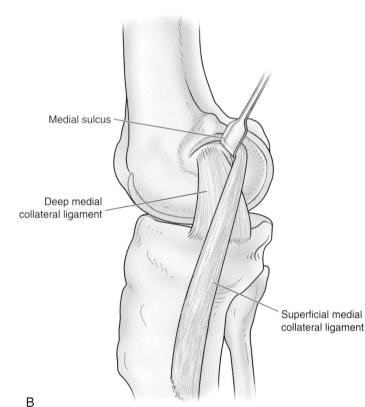

Medial sulcus

Deep medial
collateral ligament

Superficial medial
collateral ligament

B

Figure 84–12. **A,** Intraoperative photos of the medial epicondyle. **A1,** Leash of vessels over the insertion of the superficial medial collateral ligament (MCL). **A2,** Instrument placed to define the insertion of the deep MCL. **A3,** Between the two MCL insertions, at the medial sulcus, the medial epicondyle is marked in a "bull's-eye" fashion. **B,** Deep to the superficial MCL, the deep MCL overlies the medial sulcus, the palpable focus of the medial epicondyle.

ANTERIOR VERSUS POSTERIOR REFERENCING

Flexion Gap

Given the limited number of femoral component sizes available in the early days when the gap-balancing technique was developed, there was seldom an exact match between the sagittal dimension of the femoral component and the actual size of the bone, thus necessitating some compromise. With anterior referencing, the size of the component is based on the amount of the posterior femoral condyles that is removed, and therefore the flexion gap after resection will vary from anatomic if the exact amount of resected condyle is not replaced by the femoral implant. Adjustments in distal femoral resection may be necessary to balance the gaps when the posterior condyles are over-resected. Over-resection of the posterior condyles can cause flexion instability, and under-resection can lead to excessive tightness in flexion, particularly when the PCL is preserved. Conversely, with posterior referencing (Fig. 84–15), the flexion gap is con-

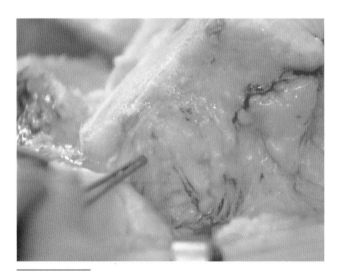

Figure 84–13. Intraoperative photo of the lateral epicondyle, the most prominent point on the lateral aspect of the distal end of the femur.

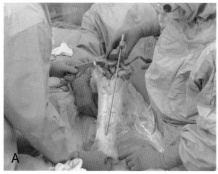
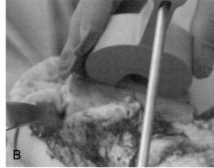
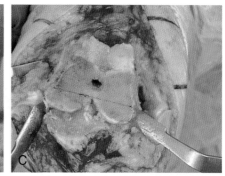

Figure 84–14. Confirming proper femoral rotation. **A,** Tibial shaft axis. **B,** Comparing the transepicondylar and tibial shaft axes. **C,** Transepicondylar axis.

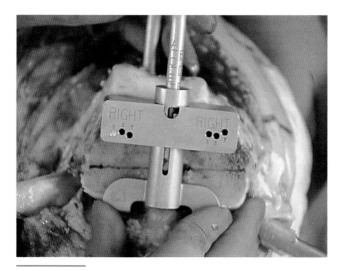

Figure 84–15. An instrument used for sagittal sizing of the femur.

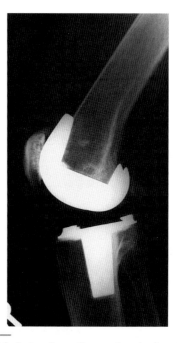

Figure 84–16. Lateral radiograph demonstrating the femoral component cemented in 3 degrees of flexion to avoid anterior notching of the femur.

stant, but there is danger of "notching" the anterior femoral cortex or having the femoral flange sit proud of the distal femoral cortex. To compensate for in-between sizing, Insall recommended downsizing components and placement of the femoral component in slight flexion (typically 3 degrees) to lessen the risk of anterior notching (Fig. 84–16). The same effect can be achieved if the instrument system creates a slightly divergent (as opposed to parallel to the anterior cortex) anterior cut, which also minimizes the risk of anterior femoral notching.

After the cut is made, the flexion gap between the surfaces of the posterior femoral condyles and proximal end of the tibia is measured. Insall's original description included spacer blocks to determine the gap size (Fig. 84–17); an alternative is to use tensor devices to measure the soft tissue tension on the medial and lateral side of the gap (Figs. 84–18 and 84–19). With the use of tensors, the proximal tibial cut is made first to properly tension the flexion space (Fig. 84–20). The size of this space corresponds to the combined thickness of the tibial and femoral components and determines the thickness of the tibial component required to stabilize the knee in flexion. If the flexion gap is asymmetric, further ligament release procedures, described later, may be necessary to establish

flexion space symmetry. Alternatively, flexion space asymmetry may be the result of improper femoral rotation, and in this case adjustment of the AP femoral cut is required to correct rotation and balance the flexion gap.

Extension Gap

As with the flexion gap, sizing of the extension gap is performed by using either spacers or a tensioning device. The distal femoral osteotomy is performed after the proximal tibial cut is completed at a predetermined level (usually 10 mm above the joint line) corresponding to the thickness of the femoral component (Fig. 84–21). The extension space so formed is then assessed with a spacer block or tensiometer, and the distal end of the femur is recut when necessary to match the flexion gap (see Fig. 84–18). In this way, the amount of additional resection can be calculated from the difference between the thickness of the

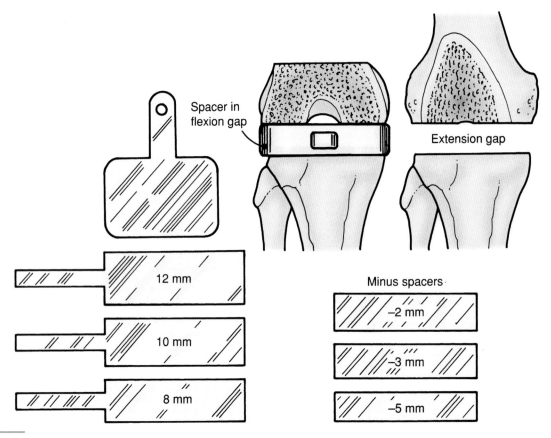

Figure 84–17. The flexion and extension gaps are assessed by a series of spacers. When the extension gap is smaller than the flexion gap, it must be equalized by resection of extra distal femoral bone. The amount needed is assessed by using the spacer system. Minus spacers are available when the flexion gap requires the thinnest (8 mm) spacer.

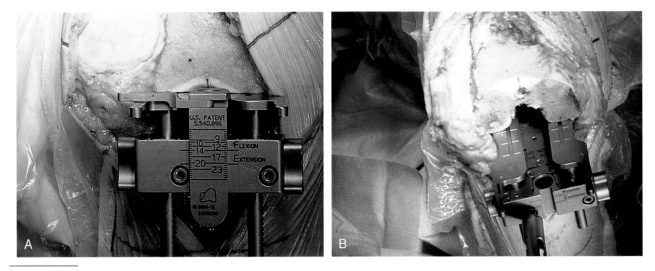

Figure 84–18. Close-up intraoperative view of a tensor. **A**, In extension. **B**, In flexion.

flexion block and the extension block. Cutting away more distal femoral bone than the femoral component will ultimately replace should be minimized because it will elevate the joint line. When a preoperative flexion contracture contributes to gap imbalance, appropriate soft-tissue balancing and posterior release should be performed before considering additional bone resection.

An alternative to using a predetermined distal femoral resection is to cut the extension gap according to the measured height of the flexion gap. The knee is extended and axial traction is applied to the limb with a mechanical device such as a tensor (see Figs. 84–18 to 84–20). With the soft tissue under tension, the level of distal femoral osteotomy is determined by the thickness of

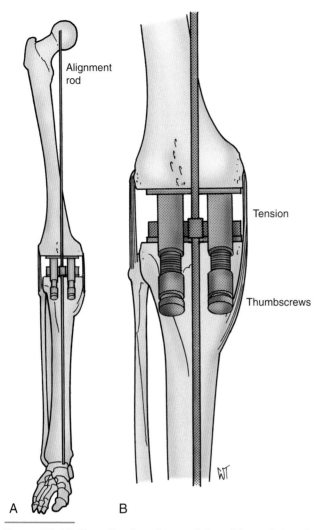

Figure 84–19. By adjusting the medial and lateral thumbscrews of the tensor, the alignment rod is brought into the mechanical axis.

spacer blocks that fit the flexion gap. A distal femoral osteotomy is performed at this level perpendicular to the mechanical axis and at a measured valgus angle relative to the anatomic axis of the femur (Figs. 84–22 to 84–24) The valgus cut on the distal end of the femur relative to the anatomic axis is the difference between the anatomic and mechanical axis, which can be measured on long-cassette radiographs. Once again, the surgeon should be cognizant of the fact that removing more distal bone than the femoral implant replaces will result in elevation of the joint line.

PROS AND CONS OF THE GAP-BALANCING TECHNIQUE

The essential philosophy of the gap technique is that it builds on the state of the soft tissues after the initial soft-tissue correction. The soft-tissue correction is performed first and the measured gap resection is performed next. This technique can be readily applied to standard primary TKA, primary TKA with severe deformity, and revision TKA. In contrast to the measured resection method described later, the amount of bone osteotomized from the femur may or may not be greater than the thickness of the femoral component. The amount of bone osteotomized from the distal end of the femur is determined by the flexion gap.

Potential pitfalls of the gap technique include the following:

1. The joint line (referenced from the femur) may be moved proximally. This problem is most likely to occur when there is a preoperative flexion contracture, when a large flexion gap mandates resection of more distal femoral bone than the femoral implant replaces, or when the chosen femoral component is smaller than the anteroposterior dimension of the femur, thereby creating a large flexion gap. Joint line alteration can

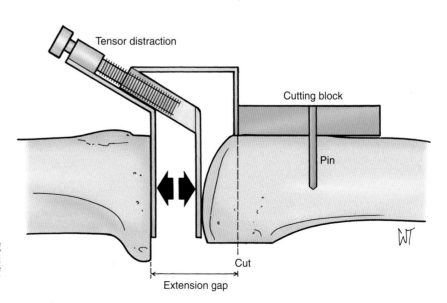

Figure 84–20. The distal femoral cutting guide is controlled by the tensor and positioned to create an extension gap of the correct dimensions.

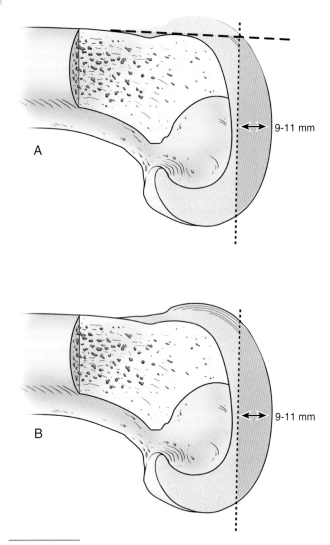

Figure 84–21. The thickness of the prosthesis, normally somewhere between 9 and 11 mm, is removed from the distal end of the femur.

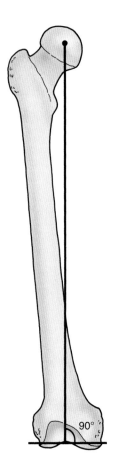

Figure 84–22. The distal femoral cut should be templated by measuring from the center of the femoral head to the center of the knee on a full-length radiograph of the femur. A second line passing into the intramedullary canal of the femur will indicate the angulation of the distal femoral cut.

be minimized by correct femoral measurement, a full range of femoral component sizes, and posterior capsulotomy to correct flexion contractures.
2. The method ensures soft-tissue balance and correct tensioning in full extension and at 90 degrees of flexion, but midrange laxity may occur when the posterior capsule is tight and the collateral ligaments are not balanced throughout the range of motion. Patients with midrange laxity may report a loose knee or lack of confidence descending stairs or walking on inclines.

Classic Measured Resection Technique

The second theory of surgical technique, the measured resection theory, begins with the philosophy of maintaining joint line position. A properly positioned joint line is key to proper cruciate ligament function and, conse-

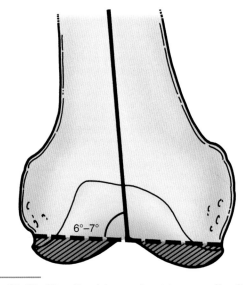

Figure 84–23. The distal femoral cut is normally aligned in 6 to 7 degrees of valgus from the intramedullary alignment rod.

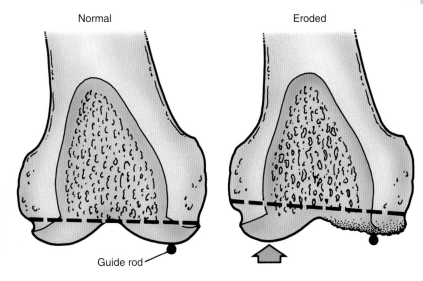

Normal   Eroded

Guide rod

Figure 84–24. Ideally, the amount of distal femoral resection should be judged from the normal side. When measurement is made from the medial femoral condyle, regardless of the pathology, extra distal femoral resection will occur.

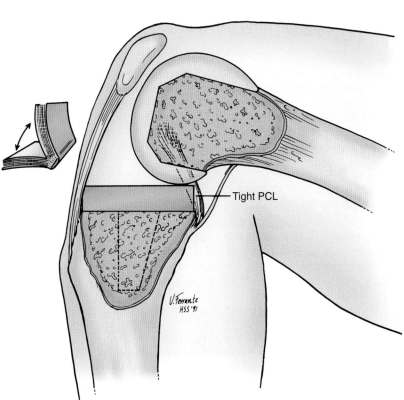

Tight PCL

Figure 84–25. An overtight posterior cruciate ligament causes "booking." There is excessive rollback of the femur, and the knee hinges open.

quently, posterior cruciate retention.[108] Hungerford developed the method of measured resection. The technique has been used in conjunction with the principles of anatomic alignment, as well as the neutral tibial cut.[71]

POSTERIOR CRUCIATE LIGAMENT

Preservation of the PCL offers many potential advantages because this ligament is an important varus-valgus stabilizer of the knee. It is a strong structure that can absorb stress that might otherwise be transmitted to the prosthesis-bone interface, it can control the rollback of the femur

on the tibia that occurs with flexion, it may be important for stair-climbing activities, and the ligament may have proprioceptive function (although abnormal proprioception will not return to normal after knee replacement).

To function properly, the PCL must be accurately tensioned during knee replacement. If the PCL is too tight, excessive tibial rollback will be promoted, thereby impeding knee flexion, causing increased posterior stress, and risking posterior polyethylene overload and anterior displacement of the femoral component. A tight PCL may also cause the knee to "open like a book" (Fig. 84–25). Recognition of excess PCL tightness is possible by observing anterior tibial component "lift-off" with trial components (Fig. 84–26). Conversely, when the PCL is too loose,

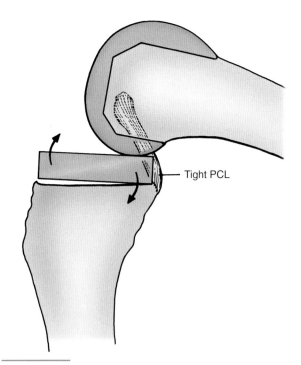

Figure 84–26. A method of demonstrating a tight posterior cruciate ligament (PCL) intraoperatively. The tibial trial component does not have undersurface fixation, and the component lifts anteriorly.

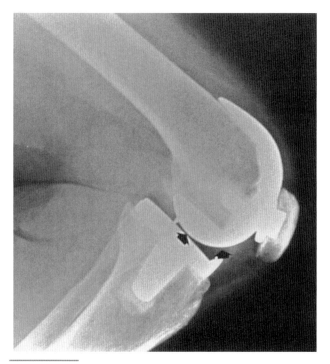

Figure 84–27. Sagittal radiograph of a "nonfunctional" posterior cruciate ligament. There has been "roll-forward" rather than "rollback" with knee flexion. The anterior margin of the femoral component abuts the anterior margin of the tibial component as it does in a total condylar-type design.

it does not control movement between the tibia and the femur (Fig. 84–27), thus allowing the femur to roll forward in flexion and limiting flexion by posterior impingement.

Proper PCL tension is dependent on maintaining the level of the joint line and the spatial relationship between the femur and tibia. The ideal PCL-retaining knee replacement would meet the following criteria:

1. The joint line or axis is restored to its prearthritic condition.
2. The shape and size of the femoral condyles are restored to re-create the natural distal femoral cam effect.
3. The tibial plateau surface is sloped approximately 10 degrees posteriorly and approximately 3 degrees medially.
4. The tibial surface offers no impedance to rotation and gliding movements.

In practice, techniques that are aimed at preserving the PCL meet these requirements to varying degrees. The "balance" of the PCL remains a subjective assessment, and proper balancing in the hands of experienced surgeons does not guarantee normal knee kinematics and tibial rollback. A few systems mimic the medial slope of the normal tibia, and some cut the tibia at right angles to its shaft. However, all measured resection knee systems share the objective of closely preserving or restoring the anatomic joint line by referencing the distal end of the femur. If this joint line preservation is achieved and the PCL is retained, the arc of motion should also be close to normal with correct ligament tensioning and optimal patellar tracking throughout the range of motion. Patellofemoral dysfunction remains the cause of most unsatisfactory knee arthroplasties. Maintenance of the anatomic joint line avoids patella baja (Fig. 84–28); Figgie et al[53] demonstrated that if the patella is not within a defined sagittal "neutral zone" (10 to 30 mm above the joint line), a greater number of patellar problems are observed (Fig. 84–29).

Successful PCL retention in TKA requires sustained function as well as proper initial balancing. Ligament-balancing techniques have been developed that permit PCL retention when the ligament is contracted but remains competent.[138,147,152] The techniques are similar to the medial release performed for balancing varus deformity. A graduated PCL release (Fig. 84–30A) is performed from the posterior aspect of the tibia with a periosteal elevator until the PCL tension is deemed appropriate (Fig. 84–30B). However, even for a skilled surgeon, it may be difficult to achieve the aims of successful PCL retention.[29] Although the PCL is typically intact in most arthritic knees,[151,153] the PCL can also degenerate and contract as part of the arthritic process,[5,88] thus rendering the ligament nonfunctional and making PCL retention not applicable in some arthritic knee deformities.[94,153] Likewise, the PCL occasionally becomes incompetent in the months or years after knee replacement and the prosthesis is rendered unstable.[126,179] Using cineradiography, Dennis et al have demonstrated paradoxical anterior sliding of the femur on the tibia in apparently well functioning knees with a retained PCL.[34]

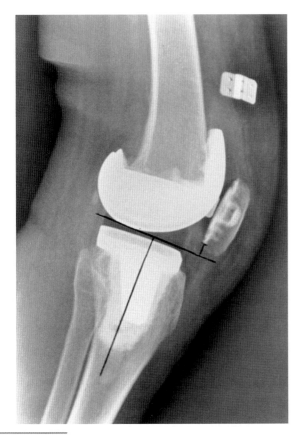

Figure 84–28. Lateral radiograph of a posterior-stabilized prosthesis showing patella baja. The distal pole of the patella lies just proximal to a projection of the joint line. Patella infra may be associated with an increased frequency of patellar symptoms.

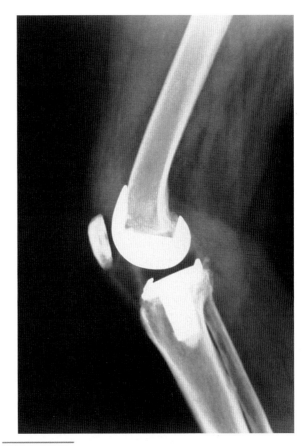

Figure 84–29. Lateral radiograph showing a satisfactory patellar position postoperatively. The patella lies in its normal position in relation to the joint line. The patellar prosthesis composite is of the correct thickness. Note the sclerosis that has developed in the remaining patellar bone. This is a common finding that develops several years postoperatively and is an example of Wolff's law.

ANTERIOR CRUCIATE LIGAMENT

The anterior cruciate ligament (ACL) is an important functional element in the normal knee, and its absence causes not only instability but also an abnormal pattern of motion, including rotational and sliding movements (e.g., pivot shift). Together with the PCL, the ACL forms a "four-bar linkage"[121] at the center of the knee, and the absence of either component destroys this mechanism. Abnormal sliding movements, in particular, can be expected when preserving only the PCL.[32,33,86,165] "Cruciate retention" refers only to the PCL in the context of TKA. The ACL is sacrificed in most modern total knee systems, with only a few knee prostheses designed to preserve both cruciate ligaments. The bicruciate-retaining meniscal-bearing Oxford knee is not recommended unless both ligaments are present.[60] In many arthritic knees, the ACL is damaged or absent, and most cruciate-preserving systems advocate removal of the ACL.

Integrating the Measured Resection and Gap Techniques

From the previous discussion, it is apparent that philosophical differences exist between the gap-balancing school of thought and the measured resection school of thought. The classic gap method emphasizes preservation of tibial bone and conforming joint surfaces and accepts, when required, proximal migration of the joint surface to balance the gaps. The classic measured resection school of thought emphasizes preservation of the joint axis and accepts less congruence of the flexion and extension gaps. Flexion contractures, when present, are corrected by a combination of posterior capsulotomy and stretching out the remaining contracture with postoperative physiotherapy.[167] In contrast, the gap technique emphasizes distal femoral bone resection in combination with posterior capsulotomy and PCL resection to accomplish intraoperative correction of flexion contractures, a principle emphasized by Insall.

The differing philosophies are also reflected in techniques and instrument systems. Although the instruments used for making bone cuts are generally similar, gap systems depend on a tensor or a series of spacers, and *adjustment* cuts for extension balance are made on the distal end of the femur. Ligament releases are generally performed before the bone cuts or perhaps after the upper part of the tibia has been osteotomized (technique using tensors or laminar spreaders). In contrast, measured resec-

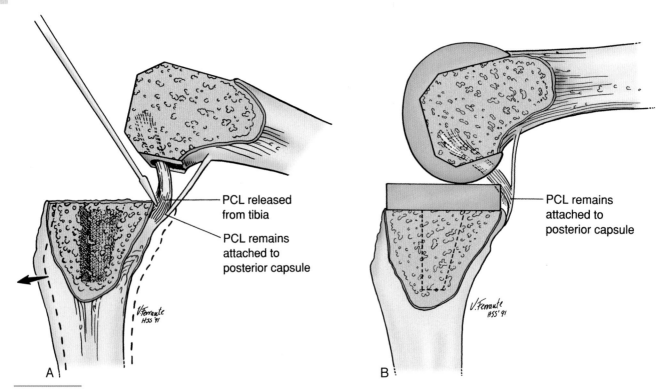

Figure 84–30. Posterior cruciate ligament (PCL) release from the posterior of the tibia lengthens a tight PCL. **A,** The release can be performed progressively until correct tension is obtained. **B,** The PCL remains attached to the posterior capsule.

tion systems osteotomize the tibia and femur independently, aiming to remove only enough bone to accommodate the components. The tensor or spacing function is performed by the components themselves, and ligament releases are performed after the trial components have been inserted to achieve balance and avoid "booking."

Despite the obvious differences in philosophy, distinctions between the gap and the measured resection techniques have blurred with the evolution of surgical techniques. Methods of PCL recession or release have made the two techniques more similar. Because PCL release opens both the flexion and the extension gaps, measured resection used with PCL release creates larger gaps, especially in flexion. In a clinical study of PCL resection, Kadoya et al[83] measured an increase in the medial and lateral flexion gaps of 4.8 and 4.5 mm, respectively, as compared with increases in the medial and lateral extension gaps of 0.9 and 0.8 mm, respectively. Using fluoroscopic analysis, several investigators have demonstrated that femoral rollback does not occur with flexion in cruciate-retaining prostheses.[86,165] In fact, some authors report femoral rollback similar to that of a natural knee when posterior-stabilized prosthetic designs are used.[32,33] Furthermore, flat tibial surfaces are not a prerequisite for PCL retention.[152] In long-term follow-up evaluations of cruciate-retaining knees with conforming articular surfaces, satisfactory results have been reported.[141,153,182] Therefore, completely flat tibial surfaces for PCL-retaining designs are not necessary, and cupping of some degree is accept-

able (provided that the PCL-driven rollback is not overly constrained). If this degree of articular conformity is permissible and compatible with PCL retention, a major objection (polyethylene wear) to retaining the PCL is negated.

The recent focus in knee replacement technique is on restoration of kinematics, not simply on the presence or absence of the PCL. More objective methods are required for deciding when the PCL is too tight or so loose that it is rendered nonfunctional. Some PCL-retaining systems have "markers" on the trial components to indicate proper kinematics. When the PCL is not fulfilling its purpose within acceptable and defined limits, PCL release may be performed, or alternatively, a posterior-stabilized design may be adopted. Most newer knee systems afford flexibility by functioning as either cruciate-retaining or cruciate-substituting systems, thereby permitting an intraoperative switch to posterior stabilization when the PCL is deemed nonfunctional or detrimental.

Current Preference in Knee Balancing

The current preference in knee ligament balancing is a modified gap technique that has elements of both the gap and the measured resection methods. Insall advocated a blend of technique whereby measured resections of both the distal end of the femur and the proximal end of the tibia are performed to avoid the need for a variable distal femoral cut. Posterior referencing of the femoral condyles allows a measured resection of the flexion gap as well. This measured resection of the flexion gap is facilitated by a larger inventory of femoral component sizes than existed when gap balancing was described and by a femoral component designed with a divergent anterior cut to minimize the risk of anterior femoral notching. Femoral component sizing and positioning remain critical to proper balancing. One should avoid allowing the femoral component to sit proud of the anterior femoral cortex, even to a minor degree (see Fig. 84–16). Because PCL release opens the flexion and extension gaps, modifications of the measured resection technique are possible. If the PCL is appropriately adjusted, strict adherence to anatomic alignment (varus tibial cut) is no longer required, and the classic alignment (perpendicular tibial cut) traditionally assigned to the gap technique can be applied. As noted previously, some degree of articular congruency that does not conflict with PCL kinematics is permissible, thus improving the prospects for longer-term polyethylene performance.

SUMMARY OF THE MODIFIED GAP TECHNIQUE

The modified gap technique can be performed by cutting either the femur or the tibia first. The femur-first technique is performed as follows:
1. Balance the ligaments.
2. Cannulate the femoral canal and cut the distal end of the femur in valgus relative to the anatomic axis (usually 4 to 6 degrees).
3. Establish proper femoral rotation (using the epicondylar axis).
4. Cut the anterior and posterior surfaces of the femur.
   a. Posterior referencing: (1) make a 3-degree flexion cut (or divergent anterior cut) and (2) correct preoperative flexion contractures by posterior release.
   b. Anterior referencing: avoid over-resection of the posterior condyles of the femur.
5. Choose the femoral component (downsize for in-between sizing).
6. Make the proximal tibial cut perpendicular to the anatomic axis.
7. Reassess ligament balance, midflexion balance, and posterior capsular tightness.
8. Adjust the distal femoral cut to deal with extension gap tightness. (Note that under-resection of the distal end of the femur is seldom needed.)
   The tibia-first technique is done as follows:
1. Balance the ligaments.
2. Cut 10 mm from the proximal end of the tibia (approximately 2 mm below the deficient side in most routine cases).
3. Balance with a tensioner.
4. Cut the distal end of the femur 10 mm.
5. Cut the anterior and posterior surfaces of the femur relative to the epicondylar axis.

PREOPERATIVE PLANNING

Full-length radiographs that show the hip, knee, and ankle joints are desirable for preoperative planning but require special equipment. Standard radiographs showing the distal femoral and proximal tibial anatomic axis serve as an acceptable alternative to long films when there is no history of previous bone instrumentation or trauma or clinical suspicion of excessive bowing. Radiographs are position sensitive, and care is required to obtain the films in neutral rotation (Figs. 84–32 and 84–33).[79] Information concerning the angle of femoral and tibial cuts and the desired entry hole position (which may not be in the bone center) is obtained. Unusual shaft bowing is noted (Fig. 84–34). Atypical anatomic variations such as an unusual canal size, angular malalignment, or previous surgery that could cause intraoperative difficulty are noted (Fig. 84–35).

EXPOSURE

Routine Exposure

MEDIAL PARAPATELLAR APPROACH

The medial parapatellar approach is the most common approach for TKA. A midline skin incision centered over the patella extends from the level of the tibial tuberosity to just above the patella. The incision is made sufficiently long to avoid traction on the skin edges during the procedure. Distally, the incision is placed approximately 1 cm medial to the tibial tubercle. The medial parapatellar arthrotomy through the capsule is made as straight as possible; it usually crosses the medial border of the patella to avoid transecting longitudinal fibers of the extensor mechanism. Proximally, the capsular incision is positioned along the medial margin of the vastus medialis within 6 to 8 mm of its edge; distally, the arthrotomy parallels the patellar tendon approximately 5 to 10 mm medial to the tibial tubercle. A medial periosteal sleeve that includes the deep MCL is elevated from the tibia to allow the proximal end of the tibia to be translated anteriorly and rotated externally. When the ACL is present, it is divided to improve the ease of this translation.

Techniques to Enhance Exposure in the Standard Medial Parapatellar Approach
1. Elevation of the deep fibers of the medial collateral ligament just below the tibial surface with posterior extension reflecting the medial capsule, the deep MCL, and the semimembranosus (Fig. 84–36).
2. Elevation of a small cuff of periosteum immediately adjacent to the patellar tendon insertion at the tibial tubercle. This technique diminishes the risk of patellar tendon avulsion during exposure.

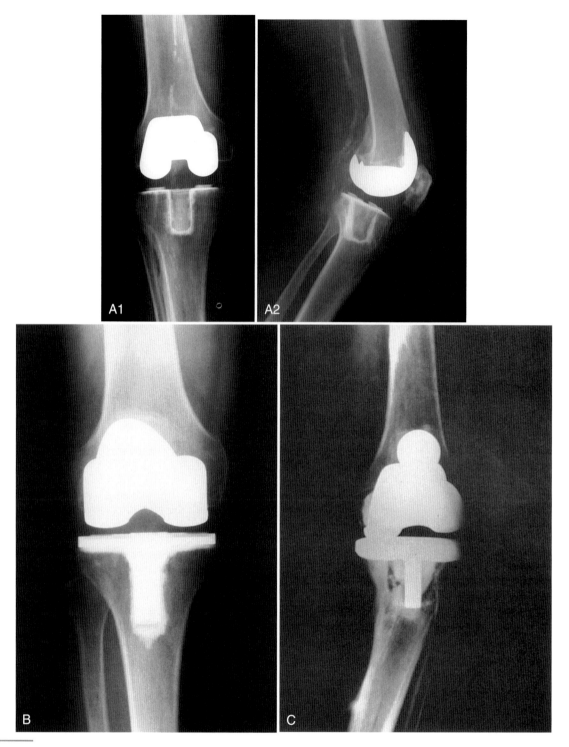

Figure 84–31. **A**, Anteroposterior and lateral radiographs of an Insall-Burstein I prosthesis at 19-year follow-up. **B**, Radiograph of a knee prosthesis that has been correctly cemented. The amount of cement is minimal. This type of cement fixation is obtained by using cement in the doughy stage. **C**, Radiograph of a knee prosthesis showing undesirable cement technique. In addition to the varus positioning, there is excessive cement in the proximal end of the tibia and around the stem.

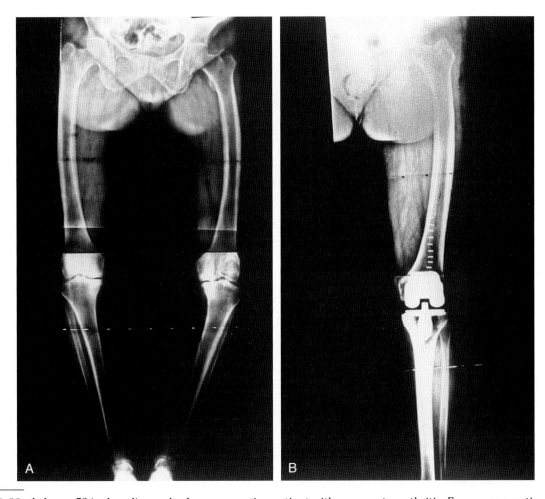

Figure 84–32. **A**, Long, 52-inch radiograph of a preoperative patient with varus osteoarthritis. From preoperative planning, a 14-degree valgus cut on the femur was predicted. **B**, Postoperative radiograph of the same patient. An extramedullary alignment check showed that the 14-degree prediction was grossly incorrect; in fact, the femur was resected at 7 degrees of valgus. The apparent lateral bowing was, in fact, excessive anterior bowing of the femur seen in a position of some external rotation.

3. Division of the lateral patellofemoral ligament, which permits slightly greater patellar eversion.
4. Excision of the fat pad. Although some surgeons perform a longitudinal split of the fat pad, we routinely excise the fat pad to improve mobilization of the patella and minimize the potential for postoperative infrapatellar scar formation.
5. Separation of the capsule from the patella at the lateral osteochondral border of the patella.

Other accepted methods of exposing the knee, such as the subvastus, vastus-splitting, trivector, and lateral parapatellar methods, as well as the newer and unproven minimally invasive methods, are discussed elsewhere in this text.

Difficult Exposure

When exposing a stiff or ankylosed knee, there is risk of avulsing the patellar ligament attachment to the tibial tubercle. If all aspects of the standard exposure are followed, with additional specific attention paid to areas of contracture, it is possible to minimize the risk of avulsion or damage to the extensor mechanism. When mobilizing the patella, it is important to perform releases to allow external rotation of the tibia so that the patella can be subluxated laterally rather than everted. Though common practice, there is no reason that the patella must be everted except during patellar preparation with the knee extended. In addition to the standard releases, which include medial dissection around to the semimembranosus bursa, excision of the fat pad, and release of the patella, one should also expose the lateral tibial plateau, remove scar, and elevate the lateral capsule to the top of Gerdy's tubercle. The lateral dissection makes room for the patella, but it should stay clear of the popliteal tendon insertion and fibular collateral ligament. Elevation of capsule around the osteoarticular border of the patella and a longitudinal incision into the infrapatellar ligament can also result in additional extensor mechanism flexibility. In more resistant cases of contracture or stiffness, more

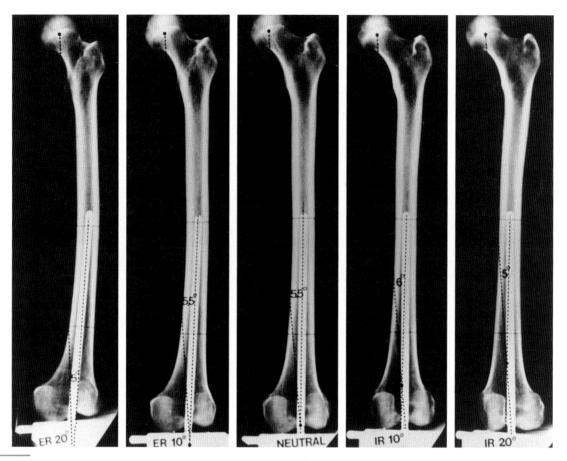

Figure 84–33. Radiographs of the femur in internal and external rotation. It can be seen that internal rotation is perceived as medial bowing and external rotation as lateral bowing. This is a normal femur, and the effect would be accentuated if the femur had excessive anterior bowing.

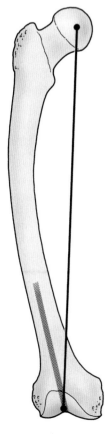

Figure 84–34. When the femur is bowed, the angle of the distal femoral cut will be increased. When templating the femur, beware of excessive valgus cuts because the bowing may represent external rotation of the femoral bone on the radiograph. An external alignment check is advisable.

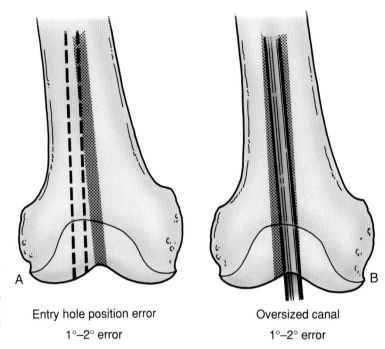

Figure 84–35. Malposition of the entry hole into the femur introduces an error in the valgus cut. **A,** A lateral entry hole increases the valgus alignment of the cut. **B,** An oversized canal allows the intramedullary rod to toggle, and a 1- to 2-degree error in both varus and valgus can be produced.

Entry hole position error
1°–2° error

Oversized canal
1°–2° error

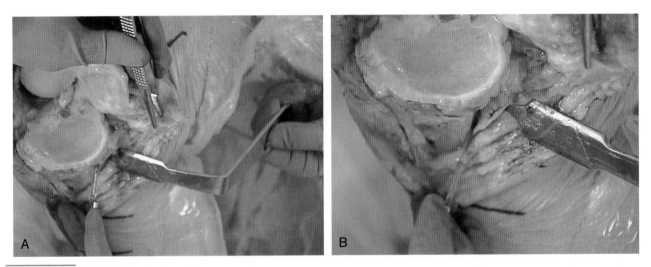

Figure 84–36. Routine exposure includes release of all soft tissues from the medial aspect of the tibia at the joint line. Medial release involves distal stripping of the superficial medial collateral ligament, which was not performed in this case. **A,** Exposure to the posteromedial aspect of the proximal end of the tibia. **B,** Close-up view.

extensile exposure is required. Difficult surgical exposures are briefly reviewed here and are discussed in detail elsewhere in this text.

RECTUS "SNIP"

The rectus snip is the extensile proximal exposure described by Insall for the medial parapatellar approach.[57] The snip is performed intraoperatively (Fig. 84–37) as needed after other methods of patellar mobilization have been completed. The medial incision for the quadriceps snip is the same as that described for the standard midline approach. At the apex of the quadriceps tendon, the arthrotomy is continued laterally across the thin proximal portion of the tendon into the vastus lateralis such that the rectus tendon is divided superficially and the trilaminar tendon extensions of the vastus muscles are divided deeply. More distally, a lateral retinacular patellar release may also be performed at this stage if it is determined that the lateral retinaculum is sufficiently tight that it pulls the patella laterally or restricts knee bending. The superior lateral genicular vessels, which run at the lower border of the vastus lateralis, need to be identified and isolated. These vessels can sometimes be saved when identified and protected during the lateral release. An important feature of this approach is that none of the structures contributing to knee extension is transversely divided.

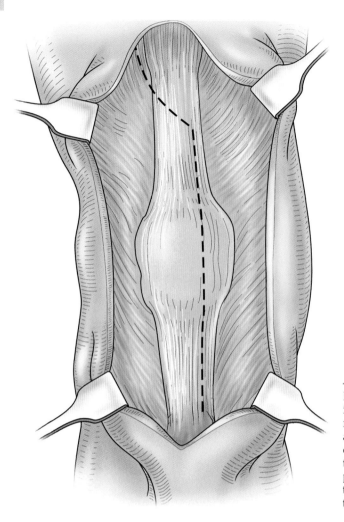

Figure 84–37. The rectus "snip." The medial parapatellar incision is continued proximally across the apex of the rectus femoris tendon into the fibers of the vastus lateralis. Division of the rectus tendon in and of itself allows elasticity and takes stress off the patellar ligament insertion into the tibial tubercle. When combined with lateral patellar release, retaining a bridge of tissue consisting of the vastus lateralis insertion into the quadriceps tendon, the result is equivalent to a quadriceps turndown.

TIBIAL TUBERCLE OSTEOTOMY

A tibial tubercle osteotomy can facilitate exposure of a stiff knee.[186] The technique requires that the fragment of bone osteotomized be sufficiently large to enhance the potential for later healing back to the tibia (Fig. 84–38). The tibial fragment is opened on a lateral soft tissue "hinge." A tibial fragment of this size may be securely reattached by wires or screws at the conclusion of the operation, whereas small fragments in osteoporotic bone afford insufficient substance for successful reattachment. Whiteside[183] reported on the use of this technique in 136 knees—both primary and revision TKAs. Complications were few, and no further release of the quadriceps mechanism was necessary in any procedure. However, Wolff and colleagues[189] reported a 23% complication rate when using a similar technique.

SUBPERIOSTEAL PEEL

In ankylosed knees, it may be necessary to perform a subperiosteal exposure of the femur or tibia. It is advisable to begin with a subperiosteal exposure of the medial aspect of the tibia to the mid-diaphysis while attempting to flex and externally rotate the knee, with care taken to not avulse the femoral attachment of the MCL. If a medial peel is not successful in creating adequate motion, the periosteum of the lower supramedial and supralateral aspect of the femur is incised, and the lower portion of the femur is "skeletonized" by subperiosteal dissection (Fig. 84–39). The entire soft-tissue envelope is peeled from the bone as a continuous sleeve and retracted posteriorly to allow the distal end of the femur to be buttonholed forward. This exposure, combined with medial subperiosteal dissection of the upper part of the tibia, allows the knee to be flexed without danger of damaging or tearing important soft-tissue structures. When the incision is closed, the soft-tissue envelope falls back around the bones. The technique is useful for long-standing ankylosis of the knee and for reimplantation after infection.[116] Extensive exposures that result in medial-lateral instability patterns may occasionally require the use of increased articular constraint.

CLOSURE

Closure should be anatomic, with effort made to restore the longitudinal alignment of the medial and lateral soft tissues along the incision. Tissues should be approximated

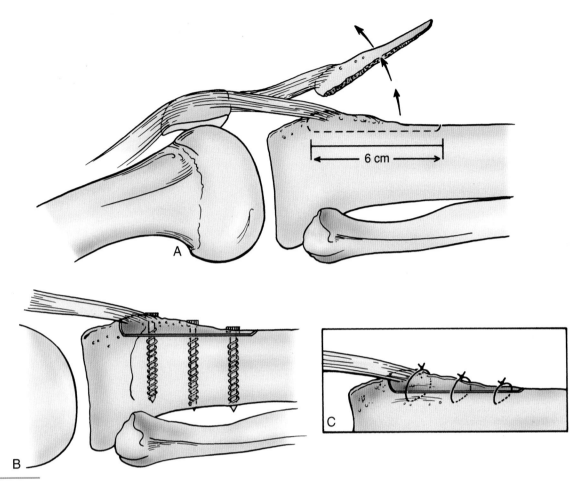

Figure 84–38. A method of exposure for difficult or ankylosed knees. **A,** The tibial tubercle is osteotomized by taking a large fragment of bone, at least 6 cm long. **B,** This allows firm reattachment with either screws or wire sutures.

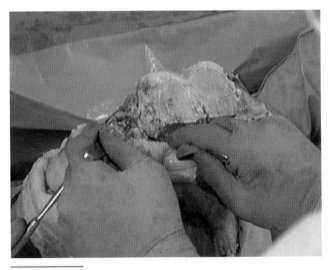

Figure 84–39. A skeletonized femur. The collateral ligaments, together with the adjacent periosteum of the distal end of the femur, have been stripped posteriorly to allow the distal end of the femur to be buttonholed anteriorly. The soft tissues remain in continuity, and after the operation has been completed, the soft-tissue sleeve remains intact, thereby providing stability. This type of exposure, combined with subperiosteal stripping of the proximal end of the tibia and quadriceps turndown or a modification thereof, is very useful in dealing with ankylosed knees and for reimplantation after infection.

without being excessively tightened or imbricated. Closure of the knee in greater than 45 degrees of flexion will help align the capsular incision, with the shape of the incision or a transverse ink or cautery mark used as a guide to alignment.[43,109] Insall routinely performed a modified vastus medialis oblique advancement in which the medial soft-tissue envelope is advanced several millimeters distally relative to the lateral soft tissues. Because the vastus medialis oblique is important in terminal extension, this advancement was meant to reduce the risk of postoperative extension lag.

TECHNIQUES AND INSTRUMENTATION

Implant systems on the market today have similarities and differ only according to the two philosophies described previously. Thus, many of the instruments used in total knee replacement are similar. The advent of interest in minimally invasive and computer-navigated approaches has led to the downsizing of standard instrumentation and the development of alternative approaches, such as making the distal femoral cut from a lateral approach. Such innovative ideas and concepts will require clinical testing and evaluation to determine their accuracy, reproducibility, and performance before widespread adoption can be advocated.

Cutting Blocks

Bone cuts may be made from the free edge of the cutting block or through slotted capture guides. The slots may afford some degree of safety by limiting the excursion of saw blades; however, in practice they obscure the saw blade tip, thus potentially increasing the risk of compromising important structures such as the MCL and sometimes leading to the creation of metal debris if the saw blade becomes confined. Although saw blades designed for the capture guides function well in the cutting slots, their cutting "teeth" are less efficient because the teeth are designed with less offset to allow the blade to pass through the cutting slot (Fig. 84–40). When capture guides are used, it is important to lubricate the surfaces and not lever the saw blade against the guide to minimize the generation of metallic debris from the saw blade rubbing the cutting block. Milling frames are particularly useful in improving the accuracy of patellar preparation. The milling frames used in some systems to make the intercondylar cut create a smooth bone surface by their rotary blade action. Rotary blades have been shown to generate less heat than standard saw blades do, thereby creating less damage to the cut bony surface.

Efficiency in femoral and tibial preparation has been advanced through improved instrumentation. Traditionally, the multiple femoral cuts were made with individual cutting blocks. Newer, universal cutting blocks allow multiple steps of bone surface preparation to be performed with a single block (Fig. 84–41). Most newer femoral cutting blocks provide slots for the anterior, posterior, and chamfer cuts, as well as guides for creation of the distal femoral lug holes. Although performing multiple femoral cuts from the same cutting block is convenient, chamfer cuts should be performed only when the final distal femoral cut is completed; otherwise they will need to be repeated each time that the distal femoral cut is repeated.

Alignment Guides

It is generally agreed that the mechanical axis of the limb should be restored. Alignment is achieved by making appropriate cuts on the femur and tibia in addition to balancing the ligaments. Standard alignment guides may be placed according to external landmarks such as the anterior superior iliac spine or the center of the hip joint[158] proximally and the ankle mortise distally (Fig. 84–42). Because these landmarks can sometimes be hard to identify, intramedullary guides have become more popular than extramedullary guides for making the distal femoral osteotomy.

Newer techniques of computer navigation involve the use of bone surface landmarks that are registered in the

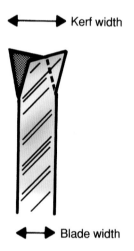

Figure 84–40. Saws used with cutting slots must have appropriately designed blades with a reduced offset of the cutting tips so that the kerf width and the slot width are nearly the same.

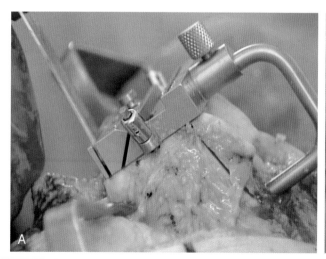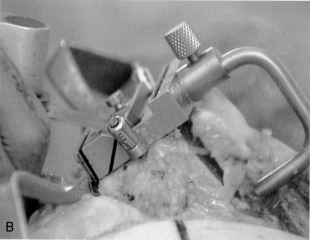

Figure 84–41. Universal femoral cutting block. **A,** Anteroposterior cuts. **B,** Chamfer cuts.

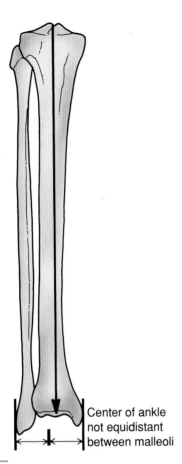

Figure 84–42. Center of the knee. The center of the talus axis lies a few millimeters medial to the center point between the malleoli.

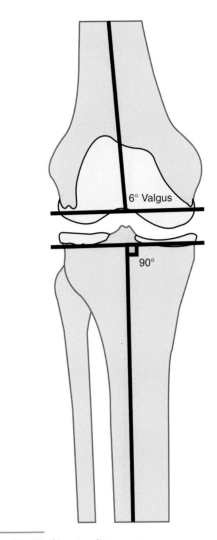

Figure 84–43. Classic alignment.

computer by means of a navigated stylus. Computer navigation may obviate the need to cannulate the medullary canal to achieve the desired mechanical alignment. Alignment is created by feeding data points into the computer with an instrumented stylus to map the bone surface. Once the bone contour is established by entering certain key points into the computer, the data are combined with data stored in the computer on standard tibial or femoral anatomy. This process of combining individual patient-derived data with stored data is called "morphing." Computer morphing generates an image or likeness of the knee on the computer screen during surgery. From this hybrid of real data and stored data, the computer will proceed to direct the surgeon regarding the accuracy of alignment.

Method of Alignment

CLASSIC METHOD

Either the tibial or the femoral osteotomy may be performed first (Fig. 84–43). The valgus cut at the distal end of the femur is in theory the difference between the anatomic and mechanical axis and is determined by using the femoral shaft as the anatomic reference. Distal femoral

valgus can vary, depending on the patient's body habitus, but it generally falls around 5 to 6 degrees of valgus. Valgus knees are generally cut in 4 to 5 degrees of valgus, whereas varus and nondeformed knees are cut at 5 to 6 degrees of valgus. In obese patients, it is important to limit the amount of valgus to 5 degrees to avoid contact between the medial knee soft tissues. The tibial cut is always made neutral to the tibial anatomic axis.[102] Hsu et al[68] confirmed that 7 degrees of femoral valgus matched with 0 degrees of proximal tibial alignment resulted in the most even load distribution across a total condylar knee prosthesis. There is ample evidence that a varus tibial cut not only results in uneven stress distribution in the proximal end of the tibia[61] but also leads to premature clinical failure. [139]

ANATOMIC METHOD

In an attempt to re-create natural knee kinematics with a PCL-retaining prosthesis, Hungerford used an anatomic method (Fig. 84–44) of lower limb alignment for TKA.[70] Femoral valgus is set at an anatomic 9 to 10 degrees, and

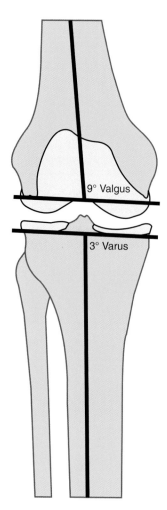

Figure 84–44. Anatomic alignment.

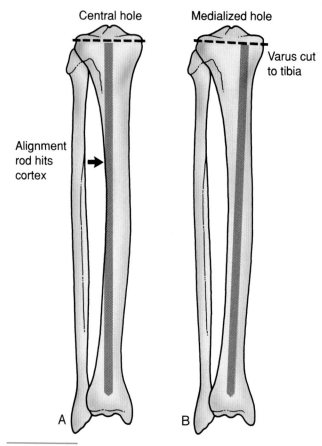

Figure 84–45. Intramedullary guides are not satisfactory when the tibia is bowed. **A**, The guide passed through a central hole abuts the lateral cortex. **B**, To pass the guide down the shaft to the ankle, the entry hole has to be medialized. This produces a varus cut in the tibia.

the tibial cut is made in 2 to 3 degrees of varus, thereby creating an anatomic 6 to 7 degrees of lower extremity valgus. Hsu et al[68] demonstrated that these angles produce even load distribution across the knee joint in a cruciate-retaining design. As noted earlier, if the surgeon is not experienced in this technique, intentional varus tibial cuts can easily result in excessive tibial varus and create uneven load distribution and ligament imbalance.

Tibial Guides

BACKGROUND

Most systems continue to use an extramedullary guide for the upper tibial osteotomy. Advocates of intramedullary tibial guides maintain that a rod of sufficient length reaching well into the tibial diaphysis will reliably align the tibial-cutting guide when there is no bow or offset of the tibial shaft. One potential pitfall of the intramedullary technique is that the shape of the tibia is inconsistent. Additionally, as for any intramedullary guide, the entry point is critical to alignment. Templating to determine the proper entry point for the tibial guide on the tibial surface

will minimize the risk of creating a varus tibial cut based on a medial entry point and a bowed tibia. A central entry hole will often cause the intramedullary rod to impact against the tibial cortex (usually lateral), and placing the entry hole so that such impact does not occur alters the angle of the proximal guide (Fig. 84–45).

The extramedullary tibial guide is placed on the leg with the use of surface landmarks. The distal end of the guide attaches above the ankle, whereas the proximal end is pinned to the center of the proximal end of the tibia, generally at the medial third of the tibial tubercle. Most guides allow adjustment at the ankle in both the mediolateral and anteroposterior direction. The center of the ankle does not exactly correspond to the midpoint between the malleoli but instead is slightly medial to this point (5 to 10 mm) (see Fig. 84–42). The anteroposterior distal guide adjustment controls the posterior slope of the proximal tibial cut. Posterior slope of the proximal end of the tibia may also be incorporated into the tibial osteotomy. As noted previously, we favor an essentially perpendicular cut relative to the tibial shaft. However, some systems, especially cruciate-retaining designs and some mobile-bearing knee designs, function more effectively with posterior slope. The 7 degrees of posterior slope is anatomic when considering the subchondral bone, but when taking the posterior menisci into consideration, the proximal tibial surface is actually perpendicular to the shaft (Fig. 84–46).

In obese patients, anteroposterior guide adjustment at the ankle may be necessary to make the guide parallel to the tibial shaft. Locating the proper proximal position of the extramedullary guide may be difficult; the natural tendency is to place the guide medially, thereby producing a varus cut. Mobilization of the infrapatellar ligament combined with a lower-profile lateral plateau cutting surface will facilitate placement of the tibial guide. By referencing off the tibial plateau center, the tibial shaft axis, and the center of the ankle, proper alignment for the proximal tibial osteotomy is usually possible. Several investigators have demonstrated that extramedullary and intramedullary systems are equally accurate in establishing tibial alignment.[31,96] However, intramedullary instrumentation forfeits some of its accuracy in the face of tibial bowing or offset of the tibial shaft, especially when used for valgus knees. Simmons et al[159] noted that the accuracy of intramedullary tibial alignment systems was 83% for varus knees versus 37% for valgus knees; they attributed the poor accuracy to the tibial bowing observed in two-thirds of valgus knees.

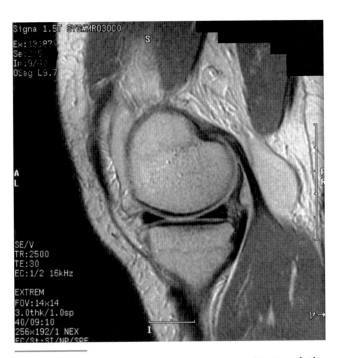

Figure 84–46. Lateral magnetic resonance image of the knee demonstrating that posterior slope is present when considering the subchondral surface; however, with the menisci intact, the 5 to 7 degrees of "physiological posterior slope" is reduced to essentially neutral.

AUTHORS' PREFERRED TECHNIQUE OF TIBIAL PREPARATION

The upper tibial osteotomy is made at right angles to the tibial shaft in the coronal plane and sloped posteriorly about 3 to 5 degrees in the sagittal plane. The extramedullary guide is provisionally secured to the tibia in alignment with the medial third of the tibial tuberosity, the tibial shaft, the center of the tibial plateau, and the middle of the ankle. Adjustments to the tibial cutting block are then performed at the ankle. The depth of proximal tibial resection is selected so that enough bone is removed to accommodate the tibial component (with a 10-mm polyethylene insert being the desired lower limit in modular tibial components and 8 mm being the lower limit with all polyethylene components). Given the few additional millimeters of laxity produced after PCL excision, 1 cm of proximal tibial bone is excised to accommodate at least a 10-mm tibial component when using a cruciate-substituting knee. The 10 mm of resection is typically measured by placing a stylus on the articular surface with the most residual cartilage; alternatively, the stylus can measure 2 mm of resection from the most eroded articular surface (Fig. 84–47). The cutting block is then fixed and the proximal tibial osteotomy is performed. Although studies have shown that resection of up to

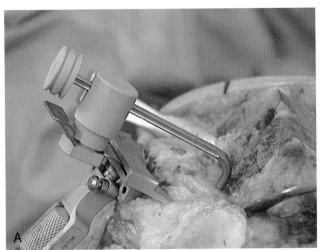
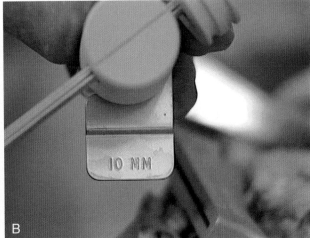

Figure 84–47. **A,** Intraoperative photo of the stylus used to determine the amount of proximal tibial bone resection. **B,** In this case, a 10-mm resection is measured off the least affected articular surface.

20 mm from the least involved side of the joint is accept-able,[58] care must be taken to avoid detaching the ITB at the level of Gerdy's tubercle.

Femoral Guides

BACKGROUND

Intramedullary femoral alignment to determine the angle of the distal femoral cut is generally favored because reliable external landmarks are not readily palpable. The thigh musculature, obesity, and surgical drapes make definition of femoral shaft orientation difficult. Multiple investigations have demonstrated that both intramedullary and extramedullary alignment systems are accurate; however, most studies suggest that intramedullary femoral alignment systems are more commonly used because of the limitations of extramedullary alignment noted previously.[23,47,105] Femoral alignment can be determined with intramedullary methods and confirmed with extramedullary methods if any uncertainty exists (e.g., unusual femoral bowing, wide intramedullary canal).

Preoperative radiographic evaluation with a three-joint view allows for identification of extra-articular deformity, such as abnormal femoral bowing. There is a strong correlation between the mechanical axis and the anatomic axis obtained with standard radiographs in the absence of extra-articular deformity (V. Kraus, unpublished data). Rotation of the femur in the preoperative full-length radiograph can create a false impression of varus or valgus bowing (Fig. 84–48). With extra-articular deformity, the starting hole position for femoral canal access can be altered slightly to properly position the intramedullary guide. However, when an extra-articular deformity prevents passage of a standard femoral guide, a modified (shorter) intramedullary alignment rod may be used, provided that the distal segment of the femoral canal that serves as a reference is oriented to achieve proper component alignment. A disadvantage of intramedullary guides is that if the angle of entry or the starting point into the canal is incorrect, the intramedullary rod may contact the femoral cortices rather than pass directly into the center of the diaphysis (see Fig. 84–35). If the rod contacts the lateral cortex, the valgus angle may be reduced, and if the medial cortex is contacted, the valgus angle may be increased.

Depending on the particular instrument system and arthritic pattern, an intramedullary rod may cause the distal femoral cutting block to contact either the medial (valgus knee) or the lateral (varus knee) condyle first. If attempts are made to fully seat the instrumentation on both condyles, errors in the distal femoral cut may occur. For example, in valgus knees (associated with lateral femoral condylar erosion), the distal femoral cutting block attachment typically contacts the medial femoral condyle first. If the surgeon allows the instrumentation to contact both condyles in this situation, the valgus angle of the distal femoral cut will be exaggerated. To avoid such errors, the surgeon must be aware of the arthritic pattern and use the intramedullary guide to establish proper posi-

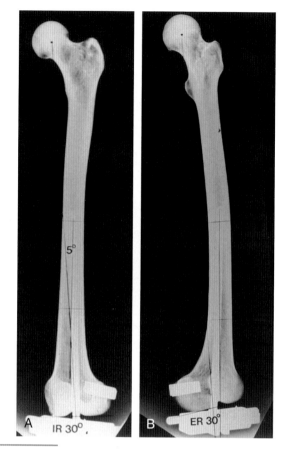

Figure 84–48. Radiographs of the femur in (**A**) internal and (**B**) external rotation. It can be seen that internal rotation is perceived as medial bowing and external rotation as lateral bowing. This is a normal femur, and the effect would be accentuated if the femur had excessive anterior bowing.

tion of the distal femoral cutting block, even if the instrumentation contacts only a single condyle (see Fig. 84–24). Asymmetric distal femoral resections are very common and serve to correct the angular deformity rather than re-create the deformity with a symmetric bone resection.

AUTHORS' PREFERRED TECHNIQUE OF FEMORAL PREPARATION

The entering hole for a femoral intramedullary guide is made about 1 cm anterior to the origin of the PCL, although this position can be adjusted to accommodate any abnormalities noted on preoperative radiographs; usually, the entry hole is directed slightly medially toward the top of the intercondylar notch (Fig. 84–49). Over-drilling the entry to 12 mm is recommended because of increased intramedullary pressure during intramedullary rod insertion; the use of a fluted rather than a round intramedullary rod has also been shown to diminish intramedullary pressure during rod insertion.[136] The distal femoral osteotomy guide is attached to the intramedullary guide at an angle derived from the preoperative radiograph, normally 5 to 7 degrees, which represents the difference between the mechanical and the anatomic axis of

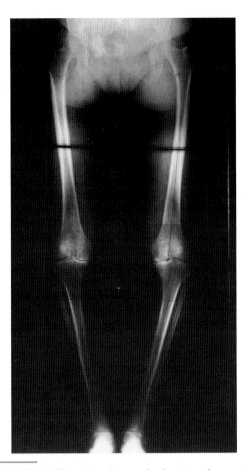

Figure 84–49. A 52-inch radiograph showing the position of entry holes from preoperative templating. Note that the femoral entry hole is slightly medial and the tibial entry hole is slightly lateral.

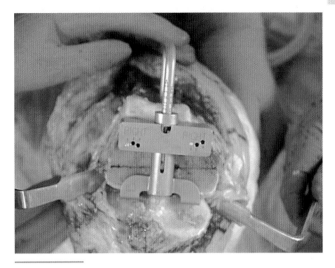

Figure 84–50. Sizing the femoral condyle.

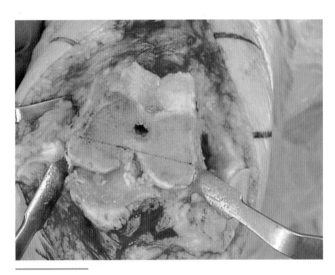

Figure 84–51. Intraoperative photograph demonstrating the epicondylar axis drawn across the cut distal femoral surface.

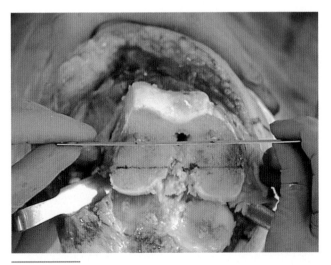

Figure 84–52. The instrumentation is aligned with the epicondylar axis (the pins are parallel to the epicondylar axis, as indicated by a ruler placed across them).

the femur. When intramedullary assessment appears unreliable, an extramedullary rod should be used to confirm that the proposed osteotomy is appropriate. When this step provides conflicting information, the preoperative radiographs should be reevaluated; rarely, intraoperative radiographic determination of the proper femoral valgus angle is necessary.

The distal femoral osteotomy is made by removing precisely the amount of bone that will be replaced by the femoral prosthesis. Some systems measure this amount from the uninvolved condyle, whereas others key off the medial femoral condyle regardless of the knee pathology (see Fig. 84–24). Generally, the surgeon can make a choice regarding the depth of the distal femoral resection. It is important to keep in mind that any resection above that being replaced by the prosthesis will result in a corresponding elevation of the joint line. Once the distal osteotomy is completed, the distal end of the femur is sized, and the anterior and posterior femoral resections are performed with appropriate templates (Fig. 84–50). Rotational alignment is adjusted when positioning the femoral template by marking the epicondylar axis on the distal femoral surface (Figs. 84–51 and 84–52).

For cruciate-substituting prostheses, the flexion and extension gaps can be measured with spacers or tensiometers, and additional distal femoral bone is removal

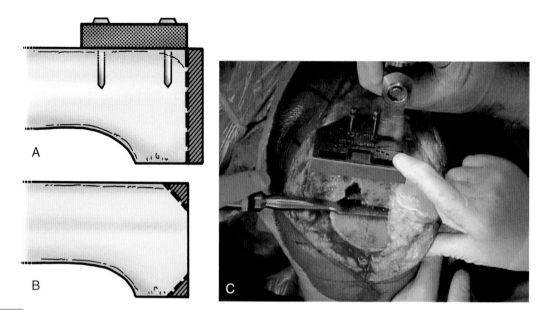

Figure 84–53. **A**, Femoral recutting should be done before the chamfer cuts are made, an important reason for incorporating spacers into the system. It is simple to remove 2 to 3 mm from the distal end of the femur. **B**, When the femur has been sculpted to receive the prosthesis, recutting is much more complex. **C**, The distal femoral recutter allowing 2, 3, and 5 mm of additional resection. (The cut tibial surface should be protected.)

when the extension gap is tighter than the flexion gap (Fig. 84–53A and B). A measured resection of the distal end of the femur will rarely warrant readjustment (typically only with severe flexion contractures). Adjustment cuts should be made before the chamfer cuts (Fig. 84–53B-D). Chamfer, notch, and fixation holes are made on the distal end of the femur (Fig. 84–54) and proximal end of the tibia (Fig. 84–55). A flexion contracture caused by posterior capsular contracture or a narrow extension gap should be corrected in favor of accepting an overly thin polyethylene liner (Fig. 84–56). Flexion of the femoral component will more readily lead to anterior impingement, and a thinner tibial insert can lead to accelerated polyethylene wear.

Rotational Positioning of Prosthetic Components

Rotational alignment of the femoral component is based on the epicondylar axis, whereas rotational alignment of the tibial component can be based on the posterior surface of the cut tibia, the anterior surface of the tibia, the tibial tubercle, and the ankle mortise. Assessment can be done with the knee in flexion, in extension, or in both as the knee is passed through a range of movement with the trial components in place.

When the tibial component rotation is determined with the knee flexed, the rotation can be related to the anterior surface of the tibia and to the position of the tibial tubercle, which should lie slightly lateral to the midposition of the component (Fig. 84–57). Reference is then made to the ankle and to the position of the malleoli, which should lie approximately 30 degrees externally rotated to the tibial component position. An alignment rod can be suspended from the tibial guide to view the relationship between the tibial component and the ankle joint. When a symmetric tibial component is used, there is often some overhang posterolaterally (Fig. 84–58) because the medial tibial plateau is larger than the lateral one; for this reason, we do not favor using the posterior margins of the tibial plateau as alignment landmarks.

Rotational alignment can also be assessed in extension, which allows the tibial component position to be related to the patellar groove of the femoral component, the tibial tubercle, and the ankle mortise. With the femoral trial prosthesis in position, a range of motion is performed and patellar tracking is observed before the final fixation holes for the tibial component are made. A tibial trial component without fixation pegs allows the component to "find" its correct position. This type of component positioning is subject to error introduced by the person holding the leg, the tourniquet on the thigh, and flexion gap tightness. Using the anatomy of the proximal end of the tibia and the ankle eliminates these potential errors in rotational positioning. Tibial tray malrotation is detrimental to patellar tracking, especially with excessive internal rotation of the tibial component. Excessive internal rotation of the tibial component increases the risk for patellar subluxation.[12] Conversely, excessive external rotation of the tibial component may also result in abnormal tracking of the patella,[124] as well as a kinematic conflict in the femorotibial articulation, such as notch-cam impingement in a cruciate-substituting design.

Mediolateral Positioning of Prosthetic Components

The medial-lateral positioning of both the femoral and tibial components is important. Generally, the components should be positioned anatomically on their respec-

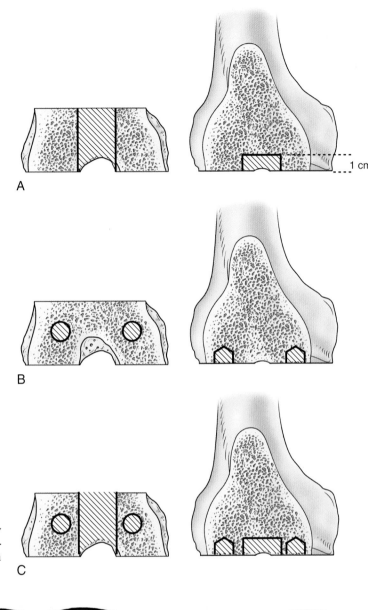

Figure 84–54. Femoral fixation can be enhanced by a central box usually found with (**A**) posterior-stabilized designs, (**B**) medial and lateral fixation lugs, or (**C**) both.

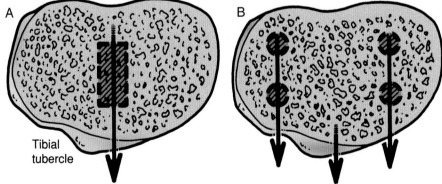

Figure 84–55. **A,** Alignment of the tibial component is projected at a point slightly medial to the tibial tubercle. **B,** Alignment of a symmetric component with the posterior margin of the tibial plateau will usually result in some internal rotation of the tibial component. One should err on the side of external rotation.

tive bones without overhang. Overhang can create pain and predispose to stiffness as a result of capsular stretching. For prostheses systems that allow separate sizing of the femur and tibia (interchangeable components), the tibial component selected will normally and quite precisely coincide with the resected tibial plateau. However, some cruciate-substituting designs have the option of some medial or lateral translation of the tibial component. This option is useful to reduce the size of marginal bony defects when present (Fig. 84–59). On the femoral side, the component should ideally coincide with the resected margin of the lateral femoral condyle. The femoral components should not be placed medially because of the consequent stress on the lateral patellar retinaculum.

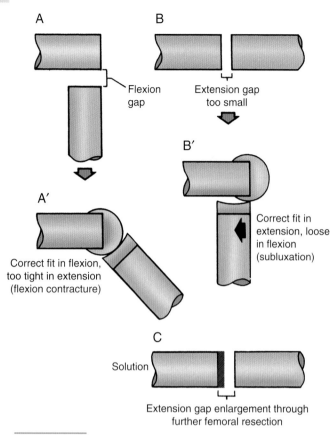

Figure 84–56. Unequal gap size is a frequent technical error. When the extension gap is too small, the knee will not fully extend; if a thinner tibial component is used, the prosthesis will be too loose in flexion. The solution is to excise more bone from the distal end of the femur.

Patellar Cuts and Cutting Guides

The goal of the patellar osteotomy is a patellar cut that results in central tracking of the patella and minimal tilt while accurately restoring patellar height (Fig. 84–60). The patellar osteotomy is perhaps the most difficult to instrument and is still often done by freehand technique with an oscillating saw used to resect the articular surface (Fig. 84–61 and 84–62).[101] Reaming or patellar milling devices[59] (Fig. 84–63) used for inset patellar components are also effective in establishing the proper resection level for onset patellar components. Caliper measurements of patellar size after resection should be equal to or slightly less than the original thickness of the patellar bone (Fig. 84–64).

Although patella resurfacing is generally recommended in patients with osteoarthrosis involving the patellofemoral joint, crystalline disease, or inflammatory arthropathy,[132] the patella does not always have to be resurfaced. Investigators have reported acceptable results without patella resurfacing,[9,10,15,16,107] especially when the patellar articular cartilage has limited articular wear. On the other hand, extreme patellar articular erosion makes use of a patellar component difficult or impossible. In these cases, contouring of the residual patellar bone ("patelloplasty") is performed. TKA without patella resurfacing in these patients has been reported with satisfactory results in short-term follow-up.[107,132] However, a study of nonresurfaced patellae with follow-up at 8.5 years showed progressive patellofemoral arthritis and maltracking in 40% of patients studied.[157]

Recent prospective, randomized trials have supported patella resurfacing. Waters and Bentley[180] randomized 514 primary TKAs to have the patella resurfaced or retained.

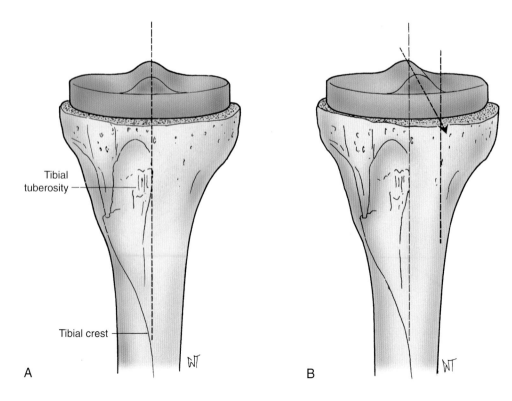

Figure 84–57. The tibial component should be aligned with the tibial tubercle. **A,** Correct position. **B,** Tibial component internally rotated on the tibia.

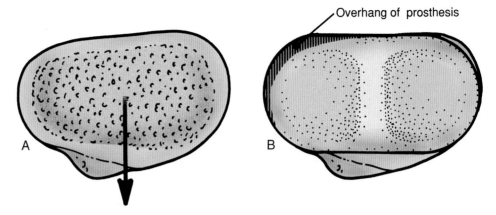

Overhang of prosthesis

Figure 84–58. **A** and **B**, With a symmetric component, some degree of posterolateral overhang of the prosthesis is expected.

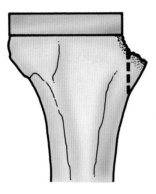

Figure 84–59. Lateralization of the tibial component can be done with cruciate-substituting designs. The tibia is deliberately undersized and placed at the lateral margin of the tibia. The medial defect is reduced, and overhanging bone can be excised vertically.

The incidence of anterior knee pain was significantly higher in the nonresurfaced group (25.1%) than in the resurfaced group (5.3%), and 10 of 11 patients undergoing secondary resurfacing for anterior knee pain experienced complete relief. A prospective randomized study by Wood et al[190] also showed a significant difference in anterior knee pain between the resurfaced and nonresurfaced groups. However, 10% of patients in the resurfacing group underwent a revision or reoperation involving the patellofemoral joint as compared with 12% in the nonresurfacing group.

Lug or fixation holes are made in the patella. Most designers currently favor three 3- to 4-mm holes placed in a triangular fashion rather than a larger, centrally placed fixation point (Fig. 84–65). A small, centralized, single-peg inset design has also functioned well.[92] A round dome patellar prosthesis should be positioned to the medial side of the oblong patellar osteotomy and is sized by the superior-inferior dimension of the bone (Fig. 84–66). The median ridge of the patella is a useful reference point for centering the component, but it should be borne in mind that the medial facet is shorter and more acutely sloped than the lateral patellar facet. Insetting designs with a diameter of 28 or 32 mm have been tried with some success (Fig. 84–67). These designs require central reaming of the patella with the periphery left intact. Inadvertent patellar fracture can be avoided by adequately

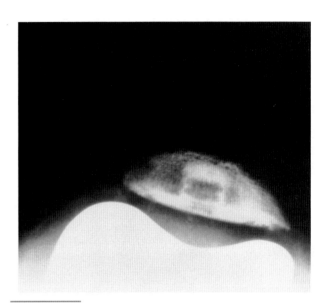

Figure 84–60. Radiograph showing a patellar component with "ideal" patellar tracking, orientation, and thickness.

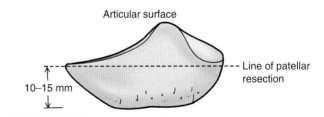

Articular surface

Line of patellar resection

10–15 mm

Figure 84–61. The line of patellar resection.

lubricating the reamer, firmly grasping the patella during reaming, and not resecting an excessive amount of patellar bone.

FITTING OF TRIAL COMPONENTS

Fitting of the trial components is done when all the initial bone cuts are completed. Stability and alignment are checked in both flexion and extension. For cruciate-substituting designs with balanced gaps, little further

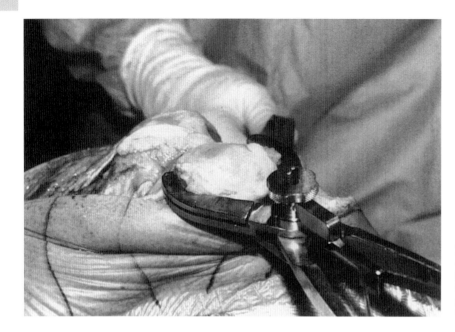

Figure 84–62. A slotted patellar cutting guide. The depth of the resection is selected by the knurl knob. The jaws grasp the patella, and the slots direct the cutting blade.

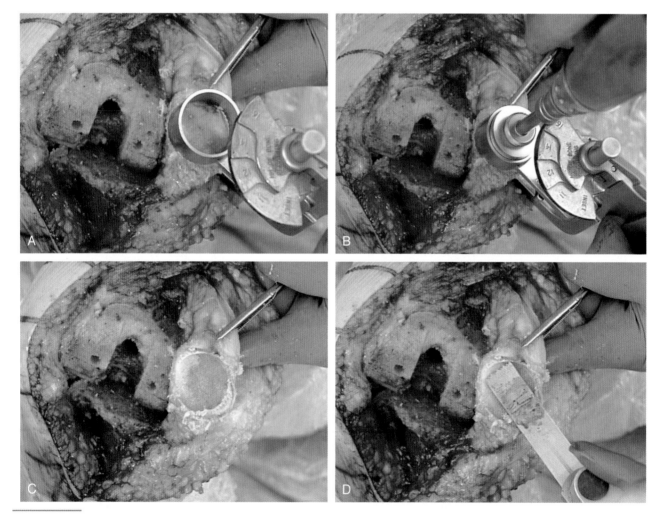

Figure 84–63. Although the reamer is traditionally used for insetting patellar components, it may also be used to create an accurate flat cut for an onset component. **A**, Patellar clamp balanced on the patella. **B**, Reamer positioned within the clamp. **C**, Patella reamed to the desired resection level. **D**, Resection completed with the saw blade.

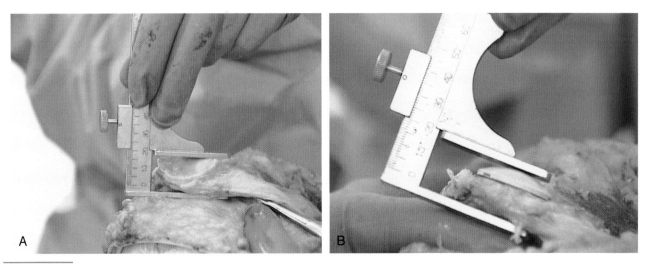

Figure 84–64. **A** and **B**, Caliper measurements of patellar thickness should be made before and after patellar osteotomy. The thickness of the patellar composite should not be increased; rather, a thickness of 2 to 3 mm less is preferred. Between 10 and 15 mm of patellar bone should remain.

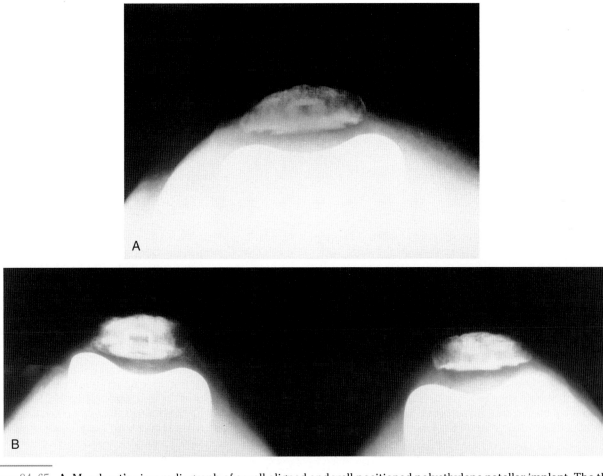

Figure 84–65. **A**, Merchant's view radiograph of a well-aligned and well-positioned polyethylene patellar implant. The thickness of the bone-polyethylene composite restores the original thickness of the patellar bone. **B**, Patellar implants inserted some years apart. On the *left*, the patellar cut was made by eye and a single-peg patellar implant was used. The patella is too thick and the patellar osteotomy is not quite symmetric. On the *right*, the arthroplasty was done more recently, a slotted patellar cutting guide was used, and a three-peg patellar implant was inserted. Although there is a slight tilt, the patellar cut is symmetric and the patellar thickness is correct.

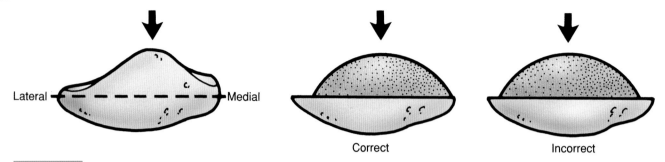

Lateral — · · · · · · — Medial

Correct

Incorrect

Figure 84–66. With a conventional patellar dome onset on the patella, the component should be medialized. This has the advantage of placing the apex of the dome in the correct position for patellar tracking but has the disadvantage of leaving peripheral lateral bone exposed.

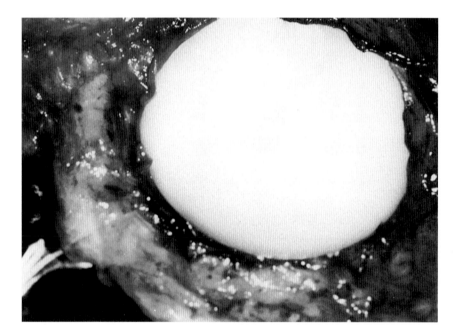

Figure 84–67. Insetting the patella allows greater thickness of polyethylene. There is a rim of peripheral exposed bone that can impinge against the femur.

adjustment should be required. For cruciate-retaining prostheses, ligament balancing is done at this stage with the use of different thicknesses of tibial trial components until satisfactory stability is achieved. When sparing the PCL, particular attention must be paid to PCL balance. Excessive tightness of the PCL can be detected by noting a tight flexion gap with excessive femoral rollback. On the contrary, a loose PCL will allow roll-forward of the femur on the tibia as the knee is flexed and result in posterior impingement. PCL recession can be accomplished by performing intrasubstance ligament lengthening or by elevating the ligament off the tibial insertion. At this stage, if optimal balance cannot be achieved, it is wise to make an intraoperative change to a PCL-substituting design.

Patellar Tracking and Position

When the correct tibial component thickness has been selected, patellar tracking is observed with the patellar component in place. The "no thumb" test is applied: the

patella should track with its medial border in contact with the femoral component throughout the range of motion without the surgeon maintaining it in this position manually (Fig. 84–68). It is permissible to take the slack out of the quadriceps tendon by applying longitudinal tension (Fig. 84–69) or by using a single stitch or towel clip to reapproximate the vastus medialis to the proximal patellar margin. If this suture ruptures or if there is any doubt about patellar tracking, a lateral retinacular release is considered. Because the "no thumb" technique may be a particularly stringent test of patellar tracking, one should consider the status of the tourniquet and other factors that might affect patellar movement during trial testing.

Testing of patellar tracking with the tourniquet deflated will give a better assessment of patellar tracking and may decrease the number of lateral releases performed.[100] Another method of checking lateral retinacular tightness is to subluxate the patellar component over the medial femoral condyle with the knee in extension. If the patella can be subluxated half of its diameter over the medial femoral condyle, the retinaculum is probably not too tight. If it is determined that the patella will not track properly

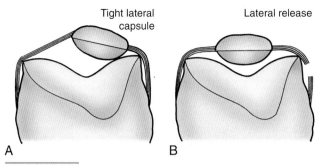

Tight lateral
capsule

Lateral release

A   B

Figure 84–68. If the patella does not track smoothly without a tendency to displace, a lateral release is performed.

with the aforementioned assessments, a lateral retinacular release is performed. After isolating the lateral superior genicular vessels (Fig. 84–70), which can be found distal to the lower border of the vastus lateralis, and protecting these vessels, a lateral retinacular release is performed approximately 1 to 2 cm from the lateral patellar margin from inside out (Fig. 84–71).

The patellar position in the sagittal plane is also important, but it is for the most part determined by the bone cuts of the femur and tibia. There is a tendency toward producing patella baja when the joint line is elevated or a thick tibial component is required. The development of postoperative patella baja may also be related to fibrosis around the infrapatellar ligament.[89]

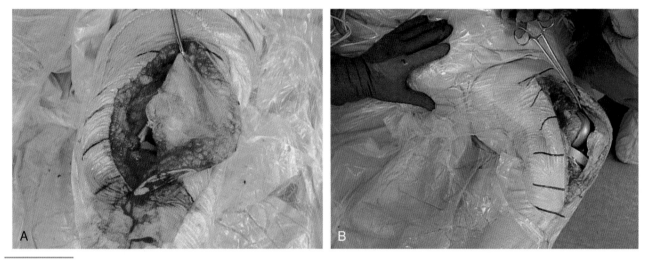

A   B

Figure 84–69. **A** and **B**, When assessing patellar traction, the "rule of no thumb" must be observed, but it is advisable to take longitudinal slack out of the extensor mechanism because on bringing the knee from flexion into extension, the patellar ligament tends to buckle and can cause a misleading lateral tilt of the patella.

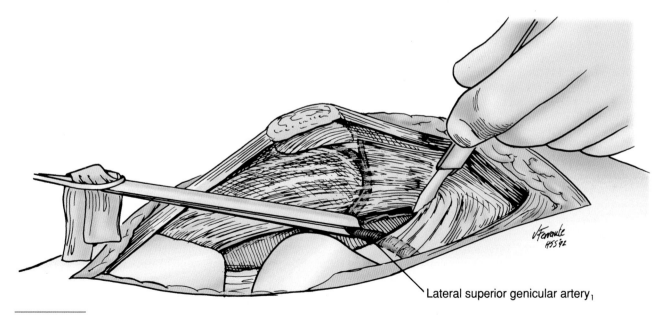

Lateral superior genicular artery

Figure 84–70. Patellar release is performed vertically about 1 inch from the lateral border of the patella from inside out while retracting and preserving the lateral genicular vessels. The release may include the lower fibers of the vastus lateralis.

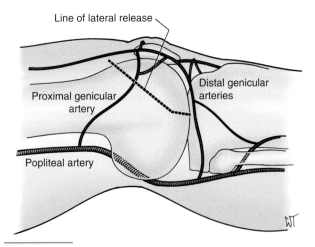

Figure 84–71. The lateral release is performed obliquely to preserve the distal genicular arteries.

CEMENTED VERSUS UNCEMENTED FIXATION

Long-term follow-up studies of cemented TKA have consistently demonstrated successful clinical results and survivorship, particularly when used in conjunction with a posterior-stabilized design (Fig. 84–31A).[28,35,149,154] Cemented designs afford the benefit that slight incongruities in the bone-prosthesis interface can be eliminated with the cement, whereas cementless prostheses require almost perfect bone cut congruency to optimize bony ingrowth with the materials available for cementless fixation. Failure of early cemented TKA designs was most likely a result of excessive prosthetic tibiofemoral constraint, concern over polymethylmethacrylate degradation, deterioration of the bone-cement interface, and resultant third-body wear. This experience led to the development of minimally constrained, PCL-retaining TKA designs that featured cementless fixation.[70] The limitation of cementless total knee design has been related to unreliable bone ingrowth secondary to incongruity, movement at the bone-prosthesis interface, or heightened requirements for both exact bone cuts and prosthetic stability for bone ingrowth to occur on the tibial side. Although the initial results of cementless and cemented TKA were comparable, a decline in satisfactory results was observed with cementless fixation.[4,117,123] Berger et al reported in 2001 that their group was abandoning cementless fixation in TKA because of an unacceptable 8% aseptic loosening rate and a 12% incidence of osteolytic lesions around screw holes.[13]

PCL retention with the thin, flat polyethylene inserts frequently used in combination with cementless designs in the past created high contact stress that resulted in polyethylene wear and osteolysis.[22,52,81,148,166] However, all failures of cementless TKA cannot be attributed to PCL retention and nonconforming polyethylene inserts alone. Cement fixation appears to provide an advantage in durability over currently available press-fit techniques. In a prospective comparison of cemented and cementless fixation with the same implant, Duffy et al[41] demonstrated better durability of femoral and tibial fixation with cemented techniques. At an average follow-up of 10 years, the survival rate of the cemented prostheses was 94% versus 72% for the uncemented group. Although these results suggest that cementless fixation alone is responsible for a higher failure rate, failure of cementless TKA is probably multifactorial. Knee implants designed for cementless use will require not only rethinking of design and instrumentation but also new materials to improve the chance for bone ingrowth.

Retrieval studies of cementless components revealed minimal bone ingrowth resulting in component loosening and migration. To enhance fixation, pegs were added to the distal femoral component and screws to the tibial component. Although femoral component fixation improved, screw osteolysis was observed under the tibial component and resulted in proximal tibial bone resorption without enhancement of bone ingrowth.[46,99] Smooth tracks on the undersurface of the tibial baseplate, screw holes in the tibial baseplate itself, and drill holes in bone serve as conduits that permit polyethylene debris to reach the cancellous tibial surface.[184] However, despite the dramatic cases of osteolysis with some cementless knee designs, the use of cement in TKA does not eliminate the risk of osteolysis. Cases of severe osteolysis have also been observed in cemented TKA.[25,62,129,133,143] Osteolysis has been related to polyethylene quality and backside wear issues accelerated by poor polyethylene locking mechanisms in cemented TKA.

Renewed efforts in cementless total knee design have resulted in the development of methods to improve bony ingrowth, including uniform porous coating of the tibial baseplate that is not recessed,[184] use of highly porous tantalum tibial baseplates, and fixation enhanced by hydroxyapatite.[125,126] Akizuki et al reported on a series of 32 hydroxyapatite-coated TKAs at 7-year follow-up. By 6 months after implantation, there were no radiographic clear zones surrounding the prostheses. Clinically, the patients were doing well without any reported revisions. One patient died 2 years after implantation of her prosthesis, and autopsy showed bone tissue at 77.7% of the interface.[3] Results by Murty et al on hydroxyapatite-coated femoral components showed 94% survivorship at 7- and 10-year follow-up.[122] Ritter and coworkers' series[141] of cemented cruciate-retaining total condylar knees and Scott's series[151] of cemented cruciate-retaining TKAs have produced results approaching those of cemented posterior-stabilized designs. Improvements in design have enhanced the results in cementless TKA as well; Whiteside's series[182] of cementless, cruciate-retaining prostheses with conforming articular surfaces and intramedullary alignment techniques common to posterior-stabilized cemented designs demonstrated outcomes matching those of cemented cruciate-substituting prostheses. Buechel et al[20] have also reported excellent results at 18 years with the use of a cementless mobile-bearing knee design. Nevertheless, until greater positive experience with cementless designs in multiple centers is available, cemented TKA will remain the gold standard against which other methods of fixation are measured.

Cement Technique

Cement fixation is achieved as polymethylmethacrylate penetrates the porous cancellous bony surfaces and creates a mechanical interlock. Pulsatile lavage is used to remove blood, fat, and debris, and proper cleaning of the cancellous bone permits uninhibited penetration of cement.[140] The cement should be applied to the bone digitally in the doughy tactile state, which allows for easy handling and manual pressurization (Fig. 84–31B and C). Insall believed centrifugation to be unnecessary in TKA because the cement layer is thin and air bubbles escape readily. Walker et al[175] determined that ideal cement penetration into bone is 3 to 4 mm; however, caution should be exercised in softer rheumatoid bone, where deeper penetration may occur. In contrast, the sclerotic surfaces frequently encountered in osteoarthritis may be drilled. Drilling of bone surfaces is performed with a 2-mm drill bit and should be limited to no more than 3 to 4 mm in depth because deeper cement penetration transfers the bone-cement interface away from the tibial surface into cancellous bone, where tibial bone strength tends to be less.

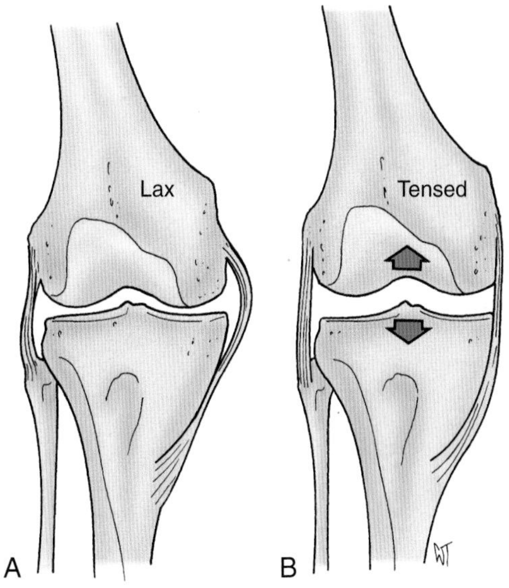

MANAGEMENT OF INSTABILITY OR DEFORMITY

Principles

In most arthritic knees, some degree of instability, deformity, contracture, or a combination of these elements will be found.[26,77] Deformity and instability can be created by asymmetric loss of articular cartilage resulting in collateral, capsular, and cruciate imbalance. Contracture of soft tissues is a secondary change that generally arises as a consequence of trauma or long-standing angular malalignment. Variations in anatomy such as tibia vara or a diminutive lateral femoral condyle can also contribute to angular abnormalities, and these abnormalities should be corrected at the time of total knee replacement. Even though some minor degree of postoperative ligament asymmetry may be tolerated, it is better to obtain near-perfect stability and avoid persistent contracture while accepting small amounts of laxity through surgical technique.

Although several investigators have suggested that residual malalignment is not detrimental to the outcome of TKA,[30,48,142,160] others have demonstrated that malalignment has a negative influence on the long-term results of TKA.* These investigations suggest that the most important factor for maintaining satisfactory long-term outcome in TKA is anatomic alignment, which depends significantly on ligamentous balance and accurate bone resection. Although the bone cuts can be made to establish anatomic alignment, proper ligamentous balance is required to maintain alignment throughout the range of motion. In a polyethylene retrieval study, Wasielewski et al[177] noted that increased wear occurred when preoperative varus or valgus was present.

---

*References 21, 61, 67, 68, 78, 98, 118, 139, 172, 188.

Figure 84–72. Symmetric instability. The ligaments, though lax, are of equal length (**A**). Both alignment and stability are restored by tensioning the ligaments (**B**).

tive varus or valgus was present. Polyethylene wear and cold flow tended to be greater in the tightest prearthroplasty compartment, most frequently when ligament releases were inadequate.

Instability of an arthritic knee may be viewed as being symmetric or asymmetric. Symmetric instability is a result of erosion of cartilage or bone without associated adaptive ligamentous changes. This type of deformity is common in early arthritis of the knee and can be corrected by active reciprocal stress during physical examination. Standard surgical techniques that create symmetric flexion and extension gaps are typically adequate to restore ligamentous balance (Fig. 84–72). Asymmetric instability, common in patients with advanced knee arthritis and those with a fixed deformity on physical examination, occurs when bone and cartilage compromise is associated with adaptive ligamentous changes (Figs. 84–73 and 84–74). These adaptive changes produce a continuum of deformity and may include contracture on the concave side of the joint with or without associated ligament laxity on the convex side of the deformed joint. Standard surgical technique and prosthesis spacing prove inadequate in balancing asymmetric instability because of fixed ligament changes. Ligament release plus ligament balancing is required to address this type of advanced deformity.

Operative management of asymmetric instability and contracture cannot be accomplished by bone cuts alone. Although postoperative bracing has been described for the management of instability after TKA, it is seldom optimal. Bracing is a treatment of ligament instability, not a treatment of ligament contracture. Two surgical methods have been described for correction of asymmetric instability. These two surgical methods are used separately or in combination, depending on the type of ligament deformity present. The first technique is a controlled ligament release from the contracted concave side of the deformity, and the second is a ligament advancement on the attenuated convex side. Ligament release of the contracted struc-

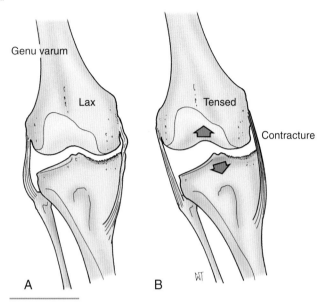

Figure 84–73. Asymmetric instability in varus. The medial ligament is shorter than the lateral ligament.

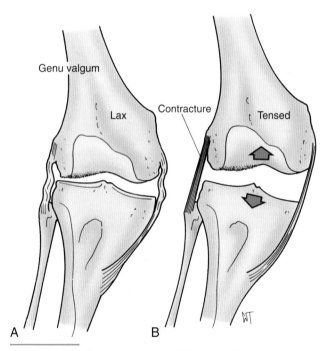

Figure 84–74. Asymmetric instability in valgus.

tures is adequate for correction of most deformities, although there are limits to the amount of correction that can be gained with ligament release. This statement is particularly true for valgus deformities, in which the amount of correction and release of structures on the lateral side of the knee is restricted by the fear of stretching the peroneal nerve. Conversely, one cannot balance a knee simply by releasing the contracted side of the knee when the opposing ligaments are stretched to the point of being incompetent. Nevertheless, every attempt should be made to balance the knee before increasing the degree of constraint in TKA, especially in younger, active patients. When a ligament is incompetent, repair of the incompe-

tent ligament or the use of a more constrained knee design will be required. When extreme deformity cannot be balanced with controlled ligament release, the options for treatment are bracing of the instability, reconstruction of the incompetent ligament, or adding increased articular constraint (such as a constrained condylar knee [CCK or TC3]) that provides for collateral ligament substitution (Figs. 84–75 to 84–77).

Asymmetric Varus Instability

PATHOPHYSIOLOGY

Varus deformity is defined by any preoperative femorotibial angle less than naturally occurring anatomic valgus. The definition is not absolute because of the variability of human limb alignment; in patients with habitual genu varum, this malalignment is typically exaggerated. Generally, TKA in patients with arthritis and habitual genu varum involves realignment to physiological valgus. Moderate to severe varus has been arbitrarily defined as greater than 15 to 20 degrees of varus deviation from the mechanical axis.[94,168]

The development of asymmetric varus instability typically follows a sequence in which loss of medial compartment bone and cartilage imparts a varus moment to the joint. The varus moment combined with the attendant periarticular inflammation associated with the arthritic process ultimately results in pathological fibrosis and contracture of the MCL. The bony deficits in a varus knee typically occur on the medial tibial plateau, although deficits may develop in both the medial aspect of the tibia and the femur in advanced disease. The MCL contracture is worsened by medial osteoarthritic overgrowth pressing outward from the joint on the ligament, thereby causing relative shortening. Eventually, the effect of contracture of the MCL is a fixed varus deformity (Fig. 84–78; see also Fig. 84–73). Simultaneously, adaptive elongating changes occur in the LCL and capsule and result in attenuation of these lateral soft-tissue structures. This combination of elements culminates in a "lateral thrust" or "varus thrust" of the knee that is observed during the stance phase of walking. Varus contracture may also be associated with a flexion contracture (described later).

MANAGEMENT OF VARUS DEFORMITY

Principles

MCL release is essential to achieve soft-tissue balance in TKA with a fixed varus deformity. Several authors have shown that residual varus deformity in TKA increases the failure rate.[21,67,68,78,98,118,172,177,188] Sambatakakis et al[146] described a radiographic "wedge sign" characteristic of incompletely corrected varus deformity hinging on a tight medial ligament; this finding has been confirmed by Laskin[94] and correlates with Insall's observation that the majority of TKA failures occur because of medial tibial collapse related to recurrence of the preoperative deformity.

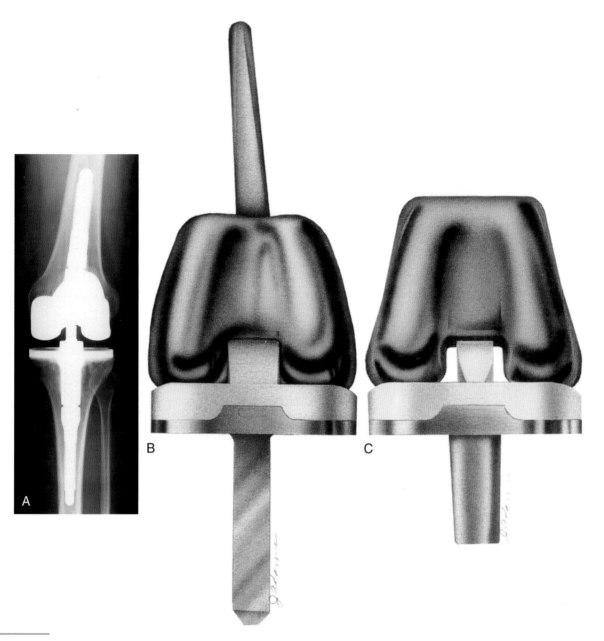

Figure 84–75. Constrained condylar knee prosthesis. **A**, Radiograph. **B**, The constrained condylar device is an unlinked constrained design that places limitations on varus-valgus deflection, anteroposterior displacement, and rotation within the flexion-extension axis of the knee. Restriction of varus-valgus deflection and rotation is provided by a large tibial spine within an intracondylar femoral box, whereas posterior subluxation is prevented by engagement of the spine on the femoral cam. **C**, Posterior-stabilized device. Nonlinked, semiconstrained posterior-stabilized devices prevent posterior subluxation via a tibial spine that engages a femoral cam. Slight rotational constraint is afforded by the degree of conformity of the femorotibial articulation. (**B** and **C**, From Scott WN: The Knee, vol 2. St Louis, Mosby–Year Book, 1994, p 1308.)

Although some investigators have reported success with PCL-balancing procedures in TKA with a fixed varus deformity,[168] other studies have demonstrated that moderate to severe varus deformity warrants PCL resection because of its contribution to varus malalignment. In fact, Alexiades et al[5] demonstrated that without the counterbalance of the ACL, the PCL tends to contract. Dennis et al[34] have shown that retaining the PCL may not result in the desired femoral rollback, nor does it prevent condylar lift-off during knee flexion. Laskin et al[94,95] (Fig. 84–79)

demonstrated that for fixed varus deformities exceeding 15 degrees, the best results in terms of pain relief, correction, and range of motion are obtained by excision of the PCL and use of a cruciate-substituting prosthesis. Teeney et al[168] noted that 40% of knees with preoperative varus tended to remain in varus; their series included more than 50% of knees with cruciate-retaining prostheses. Both Laskin[94] and Teeney et al[168] observed that the functional outcome of varus knees approached, but did not equal, the results in nondeformed knees.

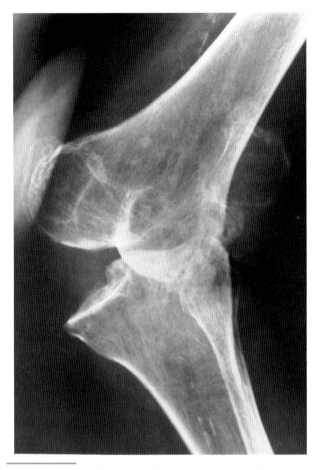

Figure 84–76. Radiograph of a very unstable valgus knee. This degree of ligamentous instability cannot be managed by any type of ligament release. Reconstruction will involve either a medial ligament tightening procedure or a constrained prosthesis.

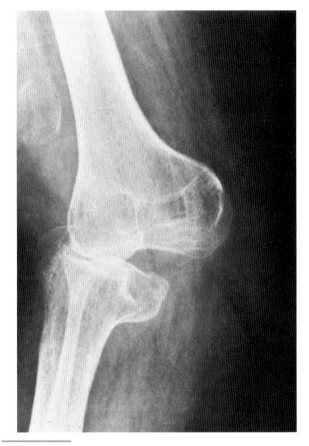

Figure 84–77. In this valgus knee, although the medial ligament is not absent, it is so elongated that soft-tissue balancing by lateral release is impractical. This is an indication for a constrained prosthesis.

Technique

Ligament balance is achieved by progressively releasing the medial soft tissues until they reach the length of the lateral ligamentous structures. The extent of the release can be monitored by periodically inserting lamina spreaders (Fig. 84–80) or using a ligament tensiometer to judge alignment with the aligning rod or plumb line. The endpoint of the release is a stable position in which a plumb line will extend from the hip through the center of the knee to the ankle joint. Computer navigation of TKA also allows the possibility of real-time assessment of knee alignment and balance during the course of ligament release. Component placement can also affect angular deformity. Dixon and Scott[36] described the use of a downsized tibial component with lateral translation of the component and removal of a portion of the medial tibial plateau to correct rigid varus deformity. If the PCL is tethering the release, it should be excised or lengthened by posterior release from the tibia. In a measured resection technique, the ligament release is performed after the bone cuts and after insertion of the trial components; for cruciate-substituting designs performed with gap balancing, the ligament releases are done before the bone cuts or after the tibial cut has been made. The cruciate-substituting

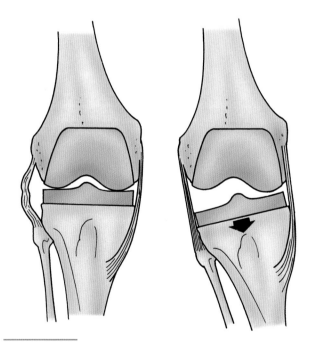

Figure 84–78. The medial ligament was not released; hence, an asymmetric instability remains.

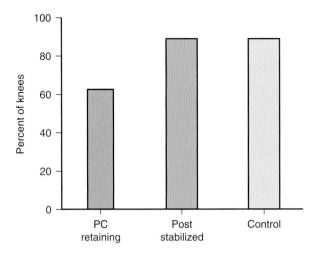

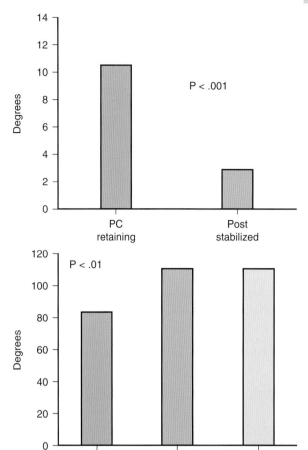

Figure 84–79. Bar graphs showing (**A**) the percentage of knees accurately aligned, (**B**) residual flexion contracture (average), and (**C**) average range of motion in knees with greater than 15 degrees of fixed varus deformity. The parameters studied were equivalent to those for a group of control knees (without significant deformity) in which a cruciate-retaining prosthesis was used. Cruciate retention in deformed knees led to less satisfactory correction of alignment and flexion contracture and inferior range of motion.

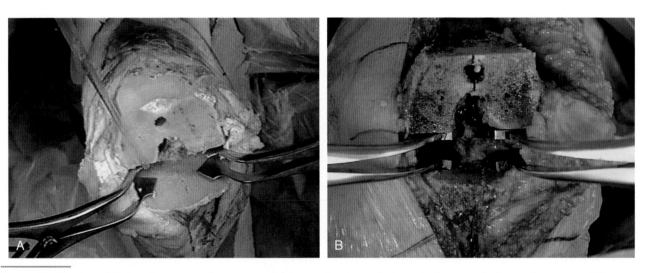

Figure 84–80. **A** and **B**, Laminar spreaders are useful in monitoring soft-tissue balance and the performance of ligament releases.

gap-balancing technique was favored by Insall for very large deformities because the laxity in the knee joint after release may occasionally dictate under-resection of the distal end of the femur to accurately balance the knee (Fig. 84–81). A full MCL release will not only correct fixed varus but also open the medial space in flexion (whereas a normal knee in flexion has more lateral than medial

laxity). Although flexion gap symmetry is influenced by the medial release, rotational alignment of the femoral component is determined relative to the femoral anatomy and *not* by the ligament release.

The medial release (Fig. 84–82) is done in steps by first removing medial osteophytes from the femur and tibia, including the protruding flare of the tibial plateau, and

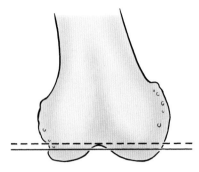

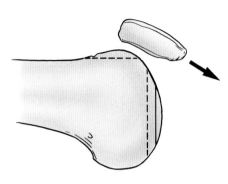

Figure 84–81. In knees with considerable ligamentous laxity, under-resection of the distal end of the femur may be preferable. The standard femoral resection will necessitate a thicker tibial component to take up the slack in the soft tissues and may cause distal migration of the patella. By under-resecting the femur, desirable patellar position is maintained.

raising a sleeve of soft tissue from the upper medial aspect of the tibia and allowing it to slide proximally. The sleeve consists of periosteum, deep medial ligament, superficial medial ligament, and the insertion of the pes anserinus tendons. More posteriorly, at the joint surface the sleeve is continuous with the semimembranosus insertion and posterior capsule. Distally, the release may include the deep fascia investing the soleus and popliteus muscles. The sleeve is made by stripping the periosteum medially from the tibia 10 to 15 cm distal to the standard arthrotomy. The knee is flexed, and the tibia is progressively externally rotated to gain posterior access. The distal attachment of the superficial medial ligament can be left intact with moderate deformities. When this is not enough, the release is continued posteriorly and distally by further subperiosteal stripping of the superficial fibers of the MCL. In this manner, correction of deformity occurs in a graduated fashion and is aided by the intermittent stretching action of a medial laminar spreader. With a progressive release, there is no discontinuity between the medial soft-tissue structures, but rather progressive separation of the periosteal layer from the tibia at a point distal to the MCL attachment to the tibia (Fig. 84–83). The result is balancing, with some overall lengthening of the limb (the amount of lengthening depends on the degree of preoperative stretching of the lateral structures). The released medial soft tissues should ideally give way gradually rather than with an obvious "pop," which would indicate that the distal insertion of the ligament has been forcibly separated from its tibial attachment or that transverse disruption of a medial structure has occurred.

To gain access with the lamina spreader, the proximal tibial osteotomy may be performed first. When varus is combined with flexion contracture, it is helpful to transversely divide the medial portion of the posterior capsule or, alternatively, elevate the capsule from both the posterior surface of the tibia and the posteromedial aspect of the femur. Laterally, the posterior capsule is often sufficiently stretched to the point that it does not contribute to a flexion contracture. Posterior osteophytes should be removed. The occasional need for under-resection of the femur should be carefully judged before too much bone is removed because the distal part of the femur can always be recut. Such a situation may arise in a varus knee when the lateral structures are stretched and the medial structures are released to balance those structures, thereby increasing the height of the extension gap.

When the proper release and balancing are performed, mobilization can be started immediately, and walking with full weightbearing is permitted as tolerated.

Ligament advancement procedures have also been described to correct varus deformity.[168] In the rare case when varus knees cannot be fully corrected with a medial release and are associated with lateral laxity, consideration may be given to lateral ligament reconstruction.

Asymmetric Valgus Instability

PATHOPHYSIOLOGY

Valgus deformity is defined as malalignment exceeding the natural femorotibial valgus orientation, typically greater than 7 to 10 degrees.[115,163,181] Krackow et al classified valgus deformity into three distinct types.[91] Type I involves lateral femoral bone loss, lateral soft-tissue contracture, and intact medial soft tissues. Type II is type I with lengthened medial soft tissues. Type III is a severe valgus deformity with malpositioning of the proximal tibial joint line (e.g., secondary to high tibial osteotomy).

In a valgus knee, the lateral soft-tissue structures, including the LCL, ITB, and lateral capsule, contract while the medial soft tissues become stretched. The lateral femoral condyle has been shown to be frequently dysplastic in valgus deformity, and therefore most of the bony deficit occurs on the femoral side.[163] However, in advanced disease, cartilage and bone erosion may be observed on the tibial side as well. In long-standing deformity, the lateral contracture and medial lengthening become permanent (see Fig. 84–74). This combination of pathologies may result in a "medial thrust" during gait. Similar to varus deformities, valgus contractures may be associated with a flexion contracture. However, presumably because of contracture of the ITB, a fixed external rotation deformity often accompanies asymmetric valgus instability, particularly in patients with inflammatory arthritis.

MANAGEMENT

Principles

Valgus release has traditionally been performed by elevating the lateral capsule, LCL, arcuate ligament, popliteus

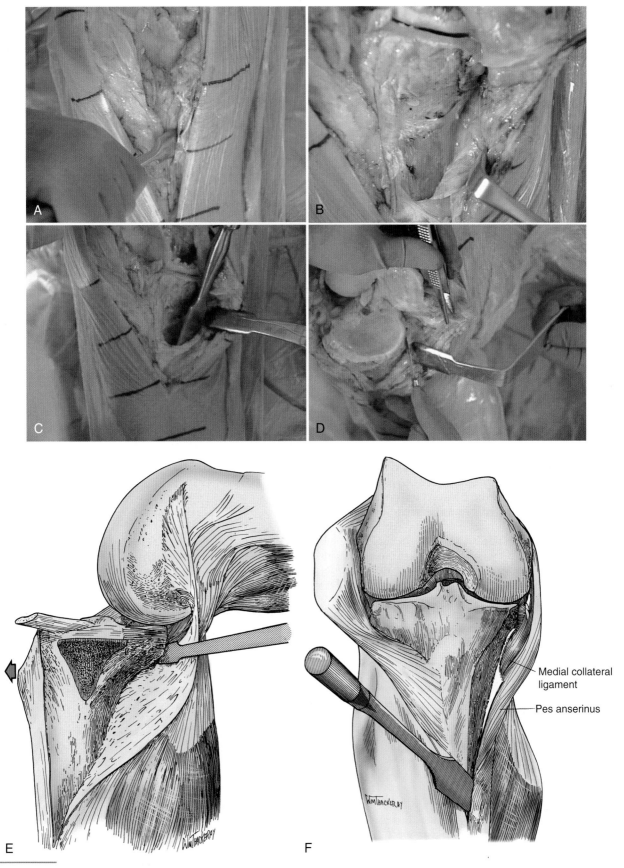

Figure 84–82. Varus release. **A** and **B**, The exposure is begun by subperiosteal stripping beneath the superficial medial collateral ligament. **C**, Completed release. Only the superficial medial collateral ligament remains intact, but this too can be detached if necessary. **D**, The tibia is externally rotated with a complete posteromedial release.

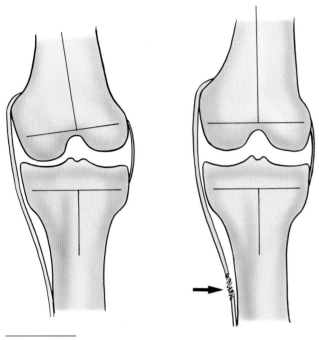

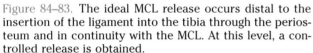

Figure 84–83. The ideal MCL release occurs distal to the insertion of the ligament into the tibia through the periosteum and in continuity with the MCL. At this level, a controlled release is obtained.

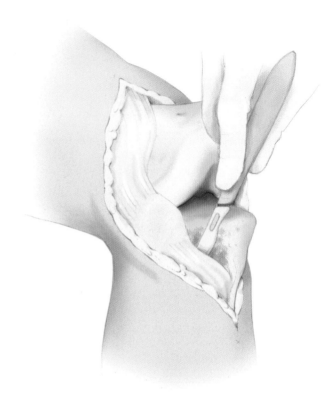

Figure 84–84. **First stage of a lateral release.** The iliotibial band is separated from its attachment to Gerdy's tubercle and the capsular attachments from the lateral margin of the tibia.

tendon, lateral femoral periosteum, distal ITB, and adjacent lateral intermuscular septum from their bony attachments. Except for the ITB, the release is performed from the lateral femoral condyle; the ITB is released from Gerdy's tubercle. Because the desired postoperative alignment is physiological valgus, some degree of lateral laxity after an extensive lateral release is typically well tolerated. The sequence of lateral release has been the focus of some controversy.[1,85,97,115,163,181] Insall described the management of lesser deformities with simple release of the ITB from its insertion on Gerdy's tubercle (Fig. 84–84). For moderate to severe fixed deformities, the lateral femoral condyle would be stripped of its soft-tissue attachments proximally for about 9 cm, and at this level the periosteum, the iliotibial tract, and the lateral intramuscular septum would be transversely divided from inside out (Figs. 84–85 and 84–86). Any part of the lateral intramuscular septum that remained attached to the distal end of the femur was divided longitudinally until the entire "flap" was free to slide. Although such an extensive release generally corrects any severity of deformity, posterolateral flexion instability may occur postoperatively.[76,115] Furthermore, case reports exist in which extensive soft-tissue stripping has devascularized the lateral femoral condyle and resulted in osteonecrosis.

Because of the risk of posterolateral instability (and osteonecrosis) after extensive soft-tissue stripping from the lateral femoral condyle, "stab-incision"[115] and "pie-crusting" techniques were developed and have become the method of choice. These techniques permit graduated intra-articular release of the posterolateral capsule and ITB. Although both techniques involve transverse punctures (pie-crusting) of the ITB well above the joint line

and some degree of transverse release of the posterolateral capsule, the stab-incision technique includes a more extensive transverse release of the arcuate complex immediately above the joint line and posterior to the ITB (Fig. 84–87). Release at the joint line leaves only the LCL for lateral restraint; perforations of the lateral capsule and ITB above the joint line in combination with a limited transverse posterolateral capsular release maintain greater soft-tissue continuity. Both techniques typically allow preservation of the popliteus tendon, thereby affording greater stability to the posterolateral corner. Whereas Miyasaka et al[115] observed a 24% incidence of posterolateral instability with extensive lateral femoral condylar release for valgus deformity, by using the stab-incision technique they limited the incidence to 6%, similar to what Insall described. Correction of valgus deformity in TKA has been associated with patellofemoral instability as a result of lateral tethering of the patella and peroneal palsy as a result of stretching of the nerve. The incidence of patellofemoral instability has been reported to be as high as 4%[97]; however, the incidence when the stab-incision technique is used and the popliteus is preserved has been reported as 0%.[115] Although the overall incidence of peroneal nerve palsy after TKA has been estimated at less than 1%, the incidence in valgus knees has been reported

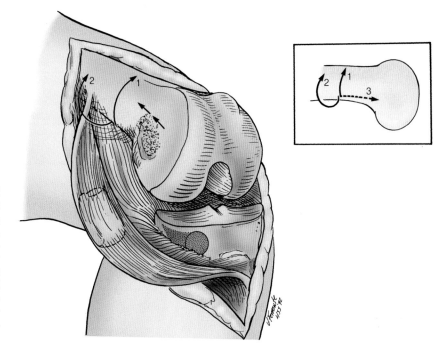

Figure 84–85. **A,** Further stages of lateral release include raising a flap from the lateral femoral condyle to a point 3 inches proximal to the joint. **B,** The periosteum is incised transversely (1), the lateral intramuscular septum and proximal iliotibial tract are divided transversely at the same level (2), and the remaining distal attachment of the lateral intramuscular septum is divided vertically and separated from the femur (3).

to be 3% to 4%.[91,163] In a recent investigation using the stab-incision technique, no cases of peroneal nerve compromise were observed.[115] In elderly patients or those with low physical demands, the use of articular constraint may avoid postoperative morbidity. In Insall's series of primary constrained implants (with up to 10 years of follow-up), there has been uniform success without prosthetic loosening, thus indicating that this approach may be a reasonable option in selected cases.[42]

Technique

Pie-Crusting Method (Insall). The knee is approached through a standard midline incision and standard medial parapatellar capsular approach. Femoral and tibial bone cuts are made to gain access and create congruent surfaces to assess gap symmetry. Because erosion occurs on the lateral femoral condyle in long-standing valgus malalignment, bone resection from the lateral condyle is often minimal. Appropriate femoral rotation is imperative to ensure proper balancing in flexion. Referencing off the posterior condyles is often not reliable because of posterior condylar erosion. Because the PCL frequently contributes to the deformity and requires resection to appropriately balance the knee, Insall recommended a posterior-stabilized design for valgus knees.[76,115] The posterolateral capsule and arcuate complex lateral to the popliteus are cut transversely at the level of the tibial cut, and titrated intra-articular and extra-articular releases of the lateral capsule at the tibial insertion and the ITB at Gerdy's tubercle are performed with a knife blade. The technique is performed by placing a moderate amount of stress in the lateral compartment with a laminar spreader or ligament tensiometer. Multiple stab incisions are made in the contracted lateral soft tissues (particularly the ITB)

within and above the joint until the deformity is corrected (see Fig. 84–87A and B). Spacer blocks are used to frequently check the balance to avoid overcorrection. As noted earlier, the popliteus and the LCL are preserved if possible to limit posterolateral instability. The technique of ligament advancement will be described later.

Correction through a Lateral Parapatellar Approach. Keblish[85] and Buechel[19] described a three-step lateral release through a lateral parapatellar approach for severe valgus deformity. The tibial tubercle is osteotomized and reflected medially while retaining a medial periosteal hinge. The infrapatellar fat pad is maintained on the patellar tendon to facilitate closing of the lateral retinacular defect. The three steps of lateral release are as follows:

1. The anterior compartment musculature and the iliotibial tract are elevated from Gerdy's tubercle to the level of the fibular head. The amount of correction is tested at this point.
2. With the knee flexed to 90 degrees, the LCL and the popliteus are elevated as a subperiosteal flap based proximally on the lateral femoral shaft. If needed, the entire periosteum is elevated. If the peroneal nerve is observed to sublux, the fibular head is resected.
3. With the knee maintained at 90 degrees of flexion, the entire periosteum of the fibular head is elevated while the peroneal nerve at the fibular neck is protected, and the fibular head is then resected. The extension position of the peroneal nerve is checked to ensure that the nerve is situated in the space created by femoral head resection.

As emphasized by Buechel,[19] the lateral instability that occurs in flexion with extensive lateral release can be corrected by compensatory external rotation of the femoral component. Patellar tracking must be carefully assessed after adjusting femoral component rotation.

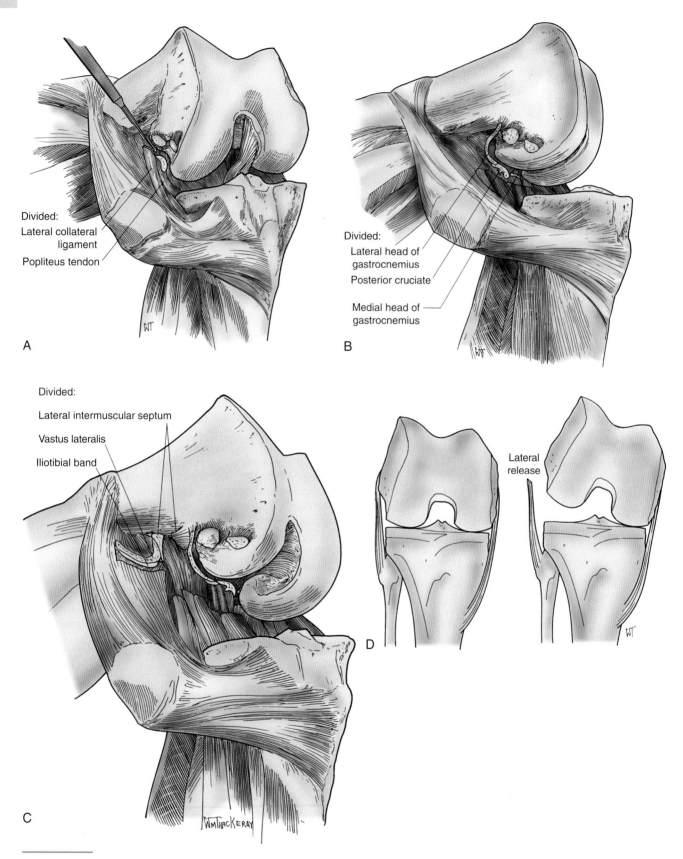

Figure 84–86. A-C, Valgus release is performed on the femur by completely releasing the soft tissues from the lateral femoral condyle and, if necessary, transversely dividing the iliotibial band. **D,** After lateral release for the correction of valgus, the knee is always inherently unstable in flexion. A lateral rotary instability may develop that will be exacerbated if there is any malrotation of the tibial component.

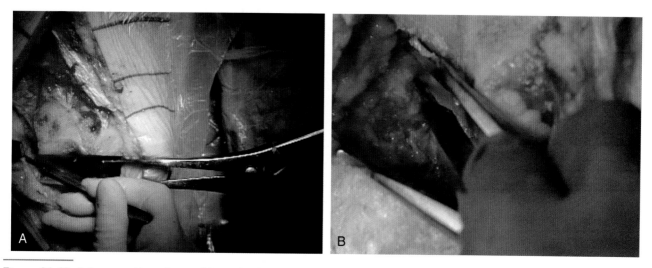

Figure 84–87. Intraoperative photo of lateral release via the "pie-crusting" technique. **A,** Joint distracted with a laminar spreader placed medially. **B,** Close-up view of multiple intra-articular punctures in the contracted lateral soft tissues proximal to the joint line.

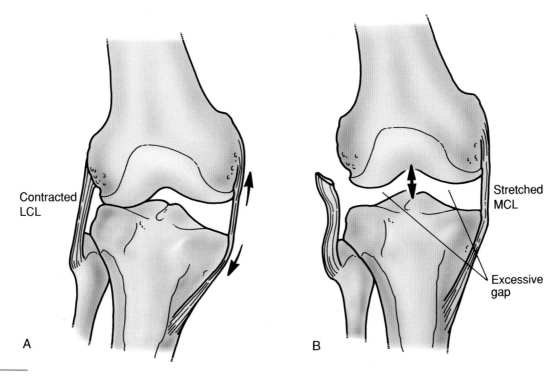

Figure 84–88. **A** and **B,** There are limits to ligament balancing. In this case, the medial collateral ligament is stretched beyond its normal length, and after lateral release, the knee will be distracted abnormally. Stabilizing this knee with thicker components involves actual lengthening of the limb, and there are clearly limits to how much lengthening can be tolerated without damage to the neurovascular structures.

Ligament Advancement or Tightening

Ligament advancement or tightening is rare in TKA. Krackow[90] has described techniques for ligament tightening for both the medial and lateral soft tissues and estimates that he has performed them in 1% to 2% of knee arthroplasties. In correction of a valgus knee, lateral ligament release may allow overlengthening of perhaps 5 mm to compensate for 5 mm of MCL stretching (Fig. 84–88).

However, when MCL elongation is 10 mm or more, it is simply not possible to achieve this much stretching by lateral release alone. The same argument can be applied to varus deformities, although there are differences (notably, the lack of a counterpart to the peroneal nerve). It is possible to overlengthen the medial side a greater amount, and provided that axial alignment is correct, some degree of lateral laxity is tolerable. As a rule of thumb, lateral laxity is acceptable if the knee alignment cannot be passively brought into varus with the knee extended. The MCL can be tightened either by proximal or by distal advancement. This type of soft-tissue reconstruction may have merit with overconstrained prostheses in younger patients. In support of Krackow's methods, Healy et al[66] reported success with lateral soft-tissue release and proximal MCL advancement with bone plug recession into the medial femoral condyle to correct valgus deformity in a small group of patients.

MEDIAL AND LATERAL PROXIMAL ADVANCEMENT

Krakow has described a method whereby the proximal attachment of the MCL to the medial femoral epicondyle is detached from the bone over a fairly wide area (Fig. 84–89).[90] The flap of tissue is advanced to a more proximal and slightly anterior position. It is secured by passing an interlocking stitch through the flap and tying it tightly over a proximally placed screw and washer; further augmentation is provided by a staple placed into the area of the original femoral condyle (Fig. 84–90). Engh and Ammeen[44] described the use of an epicondylar osteotomy with advancement of a ligament and placement of a bone block for correction of varus deformities, whereas Healy's method involves recession of the MCL attachment in its anatomic position at the medial femoral condyle rather than translocation of the proximal ligament.[66] The recessed proximal bone plug is secured over a bony bridge or button on the lateral side. For lax lateral structures, Krackow's method has been described for varus knees; reports are not available on Healy's method of proximal recession of the LCL.

Flexion Contracture

PATHOPHYSIOLOGY

Flexion contractures involve the posterior capsule, the PCL, and the musculotendinous units crossing the posterior aspect of the knee joint. In osteoarthritis, the deformity is typically limited to soft-tissue contracture associated with posterior compartment osteophytes (Fig. 84–91), whereas in inflammatory arthritis, flexion contracture may result in significant posterior femoral condylar erosion (Fig. 84–92). Extreme posterior femoral condylar erosion generally occurs in patients who have been unable to walk and have fixed flexion deformities that may exceed 90 degrees. Because of posterior condylar erosion, in addition to posterior capsular contracture, flexion contracture may be paradoxically associated with flexion instability. This situation represents a considerable technical challenge and typically warrants the application of revision TKA principles.

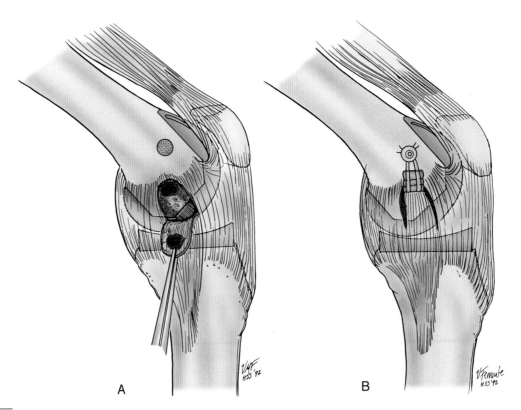

Figure 84–89. Krackow's technique of proximal medial collateral ligament (MCL) advancement. **A,** The proximal attachment of the MCL is removed en bloc without bone. A screw and washer are placed proximal and slightly anterior. **B,** With the use of a locking loop ligament fixation suture, the MCL is tightened proximally by tying the sutures around the screw and washer, which is then tightened. A second screw may be placed through the MCL's new attachment.

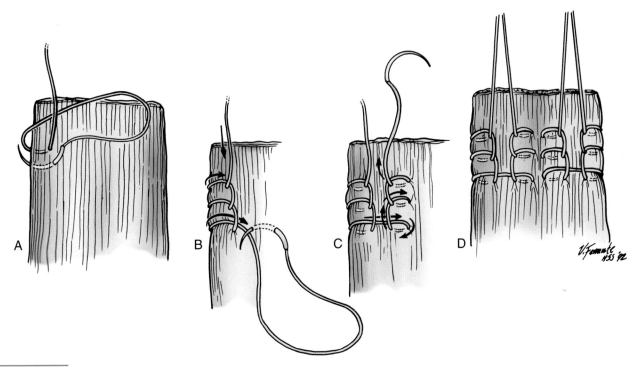

Figure 84–90. **A-D**, Krackow's locking loop ligament fixation suture.

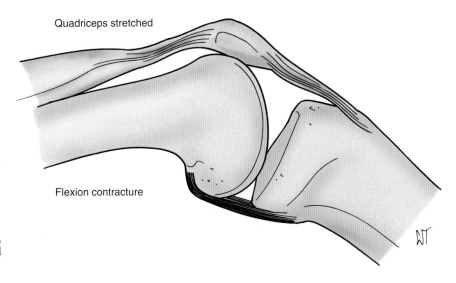

Quadriceps stretched

Flexion contracture

Figure 84–91. In a flexion contracture, the posterior capsule is shortened and adherent.

Several authors have suggested that full intraoperative correction of flexion contractures in TKA is not essential because postoperative correction is possible[54,112,167] and the clinical outcome is not affected by residual flexion contractures of up to 30 degrees.[112,169] In contrast, Firestone et al[54] reported that if a flexion contracture remains at the completion of TKA, the residual deformity will persist and worsen with time, especially if the PCL is preserved. The current consensus among knee surgeons is that flexion contractures should be corrected to the maximum extent possible at the time of TKA.

TECHNIQUE FOR RELEASE OF FLEXION CONTRACTURE

Posterior capsular release should be performed after the bone cuts. Until the bone cuts are made, posterior visualization is impeded by the posterior femoral condyles. Initially, the distal femoral and proximal tibial bone cuts should be conservative. Small flexion contractures can be reduced by removal of posterior osteophytes and elevation of the posterior capsule (Fig. 84–93).[167,169] Correction by

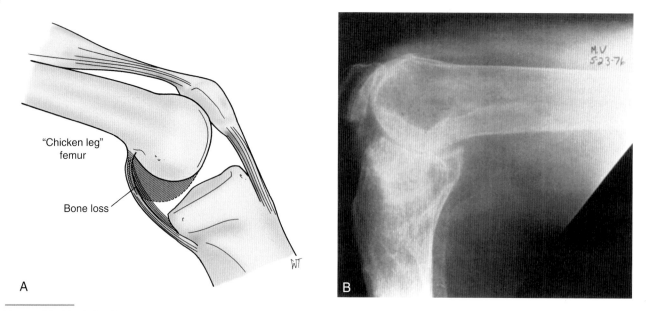

Figure 84–92. **A,** In rheumatoid arthritis, there is excessive loss of bone on the posterior aspect of the femoral condyles. **B,** Lateral radiograph showing this condition. Unless the technique recognizes and adjusts for it, flexion instability will result.

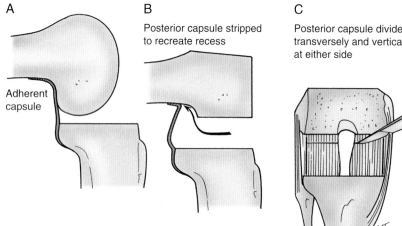
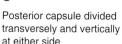
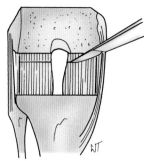

Figure 84–93. Posterior capsulotomy for flexion contracture. **A,** The posterior capsule is adherent. **B,** The original recess is reestablished. **C,** The cruciate ligaments have already been excised; only the medial and lateral parts of the posterior capsule need division. Often, the underlying gastrocnemii are adherent and must be divided as well. At the margin of the collateral ligaments, vertical incisions in the capsule must be made.

bone resection from the distal end of the femur alone unbalances the collateral ligaments such that stability in extension is provided by the tight posterior capsule, which results in kinematic abnormalities. Posterior capsulotomy is the preferred method for moderate to severe contractures and should be performed with the knee flexed. The shortened posterior capsule is first elevated from the central posterior aspect of the femur at the top of the intercondylar notch. Next, the medial and lateral capsule is elevated in a subperiosteal plane off the back of the femur. In more resistant cases, the capsule may be cut transversely and separated from the collateral structures by making vertical incisions at the medial and lateral corners. Resection of the PCL is most likely necessary and aids in division of the midline fibers. After the capsulotomy and posterior release, the trial knee components are inserted and the knee brought into as much extension as possible. If extension is still not complete, further bone can be

removed from the distal part of the femur. This procedure may necessitate the use of a constrained prosthesis when the collateral ligaments are removed from their origins because extreme cases may require resection of so much bone that the knee becomes completely unbalanced. Surgery is followed by aggressive range of motion with an emphasis on extension in the immediate postoperative period.

Extension Contracture ("Stiff Knee")

OVERVIEW

Primary TKA in stiff and ankylosed knees, though technically demanding, has been shown to provide excellent pain relief and significantly improve range of motion.[2,116,120] Stiff knees are typically defined as having less than 50 degrees of motion, whereas ankylosed knees have essentially no motion (Fig. 84–94). In the largest reported series, Montgomery et al[116] studied 82 stiff or ankylosed knees in 71 patients at an average follow-up of 5.3 years. The investigators noted an average Hospital for Special Surgery knee score improvement of 38 to 80 points and an improvement in average arc of motion of 36 to 93 degrees. All prostheses were posterior stabilized, with the majority being nonconstrained. Only one quadriceps-plasty was necessary. Peroneal nerve palsies developed in two patients with flexion-valgus deformities but resolved spontaneously, and one patient had a fracture of the inferior pole of the patella managed conservatively. This investigation is reflective of previous, smaller series,[2,120] although one series reported that quadricepsplasty was required in 42% of cases. More recently, McAuley et al[110] reported on a series of 27 arthroplasties in 21 patients with an average range of motion preoperatively of 50 degrees. Although their results reflected improvements in range of motion and quality of life, they had high complication (41%) and revision (18.5%) rates.

TECHNIQUE

The approach, as described by Montgomery et al,[116] is through a midline longitudinal incision and medial para-patellar arthrotomy. Typically, the techniques described in "Difficult Exposure" are necessary. Eversion of the patella is generally challenging and may not be possible or necessary. Early release of the lateral retinaculum and lateral patellofemoral ligaments is commonly performed. Soft-tissue releases are performed in the same fashion as they are for the varus, valgus, and flexion deformities described earlier; however, extensive soft-tissue release is routinely required. In varus knees, an extensile proximal medial tibial release is performed, whereas valgus knees are managed with a lateral release, occasionally including elevation of the LCL off the femoral side. Flexion contractures require posterior capsule release, but because of its contribution to contractures, Insall favored excision of the PCL. Occasionally, complete subperiosteal reflection of the soft tissues from the distal end of the femur (femoral

peel) is necessary (see Fig. 84–39). Adequate bone cuts are then performed to create balanced flexion and extension gaps. Despite extensive release, constrained prostheses are not typically required unless ligament stability is forfeited.

Correction of Genu Recurvatum

Genu recurvatum is an uncommon deformity and is seldom severe except in poliomyelitis or certain soft-tissue abnormalities such as Ehlers-Danlos syndrome. Operative correction is obtained by under-resection of the bone ends and the use of thicker components. However, paralytic types tend to recur. Krackow[90] has described a technique whereby the proximal ligament insertions are transferred proximally and posteriorly; such repositioning causes the collateral ligaments to tighten in extension. Postoperative bracing or the use of a heel wedge to promote a flexion moment may enhance the chance for success. Recurrent cases of recurvatum may be one of the few indications for the use of a hinged implant or a similarly constrained prosthesis. Occasionally after a previous tibial osteotomy, recurvatum will be found because of deformity of the tibia itself (tibial recurvatum) (Fig. 84–95). The anterior cor-

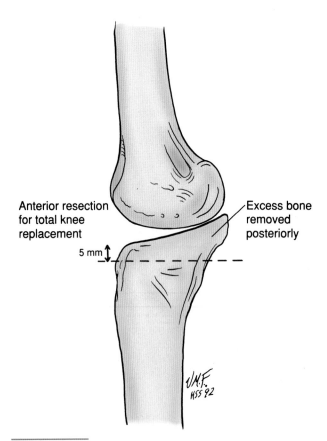

Figure 84–95. "Tibial recurvatum" after high tibial osteotomy. The osteotomy has healed with the distal fragment extended on the proximal one, which has resulted in an anterior tilt of the anterior surface. Unless care is taken when performing the tibial resection for total knee replacement, excessive bone may be removed.

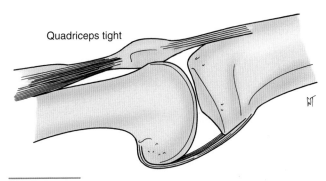

Figure 84–94. In an extension contracture, not only are there intra-articular adhesions, but the quadriceps muscle itself is also shortened and tight.

tices have impacted, and the result is an anterior slope of the tibia. This should be evident from study of the radiographs, and the level of the tibial cut should be adjusted accordingly.

MANAGEMENT OF BONE DEFECTS

Principles

Although bone defects are more common in revision TKA, they do occur in primary TKA. The etiology of bone defects in primary TKA includes erosion secondary to angular arthritic change, inflammatory arthritis, osteonecrosis, and fracture. Bone defects in primary TKA are typically asymmetric and peripheral, although contained deficiencies caused by cyst formation may occur. The base of contained and peripheral defects in primary TKA typically comprises condensed sclerotic bone, in contrast to revision surgery, in which removal of components often leaves osteopenic surfaces. A major concern with tibial defects is that subchondral bone strength diminishes substantially distal to the subchondral plate.[11,60,72] Several authors have advised that the level of lateral tibial resection should not exceed 1 cm to avoid compromising implant durability,[39,131] yet others have demonstrated that proximal tibial bone strength is adequate to 20 mm.[58]

Management

Various techniques are available to compensate for bone defects in primary TKA, including (1) translation of the component away from a defect, (2) lower tibial resection, (3) cement filling, (4) autologous bone graft, (5) allograft, (6) wedges or augments, and (7) custom implants. The use of stems in primary TKA is necessary when bone grafting is required or when the bone defect compromises fixation and renders the resurfacing component unstable without the added support of intramedullary fixation.

LOWER TIBIAL RESECTION

Lower tibial resection is often effective in eliminating bony defects (Fig. 84–96). The limit of a lower tibial resection is the insertion of the ITB and infrapatellar ligament. When more than 10 mm of bone is removed, the resection must be proximal to Gerdy's tubercle, or ITB function may be compromised. Additionally, lower tibial resection will complicate component fit because of the natural taper of the tibia and thus necessitate the use of a smaller tibial component or tapered tibial augments.

LATERAL TRANSLATION

Lateralizing a smaller tibial component size may effectively eliminate a bony defect (see Fig. 84–59) by removing any contact of the implant with the defect.[76,102] However, the largest tibial tray size and polyethylene insert should always be favored to create the largest reasonable contact surface to distribute load.

CEMENT FILLING

Lotke et al[104] and Ritter[137] demonstrated satisfactory long-term results with cement fill (Fig. 84–97), provided that the tibial bone defects are no deeper than 20 mm and involve less than 50% of either plateau. Despite these results, other authors recommend that use of cement be

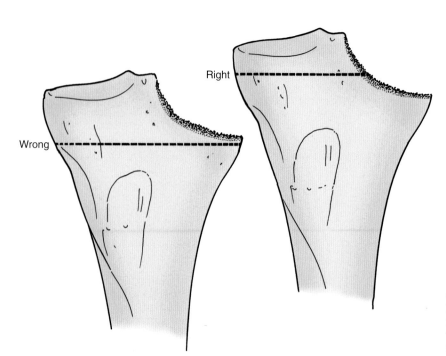

Figure 84–96. When there is asymmetric bone loss from the upper part of the tibia, the tibial resection must not be too distal but rather at the usual level.

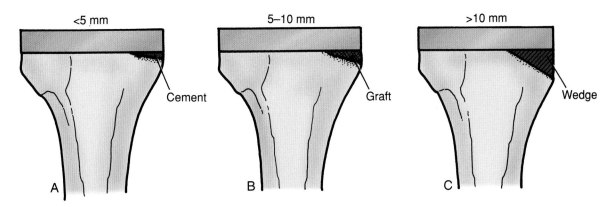

Figure 84–97. Bone defects are frequently seen in the medial aspect of the tibia. It is incorrect to make the tibial cut at the base of the defect. It is correct to resect a normal amount from the upper part of the tibia and fill the remaining defect. **A**, Small defects of less than 5 mm can be filled with cement. **B**, Defects between 5 and 10 mm are suitable for bone grafting. **C**, Defects larger than 10 mm are best treated with a metal wedge or augment.

limited to smaller peripheral defects that do not compromise tibial component support because biomechanical testing suggests that cement fill, with or without screw reinforcement, is an inferior method of defect management.[18] Clinical results have demonstrated that radiolucent lines are commonly observed under defects filled with cement.[37,77] Furthermore, larger volumes of cement introduce the risk of thermal necrosis of the cement-bone interface, and net cement shrinkage during polymerization may diminish the cement-prosthesis and cement-bone interface contact areas[18] (Fig. 84–98).

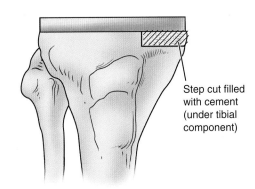

Figure 84–98. Step-cut technique for cement filling of a peripheral proximal tibial defect.

BONE GRAFTING

Both autologous bone and allograft (Figs. 84–99 to 84–101) are readily available in primary TKA. Both have demonstrated high rates of incorporation, which is particularly important in reestablishing proximal tibial bone strength and restoring bone stock should revision surgery be required. Autografting is generally favored because of its osteoinductive properties and lack of potential disease transmission. Bone graft is typically used when the size criteria for cement fill are exceeded. Dorr et al[40] identified criteria that promote improved outcome, as follows: (1) creation of a viable/bleeding bed of host bone, (2) proper fit and finish of graft in the host bed, (3) complete coverage of graft by the component to avoid graft resorption secondary to stress shielding, (4) optimal alignment of components for even load distribution, (5) limited weight-bearing when larger grafts are used to allow for graft union, and (6) protection of grafts with stems when required. Advantages of bone graft are its availability, its adaptability to size or shape of the defect, and its biological compatibility.[155]

Although contained defects are easily filled with bone graft, peripheral defects are more challenging. Several techniques have been developed that use bone available during surgery from other areas of the knee to address peripheral defects. Dorr et al[40] described success with a technique in which the peripheral defect is converted into a single oblique cut at the base of the deficiency and filled with bone from the larger distal femoral condylar resection. The graft is secured to the oblique surface by screw fixation (see Fig. 84–100). Altcheck et al[6] reported good to excellent results at an average follow-up of 4 years in 14 patients with severe angular deformity managed with this technique. All grafts consolidated without evidence of collapse, resorption, or subsidence of the prosthesis. In contrast, Laskin[93] used the resected posterior femoral condyles as bone graft to fill tibial defects and concluded after a 5-year follow-up review that the long-term prognosis for this method of bone grafting was not satisfactory.

Insall originally described the inlay autogeneic bone-grafting technique. An interference fit for a contoured bone graft is created by converting the dish-shaped peripheral defect into a trapezoidal shape (see Fig. 84–101). Because of the interlocking fit, this method of bone grafting does not require fixation. Windsor et al[187] and later Scuderi et al[155] reviewed 26 primary TKAs treated with this technique and reported 96% good to excellent results at an average follow-up of 3 years. Graft position either medially or laterally did not influence the results. With restoration of anatomic knee alignment, no tibial component loosened, and one medial bone graft collapsed.

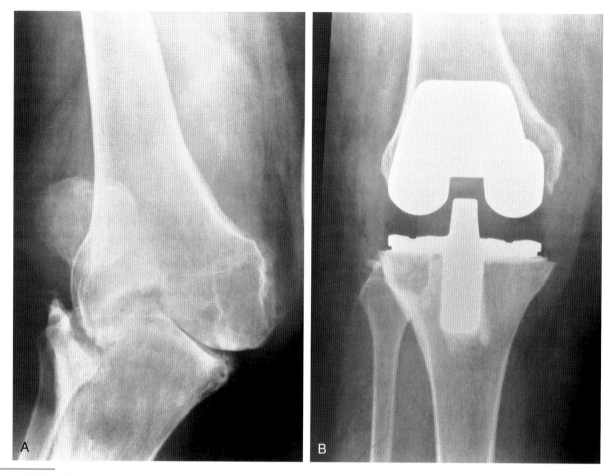

Figure 84–99. **A,** Radiograph showing a large defect in the lateral tibial plateau. **B,** Radiograph showing the appearance after packing the defect with cancellous bone graft. The graft can be either autologous or homologous.

CUSTOM PROSTHESES AND METAL WEDGE AUGMENTATION

Metal wedge augmentation permits intraoperative construction of a custom implant to address a bone defect by allowing transfer of load from the implant to the bone.[127] Custom prostheses (Figs. 84–102 to 84–105) are an option for dealing with larger defects[18]; however, custom prostheses have limitations of practicality and cost. Defects less than 25 mm can be managed effectively with metal wedge augmentation,[17] but custom prostheses may be required for larger defects. Brooks et al[18] demonstrated that metal wedge augmentation of tibial trays provided support similar to that of custom prostheses. Augments are available in triangular and rectangular shapes, in both cemented and cementless options. Although the mechanical support afforded by triangular[17] and rectangular wedges has been shown to be similar,[171] load transfer across a larger defect is probably best managed with a rectangular block[51] and stem augmentation[171] (see Fig. 84–103). Modular augments do introduce the potential for interface fretting; however, there are reports of good results using wedges attached with screw fixation.[149] In a series of 24 primary cemented TKAs with the use of metal wedge augmentation for tibial bone deficiency reported by

Pagnano et al,[127] good to excellent clinical results were achieved in 96% at an average follow-up of approximately 5 years. Radiolucent lines at the cement-bone interface beneath the metal wedge were noted in 13 of the 24 knees. The longer-term consequences of these radiolucent lines is not known.

Authors' Preferred Method for the Management of Bone Defects

TIBIAL DEFECTS

Contained Defects
When the bony defect, cavity, or cyst is enclosed within the bone, it is known as a contained defect. The treatment of choice is bone grafting with local bone graft from the osteotomies. In the rare event that local autograft is insufficient, supplementary allograft may be added.

Peripheral Defects
Peripheral defects are typically located in the posteromedial aspect of the tibial plateau. Although small and inter-

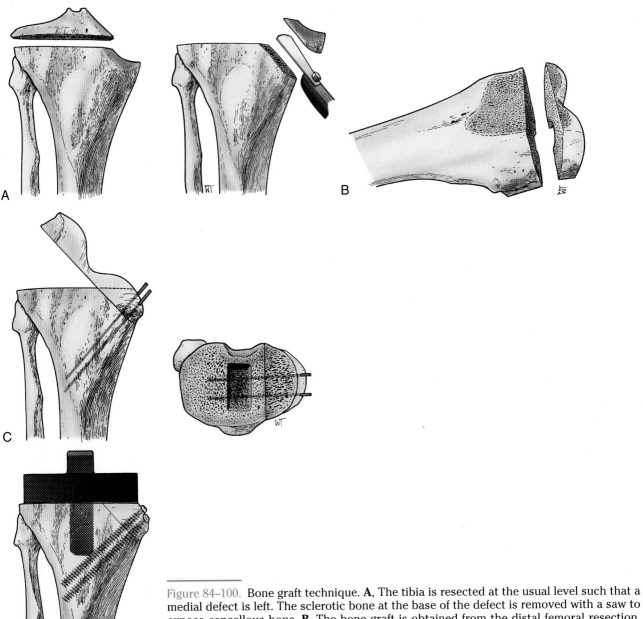

Figure 84–100. Bone graft technique. **A**, The tibia is resected at the usual level such that a medial defect is left. The sclerotic bone at the base of the defect is removed with a saw to expose cancellous bone. **B**, The bone graft is obtained from the distal femoral resection. **C**, The femoral condyle is applied to the defect temporarily with Kirschner wires. The graft is resected at the level of the tibial cut. **D**, Kirschner wires are replaced by screws, and the tibial component is set in place. (From Behrens JC, Walker PS, Shoji H: Variation in strength and structure of cancellous bone at the knee. J Biomech 7:201, 1974.)

mediate-sized defects are relatively shallow and elliptical and are bound anteriorly, medially, and posteriorly by a solid rim of cortical bone, severe defects have a steeper pitch and may involve the entire medial plateau. Several management options exist, as follows:

1. If possible, translate the tibial tray away from the location of the peripheral defect. Though simple and attractive, this method results in the use of a smaller tray that may not distribute load as effectively as a larger tibial tray (see Fig. 84–59).[69,94]

2. If not deeper than 10 mm, the defect can be eliminated by resecting the tibia at a lower level.

However, when a larger defect is present, tibial resection can be increased up to 12 to 14 mm (see Fig. 84–96).

3. Defects less than 5 mm can be managed with cement. Cement performance can be enhanced by converting the dished defect into a rectangular shape with a horizontal base and three vertical borders. The defect base should be cleaned to permit cement interdigitation (see Fig. 84–97).

4. For defects between 6 and 10 mm after the proximal tibial osteotomy is performed, bone graft is used according to the technique described by Dorr et al.[40]

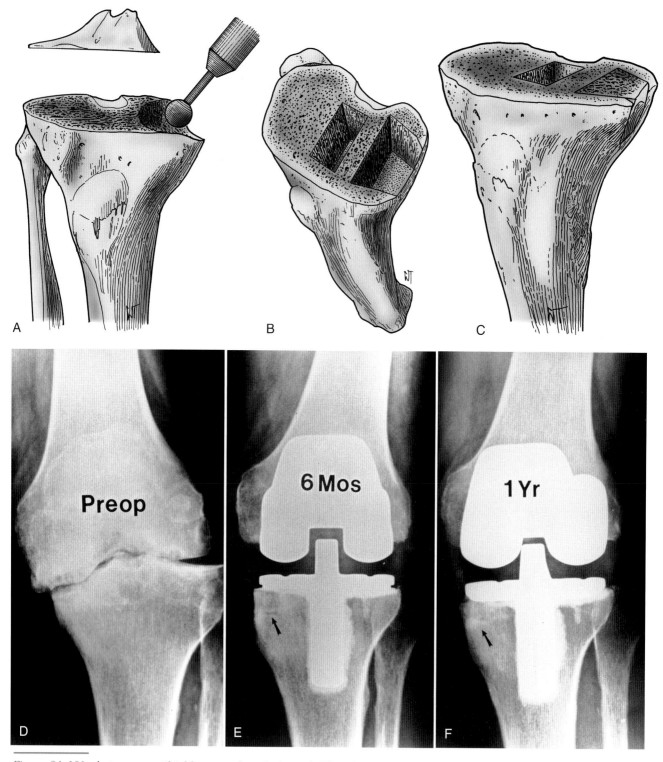

Figure 84–101. Autogenous tibial bone graft technique. **A,** The tibial defect is resected at the standard level. The remaining medial defect is reshaped with a bur. **B,** A trapezoidal defect is formed medially; usually, there is intact bone anteriorly and posteriorly to make this possible. **C,** A self-locking bone graft is fashioned to fit in the trapezoidal defect. The bone graft can be obtained from local resection in the knee; in the case of a posterior-stabilized prosthesis, bone removed from the intercondylar notch makes an ideal source. **D,** Preoperative radiograph of a medial defect. **E,** Radiograph taken 6 months after medial bone grafting via the interlocking technique. **F,** Bone graft after 1 year; the arthroplasty appears to be fully incorporated.

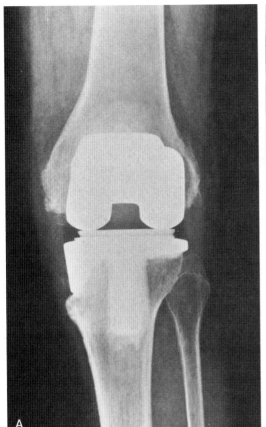

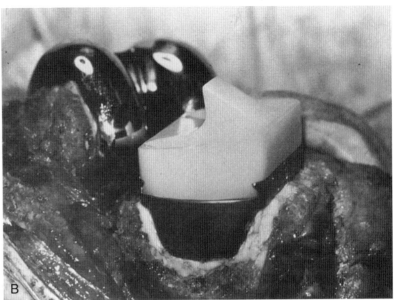

Figure 84–102. **A** and **B**, Asymmetric bone loss should be compensated for by an asymmetric tibial component.

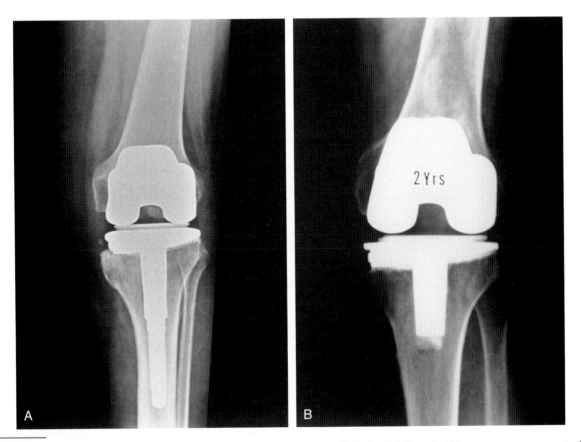

Figure 84–103. **A**, Full wedge applied to a tibial component for a medial tibial defect. In this case, an uncemented stem has been added. **B**, Full wedge applied to a tibial component. No stem extension has been added. It is not known at present whether a stem extension is necessary to resist possible shearing effects.

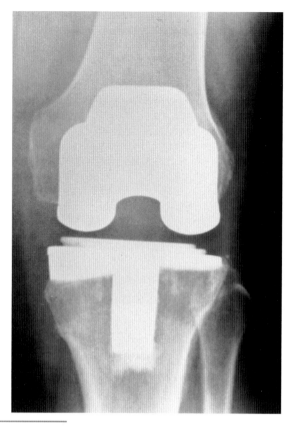

Figure 84–104. A modular medial wedge is attached to the prosthesis to fill a medial defect in the tibia.

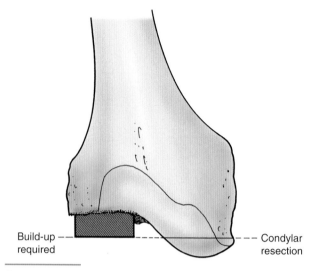

Build-up required — — Condylar resection

Figure 84–105. In some valgus knees, the level of femoral resection may pass distal to the lateral femoral condyle. Lateral augmentation of the femoral component is required.

The inlay bone-grafting method[155] is preferred because it allows for an interference fit of the graft and does not require fixation, which may interfere with tibial stem placement (see Fig. 84–101).

In situations with massive defects, alternative sources of bone graft (allograft) or metal augmentation is used. When bone can be used, the bone block is tapped into place and should fit snugly into the defect to prevent cement from entering the graft-tibia interface. In the technique of Dorr et al, the anterior and posterior margins of the defect are excised to create a single oblique cut to the base of the tibial deficiency.[40] The base of the cut should comprise a bleeding cancellous surface. To fill this defect, local autograft is obtained from the larger condyle of the distal femoral resection and rotated so that its cancellous surface is matched to the cancellous surface of the tibial defect. The junction of intact tibia and graft is occluded with supplemental bone graft to prevent cement entering the space between the graft and the tibia.

5. When inlay bone grafting with autogenous graft is not feasible, modular wedges or blocks attached to resurfacing prostheses may be used. To diminish shear force, an intramedullary stem is added to the tibial component when a full or half-oblique wedge is used.

DISTAL FEMORAL DEFECTS

Contained Defects

Contained femoral defects are managed in the same manner as contained tibial defects.

Peripheral Defects

Surface or peripheral defects of the femur are categorized as (1) affecting the chamfer cuts, (2) affecting the distal surface, or (3) major bone loss. Loss of femoral condylar bone is most frequently observed in valgus deformities when the lateral femoral condyle is dysplastic. As with the tibia, defects can be managed with cement, bone graft, and metal augments.

Femoral deficiencies can be viewed in increasing stages of bone loss.

Stage 1. Stage 1 is observed when the femoral osteotomy includes a portion of the lateral aspect of the distal end of the femur but contouring to accommodate the femoral component results in chamfer "air cuts" anteriorly and posteriorly. In our experience, cement fill is acceptable for filling the anterior and posterior spaces between the bone and prosthesis. The sclerotic bone surface should be prepared to accept cement interdigitation.

Stage 2. Stage 2 occurs when the level of the femoral osteotomy passes distal to the lateral femoral condyle even without chamfer cuts. In this situation, cement fill is typically unsatisfactory unless combined with a femoral stem extension. Even in this instance, a metal augment to the distal end of the femur is preferred.

Stage 3. Stage 3 refers to massive bone loss of one femoral condyle. Substantial bone loss can be managed with allograft or metal block augmentation, which has been shown to incorporate well but requires a period of non-weightbearing postoperatively and a femoral stem extension. The advantage of allograft is that if a revision is required, bone stock may be partially restored. Metal augments allow quicker rehabilitation without restricted weightbearing. Posterior augmentation without distal augmentation is required in cases of posterolateral deficiency. This unusual situation is encountered in rheumatoid patients with long-standing flexion contracture that results in posterior condylar erosion and in patients with combined valgus and flexion deformity. Most cases requiring posterior augmentation are also deficient distally. In general, optimizing collateral ligament stability and restoration of normal anatomy are preferable to using constrained prostheses.

INTRAOPERATIVE PROBLEMS AND THEIR SOLUTIONS

Many of the basic elements of technique, bone cutting, soft-tissue balancing, and overall alignment have already been addressed. A few intraoperative situations remain to be discussed (Fig. 84–106):

1. The flexion gap is too small to admit the thinnest tibial component. If spacers are used, this error will be identified early. It is caused by either under-resection of the proximal end of the tibia or oversizing of the femoral component. Therefore, the size of the tibial fragment should be measured, and if 7 to 8 mm has already been removed from the normal side, the problem lies in oversizing of the femur, and it will be necessary to recut the posterior femoral condyles so that one size smaller can be used.

2. The flexion gap is unequal—that is, tighter either medially or laterally. The cause is an error in the tibial cut into either varus or valgus, malrotation of the femoral component, or excessive ligament release. If the cause is either of the first two or insufficient release of a contracted structure, it should be corrected. However, sometimes the necessary medial or lateral release will cause an asymmetric flexion gap that must be accepted. A larger than normal medial gap is not of clinical consequence, but an excessive lateral gap can lead to posterolateral subluxation. The soft tissues must be given time to readhere, which means pursuing postoperative flexion rehabilitation less vigorously than normal.

3. The extension gap is larger than the flexion gap (Fig. 84–107). This situation is unusual and is created by standard bone resection in a knee with excessive ligamentous laxity. A tensor obviates this occurrence because the need for femoral under-resection will be indicated; if one has committed to a standard femoral cut, the solution is to augment the distal end of the femur (a thicker tibial component cannot be used because the flexion gap will not admit it). Augments on the distal end of the femur usually require the use of a stemmed femoral component to get proper fixation. The laxity must be symmetric and limited to

a few millimeters of passive motion. No "thrust" on weightbearing is permissible. Conversely, the components should not be so tight that they produce a flexion contracture.

4. The patella cannot be made to track despite an extensive lateral retinacular release. The causes are (1) femoral malrotation, (2) tibial malrotation, and (3) an overly thick patella. The latter two causes are readily correctable, but the first is more difficult and will result in a malfit of the femoral component. Recutting the femur in additional external rotation and adding a posterolateral augment can remedy the first situation. A stemmed component and cement are needed to give adequate fixation.

5. The alignment, fit, and motion with the trial components are satisfactory, but this is not so when the final components are inserted. There are several reasons for this:

   a. The knee does not reach full extension. The probable explanation is that the femoral component has been put on flexed so that it is sitting proud of the bone. This problem has been virtually eliminated with the use of pegs that engage the femur and ensure proper sagittal position of the femoral component. Careful placement of the final component is required when pegs are not available.

   b. The knee is too loose in extension after satisfactory trial reduction. This problem can occur even with a proper fit because the finished components are polished and become slightly less bulky than the trials; adjustment to the thickness of the tibial component will remedy the situation. A more serious occurrence is when the femoral component has been driven into soft rheumatoid or osteoporotic bone. A thicker tibial component may upset the flexion-extension balance, and a stemmed femoral component, possibly with augments, may be needed to restore the proper femoral position.

   c. The varus-valgus alignment and balance are incorrect. This situation is also due to compacting one or the other of the components (usually the femoral component) asymmetrically into soft bone. The correction is the same as previously described. When performing the final cementation, it is important to hold the leg so that it does not fall into the preoperative deformity or create component lift-off while the cement hardens.

   d. Patellar tracking is unsatisfactory. The cause is insertion of the final components in a different position from the trials. This usually happens when the bone is soft, and it is most likely to occur when a central stem tibial design is used and the tibial component is allowed to spin into internal rotation. It is, of course, correctable but can be prevented if the position of the tibial trial on the tibia is marked with methylene blue so that the surgeon can be certain that both the trial and the final components are correctly inserted.

FLEXION   EXTENSION

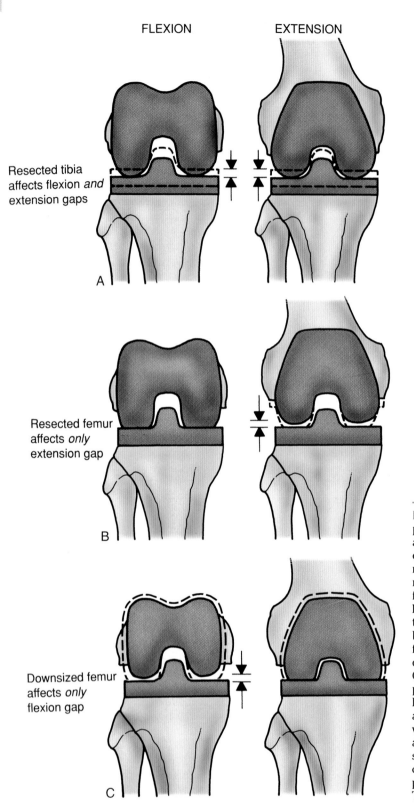

Resected tibia
affects flexion *and*
extension gaps

A

Resected femur
affects *only*
extension gap

B

Downsized femur
affects *only*
flexion gap

C

Figure 84–106. The effect of bone cuts on prosthetic fit. **A**, The level of tibial resection affects both flexion and extension gaps equally. Under-resection of the tibia will make the joint tight in both positions. Over-resection of the tibia can be compensated for by using a thicker tibial component. **B**, Distal resection of the femur affects only the extension gap, which may cause instability in extension. If the knee is too tight in flexion to admit a thicker tibial component, distal femoral buildup is the solution. **C**, Over-resection of the femur in the sagittal plane affects only the flexion gap and causes laxity in flexion. This cannot be overcome by a thicker tibial component because the knee will be too tight in extension. The solutions are to (1) restore the proper sagittal dimension of the femur by using a larger femoral component with a posterior buildup or (2) perform additional distal femoral resection. The former is preferred.

e. Excessive bleeding occurs. Opinions differ about the timing of tourniquet release or even on whether to release it at all. There have been studies that show blood loss to be similar with and without tourniquet release. Tourniquet release serves two purposes: (1) occasional profuse bleeding, usually from the lateral genicular artery, can be secured (see Fig. 84–49), and (2) blood flow may not return through an arteriosclerotic femoral artery when the tourniquet is let down.

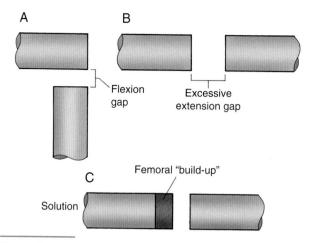

Figure 84–107. When the extension gap is too large, equalization cannot be achieved by further bone resection. The prosthesis must be built up on the femoral side.

This is usually due to clotting in the femoral artery and, if treated early, has an uneventful outcome. Release of the tourniquet alerts the surgeon to this possibility, whereas identification of this potentially catastrophic event may be delayed in the recovery room.

AFTERCARE OF TOTAL KNEE ARTHROPLASTY

At the conclusion of the operation, a bulky cotton dressing or compression stocking is applied to limit extremity swelling. A postoperative drain is left in place for approximately 24 to 36 hours. The bulky dressing is removed on the first postoperative day. Some surgeons prefer to apply a lighter dressing and initiate continuous passive motion in the recovery room, with the use of simultaneous continuous passive motion machines in bilateral cases. The patient is encouraged to flex the knee as much as is tolerated; recent investigations suggest that high flexion in the immediate postoperative period accelerates postoperative rehabilitation and is not associated with wound complications.[82]

With a cemented knee, full weightbearing under the supervision of a therapist is allowed on the first or second postoperative day. Some surgeons recommend protected weightbearing even when cement is used from the perspective of patient comfort. Progression of walking is variable and age dependent and is initially done with a walker until the patient is steady enough to use canes. General muscle exercises are performed for the feet and ankles, and isometric exercises are performed for the thigh and buttock muscles. Bicycle exercises are most useful as soon as the patient has sufficient flexion. Particularly motivated patients are placed on a "fast track" and will initiate ambulation on the afternoon of surgery. Regional anesthesia has improved pain management. The ideal block is titrated to allow motor function while moderating pain, thereby

allowing for the rapid conversion to oral pain medication and the avoidance of intravenous or intramuscular narcotics.

EMERGING TECHNOLOGIES IN SURGICAL TECHNIQUE

Minimally Invasive Total Knee Arthroplasty

Recent experience with minimally invasive surgery for unicondylar knee arthroplasty has stimulated interest in applying these basic principles to total knee replacement. The goals of minimally invasive surgery are patient satisfaction, less patient discomfort, less intraoperative blood loss, fewer inpatient days, and faster recovery, without compromising outcome. These goals are currently being investigated by using such techniques as less extensive arthrotomy, smaller cutting jigs, and instrumentation that allows for cuts to be made without everting the patella. Tria and Coon published the early results from their series of 70 minimally invasive TKAs and showed a trend toward decreased blood loss and decreased hospital stay while not observing a statistical difference in radiographic alignment of the components when compared with a group of patients who underwent standard arthrotomy.[174]

Sustained interest in this approach will require demonstration of positive treatment benefits. Future directions for investigation regarding this technique include guidelines for patient selection (e.g., degree of deformity, leg circumference, and patients who can tolerate longer surgical times), quantification of blood loss between different techniques, and development of a clinical tool to measure the hypothetical faster recovery.

Computer-Assisted Surgery

Computer-assisted navigation in TKA is an emerging technology that seeks to improve clinical outcome and implant survival by improving the reliability of bone cuts and component positioning. Computer-assisted navigation systems attempt to eliminate outliers in component positioning. Three main types of systems are available: image-free navigation, image-based navigation, and robotic systems. Image-free systems use information regarding range of motion and position of the lower extremity, gathered intraoperatively, to assist with component placement. Image-based navigation uses information obtained from preoperative computed tomography in conjunction with intraoperative fluoroscopy. Robotic systems use machines to guide the surgeon during portions of the procedure.

Over the past several years, as the technology has gone through a number of upgrades and improvements, studies have appeared in the literature in which the results of computer-assisted surgery are compared with those of conventional techniques. In a prospective randomized trial involving a comparison of these two methods in 70 patients, Chauhan et al[24] used an image-free navigation system and postoperatively evaluated alignment with a CT protocol. Their study showed statistically significant improvement in the computer-assisted group with varus/valgus and rotational alignment of the femoral component, as well as varus/valgus, rotation, and posterior slope of the tibial component. The computer-assisted surgery took an average of 13 minutes longer, but had statistically significantly less blood loss. Although studies such as this one have shown improved accuracy, the impact of computer-assisted navigation on long-term clinical outcomes and implant survival remains unproven.

References

1. Aglietti P, Buzzi R, Giron F, et al: The Insall-Burstein posterior stabilized total knee replacement in the valgus knee. Am J Knee Surg 9:8, 1996.
2. Aglietti P, Windsor RE, Buzzi R, et al: Arthroplasty for the stiff or ankylosed knee. Clin Orthop 143:115, 1979.
3. Akizuki S, Takizawa T, Horiuchi H: Fixation of a hydroxyapatite–tricalcium phosphate–coated cementless knee prosthesis. Clinical and radiographic evaluation seven years after surgery. J Bone Joint Surg Br 85:1123, 2003.
4. Albredtsson BEJ, Carlsson LV, Freeman MAR, et al: Proximally cemented versus uncemented Freeman Samuelson knee arthroplasty. A prospective randomized study. J Bone Joint Surg Br 74:233, 1992.
5. Alexiades M, Scuderi G, Vincent V, et al: A histologic study of the posterior cruciate ligament in the arthritic knee. Am J Knee Surg 2:153, 1989.
6. Altcheck D, Sculco TP, Rawlins B: Autogenous bone grafting for severe angular deformity in total knee arthroplasty. J Arthroplasty 4:151, 1989.
7. Anouchi YS, Whiteside LA, Kaiser AD, et al: The effects of axial rotational alignment of the femoral component on instability and patellar tracking in total knee arthroplasty demonstrated on autopsy specimens. Clin Orthop 287:170, 1993.
8. Arima J, Whiteside LA, McCarthy DS, et al: Femoral rotational alignment, based on the anteroposterior axis in total knee arthroplasty in a valgus knee. J Bone Joint Surg Am 77:1331, 1995.
9. Barrack RL, Bertot AJ, Wolfe MW, et al: Patellar resurfacing in total knee arthroplasty. A prospective, randomized, double-blind study with five to seven years of follow-up. J Bone Joint Surg Am 83:1376, 2001.
10. Barrack RL, Wolfe MW, Waldman DA, et al: Resurfacing of the patella in total knee arthroplasty. A prospective, randomized, double-blind study. J Bone Joint Surg Am 79:1121, 1997.
11. Behrens JC, Walker PS, Shoji H: Variation in strength and structure of cancellous bone at the knee. J Biomech 7:201, 1974.
12. Berger RA, Crossett LS, Jacobs JJ, et al: Malrotation causing patellofemoral complications after total knee arthroplasty. Clin Orthop 356:144, 1998.
13. Berger RA, Lyon JH, Jacobs JJ, et al: Problems with cementless total knee arthroplasty at 11 years followup. Clin Orthop 392:196-207, 2001.
14. Berger RA, Rubash HE, Seel MJ, et al: Determining the rotational alignment of the femoral component in total knee arthroplasty using the epicondylar axis. Clin Orthop 286:40, 1993.
15. Bourne RB, Rorabeck CH, Vaz M, et al: Resurfacing versus not resurfacing the patella during total knee replacement. Clin Orthop 321:156, 1995.
16. Boyd AD, Ewald FC, Thomas WH, et al: Long-term complications after total knee arthroplasty with or without resurfacing of the patella. J Bone Joint Surg Am 75:674, 1993.
17. Brand MG, Daley RJ, Ewald FC, et al: Tibial tray augmentation with modular metal wedges for tibial bone stock deficiency. Clin Orthop 248:71, 1989.
18. Brooks PJ, Walker PS, Scott RD: Tibial component fixation in deficient tibial bone stock. Clin Orthop 184:302, 1984.
19. Buechel FF: A sequential three-step lateral release for correcting fixed valgus knee deformities during total knee arthroplasty. Clin Orthop 260:170, 1990.
20. Buechel FF Sr, Buechel FF Jr, Pappas MJ, et al: Twenty-year evaluation of meniscal bearing and rotating platform knee replacements. Clin Orthop 388:41, 2001.
21. Cameron HU: Tibial component wear in total knee replacement. Clin Orthop 309:29, 1994.
22. Cameron HU, Hunter GA: Failure in total knee arthroplasty. Mechanisms, revisions, and results. Clin Orthop 170:141, 1982.
23. Cates HE, Ritter MA, Keating EM, et al: Intramedullary versus extramedullary femoral alignment systems in total knee replacement. Clin Orthop 286:32, 1993.
24. Chauhan SK, Scott RG, Breidahl W, et al: Computer-assisted knee arthroplasty versus a conventional jig-based technique. A randomised, prospective trial. J Bone Joint Surg Br 86:3, 2004.
25. Chiba J, Schwendeman LJ, Booth RE Jr, et al: A biomechanical, histologic, and immunohistologic analysis of membranes obtained from failed cemented and cementless total knee arthroplasty. Clin Orthop 299:114, 1994.
26. Clayton ML, Thompson TR, Mack RP: Correction of alignment deformities during total knee arthroplasties: Staged soft-tissue releases. Clin Orthop 202:117, 1986.
27. Cole JC, Lemons JE, Eberhardt AW: Gamma irradiation alters fatigue-crack behavior and fracture toughness in 1900H and GUR 1050 UHMWPE. J Biomed Res Mater 63:5, 2002.
28. Colizza WA, Insall JN, Scuderi GR: The posterior stabilized total knee prosthesis. Assessment of polyethylene damage and osteolysis after a ten year minimum followup. J Bone Joint Surg Am 77:1713, 1995.
29. Corces A, Lotke PA, Williams JL: Strain characteristics of the posterior cruciate ligament in total knee replacement. Orthop Trans 13:527, 1989.
30. Coventry MD: Two-part total knee arthroplasty: Evolution and present status. Clin Orthop 145:29, 1979.
31. Dennis DA, Channer M, Susman MH, et al: Intramedullary versus extramedullary tibial alignment systems in total knee arthroplasty. J Arthroplasty 8:43, 1993.
32. Dennis DA, Komistek RD, Colwell CE, et al: In vivo anteroposterior femorotibial translation of total knee arthroplasty: A multi-center analysis. Clin Orthop 356:47, 1998.
33. Dennis DA, Komistek RD, Hoff WA, et al: In vivo knee kinematics derived using an inverse perspective technique. Clin Orthop 331:107, 1996.
34. Dennis DA, Komistek RD, Mahfouz MR: In vivo fluoroscopic analysis of fixed-bearing total knee replacements. Clin Orthop 410:114, 2003.
35. Diduch DR, Insall JN, Scott WN, et al: Total knee replacement in young, active patients. Long-term followup and functional outcome. J Bone Joint Surg Am 79:575, 1997.
36. Dixon MC, Parsch D, Brown RR, Scott RD: The correction of severe varus deformity in total knee arthroplasty by tibial component downsizing and resection of uncapped proximal medial bone. J Arthroplasty 19:19, 2004.
37. Dorr LD: Bone grafts for bone loss with total knee replacement. Orthop Clin North Am 20:179, 1989.
38. Dorr LD, Boiardo RA: Technical considerations in total knee arthroplasty. Clin Orthop 205:5, 1986.
39. Dorr LD, Conaty JP, Schreiber R, et al: Technical factors that influence mechanical loosening of total knee arthroplasty. In Dorr LD (ed): The Knee. Baltimore, University Park Press, 1985, pp 121-135.
40. Dorr LD, Ranawat CS, Sculco TA, et al: Bone graft for tibial defects in total knee arthroplasty. Clin Orthop 205:153, 1986.
41. Duffy GP, Berry DJ, Rand JA: Cement versus cementless fixation in total knee arthroplasty. Clin Orthop 356:66, 1998.
42. Easley ME, Insall JN, Scuderi GR, Bullek DD: Primary constrained condylar knee arthroplasty for the arthritic valgus knee. Clin Orthop 380:58, 2000.
43. Emerson RH, Ayers C, Head WC, et al: Surgical closure in primary total knee arthroplasty. Flexion versus extension. Clin Orthop 331:74, 1996.
44. Engh GA, Ammeen D: Results of total knee arthroplasty with medial epicondylar osteotomy to correct varus deformity. Clin Orthop 367:141, 1999.

45. Engh GA, Dwyer KA, Hanes CK: Polyethylene wear of metal backed tibial components in total and unicompartmental knee prostheses. J Bone Joint Surg Br 74:9, 1998.

46. Engh GA, Parks NL, Ammeen DJ: Tibial osteolysis in cementless total knee arthroplasty. A review of 25 cases treated with and without tibial component revision. Clin Orthop 309:33, 1994.

47. Engh GA, Petersen TL: Comparative experience with intramedullary and extramedullary alignment in total knee arthroplasty. J Arthroplasty 5:1, 1990.

48. Faris PM, Herbst SA, Ritter MA, et al: The effect of preoperative knee deformity on the initial results of cruciate-retaining total knee arthroplasty. J Arthroplasty 7:527, 1992.

49. Faris PM, Ritter MA, Keating EM: Sagittal plane positioning of the femoral component in total knee arthroplasty. J Arthroplasty 3:355, 1988.

50. Fehring TK: Rotational malalignment of the femoral component in total knee arthroplasty. Clin Orthop 380:72, 2000.

51. Fehring TK, Peindl RD, Humble RS, et al: Modular tibial augmentations in total knee arthroplasty. Clin Orthop 327:207, 1996.

52. Feng EL, Stulberg DS, Wixon RS: Progressive subluxation and polyethylene wear in total knee arthroplasty with flat articular surfaces. Clin Orthop 299:60, 1993.

53. Figgie HE III, Goldberg VM, Heiple KG, et al: The influence of tibial-patellofemoral location on function of the knee in patients with the posterior stabilized condylar knee prosthesis. J Bone Joint Surg Am 68:1035, 1986.

54. Firestone TP, Krackow KA, Davis JD, et al: The management of fixed flexion contractures during total knee arthroplasty. Clin Orthop 284:221, 1991.

55. Freeman MAR: Arthritis of the Knee: Clinical Features and Surgical Management. New York, Springer-Verlag, 1980.

56. Gabriel SM, Dennis DA, Honey MJ, Scott RD: Polyethylene wear on the distal tibial insert surface in total knee arthroplasty. Knee 5:221-228, 1998.

57. Garvin KL, Scuderi GR, Insall JN: Evolution of the quadriceps snip. Clin Orthop 321:131, 1995.

58. Goldstein SA, Wilson DL, Sostengard DA, et al: The mechanical properties of human tibial trabecular bone as a function of metaphyseal location. J Biomech 16:965, 1983.

59. Gomes LSM, Bechtold JE, Gustilo RB: Patellar prosthesis positioning in total knee arthroplasty: A roentgenographic study. Clin Orthop 236:72, 1988.

60. Goodfellow JW, O'Connor JJ: The anterior cruciate ligament in knee arthroplasty: A risk factor with unconstrained meniscal prostheses. Clin Orthop 276:245, 1992.

61. Green GV, Berend KR, Berend ME, et al: The effects of varus tibial alignment on proximal tibial surface strain in total knee arthroplasty: The posteromedial hot spot. J Arthroplasty 17:1033, 2002.

62. Griffin FM, Insall JN, Scuderi GR: The posterior condylar angle in osteoarthritic knees. J Arthroplasty 13:812, 1998.

63. Griffin FM, Scuderi GR, Gillis AM, et al: Osteolysis associated with cemented total knee arthroplasty. J Arthroplasty 13:592, 1998.

64. Harada Y, Wevers HW, Cooke TDV: Distribution of bone strength in the proximal tibia. J Arthroplasty 3:167, 1988.

65. Harrington IJ: A bioengineering analysis of force actions at the knee in normal and pathologic gait. Biomed Eng 11:167, 1976.

66. Healy WL, Iorio R, Lemos DW: Medial reconstruction during total knee arthroplasty for severe valgus deformity. Clin Orthop 356:161, 1998.

67. Hood RW, Vanni M, Insall JN: The correction of knee alignment in 225 consecutive total condylar knee replacements. Clin Orthop 160:94, 1981.

68. Hsu HP, Garg A, Walker PS, et al: Effect of knee component alignment on tibial load distribution with clinical correlation. Clin Orthop 248:135, 1989.

69. Hsu WW, Himeco S, Coventry MB, et al: Normal axial alignment of the lower extremity and load bearing distribution of the knee. Clin Orthop 255:215, 1990.

70. Hungerford DA, Kenna RV: Preliminary experience with a total knee prosthesis with porous coating used without cement. Clin Orthop 176:96, 1983.

71. Hungerford DS, Krackow KA: Total joint arthroplasty of the knee. Clin Orthop 192:23, 1985.

72. Hvid I: Trabecular bone strength at the knee. Clin Orthop 227:210, 1988.

73. Insall JN: Technique of total knee replacement. Instr Course Lect 30:324, 1981.

74. Insall JN: Total knee replacement. In Insall JN (ed): Surgery of the Knee. New York, Churchill Livingstone, 1984, pp 587-695.

75. Insall JN: Choices and compromises in total knee arthroplasty [presidential address to The Knee Society]. Clin Orthop 226:43, 1988.

76. Insall JN: Surgical techniques and instrumentation in total knee arthroplasty. In Insall JN (ed): Surgery of the Knee. New York, Churchill Livingstone, 1993.

77. Insall JN, Hood RW, Flawn LB: The total condylar knee prosthesis in gonarthrosis. A five to nine-year followup of the first one hundred consecutive replacements. J Bone Joint Surg Am 65:619, 1983.

78. Insall JN, Lachiewicz PF, Burstein AH: The posterior stabilized condylar prosthesis: A modification of the total condylar design: Two to four year clinical experience. J Bone Joint Surg Am 64:1317, 1982.

79. Jiang CC, Insall JN: Effect of rotation on the axial alignment of the femur: Pitfalls in the use of femoral intramedullary guides in total knee arthroplasty. Clin Orthop 248:50, 1989.

80. Johnson F, Leitl S, Waugh W: The distribution of load across the knee. J Bone Joint Surg Br 62:346, 1980.

81. Jones SMG, Inder IM, Moran CG, et al: Polyethylene wear in uncemented knee replacements. J Bone Joint Surg Br 74:18, 1992.

82. Jordan LR, Siegel JL, Olivio JL: Early flexion routine. An alternative method of continuous passive motion. Clin Orthop 315:231, 1995.

83. Kadoya Y, Kobayashi A, Komatsu T, et al: Effects of posterior cruciate ligament resection on the tibiofemoral joint gap. Clin Orthop 391:210, 2001.

84. Katz MA, Beck TD, Silber JS, et al: Determining femoral rotational alignment in total knee arthroplasty: Reliability of techniques. J Arthroplasty 16:3, 2001.

85. Keblish PA: The lateral approach to the valgus knee. Surgical technique and analysis of 53 cases with over two-year followup evaluation. Clin Orthop 271:52, 1991.

86. Kim H, Pelker RR, Gibson DH, et al: Rollback in posterior cruciate ligament–retaining total knee arthroplasty. A radiographic analysis. J Arthroplasty 12:553, 1997.

87. King TV, Scott RD: Femoral component loosening in total knee arthroplasty. Clin Orthop 194:285, 1985.

88. Kleinbart FA, Bryk E, Evangelista J, et al: Histologic composition of posterior cruciate ligaments from arthritic and age-matched specimens. J Arthroplasty 11:726, 1996.

89. Koshino T, Ejima M, Okamoto R, et al: Gradual low riding of the patella during postoperative course after total knee arthroplasty in osteoarthritis and rheumatoid arthritis. J Arthroplasty 5:323, 1990.

90. Krackow KA: The Technique of Total Knee Arthroplasty. St Louis, CV Mosby, 1990.

91. Krackow KA, Jones MM, Teeny SM, et al: Primary total knee arthroplasty in patients with fixed valgus deformity. Clin Orthop 273:9, 1991.

92. Larson CM, McDowell CM, Lachiewicz PF: One-peg versus three-peg patella component fixation in total knee arthroplasty. Clin Orthop 392:94, 2001.

93. Laskin RS: Total knee arthroplasty in the presence of large bony defects of the tibia and marked knee instability. Clin Orthop 248:66, 1989.

94. Laskin RS: Total knee replacement with posterior cruciate ligament retention in patients with a fixed varus deformity. Clin Orthop 331:29, 1996.

95. Laskin RS, Rieger M, Schob C, et al: The posterior-stabilized total knee prosthesis in the knee with a severe fixed deformity. Am J Knee Surg 1:199, 1988.

96. Laskin RS, Turtel A: The use of an intramedullary tibial alignment guide in total knee replacement. Am J Knee Surg 2:123, 1989.

97. Laurencin CT, Scott RD, Volatile TB, et al: Total knee replacement in severe valgus deformity. Am J Knee Surg 5:135, 1992.

98. Lewallen DG, Bryan RS, Peterson LFA: Polycentric total knee arthroplasty. J Bone Joint Surg Am 66:1211, 1984.

99. Lewis PL, Rorabeck CH, Bourne RB: Screw osteolysis after cementless total knee replacement. Clin Orthop 321:173, 1995.

100. Lombardi AV Jr, Berend KR, Mallory TH, et al: The relationship of lateral release and tourniquet deflation in total knee arthroplasty. J Knee Surg 16:209, 2003.

101. Lombardi AV Jr, Mallory TH, Maitino PD, et al: Freehand resection of the patella in total knee arthroplasty referencing the attachments of the quadriceps tendon and patellar tendon. J Arthroplasty 13:788, 1998.

102. Lotke PA: Tibial component translation for bone defects. Orthop Trans 9:425, 1985.

103. Lotke PA, Ecker ML: Influence of positioning of prosthesis in total knee replacement. J Bone Joint Surg Am 59:77, 1977.

104. Lotke PA, Wong RY, Ecker ML: The use of methylmethacrylate in primary total knee replacements with large tibial defects. Clin Orthop 270:288, 1991.

105. Manning M, Elloy M, Johnson R: The accuracy of intramedullary alignment in total knee replacement. J Bone Joint Surg Br 70:852, 1988.

106. Maquet PGJ: Biomechanics of the Knee. New York, Springer-Verlag, 1976.

107. Marcacci M, Iacono F, Zaffagnini S, et al: Total knee arthroplasty without patellar resurfacing in active and overweight patients. Knee Surg Sports Traumatol Arthrosc 5:258, 1997.

108. Martin JW, Whiteside LA: The influence of joint line position on knee stability after condylar knee arthroplasty. Clin Orthop 259:146, 1990.

109. Masri BA, Laskin RS, Windsor RE, et al: Knee closure in total knee replacement. A randomized prospective trial. Clin Orthop 321:81, 1996.

110. McAuley JP, Harrer MF, Ammeen D, Engh GA: Outcome of knee arthroplasty in patients with poor preoperative range of motion. Clin Orthop 404:203, 2002.

111. McGraw B, McClenaghan BA, Williams HG, et al: Gait and postural stability in obese and nonobese prepubertal boys. Arch Phys Med Rehabil 81:484, 2000.

112. McPherson EJ, Cushner FD, Schiff CF, et al: Natural history of uncorrected flexion contractures following total knee arthroplasty. J Arthroplasty 9:499, 1994.

113. Messier SP: Osteoarthritis of the knee and associated factors of age and obesity: Effects on gait. Med Sci Sports Exerc 26:1446, 1994.

114. Mintzer CM, Robertson DD, Rackemann S, et al: Bone loss in the distal anterior femur after total knee arthroplasty. Clin Orthop 260:135, 1990.

115. Miyasaka KC, Ranawat CS, Mullaji A: 10- to 20-year followup of total knee arthroplasty for valgus deformities. Clin Orthop 345:29, 1997.

116. Montgomery WH, Insall JN, Haas SB, et al: Primary TKA in stiff and ankylosed knees. Am J Knee Surg 11:20, 1998.

117. Moran CG, Pinder IM, Lees TA, et al: 121 cases in survivorship analysis of the uncemented porous coated anatomic knee replacement. J Bone Joint Surg Am 73:848, 1991.

118. Moreland JR: Mechanisms of failure in total knee arthroplasty. Clin Orthop 226:49, 1988.

119. Morrison JB: Bioengineering analysis of force actions transmitted by the knee joint. Biomed Eng 3:164, 1968.

120. Muller JO: Range of motion following total knee arthroplasty in ankylosed joints. Clin Orthop 179:200, 1983.

121. Muller W: The Knee: Form, Function, and Ligament Reconstruction. New York, Springer-Verlag, 1983.

122. Murty AN, Scott G, Freeman MA: Hydroxyapatite-coated femoral components in total knee arthroplasty: Medium term results. J Arthroplasty 18:844-51, 2003.

123. Nafei A, Neilsen S, Kristensen O, et al: The press fit Kinemax knee arthroplasty. High failure rate of noncemented implants. J Bone Joint Surg Br 74:243, 1992.

124. Nagamine R, Whiteside LA, White SE, et al: Patellar tracking after total knee arthroplasty. The effect of tibial tray malrotation and articular surface configuration. Clin Orthop 304:262, 1994.

125. Onsten I, Norqvist A, Carlsson AS, et al: Hydroxyapatite augmentation of the porous coating improves fixation of tibial components. A randomized RSA study in 116 patients. J Bone Joint Surg Br 80:417, 1998.

126. Pagnano MW, Hanssen AD, Lewallen DG, et al: Flexion instability after primary posterior cruciate retaining total knee arthroplasty. Clin Orthop 356:39, 1998.

127. Pagnano MW, Trousdale RT, Rand JA: Tibial wedge augmentation for bone deficiency in total knee arthroplasty. Clin Orthop 321:151, 1995.

128. Parks NL, Engh GA, Topoleski LDT, et al: Modular tibial insert micromotion: A concern with contemporary knee implants. Clin Orthop 356:10, 1998.

129. Peters PC, Engh GA, Dwyer KA, et al: Osteolysis after total knee arthroplasty without cement. J Bone Joint Surg Am 74:864, 1992.

130. Poilvache PL, Insall HN, Scuderi GR, et al: Rotational landmarks and sizing of the distal femur in total arthroplasty. Clin Orthop 331:35, 1996.

131. Rand JA: Bone deficiency in total knee arthroplasty. Use of metal wedge augmentation. Clin Orthop 271:63, 1991.

132. Rand JA: The patellofemoral joint in total knee arthroplasty. J Bone Joint Surg Am 74:612, 1994.

133. Rhoads DD, Noble PC, Reuben JD, et al: The effect of femoral component position on patellar tracking after total knee arthroplasty. Clin Orthop 260:43, 1990.

134. Rhoads DD, Noble PC, Reuben JD, et al: The effect of femoral component position on the kinematics of total knee arthroplasty. Clin Orthop 286:122, 1993.

135. Ries MD, Guiney W, Lynch F: Osteolysis associated with cemented total knee arthroplasty. J Arthroplasty 9:555, 1994.

136. Ries MD, Rauscher LA, Hoskins S, et al: Intramedullary pressure and pulmonary function during total knee arthroplasty. Clin Orthop 356:154, 1998.

137. Ritter MA: Screw and cement fixation of large defects in TKA. J Arthroplasty 1:125, 1986.

138. Ritter MA, Faris PM, Keating EM: Posterior cruciate ligament balancing during total knee arthroplasty. J Arthroplasty 3:323, 1988.

139. Ritter MA, Faris PM, Keating EM, Meding JB: Postoperative alignment of total knee replacement. Its effect on survival. Clin Orthop 299:153, 1994.

140. Ritter MA, Herbst SA, Keating EM, et al: Radiolucency at the bone cement interface in total knee replacement. The effects of bone surface preparation and cement technique. J Bone Joint Surg Am 76:60, 1994.

141. Ritter MA, Herbst SA, Keating EM, et al: Long-term survival of a posterior cruciate–retaining total condylar total knee arthroplasty. Clin Orthop 309:136, 1994.

142. Ritter MA, Stringer EA: Predictive range of motion after total knee replacement. Clin Orthop 143:115, 1979.

143. Robinson EJ, Muluken BD, Bourne RB, et al: Catastrophic osteolysis in total knee replacement. A report of 17 cases. Clin Orthop 321:98, 1995.

144. Romness DW, Rand JA: The role of continuous passive motion following total knee arthroplasty. Clin Orthop 226:34, 1988.

145. Salter RB: The biologic concept of continuous passive motion of synovial joints: The first 18 years of basic research and its clinical application. Clin Orthop 242:12, 1989.

146. Sambatakakis A, Wilton TJ, Newton G: Radiographic sign of persistent soft-tissue imbalance after knee replacement. J Bone Joint Surg Br 73:751, 1991.

147. Sany MR, Scott RD: Posterior polyethylene wear in posterior cruciate ligament–retaining total knee arthroplasty. A case study. J Arthroplasty 8:439, 1993.

148. Schai PA, Thornhill TS, Scott RD: Total knee arthroplasty with the PFC system. Results at a minimum of ten years and survivorship analysis. J Bone Joint Surg Br 80:850, 1998.

149. Schemitsch EH, Scott RD, Ewald FC, et al: Tibial tray augmentation with modular wedges for tibial bone stock deficiency. J Bone Joint Surg Br 77(Suppl):79, 1995.

150. Scott RD: Duopatellar total knee replacement: The Brigham experience. Orthop Clin North Am 13:17, 1982.

151. Scott RD: Posterior cruciate ligament retaining designs and results. In Insall JN, Scott WN, Scuderi GR (eds): Current Concepts in Primary and Revision Total Knee Arthroplasty. Philadelphia, Lippincott-Raven, 1996, pp 37-40.

152. Scott RD, Thornhill TS: Posterior cruciate supplementing total knee replacement using conforming inserts and cruciate recession: Effect on range of motion and radiolucent lines. Clin Orthop 309:146, 1994.

153. Scott RD, Volative TB: Twelve years' experience with posterior cruciate–retaining total knee arthroplasty. Clin Orthop 205:100, 1986.

154. Scott WN, Rubinstein M, Scuderi GR: Results after knee replacement with a posterior cruciate substituting prosthesis. J Bone Joint Surg Am 70:1163, 1988.

155. Scuderi GR, Insall JN, Haas SB, et al: Inlay autogeneic bone grafting of tibial defects in primary total knee arthroplasty. Clin Orthop 248:93, 1989.

156. Sharma L, Lou C, Cahue S, Dunlop D: The mechanism of the effect of obesity in knee osteoarthritis: The mediating role of malalignment. Arthritis Rheum 43:568-575, 2000.

157. Shih HN, Shih LY, Wong YC, Hsu RW: Long-term changes of the nonresurfaced patella after total knee arthroplasty. J Bone Joint Surg Am 86:935, 2004.

158. Siegel JL, Shall LM: Femoral instrumentation using the anterosuperior iliac spine as a landmark in total knee arthroplasty. An anatomic study. J Arthroplasty 6:317, 1991.

159. Simmons ED Jr, Sullivan JA, Rackemann S, et al: The accuracy of tibial intramedullary alignment devices in total knee arthroplasty. J Arthroplasty 6:45, 1991.

160. Smith JL Jr, Tullos HS, Davidson JP: Alignment of total knee arthroplasty. J Arthroplasty 4(Suppl):S55, 1989.

161. Spyropoulos P, Pisciotta JC, Pavlou KN, et al: Biomechanical gait analysis in obese men. Arch Phys Med Rehabil 72:1065, 1991.

162. Stern SH, Insall JN: Posterior stabilized prosthesis. Results after followup of nine to twelve years. J Bone Joint Surg Am 72:1400, 1992.

163. Stern SH, Moeckel BH, Insall JN: Total knee arthroplasty in valgus knees. Clin Orthop 273:5, 1991.

164. Stiehl JB, Cherveny PM: Femoral rotational alignment using the tibial shaft axis in total knee arthroplasty. Clin Orthop 331:47, 1996.

165. Stiehl JB, Komistek RD, Dennis DA, et al: Fluoroscopic analysis of kinematics after posterior-cruciate retaining total knee arthroplasty using fluoroscopy. J Bone Joint Surg Br 77:884, 1995.

166. Swany MR, Scott RD: Posterior polyethylene wear in posterior cruciate ligament retaining total knee arthroplasty. J Arthroplasty 8:439, 1993.

167. Tanzer M, Miller J: The natural history of flexion contracture in total knee arthroplasty: A prospective study. Clin Orthop 248:129, 1989.

168. Teeny SM, Krackow KA, Hungerford DS, et al: Primary total knee arthroplasty in patients with severe varus deformity. Clin Orthop 273:19, 1991.

169. Tew M, Forster IW: Effect of knee replacement on flexion deformity. J Bone Joint Surg Br 69:395, 1987.

170. Tillett ED, Engh GA, Petersen T: A comparative study of extramedullary and intramedullary alignment systems in total knee arthroplasty. Clin Orthop 230:176, 1988.

171. Touchi H, Lock DA, Genuino VS, et al: The effect of metal wedges on the strain distribution in the proximal tibia following total knee arthroplasty. Trans Orthop Res Soc 42:731, 1996.

172. Townley CO: The anatomic total knee resurfacing arthroplasty. Clin Orthop 192:82, 1985.

173. Trent PS, Besser W, Dueland R, et al: Total knee prosthesis combining porous ingrowth and initial stabilization. Trans Orthop Res Soc 3:164, 1978.

174. Tria AJ Jr, Coon TM: Minimal incision total knee arthroplasty: Early experience. Clin Orthop 416:185, 2003.

175. Walker PS, Soudry M, Ewald FC, McVickar H: Control of cement penetration in total knee arthroplasty. Clin Orthop 185:155, 1984.

176. Wasielewski RC: The causes of insert backside wear in total knee arthroplasty. Clin Orthop 404:232, 2002.

177. Wasielewski RC, Galante JO, Leighty RM, et al: Wear patterns on retrieved polyethylene tibial inserts and their relationship to technical considerations during total knee arthroplasty. Clin Orthop 299:31, 1994.

178. Wasielewski RC, Parks NL, Williams I, et al: The tibial insert undersurface as a contributing source of polyethylene wear debris. Clin Orthop 345:53, 1997.

179. Waslewski GL, Marson BM, Benjamin JB: Early, incapacitating instability of posterior cruciate ligament–retaining total knee arthroplasty. J Arthroplasty 13:763, 1998.

180. Waters TS, Bentley G: Patellar resurfacing in total knee arthroplasty. A prospective, randomized study. J Bone Joint Surg Am 85:212, 2003.

181. Whiteside LA: Correction of ligament and bone defects in total arthroplasty of the severely valgus knee. Clin Orthop 288:234, 1993.

182. Whiteside LA: Cementless total knee replacement. Nine- to 11-year results and 10-year survivorship analysis. Clin Orthop 309:185, 1994.

183. Whiteside LA: Exposure in difficult total knee arthroplasty using tibial tubercle osteotomy. Clin Orthop 321:32, 1995.

184. Whiteside LA: Effect of porous-coating configuration on tibial osteolysis after total knee arthroplasty. Clin Orthop 321:92, 1995.

185. Whiteside LA, Arima J: The anteroposterior axis for femoral rotational alignment in valgus total knee arthroplasty. Clin Orthop 321:168, 1995.

186. Whiteside LA, Ohl MD: Tibial tubercle osteotomy for exposure of the difficult total knee arthroplasty. Clin Orthop 260:6, 1990.

187. Windsor RE, Insall JN, Sculco TP: Bone grafting of tibial defects in primary and revision total knee arthroplasty. Clin Orthop 205:132, 1986.

188. Windsor RE, Scuderi GR, Moran MC, et al: Mechanisms of failure of the femoral and tibial components in total knee arthroplasty. Clin Orthop 248:15, 1989.

189. Wolff AM, Hungerford DS, Krackow KA, et al: Osteotomy of the tibial tubercle during total knee replacement: A report of twenty-six cases. J Bone Joint Surg Am 71:848, 1989.

190. Wood DJ, Smith AJ, Collopy D, et al: Patellar resurfacing in total knee arthroplasty: A prospective, randomized trial. J Bone Joint Surg Am 84:197, 2002.

191. Wright RJ, Lima J, Scott RD, et al: Two- to four-year results of posterior cruciate–sparing condylar total knee arthroplasty with an uncemented femoral component. Clin Orthop 260:80, 1990.

192. Wright TM, Bartel DL: The problem of surface damage in polyethylene total knee components. Clin Orthop 205:67, 1986.

193. Yashar AA, Venn-Watson E, Welsh T, et al: Continuous passive motion with accelerated flexion after total knee arthroplasty. Clin Orthop 345:38, 1997.

Posterior Cruciate–Retaining Total Knee Arthroplasty

Aaron G. Rosenberg • Donald M. Knapke

In the early decades of knee arthroplasty surgery, as many as half the patients undergoing knee replacement had inflammatory arthritis (most commonly rheumatoid). Younger age, large size, osteoarthritis, and high physical activity demands all were generally not thought to be ideal indications for total knee arthroplasty (TKA). Advances in implant design, surgical technique, and rehabilitative procedures, along with careful critical assessment of results, have led to systematic improvement in TKA such that better motion and greater function can be expected for most patients undergoing TKA.

These advances have given surgeons the confidence to offer knee replacements to afflicted individuals not previously deemed sufficiently debilitated or aged to warrant the risk. Consequently, the current indications have been expanded, and orthopedic surgeons confidently offer replacement to younger and less severely affected individuals with the promise of reduced pain, restored function, and reasonable implant longevity. Indeed, contemporary TKA provides excellent pain relief and restoration of function in individuals with a multitude of painful arthritic conditions, and such implants have survival rates as high as 98% 15 years after surgery.[54]

Although multiple differing design philosophies have come and gone over the past several decades, the debate over whether to preserve the posterior cruciate ligament (PCL) in TKA continues to engage orthopedists in much the same way as the argument over which approach, anterolateral or posterior, is superior in total hip arthroplasty.

Proponents of cruciate retention have suggested that the advantages of PCL-retaining (CR) designs include more consistent preservation of the joint line, preservation of an important central stabilizing ligamentous structure, improvement in stair-climbing ability, and better conservation of bone. In addition, the potential problems unique to PCL-substituting (PS) designs, patellar clunk, post breakage, post dislocation, and post wear, are absent from CR designs. Alternatively, PS designs have been suggested to offer easier correction of deformity, a more conforming polyethylene surface that results in decreased polyethylene wear, and more reliable rollback of the femur on the tibia in flexion. Although proponents on both sides argue for better motion and better proprioception, proponents of the PS design note the more universal clinical utility of this design, which does not rely on PCL integrity, as well as the potential benefit of avoiding late posterior instability from PCL rupture, which has been reported in patients with inflammatory arthritis.[42]

INTERMEDIATE- TO LONG-TERM RESULTS OF POSTERIOR CRUCIATE–RETAINING TOTAL KNEE ARTHROPLASTY

From a clinical standpoint, many reported series of the long-term results of CR TKA continue to be excellent and have continued to improve as implant designs have solved past problems. Although the results of studies involving older-generation CR systems frequently showed 90% 10-year survivorship, these numbers have improved to 96% to 100% 10-year survivorship for newer-generation designs (Table 85–1). Such results have been demonstrated for many different CR TKA systems.*

Improvements in design features over the past several decades have included elimination of metal-backed patellae and improved patellofemoral groove designs, better understanding of modularity, and improved manufacturing and sterilization of polyethylene.[10] Newer designs offer even more promising results at intermediate-term follow-up, thus suggesting that further design modifications may continue to improve outcomes.[13]

In an extensive review of all primary TKA undertaken at the Mayo Clinic over a 22-year period, Rand et al noted several trends.[53] An overall survivorship of 84% at 15 years was a significant improvement from the 69% reported in an earlier study from the same institution.[52] Significant risk factors for failure noted in their study included younger age, male gender, noninflammatory arthritis, and the use of metal-backed patellae. They also noted the 10-year survival rate of CR TKA to be 91% as opposed to 76% with posterior-stabilized designs. Heck et al[37] reported a review presented at the 65th Annual Meeting of the American Association of Hip and Knee Surgeons. In this study of 53,750 TKAs, the annual reoperation rate was 0.0043 per year if the PCL was intact and 0.0051 per year if the PCL was substituted by the design of the prosthesis. These studies would indicate the CR implants have better long-term survivorship than PS implants do. Even if smaller series were taken into consideration, the survivorship of CR knees would at worst be equal to that of PS knees.

*References 10, 14, 15, 24, 30, 32, 34, 35, 41, 44, 50, 54, 55, 57, 67.

Table 85–1. Intermediate- to Long-Term Results of Posterior Cruciate–Retaining Total Knee Arthroplasty

STUDY	PROSTHESIS	MANUFACTURER	NUMBER OF KNEES	AVERAGE FOLLOW-UP (yr)	MEAN AGE (yr)	OSTEOARTHRITIS (%)	10 YEAR SURVIVAL (%)	REVISION OTHER THAN FOR INFECTION (%)
Schai et al[55]	PFC	J & J	155	10.5	68	62	90	13.5
Buehler et al[15]	PFC	J & J	108	9	70	72	93.4	4.6
Fetzer et al[32]	PFC	J & J	101	10.5	N/A	85%	100	1
Parker et al[50]	MG-1	Zimmer	67	12.8	66	100	90	52
Berger et al[10]	MG-II	Zimmer	109	9	72	94.4	100	1.8
Gill and Joshi[34]	Kinematic Condylar	Howmedica	216	10.1	68	88	98.2	3
Sextro et al[57]	Kinematic Condylar	Howmedica	168	15.7	65.2	64.9	96.5	7.7
Wright et al[67]	Kinemax	Howmedica	523	11.7	69	74	96.1	3.1
Laskin[41]	Genesis	S & N	46	10	69	100	96	4.2
Ritter et al[54]	AGC	Biomet	4583	N/A	65.2	64.9	98	N/A

KINEMATICS

In an unreplaced knee, the PCL serves several functions. It guides rollback of the femoral condyles on the tibial plateau during flexion, thereby allowing the posterior condyles to "clear" the posterior aspect of the tibia in high degrees of flexion and improving the mechanical efficiency of the extensor mechanism. From a stability standpoint, it prevents posterior subluxation of the tibia on the femur in flexion and provides a strong secondary role in varus/valgus stability.

The past several decades have been marked by controversy regarding the ability of the surgeon to successfully preserve the PCL in a way that is clinically meaningful. Several authors have claimed that maintaining PCL integrity during TKA (appropriate length and tension) is impossible and that the kinematic demands of PCL retention require design considerations contrary to maximizing implant longevity.[38] Yet recent research demonstrates that preservation of the PCL, combined with appropriate implant design, preserves femoral rollback.

Using three-dimensional kinematic assessment with fluoroscopic measurement, Banks et al[5] found that a group of total knee replacements with intact PCLs had essentially normal axial rotation and condylar translation whereas those with a post-cam substitution and no PCL had the smallest in vivo range of rotation and translation.

Recent work by Komistek, Dennis, and Steihl evaluated rollback of the femur on the tibia in PS and CR knees via digital analysis of video fluoroscopy of in vivo knee performance in flexion. There was no mention of surgical technique or implant design in the knees studied. Their initial studies showed a consistent pattern of anterior translation of the femur on the tibia in flexion in all the CR knees studied.[25-27,47,61,62] This finding was the reverse of the expected rollback of the femur and was called paradoxical motion (Fig. 85–1). These initial findings indicated that in the particular group of CR knees studied,

there was no evidence that the retained PCL was functioning in its expected role.

More recently, the same group studied an unselected group of CR TKA patients with the use of a specific design of implant, specific instrumentation, and specific technique to adjust PCL tension performed by a single surgeon using a standardized technique.[11] In this group of 20 patients, all but 1 demonstrated essentially normal patterns of femoral rollback.

More recent studies of the same design implanted by different surgeons[40] have revealed consistent rollback in all patients, thus indicating that these findings are not surgeon dependent but rather influenced by design and technique. It also confirmed that routine PCL preservation could be accomplished with functionally appropriate tensioning.

IMPLANT DESIGN AND SURGICAL TECHNIQUE

Further work demonstrated specific design features of the implants that appeared to be responsible for the normal kinematic patterns observed. These features included an asymmetric radius of curvature of the femoral condyles. In an unreplaced knee, the lateral condyle has a significantly increased radius of curvature when compared with the medial condyle. When guided by the development of appropriate tension on the PCL during flexion, this results in differential rollback, with greater translation on the lateral than on the medial side (Fig. 85–2). This rollback can only occur if in addition to appropriate condylar geometry, there is appropriate tension on the PCL as well as no inhibition of this motion by the interaction of the tibial articular surface. Although prosthesis design is clearly important for success with CR TKA, it must be combined with appropriate surgical technique to meet the goals of PCL retention.[9]

FEMUR POSITION ON THE TIBIA DURING A DEEP KNEE BEND

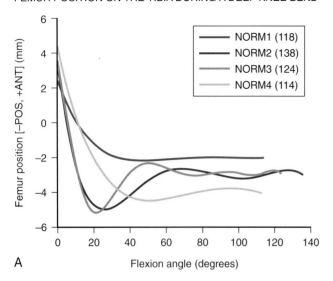

A

FEMUR POSITION ON THE TIBIA DURING A DEEP KNEE BEND

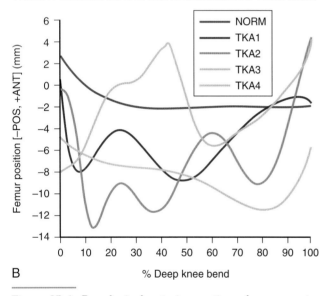

B

Figure 85–1. Paradoxical anterior motion of many posterior–cruciate retaining total knee arthroplasties. **A,** Groups of normal knees demonstrating normal femoral rollback. **B,** Groups of CR TKA demonstrating paradoxical anterior motion of femur on tibia in deep knee bend.

In PCL-preserving designs, it is clear that the contours of the femoral component must not only provide for optimal restoration of normal kinematics but also reproduce normal ligament tension. The geometry and dimensions of the femoral component need to reproduce that of the normal femur. To achieve appropriate tension on the PCL requires not only an anatomic shape of the femoral component but also a large enough number of sizes in appropriate gradations so that the anterior/posterior dimension of the femur may be accurately reproduced.

On the tibial side, several characteristics of the implant and the surgical implantation technique are required to achieve reliable PCL function. The tibial articulation must also be designed to be compatible with normal femoral rollback. In the sagittal plane, a minimally conforming

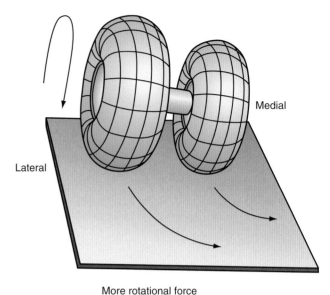

Figure 85–2. NexGen kinematics with a larger radius of curvature of the lateral condyle.

shape must allow the femur to roll back on the tibia. This slightly flattened design in the sagittal plane takes advantage of the retained ligament and allows the kinematics (rollback and rotation) to be as close to normal as possible. At the same time, significant congruence in the frontal plane allows the stress in the polyethylene to be minimized and thus reduce long-term wear.

In the process of resurfacing the tibia, the posterior slope of the articulation must be considered. If this posterior slope is not reestablished, the posterior aspect of the tibial component will be placed too far proximal, which will result in excessive tightness in the PCL during flexion. This causes excessive rollback and high pressure in the posterior part of the tibial articulation. Polyethylene wear may be increased and range of motion can also be limited. Both these situations are undesirable and can be eliminated by reproducing the normal tibial slope. If the prosthesis is designed to be inserted with a posterior inclination to the plane of resection, this must be surgically performed. Most tibial components are designed in this fashion.

PCL-RETAINING VERSUS PCL-SUBSTITUTING DESIGNS— A COMPARISON

Range of Motion

Numerous studies comparing CR and PS TKA have found no difference between the two in ultimate range of motion.[7,28]

Functional Studies

The theoretic advantage of improved proprioception by retaining the PCL has been found to be the case by Warren et al.[64] Other studies show no difference in patients' proprioception between the two types of TKA,[17,59] which may in part be due to the fact that the PCL in osteoarthritic knees has been shown to be more commonly histologically abnormal when compared with control groups.[39] This fact may render the PCL less able to provide better proprioception. Although early studies demonstrated more normal stair-climbing patterns and improvement in CR TKA,[3] several studies have shown no difference.[2,58]

Conditt et al[21] in a recent article found poorer functional scores in squatting, kneeling, and gardening in patients with PS knees. They suggested that the PCL offers better functional capacity in higher-demand activities, especially those involving deep knee flexion.

Bilateral Studies

Numerous studies have compared patients with a CR TKA on one side and a PS TKA on the other.[7,12,19,58] These studies have failed to reveal a persistent patient preference for one TKA type over the other.

Polyethylene Wear

Theoretic decreases in polyethylene wear in CR TKA secondary to the stabilizing effect of the central retained PCL have not been proved. Earlier CR designs with sharp edges and poor plastic resulted in higher rates of plastic wear. Problems with plastic include the use of excessively thin and heat-pressed plastic, as well as the addition of calcium stearate and other manufacturing and sterilization techniques. These problems have since been addressed, and increased wear rates have not been seen with newer

designs. Poor balancing in a CR TKA can result in tightness of the PCL in flexion, which can result in posterior polyethylene wear.[63] Problems of instability and post dislocation can be seen in PS TKA as well if the soft tissues are not balanced. This delineates the importance of soft-tissue balancing no matter what type of TKA is performed.

Correction of Deformity

Proponents of PS TKA have argued that larger deformities present difficult soft-tissue balancing and are more easily balanced with a PS TKA. Although this can certainly be the case, some authors have used CR TKA in the setting of significant preoperative deformity and have had good results.[31] If the deformity is severe enough, flexion/extension mismatches or collateral ligamentous insufficiency often necessitates that even PS TKA is insufficient and more constrained knee replacements or even hinged TKA is necessary (Figs. 85–3 and 85–4).

Aseptic Loosening

Rates of aseptic loosening of both CR and PS TKA remain low in modern designs, and hence no advantage for either type of TKA exists with regard to aseptic loosening rates.

Inflammatory Arthritis

In the past, many authors suggested that PS TKA was the proper choice in patients with inflammatory arthritides such as rheumatoid arthritis. This suggestion was made

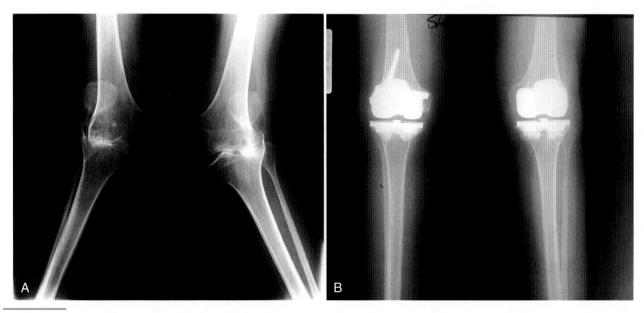

Figure 85–3. **A & B,** Correction of a large valgus deformity with a posterior–cruciate retaining total knee arthroplasty. In **A,** note bilateral severe valgus deformities, In **B,** note correction of valgus deformity with cruciate retaining total knee arthroplasty.

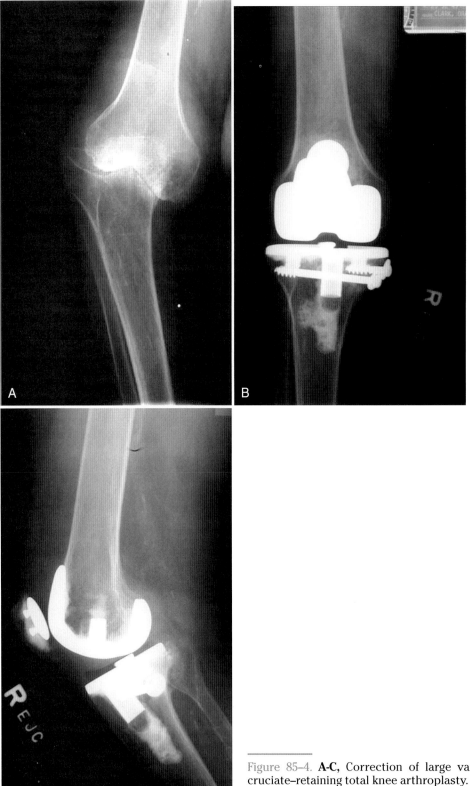

Figure 85–4. **A-C,** Correction of large varus deformity with a posterior cruciate–retaining total knee arthroplasty. **A,** Large varus deformity. AP (**B**) and lateral (**C**) films of correction of deformity with cruciate retaining total knee arthroplasty.

because of the perceived attenuation of the ligament often noted in these patients. Many authors also feared that late rupture of the PCL could lead to late posterior instability. However, Archibeck et al[4] showed 95% good or excellent results in 46 knees of rheumatoid patients treated with CR TKA at an average of 10.5 years' follow-up. Of note, in only one patient did posterior instability develop as a late complication. This study suggests that treating rheumatoid patients with knee arthritis by CR TKA yields excellent results.

POTENTIAL ADVANTAGES OF POSTERIOR CRUCIATE RETENTION

Maintenance of a Central Stabilizer

It is often said that "TKA is a soft-tissue operation." It is the contention of the CR surgeon that it is inappropriate to remove an essential soft-tissue structure when retaining it makes the soft-tissue part of the operation easier. How so? The intact PCL functions as an important secondary stabilizer. When the PCL is preserved, it not only resists posterior subluxation forces but also serves as a secondary stabilizer that resists varus/valgus instability. As opposed to the standard PS technique, which requires maintaining a relatively tight flexion gap (to prevent cam-post subluxation), CR TKA provides a natural means of balancing the flexion space on the medial and lateral sides after collateral ligament release. When large collateral ligament releases are required, there is less flexion instability than in cases in which the cruciate is removed. Consequently, flexion/extension gap balancing is simplified.

Soudry et al[60] delineated the role of the PCL in maintaining femorotibial contact points at the center of the plastic. On the contrary, when the PCL was sacrificed, contact force moved anteriorly on the plastic. Such decentralized force could predispose to plastic wear anteriorly or possibly increased loosening rates secondary to the posterior aspect of the knee being under tensile force in the PS knee.

Maintenance of Joint Line Position

Perhaps of equal importance, preservation of the PCL requires strict maintenance of the joint line. One potential problem that exists with PS knees is elevation of the joint line. Elevation greater than 8 mm has been found to significantly affect knee kinematics and has been correlated with patellofemoral symptoms and need for revision.[33] Retention of the PCL requires strict maintenance of the joint line,[29] and thus rarely is joint line elevation a problem in CR TKA.

Conservation of Bone

Another advantage of CR knees is that this design of prosthesis tends to conserve more bone. Femoral bone is conserved because no notch is needed for the spine-cam articulation. Tibial bone is conserved because no central stem is needed for CR knees in a manner similar to the stem needed for PS knees.

Patellar Clunk Syndrome

Traditional PS designs have included a rather abrupt transition from the patellofemoral groove to the intercondylar box. Although recent designs minimize such transition, PS TKA can still result in this complication. It is not generally seen in CR TKA.[1,45,49]

Avoidance of the Stress Inherent in Posterior Cruciate–Substituting Knees

In CR TKA the PCL acts as a central stabilizer to absorb force and prevent posterior subluxation. The absorption of deforming force by the ligament may protect the fixation interface from such stress and prolong long-term fixation, in addition to eliminating the need for a mechanical structure (the cam-and-post mechanism) to absorb this force. In PS TKA the spine/cam mechanism must resist posterior force, which can result in post wear.[16,51] O'Rourke et al[48] noted relatively high rates of osteolysis in PS knees at intermediate follow-up and raised the question of increased polyethylene wear from the post. Wasielewski[65] raised the possibility that shear force can be higher in PS knees and in knee replacements with more conforming polyethylene inserts, also more commonly found in PS knees. Such shear force is noted at the modular articulation with the tibial baseplate, and increases could therefore contribute to increased backside wear. Scott and Volatile likewise noted the possibility of increased loosening rates in PS TKA secondary to increased interface stress.[56] Further study in this area is certainly needed to understand the relative contribution of backside wear in TKA failure. Post wear and post fracture can also occur with PS TKA and can lead to osteolysis and/or failure of the TKA.[20,46] A poorly balanced PS TKA can result in post dislocation. These problems are not encountered in CR TKA.

Ease of Management of Supracondylar Femur Fractures

Supracondylar periprosthetic femur fractures represent what can at times be a difficult problem.[23,36] CR TKA allows easier repair of these fractures than PS TKA does. CR TKA designs are more amenable to retrograde nailing of these fractures, although newer PS TKA designs have improved in this aspect and many allow placement of a retrograde nail of sufficient diameter. Locked plates for treatment of these fractures have increased in popularity because of their ability to get these fractures to heal, even in very low supracondylar femur fractures in which a retrograde nail may not work. In osteoporotic bone, retrograde femoral nails may not obtain sufficient fixation to get the fracture to heal. CR TKA may also offer better distal femoral bone because of lack of the femoral box found in PS TKA. This extra bone can occasionally be the difference between obtaining a stable construct with a locked plate and having failure of fixation of a locked plate or necessitating treatment with a distal femoral–replacing hinged TKA.

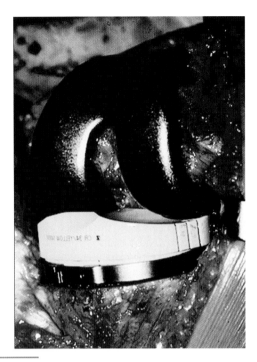

Figure 85–5. Tightness in flexion on this prosthesis can be checked at 90 degrees of flexion. Note the anterior lift-off of polyethylene insert and the anterior position of the tibia indicating excess posterior cruciate ligament tightness in flexion.

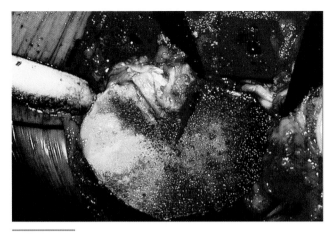

Figure 85–6. Bone block preserved for the posterior cruciate ligament.

SURGICAL TECHNIQUE

Exposure of the knee for TKA can be performed in numerous ways, including medial parapatellar, midvastus, subvastus and quadriceps-sparing techniques. Use of the "measured resection" technique is ideal in CR TKA. The method separates soft-tissue balancing from all the bone cuts. The bone is cut to orient the components for appropriate limb alignment, to maintain the joint line position, and to carefully replace equivalent thicknesses of resected bone with replacement components. These principles are necessary to obtain a balanced PCL. In replacing the femur, sizing is crucial, as is using a system with a sufficient choice of sizes to simulate all different sizes of patients' femurs. Generally speaking, when between sizes, one should choose the smaller size to avoid excessive tightness in flexion (Fig. 85–5). One must be certain to avoid internal rotation of the femoral component, a problem most commonly seen in valgus knees because of the significant lateral posterior condyle bone loss. Use of instrumentation systems that depend on the posterior condyles for rotation reference can result in internal rotation of the femoral component if the surgeon fails to notice this bone loss.

When preparing the tibia one must pay special attention to preserving the PCL during the tibial osteotomy. Some may do this by placing a retractor posteriorly during the tibial cut. Another option includes cutting around a posterior bone block (Fig. 85–6). It is equally important to re-create the posterior tibial slope to avoid excessive

tightness in flexion. When sizing the tibia it is important to pick a size that is compatible with the femoral component. One should choose as large a size as possible without any significant overhang. Rotation of the tibial component is equally important and should be centered along the medial third of the tibial tubercle or slightly more externally rotated. Such avoidance of poor tibial as well as femoral component internal rotation helps circumvent patellofemoral complications.

SOFT-TISSUE BALANCING

During CR TKA, it is essential to achieve appropriate tension in the PCL. Therefore, during the trial reduction, after preparing the femur and tibia with preservation of the PCL, the surgeon must look for signs of the ligament being either too loose or too tight. This assessment is made with the knee in flexion, the position in which the ligament is placed under tension. Tightness in flexion is evidenced by several signs[18]: the trial baseplate (if unrestricted by a post embedded in the tibia) may lift off from the tibial cut anteriorly; the femoral component may be pushed anteriorly off of the distal femoral cut as the knee is brought into flexion; rollback of the femur on the tibia may be observed to be occurring too far posteriorly with flexion, and this hinging appearance of the tibiofemoral articulation may indicate excessive tension in the PCL; and finally the ligament can also be palpated directly during the trial reduction and its tension assessed.

An insufficiently tensioned ligament can also be assessed by palpation or by attempts to perform a posterior drawer test. Of course, tightness in flexion may simply indicate an unbalanced flexion/extension gap, and thus correction of this tightness should be appraised with attention to appropriate filling of the extension gap as well. Assuming that the extension gap is well filled (there is no recurvatum or flexion contracture), one must actually assess the tension in the PCL to determine whether it is the sole contributor to flexion tightness.

If the PCL is found to be too tight with these methods of evaluation, the tibia can be subluxated anteriorly and the PCL gradually released subperiosteally from the tibial insertion. Additionally, it is important to be aware of the fact that increasing the posterior slope of the tibial cut will reduce tension on the PCL. Bellemans et al[8] demonstrated a consistent relationship between increasing tibial slope and increased flexion of the knee when preserving the PCL.

Some severe deformities may require release of the PCL. In these situations, the PCL can be recessed from its tibial insertion without compromising the patient's subjective and objective results. This technique was evaluated by Worland,[66] who found that KT-1000 readings after TKA with PCL recession were acceptable at follow-up. The advantage of this approach is that the patient's joint line is not changed and the rest of the knee kinematics is preserved. If complete release of the PCL is necessary, the surgeon has three options. Use of a standard CR articulation is possible if the flexion gap is "well filled," but this is less desirable. The second option is to use a prosthesis that is more congruent in the sagittal plane, which would be an anteriorly constrained or ultracongruent type of polyethylene insert. The third option is to convert to a posterior-stabilized prosthesis. The surgeon should assess anterior-posterior stability thoroughly at this point and select the appropriate implant.

In situations in which the surgeons wishes to convert to a PS implant after preparing for a CR implant, several considerations must be kept in mind. The most serious potential complication in converting to a PS knee is instability. Instability may occur from a combination of factors that produce a well-functioning CR knee but may sabotage conversion to a PS. These factors include the posterior tibial slope and the general principle of downsizing the femoral component when between sizes. When combined with a relative flexion collateral ligament instability, an underfilled flexion gap may result, and with flexion and varus or valgus stress (depending on the side of collateral instability), the post may slip under the cam. When converting midstream from the CR to the PS design, the surgeon must keep this potential complication in mind.

In cases in which the ligament is a part of the ligament contracture pathology (generally moderate or severe sagittal plane alignment abnormalities combined with flexion contracture) and in the revision setting, PCL substitution seems to be the most reasonable alternative. Additional settings in which PS designs are appropriate include a patellectomized knee and a knee with severe inflammatory changes that have affected the integrity of the ligament itself.[4,6]

CONCLUSION

The concept of simply resurfacing the joint and maintaining as much of the native (healthy?) structure as possible is a philosophically appealing one. However, retention of the PCL necessitates understanding the differences required in surgical technique and component design (and occasionally patient selection) for successful performance of this procedure. Multiple femoral sizes are needed to allow PCL balancing through measured resection techniques. The posterior slope must be reconstituted to allow a balanced PCL in flexion. Improvements in component design now allow improved kinematics with improved femoral rollback. These advances in design and surgical technique have created great success in previous outcome studies and lend promise to ever-improving functional outcomes for patients in the future. These improvements will help meet the increased demands for TKA in the younger, more active, more demanding patient with increased life expectancy in the near future.

References

1. Aglietti P, Buzzi R, Gandenzi A: Patellofemoral functional results and complications with posterior-stabilized total condylar knee prosthesis. J Arthroplasty 3:17-25, 1988.
2. Andriacchi TP, Galante JO: Retention of the posterior cruciate in TKA. J Arthroplasty 3(Suppl):S13-S19, 1988.
3. Andriacchi TP, Galante JO, Fermier RW: The influence of total knee-replacement design on walking and stair-climbing. J Bone Joint Surg Am 64:1328-1335, 1982.
4. Archibeck MJ, Berger RA, Barden RM, et al: Posterior cruciate ligament–retaining total knee arthroplasty in patients with rheumatoid arthritis. J Bone Joint Surg Am 83:1231-1236, 2001.
5. Banks SA, Markovich GD, Hodge WA: In vivo kinematics of cruciate-retaining and substituting knee arthroplasties. J Arthroplasty 12:297-304, 1997.
6. Bayne O, Cameron HU: Total knee arthroplasty following patellectomy. Clin Orthop 186:112-114, 1984.
7. Becker MW, Insall JN, Faris PM: Bilateral total knee arthroplasty. One cruciate retaining and one cruciate substituting. Clin Orthop 271:122-124, 1991.
8. Bellemans J, Robijns F, Duerkinckx J, et al: The influence of tibial slope on maximal flexion after total knee arthroplasty. Knee Surg Sports Traumatol Arthrosc 13:193-196, 2005.
9. Berger RA: The evolution of results of posterior cruciate retaining total knee arthroplasty. Presentation. Nineteenth Annual Vail Orthopedic Symposium, Vail, CO, January 23, 2005.
10. Berger RA, Rosenberg AG, Barden RM, et al: Long-term followup of the Miller-Galante total knee replacement. Clin Orthop 388:58-67, 2001.
11. Bertin KC, Komistek RD, Dennis DA, et al: In vivo determination of posterior femoral rollback for subjects having a Nexgen posterior cruciate–retaining total knee arthroplasty. J Arthroplasty 17:1040-1048, 2002.
12. Bolanos AA, Colizza WA, McCann PD, et al: A comparison of isokinetic strength testing and gait analysis in patients with posterior cruciate–retaining and substituting knee arthroplasties. J Arthroplasty 13:906-915, 1998.
13. Bozic KJ, Kinder J, Menegini M, et al: Implant survivorship and complication rates after total knee arthroplasty with a third-generation cemented system: 5 to 8 years followup. Clin Orthop 430:117-124, 2005.
14. Buechel FF Sr, Buechel FF Jr, Pappas MJ: Twenty year evaluation of meniscal bearing and rotating platform knee replacements. Clin Orthop 388:41-50, 2001.
15. Buehler KO, Venn-Watson E, D'Lima DD, et al: The Press-Fit Condylar total knee system: 8- to 10-year results with a posterior cruciate–retaining design. J Arthroplasty 15:698-701, 2000.
16. Callaghan JJ, O'Rourke MR, Goetz DD, et al: Tibial post impingement in posterior stabilized total knee arthroplasty. Clin Orthop 404:83-88, 2002.
17. Cash RM, Gonzalez MH, Garst J, et al: Proprioception after arthroplasty: Role of the posterior cruciate ligament. Clin Orthop 331:172-178, 1996.
18. Chmell MJ, Scott RD: Balancing the posterior cruciate ligament during cruciate-retaining total knee arthroplasty: Description of the P.O.L.O test. J Orthop Tech 4:12-15, 1996.
19. Clark CR, Rorabeck CH, MacDonald S, et al: Posterior-stabilized and cruciate-retaining total knee replacement: A randomized study. Clin Orthop 392:208-212, 2001.

20. Clarke HD, Math KR, Scuderi GR: Polyethylene post failure in posterior stabilized total knee arthroplasty. J Arthroplasty 19:652-657, 2004.

21. Conditt MA, Noble PC, Bertolusso R, et al: The PCL significantly affects the functional outcome of total knee arthroplasty. J Arthroplasty 19:107-112, 2004.

22. Cope MR, O'Brien BS, Nanu AM: The influence of the posterior cruciate ligament in the maintenance of joint line in primary total knee arthroplasty: A radiologic study. J Arthroplasty 17:206-208, 2002.

23. Dennis DA: Periprosthetic fractures following total knee arthroplasty. Instr Course Lect 50:379-389, 2001.

24. Dennis DA, Clayon ML, O'Donnel S, et al: Posterior cruciate condylar total knee arthroplasty. Clin Orthop 281:168-176, 1992.

25. Dennis DA, Komistek RD, Colwell CE, et al: MA. In vivo anteroposterior femorotibial translation of total knee arthroplasty: A multicenter analysis. Clin Orthop 356:47-57, 1998.

26. Dennis DA, Komistek RD, Mahfouz MR: In vivo fluoroscopic analysis of fixed-bearing total knee replacements. Clin Orthop 410:114-130, 2003.

27. Dennis DA, Komistek RD, Walker SA, et al: Femoral condylar liftoff in vivo in total knee arthroplasty. J Bone Joint Surg Br 83:33-39, 2001.

28. Dorr LD, Ochsner JL, Gronley J, Perry J: Functional comparison of posterior cruciate–retained versus cruciate-sacrificed TKA. Clin Orthop 236:36-43, 1988.

29. Emodi GJ, Callaghan JJ, Pedersen DR, et al: Posterior cruciate ligament function following total knee arthroplasty: The effect of joint line elevation. Iowa Orthop J 19:82-92, 1999.

30. Ewald FC, Wright RJ, Poss R, et al: Kinematic total knee arthroplasty: A 10- to 14- year prospective follow-up review. J Arthroplasty 14:473-480, 1999.

31. Faris PM, Herbst SA, Ritter MA, et al: The effect of preoperative knee deformity on the initial results of cruciate retaining total knee arthroplasty. J Arthroplasty 3:323-326, 1988.

32. Fetzer GB, Callaghan JJ, Templeton JE, et al: Posterior cruciate–retaining modular total knee arthroplasty: A 9- to 12-year follow-up investigation. J Arthroplasty 17:961-966, 2002.

33. Figgie HE 3rd, Goldberg VM, Heiple KG, et al: The influence of tibial-patellofemoral location on function of the knee in patients with the posterior stabilized condylar knee prosthesis. J Bone Joint Surg Am 68:1035-1040, 1986.

34. Gill GS, Joshi AB: Long-term results of Kinematic Condylar knee replacement. J Bone Joint Surg Br 83:355-358, 2001.

35. Gill GS, Joshi AB, Mills DM: Total condylar knee arthroplasty: 16- to 21-year results. Clin Orthop 367:210-215, 1999.

36. Haidukewych GJ, Jacofsky DJ, Hanssen AD: Treatment of periprosthetic fractures around a total knee arthroplasty. J Knee Surg 16:111-117, 2003.

37. Heck DA, Reuben JD, Stiehl JB, et al: Knee prosthetic design and reoperation. Presented at the 65th Annual Meeting of the American Academy of Orthopaedic Surgeons, New Orleans, LA, March 19-23, 1998.

38. Hirsch HS, Lotke PA, Morrison LD: The posterior cruciate ligament in total knee surgery: Save, sacrifice, or substitute? Clin Orthop 309:64-68, 1994.

39. Kleinbart FA, Bryk E, Scott WN, et al: Histologic comparison of PCLs from arthritic and age-matched knee specimens. J Arthroplasty 11:726-731, 1996.

40. Komistek RD, Mahfouz MK, Bertin KC, et al: In vivo determination of TKA kinematics: The NexGen prosthesis with and without a PCL—a multicenter analysis. J Bone Joint Surg (accepted for publication).

41. Laskin RS: The Genesis total knee prosthesis: A 10-year followup study. Clin Orthop 388:95-102, 2001.

42. Laskin RS, O'Flynn HM: The Insall Award: Total knee replacement with posterior cruciate retention in rheumatoid arthritis: Problems and complications. Clin Orthop 345:24-28, 1997.

43. Li E, Ritter MA, Mollanen T, Freeman MA: Total knee arthroplasty. J Arthroplasty 10:560-568, discussion 568-570, 1995.

44. Malkani AL, Rand JA, Bryan RS, et al: Total knee arthroplasty with the kinematic condylar prosthesis: A ten-year follow-up study. J Bone Joint Surg Am 77:423-431, 1995.

45. Maloney WJ, Schmidt R, Sculco TP: Femoral component design and patellar clunk syndrome. J Arthroplasty 17:422-426, 2002.

46. Mestha P, Shenara Y, D'Arcy JC: Fracture of the polyethylene tibial post in posterior stabilized (Insall-Burstein II) total knee arthroplasty. J Arthroplasty 15:814-815, 2000.

47. Oakeshott R, Stiehl JB, Komistek RA, et al: Kinematic analysis of a posterior cruciate retaining mobile-bearing total knee arthroplasty. J Arthroplasty 18:1029-1037, 2003.

48. O'Rourke MR, Callaghan JJ, Goetz DD, et al: Osteolysis associated with a cemented modular posterior cruciate substituting total knee design: Five to eight-year follow-up. J Bone Joint Surg Am 84:1362-1371, 2002.

49. Parker DA, Dunbar MJ, Rorabeck CH: Extensor mechanism failure associated with total knee arthroplasty: Prevention and management. J Am Acad Orthop Surg 11:238-247, 2003.

50. Parker DA, Rorabeck CH, Bourne RB: Long-term followup of cementless versus hybrid fixation for total knee arthroplasty. Clin Orthop 388:68-76, 2001.

51. Puloski SK, McCalden RW, MacDonald SJ, et al: Tibial post wear in posterior stabilized total knee arthroplasty. An unrecognized source of polyethylene debris. J Bone Joint Surg Am 83:390-397, 2001.

52. Rand JA, Illstrup DM: Survivorship analysis of TKA—cumulative rates of survival of 9200 total knee arthroplasties. J Bone Joint Surg Am 73:397-409, 1991.

53. Rand JA, Trousdale RT, Ilstrup DM, et al: Factors affecting the durability of primary total knee prostheses. J Bone Joint Surg Am 85:259-265, 2003.

54. Ritter MA, Berend ME, Meding JB, et al: Long-term followup of anatomic graduated components posterior cruciate–retaining total knee replacement. Clin Orthop 388:51-57, 2001.

55. Schai PA, Thornhill TS, Scott RD: Total knee arthroplasty with the PFC system. J Bone Joint Surg Br 80:850-858, 1998.

56. Scott RD, Volatile TB: Twelve years' experience with posterior cruciate–retaining total knee arthroplasty. Clin Orthop 205: 100-107, 1996.

57. Sextro GS, Berry DJ, Rand JA: Total knee arthroplasty using cruciate retaining kinematic condylar prosthesis. Clin Orthop 388:33-40, 2001.

58. Shoji H, Wolf A, Packard S, et al: Cruciate retained and excised total knee arthroplasty. A comparative study in patients with bilateral total knee arthroplasty. Clin Orthop 305:218-222, 1994.

59. Simmons S, Lephart S, Rubash H, et al: Proprioception following total knee arthroplasty with and without the posterior cruciate ligament. J Arthroplasty 11:763-768, 1996.

60. Soudry M, Walker PS, Reilly DT, et al: The effects of total knee replacement design on femoral-tibial contact conditions. J Arthroplasty 1:33-45, 1986.

61. Stiehl JB, Komistek RD, Cloutier JM, et al: The cruciate ligaments in total knee arthroplasty: A kinematic analysis of 2 total knee arthroplasties. J Arthroplasty 15:545-550, 2000.

62. Stiehl JB, Komistek RD, Dennis DA, et al: Fluoroscopic analysis of kinematics after posterior-cruciate–retaining knee arthroplasty. J Bone Joint Surg Br 77:884-889, 1995.

63. Swany MR, Scott RD: Posterior polyethylene wear in posterior cruciate ligament–retaining total knee arthroplasty. A case study. J Arthroplasty 8:439-446, 1993.

64. Warren PJ, Olanlokun TK, Cobb AG, Bentley G: Proprioception after knee arthroplasty. The influence of prosthetic design. Clin Orthop 297:182-187, 1993.

65. Wasielewski RC: The causes of insert backside wear in total knee arthroplasty. Clin Orthop 404:232-246, 2002.

66. Worland RL, Jessup DE, Johnson J: Posterior cruciate recession in TKA. J Arthroplasty 12:70-73, 1997.

67. Wright RJ, Sledge CB, Poss R, et al: Patient-reported outcome and survivorship after Kinemax total knee arthroplasty. J Bone Joint Surg Am 86:2464-2470, 2004.

CHAPTER 86

Posterior Cruciate Ligament–Substituting Total Knee Arthroplasty

John J. Callaghan • Steve S. Liu

Surgeons who today ascribe to posterior cruciate ligament (PCL) substitution in total knee arthroplasty base that decision on a number of beliefs and facts. They believe that the PCL is abnormal in most arthritic knees,[29] that it functions poorly in the absence of the anterior cruciate ligament (ACL), and that it is difficult to balance yet remain functionally competent.[1] In addition to these beliefs, the potential for the PCL to promote femoral rollback has not been realized in most PCL-retaining designs.

The nomenclature concerning PCL substitution can be confusing to the neophyte surgeon trying to learn about total knee arthroplasty. The original PCL-substituting design introduced at The Hospital for Special Surgery in 1978 was called the "Posterior-Stabilized" implant. However, the term *posterior stabilized* has gained widespread acceptance as a general description of PCL-substituting arthroplasties. In this chapter the term *posterior substitution* will be used when referring to a generic type of implant and *posterior stabilized* will be used in reference to the original design from The Hospital for Special Surgery design or its descendents.

EVOLUTION OF PCL-SUBSTITUTING KNEE ARTHROPLASTY BY THE INSALL GROUP

"Cruciate-sacrificing" implants preceded PCL-substituting implants in the evolution of total knee arthroplasty design. The original total condylar prosthesis was a semi-constrained, nonlinked condylar replacement. This design involved sacrifice of both cruciate ligaments. Component fixation was achieved with the use of bone cement. The femoral curvature roughly approximated that of the average knee. An anterior flange on the device allowed for articulation with an all-polyethylene patellar dome. The tibial tray had concave surfaces that provided some inherent stability of the device.[21,22] This tray had a single central intramedullary post to optimize fixation. Cruciate excision was originally undertaken to allow for extensive exposure and to afford easy correction of angular deformities. Because the surgical technique included removal of the ACL and PCL, stability depended on conformity of the tibial-femoral articular geometry in conjunction with the collateral ligaments by a mechanism that was referred to as the "uphill principle."[66] The uphill principle describes stability that results from tightening of the collateral ligaments as the femoral component tries to ride up and out of the conforming tibial well. With greater excursion of the femur, the collateral ligaments tighten and stabilize the joint. This concept depended heavily on equal tension in flexion and extension gaps to ensure stability. The femoral component was intended to stay generally in the center of the tibial well regardless of knee flexion. Femoral rollback was not intended and, in fact, it was inhibited by the design. Peter Walker was the engineer who helped develop this concept and design, along with the clinical and surgical input from John Insall and Chitranjan Ranawat.[21]

Some shortcomings of this device became apparent even though the results were predictable and durable,[18,25] and even though the clinical long-term results offer a standard of comparison for more modern knee designs.[46,49,63] Several problems became apparent with this design, including cases of insufficient flexion and posterior instability. Early reports indicated that "only" 90 degrees of flexion was attained with this design.[22,25] In cases in which the flexion gap was inadequately balanced, the tibial component had a tendency to subluxate, especially when the patients descended stairs. These findings prompted knee replacement design teams to explore PCL retention or PCL substitution.

THE POSTERIOR-STABILIZED PROSTHESIS

In May 1976, Albert Burstein, PhD, came from Case Western Reserve University in Cleveland to be chairman of The Hospital for Special Surgery Biomechanics Department. The initial attempt to use a post to prevent flexion instability had already failed. This was probably related to the hyperextension stop and the femoral polishing process around the box that led to tibial edge loading and subsequent tibial implant deformity and loosening.[53] Burstein had already studied the contact stresses on condylar surfaces. The collaboration of Burstein and Insall lasted close to 20 years. Insall had an engineering way of sorting out those solutions that were reasonable and those that were not.[4a]

In the Insall-Burstein Posterior-Stabilized prosthesis, the point of contact of the joint was shifted from the middle as it was in the original total condylar design to a more posterior position.[24] This resulted in a larger hill for the femoral component to climb before anterior displacement. The cam mechanism was specifically designed to reproduce the progressive rollback function of the posterior cruciate ligament. The tibial wedge-shaped post engaged an oval intercondylar femoral cam at approximately 70 degrees of flexion. The cam rode up the back of the post, resulting in a progressive posterior displacement of the femur. The phenomenon of rollback translates the extensor mechanism anteriorly and so increases extensor mechanism power. The femoral contact area would approach the posterior edge of the tibial component in 115 degrees of flexion, maximizing knee flexion. The tibial tray also had 3 degrees of posterior slope to help clear the posterior tibial condyles in maximum flexion. The posterior slope also acted to enhance knee stability especially in resisting posterior subluxation through the full flexion arch. The tibial component was initially all-polyethylene (Fig. 86–1). By design, the resultant joint reaction force formed by the force of the quadriceps and the force of the tibial post would be directed straight down into the tibial plateau.[5,24] In addition to the post there was an increase in anteroposterior conformity and a slight increase in mediolateral conformity when compared with the total condylar knee prosthesis. Thus, the first Insall-Burstein Posterior-Stabilized prosthesis was conceived to remove the PCL, correct deformity, reproduce femoral rollback, ensure stability in flexion, and facilitate flexion. The patella was resurfaced using an all-polyethylene dome with a central round peg. All components in this arthroplasty were implanted with the use of polymethylmethacrylate.

The significant clinical success of the Insall-Burstein Posterior-Stabilized prosthesis was not exclusively the result of posterior stabilization. The implant was developed by experienced individuals who had extraordinary surgical and engineering expertise for the era. Many features of the design, in addition to the spine-cam mechanism, contributed to its success. The first implant was placed in 1978.

There are certain features of component design that were not addressed by the Insall-Burstein Posterior-Stabilized prosthesis. The cam had no effect on knee stability in extension because it did not articulate at these lesser flexion angles. Knee stability was dependent on both the soft-tissue balance and the inherent conformity of the components. The ligament substitution mechanism did not prevent anterior tibial subluxation, nor did it substitute in any way for the collateral ligaments. Consequently, mediolateral stability of the joint was entirely dependent on intact collateral ligaments. If a knee was unstable to varus or valgus stresses, the Posterior-Stabilized prosthesis would not provide sufficient support (Fig. 86–2). These cases would need to be addressed with a more constrained implant.

Several design alterations of the Insall-Burstein Posterior-Stabilized prosthesis have been made over the years. One of the first changes involved modification of the composition of the original all-polyethylene tibial tray to include metal backing of the tibial component. This was done in the latter half of 1980 after finite element analysis demonstrated enhanced load transmission to the underlying bone with the addition of metal backing to the tibial component.[2] By 1981, the all-polyethylene tibial

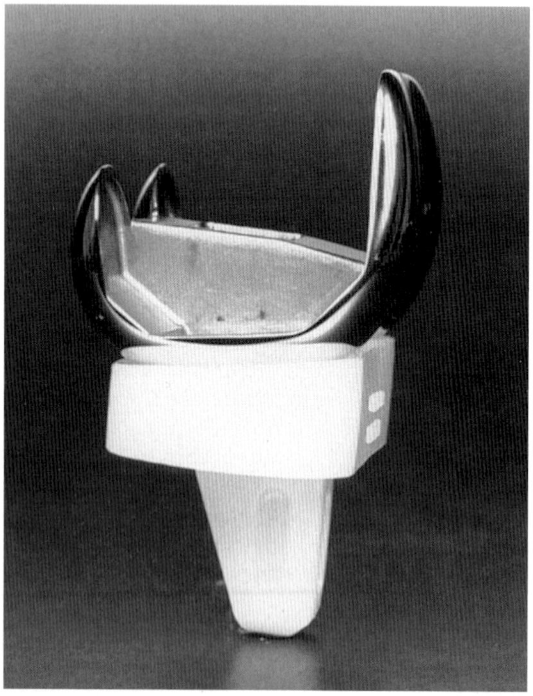

Figure 86–1. The original Insall-Burstein Posterior-Stabilized prosthesis composed of a chrome-cobalt femoral component articulating with an all-polyethylene tibial tray.

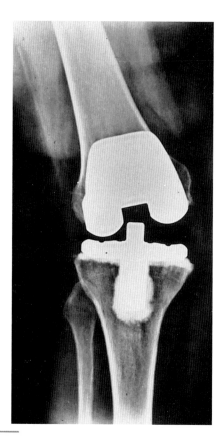

Figure 86–2. A posterior-stabilized prosthesis implanted in a patient with medial collateral ligament insufficiency. The posterior substituting mechanism does not prevent medial laxity.

component had been totally replaced by its metal-backed counterpart at The Hospital for Special Surgery.

The early 1980s also marked the advent of carbon-reinforced tibial components. Theoretically, carbon reinforcement would increase the strength of the polyethylene that composed the tibial tray. However, the clinical results with this polyethylene biomaterial proved disappointing and failure of the carbon-reinforced tibia was reported.[54-56] Thereafter, the plain (nonreinforced) polyethylene tibial tray was used routinely with the Posterior-Stabilized prosthesis.

The next major prosthetic change occurred in 1983 with the introduction of modified Posterior-Stabilized components, which was, in part, the practical result of a concern regarding the patellofemoral joint. At that time, the femoral component was altered to allow for a smoother patellofemoral transition (Fig. 86–3). This tran-

sition occurs when the patellofemoral contact point moves from the anterior flange to the distal runners as the knee goes through an arc of motion from extension to flexion. Modifications included rounding of the anterior portion of the femoral component, as well as deepening of the femoral groove in an attempt to enhance patellar tracking. Additionally, the implant was produced in various sizes. Because the original version was available in only one intermediate size, mismatches between the component and the host bone occurred; this was corrected with the introduction of multiple sizes.

INSALL-BURSTEIN II POSTERIOR-STABILIZED PROSTHESIS

The Posterior-Stabilized prosthesis continued in use without major change until the late 1980s, when the Insall-Burstein II (IB II) Posterior-Stabilized prosthesis was introduced (Fig. 86–4). This prosthesis incorporated several major changes in both component design and instrumentation. Intramedullary instruments were used for prosthetic implantation, and the original "tenser," used in the past to ensure balance between the flexion and extension gaps, was abandoned. However, the concept of ligamentous balance was not discarded, and it still remains an essential factor for successful arthroplasty. The IB II prosthesis also introduced modularity to the Posterior-Stabilized components. Thus, depending on the clinical needs of an individual case, various metallic trays, polyethylene tibial inserts, intramedullary rods, and wedges could be assembled at the time of surgery.

Additionally, the inauguration of the IB II prosthesis heralded a slight modification in the mechanism of ligament substitution. This was done in an attempt to further enhance femoral rollback and to increase knee flexion. Unfortunately, this new design required further

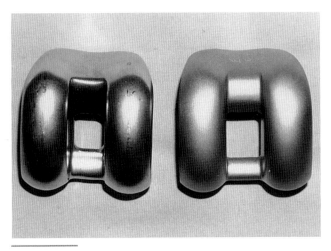

Figure 86–3. Original Insall-Burstein femoral component (**left**) and modified component (**right**). The femoral groove has been deepened and the anterior aspect more rounded.

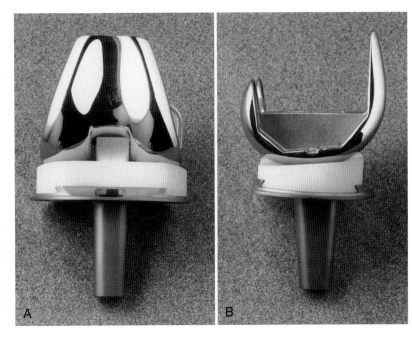

Figure 86–4. The Insall-Burstein II prosthesis. **A,** Front view. **B,** Side view. The tibial component is modular, allowing interchange of the plastic on each metallic tray. The kinematics of the design were altered slightly to improve rollback and knee flexion. Note the posterior incline to the tibial plastic, which acts to enhance knee stability.

fine-tuning secondary to reports of component dislocation.[7,35,36,41,67] Although rare, dislocations were especially worrisome in knees with a preoperative valgus deformity or in those that achieved large flexion angles.[15] Because of widespread concern regarding this problem, a modification of the tibial insert was undertaken. Changes, restricted to the tibial insert, included elevation as well as relative anterior translation of the tibial spine. These alterations served to increase the inherent stability of the device.[30,36]

Thus, the IB II prosthesis offered the advantages of a modular design while maintaining the basic mechanism of ligament substitution (Fig. 86–5). It employed essentially the same arthroplasty philosophy that had been used suc-

cessfully since the 1980s and was one of the few prosthetic designs to remain fundamentally unchanged after more than a decade in use.

NEXGEN LEGACY

Introduced in the mid 1990s, the NexGen Legacy prosthesis is the most recent evolution of the Posterior-Stabilized prosthesis lineage. The prosthesis incorporates several major design and instrumentation changes. The NexGen Legacy prosthesis includes an anatomic design with both right and left femoral components. This differs from previous Posterior-Stabilized designs, which were nonanatomic. In addition, the femoral prosthesis has a raised lateral flange and a deeper trochlear groove. These design modifications were instituted partly to further optimize patellofemoral kinematics (Fig. 86–6).

Another design modification made with the NexGen Legacy was the addition of lugs to the femoral component's condyles. These were instituted to help stabilize the prosthesis during implantation. Specifically, the femoral component lugs help prevent flexion of the femoral component during flexion. On occasion, this "femoral flex" occurred with the Insall-Burstein design and resulted, if the prosthesis was left flexed, in a gap between the component's femoral flange and the femur's anterior cortex. If correction was attempted by twisting the component into extension, the surgeon risked the possibility of creating a gap between the femur's posterior condyle and the component's posterior condyles. The advent of the lugs prevents flexion of the component during insertion, thereby preventing the femoral flex phenomenon.

The NexGen Legacy's tibial baseplates are designed to accept multiple different-sized polyethylene inserts. This contrasts to previous Posterior-Stabilized designs, in which each femoral component was paired exclusively with its size-matched tibial component. On occasion, this could lead to intraoperative difficulties if a patient's bone required different femoral and tibial component sizes. The current design of the NexGen Legacy prosthesis allows the

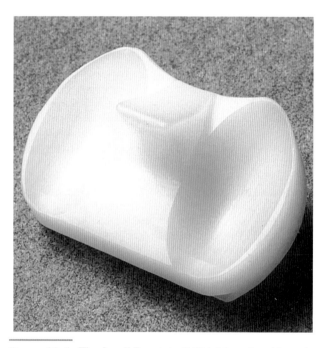

Figure 86–5. The Insall-Burstein II tibial tray has bicondylar wells that conform to the shape of the femoral component.

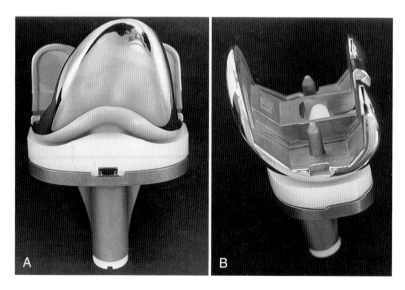

Figure 86–6. NexGen Legacy prosthesis (Zimmer, Warsaw, IN). **A,** Front view. **B,** Oblique view.

surgeon to independently pick both the femoral and the tibial components. Multiple tibial inserts are available for each tibial baseplate. The inserts are designed so that the plastic undersurface mates with the tibial baseplate while the articulating surface corresponds to the particular femoral component. This allows designers to maintain conformity at the femoral-tibial articulation while maintaining flexibility in tibial component sizing.

Finally, the spine-cam interaction was modified slightly in the NexGen Legacy prosthesis. The designers attempted to maintain the well-established benefits of PCL substitution while building increased stability into the substituting mechanism to minimize the dislocation risks associated with the previous prostheses at high flexion angles.[7,30, 35,36,41,67] Thus, the NexGen Legacy's spine-cam interaction has a similar pathway and angle of contact as the successful previous Posterior-Stabilized designs. However, the femoral cam is positioned farther posterior and proximal in the NexGen Legacy's femoral component. This increases knee stability by allowing the femoral cam to ride down the tibial spine as the knee flexes. This differentiates this implant from the previous Posterior-Stabilized designs (and most other designs), in which the femoral cam rides up along the tibial spine as the knee bends into deep flexion.[10,30] An LPS-Flex version has been developed to gain further flexion.

The instrumentation options available for implantation were also modified and increased with the NexGen Legacy prosthesis. The modifications allow for increased flexibility and surgical preference in choosing the manner to implant the prosthesis. Traditional intramedullary instrumentation, which incorporates the classic IB II surgical techniques, is available. In addition, epicondylar instruments that reference the femur's epicondylar axis to optimize femoral component rotation can be used. These instruments also permit both anterior and posterior femoral referencing to aid in positioning the femoral component. Finally, for surgeons desiring an alternative to the traditional saw-blade technique, instrumentation is available that allows for preparation of the femur and tibia using a milling technique.

CONTEMPORARY PCL SUBSTITUTION DEVICES

The success of the Insall-Burstein device led almost every other knee design team to provide PCL substitution options in their system.

Duracon PS

The Duracon PS (Howmedica, Rutherford, NJ) is an anatomic PCL-substituting design that is part of the Duracon total knee system (Fig. 86–7). The Duracon system uses a versatile tibial baseplate that accepts polyethylene inserts for either PCL substitution or PCL retention. As with other modern prostheses, one of the goals of the implant developers was optimizing articular conformity and thereby minimizing contact stresses and polyethylene wear.

The femoral component has a closed-box design, which the designers believed would prevent cement extrusion and reduce polyethylene wear particle migration. The femoral component's closed box is posteriorly located, which corresponds to the posteriorly positioned tibial post. Theoretically, this posterior placement helps preserve anterior femoral bone stock. In addition, the femoral component has a deep trochlear groove with an anatomic lateral flare. The designers believed that this would enable the patella to track naturally during knee motion.

The Duracon PS spine-cam interaction is distinctly different from other modern PCL-substituting designs. Most PCL-substituting components are designed to have the femoral cam contact the tibial spine at a knee flexion angle of 60 to 70 degrees. This results in PCL-substituting mechanisms that resemble the original Posterior-Stabilized spine-cam interaction. At lesser knee flexion angles, the spine does not contact the cam. Thus, at these lower angles, stability depends on implant conformity and soft-tissue tension. In contrast, the Duracon PS is designed for

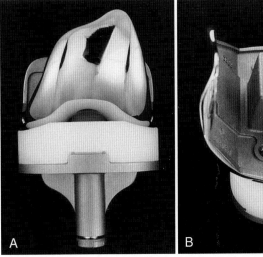
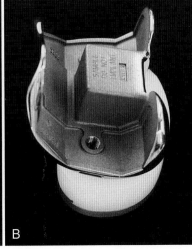

Figure 86–7. Duracon PS (Howmedica, Rutherford, NJ). **A,** Front view. **B,** Oblique view.

spine-cam interaction to begin at 10 degrees of flexion. The spine and cam then remain in contact throughout the entire range of knee motion. This spine-cam mechanism appears similar to the previous design (Kinematic Stabilizer) from the same company. The developers of these prostheses believed that spine-cam interaction throughout the knee's arc of motion would increase component stability at low flexion angles. Theoretically, this could also increase stress to the tibial spine because of the increased contact. In fact, the tibial component of the Duracon PS is reinforced with a Vitallium endoskeleton specifically to increase its strength and stability. A locking screw is used to secure the reinforced tibial post to the baseplate, thereby augmenting the basic polyethylene snap-lock mechanism.

PFC SIGMA

The PFC Sigma knee system (Johnson & Johnson, Raynham, MA) was one of the first comprehensive knee arthroplasty systems widely available. The implants are designed to take advantage of the benefits of modularity and to allow for simple intraoperative interchange between components. Specifically, the tibial tray accepts either PCL-retaining, PCL-supplementing, or PCL-substituting polyethylene tibial inserts. The tray is modular and can be augmented with tibial wedges, blocks, or various-sized tibial stems (Fig. 86–8).

The femoral component differs depending on whether it is designed for PCL-retaining or PCL-substituting knee arthroplasty. However, both the PCL-retaining and the PCL-substituting femoral components share the same coronal geometry. The implant developers used this geometry to increase contact area and protect against edge loading, thereby minimizing peak stresses. The similar coronal geometry theoretically aids in easy intraoperative switching between PCL-retaining and PCL-substituting implants.

Similar to many other modern PCL-substituting designs, the PFC Sigma femoral components are anatomic,

with parts for both right and left knees. The femoral spine interaction is similar to the original Insall-Burstein Posterior-Stabilized design. In addition, the femoral components mate either with the identical-sized tibial baseplate or with tibial trays one size larger or smaller. This permits the surgeon to upsize or downsize the tibial component by one size, allowing for a three-size spread. Conceptually, this optimizes contact at the femoral-tibial articulation, as well as between tibial baseplate and host bone.

More recently, a rotating platform version with a PCL-substituting tibial insert has become available. The femoral cam and tibial post have been modified to allow more extension before anterior cam after impingement.

Genesis II

The Genesis II total knee was designed as a comprehensive knee system with a modern PCL-substituting option. The components are anatomic and are designed to promote versatility in matching femoral and tibial component sizes. In general, the system allows the femoral prosthesis to mate with four different-sized tibial components. Additionally, the implant design incorporates several innovative features in an attempt to optimize knee kinematics. One goal was for the femoral component's trochlear groove to gently encourage lateral patellar motion as the knee comes into extension. Thus, the femoral component's trochlear groove was elongated to maximize contact with the patella throughout the arc of motion (full contact through 85 degrees of flexion). In addition, in a further attempt to facilitate patellar tracking, the trochlear groove of the Genesis II femoral component was lateralized (Fig. 86–9).

An innovative design concept employed in the Genesis II is the design of the femoral component's posterior condyles. Most conventional knee system designs require external rotation of the femoral component to achieve a trapezoidal flexion gap. External rotation of the femoral cut results in more bone resected from the posterior

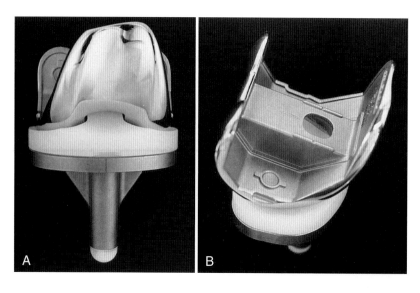

Figure 86–8. Press-Fit Condylar (Johnson & Johnson, Raynham, MA). **A,** Front view. **B,** Oblique view.

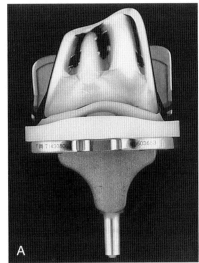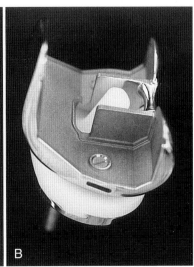

Figure 86–9. Genesis II (Smith & Nephew, Richards, Memphis, TN). **A,** Front view. **B,** Oblique view.

medial femur than from the posterior lateral femur. The asymmetric femoral bone resections help compensate for the traditional asymmetric tibial resection that occurs with a perpendicular tibial cut. This traditional cut results in more bone resected from the lateral than from the medial tibial plateau. Thus, in the traditional method of component implantation, the bone cuts counterbalance each other and result in a rectangular flexion space. Traditional components are designed for this and have symmetric posterior femoral condyles.

As opposed to traditional symmetric medial and lateral posterior condyles, the Genesis II posteromedial femoral condyle is thinner than the posterolateral condyle. This is because the femoral component is designed to be implanted with a symmetric posterior femoral cut (no external rotation of the femoral component). The Genesis II designers hoped to minimize some of the theoretical limitations associated with traditional external femoral rotation. Limitations include unnecessary anterolateral femoral bone removal, rotational malalignment of the femoral and tibial components, and excessive medial patella tracking at high flexion angles. The Genesis II asymmetric posterior femoral condyles allow for a neutral cut. Conceptually, the flexion space remains balanced because the smaller medial posterior condyle on the Genesis II femoral component compensates for the smaller posterior medial flexion space. In addition, the femoral component's built-in lateralized trochlear groove compensates for the neutral cut in extension and theoretically aids tracking of the patella.

Stability of the Genesis II PCL-substituting knee depends on both the component's articular geometry and the spine-cam interaction. The implants are designed to articulate freely through the first 60 degrees of flexion, with stability dependent on the surface geometry and soft-tissue balance. Spine-cam engagement occurs at 60 to 70 degrees of knee flexion. Theoretically, the Genesis II spine-cam interaction is designed to minimize dislocations because at high flexion angles it has greater inherent stability, as defined by the dislocation safety factor,[10,30] than does the Insall-Burstein design.

MAXIM KNEE

The Maxim Knee (Biomet, Warsaw, IN) is a PCL-substituting prosthesis that was introduced in the 1990s. The developers of the Maxim Knee attempted to design components that minimized point loading and maximized component interchangeability (Fig. 86–10). In addition, the prosthesis was designed to maximize congruity at the femoral-tibial articulation but theoretically still allow 30 degrees of rotation.

The femoral component has a "unique condylar radius design" that comprises a 1.5-in radius and a 2-in center that is constant throughout all implant sizes. This design concept is patented with matching femoral and tibial radius in the mediolateral plane. This allows for complete interchangeability among all tibial and femoral components. The Maxim Knee is anatomically designed with both right and left components.

The tibial tray has a built-in 3-degree posterior slope permitting a flat tibial bone cut. The tibial component's post is moved progressively posteriorly as the baseplate size increases. Conceptually, this modification of the spine-cam mechanism allows for a potential maximum flexion angle of approximately 130 degrees. Finally, the implant's instrumentation is posterior referencing to optimize the flexion space.

ADVANCE PS

Of the modern posterior cruciate–substituting knee designs, the ADVANCE PS knee (Wright Medical, Arlington, TN) is one of the most similar to the Posterior-Stabilized and IB II Posterior-Stabilized implants. The ADVANCE knee is a nonanatomic, symmetric knee and thus does not come with right and left components (Fig. 86–11). It maintains conformity of the articular surfaces by exclusively mating the femoral component with only one polyethylene tibial insert. However, each polyethylene insert can seat into two tibial baseplates (regular and

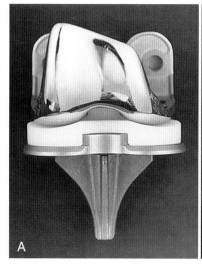 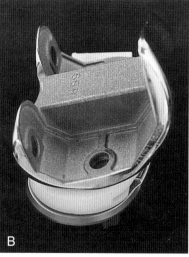

Figure 86–10. Maxim (Biomet, Warsaw, IN). **A,** Front view. **B,** Oblique view.

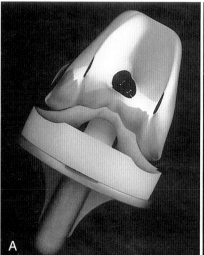 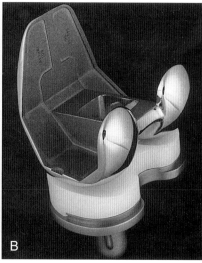

Figure 86–11. ADVANCE PS (Wright Medical, Arlington, TN). **A,** Front view. **B,** Oblique view.

"plus" size). Functionally, this allows the femoral component to be paired with either the corresponding size tibial baseplate or one a size larger.

The spine-cam mechanism resembles the one used in the Posterior-Stabilized and IB II Posterior-Stabilized designs, with some modifications. The tibial spine was moved posteriorly and is designed to engage the cam at 70 degrees. The spine-cam interaction allows for theoretical maximum flexion of more than 120 degrees for all sizes, with only a 5-degree variation across all sizes. Cam-spine congruency was designed to more uniformly distribute forces to the polyethylene as compared with the IB II prosthesis. The spine-cam mechanism was adjusted to increase resistance to dislocation at high flexion angles compared with the IB II design.

The developers attempted to optimize patellar tracking by producing a femoral implant with a deepened and posteriorly extended trochlear groove. This modification was undertaken to maximize patellar contact at high flexion angles. The femoral component's anterior flange was designed with a low profile to decrease retinacular soft-tissue tension, improve tracking of the patella, and decrease the need for lateral release.

OPTETRAK

Of the modern posterior cruciate–substituting designs, the OPTETRAK (Exactech, Gainesville, FL) knee is the other design with the most similarity to the Posterior-Stabilized and IB II Posterior-Stabilized implants. The similarity between these designs is not unexpected because some of the same engineers were involved in the development of all these prostheses. Like the ADVANCE PS, the OPTETRAK is a nonanatomic, symmetric knee and does not come with right and left components (Fig. 86–12). Conformity of the articular surface is maintained by exclusively mating the femoral component with only one polyethylene tibial insert. However, each polyethylene insert can seat into multiple tibial baseplates. Effectively, this allows most femoral components to be paired with three different-size tibial baseplates.

The spine-cam mechanism resembles the one used in the Posterior-Stabilized and IB II Posterior-Stabilized designs, with some modifications. The cam box width was reduced to minimize bone resection, and the spine-cam articulation was curved to reduce contact stress on the

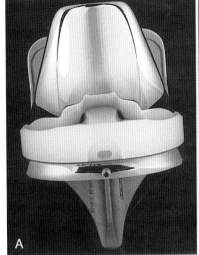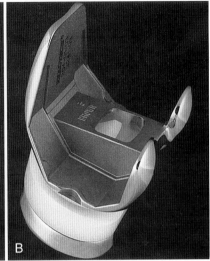

Figure 86–12. OPTETRAK (Exactech, Gainesville, FL). **A,** Front view. **B,** Oblique view.

tibial spine. Finally, the tibial spine height was designed to improve stability and minimize the risk of dislocation.

As with the ADVANCE PS knee, the designers attempted to optimize patellar tracking. This was accomplished by creating a femoral implant with a less prominent femoral flange and a deeper trochlear groove. Softening of the femoral component edges was undertaken to decrease retinacular soft-tissue tension, improve tracking of the patella, and decrease the need for lateral release.

ADVANTAGES OF PCL SUBSTITUTION

There are several potential advantages in implanting a PCL-substituting prosthesis:

1. *The surgical technique is easy to perform.* Sacrifice of the PCL is a straightforward and reproducible surgical technique. The PCL can be sharply excised from its femoral attachment. Thus, ligamentous balancing is not complicated by the possible tethering effect of this posterior structure.
2. *Minimal tibial resection is possible.* Because there is no need to balance the PCL, the surgeon is not restricted to a particular depth of tibial bone resection. It is thus possible to effect a minimal tibial resection. This allows placement of the tibial component in stronger host bone, as opposed to the weaker metaphyseal cancellous bone encountered with larger tibial resections.
3. *Knees have more normal kinematics.* PCL substitution results in total knee arthroplasty with more normal knee kinematics. Fluoroscopic studies have shown that PCL-substituting knees have femoral rollback patterns that most closely resemble those of normal knees.[12,60] Conversely, fluoroscopic analysis has shown PCL-retaining designs demonstrating erratic rollback patterns, with some PCL-retaining knee arthroplasties paradoxically rolling forward in flexion. In addition, fluoroscopic analysis of knees in

weightbearing demonstrated greater flexion with PCL-substituting designs than with PCL-retaining designs.[11]

4. *Polyethylene wear is decreased when a conforming articular surface is implanted.* Because the long-term survival of total knee prostheses is now theoretically possible, the limiting effects of polyethylene wear have become an increasing concern.[19,48,52,64,68] PCL substitution allows the implantation of a conforming articular polyethylene surface. The increased contact area provided by the conforming surface acts to decrease the stress to which the plastic is subjected. Evidence of significant polyethylene failures in PCL retaining devices with less conforming tibial articular surfaces has already been reported.[9,28,42,61]
5. *The deformity can be corrected easily.* PCL excision allows easier deformity correction in severely deformed knees.[34]

SURGICAL TECHNIQUE

The basic surgical technique for implanting PCL-substituting prostheses has been well documented.[23,26,64] The objective is to produce a knee that has equal soft-tissue tension on the medial and lateral sides in both flexion and extension. The axis of flexion is designed to be in the central portion of the knee and shared equally by both the medial and the lateral compartments.

The basic concepts behind knee arthroplasty with PCL substitution remain virtually unchanged. However, the original Posterior-Stabilized prosthesis was inserted with the use of a tenser (Fig. 86–13). This instrument applied tension to the collateral ligaments and helped align the knee. The tenser has been replaced with intramedullary instrumentation. However, it still remains imperative to pay strict attention to soft-tissue tension of the collateral ligaments.

The modern surgical technique begins with an anteroposterior radiograph of the involved extremity obtained

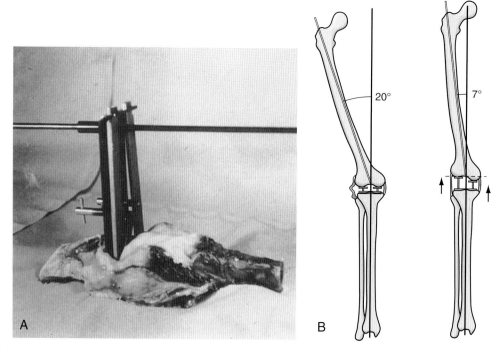

Figure 86–13. The tenser is an instrument used in ICLH arthroplasty of the knee, with which the presence or absence of soft-tissue contractures can be demonstrated at operation. Before insertion of this instrument, the cruciate ligaments are divided and the tibial plateau is sectioned at right angles to the anatomic axis of the bone. **A,** The instrument is used in the extended knee to separate first one and then the other femoral condyle from the tibia, thereby tensing the medial and lateral soft tissues in turn. A bar passes through the tibial plate at right angles to the latter. The distal end of this bar must lie over the center of the ankle. **B,** The proximal end of the bar will lie over the hip when the soft tissues are tensed only when there is neither contracture nor elongation of these tissues on either side of the joint. Thus, by tensing the tissues and noting the relationship of the proximal end of the bar to the hip, the surgeon can judge the presence and magnitude of soft-tissue contracture or elongation.

on a long film (Fig. 86–14). This radiograph is used to ensure that there are no "surprises" that would preclude the use of intramedullary instruments, as well as to help determine the angle between the anatomic and mechanical axes of the knee (Fig. 86–15). The goal of surgery is to reproduce this angle intraoperatively. This is achieved by executing tibial and femoral bone cuts, which are parallel to each other while remaining perpendicular to the mechanical axis.

The knee is exposed with a straight anterior skin incision. A straight medial parapatellar capsular incision is used for the arthrotomy. The periosteum of the proximal medial tibia is raised in a continuous layer off the tibial bone. Laterally, a small cuff of periosteum is raised in continuity with the patellar ligament to provide some protection against tibial tubercle avulsion. The patella is everted, and the knee is flexed.

With the knee in the flexed position, any remnants of the ACL are carefully excised. The tibia is now subluxed anteriorly. It is sometimes necessary, especially on varus knees, to continue the release of the structures of the proximal medial aspect of the tibia, including a portion of the semimembranosus, to allow adequate tibial subluxation.

After adequate exposure has been achieved, attention is turned to the bone cuts. Depending on surgeon's preference, the bone cuts can commence with either the tibia or the femur. The order of the cuts is not as important as is

adherence to the basic principles of knee arthroplasty in attempting to optimize alignment, balance, and stability.

The first step in cutting the distal femur is to make a small intramedullary hole. This hole should be slightly (3 to 5 mm) medial to the center of the femoral groove to allow easy drilling of the intramedullary portion of the femur. Because of concern regarding physiological changes associated with intramedullary instrumentation,[14] the hole is routinely vented. This is accomplished by overdrilling the hole (Fig. 86–16) with a step drill and using a fluted intramedullary rod. This helps reduce intramedullary pressure during the placement of subsequent intramedullary guides. The femoral alignment guide is then inserted into this intramedullary channel. It should be set at the proper valgus angle as determined by preoperative radiographs. The vast majority of knees fall between 6 and 8 degrees of anatomic valgus. On knees with a preoperative valgus alignment, the tendency is to set the guide at 5 degrees.

For most knees, the standard cutting block is attached to the intramedullary femoral alignment guide before its insertion in the femoral canal. However, for knees with a significant preoperative flexion deformity, it may be beneficial to resect an additional 3 mm of distal femoral bone. This can be accomplished by removal of the standard cutting block, which will allow for this additional distal bone resection. At this point, the femoral alignment guide

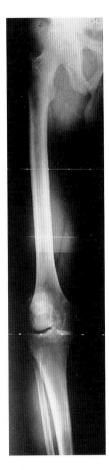

Figure 86–14. **Standing anteroposterior long radiograph of knee.**

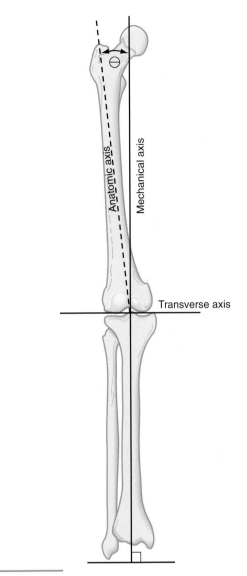

Figure 86–15. **Calculation of angle between anatomic and mechanical axes.**

is inserted into the intramedullary canal. Although this step does not set the final rotation of the femoral component, it is useful to place the guide carefully to achieve reasonable rotation of the distal femoral cut. The epicondylar axis can be used to aid in optimizing this rotation. Desired rotation is neutral to slight external rotation to ensure that the posterior femoral condylar cut will parallel the cut surface of the proximal tibia. In addition, slight external rotation will also enhance tracking of the patella (Fig. 86–17).

After the intramedullary alignment guide is placed within the femoral canal, the femoral cutting block is attached to the 0-degree distal placement guide. They are then both inserted into the intramedullary alignment guide until the cutting block rests on the anterior femoral cortex (Fig. 86–18). To further stabilize the guide, the anterior thumbscrew is hand tightened until it contacts the anterior femoral cortex. Two pins are placed in the femoral cutting block for the 0-mm resection. Finally, the distal placement guide is loosened, and a slap hammer is used to remove both the distal placement guide and the intramedullary femoral alignment guide. The distal femur is then cut through the cutting slot in the femoral cutting block.

The next step is sizing and establishing rotation of the femoral component. The anteroposterior sizing guide is used to determine which of the component sizes will give the best reconstructive result. Ideally, the body of the guide will contact the resected distal femur. Both of the guide's "feet" should rest on the posterior femoral condyles. The guide's anterior boom should contact the anterior cortex of the femur. The boom should be positioned so it does not contact abnormal bony anatomy, such as an osteophyte or a depression. The femoral size should then be read directly from the guide (Fig. 86–19). If the guide falls between sizes, the boom can be adjusted (normally by moving it medially) until the guide directly aligns with a size. This maneuver essentially allows the anteroposterior sizing guide to be used in a posterior referencing manner. By adjusting the boom, the surgeon can optimize the anteroposterior position of the implant using either strict anterior or posterior referencing or a combination of both techniques. Two headless holding pins are placed in the anteroposterior sizing guide's holes. These pins are used to establish the anteroposterior position of the femoral component as well as to place it in 3 degrees

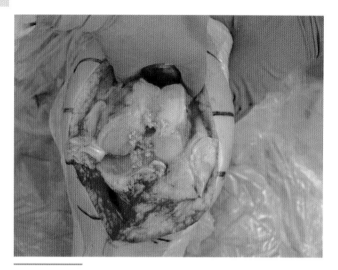

Figure 86–16. An entry hole for the intramedullary femoral rod is made with a step drill. The exact site of the entry hole is a few millimeters anterior to the insertion of the posterior cruciate ligament and situated centrally, medially, or laterally, depending on the preoperative templating on the radiograph.

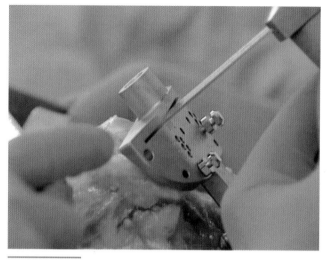

Figure 86–18. The cutting block rests on the anterior femoral cortex. Two pins are placed in the femoral cutting block to further stabilize the guide for the 0-mm resection.

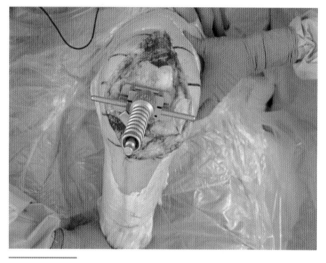

Figure 86–17. The femoral alignment guide is slightly externally rotated. Desired rotation is neutral to slight external rotation to ensure that the posterior femoral condylar cut parallels the cut surface of the proximal tibia. The epicondylar axis can be used to help optimize rotation.

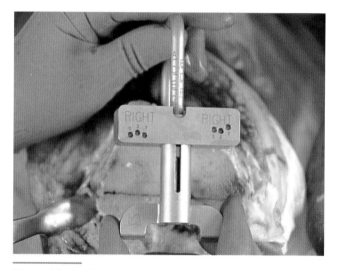

Figure 86–19. The anteroposterior sizing guide determines the size of the femoral component. The guide's "feet" should rest on the posterior femoral condyles, and the anterior boom should contact the anterior cortex of the femur. In general, the closer size is chosen, although if there is any question then the smaller size should be selected.

of external rotation (referenced from the posterior condyles). The pins should be checked to ensure that they are parallel to the epicondylar axis. If the headless pins do not align with the epicondylar axis, the pins should be fine tuned (commonly the lateral one is adjusted) so the pins and axis correspond.

At this point, the correct size 4-in-1 femoral finishing guide (as determined by the previous anteroposterior sizing guide) is placed onto the distal femur over the already-positioned headless pins (Fig. 86–20). The 4-in-1 femoral finishing guide is then pinned to the distal femur. The distal femur is then cut in a sequential order (Fig. 86–21). The most common cutting sequence is posterior

condyles, posterior chamfers, anterior condyles, and anterior chamfers. Finally, the femoral lug holes are drilled through the appropriate holes in the guide.

The next step is to cut the proximal tibia. This is done with either an extramedullary or an intramedullary guide system, depending on the surgeon's preference and the knee anatomy (Fig. 86–22). The ideal cut is 90 degrees to the long axis of the tibia in the mediolateral plane, with a slight posterior slope in the anteroposterior plane. Resection of the PCL allows for a minimal tibial resection. Therefore, in the PCL-substituting knee arthroplasty, the proximal tibial bone cut should ideally be only 5 to 9 mm below the articular surface of the normal side

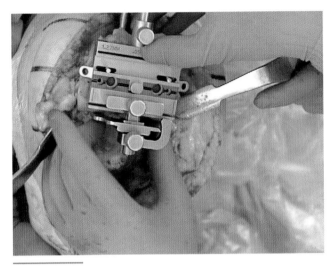

Figure 86–20. The 4-in-1 femoral finishing guide is pinned to the distal femur.

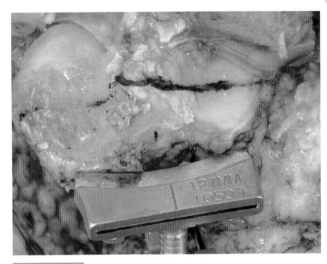

Figure 86–22. The tibial cutter is positioned to make a right-angled cut across the top of the tibia.

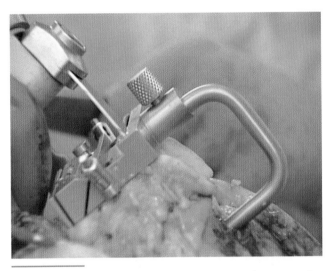

Figure 86–21. The slots are used to cut the posterior condyles, posterior chamfers, anterior condyles, and anterior chamfers. The femoral lug holes are drilled through the appropriate holes in the guide.

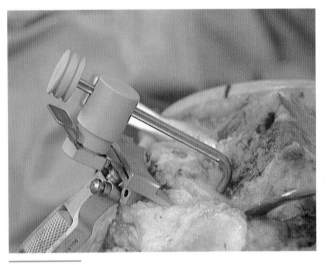

Figure 86–23. The depth of tibial resection should be between 5 and 9 mm, depending on the size of the patient and the desired thickness of the tibial component.

(Fig. 86–23). Excess tibial resection should be avoided because this will place the tibial component in a weaker cancellous bone bed.

Laminar spreaders are then inserted, and the intercondylar notch is examined. The remainder of the ACL and PCL is excised directly off their femoral attachments (Fig. 86–24). Remnants of the medial and lateral meniscus are also removed. Great care is used with meniscal excision in the region of the deep medial collateral ligament because it is vulnerable to injury at this step in the procedure.

Next, the flexion and extension gaps are carefully measured and balanced. Various spacer blocks are used in the flexed knee until proper soft-tissue balance is achieved. An alignment rod is placed through the end of a block and checked to ensure that its distal end aligns with the center of the ankle (Fig. 86–25). Malalignment of the rod is cor-

rected by adjusting the proximal tibial bone cut. With the correct size block inserted to adequately balance soft-tissue tension in flexion, the knee is brought into extension (Fig. 86–26). If it does not fully extend, the optional distal femoral resector is used to remove additional bone until full extension is achieved (Fig. 86–27). Bone from the distal femur can be resected back to the insertion of the collateral ligaments. It is imperative that additional femoral resection be undertaken if required to achieve full knee extension. The alternative choice of using a thinner tibial tray is unacceptable because it will promote laxity in flexion and increase the chance of knee dislocation.

At this point in the operative procedure, the collateral ligaments should be assessed to ensure correct knee balance. Two laminar spreaders are useful in this assessment (Fig. 86–28). In general, there are three situations that the surgeon will face:

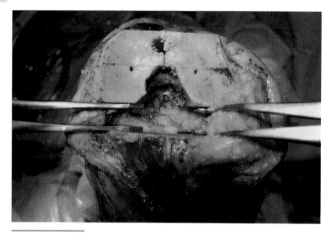

Figure 86–24. Laminar spreaders are inserted, and the intercondylar notch is examined. The cruciate ligaments and meniscal remnants are removed.

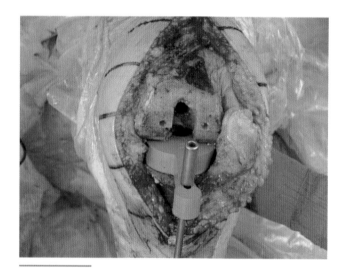

Figure 86–25. The flexion space is judged by selecting the thickest spacer that will fit comfortably between the posterior femur and the proximal tibia. The inclination of the tibial cut can be judged by passing an alignment rod through the spacer.

1. *Neutral knee:* Knees with a preoperative alignment between 0 and 10 degrees are usually relatively easy to balance. In most cases, no further releases are required other than those done initially to achieve adequate exposure.
2. *Varus knee:* In general, knees with a severe varus deformity require a more extensive medial release. An osteotome is used to subperiosteally strip the distal insertion of the superficial medial collateral ligament. If necessary, the deep portion of the medial collateral ligament and a portion of the semimembranosus insertion on the tibia are often released.
3. *Valgus knee:* Knees with greater than 10 degrees of anatomic valgus often require a release of the lateral structures. There are multiple methods for performing the ligamentous releases necessary for balancing valgus knees. Currently, a laminar spreader is used to tension the tight lateral structures. These

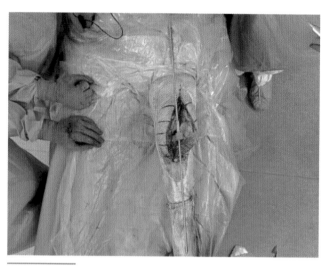

Figure 86–26. The knee is extended, using the same spacer that was used to estimate the flexion space. If the fit is excessively tight or if the knee will not come into full extension, a thinner spacer is selected to judge the amount of extra distal femoral resection required. (If necessary, minus spacers should be used.) Extremity alignment is also assessed.

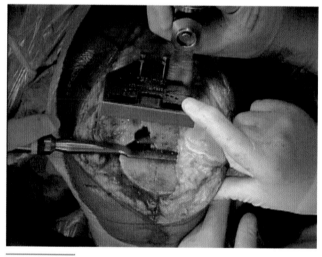

Figure 86–27. The distal femoral recutter is positioned by placing pins through appropriate holes (2, 3, or 5 mm of extra resection). The pins are placed flush against the previous distal femoral cut.

are then sequentially released using multiple stab wounds in a "pie-crusting" manner. In addition, it is usually necessary to perform a lateral retinacular release in knees with a severe valgus deformity. This can also enhance ligamentous balance.

After the soft tissues are adequately balanced, the remaining bone cuts are completed. An intercondylar notch cutting guide is now used (Fig. 86–29). This guide should be lined up with the already-drilled femoral lug holes. This serves to correctly position the guide mediolaterally. In general, the guide should be centered or placed slightly lateral to the midpoint in the mediolateral plane. The intercondylar guide should not be placed medially.

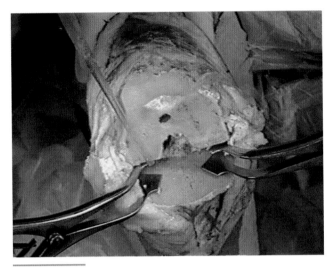

Figure 86–28. Medial and lateral laminar spreaders are useful in judging ligament balance.

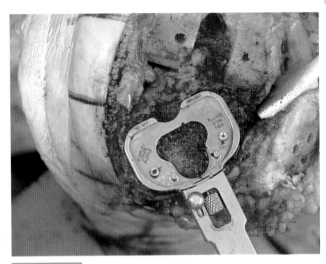

Figure 86–30. Tibial template in place. Note that correct position often results in slight overhang of the template in the posterolateral corner.

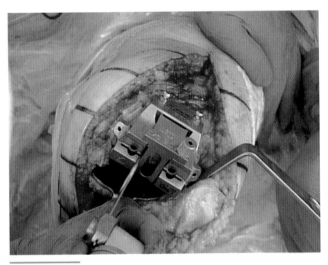

Figure 86–29. The intercondylar cutting guide applied on the distal femur. The guide should be lined up with the already-drilled femoral lug holes. In general, the guide should be centered or placed slightly lateral to the midpoint in the mediolateral plane.

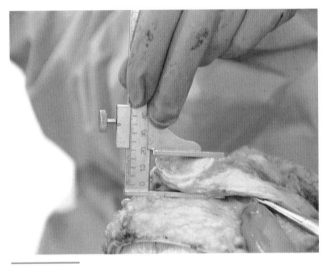

Figure 86–31. The thickness of the original patella is measured with a caliper. Note that the soft tissues surrounding the patella have been removed.

Lateral placement of the notch guide decreases the chances of intraoperative fracture of the medial femoral condyle and enhances patellar tracking. Bone from the intercondylar notch can be removed with a mill, oscillating saw, reciprocating saw, or osteotome. Optionally, if the chamfer cuts have not already been performed, the anterior and posterior chamfer cuts can also be made through slots in the intercondylar notch guide.

Attention is then returned to the tibia. The largest tibial template that fits on the resected proximal tibia without excessive overhang is chosen. The template is carefully placed to ensure correct tibial component rotation (Fig. 86–30). The template should align with the anterior aspect of the tibia, with the handle pointing slightly medial to the tubercle. Care is taken to place the template as posteriorly as possible. Correct rotation of the template,

coupled with a posterior placement, often causes slight overhang in the posterior lateral corner. After the template is positioned and pinned in place, the tibial stem hole is prepared. This is done by first drilling through the tibial drill guide and then completing tibial preparation with impaction of the appropriate-sized tibial broach.

Attention is finally turned to the patella. Synovium around the patella is carefully débrided to minimize the patella "clunk" syndrome.[20,23] This is especially important in the region of the quadriceps tendon. The width of the patella is assessed with calipers (Fig. 86–31), and the aim is to restore the prosthesis-bone composite to the same width as the preresection patellar bone (Fig. 86–32). Traditionally, the bone is prepared with the use of an oscillating saw aligned with a patellar clamp or with a patellar reaming system (Fig. 86–33).

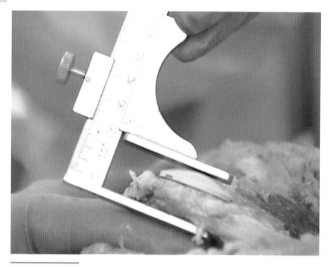

Figure 86–32. The patellar thickness with the patellar component inserted is measured with a caliper. The thickness of the patellar bone prosthesis composite should not exceed the preoperative measurement of patellar thickness.

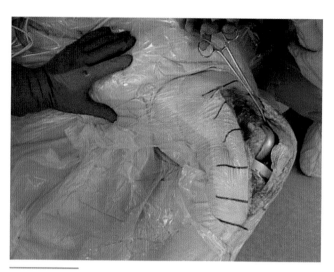

Figure 86–34. At the time of insertion of trial components, the patellar tracking should be observed. The medial edge of the patellar component should not lift away from the medial femoral runner.

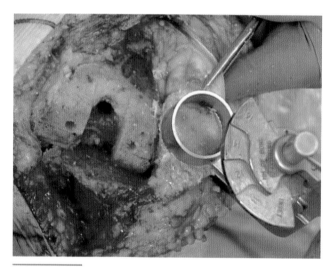

Figure 86–33. A patella reaming system for preparation of the patella.

After preparation of the host patellar bone, the appropriate-sized patellar implant is chosen. Fixation holes are then fashioned compatible with the prosthetic patellar design employed. A trial component is put in place and thickness once again assessed. This new thickness should be within 1 to 2 mm of the original width. If it is too thick, additional bone is removed.

At this point, trial components are put in place and a trial reduction is carried out. The knee is checked to ensure adequate balance of the collateral ligaments. The knee is inspected to ensure a full range of motion without excessive tightness or laxity.

Patella tracking is also examined (Fig. 86–34), making sure not to use towel clips or thumb pressure, to assess patellar stability and lateral retinacular tightness. If the patella is noted to subluxate laterally, a retinacular release

is performed. After the release is performed, the tracking of the patella is rechecked.

The trial components are removed. The tourniquet can be left inflated or released at this point. If the patella was maltracking before the tourniquet was released, the tracking should be rechecked with the tourniquet down before considering lateral retinacular release. The components are cemented in place in either one or two stages. The patellar and femoral components are cemented first. The tibial component is implanted last, using either the same batch or a second batch of cement. Pressure is maintained on the components as the cement polymerizes, and excess cement is trimmed away. The knee is then copiously irrigated and the arthrotomy carefully closed. After the skin is closed, a bulky dressing is applied, and the patient is transferred to the recovery room. Bulky dressings are especially useful if regional blocks are utilized for pain control to avoid pressure on the peroneal nerve.

CLINICAL RESULTS OF PCL-SUBSTITUTING DESIGNS

Insall-Burstein Posterior-Stabilized Prosthesis and Its Descendants: The "Insall Group" Experience

Stern and Insall reported on the 9- to 12-year results of the original Insall-Burstein prosthesis with an all polyethylene tibial component.[59] In that study, 180 knees in 139 patients were available for review, with 61% excellent, 26% good, 6% fair, and 7% poor results. Of the poor results, 14 knees required revision surgery: 9 knees were revised successfully for aseptic loosening of the femoral component (3 knees) or tibial component (6 knees), and 5 knees developed deep prosthetic infections and were treated with a 2-stage procedure. The 12-year cumulative success with an all-polyethylene tibial component was 94%.

More recently, Colizza and colleagues[8] reported on the long-term results of Insall-Burstein Posterior-Stabilized prosthesis with a metal-backed tibial component. One hundred and one knees in 74 patients were examined at a mean follow-up time of 10.8 years. The Hospital for Special Surgery results were 73% excellent, 23% good, and 4% poor. In this cohort with a nonmodular metal-backed tibial component, no cases of tibial component loosening were seen.

After the introduction of modular tibial components in 1987, recent concerns have arisen that polyethylene wear on the back side of the tibial component would lead to osteolysis. Brassard and associates[4] attempted to evaluate this concern with a long-term evaluation of the modular Insall-Burstein prosthesis. In this radiographic review, no cases of massive osteolysis were seen but the authors mentioned that three knees had local minimally progressive lesions, which were not clinically significant. This series of metal-backed tibial components had an overall incidence of tibial component radiolucent lines of 11%, compared with 49% seen with the all-polyethylene tibial component.[4,58] Therefore, the introduction of modularity to this particular implant did not appear to raise concerns about osteolysis.

In more recent long-term studies of the Insall-Burstein posterior prosthesis with a metal-backed tibial component, both best and worst case scenarios have been performed.[4,8] The best case scenario revealed a cumulative success of 96.4% at 11 years. In distinction, the worst case scenario considers knees that are lost to follow-up time as failures; this scenario yielded a cumulative success of 92.6% at 11 years.[4,8] A further testimony to implant durability is a 94% survivorship at 18 years in an active patient population younger than the age of 55 years with a posterior-stabilized prosthesis.[13]

The initial cohort of patients with the NexGen prosthesis have been reviewed. Two hundred thirty-three patients underwent 279 primary total knee arthroplasties between August 1997 and December 1999. Ten patients (10 knees) subsequently died, and 16 patients (16 knees) were excluded because of severe medical disability. Patients with severe medical conditions included those patients known to be alive with the prosthesis still in place but where no meaningful assessment of the patient's knee scores could be made after communication with a family member. Inclusion of this group of 16 patients may have lowered the overall knee scores, but the incomplete data precluded adequate analysis. An additional 12 patients (13 knees) were lost to follow-up. Thus, 195 patients (240 knees) were available for analysis. The mean age at the time of surgery was 66 years. The mean duration of follow-up time was 48 months (range, 24 to 72 months).

Preoperatively, the mean arc of motion was 107 degrees, compared with 117 degrees at the latest follow-up examination. The mean preoperative Knee Society score was 48 points, compared with 96 points at the latest follow-up examination. The mean Knee Society functional score was 83 points at the latest follow-up examination. Radiographic evaluation revealed an incidence of minor radiolucent lines of 4%, which was of no clinical significance.

No evidence of loosening, osteolysis, or polyethylene wear was seen.[57]

Insall-Burstein Posterior-Stabilized Prosthesis and Its Descendants: Other Experiences

Aglietti and coworkers reviewed their results at a minimum of 10 years with 99 posterior-stabilized prostheses. Thirty-nine knees were in patients who had died before the 10-year follow-up and 4 were removed or revised, leaving 56 knees for evaluation at an average of 12 years. There were 58% excellent, 25% good, 7% fair, and 10% poor results. Knee flexion average 106 degrees. Of the six (10%) failures, four were attributable to aseptic component loosening; none was attributable to polyethylene wear. With revision as the endpoint, 10-year survivorship was 92%.[41]

Vince and coworkers reviewed their results of the metal-backed posterior-stabilized prosthesis at a minimum of 10 years. One hundred total knee arthroplasties were performed in 86 consecutive patients by the senior author. Thirty-six were in patients who had died, and two were in patients who were infirm. Of the remaining 62 knees, 54 were directly evaluated and 8 by telephone at an average of 10.8 years. No patients were lost to follow-up. At latest follow-up, 64% were rated as excellent, 18% as good, 7% as fair, and 11% as poor, which included six failures. Flexion averaged 111 degrees. Excluding the failures, the average Knee Society clinical score was 91.6. Of the six failures, two were secondary to sepsis, two secondary to nonspecific pain, one secondary to patellar wear and fracture, and one because of aseptic tibial component loosening. Polyethylene wear was specifically examined in this study, and no implant demonstrated significant polyethylene wear or failure. There were seven patellar fractures—four required additional surgery, and the remaining three were asymptomatic and discovered incidentally at routine follow-up. Using revision as the endpoint, 12-year survivorship averaged 92%.[51]

Li and associates[43] reported their experience with an IB II prosthesis in 1999. Of 146 knees, 94 were reviewed at a mean of 10 years. The Hospital for Special Surgery scores were excellent or good in 79%, fair in 14%, and poor in 7%. The average Knee Society score was 87. Knee flexion improved from an average of 88 degrees preoperatively to 100 degrees after arthroplasty, considerably less than has been expected from this device. The 10-year survivorship was 92.35 using revision as the endpoint, and there were nine failures.

Vince and colleagues[65] followed 100 IB II prostheses prospectively. Fifty-one knees were evaluated at 10 or more years with Knee Society scores and radiographs; 14 were evaluated by telephone. An additional six knees required revision, and 29 were in patients who died. None were lost. Complete revision surgery was performed for instability (two knees), sepsis (two), loosening from osteolysis (one), and stiffness (one). Twelve patients required reoperations without revision of the tibia or femoral components: patellar revision for loosening (one), patellectomy for fracture (one), polyethylene exchange for dislocation of the spine-cam mechanism (three) and for dissociation (one), and arthroscopic resection of scar from the quadriceps tendon in six (patellar clunk). One case of tibial osteolysis occurred in the IB II. The problem of patellar fractures was decreased significantly in the IB II group, probably as a result of smoothing the anterior trochlear groove. Tibial-femoral dislocation occurred in three IB II prostheses.

Lachiewicz and coworkers[31] performed a prospective, consecutive study of 193 knees in 131 patients who were managed with the modular IB II Posterior-Stabilized total knee prosthesis by one surgeon. The mean age of the patients at the time of surgery was 68 years, and the mean duration of follow-up was 7 years (range, 5 to 14 years). Clinical evaluation was performed with use of standard knee-scoring systems. Radiographs were evaluated for the presence of radiolucent lines, osteolysis, and loosening. The overall result (as determined with The Hospital for Special Surgery scoring system) was rated as excellent for 112 knees, good for 60, fair for 15, and poor for 6. The mean postoperative flexion was 112 degrees. No clinical or radiographic loosening of the tibial component was noted. Eight knees had osteolytic lesions of the tibia. Thin, incomplete, nonprogressive radiolucent lines were noted around 30 tibial components (16%). There were three reoperations.

Oliver and colleagues[44] reported the clinical and radiographic outcome of a consecutive series of 138 hydroxyapatite-coated IB II total knee replacements with a mean follow-up of 11 years (10 to 13 years). The patients were entered into a prospective study, and all living patients (76 knees) were evaluated. The Hospital for Special Surgery knee score was obtained for comparison with the preoperative situation. No patient was lost to follow-up. Radiographic assessment revealed no loosening. Seven prostheses have been revised, giving a cumulative survival rate of 93% at 13 years.

Other PCL-Substituting Knee Results

There have been few reports on the results of PCL-substituting designs other than the Insall-Burstein Posterior-Stabilized prosthesis.

PRESS-FIT CONDYLAR PS DESIGN

Ranawat and associates[50] reviewed the results of 150 consecutive primary total knee replacements (118 patients) performed between 1988 and 1990. There were 16 bilateral procedures. All the knees in this study were PCL-substituting Press-Fit Condylar modular knees implanted with the use of cement. The predominant diagnosis was osteoarthritis in 98 patients (83%). Mean age at the time of the index procedure was 70 years (range, 29 to 85 years). One hundred twenty-five knees were observed for an adequate time interval (mean, 4.8 years; range, 3.8 to 6.2 years) for meaningful analysis. The clinical result were

excellent for 103 knees (82%), good for 13 (10%), fair for 3 (2%), and poor for 6 (5%). At the most recent follow-up, the Knee Society's[27] average functional score was 78 points (range, 0 to 100 points), and the average knee score was 93 points (range, 57 to 100 points). The mean preoperative range of motion increased from 107 degrees to 111 degrees after arthroplasty. The rate of survival was 97% in 6 years. The standard error of the mean for this calculation was 1.6%. Three revision operations were necessary: two of these were for infection, and one was for femoral-tibial instability. Patellofemoral symptoms were noted in 8% (10 knees). The authors concluded that the PCL-substituting PFC modular knee system resulted in excellent relief of pain, excellent range of motion, and restoration of function with a low prevalence of patellofemoral problems.

KINEMATIC STABILIZER PROSTHESIS

Hanssen and Rand[17] reported on the Mayo Clinic experience with the Kinematic Stabilizer prosthesis. The Kinematic Stabilizer has a central tibial post in the femoral housing restraining anterior as well as posterior motion of the tibia between 0 and 30 degrees of flexion. Past 30 degrees of flexion, as in the Insall-Burstein prosthesis, the substituting mechanism replaces only the function of the PCL in enhancing femoral rollback. Neither design substitutes for the collateral ligament. Seventy-nine arthroplasties (66 patients) with an average follow-up of 37 months were reported. There were 53 revisions and 26 primary arthroplasties in their series. Postoperatively, of the entire group, 34 knees (43%) rated excellent; 33 (42%), good; 7 (9%), fair, and 5 (6%), poor. However, in this group of arthroplasties, a majority were undergoing revision procedures. Separate analysis of the results of the 26 knees undergoing index procedures revealed 54% with excellent results, 38% good, 4% fair, and 4% poor. Postoperative motion averaged 101 degrees.

Complications of PCL Substitution

Certain complications have arisen with PCL-substituting total knee designs that can at least in part be attributed to this type of knee replacement. These include component dislocation, intercondylar fractures, patella fractures, "patella clunk" syndrome, and tibial spine wear and breakage.

DISLOCATIONS

As increasingly deep flexion was experienced with PCL-substituting designs, there were cases of the tibial spine riding underneath the femoral cam with subluxation of the flexed knee and painful locking of the joint (Fig. 86-35).[21]

A knee with a dislocated implant normally presents acutely with inability to extend. In many cases, the

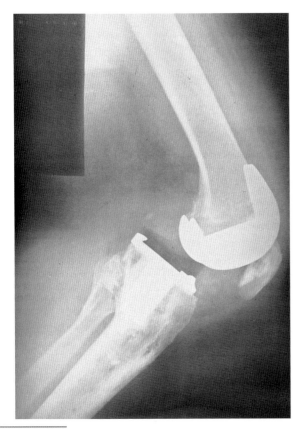

Figure 86–35. Dislocated Insall-Burstein II component.

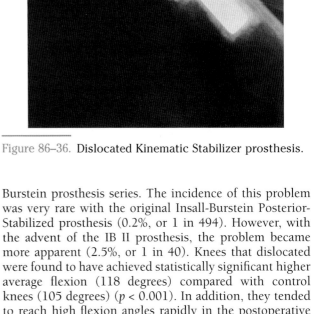

Figure 86–36. Dislocated Kinematic Stabilizer prosthesis.

patients are unable to explain the exact mechanism, or the position of the knee, when the actual dislocation occurred. In fact, this problem can occur during sleep, causing the patient to awaken with an acute inability to extend the knee. On physical examination, an obvious knee deformity is commonly found. Radiographs reveal the femoral cam translated anterior to the polyethylene tibial spine. Many times, the spine can be reduced by hyperflexion of the knee and application of an anterior drawer.

Reports of dislocations have included knees implanted with the Insall-Burstein Posterior-Stabilized prosthesis,[15,35,36] the IB II prosthesis,[7,36,41,67] the Kinemax posterior substituting prosthesis,[43] the Kinematic II Stabilizer prosthesis,[16] and other designs (Fig. 86–36).[67] It is not surprising that this problem has been seen most commonly with the Insall-Burstein and Kinematic II Stabilizer designs because they have the longest track record with the PCL-substituting concept.

Dislocations have been described in knees with a preoperative valgus alignment[7,15,16, 36,43] and in those after patellectomy.[16] Although preoperative valgus appears to increase the incidence of this problem, it can also occur in varus knees.[36,43] There is some controversy over whether the actual component dislocation occurs with the knee in mild flexion with a straight posterior mechanism or occurs at high flexion angles with a combination of posterior and rotatory stress.[35,36]

Lombardi and associates[36] analyzed the incidence of dislocations in 3032 primary knees implanted with the Insall-Burstein prosthesis series. The incidence of this problem was very rare with the original Insall-Burstein Posterior-Stabilized prosthesis (0.2%, or 1 in 494). However, with the advent of the IB II prosthesis, the problem became more apparent (2.5%, or 1 in 40). Knees that dislocated were found to have achieved statistically significant higher average flexion (118 degrees) compared with control knees (105 degrees) ($p < 0.001$). In addition, they tended to reach high flexion angles rapidly in the postoperative period. In response to this problem, the tibial plastic was modified by raising the tibial spine and moving it anteriorly (Fig. 86–37). This increased the inherent stability of the component and decreased the incidence of dislocation (0.2%, or 1 in 656).

A computer analysis of this phenomenon analyzed the propensity of PCL-substituting knee components to dislocate in the sagittal plane.[10,30] Kocmond and coworkers defined a dislocation safety factor (DSF) as the jump distance between the bottom of the femoral cam and the top of the tibial spine. The DSF was found to vary with the knee flexion angle. For knees with the Insall-Burstein PCL-substitution mechanism, the DSF increases as knee flexion increases and peaks at about 70 degrees. Knee flexion beyond this angle causes the DSF to decrease and theoretically increases the risk of dislocation. Figure 86–38 lists the DSF curves for the original Insall-Burstein Posterior-Stabilized prosthesis, the original IB II prosthesis, and the IB II prosthesis with the modified tibial insert. Many contemporary designs have attempted to minimize the risk of dislocation by ensuring a DSF equal to or

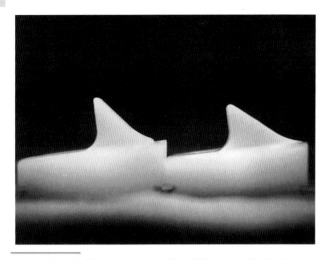

Figure 86–37. Modification of Insall-Burstein II tibial spine by anterior translation and increased height. Original Insall-Burstein plastic (**right**) and modified plastic (**left**).

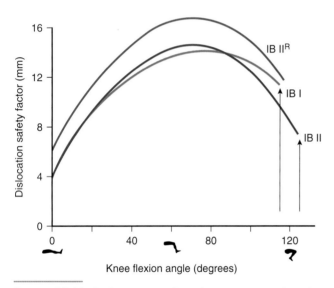

Figure 86–38. Dislocation safety factor curves for the original Insall-Burstein Posterior-Stabilized prosthesis, the original Insall-Burstein II prosthesis, and the Insall-Burstein II prosthesis with the modified tibial insert. (Redrawn from Kocmond JH, Delp SL, Stern SH: Stability and range of motion of Insall-Burstein condylar prostheses: A computer simulation study. J Arthroplasty 10:386, 1995.)

greater than that of the original Insall-Burstein Posterior-Stabilized prosthesis at high flexion angles.

The lesson with respect to arthroplasty design is simple: Sometimes very small changes, on the order of millimeters, can result in catastrophic complications. Not all spine mechanisms are the same. In general, to prevent knee dislocations, it is imperative that the surgeon balance the knee in both flexion and extension, with a special emphasis on knees with a preoperative valgus alignment. In addition, it may be undesirable to achieve large flexion angles (greater than 115 degrees) in the first postoperative week.

INTERCONDYLAR FRACTURES

Femoral fractures, although a relatively rare occurrence, can occur at the time of knee arthroplasty. Because PCL-substituting components require removal of extra bone from the intercondylar region, the possibility of distal femoral fracture with this technique is increased. Risk factors for fractures include inadequate, as well as excessive, intercondylar bone notch resection. Although it is self-evident that excessive bone removal results directly in stress risers and deficient bone, the risks associated with incomplete bone resection are not as clear-cut. Nonetheless, if insufficient notch bone is removed, the intercondylar region of the femoral component (or trial) can act like a wedge during insertion and induce a distal femoral fracture. It is imperative to remove enough bone to allow full seating of the cam. When placing the trial femoral component, forceful impaction should never be used. To ensure adequate bony resection, never undercut the femoral condyles. Although this complication has been reported,[37] the exact incidence of this phenomenon has not been well defined.

Lombardi and associates[37] reported on this complication in comparing two large series of PCL-substituting knees. In this report, 898 nonconsecutive primary knee arthroplasties performed with a PCL-substituting prosthesis were compared with a second nonconsecutive series of 532 PCL-substituting knee arthroplasties. In the second series, an intercondylar sizing guide was used to confirm the intercondylar resection size. Forty distal femoral fractures were noted in the initial series (approximate rate, 1:22; nondisplaced, 35; displaced, 5). This was in contrast to the second series, in which only one displaced fracture was noted (rate, 1:532). The rate difference between the two series was statistically significant. The authors advocate careful resection technique and intercondylar notch size verification to minimize this complication. Of note, no change in postoperative rehabilitation was required either for patients identified with a nondisplaced intercondylar fracture or for those with an intercondylar fracture treated with intraoperative stabilization.

PATELLA FRACTURES

The initial follow-up of the original Insall-Burstein Posterior-Stabilized knee demonstrated a high patella fracture prevalence. The anteroposterior dimensions and shape of the femoral component tended to be full to accommodate the spine-cam mechanism in the Insall-Burstein Posterior-Stabilized prosthesis. This pushed the patella anteriorly and presumably increased forces, which may have been responsible for a relatively higher rate of patellar fractures. In 10 cadaver knee specimens Matsuda and associates[38] demonstrated significantly higher contact stresses in the unresurfaced patella when compared with the normal knee throughout the flexion arc for several implants including the Insall-Bernstein Posterior-Stabilized. They noted that in flexion exceeding 105 degrees, patellofemoral contact occurred in two small patches. These investigators concluded that the forces could be normalized by extending the trochlear groove farther posteriorly and were less concerned with the anterior prominence of the component. The groove of the IB II was deepened to potentially decrease patella fractures and other patella problems.

Larson and Lachiewicz concluded that many patellar complications with the IB Posterior-Stabilized could be avoided by a careful surgical technique.[33] This included appropriate rotation of the femur and tibia, adequate patella resection, débridement of peripatellar synovium, and proper evaluation of patellar tracking before wound closure. They studied 118 arthroplasties at 2 to 8 years and found that no knee required reoperation for the patellofemoral joint. Mean flexion of 112 degrees was comparable to other studies with this device, and they had no cases of patellar clunk syndrome and no subluxations. There were three (2.5%) patellar fractures treated without surgery. Even this small number of fractures might be expected to improve with changes to the femoral prosthesis. They concluded that the total patellofemoral complication rate in their series was 4.2%. This was superior to the 11% that has generally been described, of which 7% were actually fractures.

PATELLAR CLUNK SYNDROME

The deeper flexion provided by the initial Insall-Burstein Stabilized Design enabled the quadriceps tendon to extend beyond the trochlear groove of the femoral component. If the anterior edge of the femoral component terminates abruptly, synovium or scar residing on the tendon falls into the intercondylar groove. If this has occurred, the same tissue must ride up out of the intercondylar area and "jump" back up onto the femoral trochlea as the patient extends the knee. Within a few months after the arthroplasty, the offending (or offended) tissue hypertrophies and becomes rubbery. This creates the painful and noisy complication that has been described as "patellar clunk." Historically, a case of patellar catching was mentioned by Insall in his original report on the posterior-stabilized knee. However, Hozack and associates[20] appear to be the first authors to define the term *patellar clunk syndrome*. They described a prominent fibrous nodule at the junction of the proximal patellar pole and the quadriceps tendon. They believed that during flexion this fibrous nodule would enter the femoral component's intercondylar notch but not restrict flexion. However, as the knee extended, the nodule would remain within the notch while the rest of the extensor mechanism slid proximally. They thought that at 30 to 45 degrees of flexion the tension on the fibrous nodule would be sufficient to cause the nodule to jerk out of the notch as it returned to its normal position. This sudden displacement would cause the audible and palpable clunk found with this entity. Treatment recommendations for patellar clunk syndrome have included physical therapy,[3] surgical removal of the nodule,[20] patellar prosthesis revision,[3,20] open resection through a limited lateral incision,[39] and arthroscopic débridement.[3,62] Pollock and coworkers[47] reviewed the prevalence of synovial entrapment with three different cam-post designs. Those with proximally positioned or wide femoral boxes were more likely to have a higher prevalence of this problem.

The largest series on treatment of patellar clunk syndrome appears to be that of Beight and colleagues.[3] They reported on 14 operative procedures (11 arthroscopic débridements and 3 patellar component revisions) performed in 12 patients. As in other reports,[20] they found a suprapatellar fibrous nodule that wedged into the intercondylar notch during flexion and dislodged as the knee extended, causing the clunk. The authors related that the symptoms resolved after nodule excision. However, four of the knees that were treated with arthroscopic débridement had recurrence of symptoms. None of the knees that underwent arthrotomy and patella button revisions had recurrence. The authors recommended a treatment protocol that commenced with a short course of nonoperative physical therapy, although they acknowledged that their results were disappointing with this. Arthroscopic débridement was suggested for knees without radiographic component abnormalities. Arthrotomy was suggested for recurrent clunks or malpositioned or loose components.

TIBIAL SPINE WEAR AND BREAKAGE

There has been a recent focus on the spine-cam mechanism in some posterior-stabilized prostheses as a source of wear debris. Mikulak and coworkers[40] reported unanticipated aseptic loosening and osteolysis with the posterior-stabilized model of the Press-Fit Condylar implant. They found that 16 of 557 (2.9%) had been revised for osteolysis from 37 to 89 months after surgery. Retrieval analysis demonstrated damage to the lateral and medial walls of the tibial spine. There was also damage to the inferior surface of the articular polyethylene inserts.

Similar findings were reported by Puloski and associates.[48] Their study, by contrast, was a retrieval analysis of a variety of failed posterior-stabilized implants. Wear was quantified on the tibial posts of all retrievals, including those revised for reinfection. They were unable to conclude that this wear mode was responsible for the failures but cautioned that the interaction between the spine and the cam is not an "innocuous articulation."

Our group has extensively studied this phenomenon. When we recognized osteolysis around IB II modular components[45] as well as Press-Fit Condylar PS modular components[6] (Figs. 86–39 and 86–40) we began performing retrieval analyses (Figs. 86–41 and 86–42). In our cases the patients were able to slightly hyperextend and most had bilateral implants. We hypothesized that impingement on the anterior post by the femoral cam caused wear damage to the post and transmitted rotational stresses to the modular inserts, generating back-side wear (Figs. 86–43 to 86–45). Avoiding flexion of the femoral component and posterior slope in the proximal tibial resection should help eliminate the problem (Figs. 86–46 and 86–47). In addition, cam-post designs should allow for hyperextension before impingement occurs.

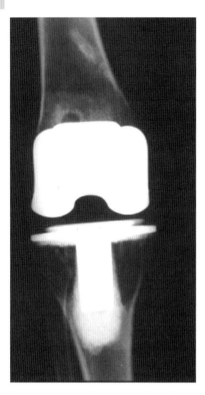

Figure 86–39. Anteroposterior radiograph of a patient with the Insall-Burstein II device taken at 5 years follow-up shows tibial osteolysis.

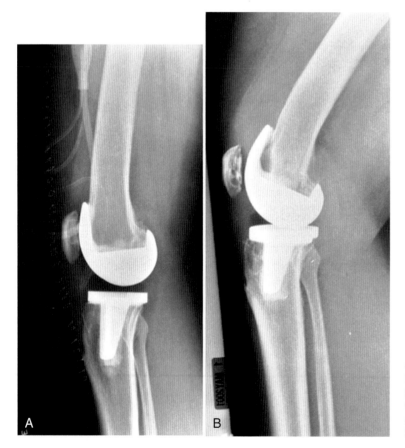

Figure 86–40. Postoperative (**A**) and 5-year follow-up lateral (**B**) radiographs of a patient with the Press-Fit Condylar posterior-stabilized device show femoral osteolysis and flexion of the femoral component.

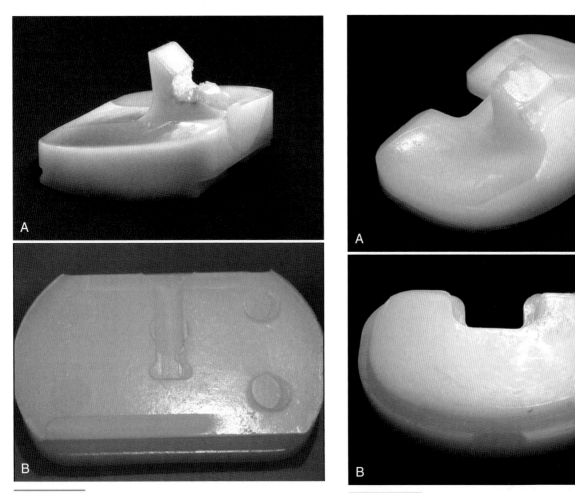

Figure 86–41. An Insall-Burstein II polyethylene retrieval shows (**A**) anterior post wear damage and (**B**) backside wear with loss of lot number markings and rotational screw hole markings.

Figure 86–42. A Press-Fit Condylar posterior-stabilized retrieval shows (**A**) anterior post wear damage and (**B**) loss of backside anterior polyethylene locking mechanism and lot number markings.

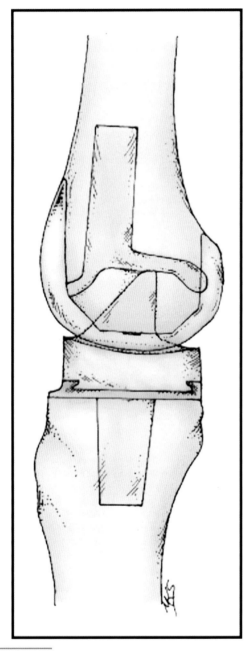

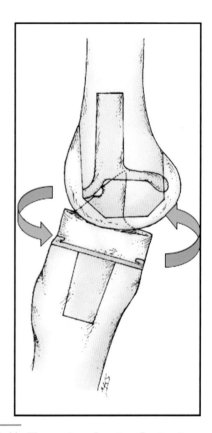

Figure 86–44. Illustration showing the impingement of the tibial post on the trochlea with the knee in hyperextension. Posterior slope of the tibial component and flexion of the femoral component can contribute to this impingement.

Figure 86–43. Illustration demonstrating the space between the polyethylene tibial post and the trochlea of the femoral component.

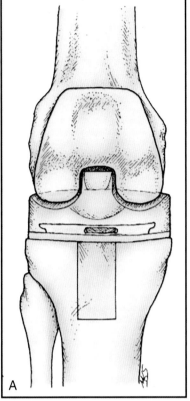
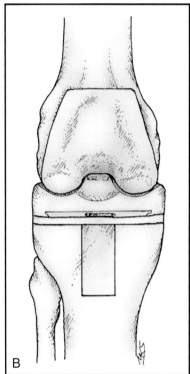

Figure 86–45. Correct positioning of the femoral and tibial component (**A**) in the coronal plane with a space between the femoral box and tibial post in the anteroposterior projection. Flexion of the femoral component and posterior slope of the tibial component, as well as a loose extension space (**B**), contribute to femoral component impingement on the tibial post.

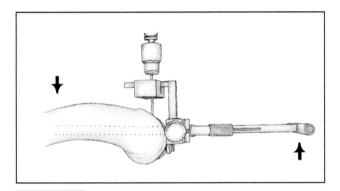

Figure 86–46. A lateral view of a femur shows an attempt to place an intramedullary guide so as to resect the distal femur in extension. The *arrows* show the need to translate the starting point anteriorly to accommodate the sagittal bow in the femur.

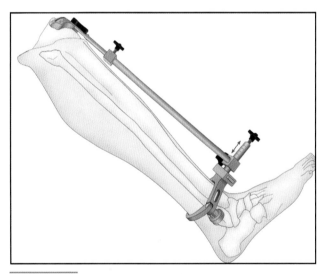

Figure 86–47. A lateral view of the tibia shows the difficulty avoiding posterior tibial slope resection.

CONCLUSION

The potential of the PCL-substitution type knee design continues to evolve. In general it has allowed the surgeon to perform a reproducible operation in almost all arthritic knees no matter what the cause of the disease and no matter how involved and complex the deformity of the knee. There is still potential for functional and clinical improvement in results with the poster newer designs that have and will in the future become available.

References

1. Arima J, Whiteside LA, Martin JW, et al: Effect of partial release of the posterior cruciate ligament in total knee arthroplasty. Clin Orthop Relat Res 353:194-202, 1998.
2. Bartel DL, Burstein AH, Santavicca EA, et al: Performance of the tibial component in total knee replacement: Conventional and revision designs. J Bone Joint Surg Am 64:1026, 1982.

3. Beight JL, Yao B, Hozack WJ, et al: The patellar "clunk" syndrome after posterior stabilized knee arthroplasty. Clin Orthop Relat Res 299:139, 1994.

4. Brassard MF, Insall JN, et al: Does modularity affect clinical success: A comparison with a minimum 10 year follow-up. Clin Orthop Relat Res 388:26, 2001.

4a. Burstein A: Personal communications, 2005.

5. Burstein AH, Insall JN: Posteriorly stabilized total knee prosthesis. US patent 4,298,992, November 10, 1981.

6. Callaghan JJ, O'Rourke MR, et al: Tibial post impingement in posterior-stabilized total knee arthroplasty. Clin Orthop Relat Res 404:83, 2002.

7. Cohen B, Constant CR: Subluxation of the posterior stabilized total knee arthroplasty: A report of two cases. J Arthroplasty 7:161, 1992.

8. Colizza W, Insall JN, Scuderi GR: The posterior stabilized total knee prosthesis: Assessment of polyethylene damage and osteolysis: Ten-year minimum follow-up. J Bone Joint Surg Am 77:1713, 1995.

9. Collier JP, Mayor MB, McNamara JL, et al: Analysis of the failure of 122 polyethylene inserts from uncemented tibial knee components. Clin Orthop Relat Res 273:232, 1991.

10. Delp SL, Kocmond JH, Stern SH: Tradeoffs between motion and stability in posterior substituting knee arthroplasty design. J Biomech 28:1155, 1995.

11. Dennis DA, Komistek RD, Stiehl JB, et al: Range of motion after total knee arthroplasty: The effect of implant design and weight-bearing conditions. J Arthroplasty 13:748-752, 1998.

12. Dennis DA, Komistek RD, Hoff WA, et al: In vivo knee kinematics derived using an inverse perspective technique. Clin Orthop Relat Res 331:107, 1996.

13. Diduch DR, Insall JN, Scott WN, et al: Total knee replacement in young active patients: Long-term follow-up and functional outcome. J Bone Joint Surg Am 79:575, 1997.

14. Fahmy NR, Chandler HP, Danylchuk K, et al: Blood-gas and circulatory changes during total knee replacement. J Bone Joint Surg Am 72:19, 1990.

15. Galinat BJ, Vernace JV, Booth RE Jr, et al: Dislocation of the posterior stabilized total knee arthroplasty: A report of two cases. J Arthroplasty 3:363, 1988.

16. Gebhard JS, Kilgus DJ: Dislocation of a posterior stabilized total knee prosthesis: A report of two cases. Clin Orthop Relat Res 254:225, 1990.

17. Hanssen AD, Rand JA: A comparison of primary and revision total knee arthroplasty using the Kinematic stabilizer prosthesis. J Bone Joint Surg Am 70:491, 1988.

18. Hernigou PH, Medevielle D, Debeyre J, et al: Proximal tibial osteotomy for osteoarthritis with varus deformity: A ten to thirteen-year follow-up study. J Bone Joint Surg Am 69:332, 1987.

19. Howie DW, Vernon-Roberts B, Oakeshott R, et al: A rat model of resorption of bone at the cement-bone interface in the presence of polyethylene wear particles. J Bone Joint Surg Am 70:257, 1988.

20. Hozack WJ, Rothman RH, Booth RE, et al: The patellar clunk syndrome. Clin Orthop Relat Res 241:203, 1989.

21. Insall JN, Ranawat CS, Scott WN, et al: Total condylar knee replacement: Preliminary report. Clin Orthop Relat Res 120:149, 1976.

22. Insall JN, Scott WN, Ranawat CS: The total condylar knee prosthesis: A report of two hundred and twenty cases. J Bone Joint Surg Am 61:173, 1979.

23. Insall JN: Technique of total knee replacement. Instr Course Lect 30:324, 1981.

24. Insall JN, Lachiewicz PF, Burstein AH: The posterior stabilized condylar prosthesis: A modification of the total condylar design, two to four year clinical experience. J Bone Joint Surg Am 64:1317, 1982.

25. Insall JN, Hood RW, Flawn LB, et al: The total condylar knee prosthesis in gonarthrosis: A five to nine-year follow-up of the first one hundred consecutive replacements. J Bone Joint Surg Am 65:619, 1983.

26. Insall JN: Total knee replacement. In Insall JN (ed): Surgery of the Knee. New York, Churchill Livingstone, 1984, p 587.

27. Insall JN, Dorr LD, Scott RD, et al: Rationale of the Knee Society clinical rating system. Clin Orthop Relat Res 248:13, 1989.

28. Kilgus DJ, Moreland JR, Finerman GA, et al: Catastrophic wear of tibial polyethylene inserts. Clin Orthop Relat Res 273:223, 1991.

29. Kleinbart FA, Bryk E, Evangelista J, et al: Histologic comparison of posterior cruciate ligaments from arthritic and age-matched knee specimens. J Arthroplasty 11:726-731, 1996.

30. Kocmond JH, Delp SL, Stern SH: Stability and range of motion of Insall-Burstein condylar prostheses: A computer simulation study. J Arthroplasty 10:383, 1995.

31. Lachiewicz PF, Soileau ES: The rates of osteolysis and loosening associated with a modular posterior stabilized knee replacement: Results at five to fourteen years. J Bone Joint Surg Am 86:525-530, 2004.

32. Landy MD, Walker PS: Wear of ultra-high molecular weight polyethylene components of ninety retrieved knee prostheses. J Arthroplasty 3(Suppl 1):573, 1988.

33. Larson CM, Lachiewicz PF: Patellofemoral complications with the Insall-Burstein II posterior-stabilized total knee arthroplasty. J Arthroplasty 14:288-292, 1999.

34. Laskin RS, Rieger M, Achob C, et al: The posterior stabilized total knee prosthesis in the knee with a severe fixed deformity. Am J Knee Surg 1:199, 1988.

35. Lombardi AV, Krugel R, Honkala TK, et al: Dislocation following primary posterior stabilized total knee arthroplasty. Presented at the 58th Annual Meeting of the American Academy of Orthopaedic Surgeons, Anaheim, CA, 1991.

36. Lombardi AV Jr, Mallory TH, Vaughn BK, et al: Dislocation following primary posterior-stabilized total knee arthroplasty. J Arthroplasty 8:633, 1993.

37. Lombardi AV Jr, Mallory TH, Waterman RA, et al: Intercondylar distal femoral fracture: An unreported complication of posterior-stabilized total knee arthroplasty. J Arthroplasty 10:643, 1995.

38. Matsuda S, Ishinishi T, Whiteside LA: Contact stresses with an unresurfaced patella in total knee arthroplasty: The effect of femoral component design. Orthopedics 23:213-218, 2000.

39. Messieh M: Management of patellar clunk under local anesthesia. J Arthroplasty 11:202, 1996.

40. Mikulak SA, Mahoney OM, dela Rosa MA, Schmalzried TP: Loosening and osteolysis with the Press-Fit Condylar posterior-cruciate-substituting total knee replacement. J Bone Joint Surg Am 83:398-403, 2001.

41. Mills HJ, McKee MD, Horne G, et al: Dislocation of posteriorly stabilized total knee arthroplasties. Can J Surg 37:225, 1994.

42. Mintz L, Tsao AK, McCrae CR, et al: The arthroscopic evaluation and characteristics of severe polyethylene wear in total knee arthroplasty. Clin Orthop Relat Res 273:215, 1991.

43. Ochsner JL Jr, Kostman WC, Dodson M: Posterior dislocation of a posterior-stabilized total knee arthroplasty: A report of two cases. Am J Orthop 25:310, 1996.

44. Oliver MC, Keast-Butler OD, Hinves BL, Shepperd JA: A hydroxyapatite-coated Insall-Burstein II total knee replacement: 11-year results. J Bone Joint Surg Br 87:478-482, 2005.

45. O'Rourke MR, Callaghan JJ, Goetz DD, et al: Osteolysis associated with a cemented modular posterior-cruciate-substituting total knee design: Five- to eight-year follow-up. J Bone Joint Surg Am 84:1362, 2002.

46. Patel DV, Aichroth PM, Wand JS: Posteriorly stabilized (Insall-Burstein) total condylar knee arthroplasty: A follow-up study of 157 knees. Int Orthop 15:211, 1991.

47. Pollock DC, Ammeen DJ, Engh GA: Synovial entrapment: A complication of posterior stabilized total knee arthroplasty. J Bone Joint Surg Am 84:2174-2178, 2002.

48. Puloski SK, McCalden RW, et al: Tibial post wear in posterior stabilized total knee arthroplasty: An unrecognized source of polyethylene debris. J Bone Joint Surg Am 83:390-397, 2001.

49. Ranawat CS, Boachie-Adjei O: Survivorship analysis and results of total condylar knee arthroplasty: Eight- to eleven-year follow-up period. Clin Orthop Relat Res 226:6, 1988.

50. Ranawat CS, Luessenhop CP, Rodriguez JA: The Press-Fit Condylar modular total knee system: Four-to-six-year results with a posterior-cruciate-substituting design. J Bone Joint Surg Am 79:342, 1997.

51. Rand JA: Comparison of metal-backed and all-polyethylene tibial components in cruciate condylar total knee arthroplasty. J Arthroplasty 8:307, 1993.

52. Revell PA, Weightman B, Freeman MAR, et al: The production and biology of polyethylene wear debris. Arch Orthop Trauma Surg 91:167, 1978.

53. Ritter MA, Campbell MS, Faris PM, et al: Long-term survival analysis of the posterior cruciate condylar total knee arthroplasty. J Arthroplasty 4:293, 1989.

54. Scott WN, Rubinstein M: Posterior stabilized knee arthroplasty: Six year experience. Clin Orthop Relat Res 205:138, 1986.

55. Scott WN, Rubinstein M, Scuderi G: Results after knee replacement with a posterior cruciate-substituting prosthesis. J Bone Joint Surg Am 70:1163, 1988.

56. Scuderi GR, Insall JN, Windsor RE, et al: Survivorship of cemented knee replacement. J Bone Joint Surg Br 71:798, 1989.

57. Scuderi GR, Clarke HD: Cemented posterior stabilized total knee arthroplasty. J Arthroplasty 19(4 Suppl 1):17-21, 2004.

58. Stern SH, Insall JN: Posterior stabilized prosthesis: Results after follow-up of nine to twelve years. J Bone Joint Surg Am 74:980, 1992.

59. Stiehl JB, Dennis DA, Komistek RD, Crane HS: In vivo determination of condylar lift-off and screw home in a mobile bearing total knee arthroplasty. J Arthroplasty 14:293, 1999.

60. Stiehl JB, Komistek RD, Dennis DA, et al: Fluoroscopic analysis of kinematics after posterior-cruciate-retaining knee arthroplasty. J Bone Joint Surg Br 77:884, 1995.

61. Tsao AK, Mintz L, McCrae CR, et al: Severe polyethylene wear in PCA total knee arthroplasties. Presented at Knee Society Meeting, Anaheim, CA, 1991.

62. Vernace JV, Rothman RH, Booth RE Jr, et al: Arthroscopic management of the patellar clunk syndrome following posterior stabilized total knee arthroplasty. J Arthroplasty 4:179, 1989.

63. Vince KG, Insall JN, Kelly MA: The total condylar prosthesis: 10 to 12 year results of a cemented knee replacement. J Bone Joint Surg Br 71:793, 1989.

64. Vince KG: The posterior stabilized knee prosthesis. In Laskin RS (ed): Total Knee Replacement. New York, Springer-Verlag, 1991, p 113.

65. Vince KG, Malo M, Thadani PJ: Posterior stabilization in total knee arthroplasty. In Callaghan JJ, et al (eds): The Adult Knee. Philadelphia, Lippincott Williams & Wilkins, 2003.

66. Walker PS, Masse Y: Principles of condylar replacement knee prosthesis design. Acta Orthop Belg 39:151-163, 1973.

67. Wang CJ, Wang HE: Dislocation of total knee arthroplasty: A report of 6 cases with 2 patterns of instability. Acta Orthop Scand 68:282, 1997.

68. Wright TM, Bartel DL: The problem of surface damage in polyethylene total knee components. Clin Orthop Relat Res 205:67, 1986.

CHAPTER 87

Mobile Bearings in Total Knee Arthroplasty

James B. Stiehl

Mobile bearings were originally introduced with the Oxford knee in 1977, which sought to improve articular congruity for improved wear characteristics using a spherical, congruous articulation while diminishing implant constraint with a floating surface.[1,17,18,30] The Oxford device pioneered by Goodfellow was a unicondylar implant that utilized a mobile plastic bearing that freely articulated on a flat metal tibial-bearing surface (Fig. 87–1). The proven advantages were a very low amount of polyethylene wear demonstrated by both laboratory and clinical studies despite a highly conforming articular design. The disadvantages primarily related to patient choice and the need for the surgeon to be able to precisely correct deformity and balance the ligaments within a narrow tolerance. This device would dislocate if there was any postoperative instability. Today, after nearly 30 years of clinical experience and very little design change, that device has been introduced into the American marketplace.

The Low Contact Stress (LCS) knee prosthesis (Depuy, Warsaw, IN) is a mobile-bearing design with modifications of the tibial component to allow for bicruciate preservation, posterior cruciate ligament (PCL) retention, or PCL sacrifice (Fig. 87–2).[7,8] The original design had a highly conforming articular surface that maintained high contact up to about 40 degrees of flexion. Unlike the Oxford unicondylar device, which was a single radius or curvature design, the LCS design had posterior condyles with decreasing and multiple radii of curvature. The other major design innovation was to make a common articulation of the femur and tibia such that these articulations remained relatively constant and highly conforming throughout the early range of motion. This was in distinction to the normal knee and most conventional fixed-bearing designs. Furthermore, a mobile-bearing patella was created to match this same geometry (Fig. 87–3). The components of this implant have remained essentially identical in geometry from the outset of original implantation in 1977. The surgical technique with the tibia-cut-first and initial flexion-block spacing has remained the standard at centers using this method.[6,21,23,33]

The potential for highly conforming mobile-bearing implants to improve the durability of total knee arthroplasty by potentially reducing polyethylene wear and osteolysis has been a desirable objective.[2,26] However, several authors have raised the concern that the introduction of additional complexity through the use of a moving bearing will also introduce new modes of device-related failure.[3,48] With the success of the LCS prosthesis,

Oxford unicondylar device, and other systems in the worldwide market, long-term studies have been made of these devices, which are summarized in this chapter. Additionally, a plethora of other mobile-bearing designs have been introduced, most of which are modifications of previously successful fixed-bearing devices. The available outcome data are lacking on most of these devices, but the efficacy can be presumed because mobile-bearing instability is a very early and manifest complication of the failed procedure. Whereas many of these designs depart from the original goal of high conformity to improve polyethylene wear, the ability to allow free implant rotation is an important design feature and this could be stated as being the most important argument for mobile bearings. The state of the art and the evolution of the mobile-bearing concept are reviewed in this chapter.

SCIENTIFIC BASIS

Kinematic Analysis

Numerous studies have been done on patients undergoing total knee arthroplasty using in vivo video fluoroscopy to assess the surface-contact kinematics during various activities such as walking, stair climbing, and performing a deep knee bend.[15,43] The LCS mobile-bearing total knee was investigated with PCL retention (meniscal bearing) or sacrifice (rotating platform) evaluating the sagittal plane kinematics.[39,40] The PCL-retaining LCS meniscal-bearing implant demonstrated consistent femorotibial contact posterior to the midsagittal tibial reference point. There was early posterior rollback up to 30 degrees, but anterior translation was noted at 60 and 90 degrees of flexion. The PCL-sacrificing LCS rotating-platform design remained virtually midline on the proximal tibia throughout range of motion. There was, however, a minor trend for early posterior rollback with anterior translation in deep flexion. It was concluded that the rotating-platform knee demonstrated a midline sagittal plane proximal tibia position throughout the deep knee bend and gait cycle that was believed to be optimal for congruency and weight-bearing. The minor early posterior femoral rollback could be attributed to the high conformity of the LCS design up to 30 degrees of flexion, whereas the anterior translation seen from 60 to 90 degrees related to the freedom due to the smaller radii of curvature of the posterior femoral condyles. The most desirable features were the midline

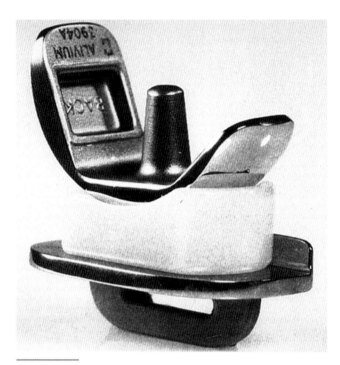

Figure 87–1. Oxford mobile-bearing unicondylar knee prosthesis designed in 1977. (From Argenson J-N, O'Connor JJ: Polyethylene wear in meniscal knee replacement. A one to nine-year retrieval analysis in Oxford. J Bone Joint Surg Br 74(2):228, 1992.)

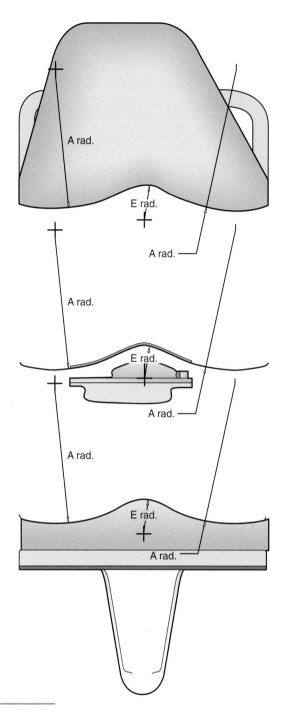

Figure 87–3. LCS design concept of common articulating surface geometries of the femur and patella to match that of the proximal tibial articular surface.

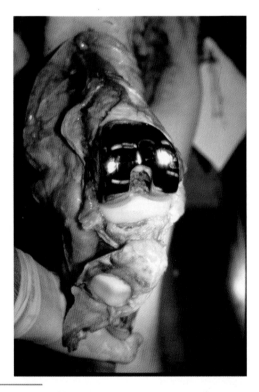

Figure 87–2. LCS rotating platform at 10-year cadaver retrieval; note pristine appearance of bearing surfaces.

position related to the design conformity and the lack of major anterior posterior translation over the proximal tibia, which could be detrimental both for tibial base plate fixation and wear. The meniscal-bearing LCS implant showed femoral tibial contact posterior to the midsagittal plane of the tibia in virtually all positions. Again there was a fairly predictable posterior femoral rollback with early flexion up to 30 degrees that could be attributed to the high conformity of the design in this position. After 60 degrees of flexion there was anterior translation of the

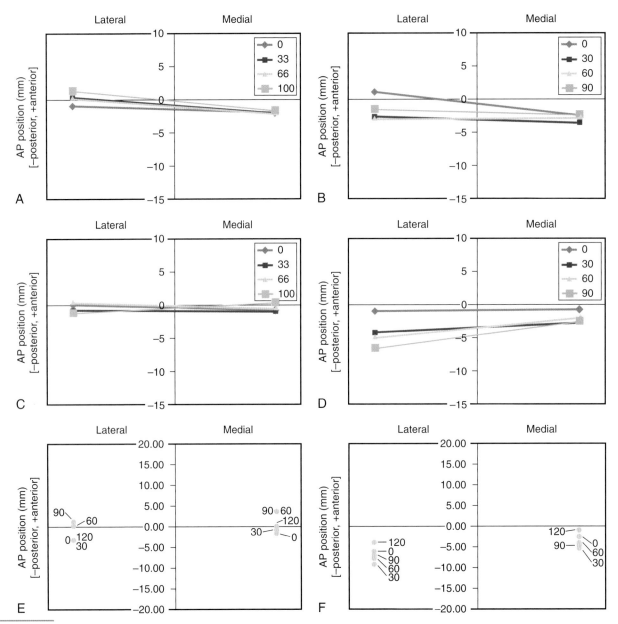

Figure 87–4. LCS kinematic analysis. **A,** LCS rotating platform in gait demonstrates centered medial pivot point and lateral posterior location at 0 degrees, followed by mild anterior movement in deep flexion. **B,** LCS rotating platform in deep knee bend demonstrates centered medial pivot with lateral anterior point at 0 degrees with posterior translation to 60 degrees followed by anterior translation at 90 degrees of flexion. **C,** LCS-PS rotating platform in gait shows a centered position on both medial and lateral surfaces dictated by the posterior stabilizer. **D,** LCS-PS rotating platform in deep flexion demonstrates predictable posterior rollback on lateral condyle with medial minor posterior translation, both dictated by posterior stabilizer. **E,** LCS AP glide demonstrates PCL-retaining kinematics in non-weightbearing with posterior starting points medial and lateral, anterior translation to 90 degrees of flexion, followed by posterior translation in deep flexion. **F,** LCS AP glide with weightbearing assessment shows posterior starting point at 0 degrees of flexion followed by further posterior translation to 90 degrees with anterior translation to 120 degrees of flexion.

condyles that persisted with flexion up to 90 degrees. This resulted from the decreased conformity of the design in higher degrees of flexion with the smaller radii of curvature of the posterior femoral condyles and from the freedom of excursion in the tracks (Fig. 87–5).

Frontal plane and screw-home in vivo kinematics were evaluated in 20 patients with the rotating-platform LCS device, and it was noted that 90% of patients had significant lift-off (>0.75 mm) during the stance phase of gait.[38] Condylar lift-off was seen in both the lateral and medial

condyles, with the maximal medial liftoff of 2.12 mm while the greatest lateral liftoff was 3.53 mm. Screw-home rotation was quite variable, and there could be internal tibial rotation in knee flexion as high as 9.6 degrees or external tibial rotation with a maximum observed of 6.2 degrees. The average screw-home rotation for the group was 0.5 degree.[25] Most designers have considered the amount of rotation necessary for fixed-bearing designs, on the order of 20 degrees, but this led to the need for relatively flat articulations and line-to-line contact. The LCS implants tested

0° flexion   90° flexion

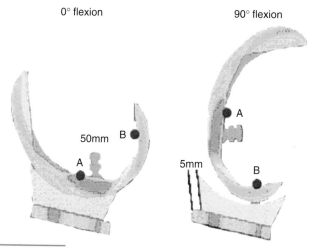

50mm

5mm

Figure 87–5. Sagittal plane geometry of the LCS design demonstrates high conformity in extension and line contact in deep flexion with diminishing multiple radii of curvature. Secondary articulating (bottom) surface moves one-tenth as much as primary surface (i.e., low stress).

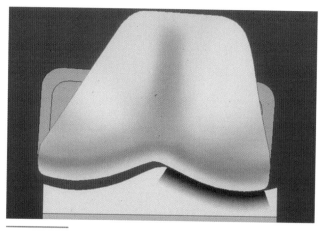

Figure 87–6. Frontal plane geometry of the LCS allows high articular contact with lateral translation noted with typical obligatory lateral liftoff seen in gait.

demonstrated the extremes of condylar rotation but an optimal performance from the design point of view because the LCS device is rotationally unconstrained. Dennis recently studied the ability of the bearings to move, finding virtually all bearings tested to show some degree of rotation. The LCS device may have substantial lift-off while remaining in virtual normal conformity (Fig. 87–6).

Haas and colleagues compared the LCS rotating-platform (LCS-RP) with a posterior-stabilized rotating-platform version (LCS-PS), evaluating both condylar lift-off and mediolateral coronal plane translation.[19] They found that the amount of mediolateral translation and condylar lift-off was statistically different for the two groups ($p < 0.05$). On average, subjects having an LCS-PS total knee arthroplasty experienced only 1.7 mm (1.1 to 2.6) of mediolateral translation. Subjects having an LCS-RP total knee arthroplasty experienced 4.3 mm (3.4 to 7.4) of mediolateral translation. This difference could be explained by the conflict of the posterior-stabilized post. On average, subjects having a LCS-PS total knee arthroplasty experienced 1.2 mm (0.6 to 2.8) of condylar lift-off during the mediolateral shift whereas subjects having an LCS-RP total knee arthroplasty experienced 2.0 mm (1.1-3.1) of condylar lift-off. The results from this study determined that during condylar lift-off, the contact of the condyle remaining on the tibia shifts away from the medial peripheral edge toward the center of the joint. The LCS-RP device allows for high conformity despite the lateral femoral displacement. With the posterior-stabilized rotating-platform tibial insert, both condylar lift-off and mediolateral translation were limited by the spine-box interference. This study was unique in that the amount of tibial translation of the rotating platform was unexpected but not surprising, given the prior results of both skeletal pin gait laboratory studies and stereoroentgenographic photogrammetry, which have shown 5 to 6 mm of translation in the normal knee.

Oakeshott and colleagues have evaluated the kinematics of the AP Glide LCS, which is a PCL-retaining device

(Fig. 87–7).[29] That device performed in many ways similar to the original meniscal-bearing LCS but with some important differences. The average range of motion of 10 patients was 119 degrees when weightbearing and 129 degrees when not weightbearing. Condylar lift-off and rotation were comparable to those in other LCS studies, but there was a range of nearly 20 degrees of tibial rotation when not weightbearing while most of the rotation during weightbearing was up to 10 degrees of external rotation. Finally, contact was significantly more anterior, with greater degrees of flexion when not weightbearing. This would highlight the potential problem of anterior impingement demonstrated by some surgeons using this implant and encourage a fairly accurate flexion space.

Wear Studies

McEwan and coworkers used an elaborate wear simulator study to compare volumetric and gravimetric wear data against cycled implants utilizing an elaborate kinematic scheme designed to duplicate in vivo usage.[25] This included a load of up to 2600 N, 60%/40% medial/lateral loading, 5 million cycles per test, irrigation with calf serum, and kinematic positioning to reflect typical total knee in vivo observations made from prior studies from Komistek and colleagues. For the high-loading scenario, the PFC Sigma fixed-bearing device produced 23 mm³ per million cycles of wear compared with the LCS-RP at 10 mm³ per million cycles ($p < 0.01$) At a reduced and controlled loading scenario, the same difference persisted with the PFC Sigma wearing of 14 mm³ per million cycles compared with the LCS-RP at 5 mm³ per million cycles ($p < 0.01$). The articulated wear patterns demonstrated a 70% area of the implant surface for the LCS design compared with 48% for the PFC device, confirming the concept of area contact for the mobile-bearing surface. Wear pattern types were similar for both implants.

A review of the literature found four other studies that reported quantitative wear measurements for knee bearings. Collier and colleagues reported an average wear rate

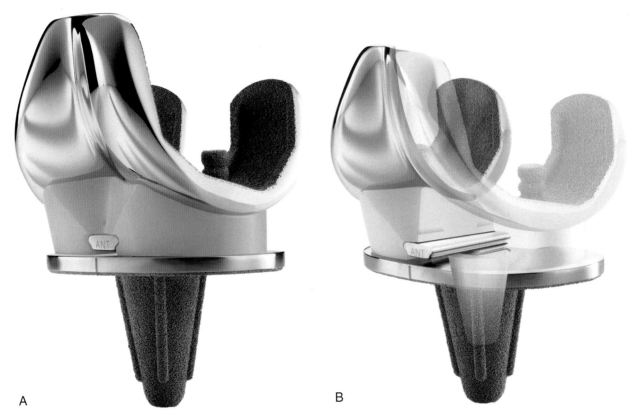

A   B

Figure 87–7. LCS AP glide prosthesis with center control arm that allows unrestricted anteroposterior motion. **A,** AP glide prosthesis. **B,** Cutaway demonstrates control arm.

of 0.09 mm/yr for 20 ethylene oxide gas–sterilized unicompartmental bearings.[12] These were of a high–contact stress design and included bearings with an original thickness of less than 6 mm. Two studies of the highly conforming Oxford unicompartmental meniscal knee bearing derived rates for bearing wear. Psychoyios and associates reported 0.036 mm/yr, and Argenson and O'Connor reported 0.026 mm/yr.[1,32] Plante-Bordeneuve and Freeman reported on 22 PCL-sacrificing total knee replacements with a high degree of tibiofemoral conformity in the sagittal plane.[31] They measured an average wear rate of 0.025 mm/yr. Evidence then indicates that a low–contact stress prosthetic knee design with a linear wear pattern can be expected to have a rate of wear less than 0.09 mm/yr. This compares favorably with the rate of approximately 0.20 mm/yr that historically has been reported for the prosthetic hip.

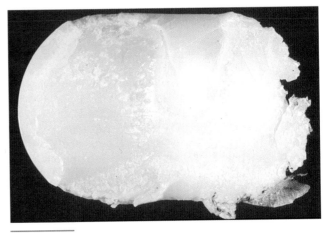

Figure 87–8. Catastrophic failure of LCS rotating platform tibial insert attributed to polyethylene breakdown from oxidation of gas in air sterilization.

Retrieval Analysis

Collier and coworkers have evaluated an extensive collection of LCS mobile-bearing devices collected over a 10-year period, including 144 meniscal bearings and 62 rotating platforms retrieved by surgeons for revision, implant failure, or other causes.[13] These devices were compared with a large database of 619 fixed-bearing total knees that had been retrieved and analyzed. The average mobile-bearing service life was 47 months, with a range

of 1 to 170 months. All the polyethylene components had been sterilized using gamma-irradiation-in-air (Fig. 87–8). They were rated for the following modes of wear: burnishing, scratching, abrasion, pitting, delamination, cracking, and cold flow. Linear wear of mobile meniscal bearings was measured based on the worst-case scenario that assumed bearing thickness to originally have been at the top of the manufacturing tolerances and the best-case scenario of a bearing thickness originating at the bottom of the manufacturing tolerances.

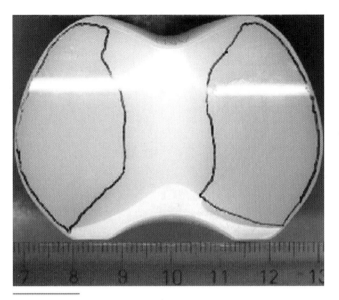

Figure 87–9. LCS rotating platform tibial insert demonstrates typical burnishing wear on upper surface.

Dislocation or subluxation was significantly more common ($p < 0.01$) for mobile bearings (20%) than fixed bearings (4%). Meniscal bearings were at greatest risk for this complication. Twenty-nine of 137 meniscal-bearing devices experienced either partial or complete extrusion of a bearing over the edge of the metal tray. In nearly half of these instances the bearing fractured (12/137). An additional 6 meniscal-bearing devices were removed for dislocation unrelated to bearing extrusion. The incidence of dislocation/subluxation for the rotating-platform design was comparable to that of fixed bearings (5%, 3/55). Three rotating bearings were noted to have twisted into a transverse orientation in vivo. Malposition was more frequently reported for mobile compared with fixed bearings (13% vs. 7%). The difference in incidence was significant ($p < 0.05$). Wear-through or fracture of the tibial and patellar bearings was also a major contributor to device failure of both mobile and fixed bearings. This usually occurred due to polyethylene fatigue. The incidence of tibial wear-through and/or fracture was 18% for both mobile bearings and fixed bearings. However, mobile patellar bearings had significantly fewer ($p < 0.01$) occurrences of wear-through and/or fracture than metal-backed fixed bearings (4% and 10% respectively). The incidence of burnishing was significantly greater in mobile bearings ($p < 0.01$) (Fig. 87–9). Fixed bearings were found to have a significantly greater incidence of abrasive wear, delamination, and cold flow ($p < 0.01$). There were no apparent differences in regard to the incidence of articular scratching, pitting, cracking, or wear-through.

Nearly all (97%) fixed bearings presented visible fretting of the polyethylene back surface. Fretting was manifested as burnishing and/or scratching. One hundred percent of the mobile bearings presented some back-surface fretting. It was usually more pronounced on the LCS device than was observed for fixed bearings. The severity was enhanced by the common observance of deep scratches concentric to the direction of bearing travel.

Because of the consistent observation that machining lines remained visible on the mobile bearings back surface, it is surmised that back-surface wear did not result in appreciable thinning of the material even in those bearings of longest duration. The mobile bearings had a significantly greater ($p < 0.01$) incidence of backside burnishing, scratching, pitting, and delamination. Oxidation proved to be more prevalent in mobile bearings (85%, 29/34) than in fixed bearings (64%, 174/273).

Fifty retrieved mobile meniscal bearings from 27 patients were measured for linear wear. The method accounted for wear on both the top and bottom surfaces. The majority (82%) of the measured bearings had an original thickness of less than 8 mm at the bottom of the articular dish. The average in-vivo duration for the bearings was 82 months. At the time of retrieval the average patient age was 70 years and the average weight was 184 pounds. Assuming a worst-case scenario in which each bearing was machined to the high end of the tolerances, the worn meniscal bearings had an average total linear wear of 0.560 mm and an average rate of wear of 0.092 mm/yr. In a best-case scenario assuming each bearing was machined to the low end of the tolerances, the bearings had an average total linear wear of −0.024 mm and an average rate of wear of −0.008 mm/yr. The appearance of negative wear is a result of 34 bearings (68%) having a measured thickness within the allotted machining tolerances. The true rate of wear fell somewhere within that range, perhaps approximating 0.05 mm/yr. The amount of wear did not correlate with in-vivo duration.

After reviewing these data, Collier and colleagues concluded that important differences between mobile and fixed bearings were observed in regard to polyethylene wear.[13] Of greatest note was the observation that mobile bearings had a lower incidence of abrasion. Abrasion is the removal of material by a grinding or rubbing process and may generate a notable topographical relief in relation to adjacent unworn areas. It is arguably the best indicator that bearing material had been steadily removed by the motion of the femoral condyles upon the bearing. The abrasion factor is important because with the advent of sterilization methods that limit bearing oxidation and its accompanying fatigue mechanisms, abrasion will likely become the wear mode of greatest concern in knee devices. For fixed-bearing designs with older polyethylene, the fatigue mechanisms of cracking and delamination dominate. Mobile bearings were found to have significantly less incidence of delamination than fixed bearings despite a much higher incidence of polyethylene oxidation. The comparative deficit of abrasion and delamination in LCS bearings could be attributed to their lower contact stress regimen. Reduced stress could also explain the lower incidence of polyethylene cold flow observed for mobile bearings. Burnishing is a similar process to abrasion, but material is removed to a lesser extent and on a fine enough scale to develop a polished surface. The higher incidence of burnishing with the LCS device may indicate that the polyethylene of the LCS device was either more abrasion resistant or that stress upon the polyethylene was comparably less.

According to Collier and colleagues, the concern that mobile bearings have a dual articulation and therefore the potential for increased debris generation appears to be mitigated by the observation that even fixed bearings fret against their metal counterfaces and produce backside wear debris.[13] When two dissimilar materials are mated together, as in a fixed-bearing system, and then stressed, it is difficult to envision that micromotion will not occur at the interface. Concern for greater debris generation because of dual articulation then appears unfounded. Mobile bearings have a reduced incidence of abrasive wear, which in the absence of fatigue is the dominating wear mechanism. Although enthusiasm for mobile meniscal bearings is tempered by the incidence of dislocation and subluxation, linear wear of these bearings was found to be almost immeasurable. Of the 50 bearings measured for wear (average duration, 82 months), 34 were found to be still within the original machining tolerances.

DESIGN CONSIDERATIONS

Surface Contact Area

Wear can be related directly to the contact stress of two articulating bodies and from the engineering literature had a direct relationship to the differences of the principal radii of curvature.[37] This obviously relates as well to the area of contact, such that two articulating surfaces with similar-conforming radii with high area of contact will have lower contact surface stress than those of dissimilar radii and much lower area contact. An interesting contradiction, however, is that the applied load relates only to the cube root of the material stiffness and area of contact such that increases in load or body weight in total knees does not dramatically increase the contact stress. Another important phenomenon relates to the fact the relationship to reduction in contact stress is not linear with increasing contact area. Gabriel and colleagues have shown that this effect is minimal below above 400 mm^2 of contact area for a total knee implant.[16]

In regard to current mobile-bearing designs, the LCS knee prosthesis, which has very high conformity in full extension, has a contact area of 902 mm^2 for the rotating platform whereas the MBK (Zimmer, Warsaw, IN) with a single radius of curvature, has 530 mm^2 of contact area (Table 87–1).[36] The latter reduction is both a function of design and the fact that a single radius of curvature in total knees must be diminished with smaller contact area as compared with the large polycentric radii of the LCS in full extension. After about 30 degrees of flexion, the LCS prosthesis reduces to near line contact. The newer Inex version (Zimmer, Warsaw, IN) of the LCS device has modified this design to increase contact area to a deeper degree of flexion. There is a large group of mobile-bearing devices available to the international orthopedic market (Fig. 87–10). Some are novel mobile-bearing designs, whereas a number are "retrofits" of prior devices that are fixed-bearing designs by origin. Early wear simulator studies have shown that the LCS design has diminished polyethylene wear compared with typical fixed-bearing designs by a factor of three. It remains to be seen if newer mobile-bearing designs with much lower contact area compared

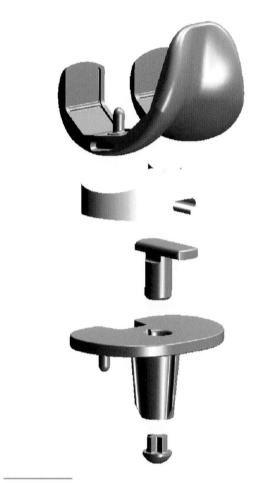

Figure 87–10. Design features of Inex mobile-bearing prosthesis that has similar articulating geometries to the original LCS prosthesis.

with the LCS design will have the favorable long-term outcome in terms of wear reduction.

Implant Stability

Implant stability may become an issue for certain designs if there is not high conformity especially in the frontal plane. This has been a problem with early designs such as the Minn prosthesis.[16] As noted from kinematic studies, the potential for abnormal motions is significant in total knee arthroplasty. Surgical technique is an important factor in this regard, because the design must be able to accommodate difficult problems in the hands of lesser-experienced surgeons.

Single versus Multiple Radii of Curvature of the Femoral Component

With the idea of maximizing of contact throughout the range of motion, engineers chose a single radius of cur-

Table 87–1. Currently Available Mobile-Bearing Total Knee Prostheses with General Features

Prosthesis	Technique	Insert Engagement	Contact Area Extension	Radius of Curvature	Anatomic Rotating Patella	Femur, Coronal Plane Conformity	Free Rotation & Translation No "Stops"
LCS Depuy	Bicruciate, PCR, PCS	Stem in stem polyethylene	902 mm^2	Multiple	Yes, Yes	Yes	Yes (all)
Rotataglide Corin	PCR, PS	2 pin on slot	NA	Single	No, No	Yes	No
HLS Tornier	PS	1 knob	NA	Multiple	No, No	Yes	No
Genesis II Smith Nephew	PCR	1 pin on slot	NA	Multiple	No, No	Yes	No
Natural Sulzer	PCR	Stem in stem polyethylene	566 mm^2	Multiple	No, No	No	No
SAL Sulzer	PCR	1 pin on slot	551 mm^2	Single	Yes, No	Yes	No
Trac Biomet	PS	Stem in stem polyethylene	NA	Dual Radius	No, No	Yes	No
MBK	PCR, PCS	2 pin on slot, bumper	530 mm^2	Single	No, No	Yes	No
AMC MKII	PCR, PS	Rim bumper	NA	Multiple	Yes, Yes	Yes	No
Legacy	PS	1 pin on slot	NA	Multiple	No, No	Yes	No
Profix	PCR	1 pin on slot	NA	Multiple	No, No	Yes	No
PFC Sigma	PS, PCR	Stem in stem polyethylene	407 mm^2	Multiple	No, No	Yes	Yes (RP)
Interax Howmedica	PCR	1 pin on slot	553 mm^2	NA	No, No	Yes	No
Oxford Biomet	NA	NA	NA	NA	No, No	Yes	No
Innex Sulzer	PCR, PCS	Stem in stem metal	NA	Multiple	No, No	Yes	Yes

vature in certain designs. This was considered reasonable because the posterior condyle seems to define a fairly circular sagittal shape and the implant would mimic this shape. The disadvantage, however, is that the total radius must be significantly smaller than that of the normal distal femoral surface, which may reduce area contact and cause a degree of instability in extension. High conformity in flexion may be desirable for contact area but leads to an inflexible articulation that must follow the kinematics of femoral tibial contact.[16] Dennis has shown that some PCL-retaining total knees that are tight in flexion cause the femoral tibial contact to remain far posterior on the proximal tibia.[14] A lesser constrained polycentric curvature has greater accommodation for this motion whereas the single radius design may "slide off the back," as was shown by the original Oxford meniscal-bearing design. A second related issue is "jumping distance" for disarticulation that must be lower for the single radius design. For the diminished polycentric radius, the condyle must "go up the hill" and travel farther to disarticulate.[16]

Similarly, certain designs have changed the center of rotation from a central position such as the LCS-RP to a more anterior position to accommodate the insert post into the tibial base stem that has been located more anteriorly. This creates an eccentric position for the rotation of the tibial insert, offsetting the insert position for a given amount of tibial rotation. Certain abnormal kinematics that have been shown to occur, such as tibial external rotation, would place the tibial insert more medial than normal, which if compounded with the normal proximal lateral translation of the femoral condyle could result in exaggerated contact on a medial tibial eminence or post.[16]

Technique

The options are bicruciate retention, PCL retention, PCL sacrifice, and PCL substitution or stabilization. Experience with the Oxford unicondylar meniscal-bearing device has shown that bicruciate retention is essential for success of this implant.[27] The LCS design experience has shown that PCL retention with the meniscal bearing is possible but must be implemented very carefully because of the risk of flexion instability. Too tight or too loose in flexion will lead to implant dislocation. The primary disadvantage of the "distal-femoral-cut-first" method is the inability to accurately adjust the flexion space on final trialing. The LCS technique has evolved into a tibial-cut-first, spacer block technique, as pioneered by Insall. This has been an important element to the long clinical success of that implant. PCL sacrifice with the tibial-cut-first technique has proven to be easy for most surgeons, reproducible, and clinically durable over the long term for the LCS device.[6,21,23,33]

PCL stabilization is a common feature of the majority of new rotating-platform designs. The primary advantage is the ability to enforce a degree of posterior femoral rollback that will improve flexion. In addition, an element of stability is added from the jumping distance of the post-cam mechanism, which ranges from 1.1 to 1.4 cm. There are, however, known liabilities of the post-cam mecha-

nism, which include decreased patellofemoral articulation of the area of the box and the potential for soft-tissue impingement or clunk in the box. The early Insall-Burstein Posterior-Stabilized prosthesis and the original LCS-RP were designed to accommodate these motions.

Mobile-Bearing Engagement

Mobile-bearing tibial inserts require certain degrees of freedom that are absent with fixed-bearing devices. The original Oxford unicondylar and LCS device clinical experience demonstrated the problem of bearing dislocation and "spin-out" associated with poor surgical technique. These problems can be diminished with capture pegs, sliding control arms (LCS AP Glide is more unconstrained than the meniscal bearing LCS), and capture rims. The downside is constraint and associated polyethylene wear that could be expected with certain "pin on slot" designs (Fig. 87–11). Also, designs that will articulate with normal motion (such as a post-cam) can be expected to wear over time. Abnormal kinematics from poor surgical technique or unaccommodated normal kinematics will likely cause exaggerated wear. An example of the latter is the TRAC II (Biomet, Warsaw, IN) total knee that is highly conforming in the coronal plane. With coronal mediolateral translation known to occur in the normal knee, this implant will wear much like a constrained condylar revision device.[36]

Patellofemoral Articulation

The patellofemoral articulation has been problematic for posterior-stabilized designs with a high incidence of patella fracture, subluxation, or implant loosening. Possible causes with some of these older designs include an

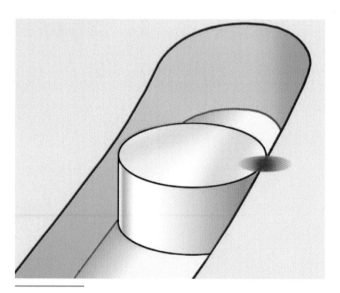

Figure 87–11. Diagram of a "pin in slot" design to demonstrate the potential high wear points of the polyethylene interface.

inherent "boxy" shape of femoral components that do not anatomically restore the patellofemoral groove. The loading forces of the patellofemoral joint are poorly understood, hence a question arises regarding the future performance of new posterior-stabilized designs in this regard. For the LCS design, patellofemoral problems are rare in most series despite a relatively thick, mobile, metal-backed patella. Several authors have suggested that the deep intercondylar groove and the anatomic shape of the LCS have been favorable for achieving more normal kinematics and longevity.[9,23,40]

SURGICAL TECHNIQUE

There are three major objectives of surgical technique in total arthroplasty. First is the need to achieve anatomic alignment of 5 to 7 degrees of valgus angulation to the mechanical axis. Second is to establish ligamentous balance by achieving careful balance of the flexion and extension gaps within 2 to 3 mm of physiologic ligament tension. Finally, is the desire to optimize the potential kinematics of the chosen prosthetic implant. The tibial-shaft-axis or tibial-cut-first technique follows the original idea of Insall that establishing the flexion gap was the most important variable in successful total condylar arthroplasty.[4] Why this approach has become an attractive surgical technique for mobile-bearing total knee arthroplasty is discussed, as is how surgical navigation will more accurately place the proximal tibial cut in total knee arthroplasty. Another option is the distal femoral measured resection method, which remains the standard method in many centers and also presents a reasonable alternative, especially with minimally invasive surgical techniques.

Tibial-Shaft-Axis Technique

The mobile-bearing total knee arthroplasty tibial-shaft-axis or tibial-cut-first method determines the proximal tibial cut utilizing either an extramedullary guide system or the making of a surgical navigated cut of the tibia perpendicular to the mechanical axis of the leg (Fig. 87–12). An intramedullary femoral rod is placed with the anteroposterior condylar cutting block. Flexion spacing is done with an anteroposterior cortical cutting block based off the anterior cortical reference. The exact dimension of the flexion space is determined with a tensor that precisely tensions and measures a rectangular flexion space (Fig. 87–13). The final assessment is done with a spacing block that also allows determination of the tibial shaft mechanical axis (Fig. 87–14). At this point the distal femoral cut is based on the anatomic axis of the femur (Fig. 87–15). Finishing cuts of the distal femur are then done, followed by the insertion of the final implant (Figs. 87–16 and 87–17).

An important step with the tibial-shaft-axis method is that primary extension ligamentous balancing must be established before the flexion space is created. This is because any ligamentous balancing done after these cuts

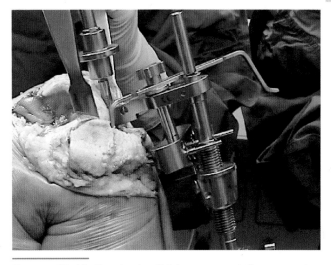

Figure 87–12. Proximal tibial extramedullary cutting device used for the Inex system "tibia-cut-first" method.

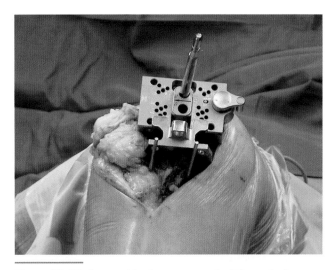

Figure 87–13. Spacer block assessment of the anterior cortical referenced anteroposterior flexion space cut block used in the Inex system.

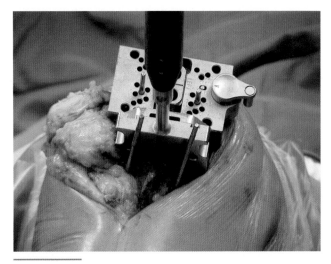

Figure 87–14. Assessment of flexion space tension and size in the Inex system.

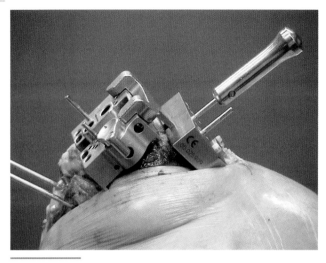

Figure 87–15. Distal femoral cut gig applied after antero-posterior cuts have been completed in the Inex system.

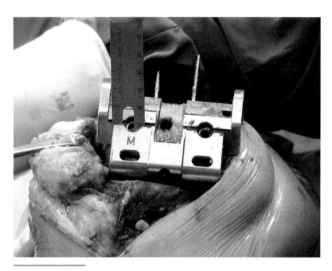

Figure 87–16. Distal femoral finishing block in the Inex system.

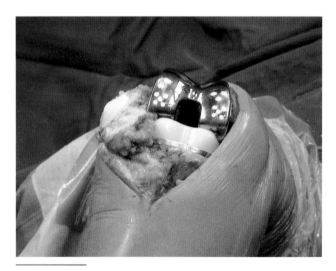

Figure 87–17. Final mobile-bearing rotating-platform Inex implants are inserted.

are made can result in the creation of a trapezoidal flexion space. Such a problem often results in bearing dislocation or "spin-out." The surgeon must have the knee balanced as his or her primary step, although some releasing such as the posterior capsule may be made after the proximal tibial cut. This can be advantageous as the posterior capsular origin on the distal femur becomes more accessible. With the knee in full extension, the ligaments should be balanced and tense. If not, additional release should be done.

OUTCOME STUDIES

LCS Original Investigational Review Board Studies

Buechel and Pappas presented their 10-year experience with the LCS knee replacement of the first 357 total knee arthroplasties in 1989.[8] There were 72 bicruciate-retaining meniscal-bearing implants, 49 PCL-retaining meniscal-bearing implants, and 137 PCL-sacrificing rotating-platform implants, with 80 revision arthroplasties. Of the entire group, there were 231 excellent results and 87 good results, with 89% of the total in these categories and the remaining in fair or poor categories. In regard to complications specific to mobile bearings, there were seven rotating-platform dislocations (3.2%) and one traumatic meniscal-bearing dislocation (0.7%). Most of the revision arthroplasties were re-revision of difficult revision cases in which there was flexion instability. Factors predisposing to mobile-bearing complications such as dislocation were stated to be malrotation of the tibial component, allowing a meniscal bearing to sublux, late rupture of the PCL, flexion-extension gap instability, and traumatic twisting of the knee joint. Three tibial components loosened (2.0%) in very heavy patients in whom the component poorly covered the proximal tibia. There were no femoral implant loosenings.

Buechel and associates reported their 11-year experience with the LCS metal-backed, rotating-bearing patellar prosthesis in 515 total knees, of which 331 had more than 24-month follow-up.[9] The overall postoperative fracture rate was 0.58%, with avascular necrosis seen in 0.38%. There was one patellar dislocation of the entire group and no polyethylene dissociations, no polyethylene wear-through, and no implant loosenings. It was postulated that the deep femoral groove engagement prevented dislocation and allowed high contact, even with subluxation.

Buechel and associates studied 373 LCS total knee replacements of their initial series surviving a minimum of 10 years.[6] Of this group, 97.9% had good or excellent with the PCL-retaining meniscal-bearing implant, 100% with the cemented rotating platform, and 97.9% with the cementless rotating platform. Meniscal-bearing dislocation occurred in 2.5% whereas 5% required meniscal-bearing exchange for wear at an average of 10.1 years. Rotating bearing dislocation was seen in 1.2%, and there were three rotating platforms revised for wear of the overall group. Kaplan-Meier survivorship for noninfected

LCS total knee replacements and mechanical loosening for any reason was 83% at 16 years for the cementless meniscal-bearing group, 97.7% for the cemented rotating-platform group, and 98.3% at 18 years for the cementless rotating-platform group.

The results of the U.S. Food and Drug Administration clinical trial in 147 meniscal-bearing and 44 rotating-platform total knees done with a cementless technique at an average of 68 months follow-up have been reported.[45] Pain was absent in 94% of meniscal-bearing knees and 93.2% of the rotating-platform knees. Range of motion averaged 120 degrees for the meniscal-bearing knees and 108 degrees for the rotating-platform knees ($p < 0.001$). The overall New Jersey Orthopaedic Score was 93.2 for the meniscal-bearing knees and 87.6 for the rotating-platform knees ($p < 0.001$). The overall survivorship was 98.1% at 7 years. The overall meniscal-bearing complication rate was 0.6%, with one fracture and one extrusion. No rotating-platform problems with bearing spin-outs were noted. The patellar complication rate was 1%.

Jordan and colleagues evaluated 473 cementless PCL-retaining meniscal-bearing LCS total knees with 2- to 10-year follow-up (average, 5 years).[21] Mechanical failure occurred in 3.6%, with meniscal-bearing fracture and dislocation in 2.5%. In 1% there was tibial subluxation resulting from ligamentous instability. Kaplan-Meier survivorship for mechanical revision for any reason was 94.6% at 8 years.

Sorrells reported the results of 525 cementless rotating-platform total knees with up to 13 years follow-up.[33] The revision rate of this entire group was 5%, and the tibial component exchange rate for polyethylene wear or instability was 2%. The survivorship for mechanical component failure was 92.9% (95% CI; range, 83% to 100%) at 13 years. Sorrels and associates reported a subgroup of this experience with 117 patients younger than 65 years (average, 56 years).[35] With average follow-up of 8.5 years, the average knee score was 91 points and the pain score was 27 (with a possible 30). The survivorship with revision for any reason was 88% at 14 years. The revision rate was 7% with four malpositioned implants, one infection, and one case of osteolysis. Bearing dislocation or "spin-out" occurred in 1 case at 3 weeks after surgery.

Callaghan and colleagues studied 114 cemented LCS-RP total knees with 9- to 12-year follow-up.[11] The average Knee Society clinical and functional scores were 90 and 75, respectively, at final follow-up. The average active range of motion was 102 degrees at final follow-up. In this series there were no cases of periprosthetic osteolysis, implant dislocation, or evidence of implant loosening and none of the patients available for follow-up have undergone revision.

Stiehl and Voorhorst studied factors affecting range of motion with the LCS total knee, evaluating the PCL-retaining or PCL-sacrificing technique in 782 total knees.[46] Postoperative motion averaged 115 degrees for the meniscal-bearing implant and 104 degrees for LCS-RP ($p < 0.05$), but the preoperative range was significantly lower for the LCS-RP. The greatest gains in motion occurred in patients with less than 90 degrees of preoperative motion, and improvement in motion was greater in patients without prior surgery.

Keblish and coworkers compared patella-resurfaced LCS total knees versus non-resurfaced LCS total knees in 52 patients with bilateral total knee arthroplasties with an average follow-up of 5.24 years.[23] Comparing the group overall, there was no significant difference with subjective preference, performance on stairs, or the incidence of anterior knee pain. However, they recommended non-resurfacing in cases with a small patella under 19 mm in thickness or in the younger active patient and resurfacing with the very large patella and in the workers' compensation case.

Keblish and coworkers reviewed their experience with the lateral parapatellar approach for the valgus deformed total knee arthroplasty in 53 patients who had undergone an LCS total knee arthroplasty.[22] The results were good to excellent in 94% of cases, and there were no failures from patellar maltracking or implant instability. They stated that lateral release, which is needed in most of these cases, is a part of the approach, allowing the medial blood supply to be preserved. More recently, a coronal Z-plasty has been recommended in which the lateral retinacular dissection is more lateral in the superficial fascia and then dissects medially through the synovium and fat pad, allowing for a significant lateral-based soft-tissue mass that allows for a watertight lateral closure. Also, the Swiss group has recommended a tibial tubercle osteotomy that allows medial eversion of the extensor mechanism.[10]

LCS International Outcome Analysis

This study included the results of 23 surgeons from around the world with extensive experience with the LCS device.[20] The surgical technique of the LCS was standardized with a tibial-cut-first method. Without exception, all surgeons utilized the recommended method. Inclusion criteria were all primary total knee arthroplasties performed before January 1, 1997, with a minimum of 5-year follow-up. Exclusion criteria were unicondylar knee replacements, revision total knee arthroplasties, and the use of all polyethylene tibial components, a late addition to the LCS system. Data collection included those parameters required for the survivorship analysis, including the dates of the operative procedure and status at last follow-up with death or revision as drop-out criteria. Demographic data included age, sex, diagnosis, involved extremity, and history of previous surgery. The type of device utilized was noted whether meniscal bearing or rotating platform, as was fixation, which was either cementless or cemented. Range of motion was recorded because this is considered to be quantifiable and routinely performed in most centers.

There were 4743 total knee arthroplasty revisions performed between February, 1981, and January, 1997.

The averaged follow-up was 5.7 years (range, 5 to 18 years). There were 1437 males and 3306 females. There were 324 bicruciate-retaining implants, 2165 PCL-retaining implants, and 2254 rotating-platform implants inserted. By diagnosis, 77.3% were osteoarthritic, 19% were rheumatoid, 2.6% were post traumatic, and 1.1% were in other categories. The overall average age at surgery was 68 years. The mean age for patients with the PCL-retaining and rotating-platform devices was 68, whereas that for those with bicruciate-retaining implants was 62 years. By diagnosis, the mean age was 69 for osteoarthritics, 64 for the other group, and 62 for post-traumatic, and rheumatoid patients. The knee was right sided in 52.2% and left sided in 47.8%.

Overall, 69% of all knees had cementless fixation whereas 31% had at least one component, either femur or tibia fixed with cement. Similarly, the patella was fixed cementless in 77% of cases. By diagnosis, for osteoarthritics, 78% of PCL-retaining knees were cementless whereas 61% were rotating-platform devices. In the rheumatoid arthritis group, 88% of the bicruciate-retaining implants were cementless. Similarly, 95% of bicruciate-retaining patellar implants were inserted cementless. By implant type, 86% of patella were cementless with bicruciate retaining; 74% were PCL retaining; and 80% were rotating platform. The overall range of motion at last follow-up examination was 110 degrees and was similar for each of the implant types. For the "other" group, the final range of motion was 118 degrees for the rheumatoid group and 98 degrees for the rotating-platform group.

With "failure" defined as revision for any reason, the survivorship was 79% (95% CI; range, 74% to 84%) at 16 years follow-up (see Figs. 87–1 and 87–2). This included a total of 259 (5.4%) of the entire cohort of patients. The survivorship for aseptic loosening was 95% (CI: 91% to 98%) (see Fig. 87–3). The overall survivorship for osteoarthritic patients was 80% at 15 years whereas that for rheumatoid patients was 85%. By implant type, the 14-year survivorship for bicruciate-retaining implants was 79%; that for PCL-retaining implants was 82%; and that for rotating-platform devices was 87%. When we look at the survivorship rates at 10 years' follow-up, the comparison is 89% for bicruciate retaining, 91% for the PCL retaining, and 94% for the rotating-platform implants. The overall 14-year survivorship for cementless fixation was 83%, and that for cemented fixation was 84%. The survivorship of knees that had patellar resurfacing when considering all causes of failure was 80% at 14 years, whereas in the unresurfaced patellar group, survivorship was 91% at 13 years. The survivorship of the patella implants for only revision of patella-related complications was 98% at 15 years.

The most common cause of revision was bearing-related issues, including chronic instability, bearing subluxation, bearing dislocation, or bearing failure in 1.3% of all patients. This was followed by implant loosening in 1.1% of cases and wear-related issues in 0.8% of cases. Chronic pain and revision for undetermined causes was noted in 0.7% of cases, and sepsis was seen in 0.5% overall. Finally, patella-related causes of failure was noted in 0.5% of cases.

COMPLICATIONS

Bearing Dislocation and Spin-out

As noted earlier, mobile-bearing dislocation is perhaps the most feared and sensational problem with these devices

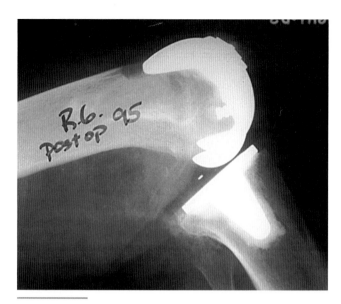

Figure 87–18. Catastrophic "spin-out" of an LCS rotating-platform device utilized in a valgus-deformed osteoarthritic knee.

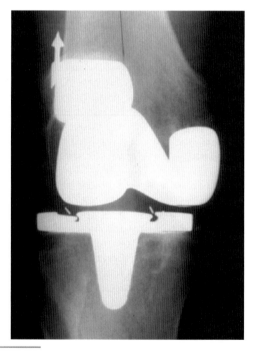

Figure 87–19. Catastrophic meniscal-bearing dislocation of LCS prosthesis.

(Figs. 87–18 and 87–19). Most surgeons have come to recognize that this relates almost solely to surgical technique. I have never seen such a complication in my own personal experience with the LCS mobile bearing but make the following caveats for prevention. Chronic flexion instability noted with many fixed-bearing devices, either PCL retaining or substituting, will usually present as an early bearing dislocation. Flexion instability must be prevented at all costs, and I would state that the flexion balance must irrevocably be within a margin of 5 mm, preferably within 3 mm. The jump distance for the LCS mobile-bearing device is about 6 mm, thus dictating these values. Thompson and associates reviewed a very large contemporary experience of a single surgeon, finding an incidence of 0.5% for the LCS-RP device.[47] There were 10 cases of "spin-out," and each case could be considered complex with a large deformity, either valgus or varus, that was not completely corrected. If these difficult cases are approached with a mobile-bearing device, the surgeon must understand that the margin for error is relatively narrow. A sensible approach would be to utilize a typical revision type of implant in these unusual cases. As for treatment, most bearing dislocations will require revision, either with thicker implants or revision to correct an imbalance or malalignment.

Malaligned Implant

Any conventional implant technique relying on extramedullary or intramedullary guides has the potential of limb malalignment. For this reason, a growing number of international surgeons have utilized computer-assisted surgical navigation to limit this possibility. Konermann and coworkers were able to demonstrate over 90% of cases within optimal alignment of ±2 degrees to the mechanical leg axis using a computer-assisted surgical navigation protocol compared with 77% done by conventional means.[24] The reason I mention this issue is that the LCS implant seems to be particularly susceptible to failure if malaligned. This may relate to the high conformity of the implant in the coronal plane, which will shift most of the force transmission to the medial compartment with varus alignment for example. Additionally, with unconstrained rotation, the tibia may rotate externally in full extension, which will exaggerate the varus malalignment. The long-term experience of Sorrels and associates has clearly addressed this problem.[34] The surgeon should be willing to revise a malaligned total knee early, before osteolysis and bone loss ensue.

Bearing Exchange

Buechel and Pappas have stated the potential of correcting bearing failure with a bearing exchange.[5] This was particularly useful with the meniscal-bearing implants that had a much higher bearing failure rate at follow-up over 10 years (Figs. 87–20). This is a very easy operation and can be done nearly as an outpatient. Reservations to this approach must be made when there is bony osteolysis and implant instability. In both of these cases, simple bearing exchange may not be suitable. Osteolysis portends implant loosening and possible infection. Instability often requires correction of ligament imbalance, something not always amenable to bearing exchange. Currently, I would reserve bearing exchange to cases of late bearing failure in the elderly and in cases such as implant anterior synovial

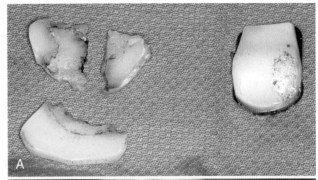

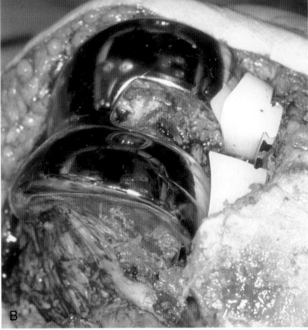

Figure 87–20. Bearing failure after 14 years in a 85-year-old patient with LCS meniscal-bearing total knee arthroplasty. **A,** Fragmentation of meniscal bearings and chronic patellar bearing wear. **B,** Bearing exchange with thicker implants in this elderly patient.

impingement in which an obvious prosthetic problem exists that may be corrected by implant exchange.

Progressive Ligament Laxity

Progressive ligament laxity after total knee arthroplasty has been poorly understood, and there are few definitive statements about the occurrence. Hamelynck studied ligamentous stability in rheumatoid patients after mobile-bearing total knee arthroplasty and found that over a long period of time the knees became more unstable.[41] However, those patients with significant early laxity from inadequate ligament balancing at the time of surgery had a much greater tendency to show progressive laxity over time. It can only be stated that the surgeon much make every effort to make the knee as closely balanced to a "perfect" stability as possible.

SPECIAL ISSUES

AP Glide Mobile-Bearing Prosthesis

The AP Glide prosthesis is a PCL-retaining variant of the LCS mobile-bearing system that has a unique control arm that allows unrestricted tibial rotation and anteroposterior translation.[28] This implant was introduced in 1995 as a more robust device for PCL retention as compared with the original meniscal-bearing device. Although numerous European centers have reported enthusiastic support for this device, two significant problems have arisen that are illustrative of the downside of this particular approach. Anterior fat pad impingement has been noted in about 5% of cases and can require revision to the more stable rotating-platform implant. The kinematic problem is excessive anterior translation that can occur if the balance in midflexion is too lax. Excision of the fat pad has been helpful in some cases but not all. The other issue with the AP Glide implant is failure from late failure of the posterior cruciate ligament. This may result from a traumatic injury, but there have been reports of idiopathic cases perhaps due to weakening of the ligament from balancing or pull off of the posterior cruciate bone block. Any surgeon interested in this design approach must be aware of these problems.

Computer-Assisted Surgical Navigation

Computer-assisted surgical navigation offers a significant tool for the surgeon who would like to try mobile bearings but is afraid of the technical challenges.[44] I have now used surgical navigation in 120 mobile-bearing total knees and have not found a single case outside of 2.5 degrees from the mechanical axis of the lower extremity. Application to the tibial-shaft-axis or tibial-cut-first technique has

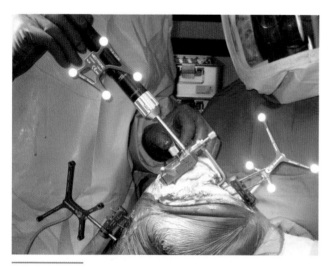

Figure 87–21. Computer-assisted surgical assessment of rotation of anteroposterior flexion cutting block used for LPS Flex-Mobile total knee prosthesis.

been quite enlightening. With tension-flexion spacing after the initial extension ligament release, at least 58% of cases will reveal femoral component rotation greater than 2 degrees from the transepicondylar axis (Fig. 87–21). This means that if the femoral component had been placed directly parallel to the transepicondylar axis, that significant flexion space imbalance may have occurred. As stated earlier, flexion space balancing with any mobile-bearing device must be precise with little room for error. I have never experienced a bearing spin-out after using the LCS-RP device for more than 10 years, but I am very meticulous with balancing ligaments. Recently, computer navigation using the Universal Total Knee application of the Medtronic Tria system has been used to assess final ligament balance. My goal is to be within 1 mm or degree of perfect in full extension and less than 3 mm or degrees at 90 degrees of flexion. These objectives are consistent to our prior fluoroscopic videokinematic studies done on excellent postoperative mobile-bearing LCS total knees where the maximal amount of component lift-off was 3.2 mm.

References

1. Argenson J-N, O'Connor JJ: Polyethylene wear in meniscal knee replacement: A one to nine-year retrieval analysis of the Oxford knee. J Bone Joint Surg Br 74:228, 1992.
2. Bartel DL, Bicknell VL, Wright TM: The effect of conformity, thickness, and material on stresses in ultra-high molecular weight components for total joint replacement. J Bone Joint Surg Am 68:1041, 1986.
3. Bert JM: Dislocation/subluxation of meniscal bearing elements after New Jersey low-contact stress total knee arthroplasty. Clin Orthop Relat Res 254:211, 1990.
4. Boldt JG, Stiehl JB, Thuemler P: Femoral rotation based on tibial axis. In Hamelynck KJ, Stiehl JB (eds): LCS Mobile Bearing Knee Arthroplasty: 25 Years of Worldwide Experience. Heidelberg, Springer Verlag, 2002, pp 175-182.
5. Buechel FF: Complications and management: Bearing exchange. In Hamelynck KJ, Stiehl JB (eds): LCS Mobile Bearing Knee Arthroplasty: 25 Years of Worldwide Experience. Heidelberg, Springer Verlag, 2002, pp 241-245.
6. Buechel FF Sr, Buechel FF Jr, Pappas MJ, D'Alessio J: Twenty-year evaluation of the New Jersey LCS rotating platform knee replacement. J Knee Surg 15:84, 2002.
7. Buechel FF, Pappas MJ: The New Jersey low-contact-stress knee replacement system: Biomechanical rationale and review of the first 123 cemented cases. Arch Orthop Traumatic Surg 105:197, 1986.
8. Buechel FF, Pappas MJ: New Jersey low contact stress knee replacement system: Ten-year evaluation of meniscal bearings. Orthop Clin North Am 20:147, 1989.
9. Buechel FF, Rosa RA, Pappas MJ: A metal-backed, rotating-bearing patellar prosthesis to lower contact stress: An 11-year clinical study. Clin Orthop Relat Res 248:34-49, 1989.
10. Burki H, VonKnoch M, Heiss C, et al: Lateral approach with osteotomy of the tibial tubercle in primary total knee arthroplasty. Clin Orthop Rel Res 362:156-161, 1999.
11. Callaghan JJ, Squire MW, Goetz DD, et al: Cemented rotating-platform total knee replacement. J Bone Joint Surg Am 82:705-711, 2000.
12. Collier JP, Mayor MB, McNamara JL, et al: Impact of gamma sterilization on clinical performance of polyethylene in the knee. J Arthroplasty 11:377-389, 1996.
13. Collier JP, Williams IR, Mayor MB: Retrieval analysis of mobile bearing prosthetic knee devices. In Hamelynck KJ, Stiehl JB (eds): LCS Mobile Bearing Knee Arthroplasty: 25 Years of Worldwide Experience. Heidelberg, Springer Verlag, 2002, pp 74-80.

14. Dennis DA, Komistek RD, Colwell CE, et al: In vivo anteroposterior femorotibial translation of total knee arthrplasty: A multicenter analysis. Clin Orthop Relat Res 356:47-57, 1998.

15. Dennis DA, Komistek RD, Hoff WA, Gabriel SM: In vivo kinematics derived using an inverse perspective technique. Clin Orthop Relat Res 331:107-117, 1996.

16. Gabriel SM, Dennis DA, Koomistek RD, et al: In vivo TKA kinematics with consequences for system stresses and strains. Proceedings of the 42nd Annual Meeting Orthopaedic Research Society, February 18-22, 1996, Atlanta, p 201.

17. Goodfellow JW, O'Connor JJ: The mechanics of the knee and prosthesis design. J Bone Joint Surg Br 60:358, 1978.

18. Goodfellow JW, O'Connor JJ: Clinical results of the Oxford knee: Surface arthroplasty of the tibiofemoral joint with a meniscal bearing prosthesis. Clin Orthop Relat Res 205:21, 1986.

19. Haas B, Stiehl JB, Komistek RD: Kinematic comparison of posterior cruciate sacrifice versus substitution in a mobile bearing total knee arthroplasty. J Arthroplasty 17:685-691, 2002.

20. Hamelynck KJ, Stiehl JB, Voorhorst PE: LCS worldwide multicenter outcome study. In Hamelynck KJ, Stiehl JB (eds): LCS Mobile Bearing Knee Arthroplasty: 25 Years of Worldwide Experience. Heidelberg, Springer Verlag, 2002, pp 212-224.

21. Jordan LR, Olivo JL, Voorhorst PE: Survivorship analysis of cementless meniscal bearing total knee arthroplasty. Clin Orthop Relat Res 338:119, 1997.

22. Keblish PA: The lateral approach to the valgus knee. Surgical technique and analysis of 53 cases with over two-year follow-up examination. Clin Orthop Relat Res 271:52-62, 1991.

23. Keblish PA, Varma AK, Greenwald AS: Patellar resurfacing or retention in total knee arthroplasty: A prospective study of patients with bilateral replacements. J Bone Joint Surg Br 76:930, 1994.

24. Konermann WH, Saur MA: Postoperative alignment of conventional and navigated total knee arthroplasty. In Stiehl JB, Knoermann WH, Haaker RG (eds): Navigation and Robotics. Heidelberg, Springer Verlag, 2004, pp 219-225.

25. McEwan HMJ, McNulty DE, Auger DD, et al: Wear-analysis of mobile bearing knee. In Hamelynck KJ, Stiehl JB (eds): LCS Mobile Bearing Knee Arthroplasty: 25 Years of Worldwide Experience. Heidelberg, Springer Verlag, 2002, pp 67-73.

26. McNamara JL, Collier JP, Mayor MB, Jensen RE: A comparison of contact pressures in tibial and patellar total knee components before and after service in vivo. Clin Orthop Relat Res 299:104, 1994.

27. Murray DW, Goodfellow JW, O'Connor JJ: The Oxford medial unicompartmental arthroplasty: A ten-year survival study. J Bone Joint Surg Br 80:983-989, 1998.

28. Oakeshott RD, Komistek RD, Stiehl JB: The A/P Glide Knee Prosthesis—Rationale, kinematics and results. In Hamelynck KJ, Stiehl JB (eds): LCS Mobile Bearing Knee Arthroplasty: 25 Years of Worldwide Experience. Heidelberg, Springer Verlag, 2002, pp 313-320.

29. Oakeshott R, Stiehl JB, Komistek RD, et al: Kinematics of a posterior cruciate retaining mobile-bearing total knee arthroplasty. J Arthroplasty 18:1029-1037, 2003.

30. O'Connor JJ, Goodfellow JW: Theory and practice of meniscal knee replacement: Designing against wear. Proc Inst Mech Eng 210:217, 1996.

31. Plante-Bordeneuve P, Freeman MA: Tibial high-density polyethylene wear in conforming tibiofemoral prostheses. J Bone Joint Surg Br 75:630-636, 1993.

32. Psychoyios V, Crawford RW, O'Connor JL: Wear of congruent meniscal bearings in unicompartmental knee arthroplasty: A retrieval study of 16 specimens. J Bone Joint Surg Br 80:976-982, 1998.

33. Sorrells RB: Primary knee arthroplasty: Long-term outcomes: The rotating platform mobile bearing TKA. Orthopedics 19:793, 1996.

34. Sorrels RB, Greenwald SA: Noncemented rotating platform total knee replacement: A five- to twelve-year follow-up study. J Bone Joint Surg 86A:2156-2162, 2005.

35. Sorrels RB, Stiehl JB, Voorhorst P: Long results of mobile bearing total knee arthroplasty in patients under 65. Clin Orthop Relat Res 390:182-189, 2001.

36. Stiehl JB: Knee kinematics and mobile bearings: New design considerations. Curr Opin Orthop 12:18-25, 2001.

37. Stiehl JB: The spectrum of prosthesis design for primary total knee arthroplasty. Instructional Course Lecture 52:397-407, 2003.

38. Stiehl JB, Dennis DA, Komistek RD, Crane HS: In vivo determination of condylar lift-off and screw-home in a mobile-bearing total knee arthroplasty. J Arthroplasty 14:293-299, 1999.

39. Stiehl JB, Dennis DA, Komistek RD, Keblish PA: Kinematic analysis of a mobile bearing total knee arthroplasty. Clin Orthop Relat Res 345:60-65, 1997.

40. Stiehl JB, Dennis DA, Komistek RD, Keblish PA: In vivo kinematics of the patellofemoral joint in total knee arthroplasty. J Arthroplasty 16:706-714 , 2001.

41. Stiehl JB, Hamelunck KJ, Briard JL: The unstable knee. In Hamelynck KJ, Stiehl JB (eds): LCS Mobile Bearing Knee Arthroplasty: 25 Years of Worldwide Experience. Heidelberg, Springer Verlag, 2002, pp 246-252.

42. Stiehl JB, Komistek RD, Dennis DA: In vivo kinematic comparison of posterior cruciate retention or sacrifice with a mobile bearing total knee arthroplasty. Am J Knee Surg 13:13-18, 2000.

43. Stiehl JB, Komistek RD, Dennis DA, Paxson RD: Fluoroscopic analysis of kinematics after posterior cruciate-retaining knee arthroplasty. J Bone Joint Surg Br 77:884-889, 1995.

44. Stiehl JB, Konermann WH, Haaker RG: Principles of computer assisted surgery. In Bellemans J, Ries M, Victor J (eds): Total Knee Arthroplasty—A Guide to get Better Performance. Heidelberg, Springer Verlag, 2005.

45. Stiehl JB, Voorhorst PE: Total knee arthroplasty with a mobile-bearing prosthesis: Comparison of retention and sacrifice of the posterior cruciate ligament in cementless implants. Am J Orthop 28:223-228, 1999.

46. Stiehl JB, Voorhorst PE, Keblish PA, Sorrells RB: Comparison of range of motion after posterior cruciate-retention or sacrifice with a mobile bearing total knee arthroplasty. Am J Knee Surg 10:216-220, 1997.

47. Thompson NW, Wilson DS, Cran GW, et al: Dislocation of the rotating platform following low contact stress total knee arthroplasty. Clin Orthop Relat Res 425:207-211, 2004.

48. Weaver JK, Derkash RS, Greenwald SD: Difficulties with bearing dislocation and breakage using a movable bearing total knee replacement system. Clin Orthop Relat Res 290:244, 1993.

CHAPTER 88

Patellar Resurfacing in Total Knee Arthroplasty

John Gallagher • Cecil Rorabeck • Robert Bourne

Total knee arthroplasty (TKA) has been performed since the 1950s,[125-127] but it was not until 1974 that the first patellar resurfacing component for TKA was introduced. Since its advent, multiple patellar resurfacing designs have become available, with two basic options—inset or onlay—existing. Traditional indications for patellar resurfacing have been based on a wide range of variables, but no single indication has been universally accepted yet. This lack of consensus has resulted in surgeons' being subdivided into those who always resurface the patella, those who never resurface, and those who sometimes do.

For surgeons performing patellofemoral resurfacing in TKA, knowledge of several key areas, including anatomy and biomechanics of the patellofemoral joint, current implant designs, and different surgical indications and techniques, helps to optimize outcomes and minimize the likelihood of complications particular to this procedure. When a TKA revision is to be performed in the setting of a previous patellar resurfacing, careful consideration must be given to the integrity of the components fixation, degree of wear, implant design, patellofemoral tracking, and quality and quantity of the remaining patellar bone stock. The advent of trabecular metal holds some promise for patellofemoral resurfacing when there has been significant loss of bone stock.

The body of knowledge on patellar resurfacing in TKA gathered since the 1970s has largely been one of equivalence between resurfacing and nonresurfacing. In more recent years, there has been a gradual trend toward favoring patellar resurfacing. Nonetheless, more randomized, blinded, controlled trials with long-term follow-up are required before the question of whether to resurface the patella or not can be answered unequivocally. Regardless of one's current belief—whether it be always to resurface, sometimes to resurface, or never to resurface the patella—there are important factors that, when considered, help to optimize patellofemoral function in TKA.

HISTORY

The first patellar resurfacing in TKA was performed in 1974 using a polyethylene dome design for the Insall-Burstein total condylar knee replacement (Zimmer, Warsaw, IN).[2] Patellar resurfacing was developed in an attempt to address residual anterior "patellofemoral" knee pain, which had occurred in 40% to 58% of these earliest TKAs, and to assist with patellofemoral tracking.[30,32,43,49,63,65,66,93,94,101,102] Initially an anterior flange on the femoral component was introduced to replace half of the patellofemoral joint. This feature did not improve the results, and subsequently a complete patellar resurfacing replacement was designed and developed.[2]

In addition to the problems experienced with residual anterior knee pain, the earliest TKA designs were associated with a high (6%) rate of patellar subluxation and dislocation, which was believed to be due to the absence of a well-defined patellar groove and a lack of provision for axial rotation of the patella.[93] Although early designs, including the total condylar knee implant, allowed only limited flexion to 90 degrees, the Insall-Burstein total condylar and posterior stabilized knee implants, introduced in 1977, allowed increased flexion and with it increased patellofemoral stress. Despite the newer designs, patellofemoral problems persisted, and although many surgeons had attributed early improved outcomes in TKA to the advent of patellofemoral resurfacing, with its growing use came increasing reports of complications particular to this new component.

Initial complication rates ranged from 4% to 50%.[20,36,52,94,99] Complications included patellar fracture, extensor mechanism disruption, patellar polyethylene wear, aseptic loosening, instability and dislocation, patellar clunk syndrome, osteonecrosis, and over-restoration or "overstuffing" of the patellofemoral joint space and catastrophic failure.* As a result of the early high complication rate, many surgeons decided not to adopt the practice of routinely resurfacing the patella, and some surgeons who had begun to do so now avoided its use.

Further advances were made, and in 1983 a deeper, more congruent patellar groove was created in these implants to enhance stability and improve tracking.[65,123] A deepened patellar sulcus and more medial placement of the patellar component were shown to reproduce more normal patellar tracking.[147] The same study showed that patellar displacement into the intercondylar notch was improved by narrowing and shortening of the notch. Another important factor was shown to be the effect of the rotational alignment of the femoral and tibial components of the knee prosthesis on patellar tracking. Rotational alignment along the epicondylar axis and lateral placement of the femoral component have been shown to improve patellar tracking in TKA.[111,123]

---

*References 1, 27, 30, 44, 45, 81-83, 93, 103, 115, 135, 136, 142, 145.

Many contemporary knee replacement prostheses now have "patella-friendly" designs with a more anatomic shaped trochlear groove and patellar button. These prostheses allow for less point loading, enhanced stability, and improved tracking of the patella regardless of whether or not the patella is resurfaced, as opposed to femoral implants with a flange designed to articulate with a nonanatomic polyethylene component.

Although many surgeons advocate patellar resurfacing as a routine part of TKA,[63,65,101] others continue to avoid resurfacing the patella, citing a high complication rate and questionable benefits associated with resurfacing. From these two camps has arisen a third, middle group of surgeons, advocating "selective resurfacing of the patella" in TKA.[36,49,72,99] This current lack of uniformity in surgical preferences for the management of the patella in TKA is a reflection of the literature until more recent years, with each camp having been able to find support in the literature for their respective positions.

ANATOMY

Patella

The patella is the largest sesamoid bone in the body, with the thickest articular cartilage of any of the joints. Its articular surface is divided into lateral and medial segments by a thick vertical median ridge, with the medial side being subdivided further into the medial facet and the most medial or "odd" facet. The larger lateral segment or facet accounts for about two-thirds of the articular surface area. The premorbid depth of articular cartilage of the patella usually is between 6 mm and 10 mm,[18] with the overall anteroposterior thickness or depth of the patella being between 21 mm and 25 mm.

All patellar implants, whether inlay or onlay, require removal of varying degrees of bone to achieve an appropriately shaped cancellous bed that allows for satisfactory positioning and fixation of the implant. Various caliper systems exist for measuring the patellar thickness. This step is helpful when trying to confirm that one has restored patellar thickness after resurfacing, but also is an invaluable tool to help avoid attempting to perform a patellar resurfacing where there is inadequate bone stock to support an implant. Most knee replacement systems can accommodate an implant with a native patellar thickness of 18 mm or more, but a thickness of less than 15 mm is a relative contraindication for resurfacing of the patella. Patellar thickness less than 15 mm may arise in patients with small body size, excessive osteochondral loss from arthritis, previous trauma or surgery, and, less commonly, patella hypoplasia.

Patellar tendon height also may be an issue when considering resurfacing. The patella itself may be located at an abnormally high (alta) or low (infra) position within the extensor mechanism.[64] Altered patellar height may occur as a result of a developmental anomaly, trauma, previous surgery, or joint line alteration after the TKA. This altered height may influence the degree of difficulty in resurfacing the patella and the subsequent stresses

imposed on the patellar implant and possibly predispose to abnormal tracking, subluxation, impingement, or recurrent dislocation.

Femur

The normal architecture of the distal femur is complex with asymmetric shape and dimensions of the femoral condyles. The medial femoral condyle is the larger of the two with a more symmetric radius of curvature. The deepest point of the trochlear groove, the sulcus, commences proximally slightly lateral to the midpoint between the condyles and migrates medially as it progresses distally. Reproducing this anatomic relationship is important for patellofemoral tracking regardless of whether or not the patella is resurfaced during TKA. Often in advanced arthritis or in a revision setting with altered anatomy, it may be difficult to achieve accurate orientation. As a guide to correct rotational placement of the femoral component, numerous axes exist, including the transepicondylar, the posterior condylar, and the anteroposterior (Whiteside line) axes (Fig. 88–1).

The epicondylar axis passes through the center of the medial and lateral epicondyles, with the posterior condylar line being a line tangent to the posteriormost surfaces

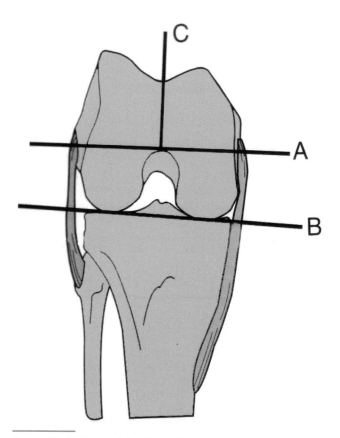

Figure 88–1. Axes of the distal femur—a guide for femoral component rotation. As a guide to correct rotational placement of the femoral component, numerous axes exist, including transepicondylar axis **(A)**, posterior condylar axis **(B)**, and anteroposterior axis (Whiteside line) **(C)**.

of both femoral condyles. In patients in whom normal knee alignment exists, the epicondylar axis in men is externally rotated relative to the posterior condylar line on average 3.5 degrees (±1.2 degrees) compared with 0 degrees (±1.2 degrees) in women.[15] With valgus osteoarthritis, and associated loss of the posterior lateral femoral condyle, the epicondylar axis may be externally rotated 10 degrees. When these epicondyles are difficult to identify, a line approximately perpendicular to this, running along the anteroposterior axis, is useful. This line runs from the center of the femoral trochlea to the midpoint of the intercondylar notch and is commonly referred to as the Whiteside line (see Fig. 88–1).[5]

The patella normally articulates with the distal femur at about 20 degrees of flexion engaging the trochlear groove and undergoing approximately 7 cm of excursion from extension to full flexion. Although the pull of the patellar tendon is vertical, the pull of the quadriceps is oblique, in line with the shaft of the femur. The combined force vector of the patella tendon and quadriceps contraction tends to draw the patella laterally. Three factors (bony, ligamentous, and muscular) discourage this lateral dislocation: the forward prominence of the lateral femoral condyle, the medial patellar retinaculum, and the lowest fibers of vastus medialis.

PATELLAR VASCULARITY

The arterial supply of the patella was well defined by Scapinelli[117] as receiving an extraosseous and intraosseous arterial inflow. A peripatellar anastomotic ring, from the supreme, superior medial, superior lateral, inferior medial, and inferior lateral geniculate arteries, constitutes the extraosseous blood supply. The intraosseous vascularity arises from a midpatellar, an apical, and a quadriceps tendon vessel. Portions of the extraosseous and intraosseous supply to the patella routinely are disrupted during a TKA, and other specific surgical maneuvers risk the loss of the remaining vascularity. Knee arthrotomy, lateral release, meniscectomy, and denervation procedures have the potential to compromise the extraosseous supply, whereas fat-pad excision and arthrotomy placement threaten the intraosseous supply. The clinical consequences of patellar devascularization have been shown with an increased incidence of patellar stress fractures, fragmentation, and loosening.[101,104]

A medial peripatellar arthrotomy routinely divides the superior medial, inferior medial, and supreme geniculate arteries. Placement of the arthrotomy, whether medial or lateral, risks disruption of a significant portion of the anastomotic ring. Cadaveric dye injections have shown that arthrotomies placed within 1 cm of the medial or lateral patellar border interrupt the intraosseous vessels.[70] Complete lateral meniscectomy may result in division of the inferior lateral geniculate artery, leaving the superior lateral vessel as the sole extraosseous blood supply to the patella. Débridement of the infrapatellar fat pad further endangers patellar vascularity by means of disruption of the radial intraosseous vessels.[70] If a lateral release is required, preservation of the superior lateral geniculate

artery is mandatory. This vessel can be isolated in the subsynovial layer 1 to 2 cm distal to the inferior border of the vastus lateralis muscle. Knees with a significant preoperative valgus deformity (typically >20 degrees), in which a lateral release can be anticipated, warrant consideration of a lateral arthrotomy for exposure.[71] This approach ensures preservation of the superior medial, inferior medial, and supreme geniculate vessels in such clinical scenarios.

Technetium-99m bone scanning has been employed to assess postoperative patellar vascularity. Wetzner and colleagues[144] examined 41 consecutive TKAs to assess the potential development of postoperative avascular necrosis of the patella. Four patellae were noted to have decreased uptake, suggesting increased risk for the development of avascular necrosis. Scuderi and associates[124] compared the clinical effect of lateral release on patellar viability after TKA. The addition of a lateral release increased the incidence of vascular compromise from 15% to 56.4%. Only one of the knees requiring a lateral release had a postoperative complication, however—a patellar fracture not requiring surgical intervention. McMahon and coworkers[90] further investigated the effect of lateral release in conjunction with infrapatellar fat-pad excision. In 70 knees undergoing TKA, excision of the infrapatellar fat pad was not identified as an independent variable for compromise of patellar vascularity.

Ritter and Campbell[112] examined the consequences of lateral release in TKA. Forty-eight patients underwent simultaneous bilateral procedures, in which one knee had a lateral release and the other did not. The knees were compared on the basis of clinical scores, radiographic findings, and technetium bone scans. No differences were noted between the two groups. No patellae developed signs of osteonecrosis. Similarly, Ritter and colleagues[113] compared 84 knees requiring lateral release and 471 without lateral release, showing no increase in prevalence of avascular necrosis, patellar component loosening, or fracture.

BIOMECHANICS

The main biomechanical function of the patella is to increase the moment arm of the quadriceps mechanism.[69] It acts as a dynamic fulcrum to transmit the forces generated by the extensor mechanism through the knee, and it provides 50% increase in knee extension strength compared with that after patellectomy.[148] The patellofemoral joint sustains some of the greatest contact pressures of all the joints in the human body. Normal walking generates approximately 50% body weight joint reaction forces, which increases to nearly eight times body weight for jumping from a small height.[109] The tremendous forces generated across the patella by even simple daily activities and its at-risk position for injury help to explain why degenerative arthritis of the patellofemoral joint is relatively common.

After successful TKA, increased ranges of flexion often are achieved, which results in increased force transmission across the patellofemoral joint.[60,61,88] The resurfaced patella also has been reported to be subjected to a 30% to

40% increase in strain and decrease in tensile strength compared with the native patella.[109]

These altered biomechanics at the patellofemoral joint have been proposed as a cause for anterior knee pain after TKA, and the decreased thickness of bone and increased strain are proposed as factors associated with increased risk of fracture with patellar resurfacing in TKA. The risk of fracture may be increased when resurfacing is combined with a lateral retinacular release, which may devascularize the extensor mechanism.[70,124]

More recent studies have shown that patellofemoral contact stresses are influenced by the design of the femoral component regardless of whether or not the patella is resurfaced.[14,29,87,89,98] In vivo and in vitro studies have shown that a deeper trochlear groove extending farther distally, with an anatomic radius of curvature, reproduces the most normal tracking by resurfaced and native patellae.[4,87,89,138] Similarly the kinematics of the tibiofemoral joint may influence patellofemoral contact force and must be considered.[92] A trochlear groove on the anterior flange that is more lateral to the midline and that gradually transitions toward the center in the distal region has been shown to approximate more closely the anatomy of the native knee and may reduce the need for a lateral retinacular release.[34]

It has been suggested that external rotation of the femoral component lateralizes the proximal end of the trochlear groove, ideally improving patellar tracking in extension. With flexion of more than 90 degrees, however, external rotation actually medializes the patellar tracking, resulting in increased patellofemoral shear stresses and potentially higher rates of wear and loosening of the patellar component and of fracture. External rotation of the femoral component increases the risk of notching on the anterolateral femoral cortex and decreases the contact between the femoral component and the anteromedial femoral cortex. To overcome this problem, the design of the femoral component in some TKA systems was modified to incorporate the external rotation into the femoral implant (Fig. 88–2). This design accommodates the resurfaced or nonresurfaced patella, and a decreased prevalence of lateral release and improved patellofemoral tracking have been noted with this design.[68]

A cadaveric study was performed with a load simulator to determine the differences in the contact and tracking characteristics of unresurfaced patellae[137] in five different TKA designs: Miller-Galante II (Zimmer), Anatomic Modular Knee (AMK) (DePuy, Warsaw, IN), Whiteside Ortholoc Modular (Dow Corning Wright, Arlington, TN), Press Fit Condylar (PFC) (Johnson & Johnson Professional, Raynham, MA), and Insall-Burstein II. Articulation of the normal patella with a prosthetic femoral component altered the normal patellofemoral contact and tracking characteristics. The exact departure depended on the design of the prosthetic trochlea. Although all of the selected prostheses showed satisfactory contact characteristics near extension, marked alterations occurred at greater flexion angles. With 90 degrees or more of flexion, there was incompatibility between the geometry of the notch of two designs of the femoral component (AMK and PFC) and the normal knee. This study showed that when determining whether or not to resurface the patella at the

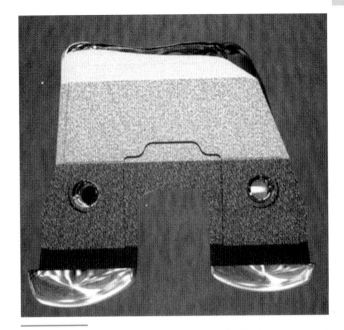

Figure 88–2. Femoral component with built-in external rotation—Genesis II total knee replacement. In the Genesis II knee implant (Smith & Nephew, Memphis, TN), a thicker lateral and a thinner medial posterior femoral condyle allow the 3 degrees of external rotation to be built into the implant rather than onto the distal part of the femur.

time of TKA, the design of the prosthetic femoral component must be taken into account.

IMPLANT DESIGNS

There are two basic contemporary designs of the patellar resurfacing implant—an inlay or onlay design.[76] The onlay designs are subdivided further into all-polyethylene components or a metal-backed component. Metal-backed patellar components were plagued by a high rate of failure in so-called first-generation designs, and although they still are used in certain knee prostheses with good results, they represent a smaller portion of the patella resurfacing implants being used in TKA.

Inlay Designs

The inlay or inset prosthesis was first designed by Freeman and colleagues.[43] It was proposed that the inset patella would result in less reduction of the overall patellar strength but would provide better resistance to shear stress. Implant shape for an inset patella is usually a small circular dome with a single fixation peg.

Two studies[37,105] have compared inlay with onlay prostheses. A comparison study of onlay and inlay patellar components with the same posterior cruciate ligament–sparing TKA was performed by Rand and Gustilo[105] in 1996. Their study showed that there was no difference in anterior knee pain or stair-climbing ability between the two groups, but that patellar tracking problems, patellar subluxation, and patellar tilt occurred less often with the inset patella. A subsequent cadaveric study by Ezzet and colleagues[37] in 2001 compared the biomechanics of an oval dome onlay component with an inlay biconvex circular dome component, using the same posterior cruciate ligament–sparing knee prosthesis. In contrast to Rand and Gustilo's study, the inset patella shifted and tilted laterally with knee flexion significantly more than the onlay patella. It is difficult to assert that the inset patella offers any clear advantage over the onlay patella with regard to tilt and subluxation. The theoretical advantage of more resistance to shear stress is tempered by the fact that it has been shown in at least one study[105] to have a higher incidence of radiolucent lines than the onlay devices.

Onlay Patella

Although the onlay patella has a long history of clinical use, the optimal shape for the component is still unknown with a variety of shapes available, including a circular or an oval-shaped dome, an oval-shaped or a dome-shaped sombrero, or a metal-backed implant. Likewise the best method of fixation has not been established, with current options being a choice between a single large central peg or three smaller peripheral pegs and cemented versus uncemented (porous metal-backed) implants.[76]

The cemented all-polyethylene onlay patella design has a successful long-standing clinical track record with a single large central peg. It has evolved to a newer three-peg fixation system with the theoretical benefits of better fixation against shear stress, reduced risk of interfering with the intraosseous blood supply, and a reduced patellar fracture risk. One study[79] showed the rate of patellar fracture being more than halved by having a three-peg design (2.1%) compared with the single-peg design (4.7%), but was unable to achieve statistical significance. The disadvantage of the three-peg designs largely revolves around the increased risk of breakage of the three fixation pegs and subsequent implant loosening, with two studies having reported such fatigue failure of the small pegs in these newer cemented, all-polyethylene patellar components.[42,59]

Metal-backed patellar onlay components have had a history with mixed results. Their design took into account several factors, including the total thickness of the implants, the thickness of the polyethylene, the modulus of elasticity of the polyethylene, the means of fixation of the polyethylene to the metal, the proportion of the polyethylene that is backed by metal, and the thickness and strength of the metal plate.[136] These components were proposed as having a theoretical benefit of uniform load transmission by the metal base plate to the underlying patellar bone and the decreased tendency of the metal-backed polyethylene to deform under stress. The theoretical benefits did not translate into improved outcomes, however—quite the opposite, with a high percentage of component failures. These failures resulted in significant joint particle debris generation, a metal-on-metal articulation, and a

metal-induced proliferative synovitis requiring a greater than 50% revision rate at 10 years.[12,78,82,100,115,132]

The newer, second-generation metal-backed implants have had much better results, with the most extensively reported of these being the rotating-bearing patella of the Low Contact Stress (LCS) (DePuy, Johnson & Johnson, Warsaw, IN) TKA system. With this device, an anatomic shaped polyethylene implant rotates freely on a polished base plate, offering a theoretical advantage of improved tracking with lower contact stress and subsequent reduced wear. The base plate of this implant is fully porous coated.[24] Good results with other metal-backed patella components also have been reported with the Natural (Intermedics, Austin, TX) and Ortholoc (Wright Medical, Memphis, TN) total knee systems.[75] Although long-term failure rates of less than 1% have been achieved,[24] their implantation is technically more demanding, requiring more precise bony preparation, and has an increased risk of bone loss or patellar fracture or both in a revision setting where there has been good bony ongrowth. Overall, despite the many studies trying to show the advantage of one patellar design over another, owing to the multiple confounding variables (including technique, preoperative diagnosis and degree of osteopenia, postoperative range of motion, and patient activity level and preservation or sacrifice of at least one of the geniculate arteries), it is impossible to advance one design (polyethylene inlay, polyethylene onlay, metal-backed onlay) over another.

SURGICAL INDICATIONS

Traditional indications for patellar resurfacing have been based on numerous factors, including age, weight, gender, patellar anatomy, quality of articular cartilage, preoperative anterior knee pain, inflammatory arthropathy, and radiographic findings. There are no absolute indications for patellar resurfacing, but numerous relative indications have been proposed (Table 88–1).*

There are situations in which it is impossible to resurface the patella, such as previous patellectomy or when siginificant erosion from wear or previous surgery has left inadequate bone stock to receive a patellar component. The cutoff for the thickness of the native patella that safely allows patellar resurfacing is determined by surgeon-related and implant-related factors, but a thickness of 18 mm or more usually is considered safe and a thickness of 15 mm or less usually is considered unsafe. Other relative contraindications for surfacing the patella are listed in Table 88–1.

Of all the indications for resurfacing, inflammatory arthritis has been the most widely accepted. Many authors have recommended routine resurfacing for all patients with rheumatoid arthritis,[11,81,99,101,120,121,131] although others offer evidence not to resurface in the same condition.[20,39,130] Overall, patients with rheumatoid arthritis as a group seem to be more satisfied with the results of TKA than patients with osteoarthritis, regardless of whether the

*References 11, 19-21, 26, 38, 39, 52, 73, 81, 99, 101, 116, 120, 121, 130-132, 134, 135, 141, 146.

patella had been resurfaced. This finding has been confirmed by the Swedish Knee Arthroplasty Register.[116]

Many surgeons have adopted a "selective resurfacing" approach,[20,73,81,99,141] in which their default technique is *not* to resurface the patella, unless their selective criteria are met (Table 88–2). Some surgeons have taken the opposite approach, "selectively nonresurface," choosing always to resurface the patella, unless their selective criteria not to resurface exist. Two different studies[73,81] have used identical criteria for selectively nonresurfacing the patella in TKA (see Table 88–2).

SURGICAL TECHNIQUES

The patella may be resurfaced using an inlay or onlay surgical technique or, alternatively, left nonresurfaced. If the patella is not resurfaced, it may undergo a "tidy up" procedure, described by some as a patelloplasty. The key technical steps of each of these three procedures are described.

Table 88–1. Relative Indications for Patellar Resurfacing and Nonresurfacing in Total Knee Arthroplasty

RESURFACING INDICATIONS	NONRESURFACING INDICATIONS
Older age	Younger age
Anterior knee pain	Noninflammatory arthritis
Inflammatory arthropathy	Thin patients
Obesity	Thin/hypoplastic patella
Female	Intraoperative preserved patellar cartilage
History of patellar subluxation and maltracking	Intraoperative congruent patellar tracking
Intraoperative patellofemoral wear	Anatomic trochlea groove on femoral implant
Intraoperative patellar maltracking	
Nonanatomic trochlea groove on femoral implant	

Inlay Patellar Resurfacing

With an inlay technique, a round all-polyethylene component is recessed into a hole reamed into the patella. Fixation is achieved using a single small polyethylene peg and cement. Before performing any bony preparation, selection of the appropriate-size component is achieved by using a series of templates and ensuring that the component will have maximal contact surface area but still be contained safely within the boundary of the articular margins. Attention is given to the location of the median ridge, and the template is centered here midway between the superior and inferior limit of the articular surface. A peripheral rim of at least 2 mm along the medial border is recommended, with most surgeons on a practical note implanting the patella button just lateral to the odd facet. The reaming jig usually has a clamp system built in, and when positioned correctly, the clamp should be tightened and held firmly to avoid loss of position.

The depth (anteroposterior thickness) of the native patella can be measured before reaming using a caliper system. To avoid overreaming (and subsequent understuffing or possibly breaching the anterior cortex), the depth-stop of the patellar reamer is set, and the patella is reamed to produce a cancellous inlay surface with a single circular peg hole. To ensure that enough bone has been removed (and to avoid subsequent overstuffing), when the reaming has been performed, the trial component is positioned, and the depth is remeasured, aiming to be within 1 mm either side of the original measure. More bone may be removed by additional increments if necessary. With the trial in place, final contouring of the surrounding osteochondral edges may be performed to avoid a step deformity between the native patella and the patella implant.

Onlay Patellar Resurfacing

Although it is recognized that some surgeons perform the flat cut freehand without the use of any jigs, it is recommended that a cutting jig be used. Proper resection

Table 88–2. Selective Indications for Patellar Resurfacing and Nonresurfacing in Total Knee Arthroplasty

	SELECTIVELY RESURFACE		SELECTIVELY NONRESURFACE	
Boyd et al[20]	Picetti et al[99]	Vince and McPherson[141]	Levitsky et al[81]	Kim et al[73]
Loss of articular cartilage	Rheumatoid arthritis	Preoperative patellofemoral symptoms	Congruent intraoperative patellofemoral tracking	Congruent intraoperative patellofemoral tracking
Exposed bone	Height >160 cm	Patellar instability	Normal patellar anatomic shape	Normal patellar anatomic shape
Gross surface irregularities	Weight >60 kg	Patellar dysmorphism	Absence of eburnated bone	Absence of eburnated bone
Tracking abnormalities	Preoperative anterior knee pain Intraoperative grade IV chondromalacia	Patellofemoral chondromalacia grade III or higher	Absence of crystalline disease	Absence of crystalline disease
			Absence of inflammatory synovial tissue	Absence of inflammatory synovial tissue

depends on adequate exposure of the articular margins, and the periarticular tissue should be released circumferentially if necessary to allow for correct positioning of the cutting jig clamp and adequate visualization of the intended osteotomy site. Due care and attention should be paid at all times to ensure protection of the patellar tendon and quadriceps mechanism. The recommended line of the osteotomy is from the medial-most edge of the patella to the level of the subchondral bone of the lateral facet. An oscillating saw is used to perform the osteotomy, aiming to leave 10 to 15 mm of residual patellar thickness, with roughly equal depth left medially and laterally.

When a flat surface is obtained, the trial templates are used to establish the implant diameter. The corresponding sized drill hole jig for either a single or three-peg component is placed flush on the cut surface, and fixation holes are drilled. The drill hole jig and the implant usually are positioned toward the medial edge of the patella, medializing the articulation and tracking of the extensor mechanism. Although this technique does not usually offer the same fine control over the exact amount of bony depth removed that the inlay technique offers, a calibrated depth measuring caliper and variable thickness implants are usually available to help restore the original anteroposterior depth of the patella.

Patelloplasty

When a decision is made not to resurface the patella, the patella may be left alone or undergo a "tidy up" procedure, or patelloplasty. Numerous different combinations of surgical steps comprise a patelloplasty. Two of the more commonly accepted techniques for performing a patelloplasty are as follows. Barrack and associates[10] advocate removal of osteophytes, smoothing of fibrillated cartilage, and drilling of eburnated bone as a reasonable approach when the patella is left unresurfaced. Keblish and colleagues[72] described more elaborate patellar preparation, including soft-tissue releases from the lateral aspect of the patella, division of the patellofemoral ligament, electrocautery of the patellar rim to provide partial denervation of the patella, and drilling of multiple sites of the patellar subchondral surface to decompress the subchondral bone.

Regardless of what patellar option is chosen, a trial reduction is performed before cementing of all components, to allow for assessment of the patellar tracking. If the patellar tracking is unsatisfactory, component repositioning or a lateral release should be considered. Usually most knee systems allow for some alteration in tibial tray rotation at this time to help optimize patellar tracking if necessary. The usual alteration if the patella was tending to sublux or dislocate laterally would be to increase the external rotation of the tibial tray; this has a net effect of internally rotating the tibial tuberosity, medializing the extensor mechanism when the tibiofemoral joint is reduced. The femoral component positioning usually cannot be changed at this stage, but if the knee system being used allows it, either external rotation or lateral displacement of the femoral component helps overcome a

tendency toward lateral subluxation. Failing all of these steps, a lateral release should be performed.

When patellofemoral tracking is satisfactory, the tibial tray rotation is marked, and the final tibial preparation is performed. If a patellar replacement is being performed, one should ensure at the time of implantation that the patellar component is fully reduced, and all excess cement around the component is removed before hardening. Care is taken also to ensure that the skin overlying the anterior surface of the patella is not caught in the patella clamp.

PATELLA-SPECIFIC COMPLICATIONS

Complications specific to the patellofemoral articulation include instability, fracture, component loosening, patellar clunk, avascular necrosis, and tendon rupture. Successful patellofemoral resurfacing requires attention devoted to the prevention of such complications.

Patellofemoral Instability

The maintenance of an efficient extensor mechanism, with a stable and well-aligned patella, is crucial to the success of any TKA. Difficulties with postoperative tilting, subluxation, and dislocation can compromise clinical outcomes with either patellar resurfacing or retention.[23] Although the incidence rate of patellar subluxation after resurfacing has been reported as 31%,[17] the incidence rate of clinically symptomatic patellar instability typically has been reported as less than 1%.[22,45,104] Intraoperative attention to technique and assessment of patellar tracking is mandatory to minimize this potential complication (Fig. 88–3). The cause of instability may be ascribed to several interrelated variables, including component malposition, soft-tissue imbalance, and limb malalignment.

Proper selection and positioning of the femoral, tibial, and patellar implants, with consideration of limb alignment and patellofemoral tracking as already discussed (see surgical technique), are essential. The femoral and tibial components must be positioned to avoid medial shift and internal rotation because both of these orientations predispose toward patellar subluxation or tilting.[54,110] Five degrees of external femoral component rotation versus a neutral or 5-degree internally rotated position has been shown to provide superior patellar tracking and knee stability.[5] Newer prosthesis designs incorporate a slight degree of external rotation into the femoral component to facilitate enhanced patellar tracking and decrease the need for additional soft-tissue balancing.[54] For similar reasons, positioning of the patellar component is biased medially, avoiding lateral placement.[48,147]

Also inherent in patellar stability is the appropriate restoration of patellar thickness.[47,57,80,85,109] The use of calipers to assess thickness accurately before and after resurfacing is recommended.[85] When appropriate thickness is restored, the incidence of associated lateral release, performed for intraoperative instability, has been reported

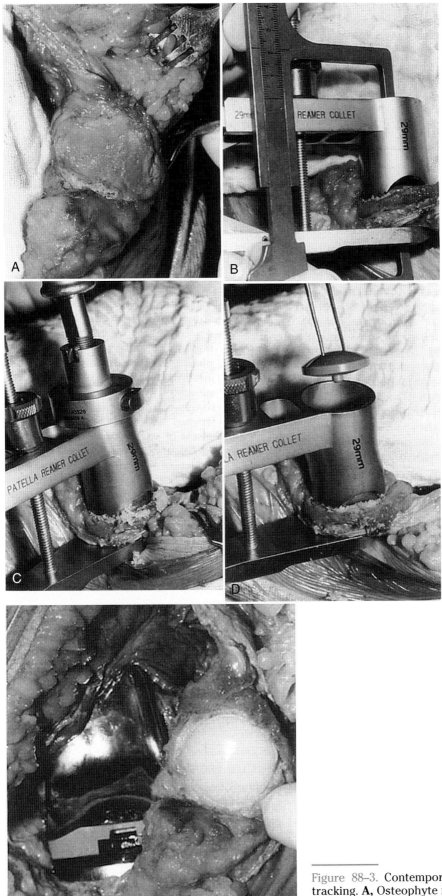

Figure 88–3. Contemporary steps to optimize patellofemoral tracking. **A,** Osteophyte removal. **B,** Patellar thickness measurement—preimplant. **C,** Precise reaming of implant recess. **D,** Patellar thickness measurement—postimplant. **E,** Medialized positioning of patellar implant.

to decrease from 55% to 12.4%.[47] Overstuffing of the knee joint in the anteroposterior plane predisposes to instability. This instability is seen clinically when a femoral implant too large in the anteroposterior dimension is used; the thickness of the patella-patellar implant composite, secondary to inadequate resection of patellar bone; or an oversized patella component is used.[22,45,91,104] With contemporary techniques, lateral retinacular release should be necessary in less than 10% of cases (see Fig. 88–3).

Postoperatively a 45-degree Merchant view is recommended to assess patellar position and fixation. An average of nearly 5 degrees of postoperative patellar tilting has been noted in midflexion with three modern knee designs, despite a satisfactory assessment of intraoperative tracking.[29] The incidence of radiographic patellar tilting has been reported as 31%, with preoperative tilting predisposing to postoperative tilting, regardless of the intraoperative management of the peripatellar soft tissues.[17]

Surgical approach to the knee does not seem to affect patellofemoral stability significantly. Clinically equivalent results, with respect to stability, have been shown with a midvastus and subvastus approach compared with a routine medial parapatellar approach.[35] Symptomatic lateral patellar instability is treated by a proximal realignment with or without component revision. Distal realignment, using a modification of the Trillat procedure, also has been employed successfully to treat recurrent patellar dislocation.[74] Combined proximal and distal realignment is not recommended because of the significant risk of subsequent patellar tendon rupture.[45]

Patellar Fracture

Fractures of the patella after TKA are uncommon.[41,46,55,114,140] Varying causes have been proposed for these fractures, such as vascular compromise, component malposition, patellar subluxation, poor component design, trauma, thermal necrosis, and increased knee flexion. Prevalence reports dealing with modern arthroplasty designs range from 0 to 6.3%.[44,46,140]

Compromise of patellar vascularity has been recognized as a significant predisposing factor for subsequent patellar fracture. Disruption of a significant portion of the patellar blood supply occurs with routine medial peripatellar arthrotomy, with fat-pad excision or lateral release representing an additional insult to the vascularity. Tria and coworkers[140] identified a statistically significant correlation between lateral release and subsequent fracture in TKA. Thermal necrosis secondary to polymethyl methacrylate fixation also has been implicated in patellar fractures.

Excessive patellar resections and insufficient patellar resections may lead to increased patellar fracture risk. A patellar resection, resulting in less than 15 mm of remaining bone, substantially weakens the host bone, increasing anterior patellar strain,[109] whereas inadequate bony resection resulting in a thicker patella–patellar implant composite also causes increased patellofemoral joint reactive forces and increased strain on the component and anterior host bone.[133] Asymmetric patellar resection leads to

eccentric loading of the patellar component and of the underlying host bone. A femoral component too large in the anteroposterior dimension, or with significant anterior translation or flexion, similarly causes increased patellofemoral joint reaction forces.

Limb malalignment can predispose to fracture owing to abnormal patellar tracking with increased contact forces. Figgie and colleagues[40] reported a significant correlation between type of fracture and limb alignment, with major discrepancies in alignment resulting in more severe fractures with less satisfactory outcomes. Deviation from standard positioning of the patellar component also increases the fracture risk because it predisposes to abnormal patellar tracking or patellar component impingement on the tibial insert, typically seen in knees with a large flexion arc.

Treatment is dictated by the extensor mechanism competence, fixation of the patellar implant, and anatomic location.[40,44,46,55,114] The natural history of patellar fractures after TKA was reviewed in detail by Goldberg and associates.[44] Four fracture configurations were identified: Type I fractures occur through the midbody or superior pole, not involving the implant, cement, or quadriceps mechanism; type II fractures disrupt the quadriceps mechanism or implant–bone–cement composite; type IIIA fractures involve the inferior pole with disruption of the patellar tendon; and type IIIB fractures are nondisplaced through the inferior pole. Knees with implant loosening, patellar dislocation, or complete quadriceps disruption (types II and IIIA) require operative intervention. The remaining fractures, type I and type IIIB, were noted to be better treated nonoperatively. Hozack and coworkers[55] also reviewed 21 fractures after TKA, showing satisfactory results with nonoperative management of nondisplaced fractures and displaced fractures without an extensor lag.

Patellar Component Loosening

Most modern patellofemoral resurfacing is accomplished with cement fixation of an all-polyethylene patellar component. Loosening is an uncommon complication; the incidence ranges from 0.6% to 1.3%.[20,23,32,86] Poor cementing technique, insults to the patellar vascularity, deficient host bone, component malposition, trauma, patellar fracture, and inadequate patellar preparation all have been implicated in patellar component loosening. Component design also has been suggested to influence loosening rates.

Although the incidence rate of patellar component loosening is low, the rate of complications related to isolated patellar revision is high. Berry and Rand[16] reported 14 significant complications in 42 knees (34%) undergoing isolated patellar revision: 5 fractures, 3 cases of patellar instability, 2 peroneal nerve palsies, 2 cases of polyethylene wear, 1 deep infection, and 1 knee with an extensor lag. Similarly, Lynch and colleagues[84] noted a 24% complication rate in 37 isolated patellar revisions. Maintenance of an intact extensor mechanism dictates treatment. Options include observation, component revision, component removal and patellar débridement, and patellectomy. Overall, satisfactory results have been obtained in 83% of knees.[16]

Patellar Clunk Syndrome

The patellar "clunk" syndrome, as described by Hozack and colleagues[56] in 1989, may be implicated as a cause of anterior knee pain in certain posterior-stabilized TKAs and other prostheses that do not support the patella adequately in deep flexion. A prominent, hyperplastic fibrous nodule forms at the junction of the proximal pole of the patella and the posterior quadriceps tendon as a result of impingement of the quadriceps tendon against the antero-superior edge of the intercondylar notch. This nodule lodges into the intercondylar notch of the femoral component during flexion and displaces with an audible catch or "clunk" as the quadriceps tendon and patella migrate proximally with extension of the knee. The presence of this clunk is noted especially in knees that have achieved a large flexion arc of motion.

Failure to elevate the quadriceps tendon sufficiently away from the femoral component by failing to reconstitute either the patella height (i.e., patella infra) or its depth (i.e., anteroposterior thickness) through the use of a relatively thin patellar component or excess bone resection has been implicated. Superior placement of the patellar component beyond the proximal border of the patella also may predispose to fibrous nodule formation.

Most knees in which a clunk develops may be asymptomatic initially, but usually progress to being symptomatic. Treatment with either open or arthroscopic débridement is indicated for knees in which symptoms persist. Although arthroscopic débridement of the nodule offers a minimally invasive means of treatment, Beight and coworkers[13] reported 4 recurrences in 11 cases. Recurrence after open arthrotomy with or without patellar component revision has not been reported.

Although reports of the patellar clunk syndrome are limited to certain posterior-stabilized prosthetic designs, Shoji and Shimozaki[129] reported 11 cases of intraoperative patellar clunk syndrome. In these cases, catching was noted with the use of a cruciate-retaining design before patellar resurfacing. The catching was eliminated by patellar resurfacing in four knees and by shaving of the superior pole of the patella in the remaining seven cases.

The development of intra-articular fibrous bands after TKA also has been noted.[139] Similar to the patellar clunk syndrome, fibrous hyperplasia occurs, resulting either in tethering the patella laterally or inferiorly or displacing the patella from the sulcus of the femoral component. Thorpe and associates[139] reported success using arthroscopic débridement.

Tendon Rupture

Rupture of either the quadriceps or the patellar tendon is an infrequent complication after TKA. Reports of incidence vary from 0.17% to 2.5%.[26,86,106,107] Lynch and colleagues[83] reported 3 quadriceps ruptures and 4 patellar tendon ruptures in 281 consecutive TKAs performed with patellar resurfacing. The use of an extensive lateral release may predispose to quadriceps tendon rupture, typically secondary to compromise of tendon vascularity. Patellar tendon rupture or avulsion may be seen in knees with significant preoperative limitations of flexion or previous surgeries. Postoperative manipulation under anesthesia to address arthrofibrosis presents an additional risk for failure of the extensor mechanism.

Treatment of patellar tendon ruptures is fraught with difficulties. Residual extensor lag, quadriceps weakness, increased risk of re-rupture, and limited flexion all have been reported after attempts at repair of such ruptures. Numerous methods of repair and/or augmentation have been reported.[106] Operative repair techniques have been described with staples, screws, autograft, allograft, and synthetic ligament augment reconstruction. The use of a medial gastrocnemius flap to provide tissue for repair and vascular ingrowth has been described.[67] Given the marginal results with either operative or nonoperative approaches, careful attention to surgical technique to avoid these complications is paramount.

REVISION SURGERY

The primary treatment options for the patella in the setting of revision surgery are determined by many factors, including whether the patella was resurfaced during the primary procedure; positioning of the femoral and tibial components; patellar tilt, tracking, and bone stock; and surgeon preference. In general, treatment options where a patellar implant exists in a revision setting include retention of the existing component, removal and insertion of another patellar prosthesis, patellar resection arthroplasty (removal of prosthesis with retention of bony shell), patellar bone grafting with autograft or allograft, and patellectomy.[8]

Results of isolated patellar resurfacing as a revision procedure are at best modest.[16,116] In a review of 2097 revision TKAs,[116] there were 198 cases that had been isolated revisions of an unresurfaced patella to a resurfaced patella. These patients were unsatisfied or uncertain about the result after 53% of these revisions, and overall their satisfaction was lower than that of patients who had undergone a complete exchange of the total knee prosthesis. The femoral and tibial components also must be revised when necessary to allow for satisfactory patellar tracking and to increase the likelihood of an acceptable outcome with any given patellar revision.

In 50% of revision knee replacements, the existing patellar component is well fixed.[8,9] A decision must be made in these circumstances as to whether the prosthetic design being used for the revision would accommodate retention of the patellar component. Laskin[77] published guidelines to help determine when it is reasonable to leave the existing patellar component, when solidly implanted in the revision TKA setting. Laskin[77] recommends leaving the patellar component when the following criteria are met: (1) The existing patellar component has little or no evidence of polyethylene surface wear, (2) the component geometry is reasonably compatible with the femoral trochlea design being implanted, and (3) the patellar prosthesis was appropriately implanted so that positioning and overall patellar height are acceptable for satisfactory patellar tracking.

If the patellar component is loose, malpositioned, or damaged, it should be revised. When the patellar component has been removed, fibrous tissue, remaining cement, polyethylene, or metal lugs should be removed. If cement or metal lugs are well fixed and would not interfere with fixation of another implant, it is acceptable to retain this material rather than risk further loss of bone stock or fracture. The quantity, quality, and location of remaining patellar bone stock should be assessed to determine whether it is sufficient to receive another implant. If 10 mm or more thickness of residual patellar bone stock exists, adequate implant fixation usually can be obtained.[33,50,77] Traditional onlay or inlay techniques can

be used, with any small areas of cavitary bone loss being used for additional cement fixation. If too much cavitary bone loss exists, the patella can be prepared to accept a biconvex polyethylene component. One study[62] showed that when using a thick but small-diameter biconvex patellar component, it was possible to reimplant with 5 mm of central bone, provided that there was good peripheral support.

Finally, in approximately 10% of revision TKAs, severe patellar bone deficiency precludes adequate fixation of another patellar implant.[50] Although previously some surgeons may have considered performing a patellectomy in this situation, this is to be strongly discouraged. Surgical alternatives include the following: patellar resection arthroplasty[7,77,96,97] or patellar bone grafting with structural or morcellized cancellous bone graft using either autograft or allograft techniques or a new development—a trabecular metal patellar implant (Fig. 88–4). Trabecular metal is a biomaterial fabricated from porous tantalum

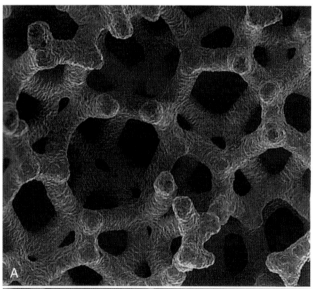

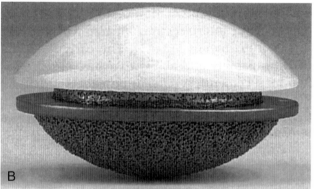

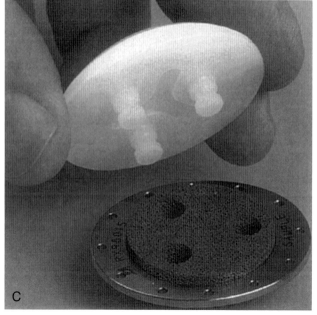

Figure 88–4. The porous tantalum patellar implant—advances in revision arthroplasty. **A,** Scanning electron micrograph of the porous tantalum (Trabecular Metal; Zimmer, Allendale, NJ). **B,** Assembled porous tantalum patellar implant–polyethylene articulating surface with the porous tantalum base. **C,** Disassembled polyethylene and base plate to reveal titanium suture ring.

(Trabecular Metal; Zimmer Trabecular Metal Technology, Inc, Allendale, NJ),[31] and the prosthesis is composed of two parts with three distinct features—a base of porous tantalum, an integral titanium alloy suture ring for initial fixation to the remnant patellar bone and tendon, and a polyethylene articulation surface.

The trabecular metal patellar implant has been designed specifically for use in patellae with severe bone deficiency. The domed porous tantalum base plate sits in a matching spherical concavity within the remnant of the patellar shell prepared by use of spherical reamers. It is secured by using multiple interrupted nonabsorbable sutures. An all-polyethylene articular component (10 mm thick) with three lugs is cemented into the flat posterior surface of the tantalum metal base plate with matching lug holes. Its use was reported in 2004 by Nasser and Poggie[95] in a series of 11 patients with severe patellar bone loss, showing stable implants with improved outcomes and high levels of patient satisfaction in 10 of the 11 patients with a mean follow-up of 32 months.

LITERATURE REVIEW OF OUTCOMES

The natural history of the patella in TKA if left nonresurfaced is an outcome that is central to deciding whether it is justified to resurface the patella at the time of TKA. Shih and colleagues[128] reported in 2003 on a retrospective review of 227 TKAs with patellae left nonresurfaced in 181 patients at an average of 8.5 years. This study showed that 60% of all these knees that underwent TKA had normal patellofemoral joints at an average of 8.5 years, without any significant progression of arthritis across the patellofemoral joint or abnormalities of patellar maltracking. Only patients with preoperative maltracking seemed to develop any progressive symptoms, raising a question of whether surgeons should be leaving the patella nonresurfaced at the time of TKA in all but these few patients.

The largest single source of data on this topic comes from the Swedish Knee Arthroplasty Register,[116] reporting on 27,372 knees undergoing joint replacement surgery between 1981 and 1995. Excluding unicompartmental knees and revision knees, 12,298 primary knee replacements were performed for osteoarthritis, with 7567 (62%) not being resurfaced and 4731 (38%) being resurfaced. In the rheumatoid group of patients, 3021 knees underwent knee replacement with most, 1813 (60%), not being resurfaced compared with 1208 (40%) that were. A comparison of patients who had their patella resurfaced with patients who had not revealed that patients who had not had their patella resurfaced generally were not as satisfied as patients who had, regardless of whether it was for osteoarthritis or rheumatoid arthritis. Looking specifically at the osteoarthritis knees, 19% of the nonresurfaced knees were considered unsatisfactory compared with 15% of the knees that were resurfaced. In the group with rheumatoid knees, 15% of the nonresurfaced knees were considered unsatisfactory compared with 12% of the resurfaced knees. These data seem to suggest a slight benefit to resurfacing the patella.

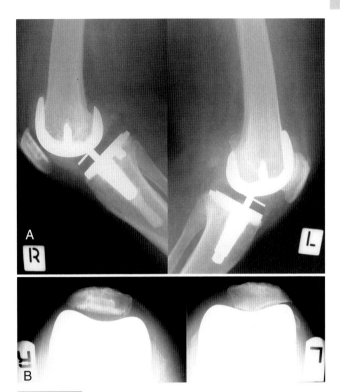

Figure 88–5. Bilateral total knee arthroplasty—contralateral controls for patellar resurfacing. Bilateral total knee replacements, with one patella resurfaced and the other left nonresurfaced. **A,** Lateral radiograph. **B,** Patellar skyline view.

In addition to this large single study, more than a dozen smaller studies* have looked at various treatment regimens for the patella in TKA. The cumulative experience of these studies, although vast, has been mostly retrospective and nonrandomized, with significant selection bias, often assessing only a single technique using subjective parameters. Despite being a substantial body of knowledge, this experience represents predominantly conflicting data with serious scientific limitations.[28]

Numerous other studies[11,36,72,81,130] in recent years have tried to overcome some of these criticisms by looking at patients who have undergone bilateral TKAs with contralateral controls (i.e., one patella resurfaced and the other nonresurfaced) (Fig. 88–5). Four of these studies[11,36,72,130] had at least 25 patients in each who had undergone such bilateral TKAs, with a cumulative tally of 112 bilateral knees between all four studies. Yet only one of these four studies, by Enis and associates,[36] showed any significant benefit from patellar resurfacing, with better pain relief and strength compared with the nonresurfaced side. The remaining three studies[11,72,130] showed no significant difference in pain relief or patient preference. These studies still were subjected to selection bias and other scientific limitations, however, which potentially could dilute the strength of any conclusions drawn.

How do we best determine whether one treatment option conveys any benefit over the other? As recom-

*References 3, 20, 38, 51-53, 73, 99, 101, 120, 122, 131, 132, 135, 141.

Table 88–3. Patellar Resurfacing versus Nonresurfacing in Total Knee Arthroplasty Randomized Controlled Trials

AUTHOR	KNEE IMPLANT USED	MINIMUM FOLLOW-UP (yr)	NO. KNEES	REVISIONS IN NONRESURFACED GROUP		REVISIONS IN RESURFACED GROUP	
				All Reasons	Patellofemoral Problems	All Reasons	Patellofemoral Problems
Bourne et al[19]	AMK	6.3	100	6	2	2	1
Feller et al[38]	PCA modular	3	40	0	0	2	0
Schroeder-Boersch et al[118,119]	Not specified	2	40	2	2	1	1
Barrack et al[6,11]	Miller Galante II	5	93	7	7	0	0
Wood et al[146]	Miller Galante II	2	198	15	15	9	9
Waters and Bentley[143]	PFC	2	474	11	11	3	3
Totals	4 types	3.4 (mean)	945 (100%)	41 (4.3%)	37 (3.9%)	17 (1.8%)	14 (1.5%)

AMK, Anatomic Modular Knee; PFC, Press Fit Condylar; PCA, Porous Coated Anatomic.

mended by Chalmers and colleagues,[28] the most reliable method of ascertaining the effectiveness of a specific intervention is via prospective, randomized double-blinded, controlled trials. There are to our knowledge only six such clinical trials[6,11,19,38,119,143,146] looking at patellar resurfacing in TKA (Table 88–3). When combined, these studies include a total of 945 knees. Although this number is a small fraction (6%) of the number (15,319) included in the Swedish Knee Arthroplasty Register,[116] these studies were well designed, with randomization of patients and blinding of the examiners and the patients to the type of patellar management used. Following are brief summaries of each of these studies.

Randomized, Controlled Trial #1

A prospective, randomized, double-blind study comparing resurfacing with nonresurfacing in a series of 100 patients using the AMK implant was reported initially in 1995 by Bourne and coworkers.[19] Outcome measures included the Knee Society clinical rating, radiographic analysis, a 30-second stair-climbing test, and measurements of quadriceps and hamstring torque. The interim 2-year analysis showed no difference in the Knee Society scores, range of motion, or stair-climbing ability. There was an increased incidence in the resurfaced knees of postoperative patellar tilting, intraoperative lateral release, and diminished pain scores. In 2004, Burnett and coworkers[25] reported on this series again with minimum follow-up of 10 years. There was a 15% overall revision rate in the nonresurfaced group and 5% in the resurfaced group. No significant difference was found regarding these revision rates or the Knee Society clinical rating scores, functional scores, patient satisfaction, anterior knee pain, or radiographic outcomes.

Randomized, Controlled Trial #2

In 1996, Feller and associates[38] reported a prospective randomized trial of 40 patients without severe deformity of the patella who underwent TKA for the treatment of osteoarthritis. This was a single-surgeon series, and the quality of the patellar articular cartilage was not a basis for exclusion from the study. For the TKAs done without resurfacing, the patelloplasty consisted of osteophyte removal only. The Porous Coated Anatomic (PCA) modular knee prosthesis (Howmedica, East Rutherford, NJ) was used in all patients, with a cemented, all-polyethylene dome patellar component used in the resurfacing group. The two groups were compared with the use of two different scoring systems—the Hospital for Special Surgery knee score and a new patellar score developed by the authors to evaluate anterior knee pain, quadriceps strength, and ability to rise from a chair and to climb stairs.

At a minimum of 3 years postoperatively, no significant difference in either score was found between the groups. There was, however, a trend toward worse scores in the resurfacing group, and the scores were lower for women and for heavier patients in both groups. The patients without resurfacing had significantly better stair-climbing ability ($p < 0.05$). There were no revisions owing to patellofemoral complications in either group. The authors concluded that in patients with osteoarthritis (without severe patellar deformity), there was no benefit to resurfacing the patella, and they did not recommend routine resurfacing of the patella in TKA.

Randomized, Controlled Trial #3

In 1997, Barrack and associates[11] reported the results of a prospective, randomized, double-blind study of 118 knees using a Miller-Galante II cruciate-retaining knee prosthesis and followed for a minimum of 2 years. There was no difference in the overall Knee Society score or the subscore for pain or function between the resurfacing and nonresurfacing group. Similarly, no difference between groups was noted with regard to patient satisfaction or the responses to a questionnaire regarding function of the patellofemoral joint. Thirty patients who had bilateral replacements with a resurfaced patella in one knee and a nonresurfaced patella in the other knee expressed no clear preference for either knee. The authors concluded that the prevalence of anterior knee pain after TKA was not influenced by whether the patella had been resurfaced. In 2001, Barrack and associates[6] reported again on this series, with lengthened follow-up to a minimum of 5 years based on data from 93 of the original 118 knees. They found no statistically significant difference in any parameter studied between the two groups and concluded that anterior knee pain was independent of whether the patella was resurfaced or not. The factors that are commonly considered valid for selective patellar resurfacing (preoperative anterior knee pain, degree of intraoperative patellar chondromalacia, and obesity) were not predictive of outcome.

Randomized, Controlled Trial #4

In 1998, Schroder-Boersch and associates[118,119] conducted a randomized trial of 40 knees, treated with or without resurfacing, followed for a minimum of 2 years. Of the 20 knees treated with nonresurfacing, 3 had a patellar subluxation, with 2 requiring revision for patellar resurfacing because of pain secondary to maltracking of the patella. Four other knees in this group had mild-to-moderate anterior pain. One resurfaced knee was revised because of aseptic loosening of the cemented patellar component. Radiographically the resurfaced knees showed less postoperative patellar tilt (mean 3.8 degrees) than did the nonresurfaced knees (mean 6.4 degrees). Patients with a resurfaced patella had better scores for pain, improved patellar tilting outcomes, and a much lower revision rate, but with low numbers in this study, the values achieved were of questionable significance.

Randomized, Controlled Trial #5

The second largest randomized, controlled clinical trial of its kind, looking at patellar resurfacing in TKA, was based on 198 osteoarthritic knees receiving a Miller-Galante II implant with a minimum 3-year follow-up. Wood and colleagues[146] reported in 2002 no difference in the Knee Society clinical rating, range of motion, or functional score between the resurfaced and nonresurfaced knees. The results with regard to postoperative knee pain and stair descent were superior, however, in the group treated with resurfacing, with 31% of the nonresurfaced knees having anterior pain compared with 16% of the resurfaced knees. The rates of revision for patellofemoral symptoms were similar, with 12% of the originally nonresurfaced knees undergoing resurfacing and 10% of the originally resurfaced knees undergoing revision. Weight, but not body mass index, was associated with pain in the nonresurfaced knees. The authors concluded that the results for anterior knee pain and stair descent favor the use of resurfacing, and that despite this difference, revision rates for patellofemoral symptoms were similar for the two techniques. Total joint loading (weight) as opposed to obesity (body mass index) also was noted to be a more accurate

factor for predicting postoperative anterior pain in the nonresurfaced knees.

Randomized, Controlled Trial #6

In 2003, Waters and Bentley[143] reported the largest to date, prospective randomized clinical trial of its kind, looking at patellar resurfacing in TKA, based on 514 consecutive TKAs using the PFC implant that were performed at the Royal National Orthopaedic Hospital in Stanmore, United Kingdom. The mean duration of follow-up was 5.3 years (range 2 to 8.5 years), and the patients were assessed double-blinded with the use of three separate scoring systems: the Knee Society score, a clinical anterior knee pain score, and the British Orthopaedic Association patient-satisfaction score. At the time of follow up, there were 474 knees, with 35 of these patients having had bilateral knee replacements, with patellar resurfacing on one side and nonresurfacing on the other.

A statistically significant difference ($p < 0.0001$) was found in the overall prevalence of anterior knee pain between the nonresurfaced group (pain in 25.1%) and the resurfaced group (pain in 5.3%). In the nonresurfaced group, there was a significantly increased requirement for additional surgery ($p = 0.0025$) with 11 patients requiring a secondary patella resurfacing, with complete relief of anterior knee pain in 10 of these 11. The overall postoperative knee scores also were lower in the nonresurfacing group, with the difference being significant among patients with osteoarthritis ($p < 0.01$). Finally, patients who underwent a bilateral knee replacement were more likely to prefer the side with the resurfaced patella, with significantly better results in these knees in terms of anterior knee pain and patient preference (chi-squared $p < 0.001$).

Although historically it was thought by some surgeons that resurfacing of the patella carried with it an unacceptable increase in the risk of new, patella-specific complications without any reasonable prospect of improved outcomes, the more recent literature tends to suggest otherwise. The two most recent and largest randomized, controlled trials performed by Wood and colleagues[146] and Waters and Bentley,[143] when combined, account for more than two-thirds (71%; 672 of 945) of all the patients involved in all six of the randomized, controlled trials assessing patellar resurfacing in TKA, with both studies showing statistically significant improved outcomes with patellar resurfacing without any significant increase in complications.

CONCLUSION

Patellar resurfacing, perhaps more than any other area of TKA, has been surrounded by controversy in the 30 years of its existence. A multitude of beliefs still exist as to what the correct approach is for the management of the patella at the time of TKA. The most clear-cut position in this regard is either always to resurface or never to resurface the patella. Even for these two camps, there remain further

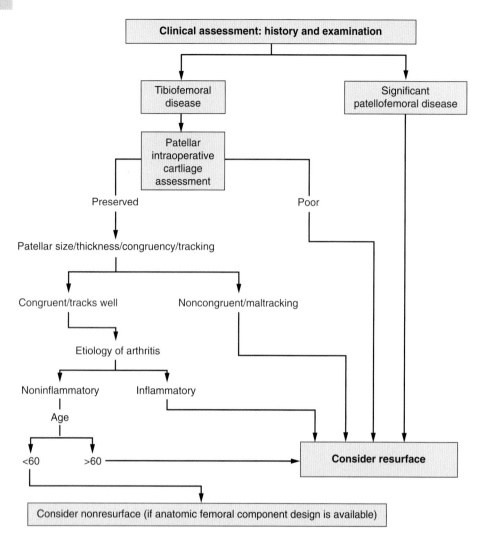

Figure 88–6. The London Health Sciences Centre approach to managing the patella in total knee arthroplasty. Decision-making algorithm for patellar resurfacing in total knee arthroplasty at London Health Sciences Centre. Selective nonresurfacing on the basis of clinical, radiographic, and intraoperative parameters.

avenues for debate. If resurfacing, the debate concerns whether to use an onlay or an inlay device and whether or not to use an all-polyethylene or metal-backed component. Surgeons who never resurface must decide whether or not to perform a patelloplasty and if so, as to what exactly a patelloplasty comprises. If one does not subscribe to either of these two approaches, there is an option to resurface the patella some of the time, which may be based solely on "instinctive reasoning" for each individual case or, alternatively, selectively resurfacing only in patients who meet strict predetermined guidelines.

Our institution's approach to the role of patellar resurfacing has been influenced by our own studies.[19,25] We currently tend to resurface the patella as a default technique, and only when certain criteria are met do we "selectively nonresurface" the patella. We prefer to use a femoral component with a patella-friendly design that caters for these occasions when we selectively nonresurface, which usually is limited to patients with insufficient bone stock to safely receive a patellar implant or in young patients with a noninflammatory arthropathy with good preservation of articular cartilage and a congruent well-tracking patella. Our decision-making algorithm for patellar resurfacing in TKA at the London Health Sciences Centre is provided in Figure 88–6.

Until more recently, there was no clear trend in the literature, allowing all groups in this debate to justify their positions on patellar resurfacing in TKA—hence the lack of uniform agreement on what single best technique to employ. The more recent literature, from the Swedish Knee registry and from the two largest and most recent randomized double-blinded, controlled studies looking at patellar resurfacing in TKA, seems to provide substantial support for the role of patellar resurfacing in TKA. These studies have shown improved outcomes with patellar resurfacing without any significant increase in the risk of complications specific to this procedure. Although it would seem that there are some clear results emerging in support of patellar resurfacing at the time of TKA, it is hoped that, with time, this position will be substantiated further with additional randomized controlled studies. This substantiation would allow for the long-standing controversy surrounding the management of the patella to pass and, it is hoped, usher in a new era with a more uniform approach to patellofemoral resurfacing in TKA.

References

1. Aglietti P, Buzzi R, Gaudenzi A: Patellofemoral functional results and complications with the posterior stabilized total condylar knee prosthesis. J Arthroplasty 3:17, 1988.
2. Aglietti P, Insall JN, Walker PS, et al: A new patella prosthesis: Design and application. Clin Orthop 107:175, 1975.
3. Anderson JG, Wixson RL, Tsai D, et al: Functional outcome and patient satisfaction in total knee patients over the age of 75. J Arthroplasty 11:831, 1996.
4. Andriacchi TP, Yoder D, Conley A, et al: Patellofemoral design influences function following total knee arthroplasty. J Arthroplasty 12:243, 1997.
5. Anouchi YS, Whiteside LA, Kaiser AD, et al: The effects of axial rotational alignment of the femoral component on knee stability and patellar tracking in total knee arthroplasty demonstrated on autopsy specimens. Clin Orthop 287:170, 1993.
6. Barrack RL, Bertot AJ, Wolfe MW, et al: Patellar resurfacing in total knee arthroplasty: A prospective randomized, double blind study with five to seven years of follow up. J Bone Joint Surg Am 83:1376, 2001.
7. Barrack RL, Matzkin E, Ingraham R, et al: Revision knee arthroplasty with patella replacement versus bony shell. Clin Orthop 356:139, 1998.
8. Barrack RL, Rorabeck CH, Engh GA: Patella options in revision total knee arthroplasty. Orthopedics 24:899, 2001.
9. Barrack RL, Rorabeck C, Partington P, et al: The results of retaining a well-fixed patellar component in revision total knee arthroplasty. J Arthroplasty 15:413, 2000.
10. Barrack RL, Schrader T, Bertot AJ, et al: Component rotation and anterior knee pain after total knee arthroplasty. Clin Orthop 392:46, 2001.
11. Barrack RL, Wolfe MW, Waldman DA, et al: Resurfacing of the patella in total knee arthroplasty: A prospective, randomized, double-blind study. J Bone Joint Surg Am 79:1121, 1997.
12. Bayley JC, Scott RD, Ewald FC, et al: Failure of the metal backed patellar component after total knee replacement. J Bone Joint Surg Am 70:668, 1988.
13. Beight JL, Yao B, Hozack WJ, et al: The patella "clunk" syndrome after posterior stabilized total knee arthroplasty. Clin Orthop 299:139, 1994.
14. Benjamin JB, Szivek JA, Hammond AS, et al: Contact areas and pressures between native patellas and prosthetic femoral components. J Arthroplasty 13:693, 1998.
15. Berger RA, Rubash HE, Seel MJ: Determining the rotational alignment of the femoral component in total knee arthroplasty using the epicondylar axis. Clin Orthop 286:40, 1992.
16. Berry DJ, Rand JA: Isolated patellar component revision of total knee arthroplasty. Clin Orthop 286:110, 1993.
17. Bindeglass DF, Cohen JL, Dorr LD: Patellar tilt and subluxation in total knee arthroplasty: Relationship to pain fixation and design. Clin Orthop 286:103, 1993.
18. Bottoni CR, Taylor DC, Arciero RA: Patellar fractures in the adult. In DeLee J, Drez D, Miller E (eds): Orthopaedic Sports Medicine—Principles and Practice, 2nd edition. Philadelphia, WB Saunders, 2003, p 1761.
19. Bourne RB, Rorabeck CH, Vaz M, et al: Resurfacing versus not resurfacing the patella during total knee replacement. Clin Orthop 321:156, 1995.
20. Boyd AD Jr, Ewald FC, Thomas WH, et al: Long term complications after total knee arthroplasty with or without resurfacing of the patella. J Bone Joint Surg Am 75:674, 1993.
21. Braakman M, Verburg AD, Bronsema G, et al: The outcome of three methods of patellar resurfacing in total knee arthroplasty. Int Orthop 19:7, 1995.
22. Briard JL, Hungerford DS: Patellofemoral instability in total knee arthroplasty. J Arthroplasty 4 (Suppl):87, 1989.
23. Brick GW, Scott RD: The patellofemoral component of total knee arthroplasty. Clin Orthop 231:163, 1988.
24. Buechel FF, Rosa RA, Pappas MJ: A metal-backed rotating-bearing patellar prosthesis to lower contact stress: An 11-year clinical study. Clin Orthop 248:34, 1989.
25. Burnett RS, Haydon CH, Rorabeck CH, et al: Patella resurfacing versus nonresurfacing in total knee arthroplasty: Results of a randomised controlled clinical trial at a minimum of 10 years' followup. Clin Orthop 428:12, 2004.
26. Cameron HU: Comparison between patellar resurfacing with an inset plastic button and patelloplasty. Can J Surg 34:49, 1991.
27. Cameron HU, Fedorkow DM: The patella in total knee arthroplasty. Clin Orthop 165:197, 1982.
28. Chalmers TC, Celano P, Sacks HS, et al: Bias in treatment assignment in controlled clinical trials. N Engl J Med 309:1358, 1983.
29. Chew JT, Stewart NJ, Hanssen AD, et al: Differences in patellar tracking and knee kinematics among three different total knee designs. Clin Orthop 345:87, 1997.
30. Clayton ML, Thirupathi R: Patellar complications after total condylar arthroplasty. Clin Orthop 170:152, 1982.
31. Cohen R: A porous tantalum trabecular metal: Basic science. Am J Orthop 31:216, 2002.
32. Dennis DA: Patellofemoral complications in total knee arthroplasty: A literature review. Am J Knee Surg 5:156, 1992.
33. Dennis DA: Removal of well-fixed cementless metal-backed patellar components. J Arthroplasty 7:217, 1992.
34. Eckhoff DG, Montgomery WK, Stamm ER, et al: Location of the femoral sulcus in the osteoarthritic knee. J Arthroplasty 11:163, 1996.
35. Engh GA, Holt BT, Parks NL: A midvastus muscle-splitting approach for total knee arthroplasty. J Arthroplasty 12:322, 1997.
36. Enis JE, Gardner R, Robledo R, et al: Comparison of patellar resurfacing versus nonresurfacing in bilateral total knee arthroplasty. Clin Orthop 260:38, 1990.
37. Ezzet KA, Hershey AL, D'Lima DD, et al: Patella tracking in total knee arthroplasty: Inset versus onset design. J Arthroplasty 16:838, 2001.
38. Feller JA, Bartlett RJ, Lang DM: Patellar resurfacing versus retention in total knee arthroplasty. J Bone Joint Surg Br 78:226, 1996.
39. Fern ED, Winson IG, Getty CJ: Anterior knee pain in rheumatoid patients after total knee replacement: Possible selection criteria for patellar resurfacing. J Bone Joint Surg Br 74:745, 1992.
40. Figgie HE III, Goldberg VM, Figgie MP, et al: The effect of alignment of the implant on fractures of the patellaafter patellacondylar total knee arthroplasty. J Bone Joint Surg Am 71:1031, 1989.
41. Firestone TP, Teeny SM, Krackow KA, et al: The clinical and roentgenographic results of cementless porous-coated patellar fixation. Clin Orthop 273:184, 1991.
42. Francke EI, Lachiewicz PF: Failure of a cemented all-polyethylene patellar component of a Press-Fit Condylar Total Knee arthroplasty. J Arthroplasty 15:234, 2000.
43. Freeman MA, Samuelson KM, Elias SG, et al: The patellofemoral joint in total knee prostheses: Design considerations. J Arthroplasty 4(Suppl):S694, 1989.
44. Goldberg VM, Figgie HE III, Inglis AE, et al: Patella fracture type and prognosis in condylar total knee arthroplasty. Clin Orthop 236:115, 1988.
45. Grace JN, Rand JA: Patellar instability after total knee arthroplasty. Clin Orthop 237:184, 1988.
46. Grace JN, Sim FH: Fracture of the patella after total knee arthroplasty. Clin Orthop 230:168, 1988.
47. Greenfield MA, Insall JN, Case GC, et al: Instrumentation of the patellar osteotomy in total knee arthroplasty: The relationship of patellar thickness and lateral retinacular release. Am J Knee Surg 9:129, 1996.
48. Gomes LSM, Bechtold JE, Gustilo RB: Patella prosthesis positioning in total knee arthroplasty: A roentgenographic study. Clin Orthop 236:72, 1988.
49. Gunston FH, MacKenzie RI: Complications of polycentric knee arthroplasty. Clin Orthop 120:11, 1976.
50. Hanssen AD: Bone grafting for severe patellar bone loss during revision knee arthroplasty. J Bone Joint Surg Am 83:171, 2001.
51. Hawker G, Wright J, Coyte P, et al: Health-related quality of life after knee replacement. J Bone Joint Surg Am 80:163, 1998.
52. Healy WL, Wasilewski SA, Takei R, Oberlander M: Patellofemoral complications following total knee arthroplasty: Correlation with implant design and patient risk factors. J Arthroplasty 10:197, 1995.
53. Heck DA, Robinson RL, Partridge CM, et al: Patient outcomes after knee replacement. Clin Orthop 356:93, 1998.
54. Hollister AM, Jatana S, Singh AK, et al: The axes of rotation of the knee. Clin Orthop 290:259, 1993.

55. Hozack WJ, Goll SR, Lotke PA, et al: The treatment of patella fractures after total knee arthroplasty. Clin Orthop 236:123, 1988.

56. Hozack WJ, Rothman RH, Booth RE Jr, et al: The patellar clunk syndrome: A complication of posterior stabilized total knee arthroplasty. Clin Orthop 241:203, 1989.

57. Hsu HC, Luo ZP, Rand JA, et al: Influence of patellar thickness on patellar tracking and patellofemoral contact characteristics after total knee arthroplasty. J Arthroplasty 11:69, 1996.

58. Hsu HP, Walker PS: Wear and deformation of patellar components in total knee arthroplasty. Clin Orthop 246:260, 1989.

59. Huang CH, Lee YM, Lai JH, et al: Failure of the all-polyethylene patellar component after total knee arthroplasty. J Arthroplasty 14:940, 1999.

60. Huberti HH, Hayes WC: Patellofemoral contact pressures: The influence of q-angle contact and tendofemoral contact. J Bone Joint Surg Am 66:715, 1984.

61. Hungerford DS, Barry M: Biomechanics of the patellofemoral joint. Clin Orthop 144:9, 1979.

62. Ikezawa Y, Gustilo RB: Clinical outcome of revision of the patellar component in total knee arthroplasty: A 2- to 7- year follow up study. J Orthop Sci 4:83, 1999.

63. Insall JN, Ranawat CS, Aglietti P, Shine J: A comparison of four models of total knee–replacement prostheses. J Bone Joint Surg Am 58:754, 1976.

64. Insall JN, Salvati E: Patella position in the normal knee joint. Radiology 101:101, 1971.

65. Insall J, Scott WN, Ranawat CS: The total condylar knee prosthesis: A report of two hundred and twenty cases. J Bone Joint Surg Am 61:173, 1979.

66. Insall J, Tria AJ, Scott WN: The total condylar knee prosthesis: The first 5 years. Clin Orthop 145:68, 1979.

67. Jaugerito JW, Dubois CM, Smith SR, et al: Medial gastrocnemius transposition flap for the treatment of disruption of the extensor mechanism after total knee arthroplasty. J Bone Joint Surg Am 79:866, 1997.

68. Kaper BP, Woolfrey M, Bourne RB: The effect of built in external femoral rotation on patellofemoral tracking in the Genesis II total knee arthroplasty. J Arthroplasty 15:964, 2000.

69. Kaufer H: Mechanical function of the patella. J Bone Joint Surg Am 53:1551, 1971.

70. Kayler DE, Lyttle D: Surgical interruption of patellar blood supply by total knee arthroplasty. Clin Orthop 229:221, 1988.

71. Keblish P: Valgus deformity in total knee replacement (TKR): The lateral retinacular approach. Orthop Trans 9:28, 1985.

72. Keblish PA, Varma AK, Greenwald A: Patellar resurfacing or retention in total knee arthroplasty: A prospective study of patients with bilateral replacements. J Bone Joint Surg Am 76:930, 1994.

73. Kim BS, Reitman RD, Schai PA, et al: Selective patellar nonresurfacing in total knee arthroplasty: 10 year results. Clin Orthop 367:81, 1999.

74. Kirk P, Rorabeck CH, Bourne RB, et al: Management of recurrent dislocation of the patella following total knee arthroplasty. J Arthroplasty 7:229, 1992.

75. Lachiewicz PF: Cement versus cementless total knee replacement: Is there a place for cementless fixation in 2001? Curr Opin Orthop 12:33, 2001.

76. Lachiewicz PF: Implant design and techniques for patellar resurfacing in total knee arthroplasty. AAOS Instr Course Lect 53:187, 2004.

77. Laskin RS: Management of the patella during revision total knee replacement arthroplasty. Orthop Clin North Am 29:355, 1998.

78. Laskin RS, Bucknell A: The use of metal backed patellar prosthesis in total knee arthroplasty. Clin Orthop 260:52, 1990.

79. Larson CM, McDowell CM, Lachiewicz PF: One-peg versus three-peg patella component fixation in total knee arthroplasty. Clin Orthop 392:94, 2001.

80. Lee TQ, Kim WC: Anatomically based patellar resection criteria in total knee arthroplasty. Am J Knee Surg 11:161, 1998.

81. Levitsky KA, Harris WJ, McManus J, et al: Total knee arthroplasty without patellar resurfacing: Clinical outcomes and long term follow up evaluation. Clin Orthop 286:116, 1993.

82. Lombardi AV Jr, Engh GA, Volz RG, et al: Fracture/dissociation of the polyethylene in metal backed components in total knee arthroplasty. J Bone Joint Surg Am 70:675, 1988.

83. Lynch AF, Rorabeck CH, Bourne RB: Extensor mechanism complications following total knee arthroplasty. J Arthroplasty 2:135, 1987.

84. Lynch JA, Baker PL, Lepse PS, et al: Solitary patellar component revision following total knee arthroplasty. Presented at AAOS, San Francisco, February 20, 1993.

85. Marmor L: Technique for patellar resurfacing in total knee arthroplasty. Clin Orthop 230:166, 1988.

86. Mason MD, Brick GW, Scott RD, et al: Three pegged all polyethylene patella: 2-6 year results. Orthop Trans 17:991, 1994.

87. Matsuda S, Ishinishi T, Whiteside LA: Contact stresses with an unresurfaced patella in total knee arthroplasty: The effect of femoral component design. Orthopedics 23:213, 2000.

88. Matthews LS, Sonstegard DA, Henke JA: Load bearing characteristics of the patello-femoral joint. Acta Orthop Scand 48:511-516, 1977.

89. McLean CA, Tanzer M, Laxer E, et al: The effect of femoral component designs on the contact and tracking characteristics of the unresurfaced patella in TKA. Orthop Trans 18:616, 1995.

90. McMahon MS, Scuderi GR, Glashow JL, et al: Scintigraphic determination of patellar viability after excision of infrapatellar fat pad and/or lateral retinacular release in total knee arthroplasty. Clin Orthop 260:10, 1990.

91. Merkow RL, Soudry M, Insall JN: Patellar dislocation following total knee arthroplasty. J Bone Joint Surg Am 67:1321, 1985.

92. Miller RK, Goodfellow JW, Murray DW, et al: In vitro measurement of patellofemoral force after three types of knee replacement. J Bone Joint Surg Br 80:900, 1998.

93. Mochizuki RM, Schurman DJ: Patellar complications following total knee arthroplasty. J Bone Joint Surg Am 61:879, 1979.

94. Murray DG, Webster DA: The variable-axis knee prosthesis: Two year follow up study. J Bone Joint Surg Am 63:687, 1981.

95. Nasser S, Poggie RA: Revision and salvage patellar arthroplasty using a porous tantalum implant. J Arthroplasty 19:562, 2004.

96. Pagnano MW, Scuderi GR, Insall JN: Patella component resection in revision and reimplantation total knee arthroplasty. Clin Orthop 356:134, 1998.

97. Parvizi J, Seel MJ, Hanssen AD, et al: Patella component resection arthroplasty for the severely compromised patella. Clin Orthop 397:356, 2002.

98. Petersilge WJ, Oishi CS, Kaufmann KR, et al: The effect of trochlear design on patellofemoral shear and compressive forces in total knee arthroplasty. Clin Orthop 309:124, 1994.

99. Picetti GD III, McGann WA, Welch RB: The patellofemoral joint after total knee arthroplasty without patellar resurfacing. J Bone Joint Surg Am 72:1379, 1990.

100. Rader CP, Lohr J, Wittmann R, et al: Results of total knee arthroplasty with a metal backed patella component. J Arthroplasty 11:923, 1996.

101. Ranawat CS: The patellofemoral joint in total condylar knee arthroplasty: Pros and cons based on five to ten year follow up observations. Clin Orthop 205:93, 1986.

102. Ranawat CS, Rose HA, Bryan WJ: Technique and results of replacement of the patellofemoral joint with total condylar knee arthroplasty. Orthop Trans 5:414, 1981.

103. Rand JA: Patellar resurfacing in total knee arthroplasty. Clin Orthop 260:110, 1990.

104. Rand JA: The patellofemoral joint in total knee arthroplasty. J Bone Joint Surg Am 76:612, 1994.

105. Rand JA, Gustilo RB: Comparison of inset and resurfacing patellar prostheses in total knee arthroplasty. Acta Orthop Belg 62(Suppl 1):154, 1996.

106. Rand JA, Morrey BF, Bryan RS: Patellar tendon rupture after total knee arthroplasty. Tech Orthop 3:45, 1988.

107. Rand JA, Morrey BF, Bryan RS: Patellar tendon rupture after total knee arthroplasty. Clin Orthop 244:233, 1989.

108. Reilly DT, Martens M: Experimental analysis of the quadriceps muscle force and patellofemoral joint reaction force for various activities. Acta Orthop Scand 43:126, 1972.

109. Reuben JD, McDonald CL, Woodard PL, et al: Effect of patella thickness on strain following total knee arthroplasty. J Arthroplasty 6:25158, 1991.

110. Rhoads DD, Noble PC, Reuben JD, et al: The effect of femoral component position on patellar tracking after total knee arthroplasty. Clin Orthop 260:43, 1990.

111. Rhoads DD, Noble PC, Reuben JD: The effect of femoral component position on the kinematics of total knee arthroplasty. Clin Orthop 286:122, 1993.

112. Ritter MA, Campbell ED: Postoperative patellar complications with or without lateral release during total knee arthroplasty. Clin Orthop 219:163, 1987.

113. Ritter MA, Keating EM, Faris PM: Clinical, roentgenographic and scintigraphic results after interruption of the superior lateral genicular artery during total knee arthroplasty. Clin Orthop 248:145, 1989.

114. Roffman M, Hirsch DM, Mendes DG: Fracture of the resurfaced patella in total knee replacement. Clin Orthop 148:112, 1980.

115. Rosenberg AG, Andriacchi TP, Barden R, et al: Patellar component failure in cementless total knee arthroplasty. Clin Orthop 236:106, 1988.

116. Robertsson O, Dunbar M, Pehrsson T, et al: Patient satisfaction after knee arthroplasty: A report on 27,372 knees operated on between 1981 and 1995 in Sweden. Acta Orthop Scand 71:262, 2000.

117. Scapinelli R: Blood supply to human patella. J Bone Joint Surg Br 49:563, 1967.

118. Schroeder-Boersch H, Scheller G, Fischer J, et al: Advantages of patellar resurfacing in total knee arthroplasty: Two-year results of a prospective randomized study. Arch Orthop Trauma Surg 117:73, 1998.

119. Schroeder-Boersch H, Scheller G, Synnatschke M, et al: Patellar resurfacing: Results of a prospective randomized study. Orthopade 27:642, 1998.

120. Scott RD: Prosthetic replacement of the patellofemoral joint. Orthop Clin North Am 10:129, 1979.

121. Scott RD, Reilly DT: Pros and cons of patella resurfacing in total knee replacement. Orthop Trans 4:328, 1980.

122. Scott WN, Kim H: Resurfacing the patella offers lower complication rates. Orthopedics 24:24, 2001.

123. Scuderi GR, Insall JN: Total knee arthroplasty: Current clinical perspectives. Clin Orthop 276:26, 1992.

124. Scuderi G, Scharf SC, Meltzer LP, et al: The relationship of lateral releases to patellar viability in total knee arthroplasty. J Arthroplasty 2:209, 1987.

125. Shetty AA, Tindall A, Ting P, et al: The evolution of the total knee arthroplasty: Part 1. Introduction and first steps. Curr Orthop17:322, 2003.

126. Shetty AA, Tindall A, Ting P, et al: The evolution of the total knee arthroplasty: Part 2. The hinged knee replacement and the semi-constrained knee replacement. Curr Orthop 17:403, 2003.

127. Shetty AA, Tindall A, Ting P, et al: The evolution of the total knee arthroplasty: Part 3. Surface replacement. Curr Orthop 17:478, 2003.

128. Shih HN, Shih LY, Wong YC, et al: Long term changes of the non-resurfaced patella after total knee arthroplasty. J Bone Joint Surg Am 86:935, 2004.

129. Shoji H, Shimozaki E: Patella clunk syndrome in total knee arthroplasty without patellar resurfacing. J Arthroplasty 11:198, 1996.

130. Shoji H, Yoshino S, Kajino A: Patellar replacement in bilateral total knee arthroplasty: A study of patients who had rheumatoid arthritis and no gross deformity of the patella. J Bone Joint Surg Am 71:853, 1989.

131. Sledge CB, Ewald FC: Total knee arthroplasty experience at the Robert Breck Brigham Hospital. Clin Orthop 145:78, 1979.

132. Soudry M, Mestriner LA, Binazzi R, et al: Total knee arthroplasty without patellar resurfacing. Clin Orthop 205:166, 1986.

133. Star MJ, Kaufman KR, Irby SE, et al: The effects of patellar thickness on patellofemoral forces after resurfacing. Clin Orthop 322:279, 1996.

134. Steinbrocker O, Traeger CH, Batterman RC: Therapeutic criteria in rheumatoid arthritis. JAMA 140:659, 1949.

135. Stern SH, Insall JN: Total knee arthroplasty in obese patients. J Bone Joint Surg Am 72:1400, 1990.

136. Stulberg SD, Stulberg BN, Hamati Y, et al: Failure mechanisms of metal-backed patellar components. Clin Orthop 236:88, 1988.

137. Tanzer M, McLean CA, Laxer E, et al: The effect of femoral component designs on the contact and tracking characteristics of the unresurfaced patella in total knee arthroplasty. Can J Surg 44:127, 2001.

138. Theiss SM, Kitziger KJ, Lotke PS, et al: Component design affecting patellofemoral complications after total knee arthroplasty. Clin Orthop 326:183, 1996.

139. Thorpe CD, Bocell JR, Tullos HS: Intra-articular fibrous bands: Patellar complications after total knee arthroplasty. J Bone Joint Surg Am 72:811, 1990.

140. Tria AJ, Harwood DA, Alicea JA, et al: Patella fractures in posterior stabilized knee arthroplasties. Clin Orthop 299:131, 1994.

141. Vince KG, McPherson EJ: The patella in total knee arthroplasty. Orthop Clin North Am 23:675, 1992.

142. Wasilewski SA, Frankl U: Fracture of polyethylene of patellar component in total knee arthroplasty, diagnosed by arthroscopy. J Arthroplasty 4(Suppl):S19, 1989.

143. Waters TS, Bentley G: Patellar resurfacing in total knee arthroplasty: A prospective, randomized study. J Bone Joint Surg Am 85:212, 2003.

144. Wetzner SM, Bezreh JS, Scott RD, et al: Bone scanning in the assessment of patellar viability following knee replacement. Clin Orthop 199:215, 1985.

145. Windsor RE, Scuderi GR, Insall JN: Patella fractures in total knee arthroplasty. J Arthroplasty 4(Suppl):S63, 1989.

146. Wood DJ, Smith AJ, Collopy D, et al: Patellar resurfacing in total knee arthroplasty. J Bone Joint Surg Am 84:187, 2002.

147. Yoshii I, Whiteside LA, Anouchi YS: The effect of patella button placement and femoral component design on patellar tracking in total knee arthroplasty. Clin Orthop 275:211, 1992.

148. Zappala FG, Taffel CB, Scuderi GR: Rehabilitation of patellofemoral joint disorders. Orthop Clin North Am 23:555, 1992.

CHAPTER 89

Fluoroscopic Analysis of Total Knee Replacement

Richard D. Komistek • Douglas A. Dennis • Mohamed R. Mahfouz

PRINCIPLES OF FLUOROSCOPY

Most previous kinematic studies involving total knee arthroplasty (TKA) have been conducted under in vitro conditions using cadavers or under noninvasive conditions using gait laboratory systems.[1,17-19,21,32,42] Unfortunately, cadaveric studies do not allow for in vivo simulations because the actuators applying the muscle loads are unable to produce in vivo motions. Gait laboratory systems are effective in determining in-plane rotation but induce significant out-of-plane rotational and translational error.[33,34] Therefore, it became imperative that a new procedure be developed if implanted joints were to be accurately analyzed.

Video fluoroscopy allows for visualization of human joints in two dimensions under dynamic, weightbearing conditions. Through the use of model-fitting techniques, it has become possible to accurately recover the three-dimensional (3-D) motions of implanted joints from the two-dimensional (2-D) video fluoroscopic images.* The initial objective of our research was to develop an automated 3-D model-fitting process that would be accurate, precise, nonbiased, and expedient and could be used on any implanted joint in the human body.[27,28,35,36]

A feature of "full-perspective" projection (x-ray) images is that objects closer to the radiation source appear larger than those that are placed farther away. This property allows measurement of out-of-plane translation (depth), as well as determination of correct poses for symmetric implant components. Because one side of the implant is positioned farther from the radiation source than the other, the portion of the implant silhouette corresponding to the nearer side will appear larger than that on the distant side.

X-Ray Image Prediction

The use of fluoroscopy has evolved from 2-D attempts[26,31] at predicting in-plane motions to 3-D techniques that recover accurate 3-D kinematics. Initial attempts at 3-D kinematics relied on library-matching techniques,[4,20,42] but more recently, a 3-D, computer-automated, iterative model-fitting technique has been developed.[27,35,36]

*References 2-5, 8-10, 12, 14, 20, 22, 27-30, 35, 36, 38-41.

To determine implanted TKA component poses from an x-ray image, the actual fluoroscope is modeled within the computer by representing its components with their computer counterparts. The radiation source is replaced by a virtual camera, the image intensifier is represented by the x-ray image itself, and patients' implants are replaced with 3-D, solid, computer-assisted design (CAD) models. Finally, the field of view of the virtual camera is set equal to the field of view of the actual fluoroscope (Fig. 89–1).

Once the fluoroscope has been modeled, viewing the CAD models through the virtual camera is equivalent to viewing the patient's anatomy through the fluoroscope. Viewing the CAD models from this perspective provides two important images that are used in the pose estimation process. The first image is a view of the CAD models superimposed (overlaid) on top of the x-ray image. This image is displayed in the graphic user interface and allows for human supervision of the pose estimation process. The second image is a synthetic x-ray image of the CAD models that consists of only their silhouettes (Fig. 89–2). This image represents a prediction of the x-ray image corresponding to the selected implant component's current 3-D position and is used in the matching process by rendering the CAD. This rendering is stored by the computer in the frame buffer as numeric values. These values are then copied into a 2-D array and stored as the synthetic x-ray image.

Modeling Methods

In our early analyses of the 3-D kinematics of TKA using video fluoroscopy, we used template matching to determine the poses of implants within x-ray images. In template matching, 3-D models of the implant components are used to create silhouette libraries (templates), which contain multiple representations of the implants at various known poses.[4,5,36,42] This method uses computer models of the implants, oriented at varying incremental degrees of out-of-plane rotations, to generate images of the implant at varying poses.[26] With the use of canonization, these images are then scaled, translated, and rotated so that all silhouettes are 15,000 pixels in size and centered in the image and the principal axis of the silhouette is aligned with the horizontal axis of the image.

The actual fluoroscopic image is then processed. The image is filtered to reduce noise, and then the contour of the implant silhouette is traced manually by a human

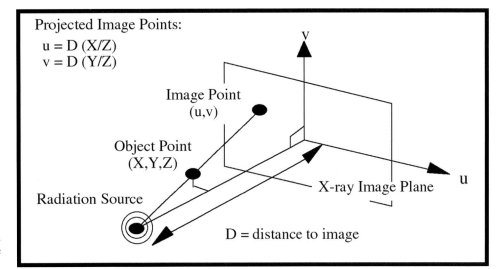

Figure 89–1. Configuration of a fluoroscope's image intensifier.

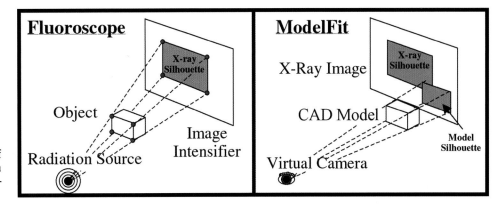

Figure 89–2. Geometry of a perspective projection model. CAD, computer-assisted design.

operator. An image is subsequently created from the traced contour of the actual implant silhouette. At this point, the x-ray contour is compared with the appropriate template and the closest match is selected from the previously developed silhouette library (it can interpolate between 1-degree images). From this match, the position of the implant components in 6 degrees of freedom can be obtained. The x-axis and y-axis rotations are obtained directly from the template image. The remaining 4 degrees of freedom are then determined from the scaling, rotation, and translation values that were required to canonize the image.

We chose to develop a model-fitting methodology because of significant limitations of using the template-matching technique.[36] Because the created library images are of the full femoral and tibial components, template matching fails if one component obstructs the other or if portions of either component are out of the field of view. The model-fitting approach requires only one femoral and one tibial component, whereas template matching requires more than 1000 femoral and tibial images in the library. These libraries are generally created at 1-degree increments; thus, actual in vivo orientations between the library orientations are determined by interpolation schemes. Most importantly, the model-fitting approach allows a human to supervise the overlay process, in contrast to the template-matching technique, which provides only numeric determination without direct visualization.[35,36] In a direct comparison, the model-fitting approach achieves significantly lower error values during the fitting process than library-matching techniques do.[35,36]

To overcome the limitations of the template-matching methods, a more accurate and reliable 3-D automated interactive kinematic analysis system (ModelFit) was developed (Fig. 89–3).[35,36] The automated method is faster than the manual technique and removes human error by using a computer algorithm to align the models with implant silhouettes. Using an energy minimization routine to maximize the correlation value, the computer very quickly and accurately determines the correct positions and orientations of the TKA implants.

An unbiased error analysis comparison was initially conducted with the same operator using the three methods (template matching, manual model fitting, and automated model fitting) and then with multiple operators using the three methods. The results from the error analysis determined that the automated model-fitting process is more accurate than the manual model-fitting or template-matching methods.[35,36] The automated method also had higher reproducibility than the manual method did: manual—1.1 mm in translation, 0.7 degree in rotation; automated—0.2 mm in translation, 0.2 degree in rotation. In addition, the automated approach was

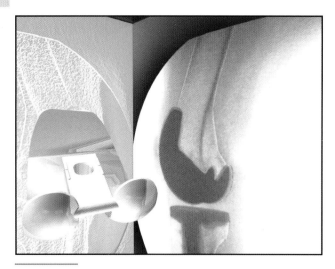

Figure 89–3. Fluoroscopy and image prediction processes.

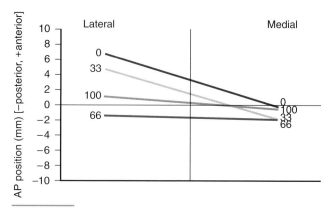

Figure 89–4. Graph showing the average medial and lateral condyle contact positions for a normal knee from heel-strike to toe-off.

statistically faster in total times ($p = 0.2$) and user times ($p = 0.005$) than the manual method.[35,36]

The model-fitting techniques developed have been used to accurately determine femoral component rotation and translation relative to the tibial component in three dimensions. After TKA implantation, patients are analyzed while performing weightbearing, dynamic activities under fluoroscopic surveillance. The video images, recorded at frame rates of either 30 or 60 Hz, are downloaded digitally onto a computer network. Initially, the 3-D femoral component is placed over the fluoroscopic image of the 2-D femoral component, and the model-fitting software package determines the best 3-D fit. Next, the 3-D tibial component is precisely positioned over the 2-D fluoroscopic image of the tibia and is fitted. Then the femoral and tibial components are grouped together and oriented with the tibia in the pure sagittal view, and the medial and lateral femorotibial condylar contact positions are determined relative to the midline of the tibia in the sagittal plane. Analysis of multiple video fluoroscopic images then allows determination of 3-D knee kinematics throughout an entire range of flexion. An extensive error analysis using a fresh cadaver was conducted to determine the relative process error. Numerous indentions were drilled into the metal femoral and tibial component to define fixed points. Then known orientations were derived for the femur relative to the tibial component. Using our model-fitting technique, the orientation was predicted and compared with the experimentally measured orientation. For all trials the error was less than 0.5 mm in translation and 0.5 degree in rotation.[35]

CLINICAL APPLICATIONS OF FLUOROSCOPY

With our automated model-fitting approach we have analyzed the kinematics for fixed posterior cruciate ligament (PCL)-retaining, mobile-bearing PCL-retaining, fixed PCL-substituting, mobile-bearing PCL-substituting, rotating-platform mobile-bearing, and anterior/posterior glide mobile-bearing TKA during deep knee bend activity and the stance phase of gait. We have routinely analyzed each implant for anteroposterior (AP) femorotibial translation, axial rotation, the incidence of femoral condylar lift-off, and the maximum range of motion. We have also determined the AP motions of normal and anterior cruciate ligament (ACL)-deficient knees with our 3-D model-fitting technique by creating 3-D models of the bones with the use of computed tomography (CT) scans.[35,36]

Anteroposterior Translation

STANCE PHASE OF GAIT

From heel-strike to toe-off, 9 of 10 subjects with a normal knee experienced posterior motion of their lateral femoral condyle, whereas the medial condyle translated posteriorly in 5 of the 10 knees (Table 89–1, Fig. 89–4). The average total condylar motion from heel-strike (0% of stance phase) to toe-off (100% of stance phase) was −5.8 mm (4.3 to −23.1 mm; SD, 8.1) and −0.4 mm (10.6 to −19.5 mm; SD, 6.6) for the lateral and medial condyles, respectively. As the direction of knee flexion angle changed from extension to flexion, the lateral condyle translated in the posterior direction. When the angle changed from flexion into extension, the lateral condyle translated anteriorly. Patients who received an ACL-retaining fixed-bearing TKA experienced somewhat differing kinematic patterns than did those with a normal knee (see Table 89–1). Eight of 15 patients experienced posterior motion of their lateral condyle from heel-strike to toe-off, whereas 11 of 15 patients exhibited posterior motion of their medial condyle. The average condylar motion (from heel-strike to toe-off) was −3.7 mm (5.7 to −23.1 mm; SD, 7.4) and −1.6 mm (18.2 to −19.5 mm; SD, 7.7) for the lateral and medial condyles, respectively.

Patients with a PCL-retaining fixed-bearing TKA experienced posterior translation of their lateral femoral condyle from heel-strike to toe-off, but less than in the normal knee or ACL-retaining fixed-bearing TKA groups

Table 89–1. Anteroposterior Translation for the Normal Knee and Fixed-Bearing ACL-Retaining TKA during Gait

	N	SUBJECTS POSTERIOR MOTION L	M	AVERAGE MOTION HS-TO (mm) L	M	>3.0 mm HS-TO* (%) M or L	>3.0 mm ANYTIME† (%) M or L	MAXIMUM MOTION (mm) M or L	STANDARD DEVIATION L	M	PIVOT POSITION LP	MP	NP
Normal knee	10	9	5	−5.8	−0.4	30	90	11.9	8.1	6.6	3	6	1
Hermes ACR	15	8	11	−3.7	−1.6	13	40	18.2	7.4	7.7	7	8	0

*Refers to greater than 3.0 mm of anterior motion for either condyle, measuring the difference between the HS and TO positions.
†Refers to greater than 3.0 mm of anterior motion for either condyle occurring anytime during the stance phase of gait.
ACR, ACL retaining; HS-TO, heel-strike to toe-off; L, lateral condyle; M, medial condyle.

Table 89–2. Anteroposterior Translation for Fixed-Bearing TKA during Gait

IMPLANT TYPE	N	SUBJECTS POSTERIOR MOTION L	M	AVERAGE MOTION HS-TO (mm) L	M	>3.0 mm HS-TO (%) M or L	>3.0 mm ANYTIME* (%) M or L	MAXIMUM MOTION (mm) M or L	STANDARD DEVIATION L	M	PIVOT POSITION LP	MP	NP
AMK PCR	5	2	4	0.4	−3.3	0	40	8.9	1.4	4.1	2	1	2
AMK PCR	5	3	1	−0.2	2.1	40	100	8.9	3.3	4.1	1	4	0
AMK PCR	5	4	0	−1.5	3.0	60	80	4.5	2.4	0.6	4	1	0
PFC PCR	15	8	5	−0.4	0.4	27	60	8.4	4.3	3.6	4	10	1
Sigma PCR	5	4	1	−4.0	−0.2	0	40	5.9	3.0	1.7	0	3	2
Apollo PCR	10	6	3	−0.5	0.7	20	40	5.6	2.6	1.6	2	7	1
Advance Medial Pivot PCR	5	3	0	−1.2	0.5	0	0	2.8	3.9	1.2	0	3	2
Advance Traditional PCR	5	3	2	0.3	0.5	40	60	5.8	3.9	1.2	1	4	0
Advantim PCR	8	6	7	−3.2	−1.8	0	50	9.5	3.1	1.6	2	4	2
NexGen PCR	20	12	15	−1.5	−1.9	30	45	6.5	4.5	3.4	10	8	2
Hermes PS	15	8	7	−0.6	−0.1	33	73	13.4	5.4	3.7	4	10	1
AMK PS	10	9	10	−4.7	3.6	0	20	6.6	2.7	2.4	3	6	1
AMK PS	5	4	2	−2.3	−0.7	0	40	5.4	3.5	3.6	2	2	1
AMK PS	4	3	1	1	4.3	75	100	13.4	4	4.8	3	1	0
AMK PS	5	4	3	0.1	0.6	20	40	7.2	2.4	3.1	4	1	0
IB2 PS	10	10	10	−5.5	−4.9	0	20	5.4	1.7	2.8	6	4	0
PFC PS	15	5	7	0.6	−0.3	27	60	8.7	4.5	4.7	3	9	3
Apollo PS	10	2.0	1.0	1.1	1.8	30	50	5.0	1.6	1.4	6.0	2.0	2.0

*Refers to greater than 3.0 mm of anterior motion for either condyle occurring at anytime during the stance phase of gait.
HS-TO, heel-strike to toe-off; L, lateral condyle; M, medial condyle; PCR, PCL retaining; PS, posterior stabilized.

(Table 89–2). Only 51 of 83 (61.4%) patients experienced posterior motion of their lateral condyle and 38 of 83 (45.8%) patients had posterior motion of their medial condyle. On average, the lateral condyles had only −1.2 mm (3.5 to −5.9 mm; SD, 3.2) of posterior motion and 0.0 mm (3.3 to −3.2 mm; SD, 2.3) of medial condylar motion from heel-strike to toe-off. From heel-strike to toe-off, 18 of 83 (21.7%) patients experienced greater than 3 mm of paradoxical anterior translation of either condyle and 52% of patients experienced greater than 3 mm at any increment of stance phase. Patients with a posterior-stabilized fixed-bearing TKA experienced motion patterns similar to those of patients with a PCL-retaining fixed-bearing TKA (see Table 89–2). Only 45 of 74 (60.8%) patients experienced posterior motion of the lateral femoral condyle from heel-strike to toe-off and 41 of 74 (55.4%) patients had posterior motion of the medial condyle. On average, the lateral femoral condyle trans-

lated posteriorly −1.3 mm (3.5 to −6.4 mm; SD, 3.2) and the medial condyle translated anteriorly 0.5 mm (4.0 to −5.5 mm; SD, 3.3) from heel-strike to toe-off. From heel-strike to toe-off, 17 of 74 (23%) patients experienced greater than 3 mm of anterior femoral translation of either condyle and 37 of 74 (50%) patients experienced greater than 3 mm at any increment of stance phase.

Only one PCL-retaining mobile-bearing TKA was analyzed during the stance phase of gait that allows the polyethylene to translate and rotate (Table 89–3). Only 5 of 10 (50%) and 4 of 10 (40%) patients experienced posterior motion of the lateral or medial condyle, respectively. On average, from heel-strike to toe-off, the lateral condyle translated in an anterior direction 0.2 mm (15.0 to −5.3 mm; SD, 5.7) and the medial condyle translated posteriorly −0.3 mm (5.1 to −11.9; SD, 4.5). From heel-strike to toe-off, 2 of 10 (20%) patients experienced greater than 3 mm of paradoxical anterior femoral translation of either

Table 89–3. Anteroposterior Translation for Mobile-Bearing TKA during Gait

IMPLANT TYPE	N	SUBJECTS POSTERIOR MOTION		AVERAGE MOTION HS-TO (mm)		>3.0 mm HS-TO (%)	>3.0 mm ANYTIME* (%)	MAXIMUM MOTION (mm)	STANDARD DEVIATION		PIVOT POSITION		
		L	M	L	M	M or L	M or L	M or L	L	M	LP	MP	NP
LCS AP Glide PCR	10	5	4	0.2	−0.3	20	50	20.9	5.7	4.5	3	7	0
LCS RP PS	10	7	1	−2.6	2.1	10	80	6.2	3.6	1.2	3	6	1
LCS RP PS	10	3	4	1.0	−0.2	10	30	3.8	1.5	2.6	5	5	0
LCS RP PS	5	2	2	−0.3	1.4	40	60	4.4	2.0	2.2	2	1	2
Sigma RP PS	10	4	3	−0.4	0.8	10	10	5.4	1.7	2.1	4	5	1
LCS RP PCS	19	8	10	0.2	−0.2	32	53	6.5	3.3	3.8	9	7	3
LCS RP PCS	5	1	2	1.0	−0.2	20	60	5.0	1.9	2.8	2	1	2
LCS RP PCS	10	7	4	−0.2	−0.2	20	40	9.3	1.9	2.8	3	7	0

*Refers to greater than 3.0 mm of anterior motion for either condyle occurring anytime during the stance phase of gait.
HS-TO, heel-strike to toe-off; L, lateral condyle; M, medial condyle; PCR, PCL retaining; PCS, PCL sacrificing; PS, posterior stabilized.

Table 89–4. Average Anteroposterior Translation for All Groups during Gait

KNEE TYPE	N	SUBJECTS POSTERIOR MOTION		AVERAGE MOTION HS-TO (mm)		>3.0 mm HS-TO (%)	>3.0 mm ANYTIME* (%)	MAXIMUM MOTION (mm)	STANDARD DEVIATION		PIVOT POSITION		
		L	M	L	M	M or L	M or L	M or L	L	M	LP	MP	NP
Normal	10	90.0	50.0	−5.8	−0.4	30	90	11.9	8.1	6.6	30.0	60.0	10.0
ACR	15	53.3	73.3	−3.7	−1.6	13	40	18.2	7.4	7.7	46.7	53.3	0.0
PCR	83	61.4	45.8	−1.2	9.9	22	52	6.7	3.2	2.3	31.3	54.2	14.5
PS	74	60.8	55.4	−1.3	0.5	23	50	8.1	3.2	3.3	41.9	47.3	10.8
PCR mobile bearing	10	50.0	40.0	0.2	−0.3	20	50	20.9	5.7	4.5	30.0	70.0	0.0
PS mobile bearing	35	45.7	28.6	−0.6	1.0	18	45	5.0	2.2	2.0	40.0	48.6	11.4
PCS mobile bearing	34	47.1	47.1	0.3	−0.2	24	51	6.9	2.4	3.1	41.2	44.1	14.7
Average of all knees		53.0	43.4	−0.5	0.2	21	50	9.5	3.3	3.1	36.9	52.8	10.3

*Refers to greater than 3.0 mm of anterior motion for either condyle occurring anytime during the stance phase of gait.
ACR, ACL retaining; HS-TO, heel-strike to toe-off; L, lateral condyle; M, medial condyle; PCR, PCL retaining; PCS, PCL sacrificing; PS, posterior stabilized.

condyle and 5 of 10 patients (50%) experienced greater than 3 mm at any increment of stance phase. The maximum amount of paradoxical anterior femoral translation was 20.9 mm but could be attributable to femorotibial rotation rather than pure translation. On average, 16 of 35 (45.7%) patients with a posterior-stabilized mobile-bearing TKA experienced posterior motion of their lateral condyle and 10 of 35 (28.6%) patients had posterior motion of the medial condyle (see Table 89–3). On average, from heel-strike to toe-off, the lateral condyle translated in the posterior direction −0.6 mm (2.7 to −4.2 mm; SD, 2.2) and the medial condyle translated anteriorly 1.0 mm (4.2 to −2.1 mm; SD, 2.0). Five of 35 (14.3%) patients experienced greater than 3 mm of paradoxical anterior femoral translation of either condyle and 15 of 35 (42.8%) patients experienced greater than 3 mm at any increment of stance phase. On average, patients with a PCL-sacrificing mobile-bearing TKA experienced kinematic patterns similar to those of patients who received a posterior-stabilized mobile-bearing TKA (see Table 89–3). Only 16 of 34 (47.1%) patients experienced posterior motion of the lateral condyle and 16 of 34 (47.1%) patients had posterior motion of the medial condyle. On average, from heel-strike to toe-off, the lateral condyle

translated 0.3 mm (5.7 to −2.7 mm; SD, 2.4) in the anterior direction and the medial condyle translated −0.2 mm posteriorly (4.3 to −5.1 mm; SD, 3.1). Nine of 34 (26.5%) patients experienced greater than 3 mm of paradoxical anterior femoral translation of either condyle and 17 of 34 patients (50%) experienced greater than 3 mm at any increment of stance phase.

A summary comparison of each study group revealed some interesting findings during the stance phase of gait (Table 89–4). Patients with a normal knee experienced the highest incidence (90%) and magnitude (−5.8 mm) of posterior motion of the lateral femoral condyle. The kinematic patterns for the fixed- and mobile-bearing posterior-stabilized TKA groups were similar, as were the kinematic patterns for the various mobile-bearing designs (PCL-retaining mobile-bearing, posterior-stabilized mobile-bearing, and PCL-sacrificing mobile-bearing TKA). On average, for all TKAs during the stance phase of gait, only 125 of 236 (53.0%) patients had posterior motion of their lateral condyle and 102 of 236 (43.2%) patients experienced posterior motion of the medial condyle. On average, the lateral condyle translated posteriorly −0.5 mm (SD, 3.3) and the medial condyle translated anteriorly 0.2 mm (SD, 3.1). Although it was expected that knees with an intact ACL and PCL (normal knees and ACL-retaining TKA groups) would demonstrate less variability in kinematic data, the opposite was observed, but this could also be attributed to bone size and each subject's specific gait motion.

No statistically significant differences between the normal knee and any of the TKA groups were noted in magnitudes of femorotibial translation during the entire stance phase of gait (heel-strike to toe-off: $p > 0.1$). However, kinematic patterns occurring during individual interval segments of the stance phase (heel-strike to 33% of stance phase, 33% to 66% of stance phase, and 66% of stance phase to toe-off) were often visibly different. Additionally, although the magnitude of AP translation during gait was similar among groups, the contact location for normal knees was typically centrally located on the tibia whereas the contact for most of the TKA groups was posterior, particular in PCL-retaining TKA.

DEEP KNEE BEND

All 10 (100%) subjects with a normal knee experienced posterior motion of the lateral condyle from full extension to 90 degrees of knee flexion, whereas 9 of 10 (90%) subjects experienced posterior motion of the medial condyle (Table 89–5, Fig. 89–5). On average, lateral condylar

motion was −19.2 mm (−5.8 to −31.6 mm; SD, 8.4) and medial condylar motion was −3.4 mm (3.3 to −11.8 mm; SD, 4.6) in the posterior direction. All subjects experienced posterior motion of both condyles from full extension to maximum flexion, but 3 of 10 (30%) subjects had greater than 3 mm of medial condyle anterior translation during any increment of knee flexion. All lateral femoral condyles experienced only posterior motion. The maximum amount of medial condyle anterior translation was 5 mm. Similar to the subjects with a normal knee, all 10 (100%) patients with an ACL-retaining fixed-bearing TKA experienced posterior motion of their lateral condyle and 9 of 10 (90%) patients had posterior motion of their medial condyle (see Table 89–5). The average amount of lateral condylar movement was −13.6 mm (−10.0 to −20.3 mm; SD, 3.7) and the average medial condylar motion was −6.1 mm (5.6 to −15.0 mm; SD, 6.3) in the posterior direction. One of 10 (10%) patients experienced paradoxical anterior femoral motion of their medial condyle greater than 3 mm from full extension to 90 degrees of knee flexion and 6 of 10 (60%) patients experienced greater than 3 mm of medial condyle anterior translation during any increment of knee flexion. Similar to the normal knee, all lateral femoral condyles demonstrated only posterior motion.

Unlike the subjects with a normal knee or an ACL-retaining fixed-bearing TKA, only 87 of 136 patients (63.9%) with a PCL-retaining fixed-bearing TKA experienced posterior motion of their lateral condyle and even fewer, 47 of 136 (34.5%), had posterior motion of their medial condyle (Table 89–6). On average, from full extension to 90 degrees of flexion, patients experienced only −1.6 mm (4.7 to −6.4 mm; SD, 3.4) of posterior motion of the lateral condyle, whereas medial condylar motion was 1.0 mm (6.3 to −4.3 mm; SD, 3.5) anteriorly, significantly less than the normal knee or ACL-retaining fixed-bearing TKA ($p < 0.01$). From full extension to 90 degrees of knee flexion, 32 of 136 (23.5%) subjects experienced greater than 3 mm of anterior translation and 95 of 136 (69.8%) subjects experienced anterior femoral translation greater than 3 mm at any flexion increment of either the medial or lateral femoral condyle. Although this group of subjects had variable kinematic patterns, there was a distinct difference between subjects with an asymmetric condylar TKA and with those with a symmetric condylar TKA. In one study, 20 of 20 subjects who had a PCL-retaining TKA with asymmetric condyles achieved posterior femoral rollback of their lateral condyle. Unlike patients who

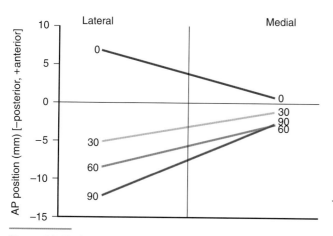

Figure 89–5. Graph showing the average medial and lateral condyle contact positions during a deep knee bend for a normal knee (0 to 90 degrees of flexion)

Table 89–5. Anteroposterior Translation for the Normal Knee and Fixed-Bearing ACL-Retaining TKA during a Deep Knee Bend

	N	SUBJECTS POSTERIOR MOTION L	SUBJECTS POSTERIOR MOTION M	AVERAGE MOTION 0-90° (mm) L	AVERAGE MOTION 0-90° (mm) M	>3.0 mm 0-90° (%) M or L	>3.0 mm ANYTIME* (%) M or L	MAXIMUM MOTION (mm) M or L	STANDARD DEVIATION L	STANDARD DEVIATION M	PIVOT POSITION LP	PIVOT POSITION MP	PIVOT POSITION NP
Normal knee	10	10	9	−19.2	−3.4	0	0.3	5	8.4	4.6	1	8	1
Axiom	10	10	9	−13.6	−6.1	10	60	8.1	3.7	6.3	1	7	2

*Refers to greater than 3.0 mm of anterior motion for either condyle occurring anytime during any increment of flexion.
L, lateral condyle; M, medial condyle.

Table 89–6. Anteroposterior Translation for Fixed-Bearing TKA during a Deep Knee Bend

IMPLANT TYPE	N	SUBJECTS POSTERIOR MOTION L	M	AVERAGE MOTION 0-90° (mm) L	M	>3.0 mm 0-90° (%) M or L	>3.0 mm ANYTIME* (%) M or L	MAXIMUM MOTION (mm) M or L	STANDARD DEVIATION L	M	PIVOT POSITION LP	MP	NP
AMK PCR	5	4	4	−6.4	−2.4	40	100	10.1	6.0	8.5	0	4	1
PFC PCR	20	11	9	−1.6	−0.2	20	65	9.4	3.4	2.8	7	10	3
PFC PCR	20	7	5	0.5	2.0	35	70	8.8	2.7	3.5	11	9	0
PFC PCR	10	9	6	−2.0	−0.3	10	80	9.2	2.9	3.5	4	5	1
Sigma PCR	20	10	5	−0.9	1.5	20	95	10.0	4.3	3.0	8	10	2
Apollo PCR	10	8	1	−2.2	2.7	30	50	5.9	2.7	2.3	4	6	0
Genesis PCR	20	14	3	−1.4	1.9	25	70	7.8	2.9	2.1	11	9	2
Advantim PCR	6	1	0	2.6	6.4	83	100	10.5	2.7	3.1	5	1	0
FS 1000 PCR	5	4	2	−1.1	0.8	20	40	4.7	2.7	1.6	0	5	0
NexGen PCR	20	19	12	−3.7	−2.6	0	45	7.2	3.2	4.7	6	13	1
Ascent PS	10	8	6	−4	−2.9	10	40	6.1	4.3	4.1	3	7	0
Maxim PS	10	8	6	−5.5	−0.8	0	60	4.8	5.9	3	1	9	0
AMK PS	5	5	4	−5.1	−1.4	0	80	5.2	4	2	0	3	2
PFC PS	20	20	5	−7.1	0.9	0	70	8.1	2.4	3.3	2	18	0
Sigma PS	12	12	7	−3.7	−0.1	0	25	5.1	2.1	2.1	1	11	0
Sigma PS	20	13	10	−0.6	−0.5	5	35	7.6	1.7	2.5	8	8	4
Sigma PS	20	19	11	−3.6	−0.4	5	45	4.7	2.8	2.6	4	15	1
Apollo PS	10	8	5	−1.3	0	0	30	4.2	1.4	1.5	6	3	1
Apollo PS	8	5	8	−2.4	−1.9	0	38	7.8	4.3	0.9	1	7	0
Scorpio PS	10	7	6	−1.6	0	20	40	8.4	3.6	4.2	3	7	0
Natural PS	8	7	8	−5.5	−3.3	0	13	5.6	3.1	2.6	3	4	1
Legacy PS	30	24	22	−3.9	−1.8	7	43	7.5	4	3.2	5	20	5

*Refers to greater than 3.0 mm of anterior motion for either condyle occurring anytime during any increment of flexion.
L, lateral condyle; M, medial condyle; PCR, PCL retaining; PS, posterior stabilized.

had a PCL-retaining fixed-bearing TKA with symmetric condyles, those with a posterior-stabilized fixed-bearing TKA experienced a higher incidence and magnitude of posterior condylar motion, but less in magnitude when compared with the normal knee (see Table 89–6). From full extension to 90 degrees of knee flexion, 136 of 163 (83.4%) patients with a posterior-stabilized fixed-bearing TKA experienced posterior motion of their lateral condyle and 98 of 163 (60.1%) had posterior motion of their medial condyle. On average, lateral condylar motion was −3.7 mm (1.5 to −9.6 mm; SD, 3.3) and medial condylar motion was −1.0 mm (3.1 to −5.9 mm; SD, 2.7) in the posterior direction. From full extension to 90 degrees of knee flexion, only 6 of 163 (3.7%) subjects experienced greater than 3 mm of anterior femoral translation and 70 of 163 (42.9%) had anterior translation greater than 3 mm at any flexion increment of either the medial or lateral femoral condyle.

Patients with a PCL-retaining mobile-bearing TKA demonstrated kinematic trends similar to those of patients who had a PCL-retaining fixed-bearing TKA with symmetric condyles (Table 89–7). Only 47 of 69 (68.1%) patients experienced posterior motion of their lateral condyle and 32 of 69 (46.4%) had posterior motion of the medial condyle. On average, from full extension to 90 degrees of flexion, the lateral condyle moved −1.3 mm (5.2 to −7.1 mm; SD, 3.5) posteriorly and the medial

condyle moved 0.4 mm (5.9 to −6.8 mm; SD, 3.8) anteriorly. Seventeen of 69 (24.6%) patients experienced greater than 3 mm of anterior translation and 41 of 69 (59.4%) experienced anterior femoral translation greater than 3 mm at any flexion increment of either the medial or lateral femoral condyle. Patients with a posterior-stabilized mobile-bearing TKA showed kinematic trends very similar to those implanted with a posterior-stabilized fixed-bearing TKA (see Table 89–7). From full extension to 90 degrees of knee flexion, 87 of 103 (84.4%) patients experienced posterior motion of their lateral condyle and 51 of 103 (49.5%) had posterior motion of their medial condyle. In 6 of the 10 studies that were conducted, the patients experienced a 95% or greater incidence of lateral condyle posterior motion. On average, the amount of posterior motion was −3.8 mm (0.3 to −9.0 mm; SD, 2.9) for the lateral condyle and −0.7 mm (4.2 to −5.7 mm; SD, 3.0) for the medial condyle. From full extension to 90 degrees of knee flexion, 7 of 103 (6.8%) patients experienced greater than 3 mm of anterior translation and 35 of 103 (34.0%) experienced anterior femoral translation greater than 3 mm at any flexion increment of either the medial or lateral femoral condyle. Fifty of 59 (84.7%) patients with a PCL-sacrificing mobile-bearing TKA experienced posterior motion of their lateral condyle and 22 of 59 (37.3%) exhibited posterior motion of their medial condyle (see Table 89–7). The average amount of motion

Table 89–7. Anteroposterior Translation for Mobile-Bearing TKA during a Deep Knee Bend

IMPLANT TYPE	N	SUBJECTS POSTERIOR MOTION L	M	AVERAGE MOTION 0-90° (mm) L	M	>3.0 mm 0-90° (%) M or L	>3.0 mm ANYTIME* (%) M or L	MAXIMUM MOTION (mm) M or L	STANDARD DEVIATION L	M	PIVOT POSITION LP	MP	NP
LCS AP Glide PCR	10	7	8	−1.4	−0.9	0	30	5.8	3.5	2.1	2	6	2
LCS AP Glide	10	7	7	−0.9	−1.8	20	70	8.4	3.2	4.6	3	4	3
LCS Meniscal Bearing PCR	13	11	5	−2.2	2.8	54	85	25.7	4.2	5.5	7	5	1
Sigma RP PCR	15	14	4	−3.3	0.7	20	53	6.0	2.8	3.4	8	6	1
MBK PCR	21	8	8	1.4	1.2	33	62	12.4	3.8	3.3	10	7	4
LCS RP PS	10	9	6	−4.9	−1.1	0	30	4.9	2.9	2.5	2	8	0
LCS RP PS	5	5	5	−5.9	−2	0	0	2.8	4.3	2.2	1	3	1
LCS RP PS	10	9	5	−2.2	−1.4	0	20	5.8	2.9	4.3	5	4	1
LCS RP PS	10	7	7	−2.7	−1.3	0	30	8.5	3.7	2.3	3	7	0
Sigma RP PS	10	9	3	−2.3	0.7	10	30	3.8	1.3	1.8	1	8	1
Sigma RP PS	20	19	4	−3.7	1.8	20	60	9.1	2.7	2.5	4	15	1
Sigma RP PS	10	7	7	−2.3	−1.5	10	30	5.7	2.2	3.1	7	3	0
Scorpio Super Flex PS	10	8	5	−2.4	−0.2	0	40	5.3	2.6	1.9	6	3	1
Legacy High Flex PS	10	6	1	−1.2	2.5	30	70	7.9	2	2.5	3	7	0
SROM RP PS	8	8	8	−11.8	−5.9	0	25	8.4	4.7	5.3	1	7	0
LCS RP PS	20	18	6	−3.1	0.8	30	65	10.2	3.3	3	11	9	0
LCS RP PS	8	6	3	−0.9	−0.5	0	63	4.5	2.4	2.5	4	4	0
LCS RP PS	17	13	6	−1.6	0.6	29	47	6.0	3.5	2.5	6	8	3
LCS RP PS	9	8	4	−2.6	1.2	11	56	7.5	2	2.9	3	6	0
LCS RP PS	5	5	3	−2.5	0.1	20	40	6.0	2.1	2.1	3	2	0

*Refers to greater than 3.0 mm of anterior motion for either condyle occurring anytime during any increment of flexion.
L, lateral condyle; M, medial condyle; PCR, PCL retaining; PS, posterior stabilized.

Table 89–8. Average Anteroposterior Translation for All Groups during a Deep Knee Bend

IMPLANT TYPE	N	SUBJECTS POSTERIOR MOTION L	M	AVERAGE MOTION 0-90° (mm) L	M	>3.0 mm 0-90° (%) M or L	>3.0 mm ANYTIME* (%) M or L	MAXIMUM MOTION (mm) M or L	STANDARD DEVIATION L	M	PIVOT POSITION LP	MP	NP
Normal	10	100.0	90.0	−19.2	−3.4	0	30	5.0	8.4	4.6	10.0	80.0	10.0
ACR	10	100.0	90.0	−13.6	−6.1	10	60	8.1	3.7	6.3	10.0	70.0	20.0
PCR	136	64.0	34.6	−1.6	1.0	28	72	8.4	3.4	3.5	41.2	52.9	7.4
PS	163	83.4	60.1	−3.7	−1.0	4	43	6.3	3.3	2.7	22.7	68.7	8.6
PCR mobile bearing	69	68.1	46.4	−1.3	0.4	25	60	11.7	3.5	3.8	43.5	40.6	15.9
PS mobile bearing	103	84.5	49.5	−3.9	−0.8	7	34	6.2	2.9	2.8	32.0	63.1	4.9
PCS mobile bearing	59	84.7	37.3	−2.1	0.4	18	54	6.8	2.7	2.6	45.8	49.2	5.1
Averages		76.9	45.6	−2.5	0.0	17	52	7.9	3.1	3.1	37.0	54.9	8.4

*Refers to greater than 3.0 mm of anterior motion for either condyle occurring anytime during any increment of flexion.
ACR, ACL retaining; L, lateral condyle; M, medial condyle; PCR, PCL retaining; PCS, PCL sacrificing; PS, posterior stabilized.

was −2.1 mm (1.5 to −8.8 mm; SD, 2.8) in the posterior direction for the lateral condyle and 0.3 mm (3.8 to −4.1 mm; SD, 0.3) in the anterior direction for the medial condyle. From full extension to 90 degrees of knee flexion, 13 of 59 (22.0%) patients experienced greater than 3 mm of anterior translation and 33 of 59 (55.9%) had an anterior slide greater than 3 mm at any flexion increment.

Similar to the gait activity, overall comparison of each group revealed some interesting phenomena (Table 89–8). The normal knee and ACL-retaining fixed-bearing TKA groups experienced very similar results and had the highest variability (widest standard deviations) of any knee group. The normal and ACL-retaining TKA groups showed the highest magnitudes of posterior femoral rollback of both the medial and lateral femoral condyles when compared with any of the other TKA groups ($p < 0.01$). Fixed-bearing posterior-stabilized TKA demonstrated greater posterior femoral rollback of the medial and lateral condyles than did fixed- or mobile-bearing PCL-retaining TKA and PCL-sacrificing mobile-bearing TKA ($p < 0.01$), but the rollback was statistically similar to that of mobile-bearing, posterior-stabilized TKA ($p > 0.5$). No statistically significant differences were observed among fixed- and mobile-bearing PCL-retaining TKA groups or PCL-sacrificing mobile-bearing TKA ($p < 0.2$). When investigating the effects of surgeon variability on AP motion patterns of subjects implanted with the same TKA design, no differences were observed ($p > 0.2$) in an analysis of the mobile-bearing TKA groups. In contrast, statistically significant differences among different surgeons was observed for subjects implanted with fixed-bearing TKA devices ($p < 0.05$).

Axial Femorotibial Rotation

GAIT

From heel-strike to toe-off, 8 of 10 (80%) subjects with a normal knee experienced normal axial rotation (tibia internally rotating with increasing knee flexion) and 8 of 10 (80%) experienced reverse rotation during at least one analyzed increment of the stance phase of gait (Table 89–9, see Fig. 89–4). The normal knee did not experience progressively increasing axial rotation during the stance phase of gait, but rather demonstrated a variable pattern that involves extension, flexion, extension, and then flexion before toe-off. This variable pattern is due to the knee flexion angle changing from flexion to extension during the stance phase of gait and leading to the presence of both internal and external rotation of the tibia during the stance phase of gait. The average amount of axial rotation from heel-strike to toe-off for all normal knees was 5.7 degrees and the average maximum axial rotation at any increment during stance phase increased to 11.1 degrees. The maximum amount of normal rotation observed for any individual knee at any analyzed increment was 24.0 degrees (tibia internal rotation) and the maximum opposite rotation observed was −10.1 degrees (tibia external rotation). Nine of 10 (90%) subjects achieved at least 5.0 degrees of normal rotation, 5 of 10 (50%) had greater than 10.0 degrees, and 5 of 10 (50%) demonstrated greater than −5.0 degrees of reverse rotation. Patients who received an ACL-retaining fixed-bearing TKA and those with an ACL-deficient (non-implanted) knee experienced less overall rotation and greater variability than the normal knee did (see Table 89–9). The average amount of axial rotation from heel-strike to toe-off for these knees was only 2.0 degrees and the average maximum amount of axial rotation at any increment of stance phase increased to only 3.5 degrees.

Patients with a PCL-retaining fixed-bearing TKA also experienced less overall rotation and greater variability than the normal knee did (Table 89–10). The average amount of axial rotation from heel-strike to toe-off for these knees was only 2.1 degrees and the average maximum amount at any increment during stance phase was 5.3 degrees. The average maximum amount of normal and reverse rotation for each fixed-bearing PCL-retaining TKA study group was 9.6 and −7.6 degrees, respectively (see Table 89–12). Patients with a posterior-stabilized fixed-bearing TKA experienced less overall rotation and greater variability than the normal or PCL-retaining fixed-

bearing TKA groups did during the stance phase of gait (see Table 89–10). The average amount of axial rotation from heel-strike to toe-off for these knees was only 1.4 degrees and the average maximum amount at any increment during stance phase increased to 4.3 degrees. The average maximum amount of normal and reverse rotation for each fixed-bearing posterior-stabilized TKA study group was 8.2 and −7.0 degrees, respectively (see Table 89–12).

Patients with a PCL-retaining mobile-bearing TKA experienced, on average, less rotation than did subjects with a PCL-retaining fixed-bearing TKA during the stance phase of gait (Table 89–11). The average amount of axial rotation from heel-strike to toe-off was only 0.1 degree and the average maximum amount of axial rotation at any increment during stance phase increased to 5.1 degrees. The maximum amount of normal and reverse rotation for any individual TKA at any analyzed increment was 9.9 and −26.6 degrees.

Patients with a posterior-stabilized mobile-bearing TKA experienced, on average, more rotation than did subjects with a posterior-stabilized fixed-bearing TKA during the stance phase of gait (Table 89–11). The average amount of axial rotation from heel-strike to toe-off was 2.2 degrees and the average maximum amount at any increment during stance phase increased to 4.7 degrees. The average maximum amount of normal and reverse rotation for each mobile-bearing posterior-stabilized TKA study group was 12.0 and −5.9 degrees, respectively (Table 89–12). Patients with a PCL-sacrificing mobile-bearing TKA experienced, on average, minimal rotation during the stance phase of gait (see Table 89–11). The average amount of axial rotation from heel-strike to toe-off was 0.0 degree and the average maximum amount of axial rotation at any increment during stance phase was 3.0 degrees. The average maximum amount of normal and reverse rotation for each mobile-bearing PCL-sacrificing TKA study group was 7.3 and −10.1 degrees, respectively (see Table 89–11).

A summary comparison of each study group revealed some interesting findings during the stance phase of gait (Table 89–12). Patients with a normal knee experienced the highest incidence (80%) and magnitude (average, 5.7 degrees; average maximum, 24.0 degrees) of axial rotation. The axial rotation patterns for the fixed- and mobile-bearing posterior-stabilized TKA groups were similar, as were the axial rotation patterns for the fixed- and mobile-bearing PCL-retaining TKA groups. Although most subjects with a PCL-sacrificing mobile-bearing TKA did experience axial rotation, the *average* rotation for this group was 0.0 degrees. On average, for all TKAs during the stance phase of gait, only 146 of 252 (57.9%) knees experienced a normal axial rotational pattern, a decrease from the normal knees, which experienced 80% normal rotation, but this difference was not statistically different ($p = 0.15$). In addition, only 86 of 252 (34.1%) TKAs experienced greater than 5.0 degrees of axial rotation at any increment, a significant decrease from that observed in normal knees (90%; $p < 0.05$). This trend continued for knees experiencing greater than 10.0 degrees of axial rotation. Only 15 of 252 (6.0%) TKAs experienced greater than 10.0 degrees of axial rotation as compared with 50% of the normal knee group ($p = 0.01$).

Table 89–9. Axial Rotation for the Normal Knee, ACL-Retaining TKA, and Nonimplanted ACL-Deficient Knee in Gait

	N	NORMAL ROTATION[1] (HS-TO) (%)	REVERSE ROTATION[2] (HS-TO) (%)	NORMAL ROTATION[3] ALL INCR. (%)	REVERSE ROTATION[4] ANY INCR. (%)	AVERAGE ROTATION (HS-TO)[5] (°)	AVERAGE MAX. ROT. ALL INCR.[6] (°)	AVERAGE MAX. REV. ALL INCR.[7] (°)	MAXIMUM NOR. ROT. ALL INCR.[8] (°)	MAXIMUM REV. ROT. ALL INCR.[9] (°)	NORMAL ROTATION[10] >5.0° (%)	NORMAL ROTATION[11] >10.0° (%)	REVERSE ROTATION[12] ≥5.0° (%)
Normal knee	10	80	20	20	80	5.7	11.1	−4.1	24.0	−10.1	90	50	50
Hermes	15	33	67	27	73	2.0	3.5	−1.6	12.0	−5.4	13	7	7
ACL deficient	5	60	40	0	100	2.0	10.4	−7.4	17.5	−19.3	80	40	40

[1]Refers to the percentage of knees experiencing normal rotation from heel-strike to toe-off.
[2]Refers to the percentage of knees experiencing reverse rotation from heel-strike to toe-off.
[3]Refers to the percentage of knees experiencing normal rotation during all increments of the stance phase of gait.
[4]Refers to the percentage of knees experiencing reverse rotation during at least one increment of the stance phase of gait.
[5]Refers to the average rotation from heel-strike to toe-off.
[6]Refers to the average maximum normal rotation each knee achieved at any increment of the stance phase of gait.
[7]Refers to the average maximum reverse rotation each knee achieved at any increment of the stance phase of gait.
[8]Refers to the maximum normal rotation each knee achieved at any increment of the stance phase of gait.
[9]Refers to the maximum reverse rotation each knee achieved at any increment of the stance phase of gait.
[10]Refers to the percentage of knees experiencing at least 5.0 degrees of normal axial rotation at any increment of the stance phase of gait.
[11]Refers to the percentage of knees experiencing at least 10.0 degrees of normal axial rotation at any increment of the stance phase of gait.
[12]Refers to the percentage of knees experiencing at least −5.0 degrees of reverse axial rotation at any increment of the stance phase of gait.

Table 89–10. Axial Rotation for Fixed-Bearing PCL-Retaining and Posterior-Stabilized TKA in Gait

IMPLANT TYPE	N	NORMAL ROTATION[1] (HS-TO) (%)	REVERSE ROTATION[2] (HS-TO) (%)	NORMAL ROTATION ALL INCR.[3] (%)	REVERSE ROTATION ANY INCR.[4] (%)	AVERAGE ROTATION (HS-TO)[5] (°)	AVERAGE MAX. ROT. ALL INCR.[6] (°)	AVERAGE MAX. REV. ALL INCR.[7] (°)	MAXIMUM NOR. ROT. ALL INCR.[8] (°)	MAXIMUM REV. ROT. ALL INCR.[9] (°)	NORMAL ROTATION[10] >5.0° (%)	NORMAL ROTATION[11] >10.0° (%)	REVERSE ROTATION[12] ≥5.0° (%)
AMK PCR	5	100	0	20	80	5.9	6.8	−0.9	10.5	−2.8	80	20	0
AMK PCR	5	40	60	0	100	−4.0	2.6	−6.3	4.3	−17.2	0	0	40
AMK PCR	5	80	20	20	80	3.1	5.4	−1.7	7.9	−3.5	40	0	0
PFC PCR	15	60	40	13	87	0.1	2.8	−3.1	9.0	−11.1	13	0	20
Sigma PCR	5	100	0	20	80	5.0	8.0	−2.8	12.2	−6.0	80	40	40
Apollo PCR	10	90	10	20	80	6.4	7.9	−2.1	16-3	−5.1	80	40	10
Advance Medial Pivot PCR	5	60	40	0	100	2.2	4.0	−1.8	5.1	−3.1	40	0	0
Advance Traditional PCR	5	60	40	0	100	0.2	5.6	−4.7	9.5	−7.9	60	0	60
Advantim PCR	8	75	25	0	100	2.3	6.2	−4.3	9.6	−6.9	38	0	13
NexGen PCR	20	55	45	0	100	−0.5	3.2	−3.7	11.2	−12.4	25	5	30
Hermes PS	15	40	60	7	93	0.5	3.6	−2.7	8.3	−5.6	27	0	13
AMK PS	10	60	40	10	90	1.3	3.9	−2.8	8.5	−6.7	30	0	10
AMK PS	5	60	40	20	80	0.7	3.1	−2.0	4.6	−5.8	0	0	20
AMK PS	4	50	50	25	75	4.4	7.4	−3.6	11.8	−8.5	75	25	50
AMK PS	5	80	20	20	80	2.0	4.0	−2.3	7.1	−7.5	20	0	20
IB2 PS	10	40	60	20	80	0.8	4.7	−2.9	8.1	−7.1	50	0	20
PFC PS	15	40	53	13	87	−0.1	3.3	−3.6	10.0	−8.2	27	7	20
Apollo PS	10	80	20	0	100	1.7	4.1	−2.9	7.2	−6.2	30	0	20

See footnotes in Table 89–9.
PCR, PCL retaining; PS, posterior stabilized.

Table 89–11. Axial Rotation for the Mobile-Bearing PCL-Retaining and Posterior-Stabilized, and PCL-Sacrificing TKA in Gait

IMPLANT TYPE	N	NORMAL ROTATION[1] (HS-TO) (%)	REVERSE ROTATION[2] (HS-TO) (%)	NORMAL ROTATION ALL INCR.[3] (%)	REVERSE ROTATION ANY INCR.[4] (%)	AVERAGE ROTATION (HS-TO)[5] (°)	AVERAGE MAX. ROT. ALL INCR.[6] (°)	AVERAGE MAX. REV. ALL INCR.[7] (°)	MAXIMUM NOR. ROT. ALL INCR.[8] (°)	MAXIMUM REV. ROT. ALL INCR.[9] (°)	NORMAL ROTATION[10] >5.0° (%)	NORMAL ROTATION[11] >10.0° (%)	REVERSE ROTATION[12] ≥5.0° (%)
LCS AP Glide PCR	10	60	40	20	80	0.1	5.1	-5.0	9.9	-26.6	40	0	40
LCS RP PS	10	100	0	0	100	5.5	8.0	-2.8	15.8	-4.9	90	30	0
LCS RP PS	10	30	70	20	80	-1.3	2.6	-3.2	8.6	-7.6	10	0	30
LCS RP PS	5	80	20	20	80	3.0	5.5	-3.1	10.9	-8.2	40	20	20
Sigma RP PS	10	40	50	0	100	1.6	2.7	-1.1	12.6	-3.0	10	10	0
LCS RP PCS	20	45	55	10	85	0.5	3.5	-2.9	9.6	-12.1	35	0	20
LCS RP PCS	5	20	80	20	80	-2.5	1.3	-4.2	3.7	-13.3	0	0	20
LCS RP PCS	10	80	20	10	90	2.1	4.3	-2.5	8.5	-4.9	40	0	0

See footnotes in Table 89–9.
PCR, PCL retaining; PCS, PCL sacrificing; PS, posterior stabilized.

Table 89–12. Summation Analysis for the Axial Rotation of All Knee Types in Gait

IMPLANT TYPE	N	NORMAL ROTATION[1] (HS-TO) (%)	REVERSE ROTATION[2] (HS-TO) (%)	NORMAL ROTATION ALL INCR.[3] (%)	REVERSE ROTATION ANY INCR.[4] (%)	AVERAGE ROTATION (HS-TO)[5] (°)	AVERAGE MAX. ROT. ALL INCR.[6] (°)	AVERAGE MAX. REV. ALL INCR.[7] (°)	MAXIMUM NOR. ROT. ALL INCR.[8] (°)	MAXIMUM REV. ROT. ALL INCR.[9] (°)	NORMAL ROTATION[10] >5.0° (%)	NORMAL ROTATION[11] >10.0° (%)	REVERSE ROTATION[12] ≥5.0° (%)
Normal	10	80	20	20	80	5.7	11.1	-4.1	24.0	-10.1	90	50	50
Fixed bearing ACR	15	33	67	27	73	2	3.5	-1.6	12	-5.4	13	7	7
ACL deficient	5	60	40	0	100	2	10.4	-7.4	17.5	-19.3	80	40	40
Fixed bearing PCR (+ PCL)	83	69	31	8	92	2.1	5.3	-3.1	9.6	-7.6	40	10	22
Fixed bearing PS	74	53	46	12	88	1.4	4.3	-2.9	8.2	-7.0	31	3	19
Mobile bearing PCR	10	60	40	20	80	0.1	5.1	-5	9.9	-26.6	40	0	40
Mobile bearing PS	35	60	37	9	91	2.2	4.7	-2.6	9.9	-5.9	37	14	11
Mobile bearing PCS	35	51	49	11	86	0.0	3.0	-3.2	7.3	-10.1	31	0	14
Average of all knees		59	40	17	83	1.9	5.9	-3.7	12.6	-11.5	37	9	20
Average of all TKA		58	41	12	88	1.2	4.5	-3.3	9.4	-11.4	34	6	18

See footnotes in Table 89–9.
ACL, anterior cruciate ligament; ACR, ACL retaining; PCL, posterior cruciate ligament; PCR, PCL retaining; PCS, PCL sacrificing; PS, posterior stabilized; TKA, total knee arthroplasty.

DEEP KNEE BEND

From full extension to 90 degrees of knee flexion, all 10 normal knees experienced normal axial rotation (tibia internally rotating with increasing knee flexion) and only 4 of 10 (40%) subjects demonstrated reverse rotation during at least one flexion increment of a deep knee bend (Table 89–13, see Fig. 89–5). The average amount of axial rotation from full extension to 90 degrees of knee flexion was 16.5 degrees and the average maximum amount of axial rotation at any flexion increment was 17.3 degrees. The maximum amount of normal and reverse rotation of any normal knee at any flexion increment was 27.7 and −7.3 degrees. All 10 knees achieved at least 5.0 degrees of normal rotation, 9 of 10 (90%) achieved greater than 10.0 degrees, and only 1 of 10 (10%) demonstrated greater than −5.0 degrees of reverse rotation. Patients who received an ACL-retaining fixed-bearing TKA also achieved excellent axial rotation patterns, whereas those with an ACL-deficient knee experienced more variable rotational patterns (see Table 89–13). Seven of 10 (70%) knees implanted with an ACL-retaining fixed-bearing TKA experienced normal rotation from full extension to 90 degrees of knee flexion and 6 of 10 (60%) experienced reverse rotation during at least one flexion increment. The average amount of axial rotation from full extension to 90 degrees of knee flexion was 8.1 degrees and the average maximum amount at any increment of a deep knee bend increased to 11.8 degrees.

Patients with a PCL-retaining fixed-bearing TKA experienced less overall rotation and greater variability than the normal knee did ($p = 0.0004$; Table 89–14). The average amount of axial rotation for all knees from full extension to 90 degrees of knee flexion was only 3.7 degrees, and this amount increased to 6.5 degrees when assessing the maximum average of all increments of flexion during a deep knee bend. The average maximum amount of normal and reverse rotation for each fixed-bearing PCL-retaining TKA study group was 13.0 and −9.7 degrees, respectively (see Table 89–14). Similar to the AP analysis, subjects who had a PCL-retaining TKA with asymmetric condyles also achieved more normal axial rotation patterns than did subjects with a PCL-retaining TKA with symmetric condyles. Patients with a posterior-stabilized fixed-bearing TKA experienced slightly less overall rotation than did subjects with a PCL-retaining fixed-bearing TKA during a deep knee bend and significantly less rotation than the normal knee ($p = 0.0004$; Table 89–14). The average amount of axial rotation from full extension to 90 degrees of flexion was 3.1 degrees and the average maximum axial rotation at any flexion increment increased to 5.5 degrees. The average maximum amount of normal and reverse rotation for each fixed-bearing posterior-stabilized TKA study group was 11.5 and −7.6 degrees, respectively (see Table 89–14).

Patients with a PCL-retaining mobile-bearing TKA experienced axial rotational patterns similar to those of subjects with a PCL-retaining fixed-bearing TKA but less than that in normal knees ($p = 0.0005$; Table 89–15). The average amount of axial rotation from full extension to 90 degrees of knee flexion was 3.9 degrees and the average maximum axial rotation at any flexion increment

increased to 7.3 degrees. The average maximum amount of normal and reverse rotation for each mobile-bearing PCL-retaining TKA study group was 15.6 and −11.4 degrees, respectively (see Table 89–15). Patients with a posterior-stabilized mobile-bearing TKA experienced, on average, statistically more rotation than did subjects with a posterior-stabilized fixed-bearing TKA ($p = 0.02$) during a deep knee bend but less than that in normal knees ($p = 0.0009$; see Table 89–15). The average amount of axial rotation from full extension to 90 degrees of knee flexion was 3.9 degrees, and this amount increased to 6.5 degrees when the average maximum amount of axial rotation at any flexion increment was determined. The average maximum amount of normal and reverse rotation for each mobile-bearing posterior-stabilized TKA study group was 12.5 and −8.9 degrees, respectively (see Table 89–15). Patients with a PCL-sacrificing mobile-bearing TKA experienced, on average, slightly less rotation during a deep knee bend than did subjects with either a PCL-retaining or posterior-stabilized mobile-bearing TKA and significantly less than normal knees ($p = 0.0003$; see Table 89–15). The average amount of axial rotation from full extension to 90 degrees of knee flexion was 3.3 degrees, and this amount increased to 5.5 degrees when the average maximum amount of axial rotation at any flexion increment was determined. The average maximum amount of normal and reverse rotation for each mobile-bearing PCL-sacrificing TKA study group was 11.4 and −5.9 degrees, respectively (see Table 89–15).

A summary comparison of each study group revealed some interesting findings during knee flexion from full extension to 90 degrees of knee flexion (Table 89–16). Patients with a normal knee experienced the highest incidence (100%) and magnitude (average, 16.5 degrees; maximum, 27.7 degrees) of axial rotation. The axial rotation patterns for the fixed- and mobile-bearing posterior-stabilized TKA groups were similar, as were the axial rotation patterns for the fixed- and mobile-bearing PCL-retaining TKA groups. Substantial variability in average and maximum axial rotation values was observed within each implant group. For example, the range of average axial rotation was −1.1 to 7.6 degrees for the PCL-retaining mobile-bearing TKA group and 1.0 to 7.2 degrees for the posterior-stabilized mobile-bearing TKA group (see Table 89–16). Similarly, the maximum amount of normal rotation ranged from 7.0 to 35.9 degrees and from 9.5 to 22.4 degrees for subjects with a PCL-retaining and posterior-stabilized mobile-bearing TKA, respectively (see Table 89–16). On average, for all TKAs during a deep knee bend, only 551 of 745 (74.0%) knees experienced a normal axial rotational pattern, a significant decrease from the normal knee group in which 100% (10 of 10) demonstrated a normal axial rotational pattern ($p = 0.001$). Also, only 425 of 745 (57.0%) TKAs experienced greater than 5.0 degrees of axial rotation at any increment, a significant decrease from the normal knee group (100%, 10 of 10; $p = 0.001$). This trend continued for the number of knees experiencing greater than 10.0 degrees of axial rotation. Only 127 of 745 (17.0%) subjects with a TKA experienced greater than 10.0 degrees of axial rotation versus 90% (9 of 10) of normal knees ($p = 0.001$).

Text continues on p. 1609

Table 89–13. Axial Rotation for the Normal Knee, ACL-Retaining TKA, and Nonimplanted ACL-Deficient Knee during a Deep Knee Bend

	N	NORMAL ROTATION[1] (90-0) (%)	REVERSE ROTATION[2] (90-0) (%)	NORMAL ROTATION ALL INCR.[3] (%)	REVERSE ROTATION ANY INCR.[4] (%)	AVERAGE ROTATION (90-0)[5] (°)	AVERAGE MAX. ROT. ALL INCR.[6] (°)	AVERAGE MAX. REV. ALL INCR.[7] (°)	MAXIMUM NOR. ROT. ALL INCR.[8] (°)	MAXIMUM REV. ROT. ALL INCR.[9] (°)	NORMAL ROTATION[10] >5.0° (%)	NORMAL ROTATION[11] >10.0° (%)	REVERSE ROTATION[12] ≥5.0° (%)
Normal knee	10	100	0	60	40	16.5	17.3	-0.3	27.7	-7.3	100	90	10
Axiom	10	70	20	40	60	8.1	11.8	-3.3	20.9	-14.1	90	40	60
ACL deficient	5	60	40	20	80	9.8	13.3	-4.3	21.2	-9.8	80	60	40

[1]Refers to the percentage of knees experiencing normal rotation from 0 to 90 degrees of knee flexion.
[2]Refers to the percentage of knees experiencing reverse rotation from 0 to 90 degrees of knee flexion.
[3]Refers to the percentage of knees experiencing normal rotation during all increments of knee flexion t.
[4]Refers to the percentage of knees experiencing reverse rotation during at least one increment of knee flexion.
[5]Refers to the average rotation from 0 to 90 degrees of knee flexion.
[6]Refers to the average maximum normal rotation each knee achieved at any increment of knee flexion .
[7]Refers to the average maximum reverse rotation each knee achieved at any increment of knee flexion.
[8]Refers to the maximum normal rotation each knee achieved at any increment of knee flexion.
[9]Refers to the maximum reverse rotation each knee achieved at any increment of knee flexion.
[10]Refers to the percentage of knees experiencing at least 5.0 degrees of normal axial rotation at any increment of knee flexion.
[11]Refers to the percentage of knees experiencing at least 10.0 degrees of normal axial rotation at any increment of knee flexion.
[12]Refers to the percentage of knees experiencing at least -5.0 degrees of reverse axial rotation at any increment of knee flexion.

Table 89–14. Axial Rotation for Fixed-Bearing PCL-Retaining and Posterior-Stabilized TKA during a Deep Knee Bend

IMPLANT TYPE	N	NORMAL ROTATION[1] (90-0) (%)	REVERSE ROTATION[2] (90-0) (%)	NORMAL ROTATION ALL INCR.[3] (%)	REVERSE ROTATION ANY INCR.[4] (%)	AVERAGE ROTATION (90-0)[5] (°)	AVERAGE MAX. ROT. ALL INCR.[6] (°)	AVERAGE MAX. REV. ALL INCR.[7] (°)	MAXIMUM NOR. ROT. ALL INCR.[8] (°)	MAXIMUM REV. ROT. ALL INCR.[9] (°)	NORMAL ROTATION[10] >5.0° (%)	NORMAL ROTATION[11] >10.0° (%)	REVERSE ROTATION[12] ≥5.0° (%)
AMK PCR	5	80	20	40	60	5.3	7.9	-1.9	14.3	-10.7	80	20	20
PFC PCR	20	75	25	15	85	1.8	5.6	-3.5	9.6	-14.2	60	0	20
PFC PCR	20	65	35	15	85	2.2	5.6	-3.4	16.9	-9.3	65	10	30
PFC PCR	10	80	20	10	90	3.0	8.1	-5.9	21.3	-15.8	70	30	40
Sigma PCR	18	89	11	22	78	3.2	4.8	-1.4	8.5	-7.4	44	0	11
Sigma PCR	9	78	11	11	89	3.8	5.1	-1.3	11.0	-3.5	44	11	0
Apollo PCR	10	90	10	20	80	6.4	7.9	-2.1	16.3	-5.1	80	40	10
Genesis PCR	10	80	20	50	50	5.4	8.5	-2.6	14.3	-14.8	70	50	20
Genesis PCR	10	100	0	20	80	5.5	8.0	-3.1	12.1	-7.7	90	20	40
Advantim PCR	6	83	17	17	83	3.0	6.6	-1.6	9.0	-4.7	83	0	0
FS 1000 PCR	5	80	20	20	80	2.3	3.5	-1.3	8.1	-4.2	20	0	35
NexGen PCR (+ PCL)	20	55	45	5	95	1.5	6.3	-5.4	13.1	-22.3	80	10	10
NexGen PCR (+ PCL)	20	90	10	30	65	4.1	6.0	-1.6	14.2	-6.7	65	10	25
NexGen PCR (– PCL)	20	40	60	5	95	-1.0	2.7	-3.4	5.8	-9.5	5	0	30
Ascent PS	10	70	30	10	90	1.2	4.5	-3.2	12.1	-8.7	30	20	0
Maxim PS	10	80	20	30	70	4.8	6.3	-1.2	11.7	-3.6	60	20	20
AMK PS	5	60	40	0	100	-1.0	3.7	-4.6	5.6	-13.7	20	0	0
PFC PS	20	100	0	50	50	10.4	11.3	-0.2	21.0	-4.8	90	60	5
PFC PS	20	85	15	45	55	4.1	5.4	-1.0	10.3	-9.1	55	5	33
Sigma PS	12	67	33	17	83	1.7	6.8	-3.7	15.1	-13.4	58	25	5
Sigma PS	20	85	15	45	55	4.1	5.4	-1.0	9.7	-9.0	60	0	33
Sigma PS	18	50	50	6	94	0.1	3.3	-3.1	8.0	-7.6	39	0	0
Sigma PS	9	67	0	11	89	2.2	3.7	-1.5	5.8	-4.6	22	0	20
Apollo PS	10	80	20	0	100	1.7	4.1	-2.9	7.2	-6.2	30	0	0
Apollo PS	8	75	25	13	88	2.6	4.9	-2.0	9.4	-4.3	50	0	0
Scorpio PS	10	70	30	20	80	2.8	6.9	-3.8	14.3	-13.2	60	30	20
Scorpio PS	10	80	20	20	80	2.8	5.0	-2.1	10.3	-8.8	40	10	20
Natural PS	8	75	25	13	75	2.6	4.0	-1.5	11.4	-3.8	25	13	0
Legacy PS	7	57	43	29	71	5.0	7.0	-2.1	13.1	-6.6	57	43	14
Legacy PS	10	90	10	40	60	4.9	6.6	-0.4	16.1	-2.8	60	20	
Legacy PS	25	72	28	12	84	1.9	3.8	-1.8	14.3	-9.7	20	8	8

See footnotes in Table 89-13.
PCL, posterior cruciate ligament; PCR, PCL retaining; PS, posterior stabilized.

Table 89–15. Axial Rotation for Mobile-Bearing PCL-Retaining, Posterior-Stabilized, and PCL-Sacrificing TKA during a Deep Knee Bend

IMPLANT TYPE	N	NORMAL ROTATION[1] (90-0) (%)	REVERSE ROTATION[2] (90-0) (%)	NORMAL ROTATION ALL INCR.[3] (%)	REVERSE ROTATION ANY INCR.[4] (%)	AVERAGE ROTATION (90-0)[5] (°)	AVERAGE MAX. ROT. ALL INCR.[6] (°)	AVERAGE MAX. REV. ALL INCR.[7] (°)	MAXIMUM NOR. ROT. ALL INCR.[8] (°)	MAXIMUM REV. ROT. ALL INCR.[9] (°)	NORMAL ROTATION[10] >5.0° (%)	NORMAL ROTATION[11] >10.0° (%)	REVERSE ROTATION[12] ≥5.0° (%)
LCS AP Glide PCR	10	60	40	0	100	0.6	4.2	-4.0	12.6	-7.7	40	10	40
LCS AP Glide PCR	10	50	50	0	100	-1.1	3.0	-4.1	7.0	-12.4	30	0	30
LCS AP Glide PCR	20	80	15	30	70	6.4	8.5	-2.1	19.9	-11.2	80	40	10
LCS AP Glide PCR	2	50	50	0	100	4.9	9.7	-7.9	14.1	-8.5	100	50	100
LCS Meniscal Bearing PCR	13	85	15	8	92	7.0	12.8	-6.4	35.9	-23.4	85	62	38
LCS Meniscal Bearing PCR	10	60	30	40	60	3.5	7.8	-2.5	10.5	-13.3	90	20	30
Sigma RP PCR	15	80	20	20	80	5.2	6.6	-1.2	13.1	-8.0	67	20	7
MBK PCR	7	100	0	71	29	7.6	8.1	0.2*	14.6	-3.8	71	29	0
MBK PCR	20	50	45	10	90	1.0	4.9	-4.9	12.5	-14.4	40	10	45
LCS RP PS	10	80	20	40	60	4.3	6.8	-2.2	12.4	-8.7	50	20	30
LCS RP PS	5	60	40	40	60	5.2	7.5	-1.8	13.9	-8.9	60	40	20
LCS RP PS	10	70	30	40	60	2.7	7.5	-4.4	14.6	-17.5	60	30	30
LCS RP PS	10	70	30	40	60	2.7	6.9	-3.7	13.1	-14.9	50	30	30
Sigma RP PS	10	100	0	30	70	4.0	4.8	-1.2	9.3	-3.6	40	0	0
Sigma RP PS	20	95	5	40	55	7.2	9.0	-1.3	22.4	-12.2	85	35	10
Sigma RP PS	10	50	50	10	90	1.0	3.7	-2.8	9.8	-9.7	40	0	20
Sigma RP PS	9	89	0	22	78	4.1	6.8	-2.2	11.2	-4.1	67	22	0
Scorpio Super Flex PS	10	80	20	20	80	4.0	7.5	-2.6	13.1	-10.2	60	30	20
Scorpio Super Flex PS	5	60	40	40	60	3.4	6.6	-2.2	9.5	-10.1	80	0	20
Legacy High Flex PS	10	90	10	30	70	4.6	5.6	-0.8	10.4	-2.9	50	20	0
Legacy High Flex PS	20	85	15	n/a†	n/a†	5.4	7.0	-3.7	13.3	-9.0	50	25	5
Legacy High Flex PS	5	40	40	0	100	1.8	5.2	-3.7	10.9	-5.1	40	20	20
Legacy High Flex PS	15	80	20	27	73	3.1	6.3	-3.6	10.9	-11.4	67	7	27
SROM RP PS	8	88	12	38	62	4.9	7.0	-1.7	13.2	-5.8	50	25	13
LCS RP PCS	10	20	80	10	90	6.4	8.5	-2.5	21.0	-6.8	80	30	20
LCS RP PCS	10	70	30	20	80	2.9	5.3	-2.2	9.6	-6.0	60	0	20
LCS RP PCS	8	50	50	13	87	0.6	4.6	-3.9	9.3	-7.2	63	0	38
LCS RP PCS	16	75	25	6	94	2.2	3.9	-1.8	14.7	-6.5	25	6	13
LCS RP PCS	2	100	0	0	100	1.1	2.8	-1.8	3.6	-1.8	0	0	0
LCS RP PCS	8	88	12	25	75	4.4	7.0	-2.4	14.5	-7.2	75	13	13
LCS RP PCS	8	38	25	25	75	1.7	3.4	-2.1	5.8	-4.6	25	0	0
LCS RP PCS	9	89	11	44	44	6.6	7.9	0.0	13.7	-8.4	67	44	11
LCS RP PCS	5	60	40	20	80	3.4	5.9	-2.5	10.1	-5.0	40	0	20

See numbered footnotes in Table 89–13.
*The average minimal rotation (reverse rotation) for each knee was positive.
†Patients were not analyzed at all increments of knee flexion.
PCR, PCL retaining; PCS, PCL sacrificing; PS, posterior stabilized.

Table 89–16. Summation Analysis for the Axial Rotation of All Knee Types during a Deep Knee Bend

IMPLANT TYPE	N	NORMAL ROTATION[1] (0-90) (%)	REVERSE ROTATION[2] (0-90) (%)	NORMAL ROTATION ALL INCR.[3] (%)	REVERSE ROTATION ANY INCR.[4] (%)	AVERAGE ROTATION (0-90)[5] (°)	AVERAGE MAX. ROT. ALL INCR.[6] (°)	AVERAGE MAX. REV. ALL INCR.[7] (°)	MAXIMUM NOR. ROT. ALL INCR.[8] (°)	MAXIMUM REV. ROT. ALL INCR.[9] (°)	NORMAL ROTATION[10] >5.0° (%)	NORMAL ROTATION[11] >10.0° (%)	REVERSE ROTATION[12] ≥5.0° (%)
Normal	10	100	0	60	40	16.5	17.3	−0.3	27.7	−7.3	100	90	10
Fixed bearing ACR	10	70	20	40	60	8.1	11.8	−3.3	20.9	−14.1	90	40	60
ACL deficient	5	60	40	20	80	9.8	13.3	−4.3	21.2	−9.8	80	60	40
Fixed bearing PCR (+ PCL)	163	79	21	20	80	3.7	6.5	−2.7	13.0	−9.7	66	13	20
Fixed bearing PCR (− PCL)	20	40	60	5	95	−1	2.7	−3.4	5.8	−9.5	5	0	25
Fixed bearing PS	212	76	23	24	75	3.1	5.5	−2.1	11.5	−7.6	52	15	12
Mobile bearing PCR	107	69	28	20	80	3.9	7.3	−4.1	15.6	−11.4	64	25	27
Mobile bearing PS	157	80	19	31	69	3.9	6.5	−2.5	12.5	−8.9	58	21	15
Mobile bearing PCS	76	63	33	18	80	3.3	5.5	−2.1	11.4	−5.9	51	12	16
Average all knees		74	24	27	69	5.7	8.5	−2.8	15.5	−9.4	58	18	18
Average all TKA		74	24	23	76	2.8	5.7	−2.8	11.6	−8.9	57	17	18

See footnotes in Table 89–13.
ACL, anterior cruciate ligament; ACR, ACL retaining; PCL, posterior cruciate ligament; PCR, PCL retaining; PCS, PCL sacrificing; PS, posterior stabilized; TKA, total knee arthroplasty.

Femoral Condylar Lift-Off

Initially, 40 subjects were analyzed under fluoroscopic surveillance to assess the incidence of femoral condylar lift-off. Twenty subjects were implanted with a fixed-bearing PCL-retaining TKA, and 20 subjects received a posterior-stabilized TKA. Thirty of the 40 (75%) subjects experienced femoral condylar lift-off during a deep knee bend. Fourteen of the 20 (70%) subjects with a PCL-retaining TKA and 16 of the 20 (80%) subjects with a posterior-stabilized TKA experienced femoral condylar lift-off at some increment of knee flexion. Condylar lift-off in these subjects most commonly occurred on the lateral side in subjects with a PCL-retaining TKA and either medially or laterally in subjects with a posterior-stabilized TKA.

A follow-up study was then conducted on 30 subjects with a posterior-stabilized TKA to determine whether femoral component alignment could contribute to condylar lift-off.[22,39] After implantation, CT scans were analyzed to determine the angle between the posterior condylar line and the transepicondylar axis. It was hypothesized that if the components were malaligned during surgery, this could contribute to condylar lift-off. The results from this study revealed that subjects with perfect alignment did not achieve condylar lift-off at any angle. Overall, the correlation between malalignment and condylar lift-off was 70%.

Although condylar lift-off occurred more frequently in our earlier studies, clinicians have focused their attention on better ligament-balancing and alignment techniques. In many of their efforts condylar lift-off has been significantly reduced. One of our best studies supporting this effort was conducted with an intraoperative pressure-sensitive trial device.[40,41] The results from this study were quite revealing. With use of the intraoperative device, only three subjects could not be perfectly balanced during surgery. Postoperatively, they were the only three subjects in the study to experience condylar lift-off, and the location and magnitude of lift-off were similar to the intraoperative information.

Range of Motion

Initially, we analyzed the in vivo, passive (non-weightbearing) and active (weightbearing) range of motion for patients with normal knees, PCL-retaining implants, and posterior-stabilized inplants.[7] All three knee subgroups demonstrated a statistically significant decline in range of motion when measured during weightbearing as compared with non-weightbearing conditions (normal, $p < 0.045$; posterior stabilized, $p < 0.001$; PCL retaining, $p < 0.001$). This reduction in motion was greatest in the PCL-retaining TKA subgroup (20-degree reduction). The normal knee subgroup exhibited flexion that was superior to that of both TKA subgroups whether measured under passive non-weightbearing ($p < 0.001$) or active weightbearing conditions ($p < 0.001$). The maximum mean postoperative flexion for PCL-retaining (123 degrees) and posterior-stabilized (127 degrees) TKA subgroups was similar when evaluated under passive non-weightbearing conditions ($p > 0.176$). When measured under weight-

bearing conditions, patients implanted with a posterior-stabilized TKA exhibited significantly greater mean flexion than did those with PCL-retaining TKA (113 versus 103 degrees, $p < 0.024$). This finding occurred despite the fact that the PCL-retaining subgroup demonstrated greater knee flexion (118 versus 108 degrees) and had higher Hospital for Special Surgery scores (65.2 versus 58.7 points) than did the posterior-stabilized subgroup preoperatively and also were of younger age (53.7 versus 65.5 years), although these differences were not statistically significant.

Follow-up studies were then conducted and revealed that certain posterior-stabilized TKA designs do not achieve more range of motion than certain PCL-retaining TKA designs do, thus leading to the assumption that not all posterior-stabilized TKA designs are similar. In addition, bearing mobility does not necessarily lead to increased range of motion. More recently, the Legacy PS High Flex fixed- and mobile-bearing TKAs have been analyzed under in vivo weightbearing range of motion.[2] Subjects in this study experienced, on average, 125 degrees (maximum, 154 degrees) and 116.3 degrees (maximum, 136 degrees) of weightbearing range of motion for the mobile- and fixed-bearing TKAs, respectively (Fig. 89–6). The subjects with these two knee designs achieved the highest weightbearing motion of all the TKAs analyzed in our previous studies.

CLINICAL SIGNIFICANCE

Anteroposterior Translation

In a normal knee, posterior femoral rollback during a deep knee bend routinely occurs and averages –19.2 mm (range, –5.8 to –31.6 mm) and –3.4 mm (range, 3.3 to –11.8 mm) for the lateral and medial femoral condyles,

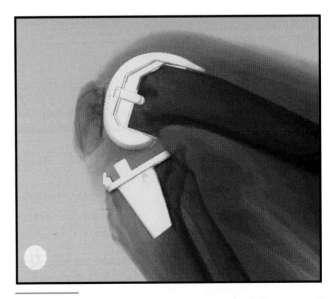

Figure 89–6. Example of a subject with a high-flexion total knee arthroplasty design achieving excellent weightbearing motion.

respectively.[24] Therefore, a medial pivot kinematic pattern is present. Numerous other kinematic evaluations have found a similar pattern and magnitude of posterior femoral rollback during deep flexion activities.[7,15,16,20,23,25,27,32,33] The magnitude of AP translation in lesser flexion activities such as gait is substantially reduced in a normal knee and in the multiple TKA designs evaluated in our studies. The highest magnitudes of AP translation were observed in the normal and ACL-retaining TKA groups ($p < 0.01$), thus emphasizing the importance of the ACL and PCL in determining AP translational kinematic patterns. The magnitudes of posterior femoral rollback during deep flexion in all TKA designs tested were less than in the normal knee. This may explain, at least in part, why knee flexion after TKA is reduced when compared with the normal knee.

During gait, fixed- and mobile-bearing posterior-stabilized TKA designs experienced kinematic patterns similar to those that lacked a cam-and-post mechanism ($p > 0.1$). This has been attributed to the fact that the cam-and-post mechanism of most posterior-stabilized TKA designs does not engage during lesser flexion activities such as gait. During a deep knee bend, however, posterior-stabilized TKA designs routinely showed greater posterior femoral rollback than did designs without a cam-and-post mechanism ($p < 0.01$). This similarly explains, at least in part, why superior weightbearing flexion is typically obtained in PCL-substituting TKA in contrast to designs that lack a cam-and-post mechanism.[11]

The anterior translation of the femur on the tibia observed in our investigation has numerous potential negative consequences. First, anterior femoral translation results in a more anterior axis of flexion, thereby lessening maximum knee flexion. Second, the quadriceps moment arm is decreased, which results in reduced quadriceps efficiency. Third, anterior sliding of the femoral component on the tibial polyethylene surface risks accelerated wear. Blunn et al,[6] in a laboratory evaluation of polyethylene wear, reported dramatically increased wear with cyclic sliding as compared with compression or rolling because of increased subsurface shear stress.

An important criterion influencing TKA kinematics is surgeon variability. In surgeon to surgeon comparisons of subjects implanted with the same fixed-bearing TKA, a statistically significant difference in AP motion patterns was observed ($p < 0.05$). For example, three different studies were done by three different surgeons, all implanting the same fixed-bearing posterior-stabilized TKA prosthesis. In two of these studies, 95% and 100% of patients experienced posterior rollback of the lateral femoral condyle, respectively, during deep flexion. In the third evaluation, only 65% of patients had posterior motion of the lateral condyle. This statistically significant variance among different surgeons was not observed in subjects implanted with mobile-bearing TKA designs. This may be attributed, at least in part, to the increased sagittal plane conformity typically found in mobile-bearing TKA designs, which provides enhanced control of kinematic patterns and therefore lessens the effect of differences in surgical technique among different surgeons.

There was also great variability among TKA types within each group (posterior-stabilized fixed-bearing TKA, PCL-retaining fixed-bearing TKA, etc.). For example, patients who had a PCL-retaining fixed-bearing TKA with asymmetric femoral condyles experienced more than twice the amount of posterior femoral motion and substantially less paradoxical anterior femoral translation than did patients who had a PCL-retaining fixed-bearing TKA with symmetric femoral condyles.[5] Although it has often been assumed that all posterior-stabilized fixed-bearing TKA designs have similar kinematic patterns, the opposite is actually true. Differing incidences and magnitudes of posterior femoral rollback were typically seen when comparing different fixed-bearing posterior-stabilized TKA designs. One fixed-bearing posterior-stabilized TKA design, for example, showed an excessively posterior contact position throughout the flexion range, thereby never achieving cam-post engagement.

Axial Femorotibial Rotation

The percentage of subjects experiencing normal rotational patterns, as well as the magnitudes of axial rotation, decreased in all TKA groups when compared with normal knee subjects during a deep knee bend maneuver ($p < 0.01$). Greater axial rotation occurred during deep flexion than during gait in all study groups. Average axial rotational magnitudes in both gait and a deep knee bend were similar among major implant categories (i.e., fixed versus mobile bearing, PCL retaining versus posterior stabilized). The present study, however, may underestimate the maximum magnitudes of axial rotation occurring during extreme flexion in posterior-stabilized TKA designs since analysis was performed only to a maximum of 90 degrees of flexion. Many posterior-stabilized implants are designed to have late (>70 degrees of knee flexion) cam-post engagement, which may result in additional axial rotation at flexion increments greater than 90 degrees.

Although average magnitudes of axial rotation in fixed-versus mobile-bearing TKA groups were similar, additional analysis suggests that the site of rotation differs. Komistek et al[28] performed in vivo video fluoroscopic analyses of two different designs of rotating-platform TKA. Tantalum beads were embedded within the mobile polyethylene bearings to determine the amount of polyethylene bearing mobility during a deep knee bend. They found that the polyethylene bearing typically rotated in conjunction with the femoral component, thus confirming the presence of bearing mobility. Similar findings were observed by D'Lima et al[13] in a cadaveric analysis of axial rotation after implantation mobile-bearing TKAs. Therefore, in rotating-platform TKA designs, axial rotation typically occurs on the inferior surface of the polyethylene bearing, whereas rotation obviously occurs on the superior surface in fixed-bearing TKAs. This may play a role in reduction of polyethylene wear after implantation of mobile-bearing TKAs. Bearing mobility should reduce shear force on the superior aspect of the polyethylene bearing, thereby lessening wear. Morra et al[37] demonstrated that low contact stress (<8 MPa) is present on the inferior surface of rotating-platform polyethylene bearings when articulating against a highly polished cobalt-chromium surface, which should minimize polyethylene wear during activities requiring axial rotation. Moreover, increased axial rotation was present in deep flexion if the ACL was intact. Average values in normal and ACL-retaining TKA subjects (16.5 and 8.1 degrees) were significantly higher than in TKA study groups in which the ACL was absent (<4.0 degrees; $p < 0.01$).

Reverse axial rotational patterns during individual increments of gait or a deep knee bend were common in all study groups but were more frequently observed after TKA. It was uncommon for subjects in any TKA group to demonstrate a progressive normal rotational pattern throughout all increments of deep flexion. Typically, alternating patterns of internal and external tibial rotation were observed as flexion increased. Reverse axial rotation is undesirable; it risks patellofemoral instability because of lateralization of the tibial tubercle during deep flexion, as well as lessening of maximum knee flexion as a result of reduced posterior femoral rollback of the lateral femoral condyle. High variability in axial rotation patterns and magnitudes was found among different TKA categories, between different implant designs within the same implant category, and among identical implant designs implanted by different surgeons. Subjects with either a posterior-stabilized or a PCL-retaining TKA with asymmetric condyles achieved more axial rotation, and the patterns were more reflective of the normal knee. This suggests that axial rotation is determined by many factors, including implant design, individual patient anatomic variances, and the surgical technique of TKA.

Femoral Condylar Lift-Off

In our studies, condylar lift-off occurred both medially and laterally in subjects with posterior-stabilized TKA but was observed predominantly on the lateral side in those implanted with PCL-retaining TKA. This may be related to the presence or absence of the cruciate ligaments. In a knee with intact cruciate ligaments, the ACL originates at the lateral femoral condyle, whereas the femoral attachment of the PCL is medial. We therefore theorize that the ACL acts as a "checkrein" limiting the presence of later femoral lift-off, with the PCL similarly resisting femoral lift-off medially. In posterior-stabilized TKA with both cruciate ligaments resected, the incidence of femoral condylar lift-off was similar both medially and laterally. In PCL-retaining TKA, femoral condylar lift-off predominantly occurred laterally, with lift-off resisted medially, possibly because of preservation of the PCL.

The incidence of condylar lift-off reported in our more recent studies is lower than the results from our earlier studies. Before the use of fluoroscopy, the incidence and magnitude of condylar lift-off were not known. The results from our in vivo fluoroscopic studies have led to many follow-up studies in which surgeons have used various ligament-balancing and component alignment techniques in an attempt to minimize the incidence and magnitude of condylar lift-off. The results from these studies have been promising because these new techniques have led to a reduced incidence of condylar lift-off.[22,29,39-41]

Range of Motion

Weightbearing range of motion was significantly diminished in all of our subjects, presumably as a result of the complex interaction of dynamic muscle forces, soft-tissue constraints, posterior soft-tissue impingement, and articular congruity. Under passive, non-weightbearing conditions, in contrast, the knee seeks the course of least resistance and may not reflect normal weightbearing articulated motion. The importance of weightbearing in kinematic evaluation of the knee is supported by the work of Hsieh and Walker, who discovered that in an unloaded knee joint, joint laxity is primarily determined by soft-tissue constraints, whereas in a loaded knee joint, the geometric conformity of the joint surfaces is the primary determinant in controlling knee joint laxity.[21]

When tested under weightbearing conditions, patients with PCL-retaining TKA with symmetric condyles exhibited significantly lower postoperative motion than did those with posterior-stabilized TKA. The inferior flexion observed with PCL-retaining TKA can be explained by the paradoxical anterior femoral translation occurring with progressive flexion, as previously discussed. This anterior translation of femorotibial contact with progressive flexion may limit maximum flexion because of anteriorization of the axis of flexion, earlier impingement of the posterior soft-tissue structures, and tightening of the extensor mechanism (from anterior femoral displacement). Alternatively, patients implanted with posterior-stabilized TKA demonstrate posterior femoral rollback, dictated by interaction of the femoral cam and tibial post mechanism of the posterior-stabilized design, regardless of weightbearing status.

More recently, the introduction of high-flexion–type TKAs has led to an increase in weightbearing range of motion when compared with traditional TKA designs. The results from these studies have also demonstrated that not all high-flexion TKA designs are similar. Often, slight modifications have been made to traditional TKAs, and therefore subjects with one of these high-flexion TKAs did not achieve an increase in their weightbearing range of motion.

SUMMARY

It must be noted that not all fluoroscopic analyses are similar. 3-D model-fitting–type analyses provide a definite advantage over traditional library-matching techniques.[36] Using a 3-D, automated model-fitting technique reduces error since the human operator only positions the implant components in their initial position and then the computer performs the mathematic process to determine the best possible fit of the 3-D CAD model onto the 2-D fluoroscopic image.[35] In addition, the automated model-fitting process can also fit occluded images and poorer-quality fluoroscopic images and does the kinematic calculations automatically so that human error is not introduced. Finally, the use of our fluoroscopic process has revealed some distinct kinematic differences between the normal knee and TKA designs. In addition, not all TKA designs are similar because subjects with certain implant designs achieve more normal kinematic patterns.

References

1. Andriacchi TP, Stanwyck TS, Galante JO: Knee biomechanics and total knee replacement. J Arthroplasty 1:211-219, 1986.
2. Argenson JN, Komistek RD, Mahfouz MR, et al: A high flexion total knee arthroplasty design replicates healthy knee motion. Clin Orthop 428:174-179, 2004.
3. Argenson JN, Scuderi GR, Komistek RD, et al: In vivo kinematic evaluation and design considerations related to high flexion in total knee arthroplasty. J Biomech 38:277-284, 2005.
4. Banks SA, Hodge WA: Implant design affects knee arthroplasty kinematics during stair-stepping. Clin Orthop 426:187-193, 2004.
5. Bertin KC, Komistek RD, Dennis DA, et al: In vivo determination of posterior femoral rollback for subjects having a Nexgen posterior cruciate–retaining total knee arthroplasty. J Arthroplasty 14:1040-1048, 2002.
6. Blunn GW, Walker PS, Joshi A, Hardinge K: The dominance of cyclic sliding in producing wear in total knee replacements. Clin Orthop 273:253-260, 1991.
7. Dennis DA, Komistek RD, Cheal EJ, et al: In vivo femoral condylar lift-off in total knee arthroplasty. J Bone Joint Surg Br 83:33-39, 2001.
8. Dennis DA, Komistek RD, Mahfouz MR: In vivo fluoroscopic analysis of fixed-bearing total knee replacements. Clin Orthop 410:114-130, 2003.
9. Dennis DA, Komistek RD, Mahfouz MR, et al: Multicenter determination of in vivo kinematics after total knee arthroplasty. Clin Orthop 416:37-57, 2003.
10. Dennis DA, Komistek RD, Mahfouz MR, et al: A multicenter analysis of axial femorotibial rotation after total knee arthroplasty. Clin Orthop 428:180-189, 2004.
11. Dennis DA, Komistek RD, Stiehl JB, et al: Range of motion following total knee arthroplasty: The effect of implant design and weight-bearing conditions. J Arthroplasty 13:748-752, 1998.
12. Dennis DA, Mahfouz MR, Komistek RD, Hoff WA: In vivo determination of normal and anterior cruciate ligament–deficient knee kinematics. J Biomech 38:241-253, 2005.
13. D'Lima DD, Trice M, Urquhart AG, Colwell CW Jr: Tibiofemoral conformity and kinematics of rotating-bearing knee prostheses. Clin Orthop 386:235-242, 2001.
14. Dorr LD, Ochsner JL, Gronley J, Perry J: Functional comparison of posterior cruciate–retained versus cruciate-sacrificed total knee arthroplasty. Clin Orthop 236:36-43, 1988.
15. Draganich LF, Andriacchi T, Anderson GBJ: Interaction between intrinsic knee mechanics and the knee extensor mechanism. J Orthop Res 5:539-547, 1987.
16. El Nahass B, Madson MM, Walker PS: Motion of the knee after condylar resurfacing. An in vivo study. J Biomech 24:1107-1117, 1991.
17. Fukubayashi T, Torzilli PA, Sherman MF, Warren RF: An in vitro biomechanical evaluation of anterior-posterior motion of the knee. Tibial displacement, rotation, and torque. J Bone Joint Surg Am 64:258-264, 1982.
18. Garg A, Walker PS: Prediction of total knee motion using a three-dimensional computer-graphics model. J Biomech 23:45-58, 1990.
19. Grood ES, Suntay WJ: A joint coordinate system for the clinical description of three-dimensional motions: Application to the knee. J Biomech Eng 105:136-144, 1983.
20. Hoff W, Komistek R, Dennis D, et al: Three-dimensional determination of femoral-tibial contact positions under in vivo conditions using fluoroscopy. Clin Biomech 13:455-470, 1998.
21. Hsieh HH, Walker PS: Stabilizing mechanisms of the loaded and unloaded knee joint. J Bone Joint Surg Am 58:87-93, 1976.
22. Insall J, Scuderi GR, Komistek RD, et al: Correlation between condylar lift-off and femoral component alignment. Clin Orthop 403:143-152, 2002.
23. Jonsson J, Karrholm J, Elmquist LG: Kinematics of active knee extension after tear of the anterior cruciate ligament. Am J Sports Med 17:796-802, 1989.
24. Karrholm J, Brandsson S, Freeman MAR: Tibiofemoral movement 4: Changes of axial tibial rotation caused by forced rotation at the weight-bearing knee studied by RSA. J Bone Joint Surg Br 82:1201-1203, 2000.
25. Karrholm J, Selvik G, Elmqvist LG, Hansson LI: Active knee motion after cruciate ligament rupture. Stereoradiography. Acta Orthop Scand 59:158-164, 1988.
26. Komistek RD, Dennis DA, Mabe JA, Walker SA: An in vivo determination of patellofemoral contact positions. Clin Biomech 15:29-36, 2000.
27. Komistek RD, Dennis DA, Mahfouz MR: In vivo fluoroscopic analysis of the normal human knee. Clin Orthop 410:69-81, 2003.
28. Komistek RD, Dennis DA, Mahfouz MR, et al: In vivo polyethylene bearing mobility is maintained in posterior stabilized total knee arthroplasty. Clin Orthop 428:207-213, 2004.
29. Komistek RD, Dennis DA, Mahfouz MR, et al: In vivo determination of three dimensional normal knee motion during five weight-bearing activities. J Bone Joint Surg Suppl IV, 2004.
30. Komistek RD, Kane TR, Mahfouz MR, et al: Knee mechanics: A review of past and present techniques to determine in vivo loads. J Biomech 38:215-228, 2005.
31. Komistek RD, Stiehl JB, Dennis DA, et al: Mathematical model of the lower extremity joint reaction forces using Kane's method of dynamics. J Biomech 31:185-189, 1998.
32. Kurosawa H, Walker PS, Abe S, et al: Geometry and motion of the knee for implant and orthotic design. J Biomech 18:487-497, 1985.
33. Lafortune MH, Cavanagh PR, Sommer HJ III, Kalenak A: A three-dimensional kinematics of the human knee during walking. J Biomech 25:347-357, 1992.
34. Levens AS, Berkeley CE, Inman V, Blosser JA: Transverse rotation of the segments of the lower extremity in locomotion. J Bone Joint Surg Am 30:859-872, 1948.
35. Mahfouz MR, Hoff WA, Komistek RD, Dennis DA: A robust method for registration of three-dimensional knee implant models to two-dimensional fluoroscopy images. IEEE Trans Med Imaging 22:1561-1574, 2003.
36. Mahfouz MR, Hoff WA, Komistek RD, Dennis DA: Effect of segmentation errors on 3D-to-2D registration of implant models in x-ray images. J Biomech 38:229-239, 2005.
37. Morra EA, Postak PD, Greenwald AS: The influence of mobile bearing knee geometry on the wear of UHMWPE tibial inserts II: A finite element study. Scientific Exhibit. Presented at the Annual Meeting of the American Academy of Orthopaedic Surgeons, 1999.
38. Ranawat CS, Komistek RD, Rodriguez JA, et al: In vivo kinematics for fixed and mobile-bearing posterior stabilized knee prostheses. Clin Orthop 418:184-190, 2004.
39. Scuderi GR, Komistek RD, Dennis DA, Insall J: The impact of femoral component rotational alignment on condylar lift-off. Clin Orthop 410:148-154, 2003.
40. Wasielewski RC, Galat DD, Komistek RD: An intraoperative pressure-measuring device used in total knee arthroplasties and its kinematics correlations. Clin Orthop 427:171-178, 2004.
41. Wasielewski RC, Galat DD, Komistek RD: Correlation of compartment data from an intraoperative sensing device with postoperative fluoroscopic kinematic results in TKA patients. J Biomech 38:333-339, 2005.
42. Whiteside LA, Kasselt MR, Haynes DW: Varus-valgus and rotational instability in rotationally unconstrained total knee arthroplasty. Clin Orthop 219:147-157, 1987.

CHAPTER 90

Cementless Total Knee Designs

Leo A. Whiteside

Cement use in total knee arthroplasty remains a controversial issue. Many cemented total knee replacement designs introduced through the years have failed and been removed from the market. Those that remain are the few select designs that have performed reasonably well because of specific design characteristics, including a well-fixed tibial component with an effective stem, multiple sizes of femoral components, a generous curvature on each femoral condyle, and a conforming polyethylene surface with a large articular contact surface area.[18] With the advent of new instruments, these cemented implants, even when placed by inexperienced arthroplastic surgeons, have had a high rate of success. Cement fixation, however, remains a source of consternation for implant designers. Attempts to produce a cemented all-polyethylene tibial component have resulted in a loosening rate in excess of 20% at 5 years,[10] and the use of cemented total knee replacement in younger, active patients results in high failure because of loosening.[25,38]

The primary goal of noncemented fixation of total joint arthroplasty is to improve the longevity of the implant. Many cementless designs were unsuccessful even at early follow-up periods, but others have been highly successful. In fact, the femoral component in almost all cementless designs reliably achieves fixation to bone and is commonly used in hybrid total knee arthroplasty.[21] The tibial component in cementless total knee arthroplasty, as in cemented arthroplasty, has been the greatest source of problems related to fixation because most designs have begun with inadequate fixation.

Quality of fixation and load transfer characteristics of the implant-bone interface are two of the most important factors in determining implant longevity. The implants must be designed to apply load in compression to ensure bone hypertrophy and avoid shear or tensile failure of the interface between the porous surface and the base metal. The fixation system must achieve the best immediate fixation possible to allow early weightbearing.

The tibial component has traditionally been considered to present the major load transfer and fixation problems. Adherence of the stem and pegs to the supporting cancellous bone may cause proximal stress shielding, as well as high shear stress at the bone-prosthesis interface and high bending stress in the stem.[32] According to Murase et al[32] in a study of cemented designs, the best configuration to achieve stability and yet avoid proximal stress shielding included a short central stem for toggle control. Tibial component fixation systems without a central stem do not achieve adequate toggle control to prevent lift-off and sinking of the tibial component in response to an eccentrically applied load.[1,23,24,40,49] Eccentric and tangential loading also causes shear stress at the interface between bone and the undersurface of the tray.[13,20,22,29,31,50]

Although fixation of the femoral component has generally not been as difficult as that of the tibial component, femoral component design is far from simple. Weight-bearing with the knee in extension can generate high shear stress at the anterior and posterior flange surfaces if the surfaces are adherent to bone.[48] Weightbearing in flexion can generate high shear stress at the distal surfaces if the bone is not seated posteriorly and the component is not fixed rigidly against shear loading.[48]

Strain gauge data and clinical radiographic data of the tibial component were in close agreement in a study by Whiteside and Pafford.[60] Low-strain readings around the peripheral rim corresponded to peripheral atrophy seen in the radiographic study, and the area of high-strain readings on the metaphyseal flare corresponded to the area where the hypertrophic cancellous bone joined the metaphyseal cortex. These findings suggested that tibial load bearing causes primarily compressive stress and that the load is transferred through the cancellous bone of the proximal end of the tibia to the cortical bone of the tibial metaphysis, to a certain extent bypassing the proximal peripheral rim of the tibia. The high strain in the anterolateral area of the tibia suggests that the surface fibers of the bone in this area deform to a greater extent than do other areas after total knee arthroplasty. This may be explained by the relatively soft central bone in the anterolateral tibial metaphysis. This softer bone should transfer relatively less of the load, thus allowing the peripheral surface bone to deform more than other areas.

In the medial condylar area, the bone is denser than in the central condylar area and is therefore more capable of transferring axial load. The radiographic study confirmed this to be a significant clinical pattern.[60] The most likely cause of sinking is inadequate stem fixation that results in compressive failure of the soft cancellous bone in the anterolateral cut surface of the tibia. The sleeve around the tibial stem appeared to control anterolateral sinking of the tibial tray. The relatively soft cancellous bone in the upper surface of the tibia[19] makes this area especially vulnerable to compressive failure, and the need for a stem on the tibial tray to protect this area is abundantly documented in the biomechanical literature. Bartel et al[1] demonstrated in a finite element analysis that prostheses without a stem are likely to sink into the soft areas of the tibial surface when the component is loaded eccentrically. Walker et al[48] and Lewis et al[24] found in separate studies that fixation of the tibial component was best achieved by a rigid tray and central metal stem. Results of the study by Bartel et al[1] also suggest that peripheral contact between the tray and the cortex of the upper part of the tibia would alleviate this problem of sinking. However, the peripheral rim of the proximal end of the tibia does not have a true cortex,[51] and the hardest bone is not arranged around the periphery but instead is usually found on both the medial and lateral posterior surfaces and medially just beneath the articular cartilage. Therefore, a finite element model that includes a substantial cortex would probably predict inappropriate benefits from rim contact with the upper tibial surface. All the tibiae in the study in which sinking of the tibial component occurred had good rim contact.

The load transfer characteristics of the femoral component observed in a clinical radiographic study[60] are predictable from the study of Walker et al[48] on fixation of the femoral component. If the anterior and posterior flange surfaces of the femoral component are bonded to bone, the femoral shaft transfers weightbearing load in the form of shear stress through the flange surfaces during weightbearing in extension, but the load can be transferred to the distal surfaces in the form of compressive stress if the anterior and posterior flange surfaces are not bonded to bone. Compressive loading is desirable because it encourages ossification at the porous metal-bone interface and promotes hypertrophy of the adjacent cancellous bone. Whiteside and Pafford found it interesting that gaps at the distal surface failed to close and developed a surrounding halo of cancellous bone atrophy, but this is not surprising because the hypertrophy produced by compressive loading on either side of the gap leads to stiffening of the bone and thus increases its ability to transfer load.[60] As the load is transferred in increasing proportion through the hypertrophic bone, the atrophic bone overlying the gap becomes less capable of bearing load, thus transferring more load to the areas that contact the metal surface. It is difficult to see how load sharing and equalization of stress could be expected to occur, and it is not surprising that gaps, when carefully scrutinized, were seldom seen to close. Current designs incorporate anterior porous coating to ensure early complete bonding of bone to metal and accept the higher shear stress on the anterior flange surfaces. This is acceptable because of improvement in the bonding strength of the porous metal surface to the bare metal. The distal stress relief that occurs because of this design feature is deemed preferable to the anterior femoral osteolysis that can occur if this surface is left unbonded to bone.

Walker et al[48] further predicted that unbonding of the posterior flange surfaces would cause stress relief of these surfaces during weightbearing in flexion. In the study by Whiteside and Pafford,[60] all the specimens showed evidence of greater hypertrophy at the posterior bevel and posterior flange surfaces than at any other surface. The observed pattern of cancellous hypertrophy suggested that the weightbearing loads were transmitted primarily in compression through the cancellous bone and through the interfaces of both components. The smooth posterior femoral flange surface did not appear to prevent posterior femoral condylar hypertrophy. The smooth flange surfaces and the smooth stem and pegs on the femoral component did not appear to bear significant axial load.

The loading pattern of the tibia during normal gait is complex. Although eccentric anterior and posterior loading occurred during weightbearing in flexion and extension in Whiteside and Pafford's study[60] no attempt was made to quantify this effect. In general, it appeared possible to achieve reliable fixation of the femoral and tibial components without clinically significant stress shielding in either the distal femur or proximal tibia.

Applying a rigid metal tray to a flat surface of cancellous bone does not provide adequate resistance to compressive failure of cancellous bone, lift-off of the opposite side, and toggling micromotion of the component. When early results showed problems with fixation, stems and peripheral screws began to appear on these implant designs. Biomechanical studies clearly indicated that peripheral screws and stems on the tibial component were highly effective and that micromotion of the tray was unacceptably large without these fixation-enhancing features.[30,47] An aspect of tibial component fixation that is commonly overlooked, but is probably the most important, is preparation of the upper tibial surface. Small surface irregularities and incongruities can have a devastating effect on fixation, but this aspect of fixation has received little attention in most cementless tibial component designs.

Biomechanical studies have shown that when tibial components are fixed to the bone surface with only short pegs, they sink on the loaded side and lift off on the opposite side.[47] Both stem and screws were effective in controlling sinking and lift-off in the study by Volz et al.[47] Radiographic and histological studies have shown that bone ingrowth into a tibial tray is infrequent,[12] which suggests that micromotion may be unacceptably large. Achieving rigid initial fixation is the most important factor in promoting bone ingrowth. Miura et al[30] evaluated the effect of screws through the tibial tray and a sleeve on the stem to improve fixation of the tibial component. Bone strength appeared to affect tibial component fixation. It was a major factor in preventing both subsidence and micromotion. Without mechanical fixation, low bone quality was associated with unacceptably large micromovement. The anterolateral portion showed the lowest bone strength in the proximal tibial surface. Hvid and Hansen also reported that bone strength at the anterolateral and intercondylar regions was very low.[17]

In the study by Miura et al,[30] screws were effective in controlling micromovement under axial and sheer loading. When components with screws were compared with those without screws, lift-off was found to be reduced more than 90%. Screws shifted the tilting center lines posteriorly. This finding suggested that the main effect of the screws was to prevent lift-off. Screws also ensured initial bone-implant contact. Miura et al reported that they frequently observed the component to settle on the tibial surface when the screws were tightened. Screws did not eliminate micromotion under axial loads, but they did change the pattern of micromotion. Without screws, micromotion was associated with lift-off and sinking, whereas with screws, sinking and lift-off were minimized, but downward bending of the tray was significantly greater. Although it is uncertain how much micromotion is acceptable while bone ingrowth occurs, it should be minimized as much as possible. A material with an elastic modulus similar to that of cancellous bone may be optimal for stress distribution beneath the tibial tray, but it may also increase the micromotion caused by bending. The results of the study by Miura et al[30] suggest that techniques to lessen bending of the tibial tray minimize micromotion. Mechanisms to prevent bending of the tibial tray might include a material with a higher elastic modulus and the addition of an arch to support the tibial tray.

The mechanical effect of a tight stem appeared in the study of Miura et al[30] to improve the keel effect by packing the surrounding soft cancellous bone and thus improving the press-fit effect, increasing the surface area, and placing the stem closer to the inner surface of the posterior cortex. Use of a tight stem alone was effective in preventing lift-off and sinking under axial loads, but the use of screws had an overriding effect on sinking and subsidence. Addition of the stem to a screwed-down tibial component had a small (but statistically significant) effect only during lift-off. The location of the tilting axis varied with each specimen and with each group. The effect of screws was to shift the tilting axis posteriorly in comparison to groups without screws. This is an important mechanical effect and is probably a result of the resistance to lift-off afforded by the screws. It is also the cause of the low subsidence found in components fixed with screws. If lift-off was unchecked, the tilting axis shifted toward the point of load application, thus decreasing the area through which the load was transferred. This increased the pressure and aggravated sinking.

Micromotion, as strictly defined in the study of Miura et al,[30] was not markedly affected by the use of screws or a tight stem. However, had micromotion been defined as the sum of subsidence (downward or upward) and recoverable motion, the effect of both screws and a stem would have been remarkable. The use of screws or a tight stem alone affected movement of the tray, but a significant additive effect of screws and a stem was also seen in minimizing lift-off.

DESIGN-RELATED FAILURE

Implant material and design features that have occurred coincidentally with cementless total knee replacement designs and are responsible for implant failure are flat polyethylene,[4] heat-pressed polyethylene,[3] and patch porous-coated surfaces.[56] The combination of these features, along with poor quality assurance of polyethylene and gamma irradiation of this material, has caused remarkable wear problems that have led to clinically significant osteolysis.[8,45,53,56] This type of wear and osteolysis is not a function of the fixation method; instead, it is caused by design features that have incidentally been associated with cementless fixation.

Tibial Component Design

An inflammatory response to particulate debris has been identified as the primary cause of osteolysis in total knee arthroplasty.[36] Debris contained within the joint minimally affects the surrounding bone, but once it gains access, the osteolytic attack is aggressive. Design features of implants that contribute to this phenomenon by the amount of particulate debris released in wear conditions include the configuration of the porous coating and other modes of joint fluid access to periprosthetic bone, the stability of the locking mechanism that secures the polyethylene articulating surface to the tibial tray, and the amount of intra-articular pressure within the joint.

Smooth metal surfaces that separate pads of porous coating have been shown in experimental and clinical studies to produce metaphyseal and diaphyseal osteolytic lesions by conducting debris into areas of bone that are not protected by the mechanisms that capture wear debris and transfer it to the local lymphatic system.[5,8,26,52,62] Although these osteolytic lesions have been ascribed to cementless fixation and to the use of screws,[8] they are rare unless the tibial component design includes patch porous coating on the undersurface of the tray, inadequate fixation of the tibial component, and mechanisms that produce large amounts of particulate debris in the knee. As has been seen in cementless total hip arthroplasty, osteolysis occurs when patches of porous coating on the implant are separated by smooth metal surfaces. These smooth metal surfaces form fibrous tissue bridges that conduct polyethylene debris and joint fluid to the diaphyseal endosteal area, where no mechanism exists to diminish the inflammatory response. Porous-coated patches on the Harris-Galante cementless total hip femoral prosthesis appeared to be the cause of a high rate of femoral diaphyseal osteolysis, regardless of the method of fixation to bone.[26,62]

This phenomenon can be explained by a study conducted by Ward et al[52] in which the porous coating around the extraosseous portion of proximal tibial prostheses was observed to seal the bone-cement interface from invasion by polyethylene debris whereas prostheses with smooth surfaces connecting the joint to the bone-cement interface had a high rate of osteolysis and loosening.

This observation was also supported in a laboratory study by Bobyn et al,[5] who reported the effect of porous coating and smooth metal surfaces on migration of particulate debris from the joint cavity in rabbits. Partially porous-coated rods readily conducted polyethylene debris from the knee joint into the medullary canal of the femur, but circumferentially porous-coated rods had bone and tissue penetration into the porous coating that acted as a barrier to migration of the polyethylene debris.

The Ortholoc Modular tibial component (Wright Medical Technology, Arlington, TN), which has patches of porous coating separated by smooth metal bridges on its undersurface, was clinically compared with the Ortholoc II tibial component (Wright Medical Technology), which has continuous porous coating on the undersurface. The rate of osteolysis was found to be statistically significantly greater in knees with the patch porous coating design (Fig. 90-1).[56] Osteolysis did not occur around the tibial stem or pegs in 675 patients whose knees were replaced with the Ortholoc II design, but three nonprogressive osteolytic lesions were found around screws on postoperative radiographs. Partial radiolucency was seen beneath the tibial surface in 27 knees. None have been revised for osteolysis.

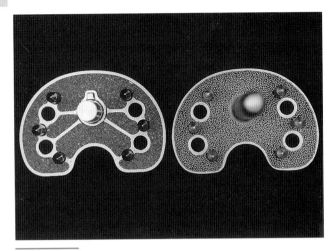

Figure 90–1. Undersurfaces of the Ortholoc Modular (*left*) and Ortholoc II (*right*) tibial components. The Ortholoc Modular has smooth metal bridges around the pegs and screw holes that converge on the central stem. Porous coating covers the entire undersurface of the Ortholoc II component. No bridges of smooth metal connect the joint cavity or screw holes to the smooth stem. (From Whiteside LA: Effect of porous-coating configuration on tibial osteolysis after total knee arthroplasty. Clin Orthop 321:93, 1995.)

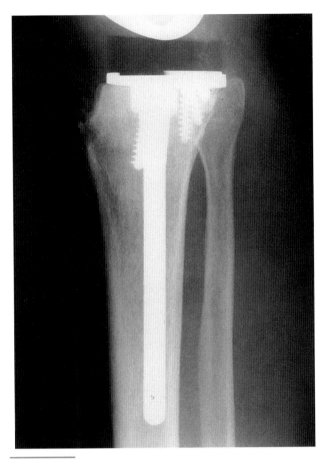

Figure 90–2. Lateral radiograph of an Ortholoc Modular tibial component 1 month after surgery. No sign of osteolysis is evident around the stem, screws, or pegs. (From Whiteside LA: Effect of porous-coating configuration on tibial osteolysis after total knee arthroplasty. Clin Orthop 321:95, 1995.)

In contrast, radiographically detectable osteolysis was seen around the tibial stem in 28 (23%) of 124 Ortholoc Modular total knee prostheses with long (150-mm) stems (Figs. 90–2 and 90–3). Of those 28, none had radiographically identifiable osteolysis around the screws or pegs, but 15 (54%) had partial radiolucent lines that extended beneath at least half the tray on either the anteroposterior or lateral view, and 4 (14%) had radiolucency beneath the entire tibial surface on either radiographic view. An additional 15 (12%) of the 124 knees had radiographically identifiable radiolucency around the stem. Radiographically detectable osteolysis was seen around the tibial stem in 19 (17%) of 112 Ortholoc Modular total knee prostheses with short (75-mm) stems. Thirty (27%) knees had radiolucent lines that extended halfway across the undersurface of the tray, and 9 (8%) knees had complete radiolucent lines under the tray on the anteroposterior or lateral radiographic view.

Two Ortholoc Modular knees (one with a short-stem prosthesis, one with a long-stem prosthesis) underwent revision for progressive osteolytic defects around the stem. The knee with a short stem had severe, persistent pain, whereas the knee with a long stem had no pain. Both knees had hypertrophic synovial tissue that filled the cyst around the stem and connected freely with the undersurface of the tibial tray and the joint cavity, following along the smooth metal surfaces between the porous-coated patches. Histological analysis of biopsy tissue revealed abundant polyethylene-laden macrophages and free polyethylene particles throughout the tissue, but no metallic debris (Fig. 90–4).

It was postulated that the gasket effect of the continuous porous coating on the Ortholoc II tibial tray prevented access of uncontained polyethylene debris and joint fluid to the surrounding bone. However, in the knees with an Ortholoc Modular component, the smooth metal bridges connecting the screw holes and joint cavity with the stem provided access for migration of fluid and debris to the diaphyseal medullary canal. In the biopsy specimens taken from the two knees that underwent revision, polyethylene debris was present around the stems and in all the osteolytic cysts.

Another group also reviewed the effect of osteolytic attack in cementless total knee arthroplasty and found that smooth metal surfaces provided little resistance to progressive invasion of osteolytic tissue whereas porous-coated metal interfaces with bone were highly resistant to osteolytic attack.[8]

Polyethylene Locking Mechanism

Design of the locking mechanism that secures the polyethylene articulating surface to the tibial component appears to be another factor in migration of debris from

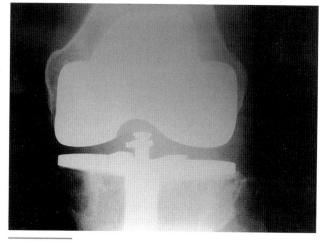

Figure 90–5. Radiograph of a knee with evidence of osteolysis in the femur and tibia. At the time of revision surgery, the locking mechanism of the polyethylene to the tibial component was found to allow at least 1 mm of micromotion between the components, thus creating a pumping action that forced joint fluid into surrounding tissue.

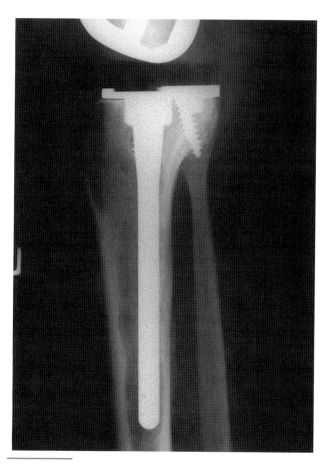

Figure 90–3. Lateral radiograph of an Ortholoc Modular tibial component with osteolysis surrounding the 150-cm stem 2 years after surgery. No evidence of osteolysis is present around the screws or pegs. (From Whiteside LA: Effect of porous-coating configuration on tibial osteolysis after total knee arthroplasty. Clin Orthop 321:95, 1995.)

the joint to surrounding bone stock. In a study of four failed knee implants (one Synatomic, three AMK; DePuy, Warsaw, IN) retrieved at the time of revision surgery for osteolysis, gross motion of more than 1 mm between the polyethylene piece and metal component was observed. Osteolysis had appeared on radiographs between 18 and 36 months after the original implantation and progressed rapidly (Fig. 90–5). At the time of revision surgery, connection between the joint cavity and the intraosseous cyst was always found at the synovial attachment to the bone in implants fixed with or without screws. The bone-cement interface was eroded severely in the two cemented tibial components. In the two cases in which the prostheses were fixed with a cementless technique, the bone-metal interface remained intact, but the synovial fluid and inflamed synovial tissue attacked the bone at the synovial attachment. Severe wear was found in three tibial components, and the cysts were filled with a thick, friable, synovial pannus. The other knee had no visible sign of wear. Pumping of the loose polyethylene appeared to create a pressure wave in the synovial fluid that was conducted directly to the capsular attachment to bone.[27]

A laboratory study was undertaken in retrieved knees whose implants were intact to simulate the piston-like motion of a loose locking mechanism and determine the amount of hydrostatic pressure generated at the interface. Polyethylene articulating components with locking tabs removed were tested first to simulate a loose locking mechanism; they were then exchanged for components with locking tabs intact to simulate a secure locking mechanism. The pressure measured beneath the anteromedial screw hole was nearly the same or higher than intra-articular pressure in the knees with a mobile polyethylene component, whereas pressure beneath the screw hole was a fraction of the intra-articular pressure in knees with a fixed polyethylene component.

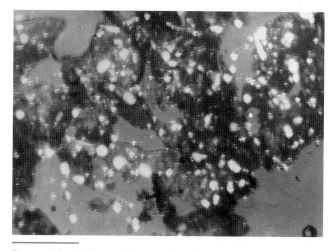

Figure 90–4. Photomicrograph of a histological section under polarized light. Abundant polyethylene-laden macrophages and free polyethylene particles are present throughout the tissue. No metal debris could be found (original magnification ×100). (From Whiteside LA: Effect of porous-coating configuration on tibial osteolysis after total knee arthroplasty. Clin Orthop 321:96, 1995.)

Intra-articular Pressure

Regarding the effect of hydraulic pressure created by a poorly fixed locking mechanism, bone cysts and tissue necrosis are thought to occur as a result of joint fluid forced under high pressure through cartilage defects into subchondral bone. Intra-articular pressure was measured in the laboratory in 10 normal knees and 10 knees retrieved at autopsy with total knee implants intact. The testing conditions were set to determine whether the pressure was high enough during range of motion and with effusion to force reactive joint fluid and particulate debris into surrounding tissue and bone and cause osteolysis. Although the normal and retrieved knees had similar trends in intra-articular pressure throughout range of motion, the retrieved knees had statistically significantly higher intra-articular pressure at every flexion angle except 30 degrees without effusion. Joint pressure was especially high in the suprapatellar and posterior regions of the retrieved knees and required significantly more time to diminish than did pressure in the normal knees.

Pressure in the retrieved knees was occasionally high enough to cause tissue necrosis and bone cysts, which may suggest a mechanism for osteolytic cyst formation around components even when wear is minimal. These findings suggest that intra-articular pressure can be transmitted to the bone-implant interface and that a poorly fixed polyethylene component can trap synovial fluid and act as a pump to generate high pressure.[7]

The amount or size of particulate debris therefore does not appear to matter as much in the progression of osteolysis as does free access to the joint. In the Ortholoc Modular knees revised for osteolysis, neither had severe polyethylene wear, and the knees with radiographically detectable osteolysis did not appear to have radiographic evidence of severe wear.[56] In the knees retrieved for gross motion between the polyethylene articulating surface and tibial tray, destruction of bone was present even without severe component wear.[27]

Patellar Design

Attempts to produce a metal-backed cementless patellar component led to further problems that were unrelated to a specific method of fixation but nonetheless were attributed to cementless technology. Wear through the polyethylene to the metal backing and subsequent contamination of the articular surface with metal and polyethylene debris led to further damage of already compromised tibial polyethylene components and also to massive osteolysis and loss of bone stock. This cascade of events is often attributed to cementless fixation of the femoral and tibial components, whereas it really indicates that the design concepts and performance of the patellar component were poor. It is clear that the patellar surface is difficult to replace with either a cemented or a cementless component, and use of a metal backing on a thin polyethylene patellar component is a treacherous undertaking.

Femoral Component Design

Fracture of the metal femoral component has rarely been a problem in the development of total knee designs, but those that fractured were usually cementless designs that generated excessive stress through an attempt to conserve bone. Stress in noncemented knees is different from that generated in knees fixed with cement,[48,60] and these differences in point and direction of load application may focus high stress on critical cross-sectional dimensions. Porous coating decreases the strength of metal implants because it thins the cross-sectional dimension, especially at corners and junction areas, where the metal may already be at critical dimensions.

When the Ortholoc II knee femoral component was designed in the mid-1980s, a double porous bead layer was applied to the inner surface for cementless fixation.[59] The design was changed soon thereafter to a single layer of beads to improve strength characteristics because within a year of implantation, the manufacturer received reports that fracture of the femoral component had occurred in the design with a double layer of beads, especially those of smaller size (Figs. 90–6 to 90–8). In the author's series of 613 Ortholoc II prostheses with a double bead layer on the femoral component, four fractures occurred. All four implants fractured at the junction between the posterior bevel and the distal surface of the medial femoral condyle.[59]

When a geometric design is shaped with a saw to fit into a curved surface that follows the normal contours of the knee surface, thin sections are formed at the corners. Thin

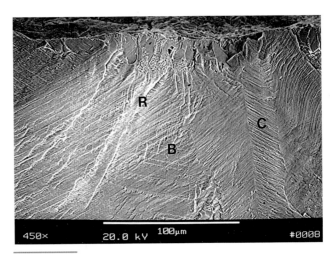

Figure 90–6. Beach marks (B) on the fractured surface of an Ortholoc II femoral component. The concentric beach mark lines converge at a point on the inner surface of the implant where the crack initiated. Radial lines (R) were found on all fractured surfaces. They are oriented in a radial pattern from the point of crack initiation on the inner beaded surface of the component. Chevron zones (C) were found consistently on the fractured surface. These markings are typical of bending fatigue failure. (From Whiteside LA, Fosco DR, Brooks JG Jr: Fracture of the femoral component in cementless total knee arthroplasty. Clin Orthop 286:74, 1993.)

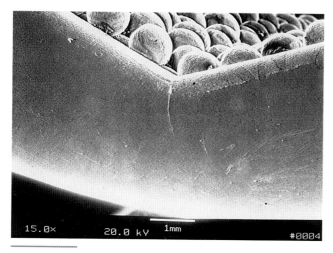

Figure 90-7. A crack originated from the inner beaded surface at the junction between the posterior bevel and the distal surface of the nonfractured lateral side in a femoral condyle. (From Whiteside LA, Fosco DR, Brooks JG Jr: Fracture of the femoral component in cementless total knee arthroplasty. Clin Orthop 286:75, 1993.)

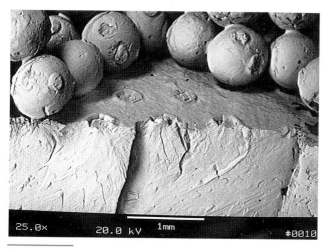

Figure 90-8. Scanning electron micrograph of the inner beaded surface. The fracture joint remnants of several bead craters can be seen. (From Whiteside LA, Fosco DR, Brooks JG Jr: Fracture of the femoral component in cementless total knee arthroplasty. Clin Orthop 286:76, 1993.)

metal at this critical area predisposes the piece to fracture, and porous coating of the inner surface requires that these critical sections be thinned even further. The sintering process can degrade the quality of the base metal itself and thus weaken the implant, and the notch effect caused by the porous coating can also be important in weakening the implant if the porous surface is loaded in tension.

Loads applied to the outer surface of the implant by body weight and muscle force cause bending moments that tend to close the implant and apply tensile stress to the outer surface. However, loads applied to the inner surface are likely to have the opposite effect. If the anterior and posterior surfaces are not allowed to adhere to

bone, load is borne on the distal surfaces preferentially.[48,60] Because the Ortholoc II femoral component was designed to avoid axial load bearing by its anterior and posterior flange surfaces, surgical technique that over-resected the distal surface in relation to the bevel surfaces could have resulted in load bearing exclusively through the inner bevel surfaces. If the implant contacted only the anterior and posterior bevel surfaces and was also not adherent to the surfaces, a wedge would be created, and the femoral component would straighten slightly with weightbearing loads. Application of these cyclic bending loads on the distal portion of the implant probably produced a bending moment that generated tensile load on the inner surfaces.

Surgical bone preparation of the femoral surface for the Ortholoc II implant apparently created a mechanical environment that exposed the porous inner surface to tensile load. Although the inner surface of the femoral component is not generally considered to be the site of significant tensile stress, the combination of cementless technique and smaller implant size predisposed the implants with a double layer of beads to fracture.

INSTRUMENTATION

The instrumentation that has made cemented arthroplasty successful for most surgeons was developed primarily to ensure correct alignment for cementless knee replacement.[16,61] Aside from instrumentation, many of the principles that resulted in successful cemented knee arthroplasty were not applied to the newer cementless components. Early in the process, developers often stated that implants designed for cemented installation could not simply be porous coated and then used for cementless fixation to bone. In fact, that was exactly what should have been done. Ignoring established criteria of successful total knee arthroplasty design led to experimentation in design that culminated in poor short-term results and catastrophic long-term results of many of the early cementless knee components. The early failure of cemented tibial components led to extensive research on fixation of the tibial component, and finally the published literature arrived at a consensus that the cancellous bone of the upper part of the tibia was incapable of supporting the tibial component unless an effective stem was incorporated in the design. Nevertheless, the majority of the early cementless designs did not have a stem and also failed to achieve adequate peripheral fixation of the tibial component to the cancellous-cortical structure of the upper tibia. It is not surprising that large numbers of these tibial components loosened and required revision arthroplasty.

RESULTS

The results of cementless total knee replacement since the mid-1980s have proved to be highly dependent on design. Prostheses with excellent fixation of the tibial component, minimal constraint at the articular surface, or both have had very low rates of loosening and have been reliable in all age groups and in cases of inflammatory as well as degenerative arthritic conditions. Fifteen-year survival rates of the Ortholoc total knee replacement[57] and the LCS[6] (DePuy) are similar in terms of loosening and wear. The Natural Knee (Intermedics Orthopaedics, Austin, TX) has also continued to deliver excellent clinical results with cementless fixation techniques.[15] The Performance total knee design (Biomet, Warsaw, IN) and the PFC total knee design (Johnson & Johnson Orthopaedics, Raynham, MA) have been reported to perform similarly when fixed with cemented or osteointegrated techniques. These five knee systems have varying combinations of excellent initial fixation, low articular surface constraint, and precise preparation of the upper tibial surface.

A study of 10-year results with the cemented and cementless technique for the AGC (Biomet) knee implant revealed no difference in loosening, pain, and knee scores with the two fixation methods. It is important to note in this study that the most difficult patients—young, active male patients—all underwent the cementless technique.[2] The PFC knee design was evaluated in a randomized, prospective study comparing cemented and cementless fixation.[28] Clinical performance was virtually identical, but radiolucent lines were found to be significantly more likely to occur in cemented components. The status of cementless total knee arthroplasty is now at the same point as cemented total knee arthroplasty was 10 to 15 years after its introduction. The design characteristics that consistently lead to success are now well known, and the surgical procedure is effective when performed by surgeons who are expert in its use.

Cemented total knee replacement is fairly consistently successful but has not yet become standardized. Some authors recommend superficial penetration of cement into the surface of the bone,[18] whereas others recommend deep penetration. Some authors recommend cementing only the tibial component,[22] whereas others recommend that all components be cemented.[18] Although many reports of excellent long-term results with cemented all-polyethylene tibial components are available in the literature, efforts to design an all-polyethylene tibial component that is reliable with full cement technique have been fraught with fixation problems. One clinical review reported that 18% of patients had to undergo revision or experienced gross loosening 1 year after surgery.[10] Although this finding may be related to the articular surface design and to the flatness of the femoral component surface, the reasons have not been fully established, and there may be other subtle features of cemented total knee replacement design that make it less than completely reliable.

Close evaluation of published long-term results indicate a rapid fall in prosthetic survival rate after 10 years in service,[33,38] especially in heavy, active patients, who begin to show radiographic evidence of failure as early as 4 years after surgery.[38] One group reported a good 10-year survival rate (approximately 94%) when revision for loosening was considered the endpoint, but when the endpoint represented moderate pain, loosening, or revision, the survival rate dropped to 84% at 10 years.[33] Worsening results in

their series over the 10-year period were caused by progressively increasing pain, instability, and deformity. This suggests that the implants gradually loosen, move, and migrate. This explanation was supported in a report on motion of the tibial component of radiographically intact cemented total condylar knee arthroplasties.[42] In this study, 27 cemented knee arthroplasties were evaluated for motion between the tibial component and bone during varus-valgus stress testing. The least amount of motion was 0.2 mm, and the greatest was 2.1 mm. All knees had detectable motion between the cement and bone.

Because the bone-cement interface is subject to progressive osteolytic attack and this attack is especially rapid in cement interfaces with cancellous bone, as is the case with the acetabular component in total hip arthroplasty,[44] it is not unlikely that the bone-cement interface in total knee arthroplasty is undermined during the first few years and develops a fibrous tissue interface without a surrounding sclerotic margin. Early studies comparing migration of cemented implants with that of cementless ones implanted by means of the radiostereophotogrammetry technique revealed less migration in cemented components. However, as these studies progress and as the more effective cementless tibial component techniques are evaluated, it appears that progressive migration is minimized as reliably with the cementless technique when a stem and screws are used.[41] Reports comparing the current cementless technique with cemented fixation of the tibial component showed progressive migration of the cemented components over the 5-year observation period, whereas the cementless implants ceased to migrate during the first year.[35]

CEMENTLESS REVISION AND BONE RECONSTRUCTION IN TOTAL KNEE REPLACEMENT

Of the few modern-design cementless implants that require revision, few need major bone grafting or cementing to restore bone stock and achieve stability.[58] The bone-implant interface has been remarkably benign, even in cases with severe patellar wear and massive contamination of the joint by metal and particulate polyethylene debris.

In patients who have massive bone loss, the cementless technique has been used successfully in revision arthroplasty of previously cemented or noncemented knees.[43,54,55,58] Bone deficit has been managed with block and morselized grafting techniques in combination with various implant systems. Even though larger defects are commonly thought to require a block allograft and a specially designed prosthesis,[46] a high rate of success has been reported with morselized graft and a regular prosthesis.[43,54,55,58]

Although it seems that bone loss around the knee joint would cause irreversible laxity and chronic instability, it is possible to restore the joint surface in relation to the ligament attachments. However, injury and chronic deformity usually do cause adaptive changes of the fibrous tissue structures about the knee, so reconstruction of the femur and tibia to their original lengths may not be possible. As in knees with prolonged flexion contracture, permanent shortening of the posterior capsular structures occurs in a failing joint to accommodate the sinking implants; therefore, restoration of the joint surfaces to their original length requires in situ reconstruction.

When total knee arthroplasty fails, the cancellous bone in the distal femur and proximal tibia has usually been damaged severely or destroyed completely such that a sclerotic shell with large peripheral deficits is left. In most cases, however, enough diaphyseal cortical structure remains intact above and below the knee that implants with long stems can be used to engage this bone. The articular surfaces can then be augmented to rest on the rim of the deficient femoral and tibial metaphyses. The capsular ligaments can be tensioned so that constrained implants are seldom necessary.

Operative Procedure

The operative procedure includes complete removal of the implant and cement, débridement of the reactive membrane, and curettage to expose viable bone at all accessible surfaces. The medullary canals of the femur and tibia are reamed to accept an implant with a stem length of at least 150 mm and are fit tightly into the diaphyseal isthmus over a 2- to 4-cm length. The metaphyseal bone surface is prepared to accept seating of the femoral and tibial components over at least 25% of the rim circumference, and an effort is made to seat the femoral component posteriorly against substantial bone structure. Three thicknesses of femoral component are generally available for each size of implant in modern revision total knee arthroplasty systems, as are tibial thicknesses from 10 to 35 mm (Fig. 90–9). Posteriorly thickened femoral components make it possible to seat the implant posteriorly on bone so that linked hinges or highly constrained systems are not necessary to achieve stability.

Bone-Grafting Procedure

Fresh frozen allograft with morsels measuring 0.5 to 1 cm in diameter is soaked for 5 to 10 minutes in normal saline with the addition of polymyxin, 500,000 U, bacitracin, 50,000 U, and cefazolin, 1 g/L. Ten milliliters of powdered demineralized cancellous bone is added to each 30 mL of fresh frozen cancellous allograft. The bone defects are packed with this mixture, and the implants are impacted to seat on the remnant of viable bone while the morselized bone graft is compacted.

Clinical Results

In a clinical review of 62 patients managed with this operative and bone-grafting treatment program, all patients except one had significant improvement in postoperative

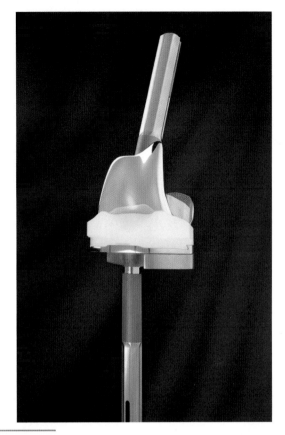

Figure 90–9. The Profix revision total knee replacement system (Smith and Nephew, Memphis, TN) features femoral and tibial components with a long stem for stability, posterodistal and distal-only wedges on the femoral component for severe structural bone loss, and conforming polyethylene with anterior buildup for anteroposterior stability.

pain scores in comparison to preoperative scores, and 82.6% of patients were pain-free at the 1-year postoperative follow-up visit (Figs. 90–10 to 90–12). Although the complication rate was high (22.5% of patients required repeated surgical treatment), only two patients required repeated revision for implant loosening. Pain was eliminated in one patient and was reduced to mild in the other.[58]

Rationale

Cancellous and cortical bone loss after failure of total knee arthroplasty necessitates replacement with allograft, and although block allografts have been advocated for such large deficits, the described morselized grafting technique obviates the more expensive, prolonged, and complicated block operation. Use of morselized allograft was developed in conjunction with stem-stabilized augmented implants that allow rigid fixation and adjustment of joint surface position, and it was found that revision for loosening was seldom needed.[54,55] The ready availability of morselized allograft and its history of clinical success led

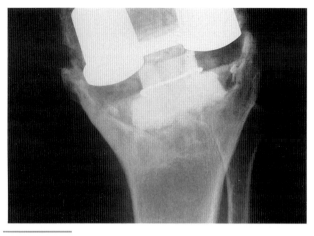

Figure 90–10. Preoperative radiograph of a left knee with a failed cemented component. Massive central and peripheral bone loss has occurred. (From Whiteside LA, Bicalho PS: Radiologic and histologic analysis of morselized allograft in revision total knee replacement. Clin Orthop 357:152, 1998.)

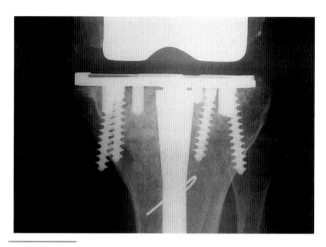

Figure 90–12. Radiograph, 7 years after surgery, of the knee shown in Figure 90–10. The graft has ossified, and trabecular bone is evident along the medial side of the tibia. (From Whiteside LA, Bicalho PS: Radiologic and histologic analysis of morselized allograft in revision total knee replacement. Clin Orthop 357:152, 1998.)

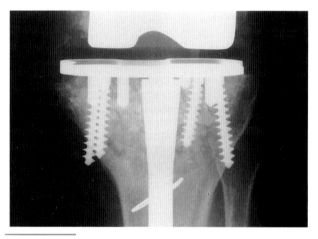

Figure 90–11. Radiograph, 1 month after surgery, of the knee shown in Figure 90–10. Tibial grafting with morselized allograft fills the defect. The lateral edge of the tibial tray is resting on bone. The stem prevents the medial edge from sinking into the allograft. (From Whiteside LA, Bicalho PS: Radiologic and histologic analysis of morselized allograft in revision total knee replacement. Clin Orthop 357:152, 1998.)

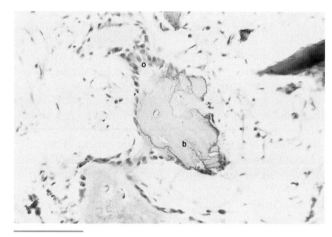

Figure 90–13. Photograph of a histological section from a 3-week postoperative biopsy specimen. Granules of demineralized bone (b) are visible and surrounded by plump osteoblasts (o) and new osteoid. Vascular stroma is present throughout the allografted area. There is no histological evidence of bone resorption (hematoxylin-eosin stain; original magnification ×160). (From Whiteside LA: Results: Cementless. In Rorabeck CH, Engh GA [eds]: Revision Total Knee Arthroplasty. Baltimore, Williams & Wilkins, 1997, p 456.)

to its use for reconstruction of bone defects. Granulated allograft bone that is smaller than the 0.5- to 1-cm pieces advocated is often resorbed and removed by the inflammatory process.[11] Pieces larger than those advocated are much more difficult to construct, slower to ossify, and slower to incorporate.[9] Rapid healing and ossification occurred in the reported series, probably because the implants were stable and the allograft was surrounded by viable bone (Figs. 90–13 to 90–16).[58]

Although morselized cancellous allograft is osteoconductive rather than osteoinductive, it can serve as a scaf-

folding for new bone formation. The demineralized bone added to the morselized allograft provides the osteoinductive stimulus and probably augments healing of failed hinge cases in which massive defects are encountered. Bone formation appears to begin early and progresses slowly through the first 18 months to 2 years. Findings from biopsy specimens taken from patients undergoing this treatment program suggest that the graft is fully mature by 3 years after surgery.[58] Most of the bone visible in the grafted areas is a combination of entombed allograft

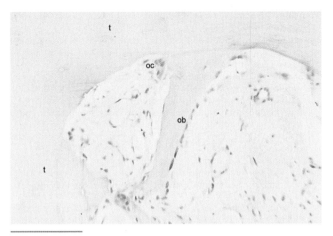

Figure 90–14. Photograph of a histological section from a 3-month biopsy specimen. Dead trabeculae (t) are still abundant. Osteoclasts (oc) and new osteoid with osteoblasts (ob) are evident adjacent to the allograft. The allografted area contains multiple sites of bone resorption. New osteoid is often found on one surface of a trabecula with osteoclastic resorption on the opposite surface. Osteoblasts at this interval are flatter and less numerous than in the 3-week biopsy specimen (hematoxylin-eosin stain; original magnification ×160). (From Whiteside LA: Results: Cementless. In Rorabeck CH, Engh GA [eds]: Revision Total Knee Arthroplasty. Baltimore, Williams & Wilkins, 1997, p 456.)

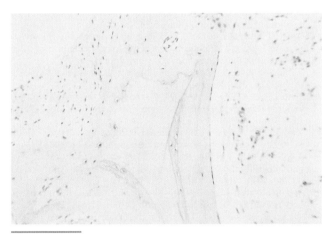

Figure 90–15. Photograph of a histological section from a 21-month biopsy specimen. Mature lamellar bone and disorganized woven bone surround the allograft. The bone remodeling rate in the allografted area has decreased significantly. Trabeculae are now completely entombed by mature or woven bone. Bone remodeling has decreased, and osteoblastic or osteoclastic activity is directed toward new bone, not toward the allograft (hematoxylin-eosin stain; original magnification ×100). (From Whiteside LA: Results: Cementless. In Rorabeck CH, Engh GA [eds]: Revision Total Knee Arthroplasty. Baltimore, Williams & Wilkins, 1997, p 457.)

trabeculae and new lamellar bone, thus indicating that bone graft healing plus maturation of morselized cancellous allograft fortified with demineralized bone powder is similar to the mechanism of fracture callus formation. Structurally reliable bone is produced to support the

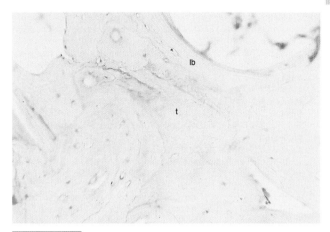

Figure 90–16. Photograph of a histological section from a 37-month biopsy specimen. Entombed trabeculae (t) are present throughout the allograft. The visible allograft is completely encased by mature lamellar bone (lb). Bone remodeling continues at normal levels. Few osteoclasts are found, and there is minimal evidence of osteoblastic activity (hematoxylin-eosin stain; original magnification ×100). (From Whiteside LA: Results: Cementless. In Rorabeck CH, Engh GA [eds]: Revision Total Knee Arthroplasty. Baltimore, Williams & Wilkins, 1997, p 457.)

implant and can be relied on in the event that a revision operation is required.

SUMMARY

After 20 years of clinical experience with cementless total knee replacement, it can be recommended without reservation. A cementless total knee replacement operation can be performed quickly and effectively, the results are reliable and durable, and complications are relatively easy to handle. Advanced biomaterials that improve osteointegration of porous interfaces will certainly broaden the scope of cementless fixation techniques in total knee arthroplasty. Hydroxyapatite added to the porous surface has already proved successful, even in implants that are not otherwise very effective.[14,34,37,39] In cases of revision total knee arthroplasty, the cementless technique can be used if certain issues are addressed. Adequate rigidity of fixation must be achieved with long-stemmed implants seated on structurally reliable bone and placed atop bone graft material with osteoinductive properties. Massive cementing is not necessary even in the presence of severe metaphyseal bone loss in the femur and tibia, provided that a rigidly fixed diaphyseal stem is used.

References

1. Bartel DL, Burstein AH, Santavirta EA, et al: Performance of the tibial component in total knee replacement. J Bone Joint Surg Am 64:1026, 1982.
2. Bassett RW: Results of 1000 Performance knees: Cementless versus cemented fixation. J Arthroplasty 13:409, 1998.

3. Bloebaum RD, Nelson K, Dorr LD, et al: Investigation of early surface delamination observed in retrieved heat-pressed tibial inserts. Clin Orthop 269:120, 1991.

4. Blunn GW, Walker PS, Joshi A, et al: The dominance of cyclic sliding in producing wear in total knee replacements. Clin Orthop 273:253, 1991.

5. Bobyn JD, Jacobs JJ, Tanzer M, et al: The susceptibility of smooth implant surfaces to peri-implant fibrosis and migration of polyethylene wear debris. Clin Orthop 311:21, 1995.

6. Buechel FF, Rosa RA, Pappas MJ: A metal-backed, rotating-bearing patellar prosthesis to lower contact stress. Clin Orthop 248:34, 1989.

7. Emoto G, DeWeese FT, Arizono T, et al: Comparison of intraarticular pressure in normal and retrieved specimens and its effect on effusion volume and flexion angle. Proc Am Acad Orthop Surg 1:249, 1999.

8. Engh GA, Dwyer KA, Hanes CK: Polyethylene wear of metal-backed tibial components in total and unicompartmental knee prostheses. J Bone Joint Surg Br 74:9, 1992.

9. Enneking WF, Mindell ER: Observations on massive retrieved human allografts. J Bone Joint Surg Am 7:1123, 1991.

10. Faris PM, Ritter MA, Meding JB, et al: Minimum two year clinical evaluation and finite element evaluation of a flat all polyethylene tibial component. Orthop Trans 19:387, 1995.

11. Friedlander GE: Current concepts review: Bone grafts. J Bone Joint Surg Am 69:786, 1987.

12. Haddad RJ, Cook SD, Thomas KA, et al: Histologic and microradiographic analysis of noncemented retrieved PCA knee components. Presented at the 53rd Annual Meeting of the American Academy of Orthopaedic Surgeons, February 20-25, 1986, New Orleans.

13. Harrington IJ: A bioengineering analysis of force actions at the knee in normal and pathological gait. Biomed Eng 11:167, 1976.

14. Hildebrand R, Trappmann D, Georg C, et al: [What effect does the hydroxyapatite coating have in cementless knee arthroplasty.] Orthopade 32:323, 2003.

15. Hofmann AA, Murdock LE, Wyatt RWB, et al: Total knee arthroplasty. Two- to four-year experience using an asymmetric tibial tray and a deep trochlear-grooved femoral component. Clin Orthop 269:78, 1991.

16. Hungerford DS, Kenna RV: Preliminary experiences with a total knee prosthesis with porous coating used without cement. Clin Orthop 176:95, 1983.

17. Hvid I, Hansen SL: Trabecular bone strength patterns at the proximal tibial epiphysis. J Orthop Res 3:462, 1985.

18. Insall JN, Tria AJ, Scott WN: The total condylar knee prosthesis: The first 5 years. Clin Orthop 145:68, 1979.

19. Johnson JA, Krug WH, Nahon D, et al: An evaluation of the load bearing capability of the cancellous proximal tibia with special interest in the design of knee implants. Trans Orthop Res Soc 8:403, 1983.

20. Kagan A: Mechanical causes of loosening in knee joint replacement. J Biomech 10:387, 1977.

21. Kenna RV, Hedley AK, Hungerford DS, et al: The PCA Total Hip System (Technical Monograph). Phoenix, Arizona, Harrington Arthritis Research Foundation, 1984.

22. Kobs JK, Lachiewicz PF: Hybrid total knee arthroplasty. Two- to five-year results using the Miller-Galante prosthesis. Clin Orthop 286:78, 1993.

23. Kostuik JP, Schmidt O, Harris WR, et al: A study of weight transmission through the knee joint with applied varus and valgus loads. Clin Orthop 108:95, 1975.

24. Lewis JL, Askew MJ, Jaycox DP: A comparative evaluation of tibial component designs of total knee prosthesis. J Bone Joint Surg Am 64:129, 1982.

25. Lonner JH, Hershman S, Mont M, Lotke PA: Total knee arthroplasty in patients 40 years of age and younger with osteoarthritis. Clin Orthop 380:85-90, 2000.

26. Maloney WJ, Jasty M, Harris WH, et al: Endosteal erosion in association with stable uncemented femoral components. J Bone Joint Surg Am 72:1025, 1990.

27. Martin JW, Whiteside LA: Osteolysis associated with mobile polyethylene components in total hip and total knee arthroplasty. Orthop Trans 21:243, 1997.

28. McCaskie AW, Deehan DJ, Green TP, et al: Randomised, prospective study comparing cemented and cementless total knee replacement. J Bone Joint Surg Br 80:971, 1998.

29. Minns RJ: Forces at the knee joint: Anatomical considerations. J Biomech 14:633, 1980.

30. Miura H, Whiteside LA, Easley JC, et al: Effects of screws and a sleeve on initial fixation in uncemented total knee tibial components. Clin Orthop 259:160, 1990.

31. Morrison JB: The mechanics of the knee joint in relation to normal walking. J Biomech 3:51, 1970.

32. Murase K, Crowninshield RD, Pedersen DR, et al: An analysis of tibial component design in total knee arthroplasty. J Biomech 16:13, 1982.

33. Nelissen RGHH, Brand R, Rozing PM: Survivorship analysis in total condylar knee arthroplasty. J Bone Joint Surg Am 74:383, 1992.

34. Nelissen RG, Valstar ER, Rozing PM: The effect of hydroxyapatite on the micromotion of total knee prostheses. A prospective, randomized, double-blind study. J Bone Joint Surg Am 80:1665, 1998.

35. Nilsson KG, Karrholm J: Increased varus-valgus tilting of screw-fixated knee prostheses: Stereoradiographic study of uncemented versus cemented tibial components. J Arthroplasty 8:529, 1993.

36. Oishi CS, Walker RH, Colwell CW Jr: The femoral component in total hip arthroplasty. J Bone Joint Surg Am 76:1130, 1994.

37. Onsten I, Nordqvist A, Carlsson AS, et al: Hydroxyapatite augmentation of the porous coating improves fixation of tibial components. A randomised RSA study in 116 patients. J Bone Joint Surg Br 80:417, 1998.

38. Ranawat CS, Flynn WF, Saddler S, et al: Long-term results of the total condylar knee arthroplasty: A 15-year survivorship study. Clin Orthop 286:94, 1993.

39. Regner L, Carlsson L, Karrholm J, Herberts P: Tibial component fixation in porous- and hydroxyapatite-coated total knee arthroplasty: A radiostereometric evaluation of migration and inducible displacement after five years. J Arthroplasty 15:681, 2000.

40. Rosenqvist R, Bylander B, Knutson K, et al: Loosening of the porous coating of bicompartmental prostheses in patients with rheumatoid arthritis. J Bone Joint Surg Am 68:538, 1986.

41. Ryd L: The role of roentgen stereophotogrammetric analysis (RSA) in knee surgery. Am J Knee Surg 5:44, 1992.

42. Ryd L, Lindstrand A, Rosenquist R, et al: Micromotion of conventionally cemented all-polyethylene tibial components in total knee replacements. Arch Orthop Trauma Surg 106:82, 1987.

43. Samuelson K: Bone grafting and noncemented revision arthroplasty of the knee. Clin Orthop 226:93, 1988.

44. Schmalzried TP, Kwong LM, Jasty M, et al: The mechanism of loosening of cemented acetabular components in total hip arthroplasty. Clin Orthop 274:60, 1992.

45. Tanner MG, Whiteside LA, White SE: Effect of polyethylene quality on wear in total knee arthroplasty. Clin Orthop 317:83, 1995.

46. Tsahakis PJ, Beaver WB, Brick GW: Technique and results of allograft reconstruction in revision total knee arthroplasty. Clin Orthop 303:86, 1994.

47. Volz RG, Nisbet J, Lee R, et al: The mechanical stability of various noncemented tibial components. Clin Orthop 226:38, 1988.

48. Walker PS, Granholm J, Lowrey R: The fixation of femoral components of condylar knee prostheses. Eng Med 11:135, 1982.

49. Walker PS, Greene D, Reilly D, et al: Fixation of tibial components of knee prostheses. J Bone Joint Surg Am 63:258, 1981.

50. Walker PS, Hajek JV: The load bearing area in the knee joint. J Biomech 5:581, 1972.

51. Walker PS, Soudry M, Ewald FC, et al: Control of cement penetration in total knee arthroplasty. Clin Orthop 185:155, 1984.

52. Ward WG, Johnson KS, Dorey FJ, et al: Extramedullary porous coating to prevent diaphyseal osteolysis and radiolucent lines around proximal tibial replacements. J Bone Joint Surg Am 75:976, 1993.

53. White SE, Tanner MG, Whiteside LA: Effects of sterilization on wear in total knee arthroplasty. Clin Orthop 331:164, 1996.

54. Whiteside LA: Cementless reconstruction of massive tibial bone loss in revision total knee arthroplasty. Clin Orthop 248:80, 1989.

55. Whiteside LA: Cementless revision total knee arthroplasty. Clin Orthop 286:160, 1993.

56. Whiteside LA: Effect of porous-coating configuration on tibial osteolysis after total knee arthroplasty. Clin Orthop 321:92, 1995.

57. Whiteside LA: Clinical results of cementless total knee replacement at 12-15 year followup. Orthop Trans 21:220, 1997.

58. Whiteside LA, Bicalho PS: Radiologic and histologic analysis of morselized allograft in revision total knee replacement. Clin Orthop 357:149, 1998.
59. Whiteside LA, Fosco DR, Brooks JG Jr: Fracture of the femoral component in cementless total knee arthroplasty. Clin Orthop 286:71, 1993.
60. Whiteside LA, Pafford J: Load transfer characteristics of a noncemented total knee arthroplasty. Clin Orthop 239:168, 1989.
61. Whiteside LA, Summers RG: Anatomical landmarks for an intramedullary alignment system for total knee replacement. Orthop Trans 7:546, 1983.
62. Woolson ST, Maloney WJ: Cementless total hip arthroplasty using a porous-coated prosthesis for bone ingrowth fixation. J Arthroplasty 7:381, 1992.

CHAPTER 91

Cemented Total Knee Replacement: The Gold Standard

Thomas K. Fehring • J. Bohannon Mason

Total knee arthroplasty (TKA) is one of the most successful surgical procedures in medical history. A condylar design with good cementing technique is considered the gold standard in TKA today. Most patients, including young patients, can expect a long service life from a cemented condylar knee replacement. Depending on the age of the patient at primary surgery, many implants function well for the remainder of the patient's life.

Despite the success of cemented condylar knee replacements, some authors have advocated a change to cementless fixation for TKA patients. This chapter looks critically at the available evidence to determine what type of fixation is best for TKA patients with respect to age and activity levels. An evidence-based analysis of the current literature regarding knee fixation should help define the role for cemented and cementless knee fixation.

EVOLUTION OF CEMENTLESS FIXATION

Cementless fixation was developed as a response to the early failures of total hip arthroplasty (THA) in young patients. Cemented THAs did poorly in this subset of patients. Dorr and colleagues[7] reported a 67% revision rate in patients younger than 45 years old undergoing cemented THAs. Ranawat and coworkers[21] reported a 30% radiographic loosening rate in patients 40 to 60 years old who had cemented THAs. Sullivan and colleagues[29] looked at 90 patients, all of whom were younger than 50 years, with an 18-year follow-up and found that 50% of the acetabular components loosened, and 8% of the stems loosened. To improve the long-term results of hip replacement, cementless fixation was offered as a potential solution. The transition from cemented THA to cementless THA in young patients has been a true success. Tapered or extensively coated cementless femoral hip implants have shown outstanding clinical results at extended follow-up. At this time, many authors opine that total hip fixation is a solved problem.

The success of cementless hip fixation in young patients led to increased interest in cementless fixation in knee replacement. Proponents of cementless fixation in TKA believe that biological fixation has the potential to achieve a more durable bond of the implant to the bone and improved success over cemented fixation. This chapter discusses the available literature, which to date fails to substantiate this claim.

ADVANTAGES OF CEMENTLESS FIXATION IN TOTAL KNEE ARTHROPLASTY

Purported advantages of cementless total knee fixation include shorter operative time, ease of revision, and improved longevity for younger patients. Reduced operative time is probably the most seductive reason for a surgeon to use this technology. By eliminating the 15 to 20 minutes per case for polymerization of the cement, the surgeon can complete the procedure in a more timely manner. In the age of diminishing reimbursement, certainly this time savings is enticing.

Another potential advantage of cementless knee fixation is ease of revision. In the absence of cement interdigitation, component removal is simplified. The interface between the host bone and the prosthesis is divided, and there is no need to remove embedded cement fragments. Additionally, where porous implants that have failed to ingrow, removal is accomplished easily with disruption of the fibrous membrane and a few blows of the mallet. The resultant bone is usually a sclerotic bed that can be prepared for revision implants with only a few millimeters of bone resection.

Our center has shown that the results of revision of a failed cementless implant to a cemented construct is similar to that of a failed cemented knee revised with cement.[9] The results were not significantly better, however, calling into question whether ease of revision for the operating surgeon translates into an improved result for the patient. In this series, the in-service life of the failed cementless group was limited. Half of the patients revised for failure of ingrowth had their revision within 2 years of the index arthroplasty, and two-thirds of these patients had no pain-free interval after the index surgery. The potential advantages of revision of cementless implants may be more imagined than real.

The main advantage of cementless fixation in young patients is the potential for improved longevity; this was a driving force behind the evolution to cementless total knee fixation in young patients. When a cementless implant becomes osseously integrated, it is extremely rare for it subsequently to loosen. This outcome is attractive for younger patients. In contrast, there is concern that the bone-cement interface has the potential for late deterioration, especially in young active patients. Although this failure mechanism is possible, it occurs infrequently. A cemented knee replacement is loaded primarily in compression—a force well tolerated at the bone-cement interface. This situation is distinctly different from that of hip replacement, in which the forces on the cement-bone interface are a combination of tension, compression, and shear. Although such forces can lead to early failure in young active hip patients, there is little evidence in the literature to substantiate that deterioration of this interface is a significant problem in young cemented knee replacement patients.

JUSTIFICATION FOR CHANGE

It has been stated that without change there can be no progress. There is frequently a price for innovation, however. For any surgeon, the driving force to change a successful procedure must be either identification of a particular problem or the potential for significant outcome improvement for the patient. Cemented total knee replacement has been an extremely successful operation. Consideration of deviation from this time-honored procedure begs the question—is there a problem with total knee fixation in young patients that justifies the risks inherent in cementless technology? An evidence-based analysis of the salient literature concerning total knee replacement should help one define whether or not a problem exists with current fixation techniques or whether there is an advantage to using cementless fixation in young patients.

LITERATURE REVIEW OF CEMENTED TOTAL KNEE ARTHROPLASTIES

If we look at the long-term results of cemented TKA in all age groups, the results are outstanding. Without stratifying for age, multiple articles that have been published cite greater than 90% success rate. Scuderi and coworkers,[27] looking at 1200 posterior-stabilized knees, had a 98% good or excellent result. Ranawat and associates,[22] looking at a 14-year survivorship of cemented TKA, had a 95% success rate. Font-Rodriguez and colleagues,[13] looking at more than 2000 posterior-stabilized metal-backed knees at 14-year follow-up, noted a success rate of 98%.

A cemented TKA performed in an elderly patient should have a service life longer than the life of the patient barring technical failure or infection. The true test of longevity comes, however, from examining the results of cemented TKA in studies stratified for age. Ranawat and colleagues[23] reported a 94% 10-year survivorship in patients younger than 55 years old using cemented fixation. Gill and associates[14] reported a 98% good or excellent result at 10 years in their cemented TKA patients younger than 55 years old. Diduch and coworkers,[6] in evaluating 118 patients younger than 55 years old, had a 94% good or excellent result at 8 years using cemented fixation. The results of cemented fixation in this demanding patient subset are encouraging and fail to substantiate the theory of cement interface deterioration over time. The long-term results of cemented TKA in young patients are superior to the results of cemented THA in similarly young patients. The

rationale that there is a mandate for change because of poor results of cemented fixation in young TKA patients is not substantiated by long-term data.

It has been said that orthopedics is the art of drawing sufficient conclusions from insufficient evidence. The evolution from cemented TKA to cementless TKA was attempted without sufficient evidence that there was a definitive problem. The evolution of cementless technology in total knee replacement may have been unnecessary. The only way question this can be addressed is a careful review of comparative literature.

COMPARATIVE LITERATURE: CEMENT VERSUS CEMENTLESS

Many articles have directly compared cemented fixation with cementless fixation in TKA. Rand and Trousdale[24] looked at more than 11,000 TKAs and performed a survivorship analysis at 10 years; 92% of TKAs were successful when cemented fixation was used, whereas only 61% were successful without cement ($p < 0.001$). Rorabeck[25] compared more than 300 hybrid or cementless TKAs with 224 cemented TKAs and found a 9.6% revision rate in the cementless group at 3 years and only a 1.8% revision rate in the cemented group. Barrack and coworkers[1] looked at 82 cementless rotating platform knees and compared them with 76 cemented rotating platform mobile-bearing knees; 8% of the cementless knees were revised, whereas no cemented knees were revised. The cementless knees also had significantly lower Knee Society scores. Gioe and colleagues[15] evaluated 5760 knees looking at various implants and methods of fixation and found that cementless TKAs had the lowest survival rate of all implants reviewed.

The designers of the Miller-Galante knee (Zimmer, Warsaw, IN), a knee that was introduced as a cementless TKA, came to the same conclusion. Berger and associates,[2] in evaluating 131 cementless TKAs at a mean follow-up of 11 years, found that 8% of the tibial components never achieved ingrowth. The authors of this article and designers of this implant commented that they have abandoned cementless fixation in TKA.[2]

HYBRID FIXATION TECHNIQUES

Two so-called hybrid techniques are currently used clinically: (1) cementation of the tibial component while leaving the femoral component cementless and (2) partial cementation of the tibial component (i.e., cementing the base plate and leaving the tibial stem cementless). Neither of these hybrid fixation methods has evidence-based literature support.

Campbell and coworkers[5] looked at 74 hybrid TKAs in which the tibia was cemented and the femur was left cementless. They found the femoral components' survivorship to be only 87%. They concluded that cementless femoral fixation is unreliable, and that this type of hybrid fixation should be abandoned. Gioe and colleagues[15] evaluated 5760 knees and found that cemented metal-backed components had a 96% survival, whereas hybrid total knee replacements had only an 89% success rate.

The clinical results of partial cementation of the tibial component have been less predictable than fully cementing the tibial component. Schaper and associates[26] noted a 1.9% loosening rate and a 93.6% satisfaction rate among the patients with tibial components that had partial cementation and no loosening and a 97.7% satisfaction rate among patients whose tibial components were fully cemented. This study is consistent with the biomechanical studies evaluating this type of construct. Bert and McShane[3] found that tibial trays treated with partial cementation had significantly more micromotion compared with a fully cemented construct. Jazrawi and colleagues[17] confirmed this in their laboratory finding that cemented metaphyseal engaging stems had significantly less tray motion than a cementless construct of the same length.

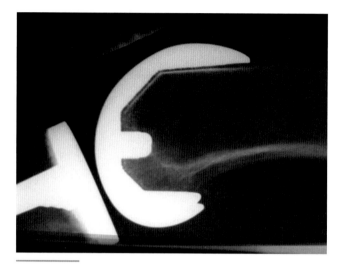

Figure 91–1. Fluoroscopic view of a cementless total knee arthroplasty depicts failure of ingrowth.

EARLY FAILURES IN TOTAL KNEE ARTHROPLASTY

Patients who have undergone TKA expect at least 10 to 15 years of in-service life before subsequent revision surgery becomes necessary. At our center, we analyzed the mechanisms of failure in patients requiring revision surgery within 5 years of the index arthroplasty.[11] From a revision TKA data set of 440 knees, 94% of which were referred from their local orthopedist, we found that 63% of patients were revised within 5 years of the index arthroplasty. The key reasons for these revisions were infection, poor surgical technique, and poor surgeon judgment. Of the early failures—the patients revised within 5 years— 37% failed because of infection; 26% failed because of instability. Thirteen percent of patients were revised within 5 years because of failure of cementless fixation. In contrast, only 3% of the early failures failed because of aseptic loosening of a cemented implant. We concluded that the dominant modes of failure within the first 5 years were infection, instability, and fibrous ingrowth of cementless implants. If all our patients in this early failure group would have been routinely cemented and had proper ligamentous balancing, the overall failure rate would have decreased 40%, and the overall number of revisions would have decreased 25%.

DIAGNOSIS OF FAILED CEMENTLESS KNEES

Results of TKA are generally good. A certain subset of patients do not do well, however, despite an excellent radiographic result. There are multiple reasons for failure of a TKA.[10] Aseptic loosening is a common cause, yet it is a diagnosis that can be elusive.[8,16,18] Plain radiographs are helpful and can be diagnostic of aseptic loosening, but even slight obliquity of the film can obscure radiolucent lines adjacent to the prosthesis.[8,19] Plain radiographs with a divergence of the beam of only 3 degrees from a plane parallel to the bone-implant interface do not detect a 2-mm lucent line beneath the tibial component.[19]

To facilitate the diagnosis of aseptic loosening, we described the use of fluoroscopic radiographs of the knee to evaluate aseptic loosening in patients with cementless TKAs. We showed how fluoroscopic guidance allows one to position the x-ray beam parallel to the bone-prosthetic interface so that the presence and extent of radiolucent lines beneath a cementless component can be measured (Fig. 91–1).[10]

In contrast to failed cemented TKA, in which cement fragmentation may be evident, and the cement-bone interface is not as close to the obscuring metal of the implant, the interface beneath a cementless implant may be more difficult to assess. The porous surface may obscure a demarcation line, and sclerosis beneath a fixed porous implant can be confused with consolidation and spot welds.

In cementless TKA, the presence of any line between implant and bone shows lack of bony incorporation in that area. If such lines are extensive or progressive, this implant is loose and may be the source of symptoms.[10] Some patients lack bony ingrowth, yet function well with a fibrously ingrown implant. If a patient presents with a painful TKA, has normal-appearing x-rays, and has start-up pain, fluoroscopic views are indicated. If fluoroscopic radiographs corroborate a problem with the interfaces, chances for successful revision are good.[9]

RESULTS OF TREATING FAILED CEMENTLESS KNEES

We have established that cementless TKAs fail at a more frequent rate than cemented TKAs; it is important to determine how patients do after they are revised to a cemented construct. We looked at a group of 27 cementless TKAs revised for lack of ingrowth and compared them with a group of 36 patients revised for aseptic loosening of cemented TKAs. We found that the cementless TKA group was being revised much earlier than the cemented group. Of the cementless patients, 52% had revision of their arthroplasty within 2 years of their index surgery. The average pain-free interval for the cementless group was only 11 months, with 63% having no pain relief after their index arthroplasty. In contrast, only 5 of 36 (14%) patients in the cemented group had revision in the first 2 years, whereas the average pain-free interval for the cemented group was 64 months.[9] We found that revision of failed cementless TKAs with a cemented implant was a reliable procedure, but the average time to revision of cementless implants was significantly less than the time to revision of cemented constructs.

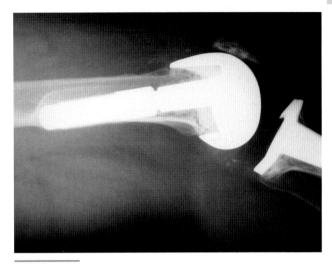

Figure 91–2. Lateral radiograph of a revision total knee arthroplasty with a cementless stem depicts femoral loosening and stem migration.

CEMENTED VERSUS CEMENTLESS FIXATION IN REVISION TOTAL KNEE ARTHROPLASTY

Stable fixation is an integral part of any TKA. Revision surgery is no exception. How to achieve such stability in a revision situation with compromised periarticular bone is controversial. To enhance stability, implants with extended stems have been used during revision knee surgery. The use of such stems transfers stress from the deficient plateau to the shaft.[28] In revision TKA, proponents of either cemented or cementless stem fixation have reported their results. Excellent midterm results have been reported using cemented stem fixation. Other authors have reported good clinical results with cementless stems.[4] Radiopaque lines commonly were seen around the cementless implants, however. Little comparative information is available in the literature to guide the surgeon doing revision TKA in determining what type of stem fixation should be used. We evaluated a group of patients to determine whether cemented or cementless stem fixation was superior in a series of revision TKA implants with metaphyseal engaging stems.[12]

We looked at 107 cemented stems and compared them with 95 press-fit metaphyseal engaging stems.[12] Using a modified Knee Society radiographic scoring system, 100 (93%) of the 107 implants with cemented stems were considered stable, 7 (7%) were categorized as possibly loose requiring close follow-up, and none were loose. Of the 95 implants with cementless stems, only 67 (71%) were categorized as stable, 18 (19%) were possibly loose requiring close follow-up, and 10 (10%) were loose (2 tibial and 8 femoral implants) (Fig. 91–2).[12] We concluded from this study that cementless metaphyseal engaging stems were unpredictable for fixation in revision TKA. These findings mirrored the study of Murray and associates,[20] who looked at 40 cemented stems and found that only 1 of them was loose at 58 months of follow-up. Our study dealt with metaphyseal engaging stems; we know of no study comparing diaphyseal engaging cementless stems with cemented constructs.

CONCLUSION

Because of the predictable durable nature of cemented total knee fixation, this method is used exclusively at our center. The morbidity associated with lack of ingrowth and subsequent early revision prevents us from using cementless fixation at this time. After the evidence-based analysis presented in this chapter, one can see that there is no justification for using cementless total knee implants in any age patient at this time.

References

1. Barrack RL, Nakamura SJ, Hopkins SG, et al: Early failure of cementless mobile-bearing total knee arthroplasty. J Arthroplasty 19(Suppl 2):101-106, 2004.
2. Berger RA, Lyon JH, Jacobs JJ, et al: Problems with cementless total knee arthroplasty at 11 years followup. Clin Orthop 392:196-207, 2001.
3. Bert JM, McShane M: Is it necessary to cement the tibial stem in cemented total knee arthroplasty? Clin Orthop 356:73-78, 1998.
4. Bertin KC, Freeman MAR, Samuelson KM, et al: Stemmed revision arthroplasty for aseptic loosening of total knee replacement. J Bone Joint Surg Br 67:242-248, 1985.
5. Campbell MD, Duffy GP, Trousdale RT: Femoral component failure in hybrid total knee arthroplasty. Clin Orthop 356:58-65, 1998.
6. Diduch DR, Insall JN, Scott WN, et al: Total knee replacement in young, active patients. J Bone Joint Surg Am 79:582, 1997.
7. Dorr LD, Kane TJ, Conaty JP: Long-term results of cemented total hip arthroplasty in patients 45 years old or younger: A 16-year follow-up study. J Arthroplasty 9:453-456, 1994.
8. Ducheyne P, Kagan A, Lacey JA: Failure of total knee arthroplasty due to loosening and deformation of the tibial component. J Bone Joint Surg Am 60:384-391, 1978.
9. Fehring TK, Griffin WL: Revision of failed cementless total knee implants with cement. Clin Orthop 356:34-38, 1998.
10. Fehring TK, McAvoy G: Fluoroscopic evaluation of the painful total knee arthroplasty. Clin Orthop 331:226-233, 1996.
11. Fehring TK, Odum S, Griffin WL, et al: Early failures in total knee arthroplasty. Clin Orthop 392:315-318, 2001.

12. Fehring TK, Odum S, Olekson C, et al: Stem fixation in revision total knee arthroplasty: A comparative analysis. Clin Orthop 416:217-224, 2003.

13. Font-Rodriguez DE, Scuderi GR, Insall JN: Survivorship of cemented total knee arthroplasty. Clin Orthop 345:79-86, 1997.

14. Gill GS, Chan C, Mills DM: 5- to 18-year follow-up study of cemented total knee arthroplasty for patients 55 years old or younger. J Arthroplasty 12:49-54, 1997.

15. Gioe TJ, Killeen KK, Grimm K, et al: Why are total knee replacements revised? Clin Orthop 428:100-106, 2004.

16. Insall JN, Hood RW, Flaun LB, et al: The Total Condylar Knee prosthesis in gonarthrosis: A five to nine year follow up of the first one hundred consecutive replacements. J Bone Joint Surg Am 65:619-628, 1983.

17. Jazrawi LM, Bai B, Kummer FJ, et al: The effect of stem modularity and mode of fixation on tibial component stability in revision total knee arthroplasty. J Arthroplasty 16:759-767, 2001.

18. King TV, Scott RD: Femoral component loosening in total knee arthroplasty. Clin Orthop 194:285-290, 1985.

19. Magee FP, Weinstein AM: The effect of position on the detection of radiolucent lines beneath the tibial tray. Trans Orthop Res Soc 11:357, 1986.

20. Murray PB, Rand JA, Hanssen AD: Cemented long-stem revision total knee arthroplasty. Clin Orthop 309:116-123, 1994.

21. Ranawat CS, Atkinson RE, Salvati EA, et al: Conventional total hip arthroplasty for degenerative joint disease in patients between the ages of forty and sixty years. J Bone Joint Surg Am 66:745-751, 1984.

22. Ranawat CS, Flynn WF Jr, Deshmukh RG: Impact of modern technique on long-term results of total condylar knee arthroplasty. Clin Orthop 309:131-135, 1994.

23. Ranawat CS, Padgett DE, Ohashi Y: Total knee arthroplasty for patients younger than 55 years. Clin Orthop 248:27-33, 1989.

24. Rand JA, Trousdale RT: Factors affecting the durability of primary total knee prostheses. J Bone Joint Surg Am 85:259-265, 2003.

25. Rorabeck CH: Total knee replacement: Should it be cemented, cementless or hybrid? Can J Surg 42:21-26, 1999.

26. Schaper LA, Badenhausen WE, Pomeroy DL, et al: Long-term clinical and radiographic results in 453 total knee arthroplasty cases using one design with three alternative methods of tibial fixation (Abstract). Sixty-sixth Annual Meeting Proceedings, American Academy of Orthopaedic Surgeons, Rosemont, IL, 1999, p 141.

27. Scuderi GR, Insall JN, Windsor RE, et al: Survivorship of cemented knee replacements. J Bone Joint Surg Br 71:798-803, 1989.

28. Stern SH, Wills D, Gilbert JL: The effect of tibial stem design on component micromotion in knee arthroplasty. Clin Orthop 345:44-52, 1997.

29. Sullivan PM, MacKenzie JR, Callaghan JJ, et al: Total hip arthroplasty with cement in patients who are less than fifty years old. J Bone Joint Surg Am 76:863-869, 1994.

CHAPTER 92

Minimally Invasive Total Knee Arthroplasty

Giles R. Scuderi • Alfred J. Tria, Jr.

Standard total knee arthroplasty (TKA) has been in development since introduction of the first total knee replacement in 1974.[4,5] The techniques of balancing the ligaments, equalizing the flexion-extension gaps, and adjusting the overall alignment have been perfected so that the long-term results are very satisfactory and are now approaching 20 years in follow-up studies.[2,6,7,9,11,13] Minimally invasive surgery (MIS) for knee arthroplasty began in the late 1990s. Repicci's work with unicondylar knee replacement encouraged further interest in both the limited surgical approach and partial knee arthroplasty.[8,10] The logical extension of his work was to apply the MIS principles to total knee surgery. Some investigators have been implanting knee replacements via limited surgical approaches for the past 15 years, but no techniques have survived the test of time or replaced the standard surgery. With the now established MIS techniques for unicondylar surgery, MIS total knee replacement has a much better foundation.

The authors have been working with MIS TKA for the past 3 years, and this chapter summarizes the early experience and results. Several minimally invasive approaches have evolved from the traditional extensile approaches and are considered part of a continuum of approaches from the limited medial parapatellar arthrotomy, limited midvastus, and limited subvastus to the quadriceps-sparing approach. These are limited extensile approaches that can easily be converted to a traditional approach if necessary. With MIS TKA, modified and smaller instrumentation has evolved that facilitates preparation of the knee. The intention of MIS TKA is to limit surgical dissection without compromising the procedure. The proposed advantages of less invasive surgery include reduced postoperative morbidity, reduced pain, reduced blood loss, and faster recovery.

Not all patients are candidates for MIS. The deformity should be limited to less than 15 degrees of varus, 20 degrees of valgus, or a flexion contracture of less than 10 degrees with a minimum range of motion of 90 degrees because knees with greater deformity require greater soft-tissue dissection and release to correct the fixed deformities. Patients with rheumatoid or inflammatory arthritis, diabetes, and previous surgery should be considered for a more traditional extensile exposure. Clinically, we have also noted that large-muscled male patients, obese patients, and patients with either a wide femur or a short patellar tendon require greater exposure.[13]

LIMITED MEDIAL PARAPATELLAR ARTHROTOMY

The limited medial parapatellar arthrotomy is a modification of the traditional approach and is popular because of its familiarity, simplicity, and excellent exposure of all three compartments of the knee. In the mini-incision technique, a 10- to 14-cm anterior midline skin incision is made from the superior pole of the patella to the tibial tubercle. The limited medial parapatellar arthrotomy extends 2 to 4 cm into the quadriceps tendon (Fig. 92–1). This technique usually allows lateral subluxation of the patella without eversion and permits adequate exposure of the joint. If the need arises, the arthrotomy can easily be extended to a more traditional approach by gradual lengthening into the quadriceps tendon.

Once the knee is exposed and the patella subluxated laterally, the bone cuts are made. There is no difference in the bone resection; however, the instrumentation has been modified to fit in a smaller space and also permit accurate bone resection. The authors use the NexGen Multi-Reference 4 in 1 Instrumentation (Zimmer, Warsaw, IN), which has been modified for the minimal-incision approach.

Careful placement of retractors protects the supporting soft-tissue structures. The incision can be moved as a "mobile window" from medial to lateral and from superior to inferior as necessary to aid in visualization without applying undue force on the skin and subcutaneous tissue. The order of the bone resection is dependent on the surgeon's preference, but the authors recommend cutting the tibia first. Once the proximal tibia bone is removed, there is laxity of the joint in both the flexion and extension gaps, thereby permitting easier exposure of the knee and placement of the femoral instrumentation.

With the knee in 90 degrees of flexion, the tibia is resected perpendicular to the mechanical axis with an extramedullary cutting guide set at the appropriate depth and slope (Fig. 92–2). The retractors are strategically placed to protect the collateral ligaments and the patellar tendon. The retractors also permit mobilization of the arthrotomy to facilitate exposure. This "mobile window" is moved medially when the medial side is resected and laterally when the lateral aspect of the tibia is cut because pulling on both the medial and lateral retractors at the same time limits exposure. To remove the resected proximal tibial bone, it may be necessary to bring the knee to

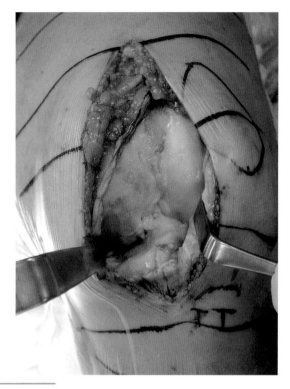

Figure 92–1. Limited medial parapatellar arthrotomy

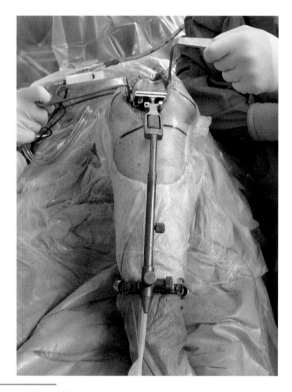

Figure 92–2. Tibial resection.

60 to 70 degrees of flexion. The bone is then brought forward through the arthrotomy with external rotation as the soft-tissue attachments are released. After removal of the proximal tibial bone, attention is directed to the femur. The knee is once again brought to 90 degrees of flexion,

and a limited amount of synovial tissue and fat is resected from the anterior cortex. Very little dissection is performed in the suprapatellar pouch in an effort to reduce bleeding and scar tissue formation. We also try to preserve the infrapatellar fat pad for the same reason. The distal end of the femur is resected with the modified intramedullary cutting guide set at the appropriate valgus alignment (Fig. 92–3A). The next step is to identify either the anteroposterior axis of the distal femur or the transepicondylar axis, which can be done with the knee flexed and careful positioning of the retractors. Once the femoral rotation is determined, the femur is sized (Fig. 92–3B). With the current inventory of femoral component sizes, it is preferable to select the component that is closest to the measured femur. After resection of the anterior and posterior portions of the femur, the menisci are removed, and if a posterior-stabilized prosthesis is being implanted, the posterior cruciate ligament is completely resected. The flexion and extension gaps are now measured and balanced with the spacer block technique (Fig. 92–3C). After balancing the knee, the final finishing cuts are made on the distal femur, and the tibia is sized and prepared to accept the final component.

The patella is prepared last. With the knee in extension or slight flexion, the patella is everted and resected at the appropriate depth with either a saw or a reamer. The entire extensor mechanism does not have to be twisted or everted. The patella can easily be prepared with minimal disruption of the extensor mechanism because the distal femoral and proximal tibial resections have been completed and there is a great deal more laxity and space in the knee joint cavity.

The provisional components are implanted in a slightly different order because of the limited exposure. The trial tibial tray is implanted first. The knee is hyperflexed and externally rotated so that the tibia is introduced forward through the arthrotomy. The tibial tray is then seated in place. The knee is brought back to 90 degrees of flexion, and with distraction of the joint, the flexion space opens and the femoral component is impacted in place. The tibial articular surface is then inserted. A trial reduction is performed and the knee assessed for balance and range of motion. If the trial tests are satisfactory, the provisional components are removed and the bone surfaces are cleaned with pulsatile lavage. The final components are cemented in sequential fashion as described earlier. All excess cement is removed and the knee is reduced (Fig. 92–4). The wound is then irrigated with an antibiotic solution. The arthrotomy is closed over a suction drain, and the subcutaneous layer and skin are closed in routine fashion.

A recent review of 118 consecutive primary TKAs performed by one of the authors (GRS) revealed that 69 procedures (58%) could be performed with a mini-incision and limited arthrotomy. The average incision length in extension for this group of patients was 4.6 inches (range, 3.75 to 5.25 inches). The remaining 49 procedures (42%) were performed with a standard incision and arthrotomy. It was statistically significant that 71% of the females had a mini-incision as opposed to 33% of the males. The mini-incision knees also had better preoperative knee flexion (117 versus 109 degrees) and an overall better arc of

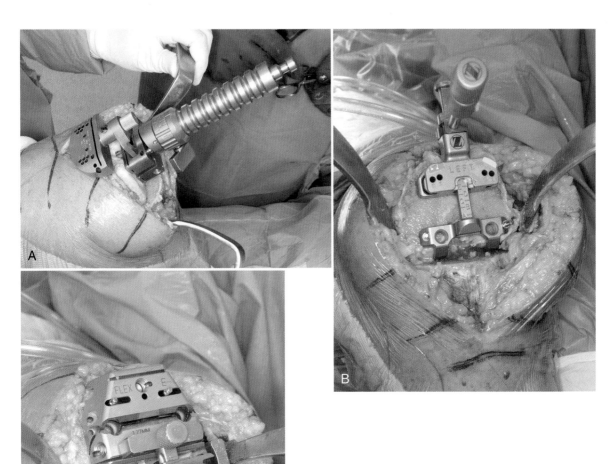

Figure 92–3. **A,** Distal femoral cutting guide. **B,** Femoral sizing guide. **C,** Femoral cutting block.

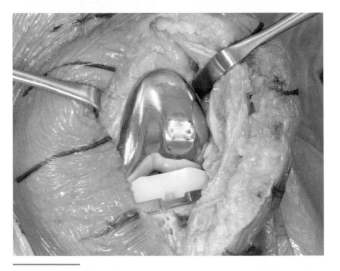

Figure 92–4. The final components inserted through a limited arthrotomy.

motion (116 versus 107 degrees). The mini-incision patients were also shorter in stature and lighter in weight with a lower body mass index and smaller femurs.

LIMITED SUBVASTUS APPROACH

The subvastus approach takes advantage of the natural planes of dissection and preserves the extensor mechanism, thereby minimizing patellofemoral instability. This approach can be used in MIS in carefully selected patients. After a 10- to 14-cm anterior midline skin incision, a medial flap is created to expose the extensor mechanism, vastus medialis, and medial retinaculum. A longitudinal incision is then made along the medial border of the patellar tendon and patella. A transverse incision is next made along the inferior border of the vastus medialis. The vastus medialis obliquus is then bluntly released from the intermuscular septum. After division of the synovium in the

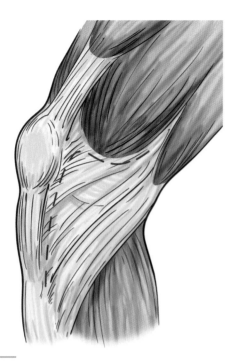

Figure 92–5. Subvastus approach.

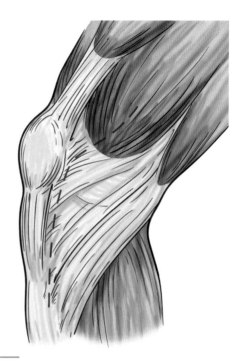

Figure 92–6. Midvastus approach.

suprapatellar pouch, the patella is subluxated laterally as the knee is brought from extension into flexion (Fig. 92–5). This approach does not violate the quadriceps tendon and exposes the knee along an intermuscular plane. After exposure of the joint, the TKA is performed in a similar fashion as described earlier for the limited medial parapatellar arthrotomy.

Proponents report exposure equivalent to that of the medial parapatellar arthrotomy but with less pain and a stronger extensor mechanism.[12] However, this approach does have its limitations and is not recommended in an obese patient, especially one with a short thigh, in heavy muscular knees with a very prominent vastus medialis, in a stiff knee with a significant flexion contracture, in a severe valgus knee, and in a knee that has previously undergone surgery. When performing this approach care must be taken in the subvastus region adjacent to the adductor tubercle because it contains the descending genicular artery and its branches, the intermuscular septal arteries, and the saphenous nerve.

LIMITED MIDVASTUS APPROACH

The midvastus approach evolved as a compromise to take advantage of the exposure of the medial parapatellar arthrotomy and the extensor mechanism benefits of the subvastus approach. As with the previously described approaches, a 10- to 14-cm anterior midline skin incision is made. A medial parapatellar arthrotomy is initiated from the tibial tubercle to the superior pole of the patella. At the superior medial border of the patella, the arthrotomy is then extended into the belly of the vastus medialis (Fig. 92–6). The fascia of the vastus medialis is incised and the muscle split in line with its fibers. The knee is brought

into flexion and the patella is subluxated laterally. Inadvertent tearing of the fascia and muscle fibers extends the exposure and has no adverse effect on the outcome. Once the knee is brought into flexion, the procedure can be performed as described earlier.

Advantages of the midvastus approach include decreased postoperative pain, preservation of patellar vascularity, improved patellar tracking, better postoperative quadriceps strength, decreased blood loss, and shorter hospital stay.[11] This approach may be difficult in a patient with an obese knee, a stiff knee with limited range of motion, a knee with robust vastus medialis, and a knee with hypertrophic osteoarthritis. The midvastus approach may be used in individuals in whom the subvastus technique may be inappropriate because of body habitus or limited preoperative motion; however, the choice is based on surgical experience.

THE QUADRICEPS-SPARING SURGICAL APPROACH

In a varus knee, a curvilinear medial incision is made from the superior pole of the patella to the tibial joint line (Fig. 92–7). The arthrotomy is in line with the skin incision and can include a transverse incision beneath the vastus medialis to increase exposure of the medial femoral condyle (Fig. 92–8). In a valgus knee, the incision may be made on the lateral side of the patella to the tibial joint line (Fig. 92–9). The arthrotomy is performed in a vertical fashion, and the iliotibial band is pealed from the tibial plateau joint line in an anterior-to-posterior direction (Fig. 92–10).

The knee is placed in full extension and the posterior surface of the patella is removed with a freehand saw cut.

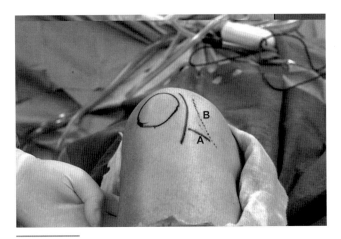

Figure 92–7. Medial incision in a right, varus knee. Line A represents the tibiofemoral joint line, and line B outlines the margin of the medial femoral condyle.

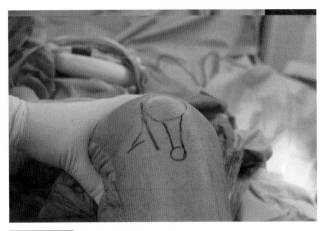

Figure 92–9. The lateral incision is almost vertical along the side of the patella and extends to the tibial joint line.

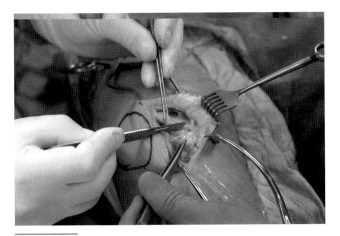

Figure 92–8. The surgical knife blade is finishing the transverse cut beneath the vastus medialis.

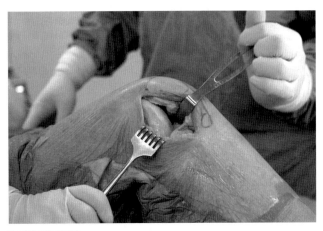

Figure 92–10. The iliotibial band is sharply elevated from the lateral side of the tibia. No transverse capsular incision is used for the lateral approach.

The patella cannot be everted for this step and is usually turned to a 90-degree angle (Fig. 92–11). The holes for the patellar prosthesis can be completed at this time, and the final thickness of the resurfaced patella can be compared with the original thickness. The authors try to decrease the thickness by 2 mm while still leaving a minimum of 10 mm of underlying bone. Early patellar resection gives the surgeon more room to work on the femoral and tibial cuts. However, it is not mandatory that the patella be resurfaced. The cut surface is protected with a thin metal button that is pinned in place.

The anteroposterior axis line (Whiteside's line) is drawn on the uncut surface of the femur. A hole is then made in the femur just above the intercondylar notch, and an intramedullary rod is set in place that references the medial femoral condyle (Fig. 92–12). A side-cutting guide is attached to the intramedullary reference rod (Fig. 92–13). The distal cut is made across both femoral condyles, and the thickness of the bone fragments is measured to be sure that the resection is accurate.

The tibial guide is centered on the tibial tubercle and fixed in place with a threaded pin. After the varus/valgus

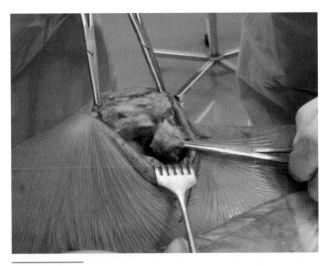

Figure 92–11. The fat pad is excised and the posterior surface of the patella is removed with a freehand oscillating saw cut.

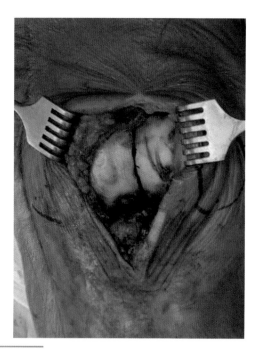

Figure 92–12. The anteroposterior axis of Leo Whiteside is marked on the surface of the femur for rotational alignment.

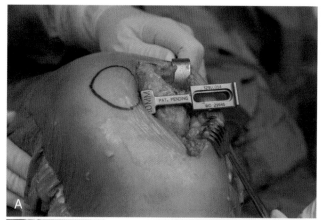

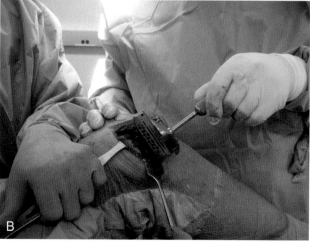

Figure 92–13. **A**, The intramedullary guide rests on the medial femoral condyle. **B**, The cutting block is attached to the intramedullary guide, and the saw cut is made from the medial side across the two distal condylar surfaces.

and flexion/extension positioning is set for the proper perpendicular tibial cut, the depth of the cut is set by referencing a depth gauge and also by checking the actual space in full extension with a spacer block (Fig. 92–14). The depth of the cut can be varied to allow for a flexion contracture. The proximal tibial cut is made by using the medial-based cutting slot on the tibial cutting guide. The cut should be made with care to avoid injury to the posterior neurovascular structures and is most often completed by dividing the tibial resection bone in three pieces.

At this point, the extension space can be evaluated with a spacer block and an extramedullary rod (Fig. 92–15). The medial and lateral collateral ligament structures should be equally balanced. If an inequality is present, the proper releases should be performed in standard fashion for varus and valgus deformities. Releases for a varus knee can be performed on the medial side of the tibia, and lateral releases for a valgus knee can also be completed through a medially based arthrotomy. Alternatively, a valgus knee can be approached through a lateral incision, but this is not absolutely necessary. Because 10 mm of bone has been removed from both the distal femur and proximal tibia, there is ample space to complete the releases and to visualize the lateral side of the knee.

The knee is now placed in 90 degrees of flexion and the femoral tower guide positioned on the distal femoral cut surface. This instrument has two footpads that reference the posterior condyles (Fig. 92–16). The tower should be parallel to the anteroposterior axis line and should be adjusted, if necessary, by rotating the footpad off the deficient condyle (Fig. 92–17). After the instrument is pinned in position, the knee is brought to full extension and a gauge attached to reference the anterior surface for determining both component sizing and the location of the external rotation cut. The proper size femoral finishing

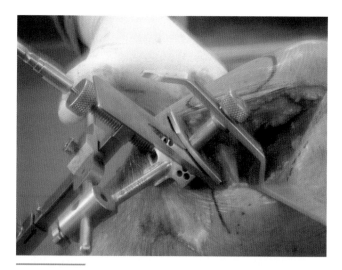

Figure 92–14. The extramedullary tibial cutting guide sets the cutting block on the medial aspect of the tibia and uses the depth gauge to measure the resection.

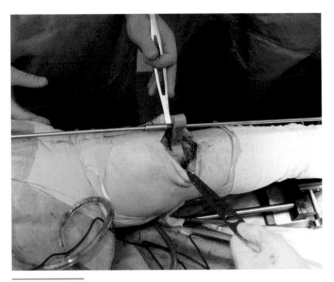

Figure 92–15. The extension space is measured with a spacer block and extramedullary rods.

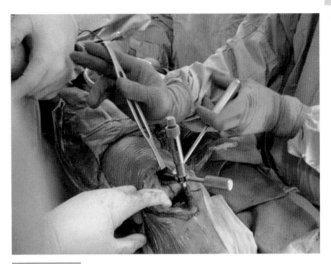

Figure 92–17. The knee is flexed 15 degrees and the probe identifies the size of the femur and the location of the anterior surface cut.

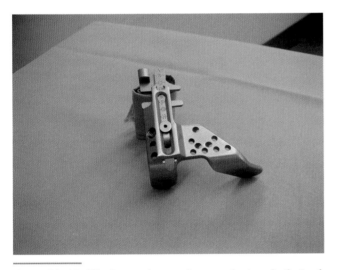

Figure 92–16. The femoral tower has two foot pads that reference the posterior aspect of each femoral condyle.

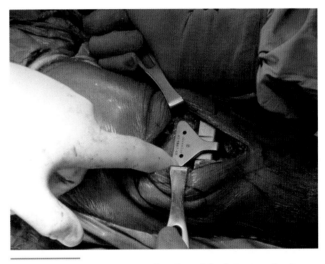

Figure 92–18. The femoral finishing block is attached to a plate that references the anterior femoral cut and is positioned in a medial-to-lateral direction in full extension.

block is then placed on the end of the femur with the knee still in full extension (Fig. 92–18). The block is attached to a reference plate that lies flat on the external rotation cut surface and is positioned in the medial-to-lateral plane. After the block is pinned in place, the peg holes and all cuts are completed with the knee in 90 degrees of flexion (Fig. 92–19). The flexion and extension spaces can now be compared and adjusted in the traditional fashion if there is a discrepancy.

The tibial cut surface is sized for placement of the tray. The tibial handle is attached to the tray (Fig. 92–20) and used to adjust the rotational alignment with reference to the tibial tubercle, the femoral notch cut, and the malleoli of the ankle. The tray is pinned in place and the cement hole and fins are completed.

The trial components are inserted with the femur first. The tibial tray is used without the stem at this juncture to save time and allow testing with more than one size tibial plastic insert. Patella tracking is confirmed at this point.

All the components are cemented with standard bone cement. The tibial tray (without the polyethylene insert) is implanted first. In the cruciate-retaining knee design, the tibia tray has four pegs and is inserted easily. In the posterior-stabilized design, the stem is difficult to insert and the knee position must be varied between 30 and 80 degrees of flexion, depending on soft-tissue tightness, with the patella subluxated to the lateral side (Fig. 92–21). The femoral component is cemented second and should be gently placed on the cut surface with impaction only after the position is completely confirmed. The patella is cemented last. The polyethylene insert is locked into position after the cementing is completed (Fig. 92–22). Range of motion, tibiofemoral tracking, and patellofemoral tracking should all be confirmed at this point.

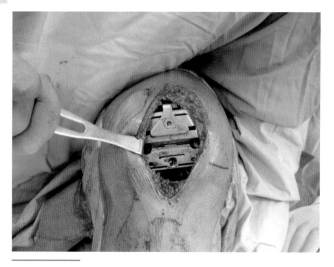

Figure 92–19. The femoral finishing cuts are made with the knee in 90 degrees of flexion.

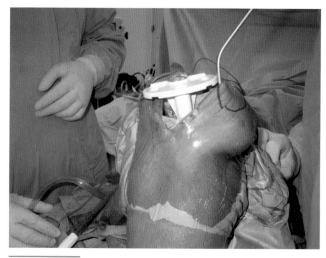

Figure 92–21. The tibial trial for the posterior-stabilized design is sometimes difficult to fit into a flexed knee.

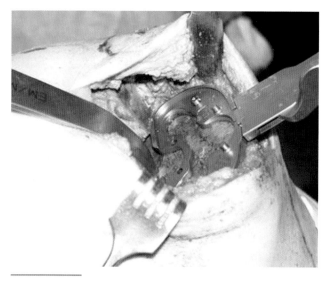

Figure 92–20. The tibia finishing guide is locked on the back of the tibia and rotated properly with respect to the tibial tubercle.

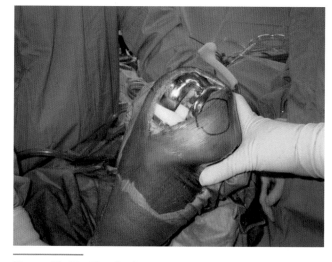

Figure 92–22. The final components with the patella subluxated to the lateral side.

Surgical drains can be used if desired. The arthrotomy is closed in standard fashion along with the skin (Fig. 92–23). It is important to secure the attachment of the vastus medialis to prevent disruption of the medial closure and subluxation of the patella.

POSTOPERATIVE MANAGEMENT

Patients begin full weightbearing ambulation and range-of-motion exercises as soon as they are alert, stable, and able to bear weight. Anticoagulation is achieved with fondaparinux (Arixtra), a pentasaccharide,[1,3] or enoxaparin (Lovenox). Patients are discharged within 2 to 4 days to a rehabilitation center. Some patients do elect to go directly home and are monitored as outpatients.

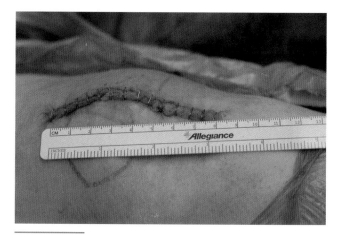

Figure 92–23. The 8-cm skin incision with the knee in full extension.

RESULTS WITH THE QUADRICEPS-SPARING TECHNIQUE

Two hundred four procedures have now been completed over the past $2^{1}/_{2}$ years. Five surgeries required extension of the capsular incision into the quadriceps tendon and were not included in the data analysis. Three knees required a larger incision to implant the femoral component. One knee was too obese, and in one case the middle geniculate artery was cut and increased exposure was required to gain control of the bleeding vessel. The average age was 67 with a range of 51 to 84 years. There were 33 bilateral procedures. Tourniquet time has gradually decreased from a starting time of 120 minutes to an average of 65 minutes now. Tourniquet time for a standard TKA is 40 minutes. Blood loss averaged 375 mL, with blood loss during standard TKA being 450 mL. One patient required manipulation of the knee under general anesthesia and has never gained more than 65 degrees of motion. The average pain score from the physical therapy department on the first postoperative visit was 5 for the quadriceps-sparing MIS patients and 7 for the standard knee surgeries. There have been one nonfatal pulmonary embolism and one nonfatal myocardial infarction. Two patients had transient arrhythmias. No infections, wound breakdown, component loosening, or reoperations have occurred.

The average length of stay is 2 days. All the postoperative radiographs were measured. Using a bracket of ±4 degrees from the perfect position, two tibial components are outside that margin with a varus position of 7 degrees. The average distal femoral valgus is 6 degrees, and the overall knee alignment is in 4 degrees of valgus. These radiograph were compared with those of a matched group of patients who underwent unilateral high-flex posterior-stabilized knee arthroplasty with the standard arthrotomy incision during the same period, and no statistically significant differences were found.

The follow-up is admittedly very short and can indicate only trends at best. However, the range of motion at the first office visit was 20 degrees greater than that of the matched group of unilateral high-flex knees, and this is statistically significant at $p < 0.05$.

CONCLUSIONS

MIS TKA is in the early stages of development. Many opponents believe that the technique is nothing more than a cosmetic modification of the standard TKA and will lead to more complications and less patient satisfaction. These criticisms must not be ignored and must also be answered with strong factual support. MIS is a surgery that is not determined by the length of the incision or the cosmetic result. The term "minimally invasive" should refer to the extent of violation of the anatomic structures about the involved joint. In the knee, the MIS approach should not violate the extensor mechanism and should not violate the suprapatellar pouch. MIS should be a capsular approach, and as such, it should produce less discomfort and faster recovery. Extensions of the arthrotomy into the quadriceps tendon or the vastus medialis are variations of the quadriceps-sparing approach. The extensions are certainly of value and should be considered a part of the continuum of TKA surgery. Perhaps the best way to proceed with the surgical technique is to progress to use of the quadriceps-sparing instruments from the standard operative approach to a mini-incision exposure and then to the true capsular incision.

References

1. Bauer KA, Eriksson BL, Lassen MR, Turpie AG: Fondaparinux compared with enoxaparin for the prevention of venous thromboembolism after elective major knee surgery. N Engl J Med 345:1305-1310, 2001.
2. Colizza W, Insall J, Scuderi G: The posterior stabilized total knee prosthesis: Assessment of polyethylene damage and osteolysis after a ten-year-minimum follow-up. J Bone Joint Surg Am 77:1716-1720, 1995.
3. Eriksson BL, Bauer KA, Lassen MR, Turpie AG: Fondaparinux compared with enoxaparin for the prevention of venous thromboembolism after hip-fracture surgery. N Engl J Med 345:1298-1304, 2001.
4. Insall J, Ranawat C, Scott WN, Walker P: Total condylar knee replacement. Preliminary report. Clin Orthop 120:149-154, 1976.
5. Insall J, Tria A, Scott W: The total condylar knee prosthesis. The first five years. Clin Orthop 145:68-77, 1979.
6. Malkani AL, Rand JA, Bryan RS, Wallrichs SL: Total knee arthroplasty with the kinematic condylar prosthesis. A ten year follow-up study. J Bone Joint Surg Am 77:423-431, 1995.
7. Ranawat C, Flynn W, Saddler S, et al: Long-term results of the total condylar knee arthroplasty. A 15-year survivorship study. Clin Orthop 286:96-102, 1993.
8. Repicci JA, Eberle RW: Minimally invasive surgical technique for unicondylar knee arthroplasty. J South Orthop Assoc 8:20-27, 1999.
9. Ritter MA, Herbst SA, Keating EM, et al: Long term survivorship analysis of a posterior cruciate retaining total condylar total knee arthroplasty. Clin Orthop 309:136-145, 1994.
11. Scott RD, Volatile TB: 12 years experience with posterior cruciate retaining total knee arthroplasty. Clin Orthop 205:100-107, 1986.
10. Romanowski MR, Repicci JA: Minimally invasive unicondylar arthroplasty: Eight-year follow-up. J Knee Surg 15:17-22, 2002.
12. Scuderi GR, Tenholder M, Capeci C: Surgical approaches in mini-incision total knee arthroplasty. Clin Orthop 428:61-67, 2004.
13. Stern SH, Insall JN: Posterior stabilized prosthesis. Results after follow-up of nine to twelve years. J Bone Joint Surg Am 74:980-986, 1992.

CHAPTER 93

Unicompartmental, Bicompartmental, or Tricompartmental Arthritis of the Knee: Algorithm for Clinical Management

Anthony H. Presutti • Richard Iorio • William L. Healy

Arthritis of the knee is a common clinical problem that affects approximately 2% of the population older than 17 years of age. Among patients 65 years of age and older, up to 10% have arthritic knee symptoms, including pain, stiffness, and limitation of activity.[55,89] Patients with arthritis are more likely to seek medical care than patients without arthritis.[53]

Arthritis of the knee presents as a spectrum of unicompartmental, bicompartmental, or tricompartmental arthritis. *Unicompartmental arthritis* is defined as degeneration of the articular cartilage of either the medial tibiofemoral joint space, the lateral tibiofemoral joint space, or the patellofemoral joint space. It may be associated with meniscus tears, instability, or malalignment.[5,53,55,89] *Bicompartmental arthritis* is usually defined as unicompartmental arthritis and patellofemoral arthritis. *Tricompartmental arthritis* involves articular cartilage deterioration of the medial tibiofemoral joint, the lateral tibiofemoral joint, and the patellofemoral joint.

The most common clinical symptom associated with arthritis of the knee is pain, which can be global or limited to one affected joint space. Associated clinical findings may include stiffness, swelling, effusion, crepitus, impingement, instability, and malalignment. Radiographic findings associated with arthritis of the knee may include joint space narrowing, squaring of the femoral condyles, subchondral sclerosis, intercondylar and joint line osteophytes, and malalignment (varus or valgus).[5,29]

In this chapter the natural history of unicompartmental, bicompartmental, and tricompartmental arthritis of the knee is reviewed and nonoperative and operative management is discussed. Early diagnosis and early treatment of arthritis of the knee may reduce pain, improve function, and improve long-term outcomes for patients with arthritis of the knee.[89] An algorithm for treatment is presented.

NATURAL HISTORY OF ARTHRITIS OF THE KNEE

The specific cause of degenerative arthritis is not clear, but it can be progressive in an active patient.[30,76] Trauma is a common cause of articular cartilage deterioration and symptomatic arthritis of the knee.* The clinical spectrum

*See references 5, 8, 29, 30, 47, 53, 55, 76, 83, 115, 127, and 152.

of arthritis of the knee can range considerably from minimal to severe symptoms, and clinical symptoms and radiographic images may not correlate. Patients with significant radiographic joint space deterioration may have minimal symptoms and vice versa.

Degenerative arthritis of the knee should be differentiated from focal articular cartilage defects in the knee.[25,81,130] In general, the size and location of articular cartilage defects in the knee determine the severity of symptoms and indications for treatment.[130] If an articular cartilage defect is greater than 2 to 3 cm², or has good peripheral "shoulders," degenerative arthritis may not develop for a long time.[25,61,130] Articular cartilage defects in which the exposed subchondral bone is not surrounded by a good peripheral "shoulder" tends to be more symptomatic and deteriorate more rapidly.[130] Symptomatic articular cartilage lesions often progress with age, and treatment of isolated lesions may minimize the development of degenerative arthritis.[25,31,38,45,130]

EVALUATION OF ARTHRITIS OF THE KNEE

A database for evaluating arthritis of the knee includes medical and orthopedic history, physical examination, and musculoskeletal imaging. History and physical examination can provide specific information regarding joint line tenderness, meniscal damage, ligament instability, and malalignment. History and physical examination should provide clear indication of whether a knee has unicompartmental, bicompartmental, or tricompartmental arthritis.[89]

Radiographic evaluation of an arthritic knee begins with an anteroposterior weightbearing radiograph of the knee in full extension.[69] A posteroanterior weightbearing radiograph with the knees flexed 40 degrees adds information about articular cartilage deterioration in a more functional position and gives better information about articular cartilage integrity in the lateral tibiofemoral compartment.[38,69] Lateral, tunnel, and tangential views of the knee provide complementary information regarding articular cartilage deterioration in the medial, lateral, and patellofemoral compartments of the knee joint.[155] Standing hip-knee-ankle radiographs allow evaluation of the mechanical axis of the limb and angular deformity of the lower limb. The mechanical axis is determined by a line drawn from the center of the femoral head to the center of the ankle.[69,155] The mechanical axis should pass through the center of, or just medial to, the center of the knee. A mechanical axis of 0 to 3 degrees of varus is considered normal.[42,69] Angular deformities of greater than or equal to 10 degrees varus or valgus are frequently associated with symptomatic arthritis of the knee.[69]

NONOPERATIVE TREATMENT

Nonoperative treatment for arthritis of the knee is palliative treatment, which is intended to alleviate symptoms. In general, nonoperative treatment does not cure arthritis of the knee. Nonoperative treatment is not specific for unicompartmental, bicompartmental, or tricompartmental arthritis of the knee except for unloader braces and orthotics, which are most commonly used for medial tibiofemoral unicompartmental arthritis of the knee.

Exercise and Physical Therapy

Stretching and strengthening exercises may reduce symptoms and improve function of an arthritic knee.[38] Stretching can prevent contracture and maintain range of motion, and strengthening can increase muscle strength and dynamic stability of an arthritic knee. Quadriceps weakness is seen in patients with knee arthritis and may be a risk factor for the disease. Patient education programs and supervised fitness sessions have been associated with improved functional status for patients with arthritic knees without worsening the arthritic symptoms.[103] Therapeutic modalities such as cold treatment, hydrotherapy, ultrasonography, iontophoresis, and massage can also help the symptoms associated with arthritis of the knee. Heat treatments are best used to decrease morning stiffness and reduce start-up discomfort.[54]

Weight Loss

Obesity is an independent risk factor for the development of knee arthritis.[177] Weight loss reduces the joint reaction forces and is a fundamental concept in the treatment of arthritic joints.[9] Women older than the age of 50 years, with malalignment, have a higher prevalence of arthritis than age-matched controls in the general, nonaffected population.[55,107] Weight loss (5.1 kg) by obese women decreases the risk of degenerative arthritis by greater than 50%.[57]

Medications

Analgesic medications such as acetaminophen provide effective pain relief and have minimal side effects. Acetaminophen is inexpensive and is available over the counter.

It also can provide predictable relief from symptoms of an arthritic knee.[23,24,111] Nonsteroidal anti-inflammatory drugs (NSAIDs) are the most common drugs used to treat osteoarthritis of the knee.[24,27,104,111] NSAIDs inhibit cyclooxygenase-1 or -2 (COX-1 or -2) and have both an anti-inflammatory and analgesic benefit for patients with arthritic knees. NSAIDs can be associated with gastrointestinal side effects. Short-term clinical trials comparing NSAIDs and acetaminophen show equal efficacy.[23] Chronic use of NSAIDs requires monitoring of the hepatic, renal, and gastrointestinal systems. NSAIDs that are COX-2 inhibitors have shown the ability to improve symptoms associated with an arthritic knee while causing fewer gastrointestinal and renal side effects.[104,111] However, the cardiovascular side effects associated with rofecoxib led to its removal from the market in September 2004. Questions are being asked about other COX-2 inhibitors currently on the market. COX-2 inhibitors are more expensive than COX-1 NSAIDs and given the uncertainty regarding their safety, the use of COX-2 inhibitors should be considered very carefully. Because of renal and hepatic side effects, monitoring of markers of liver and renal function is warranted in those patients who take these drugs for the long term.

Nutritional Supplements/ Topical Analgesics

Nutritional supplements (such as glucosamine and chondroitin sulfate) claim to be "chondral protective." Double-blind randomized trials demonstrate that glucosamine is mildly effective for relieving pain associated with osteoarthritis.[2,104,111,133,138,154] In a study by Reginster and colleagues,[153] 212 patients with arthritis of the knee were randomized to a glucosamine or a placebo group. After 3 years of treatment, the glucosamine group had less joint space narrowing and improved WOMAC scores when compared with placebo. It has not been determined whether glucosamine has a long-term benefit on the articular cartilage of an arthritic joint.[2,111] Some patients report improvement in symptoms of an arthritic knee with the use of topical agents such as methylsalicylate, capsaicin, and NSAID creams.[9]

Injections

Arthritic flares associated with pain, swelling, and effusion can be treated with aspiration of the knee and intra-articular injection of a corticosteroid. This injection is frequently combined with a local anesthetic to provide short-term relief. Corticosteroids are associated with an increased risk of damage to the articular cartilage and should not be repeated more than three to four times annually.[79] Hyaluronic acid joint injections are intended to provide "viscosupplementation" of the synovial fluid of the knee. Hyaluronic acid preparations are high-molecular-weight solutions that are intended to supplement the reduced concentration of hyaluronans seen in arthritic knees. It has been suggested that hyaluronic acid may slow the progression of arthritis of the knee and decrease inflammation in the synovial lining when compared with corticosteroid injections.[38,60] Short-term studies[38,153,154] suggest there is no advantage of hyaluronic acid injections over the use of NSAIDs. Hyaluronan has a slower onset of action, it is more expensive, and it has a higher risk of localized inflammatory response.[54] However, in patients older than 60 years of age, hyaluronic acid may provide longer-lasting pain relief than corticosteroid injections.[3,9,54,60,79,109,179] In one prospective randomized study, Leopold[108] demonstrated no difference between hyaluronic acid and corticosteroid injections in terms of pain relief or function at 6-month follow-up. The role of hyaluronic acid injections for treatment of an arthritic knee is not clear at this time.

Ambulatory Aids

Ambulatory aids can help a patient with acute exacerbations of symptoms of an arthritic knee, and they may provide an ambulatory assist with patients with end-stage arthritis of the knee.[9,38,111] A cane used in the hand opposite the affected knee can decrease the weightbearing load on the affected knee from 30% to 60%.[54,60] The use of crutches can further decrease the load transmitted through the arthritic knee.

Braces

Several types of braces are available for treatment of a degenerative knee: compressive knee sleeves, supportive braces, and joint unloading braces. Compressive knee sleeves are made of material such as polypropylene or neoprene. They provide compression to the arthritic knee, which may decrease swelling and increase proprioception to provide a feeling of increased support and stability.[38] Compressive knee sleeves do not change limb alignment, increase joint stability, or enhance mechanical function. Supportive knee braces include collateral ligament braces for varus/valgus instability, anterior cruciate ligament insufficiency braces to prevent anteroposterior and rotatory instability, and patellofemoral braces to prevent patella subluxation. Joint unloading braces apply either a varus or valgus stress at the knee, which distracts the affected arthritic joint space and unloads the affected joint during weightbearing activity.[119] Joint unloader braces are generally indicated for medial unicompartmental arthritis. One fluoroscopic gait analysis[100] demonstrated that joint unloader braces when fitted and worn properly can increase the effective joint space and decrease symptoms of an arthritic knee. Clinical failure of joint unloading braces is frequently associated with poor fit of the brace and obesity about the knee. Patient compliance and cost can also be problems with brace therapy for arthritis knees. Other studies[55,78,82,148] have shown similar efficacy of unloading braces. Braces can be difficult to wear for extended periods of time because of their size and the

Table 93–1. Outerbridge Classification of Cartilage Degeneration

Stage 1	Superficial fibrillation
Stage II	Fragmentation < 1.3 cm²
Stage III	Fragmentation > 1.3 cm²
Stage IV	Eburnation

Data from Outerbridge RE: The etiology of chondromalacia patellae. J Bone Joint Surg Br 43:752-757, 1961.

amount of force imparted to the knee.[147] Joint unloader braces are generally used to unload the medial tibiofemoral joint space. The efficacy of joint unloading braces for valgus knees has not been demonstrated.

Orthotics/Footwear Modification

Well-padded, energy-absorbing shoe soles or orthotics can decrease the load across the knee during heel strike. Ankle, hind-foot, or mid-foot deformities leading to limb malalignment can exacerbate knee arthritis. Orthotic corrections and support can improve alignment of the foot or ankle, which may in turn improve overall limb alignment.[31,111] Wedges placed on the heel or sole of the shoe can realign a foot 5 degrees in either varus or valgus direction. A lateral heel wedge will unload the medial tibiofemoral joint space.[183] A medial heel wedge will unload the lateral joint space. Studies have demonstrated the efficacy of lateral heel wedges with improvement in all grades of degenerative articular cartilage change.[95] Patients with Outerbridge II (Table 93–1) had the most relief.[141] Use of medial heel wedges for lateral tibiofemoral osteoarthritis of the knee has not been reported to our knowledge.

OPERATIVE MANAGEMENT

In contrast to nonoperative treatment for arthritis of the knee, operative treatment generally attempts to "fix" or cure the problem. Sometimes the improvement does not last a lifetime owing to the underlying arthritic problem, the patient's age, weight, and activity, and the success of the surgical procedure. Operative treatment can be specific for unicompartmental, bicompartmental, and tricompartmental arthritis of the knee.

Arthroscopy

Arthroscopy of an arthritic knee can provide diagnostic information and therapeutic intervention.[22,33,172] Outcomes after arthroscopic surgery of an arthritic knee vary, and it is difficult to correlate arthroscopic findings with outcomes of arthroscopy. However, worse outcomes have been associated with greater articular cartilage degeneration as seen on preoperative radiographs, limb malalignment, and calcium pyrophosphate deposition.[50,140,161] The utilization of arthroscopy in treating arthritic knees is controversial because arthroscopy does not appear to alter the natural history of arthritis of the knee, especially with unicompartmental disease.[161,164] Arthroscopy may decrease symptoms associated with an arthritic knee by means of lavage and dilution of inflammatory cytokines.[38,49,50] Favorable[6,22,50,91,123,167] and unfavorable[14,66,124,161] results have been reported in the orthopedic literature regarding the use of arthroscopy as a treatment for arthritis of the knee. Mosely and associates[132] studied arthroscopy used for arthritic knees by comparing a placebo group, an arthroscopic lavage group, and an arthroscopic débridement group. All three groups demonstrated a decrease in symptoms up to 2 years after intervention. The authors concluded that arthroscopy without mechanical symptoms is not indicated as a treatment for arthritis of the knee, and there may be a placebo effect with arthroscopy.

It is clear that arthroscopy can be beneficial for patients with unicompartmental arthritis who have normal or near-normal limb alignment and who have symptomatic, unstable meniscus tears or loose bone or cartilage fragments in the joint.[18,134,140,151,157,] Varus malalignment of the limb is a negative predictive factor when compared with valgus malalignment of the limb when referring to outcomes of arthroscopy for osteoarthritis of the knee.[167]

Operative Treatment of Focal Articular Cartilage Damage

Focal defects of articular cartilage in the knee have limited capacity for repair and frequently progress to clinically symptomatic osteoarthritis.[25,32,130] Subchondral fracture techniques to stimulate new fibrocartilage associated with débridement of osteophytes, excision of loose bodies, and excision of meniscal fragments can be performed with an open arthrotomy[85] or arthroscopically.[20,158] Abrasion arthroplasty, which is generally performed arthroscopically, is a modification of subchondral fracture techniques[7,85,93,98,113] in which a bur is used to stimulate bleeding that leads to fibrocartilage growth. Subchondral fracture techniques are most effective when the defects are smaller than 2 cm^2 because the mechanical properties of fibrocartilage are not as optimal for knee function as those of hyaline cartilage.

Cartilage transplantation or implantation can be useful for patients with larger focal defects of articular cartilage. Current methods of cartilage implantation include autologous osteochondral plug transfer, autologous chondrocyte implantation, and osteochondral allograft transplantation.* For these techniques to succeed a knee must be stable and reasonably well aligned. Realignment can be performed with an osteotomy,[73,139] and instability can be improved with ligament stabilization opera-

tions.[31,38,139] The utilization of cartilage transplantation and implantation techniques for unicompartmental arthritis of the knee has not been studied.

Osteotomy

Unicompartmental arthritis of the knee is frequently associated with a varus or valgus deformity. Malalignment of a limb increases stress on the damaged articular cartilage in the affected tibiofemoral compartment, which leads to joint line pain, loss of articular cartilage, and progressive deformity of the limb. The rationale of osteotomy of the knee is to realign the limb and shift the weightbearing force from damaged articular cartilage to healthy articular cartilage in the less affected tibial femoral compartment. Clinical, radiographic, and biological improvement has been documented when an osteotomy sufficiently unloads a degenerative compartment.[26,61,96]

Patient selection is critical for a successful outcome after osteotomy about the knee.[73] The best candidate for an osteotomy of the knee is a young, active patient whose life expectancy far exceeds the expected survival of a knee implant. A stable knee and a functional range of motion is required for osteotomy.[38,69] Anterior cruciate ligament insufficiency may not be a strict contraindication for osteotomy because it can be corrected at the same time as an osteotomy.[139]

The normal mechanical axis of the limb is defined as a straight line drawn from the center of the femoral head to the center of the ankle joint. This line should pass through the center, or just medial to the center, of the knee joint. Angular deformity at the knee can be measured by the angle subtended at the knee by a line through the center of the femoral head and the center of the knee and extended to the floor and a line from the center of the knee to the center of the ankle. A 0- to 3-degree varus angle is considered normal.[69,103] An osteotomy should be planned to shift the mechanical axis from the degenerative tibiofemoral compartment to the more healthy articular cartilage of the other tibiofemoral compartment in the knee. Sufficient correction is generally obtained when the angular deformity is corrected with 2 to 4 degrees of overcorrection.[84]

Proximal tibial valgus osteotomy can provide successful outcomes for patients with medial tibiofemoral unicompartmental osteoarthritis associated with a varus deformity.[38,6975,84] Patients with lateral tibiofemoral subluxation, lateral thrust, or range of motion less than 90 degrees are not ideal candidates for proximal tibial osteotomy. Mild to moderate patellofemoral degenerative changes are not a contraindication to proximal tibial osteotomy.[87] Various methods for proximal tibial osteotomy have been used, including lateral closing wedge, medial opening wedge, or dome osteotomy. Perhaps the most commonly used technique for proximal tibial osteotomy is the lateral closing wedge osteotomy, which can be stabilized with internal fixation, external fixation, or a cast. Billings and associates[19] described a technique involving an angular cutting guide and plate and screw fixation that provided reproducible angular

---

*See references 15, 21, 25, 35, 39-41, 59, 64, 65, 70, 92, 122, 128-130, 142, 165, and 182.

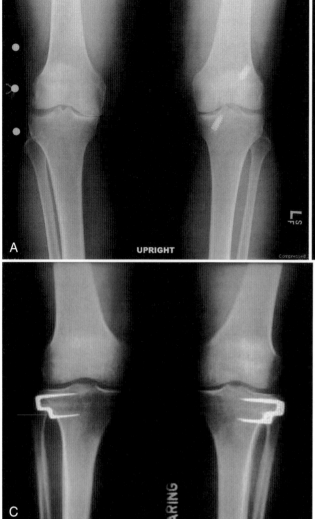

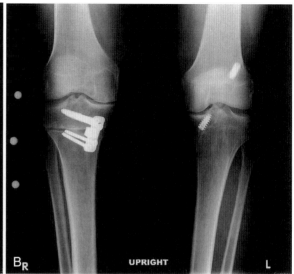

Figure 93–1. **A,** Anteroposterior standing radiograph of a 49-year-old firefighter with unicompartmental, medial tibiofemoral osteoarthritis. **B,** Postoperative standing anteroposterior radiograph demonstrating correction of varus deformity and widening of the medial tibiofemoral joint space. The patient has returned to full duty as a fireman. **C,** Postoperative standing anteroposterior radiograph of bilateral, lateral closing wedge proximal tibial osteotomies.

correction. Furthermore, stability was created at the osteotomy site, which allowed for early range of motion of the knee.

Medial opening wedge osteotomy (Fig. 93–1) can be used in treating medial compartment osteoarthritis. Fixation methods include plate and screw constructs with or without bone graft,[10] external fixation or hemicalitosis,[114] and small wire external fixation. Advantages of the opening wedge osteotomy include a simple osteotomy without removal of a wedge, no disruption of the proximal tibiofibular joint, potential decreased risk of peroneal nerve injury, prevention of patella baja, and prevention of contraction of the patella tendon with resultant loss of range of motion.

Medial opening wedge osteotomy of the proximal tibia for medial tibiofemoral osteoarthritis was successful in a series of 21 knees in 18 patients followed for an average of 78.6 months.[102] This series used porous hydroxyapatite instead of bone graft in the opening wedge space. All patients had pain relief and improvement in walking ability. No patient required conversion to total knee arthroplasty at short-term follow-up.

Proximal tibial valgus osteotomy can have problems. One study[173] has demonstrated a recurrence of varus malalignment in up to 18% of patients, progression of lateral compartment osteoarthritis in 60% of patients, and progression of medial compartment osteoarthritis in 93% of patients.[173] In patients whose osteotomy is fixed with external fixation there is increased risk for pin-tract infection, nonunion, and deep venous thrombosis.

The Mayo Clinic has a more than 40-year experience with tibial osteotomy for medial tibiofemoral osteoarthritis and varus deformities of the knee. Coventry and coworkers[44] reported on 87 osteotomies in 73 patients observed for an average of 10 years. Failure was defined as conversion to total knee replacement. Survivorship was 89% at 5 years and 75% at 10 years. Results were less good if anatomic valgus was less than 8 degrees or if the patient was more than 1.32 times ideal body weight.

Insall and colleagues[87] reported on 95 knees treated with proximal tibial valgus osteotomy observed for 8.9 years. Eighty-one knees had good to excellent results at 5 years. Sixty knees had good or excellent results at 9 years. Twenty-two knees were converted to total knee arthroplasty. Twenty-nine knees had recurrence of the varus deformity, but this was not associated with lack of "ideal" alignment. These authors found in a later study that proximal tibial valgus osteotomy met the expectations of 28 of 34 men with high-demand activities.[135]

Noyes and associates[139] looked at the results of proximal tibial valgus osteotomy associated with anterior cruciate ligament reconstruction. Ten of 15 patients reported significant improvement in symptoms. Noyes and associates[139] recommended anterior cruciate ligament reconstruction with proximal tibial valgus osteotomy for patients with medial compartment osteoarthritis and functional instability who plan to return to high demand activity such as athletics.

Holden and coworkers[80] evaluated 51 knees in 45 patients who had a proximal tibial valgus osteotomy. Seventy percent of the knees were rated as good to excellent at 10 years. Anterior cruciate ligament deficiency was associated with poor results. Poor results were also associated with age older than 50 years, previous arthroscopy, a lateral thrust on walking, preoperative flexion less than 120 degrees, insufficient valgus correction, and delayed union or nonunion of the osteotomy.[4,77,136]

When osteotomy fails, conversion to total knee arthroplasty is generally more difficult to perform than a primary total knee arthroplasty. The osteotomy shifts the articular surface of the knee in relation to the medullary canal. This can lead to bony insufficiency of the lateral aspect of the proximal tibia and alterations of the patellofemoral joint secondary to patella baja and contraction of the patella tendon. Clinical results after conversion total knee arthroplasty vary. Parvizi and coworkers[144] observed 166 knees in 118 patients. Thirteen knees were revised at a mean of 5.9 years. Loose implants were seen in 17 tibial components and 7 femoral components at the time of final follow-up. Failures were associated with male gender, increased weight, age at the time of total knee arthroplasty, coronal laxity, and preoperative malalignment. Katz and colleagues[94] compared total knee arthroplasty after osteotomy to primary total knee arthroplasty. Seventeen of 21 knee replacements after osteotomy had good to excellent results, whereas all 21 primary knee replacements had good to excellent results. Staheli and colleagues[168] had similar results. In contrast to these studies, Meding and coworkers[125] found that previous proximal tibial osteotomy had no effect on the results of posterior cruciate ligament–retaining total knee arthroplasty performed with cement fixation.

Lateral tibiofemoral unicompartmental osteoarthritis associated with valgus deformity is less common than medial tibiofemoral unicompartmental arthritis.[38,174] Lateral tibiofemoral osteoarthritis is more common in women, and the deformity includes contraction of the lateral soft tissues, medial collateral ligament laxity, and distal lateral femoral condyle hypoplasia. Joint line obliquity can be present, and it is a consideration for choice of surgical treatment.[38,74,83,134,146]

Proximal tibial varus osteotomy can be used to treat lateral tibiofemoral osteoarthritis when the valgus angular deformity is less than 12 degrees of valgus and the predicted joint line obliquity will be less than 10 degrees.[38,43,73,134] Coventry and coworkers[43] observed 31

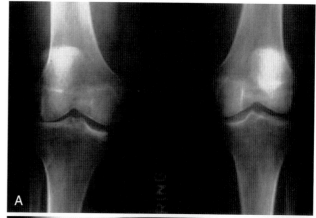

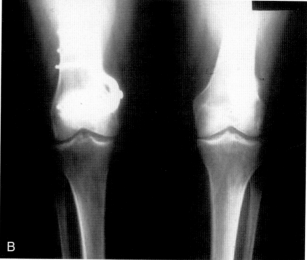

Figure 93–2. Preoperative standing anteroposterior (**A**) and postoperative standing anteroposterior (**B**) radiographs of a patient with unicompartmental, lateral tibiofemoral arthritis treated with distal femoral varus osteotomy. Note correction of the valgus deformity with widening of the lateral tibiofemoral joint space.

patients for an average of 9.4 years. Twenty-four knees had no to mild pain at last follow-up, and six were converted to total knee arthroplasty. Marti and associates[118] used a lateral opening wedge osteotomy in 36 patients. Thirty reported good to excellent results at 11 years.

Distal femoral varus osteotomy (Fig. 93–2) is indicated for larger valgus deformities associated with lateral tibiofemoral osteoarthritis.[34,51,72,121,134,] Healy and coworkers[72] reported on 23 knees followed for an average of 4 years. Nineteen knees had good to excellent results. Rheumatoid arthritis and poor preoperative range of motion were associated with a poor outcome. Long-term survival of distal femoral varus osteotomy has been reported to be 64% at 10 years.[58] Wang and Hsu[178] reported on their experience. Eighty-three percent had a satisfactory outcome with 10-year survival reported at 87%. Three of 33 knees were converted to total knee arthroplasty. Patients with severe deformity can have combined femoral and tibial osteotomies to compensate for excessive bone loss or excessive joint line obliquity.[134]

Unicompartmental Knee Arthroplasty

Unicompartmental knee arthroplasty (Fig. 93–3) is indicated for the treatment of painful unicompartmental arthritis when cartilage-sparing operations and osteotomy are not indicated. Patient selection is critical for successful unicompartmental knee arthroplasty. Ideal patients participate in low demand activities and have a stable knee with less than 15-degree flexion contracture, minimal malalignment, and minimal involvement of the contralat-

eral tibiofemoral compartment and the patellofemoral compartment.[175,176] Unicompartmental knee arthroplasty has been more commonly offered to patients with osteoarthritis and osteonecrosis[69] whereas patients with inflammatory arthritis are generally not candidates for unicompartmental arthroplasty.[176]

Early results of unicompartmental arthroplasty were not particularly good.[68,88,105,117] However, improved patient selection, improved surgical technique, and improved implants have led to improved results for unicompartmental knee arthroplasty. Best results have been obtained

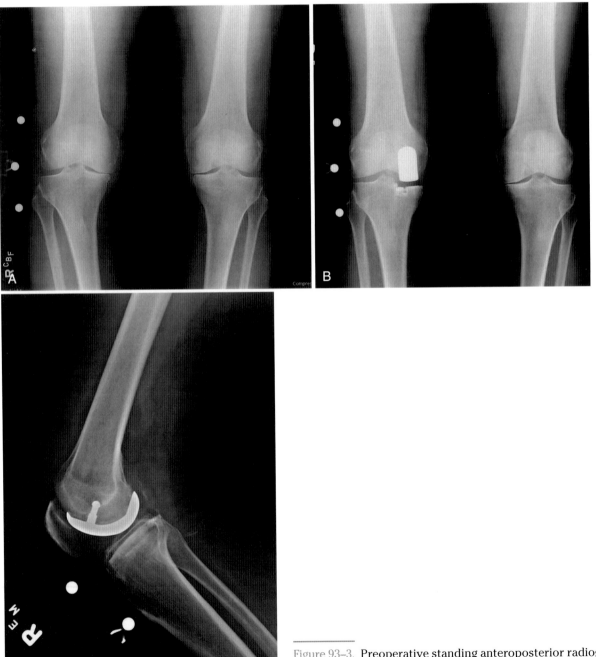

Figure 93–3. Preoperative standing anteroposterior radiograph (**A**) demonstrating unicompartmental, medial tibiofemoral arthritis treated with unicompartmental knee arthroplasty. Postoperative standing anteroposterior (**B**) and lateral (**C**) radiographs at 6 years.

when the postoperative mechanical axis is in the center of the knee or slightly medial to the knee after compartment resurfacing. Overcorrection or undercorrection is associated with early failure.[97] Patients with lateral compartment osteoarthritis should be corrected so that the mechanical axis passes through the lateral compartment.[86,105,163] Potential factors associated with less good results after unicompartmental knee arthroplasty include use, high demand activity, inadequate implant fixation, poor implant design, and insufficient polyethylene thickness.* Unicompartmental knee arthroplasty has several advantages over total knee arthroplasty, including a less extensive surgical approach,[159] avoidance of patellar resurfacing, minimal to no transfusion,[150] and potential greater range of motion.[36,137,160] Unicompartmental arthroplasty patients also have a shorter postoperative recovery time and faster return to work or preoperative activity. Furthermore, revision to a total knee arthroplasty is less difficult than revision of a total knee arthroplasty.[160]

More recent results of unicompartmental arthroplasty are more encouraging. Scott and colleagues[163] reported 85% survivorship for 10 years with revision total knee arthroplasty as the endpoint. Stockelman and Pole[171] reported 43 satisfactory results with four revisions at an average of 7.4 years after the original unicompartmental knee arthroplasty. Berger and associates[16] reported 98% survivorship at 10 years. Christensen[37] reported 7 of 575 unicompartmental knee replacements required conversion to a total knee arthroplasty at 2 to 10 years. Pennington and associates[145] reported 92% survivorship at 11 years in patients who were younger than 60 years of age when they had a unicompartmental knee replacement operation. Argenson and coworkers[12] report 94% survivorship for unicompartmental arthroplasty at 10 years.

Conversion of a failed unicompartmental arthroplasty to total knee arthroplasty can be associated with technical difficulties at the time of surgery. Potential problems include difficulty with the exposure and bony defects that may require augmentation with bone graft, cement, or metal augments. Depending on the extent of the bony deficiency, femoral or tibial implants may require an intramedullary stem for stability (this occurs more frequently in the tibia). Barrett and Scott[13] suggest that the technique of the original unicompartmental arthroplasty influences the outcome of the revision operation. If minimal bone was resected at the time of unicompartmental arthroplasty, primary knee replacement implants can generally be utilized.[13] Revision of unicompartmental knee arthroplasty can be as successful as a primary total knee replacement operation.[13]

When patients present with painful unicompartmental arthritis of the knee, it is not clear whether osteotomy or unicompartmental knee arthroplasty provides a better, more durable outcome. Broughton and coworkers[28] compared 42 unicompartmental knee replacements and 49 proximal tibial valgus osteotomies at 5 to 10 years of follow-up. Thirty-two of 42 unicompartmental knees had a good result, and 21 of 49 proximal tibial valgus osteotomies had a good result. These authors concluded that the results of unicompartmental knee replacement were better than those of proximal tibial osteotomy. Ivarsson and Gillquist[90] report that patients with a unicompartmental knee replacement have better gait velocity and superior muscle strength compared with those with an osteotomy. Schai and associates[162] looked at short term (2 to 6 year) data on 28 unicompartmental knee arthroplasties. Twenty-five knees had satisfactory pain relief, and only two knees were revised to total knee arthroplasty. They concluded that unicompartmental knee arthroplasty yields results similar to osteotomy but inferior to total knee arthroplasty. Weale and colleagues[180] reported that patient-perceived outcomes, pain scores, and functional results were equivalent at short-term follow-up when unicompartmental knee replacement and total knee arthroplasty were compared. Laurencin and coworkers[106] compared patients with a unicompartmental arthroplasty on one knee and a total knee arthroplasty on the contralateral knee. Ten of 23 preferred the unicompartmental knee arthroplasty. Three of 23 preferred the total knee arthroplasty, and the remainder had no preference.

The increasing popularity of minimally invasive or minimal-incision techniques emphasizes small incisions in the skin and in the joint capsule. The intent of minimal-incision techniques is to decrease the amount of tissue disruption, which may lead to less postoperative pain and faster knee rehabilitation. Long-term studies are not available. Short-term studies suggest[137,160] that patients with unicompartmental arthroplasty have better range of motion and walk sooner than those patients with total knee arthroplasty.

Patellofemoral Arthroplasty

The treatment of unicompartmental arthritis involving the patellofemoral joint presents it own challenges. Up to 24% of women and 11% of men older than 55 years of age have symptomatic knee arthritis of the patellofemoral compartment.[120] Any planned surgical intervention should be limited only to those patients who have failed an exhaustive course of nonoperative management. This should include activity modification, isometric quadriceps strengthening, bracing, and/or NSAIDs. Should these methods fail then surgical intervention becomes a consideration.

For those patients with osteoarthritis secondary to malalignment/maltracking (excessive Q angles) surgical management can involve arthroscopic débridement and lateral release, proximal and distal soft-tissue realignment, anteriorization/anteromedialization of the tibial tubercle, and even patellectomy.[1,62,63] Patients without an anatomic abnormality who have arthritis isolated to the patellofemoral joint present a specific challenge. Surgical options can include patellofemoral arthroplasty and total knee arthroplasty.

Patellofemoral arthroplasty initially had poor results.[112,166,174,181] Implant design changes and a greater understanding of the patellofemoral articulation and soft-tissue balancing have improved the results. Merchant[126] reported his early results with patellofemoral arthroplasty: 93% (14 of 15) of his patients reported good-to-excellent

---

*See references 17, 52, 71, 85, 99, 105, 117, 143, 156, and 162.

results at an average of 3.75 years after surgery. No major complications were noted and no component failures were noted. Lonner[110] noted 96% (24 of 25) good-to-excellent results at 6 months (1 month to 1 year) with patellofemoral arthroplasty. He states that newer designs have led to a decrease in patellofemoral complications (17% to 4%). According to Lonner, tibiofemoral degeneration is now the major source of failure with patellofemoral arthroplasty. Kooijman and coworkers[101] observed 56 knees for an average of 17 years (range, 15 to 21 years). Eighty-six percent of patients reported good-to-excellent results at 17 years. Loosening was seen in 2% of the prostheses, and 12 knees had further surgery (high tibial osteotomy, total knee arthroplasty) at an average of 15.6 years. Argenson[11] has followed 57 patellofemoral arthroplasties and notes a 58% survivorship at 16 years; 14 have been revised, 11 for femoral component loosening and 4 for stiffness. Patellofemoral arthroplasty is usually reserved for middle-aged patients (<55 years) with isolated patellofemoral arthrosis. Patients who are older will benefit from total knee arthroplasty. Mont[131] followed 30 knees for an average of 81 months (range, 48 to 133 months), with 28 excellent, one good, and one poor result reported. The poor result was due to an extensor mechanism rupture. The authors conclude that total knee arthroplasty is a viable treatment in patients with isolated patellofemoral arthritis older than 55 years of age. They also concluded the beneficial results of total knee arthroplasty in patients older than age 55 years outweigh the benefits of other surgical options (e.g., proximal/distal realignment, patellectomy) in patients with isolated patellofemoral arthritis.

Total Knee Arthroplasty

Total knee arthroplasty (Fig. 93–4) represents the gold standard for surgical management of unicompartmental, bicompartmental, and tricompartmental osteoarthritis of the knee in older patients.[116,149,150,157,170] Total knee arthroplasty also provides predictably successful outcomes in younger patients.[46,48,67,169] When a patient with a painful arthritic knee has failed to improve his or her symptoms with nonoperative treatment, total knee arthroplasty can provide a predictably successful result. The results of total knee arthroplasty are equivalent in patients with unicompartmental arthritis, bicompartmental arthritis, or tricompartmental osteoarthritis of the knee.

CONCLUSION

As this century progresses, osteoarthritis of the knee will become more common. Many effective nonoperative and operative options exist for treatment of knee arthritis (Fig. 93–5). These usually begin with nonoperative modalities: weight loss, physical therapy, medication (NSAID and non-NSAID), nutritional supplements, canes, crutches, braces, and orthotics. If nonoperative modalities fail, and if the patient is a candidate for operative intervention, then arthroscopy, osteotomy, unicompartmental arthroplasty, and total knee arthroplasty may be successful.

Arthroscopic surgery is usually reserved for unicompartmental arthritis with mechanical symptoms (catching, clicking, locking). Patients should understand that although arthroscopic surgery can relieve mechanical symptoms, the pain that is due to arthritis may or may not be improved.

Osteotomy provides an attractive, biological surgical treatment for unicompartmental arthritis of the knee. Historically, osteotomy was reserved for younger active patients, but as people live longer and remain active longer, the indications may expand. In the properly selected patients, osteotomy is very effective; and in the event of failure, it can be converted to a total knee arthroplasty.

Unicompartmental arthroplasty was initially reserved for older, sedentary patients; but like osteotomy, its indications are being expanded. Changes in implant design and surgical technique have improved unicompartmental knee arthroplasty such that it has become a very successful treatment. Conversion to a total knee arthroplasty has been shown to be equivalent to a primary total knee arthroplasty in most cases.

Total knee arthroplasty is a predictable and successful operative treatment for unicompartmental, bicompartmental, and tricompartmental osteoarthritis of the knee. It was once reserved for older patients, but it is becoming more frequent in younger patients. When other operative treatments are used as "first-line" or "bridge" operative treatments for arthritis of the knee, total knee arthroplasty can be a successful "back-up" treatment. It is imperative the surgeon consider his or her skills along with patient demands when deciding on an operative intervention.

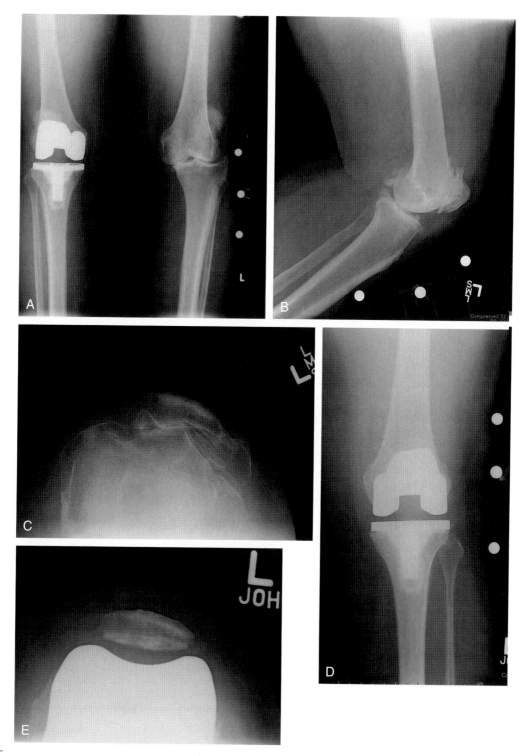

Figure 93–4. Standing anteroposterior (**A**), lateral (**B**), and patellofemoral (**C**) radiographs of a left knee showing tricompartmental osteoarthritis. Postoperative standing anteroposterior (**D**) and patellofemoral (**E**) radiographs show well-positioned and well-fixed cemented total knee arthroplasty.

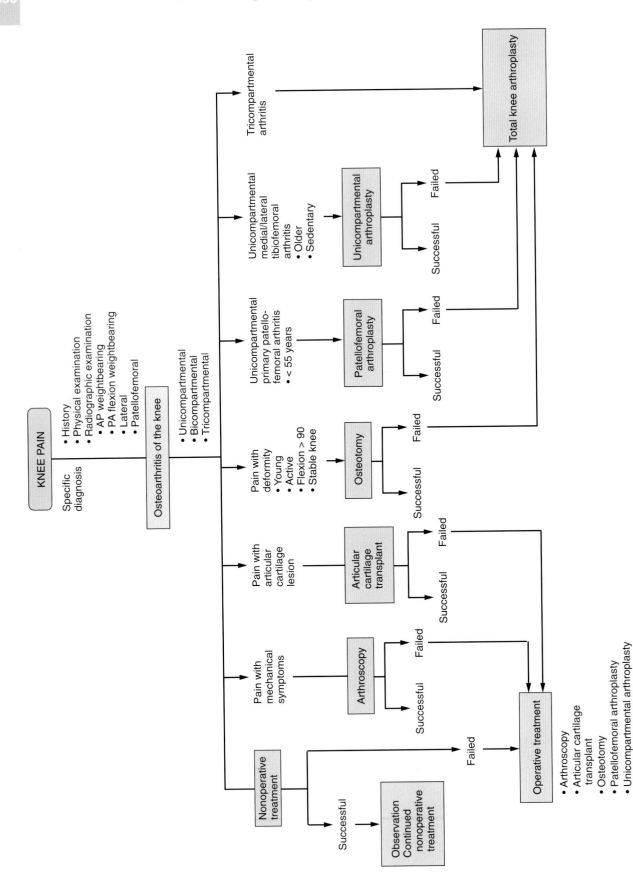

Figure 93–5. An algorithm presenting general guidelines for the nonoperative and operative management of unicompartmental, bicompartmental, and tricompartmental osteoarthritis of the knee.

References

1. Ackroyd CE, Polyzoides AJ: Patellectomy for osteoarthritis: A study of eighty-one patients followed from two to twenty-one years. J Bone Joint Surg Br 60:353-357, 1978.
2. Adams ME: Hype about glucosamine. Lancet 354:353-354, 1999.
3. Adams ME, Atkinson MH, Lussier AJ, et al: The role of viscosupplementation with hyalin G-F 20 (Synvisc) in the treatment of osteoarthritis of the knee: A Canadian multicenter trial comparing hyalin G-F 20 alone, hyalin G-F 20 with non-steroidal anti-inflammatory drugs (NSAIDs) and NSAIDs alone. Osteoarthritis Cartilage 3:213-225, 1995.
4. Aglietti P, Rinonapoli E, Stringa G, Taviani A: Tibial osteotomy for the varus osteoarthritic knee. Clin Orthop Relat Res 176:239-251, 1983.
5. Ahlbäck S: Osteoarthrosis of the knee: A radiographic investigation. Acta Radiol Diagn (Stockh) Suppl 277:7-72, 1968.
6. Aichroth PM, Patel DV, Moyes ST: A prospective review of arthroscopic débridement for degenerative joint disease of the knee. Int Orthop 15:351-355, 1991.
7. Akizuki S, Yasukawa Y, Takizawa T: Does arthroscopic abrasion arthroplasty promote cartilage regeneration in osteoarthritic knees with eburnation? A prospective study of high tibial osteotomy with abrasion arthroplasty versus high tibial osteotomy alone. Arthroscopy 13:9-17, 1997.
8. Allen PR, Denham RA, Swan AV: Late degenerative changes after meniscectomy: Factors affecting the knee after operation. J Bone Joint Surg Br 66:666-671, 1984.
9. Altman RD, et al. (American College of Rheumatology Subcommittee on Osteoarthritis Guidelines): Recommendations for the medical management of osteoarthritis of the hip and knee (2000 update). Arthritis Rheum 43:1905-1915, 2000.
10. Amendola A, Fowler P, Puddu G: Opening wedge high tibial osteotomy: Rational and surgical technique. Video presented at the 65th Meeting of the American Academy of Orthopaedic Surgeons, New Orleans, March 19-23, 1998.
11. Argenson JN: Patellofemoral replacement: Long-term results. Presented at the Knee Society Meeting, 2005 Annual Meeting of the American Academy of Orthopaedic Surgeons, Washington, DC.
12. Argenson JN, Chevrol-Benkeddache Y, Aubaniac JM: Modern unicompartmental knee arthroplasty with cement: A three to ten-year follow-up study. J Bone Joint Surg Am 84:235-239, 2002.
13. Barrett WP, Scott RD: Revision of failed unicondylar UKA. J Bone Joint Surg Am 69:1328-1335, 1987.
14. Baumgaertner MR, Cannon WD Jr, Vittori JM, et al: Arthroscopic débridement of the arthritic knee. Clin Orthop Relat Res 253:197-202, 1990.
15. Beaver RJ, Mahomed M, Backstein D, et al: Fresh osteochondral allografts for post-traumatic defects in the knee: A survivorship analysis. J Bone Joint Surg Br 74:105-110, 1992.
16. Berger RA, Nedeff DD, Barden RM, et al: Unicompartmental knee arthroplasty: Clinical experience at 6- to 10-year follow-up. Clin Orthop Relat Res 367:50-60, 1999.
17. Bernasek TL, Rand JA, Bryan RS: Unicompartmental porous coated anatomic TKA. Clin Orthop Relat Res 236:52-59, 1988.
18. Bert JM, Maschka K: The arthroscopic treatment of unicompartmental gonarthrosis: A five-year follow-up study of abrasion arthroplasty plus arthroscopic débridement and arthroscopic débridement alone. Arthroscopy 5:25-32, 1989.
19. Billings A, Scott DF, Camargo MP, Hoffman AA: High tibial osteotomy with a calibrated osteotomy guide, rigid internal fixation, and early motion: Long-term follow-up. J. Bone Joint Surg Am 82:70-79, 2000.
20. Blevins FT, Steadman JR, Rodrigo JJ, Silliman J: Treatment of articular cartilage defects in athletes: An analysis of functional outcome and lesion appearance. Orthopedics 21:761-768, 1998.
21. Bobic V: Arthroscopic osteochondral autograft transplantation in anterior cruciate ligament reconstruction: A preliminary clinical study. Knee Surg Sports Traumatol Arthrosc 3:262-264, 1996.
22. Bonamo JJ, Kessler KJ, Noah J: Arthroscopic meniscectomy in patients over the age of 40. Am J Sports Med 20:422-429, 1992.
23. Bradley JD, Brandt KD, Katz BP, et al: Comparison of an antiinflammatory dose of ibuprofen, an analgesic dose of ibuprofen, and acetaminophen in the treatment of patients with osteoarthritis of the knee. N Engl J Med 325:87-91, 1991.
24. Brandt KD: Should osteoarthritis be treated with nonsteroidal anti-inflammatory drugs? Rheum Dis Clin North Am 19:697-712, 1993.
25. Brittberg M, Lindahl A, Nilsson A, et al: Treatment of deep cartilage defects in the knee with autologous chondrocyte transplantation. N Engl J Med 331:889-895, 1994.
26. Brocklehurst R, Bayliss MT, Maroudas A, et al: The composition of normal and osteoarthritic articular cartilage from human knee joints. With special reference to unicompartmental replacement in osteotomy of the knee. J Bone Joint Surg Am 66:95-106, 1984.
27. Brooks PM, Day RO: Nonsteroidal anti-inflammatory drugs—differences and similarities. N Engl J Med 324:1716-1725, 1991.
28. Broughton NS, Newman JH, Baily RA: Unicompartmental replacement and high tibial osteotomy for osteoarthritis of the knee: A comparative study after 5-10 years' follow-up. J Bone Joint Surg Br 68:447-452, 1986.
29. Buckwalter JA, Einhorn TA, Simon SR: Orthopaedic Basic Science, 2nd ed. Chicago, American Academy of Orthopaedic Surgeons, 2000.
30. Buckwalter JA, Lane NE: Athletics and osteoarthritis. Am J Sports Med 25:873-881, 1997.
31. Buckwalter JA, Mankin HJ: Articular cartilage: Degeneration and osteoarthritis, repair, regeneration, and transplantation. Instr Course Lect 47:487-504, 1998.
32. Buckwalter JA, Mow VC, Ratcliffe A: Restoration of injured or degenerated articular cartilage. J Am Acad Orthop Surg 2:192-201, 1994.
33. Burks RT: Arthroscopy and degenerative arthritis of the knee: A review of the literature. Arthroscopy 6:43-47, 1990.
34. Cameron HU, Botsford DJ, Park YS: Prognostic factors in the outcome of supracondylar femoral osteotomy for lateral compartment osteoarthritis of the knee. Can J Surg 40:114-118, 1997.
35. Campanacci M, Cervellati C, Donati U: Autogenous patella as replacement for a resected femoral or tibial condyle: A report on 19 cases. J Bone Joint Surg Br 67:557-563, 1985.
36. Chesnut WJ: Preoperative diagnostic protocol to predict candidates for unicompartmental arthroplasty. Clin Orthop Relat Res 273:146-150, 1991.
37. Christensen NO: Unicompartmental prosthesis for gonarthrosis: A nine-year series of 575 knees from a Swedish hospital. Clin Orthop Relat Res 273:165-169, 1991.
38. Cole BJ, Harner CD: Degenerative arthritis of the knee in active patients: Evaluation of management. J Am Acad Orthop Surg 7:389-402, 1999.
39. Convery FR, Akeson WH, Amiel D, et al: Long-term survival of chondrocytes in an osteochondral articular cartilage allograft: A case report. J Bone Joint Surg Am 78:1082-1088, 1996.
40. Convery FR, Botte MJ, Akeson WH, Meyers MH: Chondral defects of the knee. Contemp Orthop Relat Res 28:101-107, 1994.
41. Convery FR, Meyers MH, Akeson WH: Fresh osteochondral allografting of the femoral condyle. Clin Orthop Relat Res 273:139-145, 1991.
42. Cooke TD, Scudamore RA, Bryant JT, et al: A quantitative approach to radiography of the lower limb: Principles and applications. J Bone Joint Surg Br 73:715-720, 1991.
43. Coventry MB: Proximal tibial varus osteotomy for osteoarthritis of the lateral compartment of the knee. J Bone Joint Surg Am 69:32-38, 1987.
44. Coventry MB, Ilstrup DM, Wallrichs SL: Proximal tibial osteotomy: A critical long-term study of eighty-seven cases. J Bone Joint Surg Am 75:196-201, 2003.
45. Curl WW, Krome J, Gordon ES, et al: Cartilage injuries: A review of 31,516 knee arthroscopies. Arthroscopy 13:456-460, 1997.
46. Dalury DF, Ewald FC, Christie MJ, Scott RD: Total knee arthroplasty in a group of patients less than 45 years of age. J Arthroplasty 10:598-602, 1995.
47. Daniel DM, Stone ML, Dobson BE, et al: Fate of the ACL-injured patient: A prospective outcome study. Am J Sports Med 22:632-644, 1994.
48. Diduch DR, Insall JN, Scoitt WN, et al: Total knee arthroplasty in young active patients: Long-term follow-up and functional outcome. J Bone Joint Surg Am 79:575-582, 1997.
49. Doherty M, Richards N, Hornby J, Powell R: Relation between synovial fluid C3 degradation products and local joint inflammation

in rheumatoid arthritis, osteoarthritis, and crystal associated arthropathy. Ann Rheum Dis 47:190-197, 1998.

50. Edelson R, Burks RT, Bloebaum RD: Short-term effects of knee washout for osteoarthritis. Am J Sports Med 23:345-349, 1995.

51. Edgerton BC, Mariani EM, Morrey BF: Distal femoral varus osteotomy for painful genu valgus: A five- to 11-year follow-up study. Clin Orthop Relat Res 288:263-269, 1993.

52. Engh GA, McAuley JP: Unicondylar arthroplasty: An option for high-demand patients with gonarthrosis. Instr Course Lect 48:143-148, 1999.

53. Epstein W, Yelin EK, Nevitt K, Kramer JS: Arthritis: A major health problem of the elderly. In Moskowitz RW, Haug MR (eds): Arthritis in the Elderly. New York, Springer, 1986, pp 5-17.

54. Evans RM, Brown E: Managing Osteoarthritis: Diagnosis and Principles of Care. Chicago, American Medical Association, 1998.

55. Felson DT, Anderson JJ, Naimark A, et al: Obesity and knee osteoarthritis: The Framingham Study. Ann Intern Med 109:18-24, 1988.

56. Felson DT, Naimark A, Anderson J, et al: The prevalence of knee osteoarthritis in the elderly: The Framingham Osteoarthritis Study. Arthritis Rheum 30:914-918, 1987.

57. Felson DT, Zhang Y, Anthony JM, et al: Weight loss reduces the risk for symptomatic knee osteoarthritis in women: The Framingham Study. Ann Intern Med 116:535-539, 1992.

58. Finkelstein JA, Gross AE, Davis A: Varus osteotomy of the distal part of the femur: A survivorship analysis. J Bone Joint Surg Am 78:1348-1352, 1996.

59. Flynn JM, Springfield DS, Mankin HJ: Osteoarticular allografts to treat distal femoral osteonecrosis. Clin Orthop Relat Res 303:38-43, 1994.

60. Frizziero L, Pasquali Ronchetti I: Intra-articular treatment of osteoarthritis of the knee: An arthroscopic and clinical comparison between sodium hyaluronate (55-730 kDa) and methylprednisolone acetate. J Orthop Traumatol 3:89-96, 2003.

61. Fujisawa Y, Masuhara K, Shiomi S: The effect of high tibial osteotomy on osteoarthritis of the knee: An arthroscopic study of 54 knee joints. Orthop Clin North Am 10:585-608, 1979.

62. Fulkerson JP: Anteromedialization of the tibial tuberosity for patellofemoral malalignment. Clin Orthop Relat Res 177:176-181, 1983.

63. Fulkerson JP, Kalenak A, Rosenberg TD, et al: Patellofemoral pain. Instr Course Lect 41:57-71, 1992.

64. Garrett JC: Fresh osteochondral allografts for treatment of articular defects in osteochondritis dissecans of the lateral femoral condyle in adults. Clin Orthop Relat Res 303:33-37, 1994.

65. Ghazavi MT, Pritzker KP, Davis AM, Gross AE: Fresh osteochondral allografts for post-traumatic osteochondral defects of the knee. J Bone Joint Surg Br 79:1008-1013, 1997.

66. Gibson JN, White MD, Chapman VM, Strachan RK: Arthroscopic lavage and débridement for osteoarthritis of the knee. J Bone Joint Surg Br 74:534-537, 1992.

67. Gill GS, Chan KC, Mills DM: Five to 8 year follow-up study of cemented total knee arthroplasty for patients 55 years old or younger. J Arthroplasty 12:49-54, 1997.

68. Goodfellow JW, Tibrewal MB, O'Connor JJ: Unicompartmental Oxford meniscal knee arthroplasty. J Arthroplasty 2:1-9, 1987.

69. Grelsamer RP: Unicompartmental osteoarthrosis of the knee. J Bone Joint Surg Am 77:278-292, 1995.

70. Hangody L, Kish G, Karpati Z, et al: Mosaicplasty for the treatment of articular cartilage defects: Application in clinical practice. Orthopedics 21:751-756, 1998.

71. Harilainen A, Sandelin J, Ylinen P, Vahvanen V: Revision of the PCA unicompartmental knee: 52 arthrosis knees followed 2-5 years. Acta Orthop Scand 64:428-430, 1993.

72. Healy WL, Anglen JO, Wasilewski SA, Krackow KA: Distal femoral varus osteotomy. J Bone Joint Surg Am 70:102-109, 1988.

73. Healy WL, Barber TC: The role of osteotomy in the treatment of osteoarthritis of the knee. Am J Knee Surg 3:97-109, 1990.

74. Healy WL, Iorio R, Lemos DW: Medial reconstruction during TKA for severe valgus deformity. Clin Orthop Relat Res 356:161-169, 1998.

75. Healy WL, Riley LH: High tibial valgus osteotomy: A clinical review. Clin Orthop Relat Res 209:227-233, 1986.

76. Hernborg JS, Nilsson BE: The natural course of untreated osteoarthritis of the knee. Clin Orthop Relat Res 123:130-137, 1977.

77. Hernigou P, Medevielle D, Debeyre J, Goutallier D: Proximal tibial osteotomy for osteoarthritis with varus deformity: A ten to thirteen-year follow-up study. J Bone Joint Surg Am 69:332-354, 1987.

78. Hewett TE, Noyes FR, Barber-Westin SD, Heckmann TP: Decrease in knee joint pain and increase in function in patients with medial compartment arthrosis: A prospective analysis of valgus bracing. Orthopedics 21:121-138, 1998.

79. Hochberg MC, Altman RD, Brandt KD, et al: Guidelines for the medical management of osteoarthritis: II. Osteoarthritis of the knee. American College of Rheumatology. Arthritis Rheum 38:1541-1546, 1995.

80. Holden DL, James SL, Larson RL, Slocum DB: Proximal tibial osteotomy in patients who are fifty years old or less: Long-term follow-up study. J Bone Joint Surg Am 70:977-982, 1988.

81. Homminga GN, Bulstra SK, Bouwmeester PS, van der Linden AJ: Perichondral grafting for cartilage lesions of the knee. J Bone Joint Surg Br 72:1003-1007, 1990.

82. Horlick S, Loomer R: Valgus knee bracing for the osteoarthritic knee. Clin J Sports Med 3:251-255, 1993.

83. Howell DS, Treadwell DV, Tripple SB: Idiopathogenesis of osteoarthritis. In Moskowitz RW, Howell DS, Goldberg VM, et al (eds): Osteoarthritis: Diagnosis and Management, 2nd ed. Philadelphia, WB Saunders, 1984, p 129.

84. Hutchison CR, Cho B, Wong N, et al: Proximal valgus tibial osteotomy for osteoarthritis of the knee. Instr Course Lect 48:131-134, 1999.

85. Insall J: The Pridie débridement operation for osteoarthritis of the knee. Clin Orthop Relat Res 101:61-67, 1974.

86. Insall J, Aglietti P: A five to seven-year follow-up of unicondylar arthroplasty. J Bone Joint Surg Am 62:1329-1337, 1980.

87. Insall JN, Joseph DM, Msika C: High tibial osteotomy for varus gonarthrosis: A long-term follow-up study. J Bone Joint Surg Am 66:1040-1048, 1984.

88. Insall JN, Walker PS: Unicondylar knee replacement. Clin Orthop Relat Res 120:83-88, 1976.

89. Iorio R, Healy WL: Unicompartmental arthritis of the knee. J Bone Joint Surg Am 85:1351-1364, 2003.

90. Ivarsson I, Gillquist J: Rehabilitation after high tibial osteotomy and unicompartmental arthroplasty: A comparative study. Clin Orthop Relat Res 266:139-144, 1991.

91. Jackson RW, Rouse DW: The results of partial arthroscopic meniscectomy in patients over 40 years of age. J. Bone Joint Surg Br 64:481-485, 1982.

92. Jacobs JE: Patellar graft for severely depressed comminuted fractures of the lateral tibial condyle. J Bone Joint Surg Am 47:842-847, 1965.

93. Johnson LL: Arthroscopic abrasion arthroplasty historical and pathologic perspective: Present status. Arthroscopy 2:54-69, 1986.

94. Katz MM, Hungerford DS, Krackow KA, Lennox DW: Results of TKA after failed proximal tibial osteotomy for osteoarthritis. J Bone Joint Surg Am 69:225-232, 1987.

95. Keating M, Faris P, Ritter MA, Keane J: Use of lateral heel and sole wedges in the treatment of medial osteoarthritis of the knee. Orthop Rev 921-924, 1993.

96. Keene JS, Dyreby JR Jr: High tibial osteotomy in the treatment of osteoarthritis of the knee: The role of preoperative arthroscopy. J Bone Joint Surg Am 65:36-42, 1983.

97. Kennedy WR, White RP: Unicompartmental arthroplasty of the knee: Postoperative alignment and its influence on overall results. Clin Orthop Relat Res 221:278-285, 1987.

98. Kim HK, Moran ME, Salter RB: The potential for regeneration of articular cartilage in defects created by chondral shaving and subchondral abrasion: An experimental investigation in rabbits. J Bone Joint Surg Am 73:1301-1315, 1991.

99. Knight JL, Atwater RD, Guo J: Early failure of the porous anatomic cemented UKA: Aids to diagnosis and revision. J Arthroplasty 12:11-20, 1997.

100. Komistek RD, Dennis DA, Northcut EJ, et al: An in vivo analysis of the effectiveness of the osteoarthritic knee brace during heel-strike of gait. J Arthroplasty 14:738-742, 1999.

101. Kooijman HJ, Driessen APPM, vanHorn JR: Long-term results of patellofemoral arthroplasty. J Bone Joint Surg Br 85:836-840, 2003.

102. Koshino T, Murase T, Saito T: Medial opening wedge high tibial osteotomy with use of porous hydroxyapatite to treat medial com-

partment osteoarthritis of the knee. J Bone Joint Surg Am 85:78-85, 2003.

103. Kovar PA, Allegrante JP, MacKenzie CT, et al: Supervised fitness walking in patients with osteoarthritis of the knee: A randomized, controlled trial. Ann Intern Med 116:529-534, 1992.

104. Lane JM: Anti-inflammatory medications: Selective cox-2 inhibitors. J Am Acad Orthop Surg 10:75-78, 2002.

105. Laskin RS: Unicompartmental tibiofemoral resurfacing arthroplasty. J Bone Joint Surg Am 60:182-185, 1978.

106. Laurencin CT, Zelicof SB, Scott RD, Ewald FC: Unicompartmental versus TKA in the same patient: A comparative study. Clin Orthop Relat Res 273:151-156, 1991.

107. Leach RE, Baumgard S, Broom J: Obesity: Its relationship to osteoarthritis of the knee. Clin Orthop Relat Res 93:271-273, 1973.

108. Leopold SS, Redd BR, Warme WJ, et al: Corticosteroid compared with hyaluronic acid injections for the treatment of osteoarthritis of the knee: A prospective, randomized trial. J Bone Joint Surg Am 85:1197-1203, 2003.

109. Lohmander LS, Dalen N, Englund G, et al: Intra-articular hyaluranon injections in the treatment of osteoarthritis of the knee: A randomized, double blind, placebo controlled multicentre trial. Hyaluronan Multicentre Trial Group. Ann Rheum Dis 55:424-431, 1996.

110. Lonner JH: Patellofemoral arthroplasty: Pros, cons, and design considerations. Clin Orthop Relat Res 428:158-165, 2004.

111. Lozada CJ, Altaman RD: Recent advances in the management of osteoarthritis. In Kelly AN, Harris ED Jr, Ruddy S, Sledge CB (eds): Textbook of Rheumatology. Philadelphia, WB Saunders, 1998, pp 1-8.

112. Lubinus HH: Patella glide bearing replacement. Orthopaedics 2:119, 1979.

113. Magnuson PB: Technique of débridement of the knee joint for arthritis. Surg Clin North Am 26:249-266, 1946.

114. Magyar G, Ahl TL, Vibe P, et al: Open wedge osteotomy by hemicallostasis of the closing wedge technique for osteoarthritis of the knee. J Bone Joint Surg Br 81:449-551, 1999.

115. Maletius W, Messner K: The effect of partial meniscectomy on the long-term prognosis of knees with localized, severe chondral damage: A twelve- to fifteen-year followup. Am J Sports Med 24:258-262, 1996.

116. Malkani AL, Rand JA, Bryan RS, Wallrichs SL: Total knee arthroplasty with Kinematic condylar prosthesis: A ten-year follow-up study. J Bone Joint Surg Am 77:423-431, 1995.

117. Marmor L: Unicompartmental knee arthroplasty: Ten to thirteen-year follow-up study. Clin Orthop Relat Res 226:14-20, 1988.

118. Marti RK, Verhager RAW, Kerkhoffs GMMJ, Moojen TM: Proximal tibial varus osteotomy: Indications, techniques, and five to twenty-one year results. J Bone Joint Surg Am 83:164-170, 2001.

119. Matsuno H, Kadowaki KM, Tsuji H: Generation II knee bracing for severe medial compartment osteoarthritis of the knee. Arch Phys Med Rehabil 78:745-749, 1997.

120. McAlindon RE, Snow S, Cooper C, et al: Radiographic patterns of osteoarthritis of the knee joint in the community: The importance of the patellofemoral joint. Ann Rheum Dis 51:844-849, 1992.

121. McDermott AG, Finkelstein JA, Farine I, et al: Distal femoral varus osteotomy for valgus deformity of the knee. J Bone Joint Surg Am 70:110-116, 1988.

122. McDermott AG, Langer F, Pritzker KP, Gross AE: Fresh small-fragment osteochondral allografts: Long-term follow-up study on first 100 cases. Clin Orthop Relat Res 197:96-102, 1985.

123. McGinley BJ, Cushner FD, Scott WN: Débridement arthroscopy: 10-year follow-up. Clin Orthop Relat Res 367:190-194, 1999.

124. McLaren AC, Blokker CP, Fowler PJ, et al: Arthroscopic débridement of the knee for osteoarthrosis. Can J Surg 34:595-598, 1991.

125. Meding JB, Keating EM, Ritter MA, Faris PM: Total knee arthroplasty after high tibial osteotomy. Clin Orthop Relat Res 375:175-184, 2000.

126. Merchant AC: Early results with a total patellofemoral joint replacement arthroplasty prosthesis. J Arthroplasty 19:829-836, 2004.

127. Messner K, Maletius W: The long-term prognosis for severe damage to weight-bearing cartilage in the knee: A 14-year clinical and radiographic follow-up in 28 young athletes. Acta Orthop Scand 67:165-168, 1996.

128. Meyers MH, Akeson W, Convery FR: Resurfacing of the knee with fresh osteochondral allograft. J Bone Joint Surg Am 71:704-713, 1989.

129. Minas T: The role of cartilage repair techniques, including chondrocyte transplantation, in focal chondral knee damage. Instr Course Lect 48:629-643, 1999.

130. Minas T, Nehrer S: Current concepts in the treatment of articular cartilage defects. Orthopedics 20:525-538, 1997.

131. Mont MA, Haas S, Mullick T, et al: Total knee arthroplasty for patellofemoral arthritis. J Bone Joint Surg Am 84:1977-1981, 2002.

132. Moseley JB Jr, O'Malley K, Petersen NJ, et al: A controlled trial of arthroscopic surgery for osteoarthritis of the knee. N Engl J Med 347:81-88, 2002.

133. Muller-Fassbender H, Bach GL, Haase W, et al: Glucosamine sulfate compared to ibuprofen in osteoarthritis of the knee. Osteoarthritis Cartilage 2:61-69, 1994.

134. Murray PB, Rand JA: Symptomatic valgus knee: The surgical options. J Am Acad Orthop Surg 1:1-9, 1993.

135. Nagel A, Insall JN, Scuderi GR: Proximal tibial osteotomy: A subjective outcome study. J Bone Joint Surg Am 78:1353-1358, 1996.

136. Naudie D, Bourne RB, Rorabeck CH, Bourne TJ: The Insall Award. Survivorship of the high tibial valgus osteotomy: A 10- to 22-year follow-up study. Clin Orthop Relat Res 367:18-27, 1999.

137. Newman JH, Ackroyd CE, Shah NA: Unicompartmental or total knee replacement? Five-year results of a prospective, randomised trial of 102 osteoarthritic knees with unicompartmental arthritis. J Bone Joint Surg Br 80:862-865, 1998.

138. Noack W, Fischer M, Forster KK, et al: Glucosamine sulfate in osteoarthritis of the knee. Osteoarthritis Cartilage 2:51-59, 1994.

139. Noyes FR, Barber SD, Simon R: High tibial osteotomy and ligament reconstruction in varus angulated, anterior cruciate ligament-deficient knees: A two- to seven-year follow-up study. Am J Sports Med 21:2-12, 1993.

140. Ogilvie-Harris DJ, Fitsialos DP: Arthroscopic management of the degenerative knee. Arthroscopy 7:151-157, 1991.

141. Outerbridge RE: The etiology of chondromalacia patellae. J Bone Joint Surg Br 43:752-757, 1961.

142. Outerbridge HK, Outerbridge AR, Outerbridge RE: The use of a lateral patella autologous graft for the repair of a large osteochondral defect in the knee. J Bone Joint Surg Am 77:65-72, 1995.

143. Palmer SH, Morrison PJ, Ross AC: Early catastrophic tibial component wear after UKA. Clin Orthop Relat Res 350:143-148, 1998.

144. Parvizi J, Hanssen AD, Spangehl MJ: Total knee arthroplasty following proximal tibia osteotomy: Risk factors for failure. J Bone Joint Surg Am 86:474-479, 2004.

145. Pennington DW, Sweinckowski JJ, Lutes WB, Drake GN: Unicompartmental knee arthroplasty in patients sixty years of age or younger. J Bone Joint Surg Am 85:1968-1973, 2003.

146. Phillips MI, Krackow KA: Distal femoral varus osteotomy: Indications and surgical technique. Instr Course Lect 48:125-129, 1999.

147. Pollo FE: Bracing and heel wedging for unicompartmental osteoarthritis of the knee. Am J Knee Surg 11:47-50, 1998.

148. Pollo FE, Otis JC, Backus SI, et al: Reduction of medial compartment loads with valgus bracing of the osteoarthritic knee. Am J Sports Med 30:414-421, 2002.

149. Ranawat CS, Flynn WF Jr, Saddler S, et al: Long-term results of the total condylar knee arthroplasty: A 15-year survivorship study. Clin Orthop Relat Res 286:94-102, 1993.

150. Ranawat CS, Padgett DE, Ohashi Y: Total knee arthroplasty for patients younger than 55 years. Clin Orthop Relat Res 248:27-33, 1989.

151. Rand JA: Role of arthroscopy in osteoarthritis of the knee. Arthroscopy 7:358-363, 1991.

152. Rangger C, Klestil T, Gloetzer W, et al: Osteoarthritis after arthroscopic partial meniscectomy. Am J Sports Med 23:240-244, 1995.

153. Reginster JY, Deroisy R, Rovati LC, et al: Long-term effects of glucosamine sulfate on osteoarthritis progression: A randomized, placebo-controlled clinical trial. Lancet 357:251-256, 2001.

154. Reichelt A, Forster KK, Fischer M, et al: Efficacy and safety of intramuscular glucosamine sulfate in osteoarthritis of the knee: A randomized, placebo-controlled, double blind study. Arzneimittelforschung 44:75-80, 1994.

155. Resnick D, Vint V: The "tunnel" view in assessment of cartilage loss in osteoarthritis of the knee. Radiology 137:547-548, 1980.

156. Riebel GD, Werner FW, Ayers DC, et al: Early failure of the femoral component in UKA. J Arthroplasty 10:615-621, 1995.

157. Ritter MA, Herbst SA, Keating EM, et al: Long-term survival analysis of a posterior cruciate-retaining total condylar TKA. Clin Orthop Relat Res 309:136-145, 1994.

158. Rodrigo JJ, Steadman JR, Silliman JF, Fustone HA: Improvement of full thickness chondral defect healing in the human knee after débridement and microfracture using continuous passive motion. Am J Knee Surg 7:109-116, 1994.

159. Romanowski MR, Repicci JA: Minimally invasive unicondylar arthroplasty: Eight year follow-up. Am J Knee Surg 15:17-22, 2002.

160. Rougraff BT, Heck DA, Gibson AE: A comparison of tricompartmental and unicompartmental arthroplasty for the treatment of gonarthrosis. Clin Orthop Relat Res 273:157-164, 1991.

161. Salisbury RB, Nottage WK, Gardner V: The effect of alignment on results in arthroscopic débridement of the degenerative knee. Clin Orthop Relat Res 198:268-272, 1985.

162. Schai PA, Suh JT, Thornhill TS, Scott RD: Unicompartmental knee arthroplasty in middle-aged patients: A 2- to 6-year follow-up evaluation. J Arthroplasty 13:365-372, 1998.

163. Scott RD, Cobb AG, McQueary FG, Thornhill TS: Unicompartmental knee arthroplasty: Eight- to 12-year follow-up evaluation with survivorship analysis. Clin Orthop Relat Res 271:96-100, 1991.

164. Sharkey PF: The case against arthroscopic débridement of the osteoarthritic knee. Arthroscopy 6:169-170, 1990.

165. Shelton WR, Treacy SH, Dukes AD, Bomboy AL: Use of allografts in knee reconstruction: I. Basic science aspects and current status. J Am Acad Orthop Surg 6:165-168, 1998.

166. Smith AM, Peckett WRC, Butler-Manuel PA, et al: Treatment of patellofemoral arthritis using the Lubinus patellofemoral arthroplasty: A retrospective review. Knee 9:27, 2002.

167. Sprague NF 3rd: Arthroscopic débridement for degenerative knee joint disease. Clin Orthop Relat Res 160:118-123, 1981.

168. Staheli JW, Cass JR, Morrey BF: Condylar TKA after failed proximal tibial osteotomy. J Bone Joint Surg Am 69:28-31, 1987.

169. Stern SH, Bowen MK, Insall JN, Scuderi GR: Cemented TKA for gonarthrosis in patients 55 years old or younger. Clin Orthop Relat Res 260:124-129, 1990.

170. Stern SH, Insall JN: Posterior stabilized prosthesis: Results after follow-up of nine to twelve years. J Bone Joint Surg Am 74:980-986, 1992.

171. Stockelman RE, Pohl KP: The long-term efficacy of unicompartmental arthroplasty of the knee. Clin Orthop Relat Res 271:88-95, 1991.

172. Stuart MJ: Arthroscopic management for degenerative arthritis of the knee. Instr Course Lect 48:135-141, 1999.

173. Stuart MJ, Grace JN, Ilstrup DM, et al: Late recurrence of varus deformity after proximal tibial osteotomy. Clin Orthop Relat Res 260:61-65, 1990.

174. Tauro B, Ackroyd CE, Newman JH, et al: The Lubinus patellofemoral arthroplasty, a five to ten year prospective study. J Bone Joint Surg Br 83:696, 2001.

175. Thornhill TS: Unicompartmental knee arthroplasty. Clin Orthop Relat Res 205:121-131, 1986.

176. Thornhill TS, Scott RD: Unicompartmental TKA. Orthop Clin North Am 20:245-256, 1989.

177. van Saase JL, Vandenbroucke JP, van Romunde LK, Valkenburg HA: Osteoarthritis and obesity in the general population: A relationship calling for an explanation. J Rheumatol 15:1152-1158, 1988.

178. Wang JW, Hsu CC: Distal femoral varus osteotomy for osteoarthritis of the knee. J Bone Joint Surg Am 87:127-133, 2005.

179. Watterson JR, Esdaile JM: Viscosupplementation: Therapeutic mechanisms and clinical potential in osteoarthritis of the knee. J Am Acad Orthop Surg 8:277-284, 2000.

180. Weale AE, Halabi OA, Jones PW, White SH: Perceptions of outcomes after unicompartmental and total knee replacements. Clin Orthop Relat Res 382:143-153, 2001.

181. Weaver JK, Weider D, Derkash RS: Patellofemoral arthritis resulting from malalignment: A long-term evaluation of treatment options. Orthop Rev 20:1075-1081, 1991.

182. Yamashita F, Sakakida K, Suzu F, Takai S: The transplantation of an autogeneic osteochondral fragment for osteochondritis dissecans of the knee. Clin Orthop Relat Res 201:43-50, 1985.

183. Yasuda K, Sasaki T: The mechanics of treatment of the osteoarthritic knee with a wedged insole. Clin Orthop Relat Res 215:162-172, 1987.

CHAPTER 94

Computer-Assisted Knee Surgery: An Overview

Mahmoud A. Hafez • Branislav Jaramaz • Anthony DiGioia III

HISTORY OF COMPUTER-ASSISTED SURGERY

Throughout history, physicians have tried to improve visibility of the inside of the human body to understand the complexity of normal and diseased body structures. Dissection of the human body began several thousand years ago. The next milestone in improving visibility did not occur until the 19th century, when Roentgen discovered the x-ray and introduced plane radiography. Surgeons in different specialties, especially orthopedics, have succeeded in transferring the powerful images of radiography to operating rooms via x-ray fluoroscopy. The advent of the computer and subsequently computed tomography (CT) in late 20th century opened a new horizon of better accuracy and visibility. Surgeons tried to transfer the operating room to the CT scan suite and vice versa to enable image-guided surgery in real time, but their attempts were not successful. The introduction of position-tracking devices made the application of image-guided surgery possible by linking the different steps of imaging, planning, and surgical implementation, even when performed at different times. Although orthopedics is more suited to computer-assisted surgery (CAS), intracranial neurosurgery perhaps has a greater demand for visibility and accuracy, which may explain why CAS initially started in neurosurgery.

Attempts to achieve accurate localization of brain tissue started long before the advent of CT. Clarke and Horseley[15] in 1906 reported a method and an instrument aimed at achieving accurate localization and precise orientation of brain tissue for the purpose of stimulation and electrolysis. This method was based on the principles of stereotaxis. Modern computer-assisted techniques in the form of robotics and navigation started in the 1980s with several neurosurgical applications. The technology was subsequently transferred from neurosurgery to orthopedics in the area of spine[92] and then gradually to hip and knee surgery. Practical application of CAS in orthopedics started in the early 1990s when robotic techniques were used for femoral canal preparation in total hip arthroplasty.[73] The technical development gradually moved from active robotics toward passive navigation systems.[2,26,54,61,70,104] The earliest navigation systems were image based and used CT scans, followed by systems that allowed navigation by intraoperative fluoroscopy or without any previous imaging (image-free). In a development parallel to robotics and navigation, computer-assisted design and manufacturing (CAD/CAM) technology started as early as the late 1970s and resulted in CAD/CAM applications in which CT data were used to produce anatomic models and custom prostheses.[11,31,64] This technology has developed further to a new modality of patient-specific templating using the technique of rapid prototyping.[9,35,80]

DEFINITION OF COMPUTER-ASSISTED SURGERY

The early CAS techniques were focused on tumor location in neurosurgery based on the principles of stereotaxis, which is defined as "the location of bodily structures using a fixed coordinate system." CAS systems in orthopedics have been significantly developed and expanded and gradually became distinguished from CAS applications in other surgical specialties. The term computer-assisted orthopedic surgery (CAOS) is now used by many orthopedic surgeons and engineers who work in this field. At present, the broad-based applications of CAOS extend far beyond the narrow definition of stereotaxis. This enormous expansion, over a relatively short period, has embraced different aspects and modes of surgical practice, such as planning, simulation, guidance, surgical assistance, automation, telesurgery, and training. Therefore, a definition of CAOS must include the application of computer-enabled technology at any stage (preoperative, intraoperative, and postoperative) in the surgical management of orthopedic conditions with the use of various systems (active, semi-active, passive, or hybrid) performed for several applications (planning, simulation, guidance, robotic, telesurgery, and/or training).

THE RATIONALE FOR COMPUTER-ASSISTED ORTHOPEDIC SURGERY IN KNEE SURGERY

The main rationale behind using CAOS techniques in knee surgery is to address limitations of the conventional techniques and also facilitate the use of new and more demanding procedures. There is also an increasingly apparent need to improve training methods to cope with the growing number of difficult procedures, such as less invasive arthroplasty, for example. In addition, objective measures to evaluate surgical performance and outcomes are needed.

It is widely agreed that the success or failure of knee procedures such as total knee arthroplasty (TKA),[29,88] osteotomy,[14,18] and ligament reconstruction[33,102] is dependent on the accuracy and precision of the surgical technique. One might argue that the reported survival rate of TKA is as high as 95% at 15 years,[42,49,85] so why bother about improving these outcomes? In fact, the reported high success rate is questionable for several reasons, such as lack of standardization of outcome measures, use of revision or radiographic measures as endpoints,[66] loss of follow-up,[65] reporting surgeons' views,[37] reporting of small series performed by senior surgeons in specialized centers, and biased literature. The majority of outcome studies did not include kinematic assessment and also relied on short, knee radiographs, which have limited accuracy.[12,45,72] Moreover, this high success rate is related to primary TKA in elderly patients. Relatively higher failure rates of TKA have been reported[22,81,87] in young active patients, revision surgery, and complicated cases.

Surgical techniques require a high degree of accuracy and reproducibility, both preoperatively and intraoperatively. Conventional preoperative planning relies on plane radiographs, which have four main limitations: accuracy of alignment measurements, visualization, accuracy in sizing implants, and accuracy in measuring the orientation of implants (especially rotational alignment). Several authors[43,50,53,56,63] have reported the inaccuracy of plane radiographs in measuring leg alignment. Plane radiographs are sensitive to changes in leg position (rotation and flexion). Ten degrees of knee flexion and 20 degrees of external to 25 degrees of internal rotation can cause statistically significant differences in measurements of knee alignment.[56] Internal rotation of the femur can be perceived as medial bowing and external rotation as lateral bowing, and this effect can be accentuated if the femur already had excessive bowing. Lack of visibility is another limitation. Short knee radiographs do not reveal abnormalities or normal variations of bones and joints away from the knee. Even with complete series and whole-leg radiographs, the images are still two-dimensional (2-D) whereas surgery is performed on three-dimensional (3-D) structures. The ability to correlate between preoperative 2-D radiographic data and intraoperative 3-D anatomy depends on the surgeon's experience. Accurate preoperative planning in revision arthroplasty is essential and should be performed with good-quality imaging that allows identification of bony defects and preparation for their appropriate treatment: bone graft, cement, or metal augmentation. The accuracy of measuring implant sizes is limited and its benefit is questionable. In one report, prediction of implant size from preoperative radiographs was accurate in 57% of cases, and measurement of implant size from postoperative radiographs was accurate in 41% of cases.[40]

Intraoperative surgical performance can also be improved. Most reconstructive procedures around the knee, such as arthroplasty, osteotomy, and ligament reconstruction, are technically demanding. Errors in surgical technique can have adverse effects on function and survival and lead to early failure and poor outcomes. Arthro-

plasty in particular involves several technical steps that are dependent on each other, such as measurement of alignment, bone cutting, soft-tissue balancing, and fixation of the implants to bone. Bone cutting can affect soft-tissue tension, and soft-tissue release can affect bone cutting. Because the knee is a 3-D structure, working in one plane (or one parameter), whether on bone or soft-tissue structures, can affect certain parameters in other planes. Currently, surgeons rely on conventional guides and instruments that have some degree of freedom and require a significant level of personal judgment ("eyeballing"). Several authors[20,71,83,97] have reported the limitations in accuracy of both intramedullary and extramedullary TKA instruments, especially for bone cutting and alignment of implants. Use of alignment guides involves violation of the intramedullary canals and may also lead to a higher risk for bleeding, infection, fat embolism, and fracture. Moreover, there is a current trend toward optimizing kinematics after TKA and reconstruction of the anterior cruciate ligament (ACL), which could be difficult to achieve with conventional techniques.

Intraoperative visualization of the bony and soft-tissue anatomy is another limitation of conventional techniques. The knee has a complex 3-D anatomy and kinematics, so bone cutting and soft-tissue balancing should be done in 3-D fashion. Unforeseen circumstances or errors during surgery require intraoperative measurements and decision making. The accuracy of visual inspection by surgeons is limited, especially when using ill-defined and inconsistent operative landmarks such as the epicondylar axis or the femoral and tibial tunnels for ACL reconstruction. These errors are even greater when dealing with obese patients or those with bone abnormalities. Certain errors such as flexion deformity of the limb or the components are difficult to visually appreciate in the operating room. A 5- to 10-degree flexion deformity of the femoral component in TKA may not be appreciated by the surgeon.[97] The introduction of minimally invasive surgery (MIS) for TKA has prompted some surgeons to draw attention to its reduced intraoperative visibility and consequently its higher risk for errors and complications.[25] Recently, some surgeons have attempted to use arthroscopy as a visualization tool to improve visibility in MIS for unicompartmental arthroplasty (UKA),[82] but this procedure is still at the experimental stage, is technically demanding, and may increase operative time.

Moreover, surgical techniques are becoming more complicated, with the trend toward less invasive and MIS techniques and the introduction of new procedures such as patellofemoral arthroplasty, cartilage repair, and double-bundle ACL reconstruction. In addition, the indications for successful procedures such as TKA have been extended to include complicated cases of postpatellectomy knees, arthrodesis, hemophilia, Charcot joints, young active patients, and failed revision. Conventional techniques may not be able to cope with this increasing demand for accuracy in these new procedures.

CAOS is an enabling technology that has the potential to enhance and improve on conventional techniques. Orthopedics and the knee joint in particular are uniquely suited for CAOS applications. Orthopedics by definition and nature is meant to correct bony abnormalities anatomically (structurally). Correction and reconstruction involve a great deal of preparation (cutting, drilling, reaming, fixation), which requires accurate planning and measurement and precise execution. Bone is a relatively nondeformable structure and is easily imaged in comparison to visceral structures and other soft tissues. Because of this inherent rigidity of bone, its location during surgery can be correlated repeatedly and consistently to a preoperative computer model.[27] The knee joint in particular is a fitting target for CAOS because it is a common site of diseases and injuries and it accommodates the highest number of surgical procedures per single joint, including different soft-tissue procedures for ligaments, menisci, and cartilage and several bony procedures such as osteotomy, arthrodesis, and arthroplasty (total, unicompartmental, and patellofemoral). Some of these techniques could be performed arthroscopically or by newer less invasive and minimally invasive techniques. The knee has the most complex anatomy and biomechanics, and procedures on it require a high degree of accuracy and reproducibility. Restoring normal function of the knee joint is difficult because of the complex kinematics and the interactions between bone, articular surfaces, ligaments, tendons, and other soft-tissue structures.

CAOS has several potential advantages. It permits accurate preoperative planning of surgery that can be transformed into precise surgical implementation. It allows interaction between computer capabilities and surgeons' expertise in the hope that when combined together, the performance of any surgical task can be improved. In TKA, CAOS can eliminate the use of alignment guides and intramedullary perforation and may decrease blood loss.[12] CAOS allows accurate intraoperative measurement of alignment, range of motion, and stability and permits one to relate postoperative follow-up to surgical techniques, thereby enhancing documentation and research. In addition, it can provide an inexpensive, readily available tool for training. CAOS can also improve the visibility and accuracy of MIS techniques and may allow the introduction of new techniques that were not possible in the past. Furthermore, CAOS has the potential to continuously improve the surgical process by closing the loop in surgical practice: linking preoperative planning to intraoperative performance and surgeons' performance to postoperative outcome.[24] However, as with any new technology or approaches, there can also be challenges and changes in practice, which will be discussed later in the chapter.

CLASSIFICATION AND CHARACTERISTICS OF COMPUTER-ASSISTED ORTHOPEDIC SURGERY SYSTEMS

A simple and clinically based classification system for CAOS was presented by Picard et al.[77] They classified CAOS into active, semi-active, or passive systems and by the imaging requirements: image-free and preoperative or intraoperative image-based, thus creating a 3×3 classification matrix (Table 94–1). The technical differences between the currently available CAOS systems are summarized in Table 94–2 and discussed later in this chapter.

Active Systems

Active robotic systems have the capability of performing a part or all of the bone preparation steps (drilling, cutting) autonomously, but under the surgeon's supervision and control. A computer monitor displays in real time the 3-D pictures of the surgical performance. These robotic systems require preoperative imaging (typically CT scans) and intraoperative registration to establish a relationship between the preoperative images and intraoperative anatomy. Rigid fixation of the robot and the knee to the operating table is always required, and some systems require tracking to control for any micromotion of the leg during robotic surgery. Robotic systems are bulky and interrupt the normal flow of the surgical procedure. Registration and other technical issues will be discussed in detail later in this chapter. The first clinically used orthopedic robot was ROBODOC, which was initially used for total hip arthroplasty[73] and then adapted for TKA.[7] CASPAR[19,90] and ACROBOT[16,44] are other orthopedic robotic systems that were initially used for TKA. There are new image-free robotic systems that are still in the developmental stage.

Semiactive Systems

Semi-active robotic systems do not autonomously perform the surgical task. Control here is shared between the surgeon and the robot. Consequently, the actions are performed by surgeons and guided or restricted by the system. A computer monitor displays in real time the 3-D

Table 94–1. Classification of Computer-Assisted Orthopedic Surgery Systems

	PREOPERATIVE IMAGE	INTRAOPERATIVE IMAGE	IMAGE-FREE
Active	Available[1]	Not available	In development[5]
Semi-active	Available[2]	Not available	In development[6]
Passive	Available[3]	Available[4]	Available[7]

Examples: 1, active robots; 2, active constrained robots; 3, computed tomography–based navigation and templating systems; 4, fluoroscopically based navigation systems; 5, bone-attached robots; 6, hand-held robots; 7, image-free navigation systems.

Table 94–2. Comparison between the Currently Available Computer-Assisted Orthopedic Surgery Systems

| | | NAVIGATION | | | PATIENT-SPECIFIC TEMPLATES |
| | | Imaged Based | | Image-Free | |
	ROBOTICS	CT	Fluoroscopy		
Data source or imaging	Preoperative CT	Preoperative CT	Intraoperative x-ray	Intraoperative collection of kinematic and morphological data	Preoperative CT
Planning	Preoperative 3-D	Preoperative 3-D	No preoperative planning but intraoperative 2-D assessment		Preoperative 3-D
Spatial arrangement in OR	Robot, leg holder, and clamps	Navigation cart, tracking devices			None
Registration and tracking	Registration ± tracking	Both required	Tracking		Not required
Intraoperative measurement and adjustment of planning	No	Yes			No

CT, computed tomography; 2-D, two-dimensional; 3-D, three dimensional; OR, operating room.

pictures of the surgical actions. Like active robotic systems, semi-active systems typically require imaging and intraoperative registration. Although the ACROBOT of Davies et al[16,44] is considered to be an active robotic system when it is in autonomous mode, it can be an example of a semi-active robotic system when it is in hands-on mode. It applies the principle of "active constraint" in which it allows the surgeon to move the robotic end effector (mill or cutter), but it restricts the surgeon's movement when it goes beyond the preplanned limits. Certain new designs under development combine some features of robotic and navigation systems (hybrid systems) and may come under the category of semi-active.[8,79,84,103]

Passive (Navigation) Systems

Currently two types of passive systems are available: the commonly used "navigation" and the "patient-specific templating" systems. These systems do not perform the surgical action by themselves and allow surgeons to have full control. Their main role is to provide information and/or guidance during the procedure. From a control and safety point of view, passive systems are generally more acceptable by the Food and Drug Administration than active robotics are.

Navigation systems (Fig. 94–1) are by far the most common CAOS system in current use. They are further classified into image based with the use of preoperative CT or intraoperative fluoroscopy, or image free with reliance on intraoperative collection of data by the surgeon. CT-based navigation systems can provide full functionality, but they require preoperative CT scans (Fig. 94–2). Fluoroscopic navigation systems (Fig. 94–3) are amenable to procedures that already use fluoroscopy, as is the case in trauma surgery, but not for procedures in which fluoroscopy is not routinely required, such as TKA. Image-

free navigation systems (Figs. 94–4 and 94–5) provide the opportunity to navigate without previous imaging. However, overall accuracy depends on the intraoperative data collection (see the later section "What Are the Potential Errors and Pitfalls?"). All forms of navigation systems require intraoperative tracking (Table 94–3) and registration to the patient's anatomy (see "Technical Considerations"). Image-based navigation can allow some limited preoperative or intraoperative planning and surgical simulation. Image-free navigation systems lack the 3-D patient-specific anatomic data and rely on a generic model of bone that is represented by the key anatomic landmarks of average bone geometry. Some recent implementations augment this information, with models based on statisti-

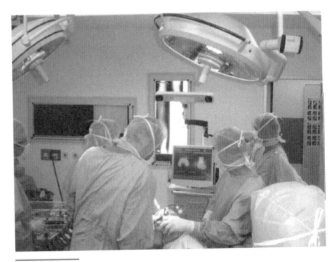

Figure 94–1. The use of a navigation system in total knee arthroplasty. Typical navigation arrangement in the operating room. (From Stiehl JB, Konermann WH, Haaker RG [eds]: Navigation and Robotics in Total Joint and Spine Surgery. Berlin, Springer, 2004.)

Figure 94–2. Total knee arthroplasty by a computed tomography–based navigation system. It offers the opportunity for preoperative planning, which is useful in the case of severe bone loss. Orientation of the implant and the need for bony or metal augmentation can be accurately planned. (From Stiehl JB, Konermann WH, Haaker RG [eds]: Navigation and Robotics in Total Joint and Spine Surgery. Berlin, Springer, 2004.)

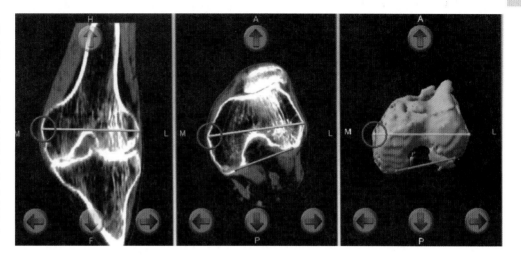

cal data (bone morphing). All navigation systems share the capability of providing valuable intraoperative information with feedback and assessment of performance in real time. They have the potential to improve the accuracy and reproducibility of surgery and reduce the number of outliers. These systems may eliminate the use of intramedullary guides in TKA and can potentially reduce blood loss and the need for blood transfusion.[12] In a reduced capability, navigation systems can be used merely as a planning platform at the preoperative stage or as a measurement tool at the intraoperative stage. Stulberg[97] also used an image-free navigation system as a measurement tool to assess the accuracy of conventional instrumentation. Navigation systems can provide complete

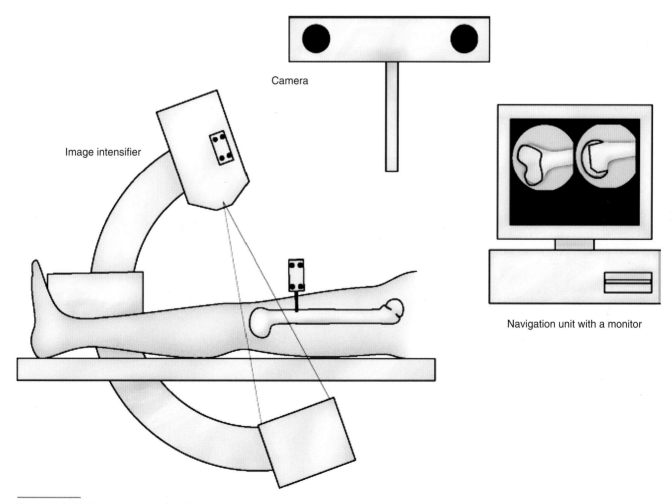

Figure 94–3. Components of a fluoroscopy-based navigation system.

SYSTEM COMPONENTS

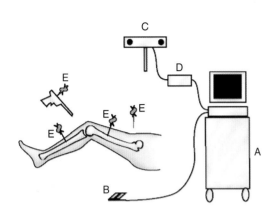

A – Surgical navigation station; B – foot pedal (input device);
C – position tracker (localizer); D – localizer interface unit;
E – tracking markers

LANDMARK LOCALIZATION

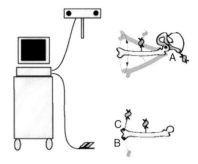

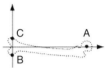

The landmark points are defined either by the analysis of
joint kinematics (A) or directly with a tracked point probe (B, C).

Such defined landmark points are then used to define the
anatomic reference system.

Figure 94–4. Schematic representation of tracking and registration for an image-free navigation system.

documentation of the surgical procedure, which can be used for outcome analysis and research purposes. As training tools, navigation systems can provide instantaneous feedback to surgeons while teaching and identifying errors or weaknesses as they occur.

The *patient-specific templating technique* (Fig. 94–6) using rapid prototyping technology is another passive modality of CAOS but currently has limited application. This technique provides 3-D patient-specific templates based on preoperative planning. The planning is typically based on CT and involves the design of templates that uniquely match the surface geometry of individual bony structures. Computer-assisted template designs are then transferred to physical templates with the use of rapid prototyping machines. Rapid prototyping refers to a class of technologies that can automatically con-

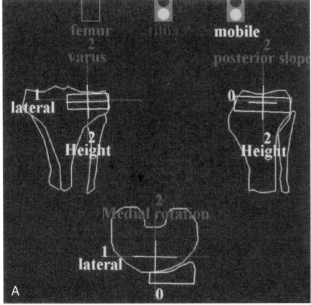

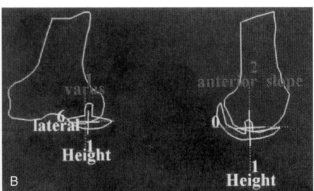

Figure 94–5. Unicompartmental knee arthroplasty by an image-free navigation system. Intraoperative information is displayed about tibial (**A**) and femoral (**B**) implant orientation. (From Stiehl JB, Konermann WH, Haaker RG [eds]: Navigation and Robotics in Total Joint and Spine Surgery. Berlin, Springer, 2004.)

Table 94–3. Types of Tracking Devices

	SENSORS	ADVANTAGES	DISADVANTAGES
Active optical	Infrared light–emitting diodes	Very accurate and fast	Direct line of sight is needed; wires or batteries are needed
Passive optical	Reflective markers	No wires or batteries	Direct line of sight is needed, possibly less accurate and not as fast
Electromagnetic	Magnetic sensors	Line of sight not needed, less invasive	Sensitive to ferromagnetic items and other electromechanical tools such as battery-operated devices. Possibly less accurate and less fast

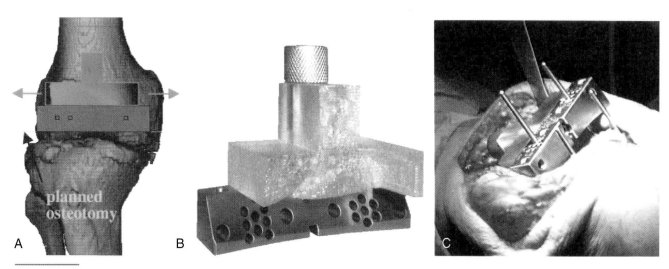

Figure 94–6. Templating technique for total knee arthroplasty: virtual model (**A**), physical template attached to a conventional femoral cutting block (**B**), and an intraoperative image with the template and cutting block attached to the bone (**C**). ((From Stiehl JB, Konermann WH, Haaker RG [eds]: Navigation and Robotics in Total Joint and Spine Surgery. Berlin, Springer, 2004.)

struct a physical model from CAD data and act as a 3-D printer. Rapid prototyping machines join together liquid, powder, or sheet material to form complex 3-D models.

The clinical application of rapid prototyping in surgery is still in its infancy.[60] The majority of clinical reports come from dentistry and maxillofacial surgery.[39] At present, clinical orthopedic applications of this technique are limited in number and confined to the production of models and guides.[9,30,80] Radermacher et al[80] pioneered the introduction of this technique in orthopedics and used it in spine, pelvis, and knee surgery. Brown et al[9] have used this technique exclusively in trauma and reported the results of 117 cases. Recently, a new generation of templating techniques was developed[13,35] in which the templates serve as instruments and can completely replace conventional instrumentation for TKA (see "Future Directions"). The terminology of this technique is not well established. The term "rapid prototyping" is generally used when the technique is applied solely to the production of anatomic models of CT images without preoperative planning, whereas the term "templating" is used when there is surgical planning. The term "individual" or "custom" is a variation of the term "patient specific." Patient-specific templating techniques differ from navigation and robotics in that they confine computer-assisted work to the preoperative stage and require no intraoperative setup, additional space in the operating room, tracking, or registration. Therefore, they may be more user-friendly to surgeons who do not accept the presence of CAOS systems in the operating room. The main criticisms of this approach are preoperative preparation of the templates, the use of CT scanning (cost and radiation), and most important, inability of the surgeon to make intraoperative adjustments to the preoperative plan.

TECHNICAL CONSIDERATIONS

Surgical Technique (Technical Steps)

Robotic and navigation systems can initially appear to be relatively complex tools, especially to novices. However, surgeons need to look at these new technologies as tools. Surgeons must understand the different components of the systems—both hardware and software. The technical steps are variable and depend on the system used and the type of procedure. However, four important steps are common to all types of navigation and robotic systems (modified from DiGioia[23]).

1. Data (image) acquisition and planning can be either preoperative, as in CT-based robotic and navigation systems, or intraoperative, as in image-free or fluoroscopy-based navigation systems. For CT-based approaches, the CT scan protocols usually involve scanning with 1 mm between slices in critical areas (around the knee, hip, and ankle joints) and 5- to 10-mm slices in noncritical areas (femoral and tibial shafts). The CT images are segmented to isolate bone from soft tissues and reconstruct a 3-D model of bone. The planner includes the CAD files of the implant geometries. The surgeon can plan the procedure, simulate the surgery, and evaluate the outcome. The plan can be modified, and once a satisfactory result is achieved, the final plan is stored in the system. The intraoperative planning in image-free navigation systems is not as detailed as preoperative planning because of the intraoperative time constraint and the lack of detailed 3-D patient-specific data. These systems typically have a default plan (based on standard techniques) that could be modified by the surgeon. For fluoroscopy-based navigation, the fluoroscopic images are obtained in the operating room, and then the surgeon plans the surgical act, for example, identifying the trajectory for insertion of the fixation screws while the navigation system displays the images in real time.

2. Registration (see Fig. 94–4) may be a foreign term to surgeons, but in fact it is a process that is routinely done by surgeons during surgical interventions when they relate the radiographic images to the patient's anatomy in the surgical field. It was first used for CT-based systems to relate the preoperative images to the patient's anatomy on the operating table. There are different registration techniques based on the variation in data acquisition and imaging for various CAOS systems. For image-based navigation, surface registration is the gold standard whereby the surgeon collects a cloud of points by touching the bone surfaces with a tracked probe. The unique shape of the bone is then matched with the preoperative image and planning to the position of the patient on the operating table. In fluoroscopy-based navigation, the registration process is automatic, as long as the bone is tracked when the images are obtained. In a more general sense, registration in image-free navigation would mean relating the patient's anatomy to generic models of the femur or tibia. For instance, the system prompts the surgeon to visually select bony landmarks on the patient or to collect centers of rotation of the joints through kinematic testing, and then these data will be related to the generic models of bone that are stored in the system.

3. Tracking (see Fig. 94–3) means real-time updates about the position and orientation of the bone and instruments (guides, jigs, saw, etc.) and their movement. There are different types of tracking devices, and their pros and cons are listed in Table 94–3. Currently used tracking devices are of the optical (active and passive) variety. Electromagnetic tracking is still at the experimental stage, but there is enthusiasm to use it clinically because it requires no tracking camera or line of sight (explained in more details later under "Future Directions"). The components of optical tracking are the tracking camera and trackers (beacons), which need to be attached to instruments or guides and also to the bone. Trackers require rigid fixation to bone (tibia and femur) through pins or clamps (hence the term *rigid bodies*). In TKA, they are usually inserted percutaneously about a handbreadth from the knee joint or can be inserted through the wound. The tracking process relies on rigid fixation of the trackers, and if they move, the registration process has to be repeated. The concepts of registration and tracking are similar to the principles of the global positioning system (GPS) that we use in our cars.

4. Intraoperative measurement and feedback (Fig. 94–7) to the surgeon are displayed in real time on a computer monitor. There is typically continuous reporting and tracking of the position and movement of bone and instruments. This also includes correlation with the preplanned strategy. For instance, in TKA, the system allows the surgeon to measure alignment, rotation, and the level of bone resection before the actual bone cutting by attaching tracking probes to the conventional cutting blocks; these measurements are then correlated with the preplanned strategy. Some systems can guide the surgeons during soft-tissue balancing by providing data on valgus-varus and flexion-extension positions, as well as the gap balance in flexion and extension.

Accuracy Validation and Standardization of Computer-Assisted Orthopedic Surgery

Like any other medical device or instrument, CAOS systems carry the risk of errors and they need to be validated. The increasing use of navigation systems, the introduction of new approaches and technology, and the current enthusiasm to use CAOS tools in minimally invasive techniques are additional reasons for standardization and validation of such systems. This will also enable surgeons to evaluate the performance, suitability, and differences between systems.

Extensive testing and validation of accuracy should be done before the introduction of any new computer-assisted system. Manufacturers usually conduct laboratory testing and possibly clinical trials for their systems before they obtain the necessary approval for marketing and wide clinical use. However, deeper and probably more objective validation and assessment of accuracy are required. To our knowledge, no standard minimum accuracy requirements for CAOS systems have yet been developed. There is also no standard methodology for validating such systems. Mor et al[62] described a methodology for testing the accuracy of an image-guided system that could be generalized and used for other CAOS systems. They divided the validation process into two categories: overall (end-to-end) evaluation and subsystem (step-to-step) evaluation. Both categories are important, but overall evaluation is of more importance to surgeons because they are more concerned

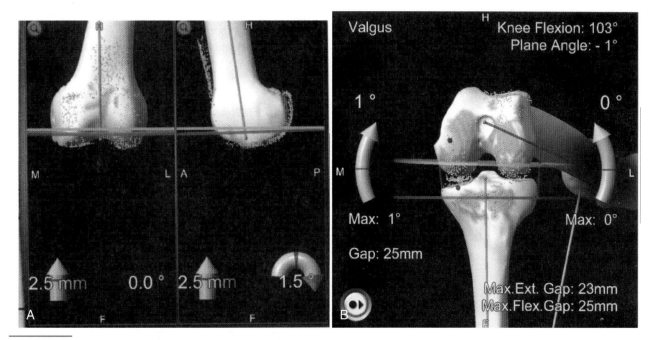

Figure 94–7. Intraoperative measurements and feedback by a navigation system for total knee arthroplasty. **A,** Intraoperative navigation screen shot with measurement of the distal femoral cut. **B,** Intraoperative navigation screen shot with measurement of soft-tissue balance in flexion at real time. (From Stiehl JB, Konermann WH, Haaker RG [eds]: Navigation and Robotics in Total Joint and Spine Surgery. Berlin, Springer, 2004.)

about the final surgical outcome, whereas manufacturers and researchers would be more interested in identifying and rectifying errors arising from individual components of a system.

OVERALL SYSTEM ACCURACY

This evaluation addresses the end result of the procedure. Therefore, it is the summative accuracy of all technical steps, including surgeons' performance. This type of evaluation may not identify the source of errors and may overlook certain errors. For example, the overall evaluation may show accurate alignment of the knee, but in fact this alignment could be the result of a combination of equal and contrasting errors such as a valgus femoral cut and a varus tibial cut. Overall system accuracy should be both laboratory and clinically based. Bench top laboratory testing represents the best-case scenario for the accuracy of the system since testing conditions can be optimized, within reason. Clinical testing is more representative of real-life circumstances, and randomized controlled trials should be considered whenever possible, including comparative trials against conventional techniques and comparative trials between different systems. Some authors have also questioned the accuracy of plane radiographs and their use in measuring alignment and have suggested that more accurate methods, such as CT-based techniques, be used to evaluate CAOS systems.[12,72] Additional surgical outcomes, such as complications traceable to the CAOS systems and operative time, should also be addressed to present a complete clinical picture to the practicing surgeon.

SUBSYSTEM ACCURACY

This evaluation addresses the performance of each individual component of a CAOS system in a laboratory environment (i.e., trackers, registration, imaging, surgeon) and describes the error distribution generated by that particular component. Examples of subsystems might include the tracking system, kinematic and morphological data collection, and/or registration. Subsystem results can also be combined statistically to calculate expected outcomes of the overall system or combinations of different subsystems.

Currently, there are no standard minimal clinical accuracy requirements for CAOS systems. Each surgical procedure has its own accuracy requirement. For example, surgeons may accept a coronal alignment for TKA within 3 degrees of error but may require a smaller margin of error (1 mm and 1 degree) for pedicle screw insertion and accept a higher degree of error for version and abduction of acetabular cup position (5 and 10 degrees). It is important to note that these accuracy requirements are likely to change when CAOS systems become standard practice and allow more accurate surgical performance, possibly within an error of 1 mm and 1 degree.

What Are the Potential Errors and Pitfalls?

Errors could be "inherent" to the system or "operator dependent" and caused by human-machine interactions. Errors can occur at any step of the procedure: imaging, planning, data collection and landmark identification, tracking, registration, and surgical performance.

IMAGING

Surgeons are aware of the higher accuracy and the 3-D capabilities of CT images versus plane radiography. Some surgeons, including the authors, believe that CT-based navigation is the gold standard as far as accuracy and functionality are concerned. Fluoroscopic images are 2-D and may have limited accuracy in the localization of anatomic landmarks. Surgeons have to identify the landmarks on the two images (anteroposterior and lateral). Errors in identifying landmarks, such as the posterior condyles or epicondylar eminences, will lead to errors in navigation. Another source of error from fluoroscopy-based navigation is that surgeons may have the impression that they are navigating directly on patients' anatomy but in fact are navigating on the 2-D images collected during surgery. Therefore, the risk is that the 2-D images may not accurately reflect the true 3-D anatomy and thus lead to navigational errors.

DATA COLLECTION

Image-free navigation relies on collecting kinematic and/or morphological data as a substitute for the imaging data. Surgeons must remember that navigation systems cannot determine whether the collected (input) data are correct or incorrect; consequently, errors during data collection (operator-dependent errors) will result in inaccurate navigational information provided to the surgeon. This shortcoming may lead to false reassurance and/or inappropriate decision making by surgeons based on the information given by the system. This scenario can be summarized as "error in, error out," commonly referred to as "garbage in, garbage out," which can occur on any medical device. Some authors have reported the low reproducibility of identifying the epicondylar axis during TKA surgery.[46] Errors may occur during component sizing, and it has been reported that navigation systems tend to oversize the femoral component.[59] Other examples of issues in TKA have included setting tibial rotation, posterior slope, and notching of the anterior femoral cortex when navigating in the sagittal plane.

TRACKING

Table 94–3 outlines the different tracking devises and their pros and cons. Current tracking devices require rigid fixation with pins, clamps, or metallic anchors to the bone. In osteoporotic bone, the pins can easily get loose and result in navigation errors in tracking and registration. Optical tracking techniques require line of sight between the camera and the tracked object and can be affected by operating rooms lights. Electromagnetic systems do not require line of sight, but their accuracy is affected by the presence of ferromagnetic metallic objects. Several authors[55,106] have investigated sources of error in different tracking systems and ways to improve accuracy.

REGISTRATION

To understand the pitfalls and identify possible errors, it is important for surgeons to know the theory and practice of registration. Occasionally, CAOS systems may fail to register, and in this case the surgeon needs to collect new data, which is easily recognizable. Registration may occur but be inaccurate, so it is important to validate and recheck the registration throughout the surgery. However, more worrisome are errors that may occur as a result of pin movement or inaccurate collection of anatomic landmarks. There is also a learning curve with this process. Several authors[1,3,100] have looked at different methods of registration and analyzed the sources of error and ways to avoid them. Surgeons familiar with navigation techniques have reported that it could take up to 10 procedures to perform reliable registration in TKA.[99]

ERRORS DURING SURGICAL PERFORMANCE

Some surgical actions such as bone cutting and drilling are not usually navigated. Errors may occur during these steps, and neither the system nor the surgeon is aware of them. Plaskos et al[78] conducted a study to identify the errors generated by bone cutting during TKA. They tracked the position of the saw guide before and after the cut was performed and the final orientation of the cut plane on the tibia or femur. They determined that bone cutting can be a significant source of error for alignment of the knee implant and that guide movement during cutting increases other contributions to bone-cutting errors. They therefore conclude that bone-cutting errors may be a factor in some of the poor results reported for computer-assisted TKA. Deflection of the saw blade and poorly fitting guides can be another source of error. Other factors that may influence the accuracy of bone cutting are surgeons' experience and the use of slotted cutting guides.[78]

CLINICAL APPLICATIONS

The clinical application of CAS in orthopedics was relatively late in comparison to the early adoption rates in neurosurgery. Nevertheless, this delay has now been compensated by the ever-growing number of applications and the variety of approaches of CAOS. The application of many CAOS techniques has moved from the bench top study laboratory phase to clinical use. Some techniques are now routinely used in many centers in Europe, North America, Japan, and Australia. By far, navigation techniques are the most commonly used modality of CAOS.

Indications

There is a consensus that proper patient selection in arthroplasty, osteotomy, and ligament reconstruction is an important factor for a successful outcome. The same basic principle must also always be applied to the use of CAOS in these conditions. Although some surgeons use CAOS routinely, it is still too early to consider CAOS a standard technique in knee surgery. Current CAOS systems involve longer operative times and introduce new equipment to the operating room. Although image-free navigation for knee surgery has led the way in the early adoption of this technology, it may not be suitable for all MIS approaches or obese patients because in these cases, identification of landmarks or point collection may not be accurate. Patients with severe osteoporosis may not be suitable because it is difficult to achieve rigid fixation of tracking pins in soft bones. The indications for using CAOS techniques have to be considered, along with the limitations and drawbacks, as discussed later.

Procedures

ARTHROPLASTY (TOTAL KNEE AND UNICOMPARTMENTAL)

TKA is currently the most common procedure performed with the use of navigation techniques[51] (see Figs. 94–1, 94–2, and 94–7). Several clinical studies[3,4,12,67,75,91,94,102,105] were published in the last few years; some were randomized trials comparing navigation systems with conventional techniques. Chauhan et al[12] conducted a randomized controlled trial involving 70 patients in which image-free navigation was compared with conventional techniques. Their assessment was based on postoperative CT scanning, and they reported statistically significant ($p < 0.05$) improvement in alignment of components with CAS techniques. Improvement was noted in femoral varus/valgus angulation, femoral rotation, tibial varus/valgus angulation, tibial posterior slope, tibial rotation, and femorotibial mismatch. They also reported a reduced need for blood transfusion in the navigation arm of the study. In a clinical study of 109 TKA procedures, Amiot and Poulin[3] found that 96% of implants were installed with a hip-knee-ankle angle of 180 ± 3 degrees. Victor and Hoste[105] in a randomized controlled trial of 100 patients showed that image-based navigation resulted in lower variability in coronal alignment. Stockl et al[94] in a randomized controlled trial of 64 TKA procedures reported that the navigation technique improved the accuracy of alignment, rotation, and flexion. Perlick et al[75] compared CT-based navigation with conventional technique in 100 patients and showed that alignment was within 3 degrees in 46 of 50 TKAs by the navigation system versus only 36 of 50 by the conventional technique. Stulberg used an image-free navigation system as a measurement tool to assess the accuracy of conventional instrumentation

and found that only 20% of conventional TKAs had all the measured steps within 3 degrees of the optimal position.

Sikorski[91] reported the results of using CT-based navigation in performing allograft-augmented revision TKA in 14 patients. The position of the implants was monitored by the computer system and adjusted while the cement was setting. He reported errors in femoral rotation and a mismatch between the femoral and tibial components. However, the author concluded that the final alignments were comparable in accuracy with those after primary TKA and the results are promising.

In a comparative clinical trial of image-based versus image-free navigation, Bathis et al[4] performed 130 TKAs and used long-leg coronal and lateral radiographs to determine postoperative leg alignment and component orientation. Sixty of 65 patients in the CT-based group and 63 of 65 in the CT-free group had a postoperative leg axis between 3 degrees of varus and valgus. No significant differences were found for varus/valgus orientation of the femoral and tibial components.

Application of navigation techniques in UKA is less popular than in TKA, but the published reports showed favorable results. Jenny et al[47] used an image-free navigation system in 30 cases of medial UKA and compared their results with a matched 30 cases performed by the conventional technique. The navigated group showed better results in frontal mechanical femorotibial angle, frontal and sagittal orientation of the femoral and tibial components, and the height of the joint space. Cossey et al[17] compared 15 conventional UKA procedures with 15 navigated UKA procedures; the latter resulted in more accurate and reproducible limb alignment.

Templating or rapid prototyping techniques were also used clinically in TKA. Fortheine et al[30] reported the clinical application of templating techniques in 10 TKAs. The designed templates were used as guides to align the conventional cutting blocks. Although they dispensed with the intramedullary alignment guides, the templates did not replace the rest of the conventional instruments (see Fig. 94–6).

Several authors have reported encouraging results in their first experience with robotic TKA. Siebert et al[90] reported the first clinical trial using an active robotic system (CASPAR) in 70 primary TKAs and showed the accuracy of alignment to be within 1 degree. Decking et al[19] used the same system in 13 patients and showed alignment accuracy to be within 1.2 degrees (Fig. 94–8). Borner et al[7] reported the clinical use of another active robotic system (ROBODOC) in TKA and stated that 500 procedure were performed from March 2000 to January 2002 with an average operative time of 90 to 100 minutes (Fig. 94–9). Jakopec et al[44] reported alignment accuracy of 1 mm while using an active-constraint robot (ACROBOT) for TKA. Cobb et al[16] reported the results of 6 UKAs performed with the same system; postoperative CT showed accuracy to be within 2 degrees and 2 mm (Fig. 94–10). Some hybrid systems that combine both navigation and robotic systems have been specifically designed and used for soft-tissue balancing during TKA.[84]

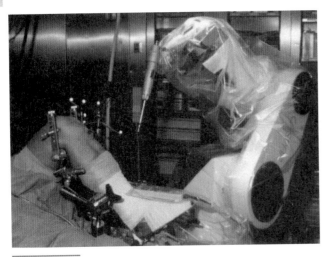

Figure 94–8. Using an active robotic system in knee surgery. The robotic arm moves with 6 degrees of freedom. It is sterilely draped and equipped with a high-speed milling tool. Relative motion between the robot and the knee joint is minimized. (From Stiehl JB, Konermann WH, Haaker RG [eds]: Navigation and Robotics in Total Joint and Spine Surgery. Berlin, Springer, 2004.)

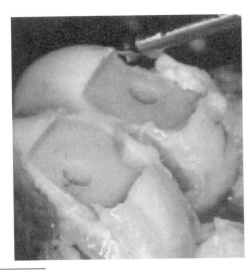

Figure 94–9. Robotic milling tool, another active robotic system for cutting the distal end of the femur. (From Stiehl JB, Konermann WH, Haaker RG [eds]: Navigation and Robotics in Total Joint and Spine Surgery. Berlin, Springer, 2004.)

SOFT-TISSUE PROCEDURES: LIGAMENT RECONSTRUCTION

CAOS systems provide a powerful tool to complement arthroscopic techniques in knee surgery. Arthroscopy can visualize soft tissues inside the joint cavity but not bony structures. Surgeons generally use fluoroscopy for image guidance during arthroscopic posterior cruciate ligament reconstruction. CAOS can potentially replace fluoroscopy and reduce the risk of radiation exposure. Accuracy, intraoperative feedback, and documentation are other advantages of CAOS. CAOS has been used in an attempt to

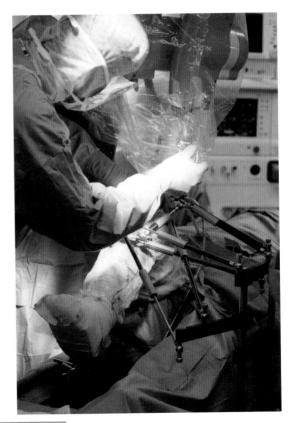

Figure 94–10. Active-constraint robot in clinical use for knee surgery. The surgeon is holding the robotic end (cutter). (Courtesy of Professor B. Davies, Imperial College, London.)

improve the accuracy of ACL reconstruction, especially placement of the femoral and tibial tunnels. Several authors have reported accurate results with the use of experimental computer-assisted ACL reconstruction.[10,86] Eichhorn[28] described the surgical techniques for clinical use of an image-free navigation system for ACL reconstruction (Fig. 94–11). Authors are just now reporting their first clinical trials with different navigation systems for ACL reconstruction. De Rycke[21] conducted a feasibility study in which a navigation system was used in 91 ACL reconstructions. The system requires digitized radiographs of the knee in two planes. It was feasible to perform the navigated surgery in a regional hospital, but the author reported a long learning curve and 10 minutes added operative time. Wiese et al[107] reported the clinical results of a multicenter study involving the use of a navigation system in 100 ACL reconstructions with a patellar tendon graft. The additional operating time was 15 minutes, but with no added complications when compared with conventional techniques. Although the early clinical results were comparable, the navigated group demonstrated more accurate and reproducible positioning of the graft as measured on radiographs. The authors considered the technique to be practical, with the potential to be accepted as routine practice.

Gotzen et al[32] used a robotic system (CASPAR) in 43 ACL reconstructions with a historical control consisting of 151 conventional procedures. The robotic system failed

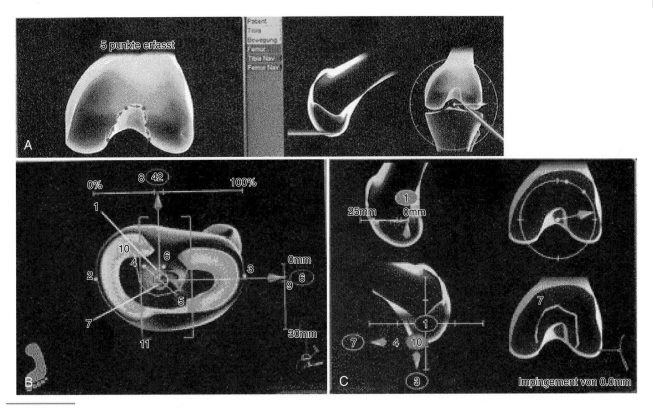

Figure 94–11. Anterior cruciate ligament reconstruction with an image-free navigation system. **A,** Acquisition of data from the femoral notch. **B,** Tibial navigation screen. **C,** Femoral navigation screen. (From Stiehl JB, Konermann WH, Haaker RG [eds]: Navigation and Robotics in Total Joint and Spine Surgery. Berlin, Springer, 2004.)

to provide better clinical results in spite of the accurate planning. The authors stopped the trial because the cost and complexity had overcome the benefits. Although there is a demand for accuracy and reproducibility in ACL reconstruction, CAOS applications have not yet been popularized. In our view, the main obstacles are the invasiveness of the procedure, introduction of the hardware, and relatively significant change in standard practice by robotic systems as weighed against the clinical benefits.

OSTEOTOMY

Keppler et al[48] used a navigation system to perform high tibial opening wedge osteotomy on plastic, cadaveric tibiae, and then patients (Fig. 94–12). The clinical experience confirmed the accuracy of results obtained in experimental surgery, with 80% of patients achieving the desired alignment. Some authors have reported the development and laboratory experiments of robotic techniques for upper tibial osteotomy.[76]

FRACTURES AROUND THE KNEE

CAOS systems have been used in patients with orthopedic trauma at different anatomic sites (spine, pelvis, extremities). The knee procedures may include fixation of long-bone fractures around the knee, such as intramedullary nailing or limited invasive plating.[34] Fluoroscopy-based navigation systems are best suited for

trauma application because of the fact that intraoperative fluoroscopy is routinely used in trauma surgery and thus no additional imaging is required. The number of orthopedic procedures that require fluoroscopy is increasing as a result of the trend to use percutaneous techniques. Consequently, the risk of radiation exposure is increasing, and there are some alarming reports in the literature.[38,96] Fluoroscopically based navigation can potentially reduce radiation exposure by orthopedic surgeons, nursing staff, and patients because such navigation techniques require a limited number of radiographic images.

MINIMALLY INVASIVE SURGERY AND COMPUTER-ASSISTED ORTHOPEDIC SURGERY

Currently, enthusiasm is growing among patients, surgeons, and health care providers for MIS techniques in joint arthroplasty and other procedures. There are very optimistic views arguing that the success of minimally invasive laparoscopic and arthroscopic surgery could be transferred to joint replacement. MIS has been applied in the past to different orthopedic subspecialties such as trauma and spine procedures. When compared with conventional techniques, MIS has the potential to provide a better short-term outcome with earlier recovery, shorter hospital stay, and fewer short-term complications such as bleeding, stiffness, and pain. Patients are usually satisfied with the better cosmesis, shorter hospital stay, and potential earlier return to work and activities.

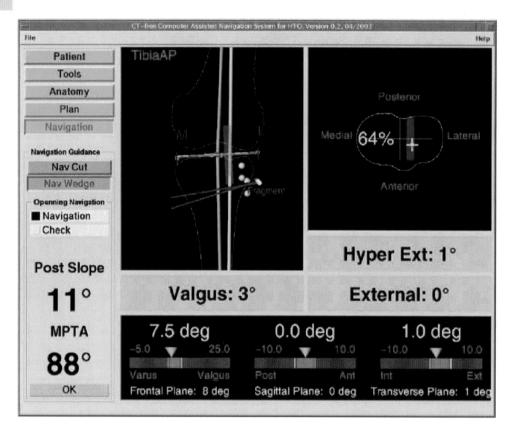

Figure 94–12. Upper tibial osteotomy by a fluoroscopically based navigation system. The wedge is opened under navigational guidance. The navigated parameters include wedge size in the frontal, sagittal, and transverse plane (*bottom of window*). The collinear parameters include different angles. The position of the weightbearing axis is shown at the *top right*, and the three-dimensional view of the wedge and mechanical axes is shown at the *top left*. (From Keppler P, Gebhard F, Grützner PA, et al: Computer aided high tibial open wedge osteotomy. Injury 35[Suppl 1]:68-78, 2004.)

However, MIS techniques are difficult to perform; visibility is reduced throughout the procedure, and anatomic landmarks are more difficult to localize. Bone cuts are done somewhat blindly with a higher potential risk for error. There is also difficulty in inserting instruments and implants. Although the reduced size guides are more convenient to use, this convenience may come at the expense of accuracy. The reduced exposure is also associated with reduced visibility and a subsequently higher risk for complications and inaccuracy.[24]

The main questions for MIS are whether it is possible to achieve a satisfactory long-term outcome that is comparable to that produced by conventional techniques and whether the short-term benefits from MIS can be justified by the increased difficulty of the technique, longer operative time, and potential for less accuracy. A few authors have reported good short-term results of such techniques.[101] However, long-term outcomes will not be known for several years. The use of CAOS tools in MIS techniques may improve visibility and accuracy. The new trend of "MIS meets CAOS" advocated by DiGioia et al[25] is currently being considered and applied by a few surgeons who have used navigation techniques in hip and knee surgery.[69,74,98]

Training

Increasing emphasis is being placed on teaching and evaluation of technical skills during surgical training.[52] Current methods of training are still very traditional, and it is unlikely that they can keep pace with the speed of the technology and the frequent introduction of new techniques. What surgeons learn during training quickly becomes obsolete. Yet once in independent practice, they rarely have the opportunity to learn new procedures under such close supervision as they had during training. Operating rooms are not always the optimal environment for learning or teaching. Operating under the guidance of a more experienced surgeon does not allow repetitive actions or proper feedback and also provides no analysis or correction of errors. Real-time teaching is an important part of training that this experience does not allow. The broad applications of MIS in general surgery (laparoscopy) were associated with the introduction of surgical simulators that permit real-time feedback and also allow errors to occur and be evaluated. Orthopedic surgeons can benefit from the transfer of such experience to MIS techniques in knee surgery. Navigational techniques can be used as information systems for training workshops on sawbones and cadavers. Several modalities can be used for training, such as surgical simulators, image overlay[57,68] (see Fig. 94–16), and virtual-reality arthroscopy.[57,89]

Limitations and Drawbacks of Computer-Assisted Surgery

Although navigation and robotic techniques have been applied to several procedures in knee surgery in developed countries, their broad application is limited by complexity, cost, setup time, and a long learning curve. Some CAOS systems require preoperative imaging (usually CT scanning) or intraoperative radiographs, which may not be routine requirements, hence the drawback of additional time, cost, and radiation risk. However, new CT scanners are faster and possibly less expensive, and new techniques may reduce the risk of radiation exposure. Henckel et al[41] reported a protocol to produce a low-cost, low-radiation knee CT scan (0.1 mSv) and stated that an accurate routine x-ray series might result in a higher radiation dose than if CT were used according to this protocol.

Navigation techniques still rely on conventional instruments for making the various bone cuts, and they may even require additional instruments and insertion of tracking pins. This double-instrumentation system (navigation and conventional) may overload hospital inventory, adversely affect operating room ergonomics,[95] and prolong operative times. Longer operating time, especially at the early stages of the learning curve, may lead to some complications such as increased blood loss or infection. In addition, the cost of navigation and robotics systems is a major concern for health care providers, and cost-effectiveness analysis may be required before universal acceptance of such systems. Future CAOS systems should be designed to be easy to use in all steps and to save on operative time by replacing the conventional mechanical instruments. It is of importance to document improvement in clinical outcomes achieved by these systems.

FUTURE DIRECTIONS

CAOS systems are already very powerful tools, yet they have even more potential for development and new applications. If orthopedics is currently leading the way in CAS in the near future, we envisage that knee surgery will also be leading the way in CAOS. Knee surgery has already attracted a wide variety of CAOS techniques and applications. MIS and the introduction of more demanding techniques will attract even more applications and perhaps lead to the development of more complete CAOS systems. This section discusses some of these future directions.

Technical Advancement

NEW IMAGING MODALITIES

There is a need to reduce the risk of radiation exposure from both CT and plane radiography. Therefore, the trend is to use other available imaging modalities such as magnetic resonance imaging (MRI) or ultrasound. Ultrasonography is noninvasive, inexpensive, portable, and readily available. It has already been used for registration purposes in some CAOS techniques.[1] Echo-morphing technology[93] is similar to bone morphing, but it uses an ultrasound probe to collect data for bony landmarks and surfaces. In these applications, ultrasound can be applied to the skin without bony exposure, which is a requirement in MIS techniques. MRI is expensive and not portable, but it is radiation-free and provides better definition of soft-tissue structures such as ligaments. MRI has the potential to replace CT, particularly for soft-tissue procedures such as ligament reconstruction. It is used routinely as a diag-

nostic procedure on the knee. Thus, computer-assisted ACL reconstruction can be performed with no extra imaging. However, segmentation of bone with MRI is more difficult than with CT images. 3-D fluoroscopy is a new imaging modality that has recently been introduced. It can reconstruct 3-D images from a series of 2-D fluoroscopic views with reduced risk of radiation exposure. It has the potential to replace CT in some conventional and computer-assisted applications.

NEW TRACKING DEVICES

New devices are likely to appear in the near future that will replace or augment current optical trackers. These new trackers eliminate the need for the relatively invasive process of inserting rigid pins into bone and the need for a contentious line of sight. Electromagnetic trackers have already been used in experimental settings and appear to be more convenient than optical trackers. They may require percutaneous insertion of small metallic pieces (similar to soft-tissue anchors) that are attached to wires. However they do not require a tracking camera or line of sight. Researchers are also investigating the feasibility of using ultrasound for tracking purposes to eliminate the relatively invasive current techniques that require pin insertion and continuous line of site. Ultrasound has the advantage that it may not require rigid fixation and can be applied superficially to the skin. It can also provide more complete spatial anatomy with imaging data that are midway between 2-D and 3-D.

New Approaches in Computer-Assisted Orthopedic Surgery Systems

HAND-HELD ROBOTIC TOOLS

Hybrid systems combine features and some advantages from both active and passive approaches. One of these systems is the "Precision Freehand Sculptor,"[8] which is a hand-held tool with a rotating bur that helps the surgeon perform accurate bone removal (and make unique shapes) based on preoperative planning (Fig. 94–13). This system resembles navigation in that it requires tracking and allows the performance of freehand action, but it is robotic because it actively controls the bone cutting. The surgeon has full control of the tool's position while holding the device. The bur removes only the bone that was planned to be removed because the bur retracts when placed beyond the planned cutting zone. These actions are tracked and displayed on a computer screen in real time. The working end of the tool is close to the size of any arthroscopic bur, and it allows bone cutting and the preparation of any unique shape to be performed through a small incision. This tool shows promise to improve other bone-sculpting procedures, such as necessary in TKA, UKA, patellofemoral arthroplasty, bone tunnel placement or notchplasty, and single- or double-bundle ACL reconstruction.

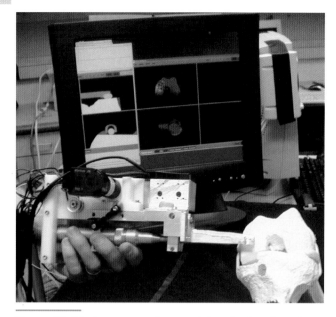

Figure 94–13. Prototype of a precision freehand sculptor while performing unicondylar knee replacement.

BONE-MOUNTED ROBOTS

A miniature bone-attached robotic system for joint replacement is being developed and tested in the laboratory for preparation of the femur in patellofemoral arthroplasty (Fig. 94–14).[108] In this approach, the robotic tool is actually attached to the femur with three pins and directs a conventional cutting bur. The system can be used in an image-based or image-free fashion in as much as it directly palpates the bone surfaces in the robot coordinate system, thereby eliminating the need for bone imaging or tracking in the operating room. Planning can be performed preoperatively or intraoperatively. Bench top experiments have supported the feasibility of this new concept, and current work is focusing on reducing the size of the robotic appa-

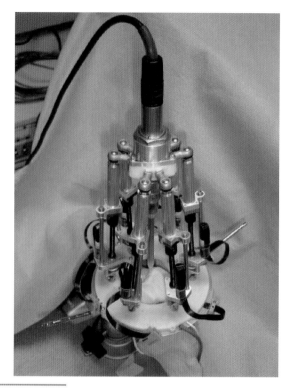

Figure 94–14. Bone-mounted robot for patellofemoral arthroplasty.

ratus. The system has the potential to improve the accuracy and reproducibility of many "bone-sculpting" procedures and reduce operating time.

PATIENT-SPECIFIC INSTRUMENTS FOR TOTAL KNEE ARTHROPLASTY

This technique falls into the passive category of CAOS (Fig. 94–15). Conceptually it is a new generation of the

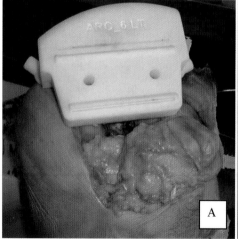
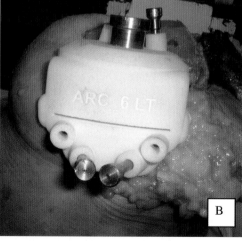

Figure 94–15. Patient-specific instrumentation for total knee arthroplasty (TKA). In experimental cadaveric TKA, femoral (**A**) and tibial (**B**) templates are used that match the individual bony surfaces in a single unique position; the device is then secured to the bone by pins. There are several slots and holes to allow all bone cuts and other preparations such as lugholes, tibial stem, and tibial keel. Note that no tracking, registration, or intramedullary perforation is required.

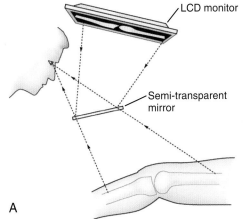

LCD monitor

Semi-transparent mirror

A

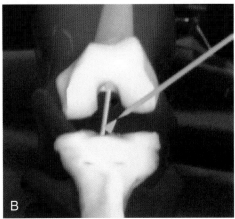

B

Figure 94–16. Image overlay. **A,** Schematic of the image overlay showing the basic operating components. **B,** Picture of what the surgeon sees during anterior cruciate ligament reconstruction.

templating techniques that were described earlier. The technique is currently confined to TKA and is still at the experimental stage with no clinical validation yet. The main unique feature of this technique in comparison to previous templating techniques is that the templates here are designed as instruments rather than guides and work as cutting blocks that can completely replace conventional instrumentations. According to authors,[13,35,36] the disadvantage of using CT scans was outweighed by the benefits in that the templates could eliminate the drawbacks of conventional instrumentation, such as cost, complexity, setup time, and perforation of intramedullary canals. This technique does not require intraoperative tracking or registration, but it cannot work as an intraoperative measurement tool. Hafez et al[35,36] reported the use of this technique in 45 TKAs (16 cadaveric and 29 plastic knees), including a comparative trial against 6 conventional TKAs (plastic knees). They stated that all operations were performed without resorting to conventional instruments and the operative time was halved. Six random postoperative CT scans of cadaveric knees were compared with the corresponding preoperative planning and showed that the mean error for femoral and tibial coronal and sagittal alignment was within 1.7° and the mean error for bone resection was within 0.75 mm. The maximum error was within 2.3° for alignment and 1.2 mm for bone resection.

IMAGE OVERLAY

This technology allows surgeons to visualize the patient's anatomy during surgery, without direct exposure, and provides other supplementary information vital to the execution of operative procedures, both delivered within the field of surgical action. Image overlay is a device built to fuse a surgeon's view of a patient together with graphic images from preoperative medical data and/or computer-generated 3-D graphics (Fig. 94–16). This device has great promise for enabling various telemedicine applications, as well as providing navigational guidance to surgeons in nontelemedicine applications. Some other alternative devices, such as a retinal scanning display, are also under investigation.[6]

New Procedures

DOUBLE-BUNDLE ANTERIOR CRUCIATE LIGAMENT RECONSTRUCTION

Anatomic double-bundle reconstruction of ACL has recently received increased attention,[5,58] but long-term outcome results are lacking. This procedure is more technically demanding than conventional techniques and requires accurate and reproducible placement of double femoral and double tibial tunnels. Navigation systems and hybrid tools may play a role in guiding the surgeon to accurately identify tunnel locations and their direction and perform in vivo kinematic measurements of stability. They have the potential to provide intraoperative feedback and measurement of the outcome.

BIOLOGICS

More than any other joints, articular cartilage abnormalities in the knee have attracted several biological solutions such as osteochondral autografts and autologous chondrocyte transplantation. These techniques are technically demanding and may benefit from the application of computer-assisted techniques that allow accurate planning and precise performance. The future is likely to feature combined use of CAOS with tissue engineering and biological resurfacing of bone and cartilage.

The Operating Room of the Future

As CAOS systems become more stable and popular, new operating rooms will be designed that incorporate these advanced navigation, robotic, and imaging systems into routine surgical practice. Several modifications are required to accommodate other new technologies and improve ergonomics.[95] The design should allow the integration of preoperative or perioperative imaging with operative performance. Optimally, the environment should encourage the application of telesurgery, virtual reality, and teaching.

CONCLUSION

CAOS technology is the "surgical toolbox of the future" and represents a spectrum of devices that include robotic, navigation (image based or image-free), templating, and hybrid tools. CAOS tools will enable more accurate and less invasive surgical techniques. They can provide "x-ray vision" without using x-ray machines, thereby eliminating radiation exposure. CAOS tools will also be used as the surgical trainers of the future by coupling simulations with real-time evaluation of surgical performance. CAOS can "close the loop" in surgical practice by measuring and directly relating surgical techniques to patient outcomes.

TKA is currently the most common procedure performed with the use of navigation techniques, and knee surgery is well suited for CAOS and may lead the way for clinical applications. Surgeons are also recognizing that CAOS technologies are an important part of the less invasive and MIS techniques. When "MIS meets CAOS," there is great potential to have an impact on daily clinical practice in the same way that arthroscopic technologies have revolutionized the way we currently practice. CAOS-based tools and systems coupled with redesigned implants and mechanical tools will enable the development of less invasive and MIS techniques for joint arthroplasty and eventually "biological" implants.

However, CAOS systems need to be validated and standardized. Surgeons should be aware of potential errors and pitfalls during the clinical application of these systems. Structured training should be available to surgeons before leaping to clinical practice. Currently, CAOS has several limitations. Clinical application is confined to senior surgeons and certain centers. Broad application of CAOS is limited by complexity, cost, setup time, and a long learning curve. CAOS systems are sophisticated tools and can be cumbersome. Improvements in clinical outcome have to be documented, and cost-effectiveness has to be analyzed before standardization of such systems. The technology and approaches are evolving, and the future will bring new CAOS systems that could be widely accepted.

References

1. Amin DV, Kanade T, DiGioia AM III, et al: Ultrasound registration of the bone surface for surgical navigation. Comput Aided Surg 8:1-16, 2003.
2. Amiot LP, Labelle H, Deguise JA, et al: Computer assisted pedicle screw fixation: A feasibility study. Spine 20:1208-1212, 1995.
3. Amiot LP, Poulin F: Computed tomography–based navigation for hip, knee, and spine surgery. Clin Orthop 421:77-86, 2004.
4. Bathis HL, Perlick, Tingart M, et al: Radiological results of image-based and non–image-based computer-assisted total knee arthroplasty. Int Orthop 28:87-90, 2004.
5. Bellier G, Christel P, Colombet P, et al: Double-stranded hamstring graft for anterior cruciate ligament reconstruction. Arthroscopy 20:890-894, 2004.
6. Blackwell M, Morgan F, DiGioia AM III: Augmented reality and its future in orthopaedics. Clin Orthop 354:111-122, 1998.
7. Borner M, Wiesel U, Ditzen W: Clinical experiences with ROBODOC and the Duracon total knee. In Stiehl JB, Konermann WH, Haaker RG (eds): Navigation and Robotics in Total Joint and Spine Surgery. Berlin, Springer, 2004, pp 362-366.
8. Brisson G, Kanade T, DiGioia AM III, et al: Precision handheld sculpting of bone. Presented at a Conference on Computer-Assisted Orthopedic Surgery, Marbellar, Spain, 2003, pp 36-37.
9. Brown GA, Firoozbakhsh K, DeCoster TA, et al: Rapid prototyping: The future of trauma surgery. J Bone Joint Surg Am 85(Suppl 4):49-55, 2003.
10. Burkart A, Debski R, Rudy T, et al: A comparison of precision for ACL tunnel placement using traditional and robotic technique. Comput Aided Surg 6:270-278, 2002.
11. Burri C, Claes L, Gerngross H: Total "internal" hemipelvectomy. Arch Orthop Trauma Surg 94:219-226, 1979.
12. Chauhan SK, Scott RG, Breidahl W, et al: Computer-assisted knee arthroplasty versus a conventional jig-based technique. A randomized, prospective trial. J Bone Joint Surg Br 86:372-377, 2004.
13. Chelule K, Seedhom BB, Hafez MA, et al: Computer-assisted total knee replacement. Osteoarthritis Cartilage 11(Suppl A):S11, 2003.
14. Chillag KJ, Nichollas PJ: High tibial osteotomy: A retrospective analysis of 30 cases. Orthopedics 7:1821, 1984.
15. Clarke RH, Horsley V: On a method of investigating the deep ganglia and tracts of the central nervous system (cerebellum). BMJ 2:1799-1800, 1906.
16. Cobb J, Henckel J, Richards R, et al: Robot assisted minimally invasive unicompartmental knee arthroplasty results of first clinical trial. Comput Aided Surg 9:88, 2004.
17. Cossey AJ, Spriggins AJ: The use of computer-assisted surgical navigation to prevent malalignment in unicompartmental knee arthroplasty. J Arthroplasty 20:29-34, 2005.
18. Coventry MB, Ilstrup DM, Wallrichs SL: Proximal tibial osteotomy. A critical long-term study of eighty-seven cases. J Bone Joint Surg Am 75:196-201, 1993.
19. Decking J, Theis C, Achenbach T, et al: Robotic total knee arthroplasty. Acta Orthop Scand 75:573-579, 2004.
20. Delp SL, Stulberg SD, Davies BL, et al: Computer-assisted knee replacement. Clin Orthop 354:49-56, 1998.
21. De Rycke J: Clinical experiences for ACL-repair with the system. In Stiehl JB, Konermann WH, Haaker RG (eds): Navigation and Robotics in Total Joint and Spine Surgery. Berlin, Springer, 2004, pp 397-399.
22. Diduch DR, Insall JN, Scott WN, et al: Total knee replacement in young, active patients. Long-term follow-up and functional outcome. J Bone Joint Surg Am 79:575-582, 1997.
23. DiGioia AM III: Surgical Navigation and Robotics for Adult Reconstruction and Trauma. Instructional Course Lecture, American Academy of Orthopaedic Surgeons, 2002.
24. DiGioia AM III, Blendea S, Jaramaz B: Computer-assisted orthopaedic surgery: Minimally invasive hip and knee reconstruction Orthop Clin North Am 35:183-189, 2004.
25. DiGioia AM III, Jaramaz B: Closing the loop in surgical practice. Lancet 354(Suppl 4):46, 1999.
26. DiGioia AM III, Jaramaz B, Blackwell M: The Otto Aufranc Award. Image guided navigation system to measure intraoperatively acetabular implant alignment. Clin Orthop 355:8-22, 1998.
27. DiGioia AM III, Jaramaz B, Colgan BD: Computer assisted orthopaedic surgery; image guided and robotic assistive technologies. Clin Orthop 354:8-16, 1998.
28. Eichhorn HJ: Image-free navigation in ACL replacement with the OrthoPilot system. In Stiehl JB, Konermann WH, Haaker RG (eds): Navigation and Robotics in Total Joint and Spine Surgery. Berlin, Springer, 2004, pp 387-396.
29. Fehring TK, Odum S, Griffin WL, et al: Early failure in total knee arthroplasty. Clin Orthop 392:315-318, 2001.
30. Fortheine F, Ohnsorge JAK, Schkommodau E, et al: CT-based planning and individual template navigation in TKA. In Stiehl JB, Konermann WH, Haaker RG (eds): Navigation and Robotics in Total Joint and Spine Surgery. Berlin, Springer, 2004, pp 336-342.
31. Giliberty RP, Epstein HY, Faegenburg D: A prototype femoral stem using CAT and CAD/CAM. Orthop Rev XII-8:59-63, 1983.
32. Gotzen L, Pashmineh-Azar A, Ziring E: Clinical experiences with CASPAR-assisted ACL reconstruction. In Stiehl JB, Konermann WH, Haaker RG (eds): Navigation and Robotics in Total Joint and Spine Surgery. Berlin, Springer, 2004, pp 412-422.
33. Greis PE, Johnson DL, Fu FH: Revision anterior cruciate ligament surgery: Causes of graft failure and technical considerations of revision surgery. Clin Sports Med 12:839-852, 1993.

34. Grützner PA, Suhm N: Computer aided long bone fracture treatment. Injury 35(Suppl 1):57-64, 2004.

35. Hafez MA: Patient-Specific Templating and Instrumentation for TKA Based on Computer Assisted Preoperative Planning [MD thesis]. University of Leeds, UK, 2005.

36. Hafez MA, Chelule KL, Seedhom BB, et al: Computer assisted total knee replacement: Could a two-piece custom template replace the complex conventional instrumentation. Comput Aided Surg 9:93-94, 2004.

37. Hafez MA, Edge AJ, Morris R: Long-term results of total knee replacement: Surgeon's versus patient's assessment J Bone Joint Surg Br 86(Suppl 1):17, 2004.

38. Hafez MA, Smith RM, Matthews S, et al: Radiation exposure to the hands of orthopaedic surgeons: Are we underestimating the risk? Arch Orthop Trauma Surg 125:330-335, 2005.

39. Harris J, Rimell J: Can rapid prototyping ever become a routine feature in general dental practice? Dent Update 29:482-486, 2002.

40. Heal J, Blewitt N: Kinemax total knee arthroplasty: Trial by template. J Arthroplasty 17:90-94, 2002.

41. Henckel J, Cobb JP, Richards R, et al: Computer-assisted arthroplasty: Appropriate imaging for assessment of implant position. Comput Aided Surg 9:105, 2004.

42. Hofmann AA, Evanich JD, Ferguson RP, et al: Ten- to 14-year clinical followup of the cementless Natural Knee system. Clin Orthop 388:85-94, 2001.

43. Ilahi OA, Kadakia NR, Huo MH: Inter- and intraobserver variability of radiographic measurements of knee alignment. Am J Knee Surg 14:238-242, 2001.

44. Jakopec M, Harris SJ, Rodriguez Y, et al: The first clinical application of a "hands-on" robotic knee surgery system. Comput Aided Surg 6:329-339, 2001.

45. Jazrawi LM, Birdzell L, Kummer FJ, et al: The accuracy of computed tomography for determining femoral and tibial total knee arthroplasty component rotation. J Arthroplasty 15:761-766, 2000.

46. Jenny JY, Boeri C: Low reproducibility of the intra-operative measurement of the transepicondylar axis during total knee replacement. Acta Orthop Scand 75:74-77, 2004.

47. Jenny JY, Boeri C: Implantation of unicondylar prosthesis using the OrthoPilot system: One way towards a minimally invasive operation. In Stiehl JB, Konermann WH, Haaker RG (eds): Navigation and Robotics in Total Joint and Spine Surgery. Berlin, Springer, 2004, pp 345-351.

48. Keppler P, Gebhard F, Grützner PA, et al: Computer aided high tibial open wedge osteotomy. Injury 35(Suppl 1):68-78, 2004.

49. Khaw FM, Kirk LM, Gregg PJ: Survival analysis of cemented press-fit condylar total knee arthroplasty. J Arthroplasty 16:161-167, 2001.

50. Kinzel V, Scaddan M, Bradley B, et al: Varus/valgus alignment of the femur in total knee arthroplasty. Can accuracy be improved by preoperative CT scanning? Knee 11:197-201, 2004.

51. Kinzl L, Gebhard F, Keppler P: Total knee arthroplasty—navigation as the standard. Chirurg 75:976-981, 2004.

52. Kohls-Gatzoulis JA, Regehr G, Hutchison C: Teaching cognitive skills improves learning in surgical skills courses: A blinded, prospective, randomised study. Can J Surg 47:277-283, 2004.

53. Koshino T, Takeyama M, Jiang LS, et al: Underestimation of varus angulation in knees with flexion deformity. Knee 9:275-279, 2002.

54. Lavallee S, Troccaz J, Sautot P, et al: Computer assisted spine surgery using anatomy-based registration. In Taylor R, Lavallee S Burdea G, Mosges R (eds): Computer Integrated Surgery. Cambridge, MA, MIT Press, 1996, pp 425-429.

55. Li Q, Zamorano L, Jiang Z, et al: Effect of optical digitizer selection on the application accuracy of a surgical localization system—a quantitative comparison between the OPTOTRAK and flashpoint tracking systems. Comput Aided Surg 4:314-321, 1999.

56. Lonner JH, Laird MT, Stuchin SA: Effect of rotation and knee flexion on radiographic alignment in total knee arthroplasties. Clin Orthop 331:102-106, 1996.

57. Mabrey JD, Gillogly SD, Kasser JR, et al: Virtual reality simulation of arthroscopy of the knee. Arthroscopy 18:E28, 2002.

58. Marcacci M, Molgora AP, Zaffagnini S, et al: Anatomic double-bundle anterior cruciate ligament reconstruction with hamstrings. Arthroscopy 19:540-546, 2003.

59. Matsumoto T, Tsumura N, Kurosaka M, et al: Prosthetic alignment and sizing in computer-assisted total knee arthroplasty. Int Orthop 28:282-285, 2004.

60. McGurk M, Amis AA, Potamianos P, et al: Rapid prototyping techniques for anatomical modeling in medicine. Ann R Coll Surg Engl 79:169-174, 1997.

61. Merloz P, Tonetti J, Eid A: Computer assisted spine surgery. Clin Orthop 337:86-96, 1997.

62. Mor AB, Jaramaz B, DiGioia AM: Accuracy and validation. In DiGioia AM, Jaramaz B, Picard F, Notle L (eds): Computer and Robotic Assisted Knee and Hip Surgery. Oxford, Oxford University Press, 2004, pp 307-316.

63. Moreland JR, Bassett LW, Hanker GJ: Radiographic analysis of the axial alignment of the lower extremity. J Bone Joint Surg Am 69:745-749, 1987.

64. Murphy SB, Kijewski PK, Simon SR: Computer-aided simulation, analysis, and design in orthopedic surgery. Orthop Clin North Am 17:637-649, 1986.

65. Murray DW, Britton AR, Bulstrode CJ: Loss to follow-up matters. J Bone Joint Surg Br 79:254-257, 1997.

66. Murray DW, Frost SJD: Pain in the assessment of total knee replacement. J Bone Joint Surg Br 80:426-431, 1998.

67. Nabeyama R, Matsuda S, Miura H, et al: The accuracy of image guided knee replacement based on computed tomography. J Bone Joint Surg Br 86:366-371, 2003.

68. Nikou C, DiGioia AM, Blackwell M, et al: Augmented reality imaging technology for orthopaedic surgery. Op Tech Orthop 10:82-86, 2000.

69. Nogler M: Navigated minimal invasive total hip arthroplasty. Surg Technol Int 12:259-262, 2004.

70. Notle LP, Zamorano LJ, Visarius H, et al: Clinical evaluation of a system for precision enhancement in spine surgery. Clin Biomech 10:293-303, 1995.

71. Novotny J, Gonzalez MH, Amirouche FM, et al: Geometric analysis of potential error in using femoral intramedullary guides in total knee arthroplasty. J Arthroplasty 16:641-647, 2001.

72. Oberst M, Bertsch C, Wurstlin S, et al: CT analysis of leg alignment after conventional vs. navigated knee prosthesis implantation. Initial results of a controlled, prospective and randomized study. Unfallchirurg 106:941-948, 2003.

73. Paul HA, Bargar WL, Mittlestadt B, et al: Development of a surgical robot for cementless total hip arthroplasty. Clin Orthop 285:57-66, 1992.

74. Perlick L, Bathis H, Tingart M, et al: Minimally invasive unicompartmental knee replacement with a nonimage-based navigation system. Int Orthop 28:193-197, 2004.

75. Perlick L, Bathis H, Tingart M, et al: Navigation in total-knee arthroplasty: CT-based implantation compared with the conventional technique. Acta Orthop Scand 75:464-470, 2004.

76. Phillips R, Hafez MA, Mohsen AM, et al: Computer and robotic assisted osteotomy around the knee. Stud Health Technol Inform 70:265-271, 2000.

77. Picard F, Moody JE, DiGioia AM III, et al: Clinical classification of CAOS systems. In DiGioia AM, Jaramaz B, Picard F, Notle L (eds): Computer and Robotic Assisted Knee and Hip Surgery. Oxford, Oxford University Press, 2004, pp 43-48.

78. Plaskos C, Hodgson AJ, Inkpen K, et al: Bone cutting errors in total knee arthroplasty. J Arthroplasty 17:698-705, 2002.

79. Plaskos C, Stindel E, Cinquin P, et al: Praxiteles: A universal bone-mounted robot for image-free knee surgery, report on first cadaver study. Comput Aided Surg 9:94, 2004.

80. Radermacher K, Portheine F, Anton M, et al: Computer assisted orthopaedic surgery with image-based individual templates. Clin Orthop 354:28-38, 1998.

81. Rand JA, Trousdale RT, Ilstrup DM, et al: Factors affecting the durability of primary total knee prostheses. J Bone Joint Surg Am 85:259-365, 2003.

82. Randle R: Arthroscopic unicompartmental replacement. Presented at the Minimally Invasive Joint Replacement Conference, September 2004, Houston.

83. Reed SC, Gollish J: The accuracy of femoral intramedullary guides in total knee arthroplasty. J Arthroplasty 12:677-682, 1997.

84. Ritschl P, Machacek J, Fuiko R, et al: The Galileo system for implantation of total knee arthroplasty: An integral solution comprising

navigation, robotics and robot-assisted ligament balancing. In Stiehl JB, Konermann WH, Haaker RG (eds): Navigation and Robotics in Total Joint and Spine Surgery. Berlin, Springer, 2004, pp 281-286.

85. Ritter MA, Berend ME, Meding JB, et al: Long-term followup of anatomic graduated components posterior cruciate–retaining total knee replacement. Clin Orthop 388:51-57, 2001.

86. Sati M, Staubli H, Bourquin Y, et al: Real-time computerized in situ guidance system for ACL graft placement. Comput Aided Surg 7:25-40, 2002.

87. Scuderi GR: Revision total knee arthroplasty: How much constraint is enough? Clin Orthop 392:300-305, 2001.

88. Sharkey PF, Hozack WJ, Rothman, RH, et al: Insall Award paper. Why are knee replacements failing today? Clin Orthop 404:7-13, 2002.

89. Sherman KP, Ward JW, Wills DP, et al: Surgical trainee assessment using a VE knee arthroscopy training system (VE-KATS): Experimental results. Stud Health Technol Inform 81:465-470, 2001.

90. Siebert W, Mai S, Kober R, et al: Technique and first clinical results of robot-assisted total knee replacement. Knee 9:173-180, 2002.

91. Sikorski JM: Computer-assisted revision total knee replacement. J Bone Joint Surg Br 86:510-514, 2004.

92. Soni AH, Gudavalli MR, Herndon WA, et al: Application of passive robot in spine surgery. Presented at the Eighth Annual Conference of the IEEE/Engineer Biology and Medical Society, 1986, pp 1186-1191.

93. Stindel E, Briard JL, Lavallee S, et al: Bone morphing: 3-D reconstruction without pre- or intraoperative imaging—concept and applications. In Stiehl JB, Konermann WH, Haaker RG (eds): Navigation and Robotics in Total Joint and Spine Surgery. Berlin, Springer, 2004, pp 39-45.

94. Stockl B, Nogler M, Rosiek R, et al: Navigation improves accuracy of rotational alignment in total knee arthroplasty. Clin Orthop 426:180-186, 2004.

95. Stone R, McCloy R: Ergonomics in medicine and surgery BMJ 328:1115-1118, 2004.

96. Storm HH: Radiation-induced acute myeloid leukaemia and other cancers in commercial jet cockpit crew: A population-based cohort study. Lancet 354:2029-2031, 1999.

97. Stulberg SD: How accurate is current TKR instrumentation? Clin Orthop 416:177-184, 2003.

98. Stulberg SD: The rationale for using computer navigation with minimally invasive THA. Orthopedics 27:942-946, 2004.

99. Stulberg SD, Loan P, Sarin V: Computer-assisted navigation in total knee replacement: Results of an initial experience of thirty-five patients. J Bone Joint Surg Am 84(Suppl 2):90-98, 2002.

100. Sugano N, Sasama T, Sato Y, et al: Accuracy evaluation of surface-based registration methods in a computer navigation system for hip surgery performed through a posterolateral approach. Comput Aided Surg 6:195-203, 2001.

101. Tria AJ Jr, Coon TM: Minimal incision total knee arthroplasty: Early experience. Clin Orthop 416:185-190, 2003.

102. Vergis A, Gillquist J: Graft failure in intra-articular anterior cruciate ligament reconstructions: A review of the literature. Arthroscopy 11:312-321, 1995.

103. Viant WJ, Phillips R, Bielby MS, et al: Computer assisted positioning of cannulated hip screws. In Lemke HU, Vannier MW, Inamura K, Farman AG (eds): Computer Assisted Radiology and Surgery (CARS). Amsterdam, Elsevier, 1999, pp 751-755.

104. Viant WJ, Phillips R, Griffiths JG, et al: A computer assisted orthopaedic surgical system for distal locking of intramedullary nails. Proc Inst Mech Eng 211:293-300, 1997.

105. Victor J, Hoste D: Image-based computer-assisted total knee arthroplasty leads to lower variability in coronal alignment. Clin Orthop 428:131-139, 2004.

106. Wagner A, Schicho K, Birkfellner W, et al: Quantitative analysis of factors affecting intraoperative precision and stability of optoelectronic and electromagnetic tracking systems. Med Phys 29:905-912, 2002.

107. Wiese M, Rosenthal A, Bernsmann K: Clinical experiences using the system. In Stiehl JB, Konermann WH, Haaker RG (eds): Navigation and Robotics in Total Joint and Spine Surgery. Berlin, Springer, 2004, pp 400-404.

108. Wolf A, Jaramaz B, Lisien B, et al: MBARS: Mini bone attached robotic system for joint arthroplasty. Int J Med Robot Comput Assist Surg 1:101-121, 2005.

CHAPTER 95

Computer-Navigated Total Knee Arthroplasty

S. David Stulberg

Computer-assisted surgery (CAS) is beginning to emerge as one of the most important technologies in orthopedic surgery, and many of the initial applications have focused on adult reconstructive surgery of the knee. The goals of this chapter are to (1) provide a brief history of CAS of the knee and the evolution of basic concepts, (2) present the rationale for the use of CAS in knee surgery, (3) describe the hardware and software components of CAS systems, (4) illustrate the most common CAS techniques used for knee reconstruction surgery, (5) summarize the early results with CAS knee reconstruction systems, and (6) present CAS applications in knee surgery that will be available in the near future.

HISTORY OF COMPUTER-ASSISTED KNEE SURGERY AND EVOLUTION OF BASIC CONCEPTS

Although a large volume of important work that became the foundation for computer-assisted knee surgery was being carried out throughout the 20th century, the initial clinical applications for knee surgery began in the 1980s.[79] In 1986, Kaiura from the University of Washington presented a master's thesis on robotic-assisted total knee arthroplasty (TKA).[24,44] This work led to design of one of the first computer robotic assistive systems for TKA. This system was described by Matsen and coworkers in 1993.[62,103] In the early 1990s, Kienzle, Stulberg, and coworkers also described a computer-assisted robotic total knee replacement system.[45,100] The desired position of the femoral and tibial cutting blocks was determined on a three-dimensional model derived from a computed axial tomographic scan obtained preoperatively. The robot was secured to the operating table and to the bones and then positioned a drill to make holes for the pins over which the femoral and tibial cutting blocks were placed. The surgeon then performed the cuts with a standard oscillating saw. The accuracy of block placement with this system was within 1 mm and 1 degree. This work also introduced a method for determining the center of the femoral head by means of a kinematic registration technique. This technique has subsequently been incorporated in all current navigation systems. Dynamic reference frames that were tracked by a camera were placed on the femur, and the hip was put through a range of motion. The center of the sphere described during the circumduction maneuver represented the center of the femoral head.

By the early 1990s, the principles on which current computer-assisted total knee replacement systems are based had been established and validated, and important steps had been taken to identify ways in which critical anatomic landmarks for knee surgery could be accurately acquired. It was, however, apparent to those working on these projects, especially to orthopedic surgeons, that robotic-based computer-assisted systems were too cumbersome, complex, and potentially too unsafe to be of substantial usefulness in the foreseeable future to an active knee replacement surgeon.

Surgical navigation systems, however, appeared at that time to offer an attractive alternative to a field such as knee surgery, which could benefit from the accuracy provided by computer-assisted techniques without having to deal with the drawbacks and complexity of robots. These systems allowed intraoperative tracking of the position of surgical tools and the bones to which they are attached. The surgeon, not a robot, could control all phases of the procedure.

The rapid evolution of surgical navigation systems to support the performance of knee surgery was made possible by the availability, in the early 1990s, of optical and electromagnetic tracking systems (Fig. 95–1A and B). Optical tracking systems have played a special role in the development of surgical navigation systems for knee surgery because of their accuracy and reliability. These tracking systems (also referred to as optical localizers) have charge-coupled devices (CCDS, or cameras) mounted on a rigid frame. These cameras measure the position and orientation of multiple tracking markers (also called trackers or rigid bodies). Each tracker incorporates a set of light-emitting diodes (LEDs), or reflective spheres mounted in precise relative positions. These trackers can be affixed to bones, tools, and implants. The optical tracker is therefore able to monitor the precise position of these objects at any point during the surgical procedure.

During the first half of the 1990s, a great deal of basic research was performed to develop surgical navigation systems using these optical tracking systems.[79] The first clinical applications incorporating these efforts began in 1995 in spine surgery. Although these applications were based on the acquisition of anatomic information by means of preoperative imaging techniques, they were the basis for the development in the late 1990s of the image-free systems currently most widely used in knee surgery.

Four types of surgical navigation models are used in computer-assisted orthopedic surgery: (1) preoperative

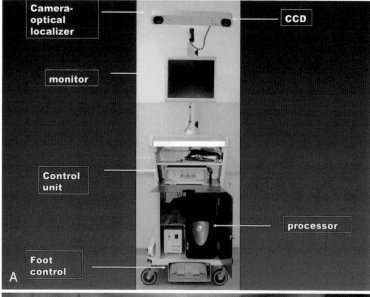

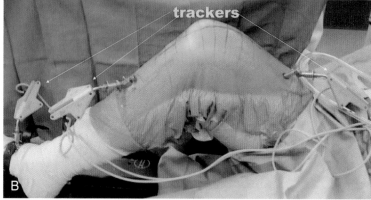

Figure 95–1. **A,** Typical image-free computer-assisted hardware system consisting of an optical tracker with charged-coupled devices (CCD, the "cameras"), a computer monitor, control unit and processor, and a foot control system for communication between the surgeon and the system. **B,** Active trackers (also called rigid bodies or fiducials) attached to bicortical screws rigidly fixed to the femur and tibia.

image based (e.g., computed tomography scans),[46,52] (2) intraoperative image based (e.g., fluoroscopy),[60,61] (3) image-free, and (4) individual templating.[22,52,66,82,96] The anatomic information on which the surgical plan is made is acquired differently in each model. Although each model has its advantages and drawbacks, the image-free method for acquiring critical anatomic information has proved to be most amenable to the current methods used to perform knee surgery. This method was first used clinically in 1993 to place grafts during anterior cruciate ligament (ACL) surgery.[79] Image-free navigation was subsequently applied to TKA surgery by Picard and Leitner.[57] The first image-free computer-assisted TKA was performed in Grenoble, France, by Saragaglia and Picard in 1997.[78] The system used became the first commercially available image-free navigation system for knee reconstructive surgery (the OrthoPilot).[77] This system identified critical anatomic landmarks using both kinematic (e.g., femoral circumduction, as described by Kienzle, Stulberg, et al, 1989[45]) and surface registration techniques. Krackow[51] and others have subsequently developed surgical navigation systems based on these concepts. There are now a large number of image-free navigation systems available for use with virtually every total knee system.

Although the foundations for the computer-assisted systems currently being used in knee surgery began being laid almost a century ago, actual systems available for clinical use have been available for less than 10 years. The rapid emergence of these systems suggests that the current models will undergo substantial evolution and modification in the next few years.

RATIONALE FOR THE USE OF COMPUTER-ASSISTED SURGERY IN KNEE RECONSTRUCTION

Successful surgical reconstruction of the knee requires proper patient selection, appropriate perioperative management, correct implant selection, and accurate surgical technique. The consequences of performing a knee reconstruction inaccurately have been well documented for TKA, unicondylar arthroplasty, ACL reconstruction, and high tibial osteotomy.*

Although mechanical instrumentation has significantly increased the accuracy and reliability with which knee reconstructions are performed, errors in implant and limb

*References 1-3, 6, 9, 15, 16, 20, 21, 26, 28, 29, 31-34, 39, 41, 54-56, 58, 65, 68-70, 75, 76, 83-86, 92, 95, 111, 112, 114, 116, 117.

alignment continue to occur, even when the procedures are performed by experienced surgeons. Moreover, the accuracy with which these procedures are performed is dependent on the knowledge and experience of the surgeon and the frequency with which the surgeon performs the procedures. CAS techniques have been developed to address the inherent limitations of mechanical instrumentation. The goals of integrating CAS with knee reconstruction techniques are to increase the accuracy of these procedures and reduce the proportion of alignment outliers that occur when these procedures are performed.

Errors can occur at numerous points during the performance of a knee reconstruction. Placement of the cutting blocks or ligament alignment jigs may be inaccurate. Attachment of these tools to bone may produce an error in their placement. The actual performance of the cut or drilling of the hole may be inaccurate (e.g., the saw blade may deflect). The final insertion of the implant may be inaccurate. Mechanical instrumentation does not provide a method for checking the accuracy of each of these steps of a knee reconstructive procedure. Another goal of integrating CAS with knee reconstruction is to provide the surgeon with a means to measure the accuracy with which each step of the procedure is performed.

Knee reconstructive procedures attempt to align limbs and implants correctly. They also seek to restore appropriate kinematic relationships and ligamentous stability to the knee.

Mechanical instrumentation cannot measure the precision with which knee kinematics and ligament stability are restored. CAS techniques make it possible to determine the presurgical kinematic relationships and ligamentous stability of the knee and help guide the surgeon to restore the desired kinematic relationships and ligamentous balance.

Finally, CAS provides a unique and unprecedented opportunity to train residents and orthopedic surgeons to perform knee reconstruction procedures accurately.[68,106,113] The use of CAS as a training tool is in its infancy. However, applications have been developed and are now being used to allow surgeons to carry out self-assessment evaluations of their surgical skills for performing TKA and ACL surgery. Applications are also being developed to test the skills of surgeons and residents to learn various knee reconstruction procedures. It may be that the most compelling rationale for applying CAS to knee reconstruction will prove to be the potential to revolutionize the way that surgeons develop and evaluate their surgical skills.

HARDWARE AND SOFTWARE REQUIREMENTS FOR SURGICAL NAVIGATION

A detailed description of the hardware and software needed to perform computer-assisted reconstructive knee surgery is beyond the scope of this chapter. However, it is important that knee surgeons understand the basic components of a computer-assisted orthopedic system so that they can use the system correctly, safely, and efficiently and can make intelligent choices regarding the appropriateness of various systems for their surgical needs.

Hardware devices common to CAS systems are (1) imaging devices; (2) computers, peripherals, and interfaces to allow them to function in the operating room; and (3) localizers and trackers (see Fig. 95–1A and B).

The imaging devices that are currently available for use with computer-assisted orthopedic surgery systems include computed tomography, magnetic resonance imaging, and fluoroscopy machines. These devices are used to acquire the anatomic information on which a presurgical or intraoperative surgical plan is formulated. This plan becomes the basis for placing cutting tools intraoperatively and for establishing the alignment and stability of the knee. Though potentially extremely useful for knee reconstruction surgery, especially for robotic or customized surgery, imaging devices as currently used with CAS knee systems have been perceived by surgeons as adding additional and cumbersome steps to well-established knee procedures without providing significant benefits. Consequently, image-free computer-assisted systems have emerged as the most desired form of CAS for knee reconstruction. As a result, the role of imaging when image-free CAS systems are used remains largely identical to its role when CAS is not used. Imaging is used preoperatively to develop a plan (e.g., applying a goniometer on a long, standing anteroposterior radiograph to determine the desired frontal alignment) and postoperatively to assess the results of the procedure.

The computers used in CAS are obviously the core of these systems. They integrate information from medical images, implant data, intraoperative tracking, and surgical plans to guide the surgeon in the performance of a knee procedure. The speed of computing, memory, storage capacity, and communication ability with peripherals have reached a level where even midrange, less expensive personal computers can satisfy the needs of image-free CAS knee applications. All current CAS knee applications use a range of platforms based usually on either the UNIX or Windows operating systems. It is likely that applications will soon be written on the open Linux operating system. The computers are currently mounted on transportable carts (or operating room booms) that include the computer, monitor, key board, mouse, power transformer and isolation unit, and tracker controller unit with ports to plug in the tracker and tracking markers. Communication between the surgeon and computer is necessary for continuous monitoring of the procedure. This communication can be achieved with single or double foot pedals, keypads, touch screens, pointer-integrated controls, or voice-activated controls (see Fig. 95–1A).

A CAS knee navigation system can be thought of as an aiming device that enables real-time visualization of surgical action with an image of the operated structures. For this navigation to occur, it is necessary that the position and orientation of an instrument be visualized with respect to the anatomic structures to which it is attached. Although this objective could be met by attaching tools to a rigid, multilinked arm attached to a pedestal, such a device would be unsuitable for knee surgery, where the limb must be freely moved. Therefore, contactless systems are used to communicate between the extremity and the computer system. Information can be transmitted by infrared light, electromagnetic fields, or ultrasound. Each method has its advantages and drawbacks. All these methods allow several objects (e.g., two bones) to be viewed simultaneously.

Optical localization via infrared light is currently the most widely used method of communication between the operated extremity and computer. Two types of optical tracking are used, active and passive. Systems with active tracking use markers (also called trackers or rigid bodies) with LEDs that send out light pulses to a camera (optical localizer). Three or (for redundancy) more of these LEDs are attached to screws or wires that are rigidly attached to the femur and tibia. The camera system to which the light is sent consists of two planar or three linear CCDs that are rigidly mounted onto a solid housing (the Polaris System, Northern Digital, is a commonly used camera system). Passive systems use reflecting spheres placed on tracking markers that are attached to screws or pins rigidly implanted in the femur and tibia. Infrared flashes sent by LED arrays on the camera housing illuminate the spheres. The two planar or three linear CCDs observe the reflections and interpolate the spatial location of each light source. It is important for surgeons and their staff to realize that the arrays on the tracking markers, whether active or passive, are specific to each CAS system. One company's trackers cannot be used on another company's CAS system, even though the trackers may appear to be similar (see Fig. 95–1A and B).

The advantages of optical localizing systems are that they are reliable, flexible, and highly accurate and have good operating room compatibility. A disadvantage of these systems is that it is necessary to provide free line of sight between the LED/spheres and the CCD arrays on the camera (optical localizer). Active trackers may require cables to power and synchronize the LEDs. These cables may be cumbersome. Active trackers can be driven by batteries, which eliminates the need for cables, but these batteries require recharging, thus making their use for sequential procedures more difficult. Passive trackers do not require cords. However, automatic tool identification is more difficult for passive systems because all spheres in view reflect the light flashes equally. Unique identification of each tracker is possible with the sequentially pulsed LEDs of active trackers. The reflecting spheres must constantly be kept clean to obtain accurate signal transmission. Moreover, the spheres are disposable and therefore a source of additional per-case expense.

Magnetic fields can be used to measure the position and orientation of objects in space. A generator coil is used to erect a homogeneous magnetic field. Specially designed "coils" can be implanted into the femur and tibia or attached to tools. These coils measure the changes in magnetic field characteristics during performance of the procedure. The computer can integrate these changes with the implant data and surgical plans to guide the surgeon in the performance of a knee procedure. These systems have a number of potential advantages. The equipment

("coils") attached to the bones and tools can be small, and the accuracy of many systems is very good. The need for a camera and its associated "line-of-sight" requirement is eliminated. However, the presence of ferromagnetic items such as implants, instruments, and operating room equipment made of steel can disturb precise measurements dramatically and in *unpredictable* ways. Moreover, the coils are disposable and therefore a source of additional per-case expense.

Ultrasonic-based navigation systems measure the duration that a sound impulse needs to travel between the emitter and microphone. Calculation of the position of each tracked object is based on the speed of sound. Though technically feasible, these systems require delicate calibration. Precision depends on the speed of sound, which may vary with differences in temperature. Sterilization of ultrasonic equipment can also be difficult.[59]

The function of software in CAS systems is to integrate medical images and mathematic algorithms with surgical tools and surgical techniques. A relatively small number of software components underlie most CAS image-free systems. These components include registration, navigation, procedure guidance, and safety.

Image-free CAS knee systems use as their preoperative plan the concepts of limb and implant alignment that are currently used with manual instrumentation (e.g., restoration of the mechanical axis). To accomplish this plan, anatomic and kinematic information about a patient must be transmitted to the software on the computer and geometrically transformed by registration algorithms. Because bones are rigid and assumed to be unlikely to deform during the procedure, the algorithms used are termed *rigid*. These algorithms also require that the trackers attached to bones do not move during the procedure. Fiducial-based registration is a type of rigid registration. Therefore, the objects to which the LEDs are attached may be referred to as fiducials, trackers, or rigid bodies. Fiducial registration requires that at least three sets of markers be implanted into each bone or attached to each tool to determine the object's position and orientation. Therefore, each tracker must have at least three LEDs or reflecting spheres. Some CAS knee systems currently use shaped-based registration as an alternative to fiducial-based registration. These systems measure the shape of the bone surface intraoperatively and match the acquired shape to a surface model created from medical images stored in the computer. The registration process for image-free knee navigation systems requires that information be acquired via kinematic techniques (e.g., circumducting the leg to determine the center of the femoral head) or surface registration techniques (e.g., touching bone landmarks with a probe).

Once the software takes anatomic and kinematic input from the extremity and geometrically transforms it, the surgeon is presented with a user interface that depicts in sequence the steps of the knee procedure. One of the most important objectives of software development in CAS knee applications is to depict procedure sequences that are familiar to surgeons and with which they have previously become comfortable with the use of manual instrumentation.

A TYPICAL IMAGE-FREE COMPUTER-ASSISTED SURGICAL TECHNIQUE FOR TOTAL KNEE ARTHROPLASTY

CAS technologies require that surgeons incorporate new tools into surgical routines with which they are experienced and comfortable. In fact, the most successful application of CAS occurs when surgeons are very familiar with all aspects of the procedure in which CAS is used. Although the details of CAS application for one knee procedure (e.g., TKA) vary from those of another knee procedure (e.g., ACL reconstruction), the basic principles and intraoperative steps are very similar for all of them. Because the TKA image-free CAS application is currently the most rapidly developing and most widely used, a brief description of a typical computer-assisted TKA will be described. It is important for surgeons to understand that the goal of CAS is to increase the accuracy and reproducibility with which the objectives of current mechanical alignment systems are achieved.

Image-free CAS techniques do not require any special preoperative planning. The methods that surgeons normally use to determine the desired frontal and sagittal limb and implant alignment and implant size can be used to guide intraoperative use of the CAS system. Mechanical alignment and CAS techniques use similar approaches for patient positioning and surgical exposure. Leg holders and pneumatic tourniquets, which are routinely used with mechanical instrumentation, can also be used with CAS.

The initial step in computer-assisted TKA is placement of screws or pins in the distal femur and proximal tibia, to which are attached the trackers (see Fig. 95–1B). They are placed outside the skin incision in a position that avoids injury to neurovascular structures and allows clear visualization of the trackers by the camera. Once the skin incision is made and the distal femur and proximal tibia are exposed, the anatomic landmarks critical for CAS-guided navigation are located. The center of the femoral head is determined with a kinematic registration technique (Fig. 95–2A and B). The hip is circumducted in a path guided by the visual cues displayed on the computer screen. The centers of the knee and ankle joint can be established by kinematic (Fig. 95–2C to F) or surface (Fig. 95–3A to I) registration techniques or by a combination of both. The other anatomic landmarks located with a CAS probe are (1) the distal end of the femur (Fig. 95–3D and E), (2) the posterior condylar line (Fig. 95–3D and E), (3) the anterior femoral cortex (Fig. 95–3F), (4) the epicondylar axis, and (5) the medial and lateral tibial articular surfaces (Fig. 95–3G to I). Presurgical frontal and sagittal alignment, medial-lateral laxity in flexion and extension, and range of motion can then be measured and recorded (Fig. 95–4).

Both ligament-balancing techniques (similar to those first described by Insall[30]) and anatomic approaches[29] can be used with computer-assisted TKA techniques. As with mechanically based techniques, the CAS anatomic procedures can begin with either the femoral or the tibial prepa-

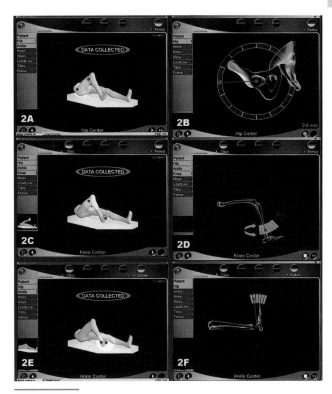

Figure 95–2. Computer interfaces illustrating the motion necessary to acquire adequate kinematic information to establish the location of the center of the hip joint (**2A** and **2B**), the knee joint (**2C** and **2D**), and the ankle joint (**2E** and **2F**).

ration. In the example illustrated, the distal end of the femur is first resected by placing a distal femoral cutting block with attached tracker on the anterior cortex of the femur. The proximal-distal, varus-valgus, and flexion-extension position of this block is guided by the CAS system (Fig. 95–5A and B). CAS determination of femoral implant size and anterior-posterior placement can be made by using either anterior or posterior referencing techniques. Rotation of the femoral component can be established with CAS by using the posterior condylar line, the epicondylar line, or the patellar groove (Whiteside's line). A single navigation tool can be used to establish all these femoral alignment and sizing objectives (Fig. 95–6A and B). The tibial cutting block, to which a tracker is attached, is placed in the desired position of varus-valgus and flexion-extension and at the desired resection level guided by the CAS system (Fig. 95–7A and B).

Once the femoral and tibial resections are completed, a trial reduction is carried out. The polyethylene insert that best balances the knee in flexion and extension is selected. The navigation system is used to measure the final alignment of the extremity, the amount of medial-lateral laxity in extension and flexion, and the final range of motion. The system can be used to guide the release of tight soft tissues medially, laterally, and posteriorly if necessary to establish a balanced, well-aligned knee. After the actual implants are inserted, the navigation system is used to

Text continued on p. 1684

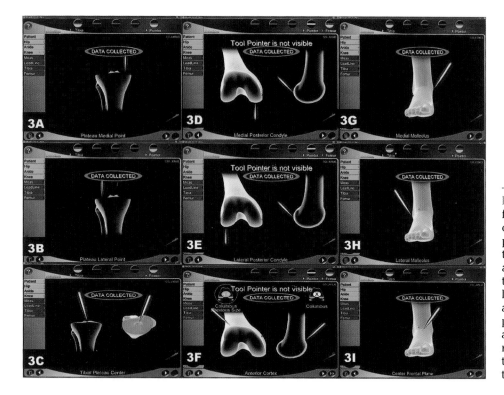

Figure 95–3. Computer interfaces illustrating the position of the surface registration pointer necessary to acquire the tibial medial and lateral articular surfaces and the tibial midpoint (**3A** to **3C**), the location of the distal femoral articular surfaces and the posterior condylar line (**3D** and **3E**), the location of anterior femoral cortex (**3F**), and the location of the center of the ankle joint (**3G** to **3I**).

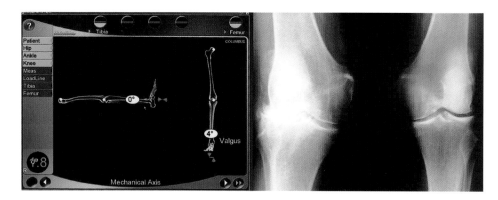

Figure 95–4. The presurgical alignment depicted on the computer screen correlates with the alignment seen on the standing preoperative radiograph.

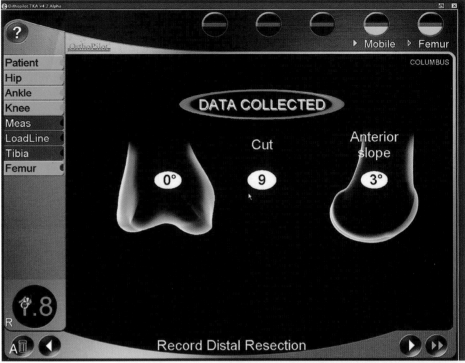

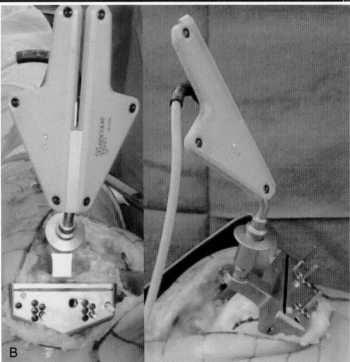

Figure 95–5. Resection of the distal end of the femur. **A,** Computer interface indicating the position of the distal femoral cutting block with regard to the frontal (0 degrees) and sagittal (3 degrees of anterior slope) mechanical alignment and the depth of resection (9 mm). **B,** Frontal and sagittal position of the distal femoral cutting block with attached tracker.

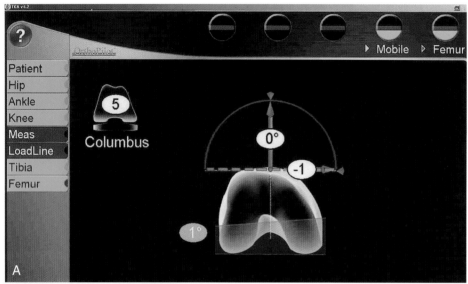

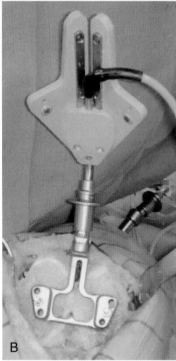

Figure 95–6. Establishing the position of the 4 in 1 femoral cutting block. **A,** Computer interface indicating rotation (0 degrees relative to Whiteside's line) of the cutting block and anterior-posterior position of (in this case, the number 5) the femoral component (1 mm above the anterior cortex). **B,** Navigation tool with attached tracker to establish rotation and anterior-posterior position of the 4 in 1 femoral cutting block.

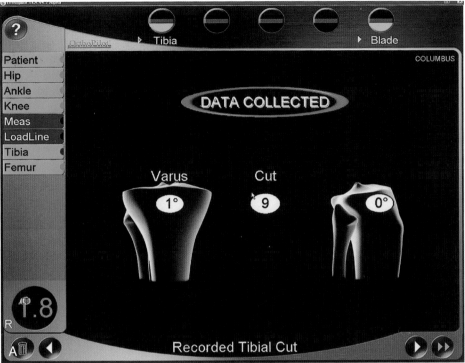

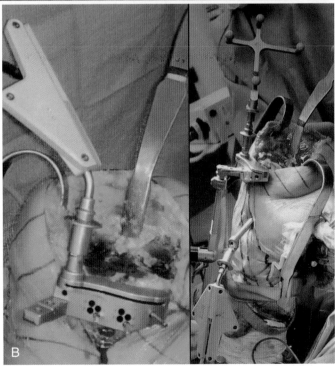

Figure 95–7. Resection of the proximal end of the tibia. **A,** Computer interface indicating the position of the proximal tibial cutting block with regard to frontal (1 degree of varus) and sagittal (0 degrees) mechanical alignment and the depth of resection from the least involved tibial surface (9 mm). **B,** Frontal and sagittal position of the proximal tibial cutting block with attached tracker.

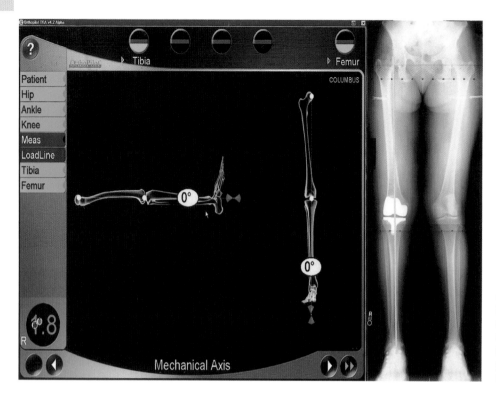

Figure 95–8. The final frontal and sagittal alignment depicted on the computer screen correlates with the postoperative standing long radiograph.

measure the final frontal and sagittal alignment of the extremity, the final medial-lateral stability, and the final range of motion (Fig. 95–8).

CLINICAL RESULTS OF COMPUTER-ASSISTED SURGERY FOR KNEE RECONSTRUCTION

Total Knee Arthroplasty

Since performance of the first image-free computer-assisted TKA in 1997, a number of centers have evaluated the clinical safety, efficacy, and usefulness of a variety of CAS image-free systems. These reports have described the (1) accuracy of limb and implant alignment associated with the use of these systems, (2) the accuracy of these systems relative to mechanical alignment systems, and (3) the usefulness of this technology as a measurement tool for assessing the accuracy with which each step of the TKA procedure is performed.

The initial studies by the developers of the various image-free TKA systems consistently report the following:
1. The systems are safe. Only rare complications directly attributable to use of the systems have been reported. Their use does not increase the incidence of complications such as deep vein thrombosis, wound-healing problems, or excessive bleeding and does not alter the perioperative management or course.
2. Limb alignment in the frontal plane is as accurate or more accurate with CAS TKA systems than with mechanical systems.
3. Limb alignment in the sagittal plane is more accurate with CAS TKA systems than with mechanical systems. Limb alignment in the sagittal plane is difficult to visually assess accurately intraoperatively.
4. Individual implant alignment is more accurate with CAS TKA than with mechanical systems.
5. There are fewer limb and implant "outliers" (i.e., alignment results outside the desired range) with CAS TKA systems than with mechanical systems.
6. The number of cases needed to become proficient in the use of CAS TKA (the CAS TKA "learning curve") is decreasing as systems evolve and seems to be 10 to 20.
7. The average increase in operating time when CAS is used is 15 to 30 minutes and decreases rapidly with increased frequency of use.

None of these studies by the developers is randomized. Most use historical controls to compare CAS TKA with mechanical TKA results.*

An increasing number of studies of CAS TKA systems performed by nondevelopers are beginning to appear in the literature. These studies, in general, confirm the findings of the developers.†

Studies using CAS intraoperatively to examine the accuracy with which each step of manual TKA procedures is performed have reported the following[11,50,99-103]:
1. Intramedullary femoral and extramedullary tibial instrumentation is consistent (within 3 degrees) and accurate in the frontal plane, but inconsistent and inaccurate in the sagittal plane.
2. It is difficult to accurately and consistently palpate the posterior femoral condyles and epicondyles with

*References 8, 10, 12, 19, 23, 25, 35, 36, 48, 49, 51, 64, 65, 67, 68, 71, 72, 80, 87- 89, 91, 93, 94.
†References 4, 5, 7, 27, 53, 63, 73, 97, 98, 105-110, 118, 119.

either mechanical or CAS instrumentation. Therefore, the femoral posterior condylar axis and the epicondylar axis are difficult to precisely define in an arthritic knee during the performance of TKA.

3. When cutting blocks are attached to bones with pins inserted manually, substantial movement of the block occurs. This movement is eliminated when pins are inserted with power.

4. Saw blades deflect into extension by 1 to 2 degrees when the distal femur and proximal tibia are resected with a stiff saw blade, even when it fits precisely within a cutting slot. This deflection significantly increases when the saw blade does not fit in the slot precisely, is flexible, or is used on a block without a slot.

5. Resecting the femur or tibia from a position other than the frontal midline (e.g., as in certain "quadrant-sparing" procedures) may introduce significant error, especially if the cutting blocks are placed in a posteriorly sloped position.

Unicompartmental Arthroplasty, Anterior Cruciate Ligament Reconstruction, High Tibial Osteotomy

The application of CAS to unicompartmental knee arthroplasty (UKA), ACL reconstruction, and high tibial osteotomy (HTO) is still in a relatively early stage of development. However, initial reports by the developers of these applications are extremely encouraging.* As with CAS TKA studies, these initial reports indicate that the overall accuracy of implant and limb alignment is improved, the accuracy of individual implant alignment is increased, and the incidence of "outliers" is reduced when CAS techniques are used. Acceptance of these CAS applications for knee surgery is likely to be more widespread in the next few years.

THE FUTURE OF COMPUTER-ASSISTED SURGERY IN KNEE RECONSTRUCTION

There is surprisingly wide acceptance of the idea that at some point in the future, navigation systems will be an accepted part of the knee surgeon's armamentarium. However, until the systems become more surgeon friendly, less cumbersome, more efficient, and less expensive, the widespread acceptance of CAS by knee surgeons may be limited. Many developments currently in progress may accelerate this acceptance.

CAS systems now exist and will continue to be refined to allow multiple knee procedures (i.e., TKA, UKA, ACL reconstruction, HTO) to be performed by a single CAS unit with a common set of computer hardware and software and a common user interface. These knee suites will facilitate the use of a single CAS system by surgeons performing a wide range of knee procedures.[102] The effort

needed to learn how to use one system for one application will not need to be repeated when the system is used for other knee applications. The use of a single CAS system to perform multiple knee procedures will also make more justifiable the substantial financial outlay required for the units.

The price of the hardware components of CAS systems is also likely to decrease significantly. As the number of users of CAS technologies increases, the source of hardware components (e.g., optical trackers) will increase and thus put downward pressure on prices. The consolidation of orthopedic companies has resulted in each offering the full array of knee procedures, from arthroscopy to complex arthroplasty reconstructions. As these companies integrate and support the CAS systems for these procedures, the cost of these units to hospitals should also drop.

Developments that are most likely to increase the use of CAS systems by knee surgeons are those that further integrate surgeons' current techniques with navigation techniques. Wireless systems using a technology such as electromagnetism would eliminate the current aggravations of having to maintain line of sight between the computer and operated extremity, decrease the bulkiness of current navigation equipment, and reduce concern regarding intraoperative tracker movement, bone fracture, or neurovascular injuries. However, as these systems become available, their safety and accuracy must be confirmed. These systems must be equal in safety and accuracy to the optical systems currently available.

Perhaps the most immediate benefit of CAS knee systems will be the development of more accurate mechanical tools. The influence of CAS on mechanical instrumentation is already being felt. Most knee surgery systems now require that cutting blocks be affixed to bone with power-driven pins. Anterior referencing for the establishment of femoral rotation is increasing in popularity. Jigs are being developed to improve the positioning of cutting blocks in the sagittal plane, the source of the most consistent error in TKA implant and limb alignment.

Finally, the widespread interest in minimally invasive arthroplasty surgery is focusing surgeons' attention on the importance of retaining accurate implant and limb alignment as exposure of surgical anatomy is reduced.[115] Techniques using nonfrontal resection planes (e.g., the "quadrant-sparing" medial approach) are making clear how the position of an implant in one plane critically affects its position in all other planes.[104] CAS systems have the potential for greatly facilitating the evolution of minimally invasive knee surgery. However, the CAS hardware and software must be configured to safely, accurately, and efficiently support the minimally invasive systems that are being developed.

References

1. Aglietti P, Buzzi R: Posteriorly stabilized total-condylar knee replacement. J Bone Joint Surg 211-216, 1988.
2. Ayers DC, Dennis DA, Johanson NA, et al: Common complications of total knee arthroplasty. J Bone Joint Surg Am 79:278-311, 1997.
3. Bargren JH, Blaha JD, Freeman MAR: Alignment in total knee arthroplasty: Correlated biomechanical and clinical observations. Clin Orthop 173:178-183, 1983.

*References 13, 14, 17, 18, 37, 38, 40, 42, 43, 47, 74, 81, 90.

4. Bathis H, Perlick L, Luring C, et al: [CT-based and CT-free navigation in knee prosthesis implantation. Results of a prospective study.] Unfallchirurg 106:935-940, 2003.

5. Bathis H, Perlick L, Tingart M, et al: Radiological results of image-based and non–image-based computer-assisted total knee arthroplasty. Int Orthop 28:87-90, 2004.

6. Berger RA, Crosset LS, Jacobs JJ: Malrotation causing patellofemoral complications after total knee arthroplasty. Clin Orthop 356:144-153, 1998.

7. Bohler M, Messner M, Glos W, Riegler M: Computer navigated implantation of total knee prostheses: A radiological study. Acta Chir Aust 33(Suppl):63, 2000.

8. Briard JL, Stindel E, Plaweski S, et al: CT free navigation with the LCS Surgetics Station: A new way of balancing the soft tissues in TKA based on bone morphing. In Steihl JB, Konermann WH, Haaker RG (eds): Navigation and Robotics in Total Joint and Spine Surgery. Berlin, Springer-Verlag, 2004, pp 274-280.

9. Cartier P, Sanouillier JL, Frelsamer RP: Unicompartmental knee arthroplasty surgery. 10-year minimum follow-up period. J Arthroplasty 11:782-788, 1996.

10. Clemens U, Konermann WH, Kohler S, et al: Computer-assisted navigation with the OrthoPilot system using the search evolution TKA prosthesis. In Steihl JB, Konermann WH, Haaker RG (eds): Navigation and Robotics in Total Joint and Spine Surgery. Berlin, Springer-Verlag, 2004, pp 236-241.

11. Currie J, Varshney A, Stulberg SD, et al: The reliability of anatomic landmarks for determining femoral implant rotation in TKA surgery: Implications for CAOS TKA. Presented at the Annual Meeting of the Mid-America Orthopaedic Association, 2005, Amelia Island, FL.

12. Delp SL, Stulberg SD, Davies B, et al: Computer assisted knee replacement. Clin Orthop 354:49-56, 1998.

13. DeRycke J: Clinical experiences for ACL-repair with the SurgiGATE system. In Steihl JB, Konermann WH, Haaker RG (eds): Navigation and Robotics in Total Joint and Spine Surgery. Berlin, Springer-Verlag, 2004, pp 397-399.

14. Dessenne V, Lavallee S, Julliard R, et al: Computer assisted anterior cruciate ligament reconstruction: First clinical tests. J Image Guided Surg 1:59-64, 1995.

15. Dorr LD, Boiardo RA: Technical considerations in total knee arthroplasty. Clin Orthop 205:5-11, 1997.

16. Ecker ML, Lotke PA, Windsor RE, et al: Long-term results after total condylar knee arthroplasty. Significance of radiolucent lines. Clin Orthop 216:151-158, 1987.

17. Eichorn H-J: Image-free navigation in ACL replacement with the OrthoPilot system. In Steihl JB, Konermann WH, Haaker RG (eds): Navigation and Robotics in Total Joint and Spine Surgery. Berlin, Springer-Verlag, 2004, pp 387-396.

18. Ellis RE, Rudan JF, Harrison MM: Computer-assisted high tibial osteotomies. In DiGioia AM, Jaramaz B, Picard R, Nolte PL (eds): Computer and Robotic Assisted Knee and Hip Surgery. Oxford, Oxford University Press, 2004, pp 197-212.

19. Fadda M, Bertelli, D, Martelli S, et al: Computer assisted planning for total knee arthroplasty. In Proceedings of the First Joint Conference on Computer Vision, Virtual Reality and Robotics in Medicine and Medial Robotics and Computer Assisted Surgery. Grenoble, France, Springer, 1997, pp 619-628.

20. Fehring TK, Odum S, Griffin WL, et al: Early failures in total knee arthroplasty. Clin Orthop 392:315-318, 2001.

21. Feng EL, Stulberg SD, Wixson RL: Progressive subluxation and polyethylene wear in total knee replacements with flat articular surfaces. Clin Orthop 299:60-71, 1994.

22. Froemel M, Portheine F, Ebner M, Radermacher K: Computer assisted template based navigation for total knee replacement. Presented at the North American Program on Computer Assisted Orthopaedic Surgery, July 6-8, 2001, Pittsburgh.

23. Fuiko R, Kotten B, Zettl R, Ritschl P: [The accuracy of palpation from orientation points for the navigated implantation of knee prostheses.] Orthopade 33:338-343, 2004.

24. Garbini JL, Kaiura RG, Sidles JA, et al: Robotic instrumentation in total knee arthroplasty. Presented at the 33rd Annual Meeting of the Orthopaedic Research Society, January 19-22, 1987, San Francisco.

25. Garg A, Walker PS: Prediction of total knee motion using a three-dimensional computer graphics model. J Biochem 23:45-58, 1990.

26. Goodfellow JW, O'Connor JJ: Clinical results of the Oxford knee. Clin Orthop 205:21-24, 1986.

27. Hart R, Janecek M, Chaker A, Bucek P: Total knee arthroplasty implanted with and without kinematic navigation. Int Orthop 27:366-369, 2003.

28. Hsu HP, Garg A, Walker PS, et al: Effect of knee component alignment on tibial load distribution with clinical correlation. Clin Orthop 248:135-144, 1989.

29. Hungerford DS, Kenna RV: Preliminary experience with a total knee prosthesis with porous coating used without cement. Clin Orthop 255:215-227, 1990.

30. Insall JW: Surgical approaches to the knee. In Insall JN (ed): Surgery of the Knee. New York, Churchill Livingstone, pp 4-54.

31. Insall JN, Binzzir R, Soudry M, Mestriner LA: Total knee arthroplasty. Clin Orthop 192:13-22, 1985.

32. Insall JN, Ranawat CS, Aglietti P, Shine J: A comparison of four models of total knee-replacement prosthesis. J Bone Joint Surg Am 58:754-765, 1976.

33. Jeffcote B, Shakespeare D: Varus/valgus alignment of the tibial component in total knee arthroplasty. Knee 10:243-247, 2003.

34. Jeffery RS, Morris RW, Denham RA: Coronal alignment after total knee replacement. J Bone Joint Surg Br 73:709-714, 1991.

35. Jenny JY, Boeri C: Computer-assisted total knee prosthesis implantation without preoperative imaging. A comparison with classical instrumentaiton. Presented at the Fourth Annual North American Program on Computer Assisted Orthopaedic Surgery, 2000, Pittsburgh.

36. Jenny JY, Boeri C: Navigated implantation of total knee prostheses: A comparison with conventional techniques. Orthop Ihre Grenzgeb 139:117-119, 2001.

37. Jenny JY, Boeri C: Implantation d'une prothese totale de genou assistee par ordinateur. Etude comparative cas-temoin avec une instrumentaiton traditionnelle. Rev Chir Orthop 87:645-652, 2001.

38. Jenny JY, Boeri C: Unicompartmental knee prosthesis. A case-control comparative study of two types of instrumentation with a five year follow-up. J Arthroplasty 17:1016-1020, 2002.

39. Jenny JY, Boeri C: Low reproducibility of the intra-operative measurement of the transepicondylar axis during total knee replacement. Acta Orthop Scand 75:74-77, 2004.

40. Jenny JY, Boeri C: Unicompartmental knee prosthesis implantation with a non–image based navigation system. In DiGioia AM, Jaramaz B, Picard R, Nolte PL (eds): Computer and Robotic Assisted Knee and Hip Surgery. Oxford, Oxford University Press, 2004, pp 179-188.

41. Jiang CC, Insall JN: Effect of rotation on the axial alignment of the femur. Clin Orthop 248:50-56, 1989.

42. Julliard R, Lavallee S, Dessenne V: Computer assisted anterior cruciate ligament reconstruction of the anterior cruciate ligament. Clin Orthop 354:57-64, 1998.

43. Julliard R, Plaweski S, Lavallee S: ACL Surgetics: An efficient computer-assisted technique for ACL reconstruction. In Steihl JB, Konermann WH, Haaker RG (eds): Navigation and Robotics in Total Joint and Spine Surgery. Berlin, Springer-Verlag, 2004, pp 405-411.

44. Kaiura RG: Robot Assisted Total Knee Arthroplasty Investigation of the Feasibility and Accuracy of the Robotic Process. Master's Thesis, Mechanical Engineering, University of Washington, 1986.

45. Kienzle TC, Stulberg SD, Peshkin M, et al: A computer-assisted total knee replacement surgical system using a calibrated robot. Orthopaedics. In Taylor RH, et al (eds): Computer Integrated Surgery. Cambridge, MA, MIT Press, 1996, pp 409-416.

46. Kinzel V, Scaddan M, Bradley B, Shakespeare D: Varus/valgus alignment of the femur in total knee arthroplasty. Can accuracy be improved by pre-operative CT scanning? Knee 11:197-201, 2004.

47. Klos TVS, Habets RJE, Banks AZ, et al: Computer assistance in arthroscopic anterior cruciate ligament reconstruction. In DiGioia AM, Jaramaz B, Picard R, Nolte PL (eds): Computer and Robotic Assisted Knee and Hip Surgery. Oxford, Oxford University Press, 2004, pp 229-234.

48. Konermann WH, Kistner S: CT-free navigation including soft-tissue balancing: LCS-TKA and Vector Vision Systems. In Steihl JB, Konermann WH, Haaker RG (eds): Navigation and Robotics in Total Joint and Spine Surgery. Berlin, Springer-Verlag, 2004, pp 256-265.

49. Konermann WH, Sauer MA: Postoperative alignment of conventional and navigated total knee arthroplasty. In Steihl JB, Koner-

mann WH, Haaker RG (eds): Navigation and Robotics in Total Joint and Spine Surgery. Berlin, Springer-Verlag, 2004, pp 219-225.

50. Koyonos L, Granieri M, Stulberg SD: At what steps in performance of a TKA do errors occur when manual instrumentation is used. Presented at the Annual Meeting of the American Academy of Orthopaedic Surgeons, 2005, Washington, DC.

51. Krackow K, Serpe L, Phillips MJ, et al: A new technique for determining proper mechanical axis alignment during total knee arthroplasty. Orthopedics 22:698-701, 1999.

52. Kuntz M, Sati M, Nolte LP, et al: Computer assisted total knee arthroplasty. Presented at the First International Symposium on Computer-Assisted Orthopaedic Surgery, February 17-19, 2000, Davos, Switzerland.

53. Lampe F, Hille E: Navigated implantation of the Columbus total knee arthroplasty with the OrthoPilot System: Version 4.0. In Steihl JB, Konermann WH, Haaker RG (eds): Navigation and Robotics in Total Joint and Spine Surgery. Berlin, Springer-Verlag, 2004, pp 248-253.

54. Laskin RS: Total condylar knee replacement in rheumatoid arthritis. A review of one hundred and seventeen knees. J Bone Joint Surg Am 63:29-35, 1981.

55. Laskin RS: Alignment of the total knee components. Orthopedics 7:62, 1984.

56. Laskin RS, Turtel A: The use of an intramedullary tibial alignment guide in total knee replacement arthroplasty. Am J Knee Surg 2:123, 1989.

57. Leitner F, Picard F, Minfelde R, et al: Computer-assisted knee surgical total replacement. In Proceedings of the First Joint Conference on Computer Vision, Virtual Reality and Robotics in Medicine and Medial Robotics and Computer Assisted Surgery. Grenoble, France, Springer, 1997, pp 629-638.

58. Lootvoet L, Burton P, Himmer O, et al: Protheses unicompartimentales de genou: Influence du positionnement du plateau tibial sur les resultants fonctionnels. Acta Orthop Belg 63:94-101, 1997.

59. Macher C, Liebing M, Lazovic D, Overhoff HM: Pilot study of total knee arthroplasty planning by use of 3-D ultrasound image volumes. Stud Health Technol Inform 77:1175-1179, 2000.

60. Mahfouz MR, Hoff WA, Komistek RD, Dennis DA: A robust method for registration of three-dimensional knee implant models to two-dimensional fluoroscopy images. IEEE Trans Med Imaging 22:1561-1574, 2003.

61. Martelli M, Marcacci M, Nofrini L, et al: Computer- and robot-assisted total knee replacement: Analysis of a new surgical procedure. Ann Biomed Eng 28:1146-1153, 2000.

62. Matsen FA, Garbini JL, Sidles JA: Robotic assistance in orthopaedic surgery. A proof of principle using distal femoral arthroplasty. Clin Orthop 296:178-186, 1993.

63. Mattes T, Puhl W: Navigation in TKA with the Navitrack System. In Steihl JB, Konermann WH, Haaker RG (eds): Navigation and Robotics in Total Joint and Spine Surgery. Berlin, Springer-Verlag, 2004, pp 293-300.

64. Miehlke RK, Clemens U, Jens J-H, Kershally S: Navigation in knee arthroplasty: Preliminary clinical experience and prospective comparative study in comparison with conventional technique. Orthop Ihre Grenzgeb 139:1109-1129, 2001.

65. Miehlke RK, Clemens U, Kershally S: Computer integrated instrumentation in knee arthroplasty: A comparative study of conventional and computerized technique. Presented at the Fourth Annual North American Program on Computer Assisted Orthopaedic Surgery, 2000, Pittsburgh, pp 93-96.

66. Nishihara S, Sugano N, Ikai M, et al: Accuracy evaluation of a shape-based registration method for a computer navigation system for total knee arthroplasty. J Knee Surg 16:98-105, 2003.

67. Nizard R: Computer assisted surgery for total knee arthroplasty. Acta Orthop Belg 68:215-230, 2002.

68. Noble PC, Sugano N, Johnston JD, et al: Computer simulation: How can it help the surgeon optimize implant position? Clin Orthop 417:242-252, 2003.

69. Nuno-Siebrecht N, Tanzer M, Bobyn JD: Potential errors in axial alignment using intramedullary instrumentation for total knee arthroplasty. J Arthroplasty 15:228-230, 2000.

70. Oswald MH, Jacob RP, Schneider E, Hoogewoud H: Radiological analysis of normal axial alignment of femur and tibia in view of total knee arthroplasty. J Arthroplasty 8:419-426, 1993.

71. Perlick L, Bathis H, Luring C, et al: CT based and CT-free navigation with the BrainLAB VectorVision System in total knee arthroplasty. In Steihl JB, Konermann WH, Haaker RG (eds): Navigation and Robotics in Total Joint and Spine Surgery. Berlin, Springer-Verlag, 2004, pp 304-310.

72. Perlick L, Bathis H, Tingart M, et al: [Usability of an image based navigation system in reconstruction of leg alignment in total knee arthroplasty—results of a prospective study.] Biomed Tech (Berl) 48:339-343, 2003.

73. Perlick L, Bathis H, Tingart M, et al: Navigation in total-knee arthroplasty: CT-based implantation compared with the conventional technique. Acta Orthop Scand 75:464-470, 2004.

74. Peterman J, Kober R, Heinze, R, et al: Computer-assisted planning and robot assisted surgery in anterior cruciate ligament reconstruction. Op Tech Orthop 10:50-55, 2000.

75. Petersen TL, Engh GA: Radiographic assessment of knee alignment after total knee arthroplasty. J Arthroplasty 3:67-72, 1988.

76. Piazza SJ, Delp SL, Stulberg SD, Stern SJ: Posterior tilting of the tibial component decreases femoral rollback in posterior-substituting knee replacement. J Orthop Res 16:264-270, 1998.

77. Picard F, Leitner F, Raoult O, Saragaglia D: Computer assisted knee replacement. Location of a rotational center of the knee. Total knee arthroplasty. Presented at the First International Symposium on Computer-Assisted Orthopaedic Surgery, February 17-19, 2000, Davos, Switzerland.

78. Picard F, Leitner F, Raoult O, et al: Clinical evaluation of computer assisted total knee arthroplasty. Presented at the Second Annual North American Program on Computer Assisted Orthopaedic Surgery, 1998, Pittsburgh, pp 239-249.

79. Picard F, Moody JE, DiGioia, AM, et al: History of computer-assisted orthopaedic surgery of hip and knee. In DiGioia AM, Jaramaz B, Picard R, Nolte PL (eds): Computer and Robotic Assisted Knee and Hip Surgery. Oxford, Oxford University Press, 2004, pp 1-22.

80. Picard F, Moody JE, DiGioia AM, et al: Knee reconstructive surgery: Preoperative model system. In DiGioia AM, Jaramaz B, Picard R, Nolte PL (eds): Computer and Robotic Assisted Knee and Hip Surgery. Oxford, Oxford University Press, 2004, pp 139-156.

81. Picard, F, Moody JE, DiGioia AM, et al: ACL reconstruction—preoperative model system. In DiGioia AM, Jaramaz B, Picard R, Nolte PL (eds): Computer and Robotic Assisted Knee and Hip Surgery. Oxford, Oxford University Press, 2004, pp 213-228.

82. Radermacher K, Staudte HW, Rau G: Computer assisted orthopaedic surgery with image-based individual templates. Clin Orthop 354:28-38, 1998.

83. Ranawat CS, Boachie-Adjei O: Survivorship analysis and results of total condylar knee arthroplasty. Clin Orthop 226:6-13, 1988.

84. Rand JA, Coventry MB: Evaluation of geometric total knee arthroplasty. Clin Orthop 232:168-173, 1988.

85. Ritter MA, Faris PM, Keating EM, Meding JB: Post-operative alignment of total knee replacement. Its effect on survival. Clin Orthop 299:153-156, 1994.

86. Ritter M, Merbst WA, Keating EM, Faris PM: Radiolucency at the bone-cement interface in total knee replacement. J Bone Joint Surg Am 76:60-65, 1991.

87. Saragaglia D, Picard F: Computer-assisted implantation of total knee endoprosthesis with no pre-operative imaging: The kinematic model. In Steihl JB, Konermann WH, Haaker RG (eds): Navigation and Robotics in Total Joint and Spine Surgery. Berlin, Springer-Verlag, 2004, pp 226-233.

88. Saragaglia D, Picard F, Chaussard C, et al: Computer-assisted knee arthroplasty: Comparison with a conventional procedure: Results of 50 cases in a prospective randomized study. Rev Chir Orthop Reparatrice Appar Mot 87:215-220, 2001.

89. Saragagaglia D, Picard F, Chaussard D, et al: Computer assisted total knee arthroplasty: Comparison with a conventional procedure. Results of 50 cases in a prospective randomized study. Presented at the First Annual Symposium on Computer-Assisted Orthopaedic Surgery, February 17-19, 2001, Davos, Switzerland.

90. Sati M, Staubli HU, Bourquin Y, et al: CRA hip and knee reconstructive surgery: Ligament reconstructions in the knee—intraoperative model system (non–image based). In DiGioia AM, Jaramaz B, Picard R, Nolte PL (eds): Computer and Robotic Assisted Knee and Hip Surgery. Oxford, Oxford University Press, 2004, pp 235-256.

91. Siebert W, Mai S, Kober R, Heeckt PF: Technique and first clinical results of robot-assisted total knee replacement. Knee 9:173-180, 2002.

92. Sharkey PF, Hozack WJ, Rothman RH, et al: Why are total knee arthroplasties failing today? Clin Orthop 404:7-13, 2002.

93. Sparmann M, Wolke B: [Value of navigation and robot-guided surgery in total knee arthroplasty.] Orthopade 32:498-505, 2003.

94. Sparmann M, Wolke B: Knee endoprosthesis navigation with the Stryker System. In Steihl JB, Konermann WH, Haaker RG (eds): Navigation and Robotics in Total Joint and Spine Surgery. Berlin, Springer-Verlag, 2004, pp 319-323.

95. Stern SH, Insall JN: Posterior stabilized prosthesis: Results after follow-up of 9-12 years. J Bone Joint Surg Am 74:980-986, 1992.

96. Stindel E, Briard JL, Merloz P, et al: Bone morphing: 3D morphological data for total knee arthroplasty. Comput Aided Surg 7:156-168, 2002.

97. Stockl B, Nogler M, Rosiek R, et al: Navigation improves accuracy of rotational alignment in total knee arthroplasty. Clin Orthop 426:180-186, 2004.

98. Strauss JM, Ruther W: Navigation and soft tissue balancing of LCS total knee arthroplasty. In Steihl JB, Konermann WH, Haaker RG (eds): Navigation and Robotics in Total Joint and Spine Surgery. Berlin, Springer-Verlag, 2004, pp 266-273.

99. Stulberg SD: CAS-TKA reduces the occurrence of functional outliers. Presented at the Annual Meeting of the Mid-America Orthopaedic Association, 2005, Amelia Island, FL.

100. Stulberg SD: Factors affecting the accuracy of minimally invasive total knee arthroplasty. Presented at the Annual Meeting of the American Academy of Orthopaedic Surgeons, 2005, Washington, DC.

101. Stulberg SD: Instructional course lecture on computer assisted surgery for hip and knee reconstruction. Presented at the Annual Meeting of the American Academy of Orthopaedic Surgeons, 2005, Washington, DC.

102. Stulberg SD, Eichorn J, Saragaglia D, Jenny J-Y: The rationale for and initial experience with a knee suite of computer assisted surgical applications. Presented at the Third International Symposium on Computer-Assisted Orthopaedic Surgery, June, 2003, Marbella, Spain.

103. Stulberg SD, Kienzle TC: In Taylor R, Lavalee S, Burdea S, Mosges R (eds): Computer Integrated Surgery, Technology and Clinical Applications. Cambridge, MA, MIT Press, 1995, pp 374-380.

104. Stulberg SD, Koyonos L, McClusker S, Granieri M: Factors affecting the accuracy of minimally invasive TKA. Presented at the Annual Meeting of the American Academy of Orthopaedic Surgeons, 2005, Washington, DC.

105. Stulberg SD, Loan P, Sarin V: Computer-assisted navigation in total knee replacement: Results of an initial experience in thirty-five patients. J Bone Joint Surg Am 84(Suppl 2):90-98, 2002.

106. Stulberg SD, Picard F, Saragaglia D: Computer assisted total knee arthroplasty. Operative techniques. Orthopedics 10:25-39, 2000.

107. Stulberg SD, Saragaglia D, Miehlke R: Total knee replacement: Navigation technique—Intra-operative model system. In DiGioia AM, Jaramaz B, Picard R, Nolte PL (eds): Computer and Robotic Assisted Knee and Hip Surgery. Oxford University Press, 2004, pp 157-178.

108. Stulberg SD, Sarin V: The use of a navigation system to assist ligament balancing in TKR. Presented at the Fifth Annual North American Program on Computer-Assisted Orthopaedic Surgery, July 6-8, 2001, Pittsburgh.

109. Stulberg SD, Sarin V, Loan P: The use of computer assisted navigation in TKR: Results of an initial experience in 35 patients. Presented at the Fifth Annual North American Program on Computer Assisted Orthopaedic Surgery, July 6-8, 2001, Pittsburgh.

110. Stulberg SD, Sarin V, Loan P: X-ray vs. computer assisted measurement techniques to determine pre and post-operative limb alignment in TKR surgery. Presented at the Fifth Annual North American Program on Computer Assisted Orthopaedic Surgery, July 6-8, 2001, Pittsburgh, PA.

111. Teter KE, Bergman D, Colwell CW: Accuracy of intramedullary versus extramedullary tibial alignment cutting systems in total knee arthroplasty. Clin Orthop 321:106-110, 1995.

112. Tew M, Waugh W: Tibiofemoral alignment and the results of knee replacement. J Bone Joint Surg Br 67:551-556, 1985.

113. Tibbles L, Lewis C, Reisine S, et al: Computer assisted instruction for preoperative and postoperative patient education in joint replacement surgery. Comput Nurs 10:208-212, 1992.

114. Townley CD: The anatomic total knee: Instrumentation and alignment technique. In The Knee: Papers of the First Scientific Meeting of the Knee Society. Baltimore, University Press, 1985, pp 39-54.

115. Tria AJ Jr: Minimally invasive total knee arthroplasty: The importance of instrumentation. Orthop Clin North Am 35:227-234, 2004.

116. Vince KIG, Insall JN, Kelly MA: The total condylar prosthesis. 10 to 12 year results of a cemented knee replacement. J Bone Joint Surg Br 71:793-797, 1989.

117. Wasielewski RC, Galante JO, Leighty R, et al: Wear patterns on retrieved polyethylene tibial inserts and their relationship to technical considerations during total knee arthroplasty. Clin Orthop 299:31-43, 1994.

118. Wiese M, Rosenthal A, Bernsmann K: Clinical experience using the SurgiGATE System. In Steihl JB, Konermann WH, Haaker RG (eds): Navigation and Robotics in Total Joint and Spine Surgery. Berlin, Springer-Verlag, 2004, pp 400-404.

119. Wixson RL: Extra-medullary computer assisted total knee replacement: Towards lesser invasive surgery. In Steihl JB, Konermann WH, Haaker RG (eds): Navigation and Robotics in Total Joint and Spine Surgery. Berlin, Springer-Verlag, 2004, pp 311-318.

CHAPTER 96

Computer-Assisted Total Knee Replacement

Sandeep Munjal • Kenneth A. Krackow

It is clear that accuracy of performance in total knee arthroplasty (TKA) is paramount. Components must be placed as precisely as possible—each correctly positioned in all 6 degrees of freedom. The soft-tissue connections, capsule, and ligaments need to be considered during placement of the components so that stability will be present and range of motion will be as full as possible. Given the capabilities of infrared, ultrasound, and electromagnetic position detection instrumentation and the speed, memory capacity, and computational capability of modern digital computers, these aspects of total knee replacement are ripe for assistance by computer. As orthopedic surgeons review personal experience and journal articles citing 90% to 95% good and excellent clinical results in 10- to 15-year time frames, there is the tendency to think that our mechanical instruments are adequate. However, errors in component rotation, postoperative instability, and patients not satisfied with limitations of motion are common. In addition, if surgeons are not obtaining and measuring postoperative long, standing, weightbearing radiographs, it is inappropriate to conclude that even axial alignment is as good as it should and can be. The first publication of a completely navigated, computer-assisted total knee replacement appeared in September 1998.[4] Today, a number of different computer-assisted navigation systems are available from a variety of manufacturers.

TERMS

CAOS is the acronym for computer-assisted orthopedic surgery. Many of the systems developed use the term *navigation*, which implies the use of computerized motion-tracking systems to guide the performance of an operation by assisting in placement of hardware, positioning of screws and cuts, and other functions. Computer-assisted navigation involves the following three steps.

Data Acquisition

Data can be acquired in three different ways: fluoroscopically, guided by computed tomography (CT)/magnetic resonance imaging (MRI), or via imageless systems. The data are then used for registration and tracking. Image-guided systems are somewhat self-explanatory. Image-less systems rely on other information, such as centers of rotation of the hip, knee, or ankle, or visual information, such as anatomic landmarks.

Registration

Registration refers to relating images (e.g., radiographs, CT, MRI, or patients' three-dimensional anatomy) to the anatomic position in the surgical field. Registration techniques required the placement of pins or "fiduciary markers" in the target bone. More recently, a surface-matching technique is used in which the shapes of the bone surface model generated from preoperative images are matched to surface data points collected during surgery.

Tracking

Tracking refers to the sensors and measurement devices that can provide feedback during surgery regarding the orientation and relative position of tools to bone anatomy. For example, optical or electromagnetic trackers are attached to regular surgical tools, which can then provide real-time information related to the position and orientation of the tool's alignment with respect to the bony anatomy of interest.

With regard to orthopedic procedures, computer-assisted navigation is most commonly performed as an adjunct to fixation of pelvic, acetabular, or femoral fractures and as an adjunct to hip and knee arthroplasty procedures.

OVERVIEW

Total knee replacement CAOS equipment allows one to follow the position and movement of any labeled item in the field of view, such as bone, instrument, or implant. The position of objects in the surgical field is shown by markers attached to the different objects, instruments mostly. Markers themselves work by emitting infrared light seen by an infrared detector. The detector "triangulates" to obtain the x, y, z coordinates of each marker in the field of view.

The detector is intimately linked to a computer that analyzes the information collected. The computer is programmed so that instruments and any other item in the surgical field "marked" with infrared emitters can be tracked. Furthermore, the computer can be programmed to know the shape and position of any particular instrument, pointer, or prosthesis. Positional accuracy is typically 0.5 to 1.0 mm., and angular accuracy is generally within 1.0 degree. Interaction is essentially simultaneous.

It is possible to track positions of the markers relative to each other. Furthermore, the equipment can follow the respective motions of each major piece in a surgical field. For bones, it is the size, shape, and position that are important. Therefore, the surgeon needs to "register" each one. Registration can be accomplished with an instrumented pointer to specify the location of the landmarks of each bone so that the computer can track its position, surfaces, and rotational alignment features.

Complete registration of the femur and tibia allows access to tibiofemoral angles, distraction and other displacements, flexion angles, and internal-external rotation—in all the 6 degrees of freedom. The system can study motion patterns and thereby calculate and display the kinematics of what is happening. One can solve for axes of flexion-extension movement under varying conditions and plot outlines of clouds of points that allow one to view surfaces and boundaries on display screens.

OPTIMIZING ALIGNMENT

Correct alignment of the component and soft-tissue balancing have been cited as two of the most important aspects of successful knee arthroplasty.[1,5,7,11,15,17,18,23] Alignment depends on many factors, including accurate preoperative planning, normal bone morphology to which standardized instruments are applied, and accurate skillful placement of these instruments. Incorrect alignment caused by variation in any of these factors can lead to abnormal wear, premature mechanical loosening of components, and patellofemoral problems.

Conventional instrument systems have limited accuracy in determining the crucial landmarks needed for alignment in TKA. With respect to coronal and sagittal alignment, the center of the ankle and the center of the hip are the crucial landmarks. Variability in bone geometry is the main cause for incorrect location of these landmarks with the use of intramedullary guiding systems.[12,21] Navigation systems use mathematic algorithms to determine the kinetic center of rotation of the hip. Assuming that the hip is a perfect ball-in-socket joint, this kinematic center is expected to coincide with the anatomic center of the hip.

An algorithm used in our institution for determining the center of the femoral head was tested by three different surgeons on eight different cadaveric hips for interobserver and intraobserver consistency. The calculated centers were then compared with a direct measurement made after disarticulating the hip and using the stylus/pointer to digitize the observed center of the femoral head. The dislocated hip, specifically, the femoral head, was carefully inspected and an equator drawn freehand. A sagittal saw was then used to cut the femoral head in half, and the midpoint of the remaining surface was digitized in the femoral reference frame. The average error was on the order of 2 to 3 mm. This error applied to a 40-cm long femur yielded a potential angular error of less than 0.55 degree for the orientation of the mechanical axis. The y-coordinate estimates in the intraobserver calculations were significantly different in both cases between investigators ($p = 0.01$) as determined by a paired Student t-test. However, this difference did not lead to a significantly different clinical angular result. Furthermore, these results were obtained in an initially less accurate setting—one without separate tracking of the pelvis. Tracking true femoral-pelvic motion has brought the variation down to less than 1 mm.[9]

Traditionally, surgeons performing TKA have been concerned with optimizing the axial alignment of the lower extremity, that is, varus and valgus. However, as the influence of alignment on survivorship became known, greater consideration for the rotational and medial-lateral positioning of components developed. With the advent of navigation systems and their implementation for use in TKA, better positioning of components is expected with fewer outliers. This chapter's method of optimizing alignment uses the Stryker Navigation Knee Track Module (Stryker Navigation Systems, Stryker Howmedica Osteonics, Allendale, NJ) developed originally by the senior author (K.A.K).

An infrared sensor array located at the side of the operating room table is used to localize emitters placed at specific locations on the lower extremity of the patient. Initially, a tracking pin was placed in the patient's ipsilateral iliac crest for the purpose of determining solely the relative femur-to-pelvis motion. Later, routines were developed that eliminate the need for the pelvic marker. These routines function with no loss of accuracy in determination of alignment.

After surgical exposure of the knee, the distal femoral and proximal tibial pins are placed. These pins function as anchors for the infrared tracker-emitters. With the infrared emitters placed onto the tracking pins, the lower extremity can be manipulated in a circular fashion about the hip. The center of the femoral head is calculated via a subroutine that assumes that the head of the femur is spherical. Two-hundred fifty data points are collected in 20 seconds as the surgeon moves the lower extremity about the hip joint in a gentle spherical arc. The method of least squares is used to find the best-fit sphere given the data points collected.[6] The center estimate is then determined by using an iterative Gauss-Newton algorithm to solve the true nonlinear system. This algorithm runs through 200 iterations to ensure convergence. Finally, the center point is transformed into the femoral reference frame. Using the pointing device, the geometry of the distal end of the femur is digitized. One must identify the medial and lateral epicondyles, the center of the knee, the anteroposterior axis of Whiteside,[22] and the condylar surfaces. Likewise, the geometry of the proximal end of the tibia is digitized as the surgeon identifies the sulcus between the tibial spines representing the initial center of the proximal tibia, a vector for neutral anteroposterior tibial rotation, the medial and lateral malleoli, and the center of the ankle. The center of the ankle is indicated by direct pointing. The vector of the instrument pointing is projected to the intermalleolar axis as that axis lies in a plane including the center point of the proximal tibia together with the points for the two malleoli.

Given all the defined points, the tibiofemoral and mechanical axes can be determined before any bone cuts have been made. Additionally, this navigation system is able to intraoperatively identify the real-time relative position of the tibia with respect to the femur. That is, one is able to precisely determine the tibiofemoral angle, the flexion-extension position, and the amount of relative internal or external rotation of the tibia with respect to the femur. In addition, changes in the relative tibiofemoral compression-distraction and mediolateral or anteroposterior displacements can be determined by calculating the change in the directional vector from the tibial to the femoral reference frames.

The potential for "instrument error" still exists with any such system. However, this infrared, computer-based system has an error ranging from 0.1 to 1 mm for each of the three positional coordinates. This error is considerably less than that in older mechanical systems.

Having created this registration, the specific locations of the femur and tibia relative to the total knee component positions are discernible at any time. It is possible to assess the position of any jig, any resulting cut, the resting position of a trial component, and the final components. Furthermore, the relative position of both the tibia and femur each to the other is always being determined. Thus, one can measure flexion-extension, rotational, and varus-valgus orientations, as well distractions, which represent the size of the tibiofemoral gaps throughout the entire flexion-extension cycle. All measurements are fast and can be done without attaching additional mechanical instruments to the bones. The surgeon is able to obtain more accurate alignment of the lower extremity than previously achieved without the use of such devices.[2,3,8,10,13,14,16,19,20] Additionally, knowledge of flexion-extension gaps at all ranges of knee flexion—both their size and symmetry—allows for more accurate ligament-balancing techniques.

Computer-assisted knee navigation is currently available for routine use. The benefits of computerized navigation are accurate positioning of jigs, the ability to correctly establish femoral component rotation, instantaneous feedback on overall alignment, and the ability to avoid implantation of malpositioned components. Overall, computer assistance results in decreased variability and the elimination of outliers. As of this writing, early 2005, more than 300 computer-assisted primary TKAs have been performed. Many thousands more have been performed worldwide with a variety of systems.

CLINICAL CHALLENGES

We look to computer assistance to improve the quality of our TKA results. In presenting this topic to hundreds of orthopedic surgeons, many are inclined to think only about potential improvement in overall alignment and to believe that their results in this regard are essentially adequate all the time. However, very few routinely obtain and, when they do, accurately measure these results. In addition, Stulberg et al have shown that long, standing lower extremity films are highly subject to rotational and projectional inaccuracy.[20] Possibly, such complacency commonly stated is unwarranted.

In addition, one ought to look beyond the issue of alignment and recognize the potential for improvement in ligament release and assessment of ligamentous stability. In addition, placement of the femoral component in the optimum relationship of extension to the functional axis of flexion can be performed to provide maximum range of motion and stability throughout that arc. We can also turn to navigation equipment to indicate proper component sizing, as well as placement.

It is critical that the surgeon be provided with and master the complete description of how a chosen system works. Only then will one be able to understand the potential for errors and other problems, be more alert for them, and know how to work around them. For example, it is necessary to understand how the system defines bony landmarks and axes and essentially to have a visual appreciation of what is going on.

As with any new operative technique, it is incumbent on the surgeon to also practice the use of these devices in mock settings. This will prevent excessive operative, tourniquet, and anesthetic times, thus reducing complications.

SURGICAL TECHNIQUE

A surgeon's first response to the concept of CAOS may be loss of autonomy. However, it is our view that a system *need not* and *should not* be designed to this end. For example, the system described here allows the surgeon to use the computer to "see" beyond the human eye and view the knee as having full kinematic dimensions. The best way for the reader to understand what assistance this particular navigation system provides is to actually work through a TKA procedure.

An infrared sensor array located at the side of the operating room table is used by the system to localize emitters placed at specific locations on the lower extremity of the patient (Fig. 96–1).

Originally, but not currently necessary, a tracking pin was placed in the patient's ipsilateral iliac crest for the purpose of tracking pure femoral-pelvic relative motion.

After routine exposure, distal femoral and proximal tibial bony tracking pins are placed (Fig. 96–2), and infrared emitters are placed on those tracking pins (Fig. 96–3).

With the pointing device, the geometry of the distal end of the femur is digitized. One identifies the medial and lateral epicondyles, the center of the knee, and the anteroposterior axis of Whiteside[22] and maps the condylar surfaces (Figs. 96–4 and 96–5).

The center of the femoral head is calculated via a subroutine that assumes that the head of the femur is essentially spherical. Data points are collected in about 20 seconds as the surgeon moves the lower extremity about the hip joint in a gentle spherical arc.

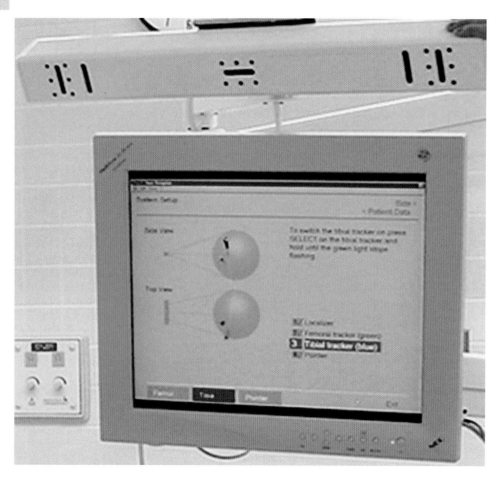

Figure 96–1. Infrared sensor.

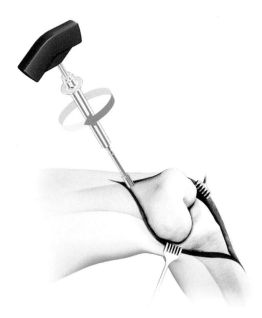

Figure 96–2. Position the anchoring pin within the incision in a region of the epiphyseal growth plate proximal to the medial anterior cortex.

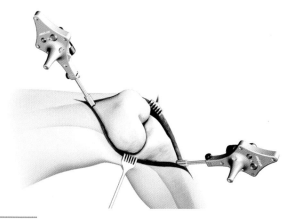

Figure 96–3. After pin fixation, mount the femoral tracker to the femoral pin and the tibial tracker to the tibial pin.

Likewise, the geometry of the proximal end of the tibia is digitized. The surgeon identifies the sulcus between the tibial spines as an initially estimated midpoint of the upper part of the tibia. The surgeon also indicates the location of the medial and lateral malleoli and, last, points to the center of the ankle.

Given all the defined points, the tibiofemoral and mechanical axes can be determined before any bone cuts have been made. Additionally, this navigation system is able to intraoperatively identify the real-time relative position of the tibia with respect to the femur. That is, one is able to precisely determine the tibiofemoral angle, the flexion-extension position, and the amount of relative internal or external rotation of the tibia with respect to the femur. In addition, changes in relative tibiofemoral compression-distraction and mediolateral or anteroposterior displacements can be determined by calculating the change in the directional vector from the tibial to the femoral reference frames (Fig. 96–6)

The operating surgeon is able to use jigs from any specific instrument system to make accurate cuts (Fig. 96–7). The position of the jig is checked (Fig. 96–8); the position of any resulting cut is also checked. Moreover, even the resting position of the trial and final components can be determined (Figs. 96–9 and 96–10). We routinely "navigate" the final cementation to be certain that the femoral and tibial components come to rest at the desired angle and level.

Comparison with Traditional Techniques

When comparing this type of system with traditional techniques, one can easily see that the only "surgical" difference is placement of the tracking pins. These pins have not been associated with any complications such as excessive blood loss or bone fracture. There is a small amount of time needed for the registration, and this together with placement of the pins requires about 5 minutes. Additional time is largely due to one's efforts to improve the accuracy of jig position and the final bone cuts. Many of the checking steps (i.e., checking alignment and cut/jig position) actually occur more quickly. The "time" is not in checking; it is in achieving greater accuracy.

DISCUSSION

Two of the most important concepts for surgeons to grasp are the limits of computer assistance and the specifics of what the computer is doing.

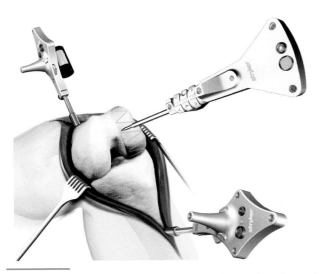

Figure 96–4. The system analyzes the digitized surface of the condyles to determine the most distal point separately for the medial and the lateral side.

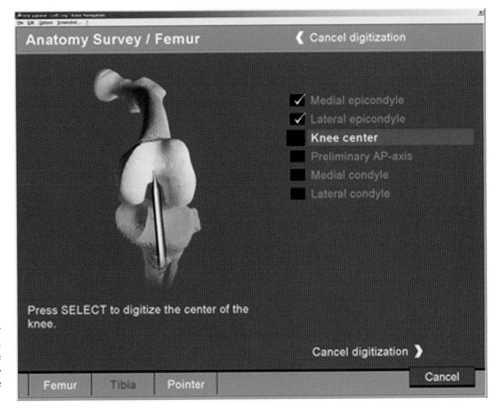

Figure 96–5. Anatomy survey of the femur. The surgeon is prompted to digitize the center of the knee after successful digitization of the epicondyles.

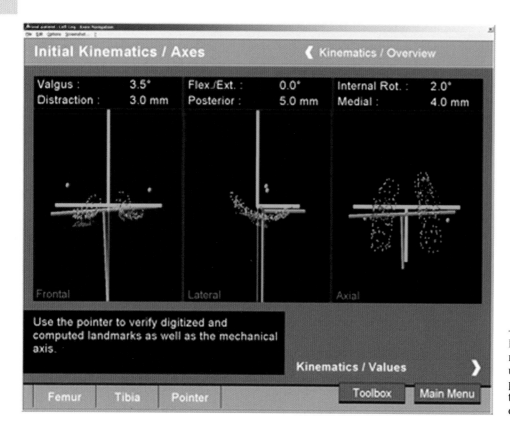

Figure 96–6. The initial kinematic axis dialog enables the user to assess the patient's precut condition relative to the mechanical axis defined during the anatomy survey.

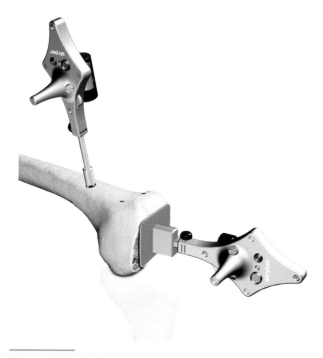

Figure 96–7. A final check is performed by placing the resection plane probe flush with the resected distal plane.

The operating surgeon must understand that the computer is only providing information or feedback based on the computer code that has been specifically programmed. In referring to or locating a point, axis, or whatever, we have to be able to program an absolutely reliable method or methodology for determining that point or axis. If the methodology or computer code is not so precise, the computer cannot be so precise. Expecting the computer to recognize the epicondylar axis when we have no "ironclad" way ourselves exposes the true limitations of any computer-assisted process. Although the computer might be willing to give an "answer," it cannot be expected to "just go in and do it."

We must understand the surgeon's interaction to either directly provide information about where bone is, including the center of the femoral head, end of the femur, proximal tibia, end of the tibia, rotational attitudes, and so forth, or go through the various routines so that the computer itself can locate these features. Specifically, as mentioned previously, the easiest feature to locate is the center of the femoral head by moving the femur around and solving for the center of the femoral head.

In developing computer-assisted surgical techniques, innovators and researchers must be sure of the validity of their measurements, inter-rater reliability, and reproducibility. Prospective users of computer-assisted techniques must be sure that each of these issues has been addressed before subjecting patients to these techniques. The individual steps of the computer-assisted process must be evaluated in a stepwise fashion to ensure the expected results.

Any new surgical technique or protocol needs to pass through a period of introspective questioning by interested surgeons. Questions that must be asked include the level of risk for infection, bleeding, and postoperative pain, as well as whether the new process should add to or improve on the current methodology. With TKA, "improvements" in technique or prostheses must also address the issues of proper alignment, durability, accu-

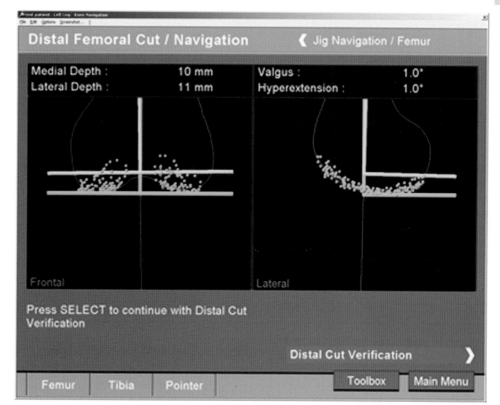

Figure 96–8. The jig navigation graphics allows the surgeon to make "real-time" minor angular adjustments to the cutting jig in both the frontal (varus/valgus) and lateral (flexion/extension) planes of the computed mechanical axis.

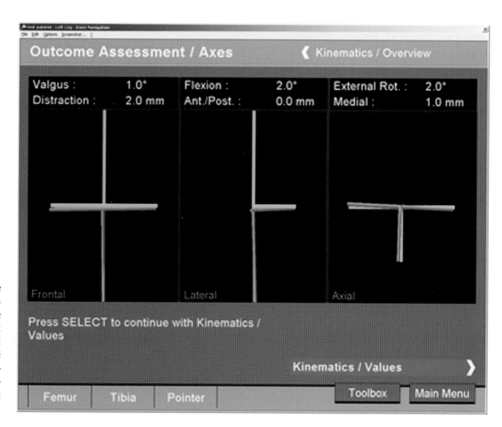

Figure 96–9. The outcome assessment axes dialog is provided to assess the patient's postcut alignment relative to the mechanical axis defined during the anatomy survey after prosthesis cementation/implantation and removal of the pneumatic tourniquet.

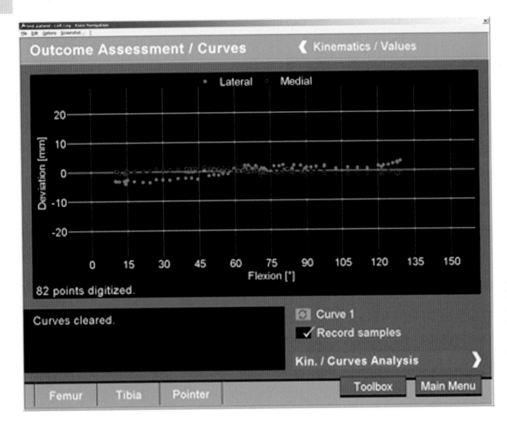

Figure 96–10. The outcome assessment curves dialog displays the final relationship (magnitude of the gap and angulation) of the medial and lateral compartments. These curves represent the femoral and tibial implants' final positional alignment.

racy, and surgical reproducibility. CAOS attempts to achieve improvement in the quality of the operation performed through intraoperative feedback to the operating surgeon.

Concern regarding appropriate alignment and ligament balancing can be assessed and corrected intraoperatively and with great precision. Whereas previously the operating surgeon relied on knowledge of deformity correction with various releases, the process can be monitored with use of the computer. Exact measurements of flexion-extension gaps, varus and valgus deformity, and tibial rotation can be patient specific and observed in real time.

At the same time, this entire process must be relatively convenient to perform. An additional degree or two of improved alignment need not sacrifice physician and patient comfort. The process should not infringe on the typical protocol of knee arthroplasty. Instead, it should simply assist the surgeon to perform more efficiently. In summary, a new methodology should improve on the existing process.

SUMMARY

Change is inevitable, and resistance, at least *total* resistance, is frequently futile. CAOS introduces a change in our traditional methods of surgery. Many operating surgeons will oppose the change and insist that it will inevitably lead to loss of autonomy or think that it is not worth the cost or trouble. However, we believe that educating ourselves about new technology will allow us to evolve into better surgeons and provide better outcomes for our patients.

References

1. Bargren JH, Blaha JD, Freeman MA: Alignment in total knee arthroplasty: Correlated biomechanical and clinical observations. Clin Orthop 173:178-183, 1983.
2. Chauhan SK, Scott RG, Breidahl W, Beaver RJ: Computer-assisted knee arthroplasty versus a conventional jig-based technique. A randomised, prospective trial. J Bone Joint Surg Br 86:372-377, 2004.
3. Chauhan SK, Scott RG, Lloyd SJ, et al: A prospective randomized controlled trial of computer assisted versus conventional knee replacement. In Langlotz FL, Davies BL, Bauer A (eds): Computer Assisted Orthopedic Surgery, Third Annual Meeting of CAOS International Proceedings. Darmstadt, Germany, Steinkopff Verlag, 2003, pp 52-53.
4. Delp SL, Stulberg SD, Davies B, et al: Computer assisted knee replacement. Clin Orthop 354:49-56, 1998.
5. Dorr LD, Boiardo RA: Technical considerations in total knee arthroplasty. Clin Orthop 205:5-11, 1997.
6. Forbes A: Robust circle and sphere fitting by least squares. Natl Phys Lab Rep 153:1-22, 1989.
7. Jeffery RS, Morris RW, Denham RA: Coronal alignment after total knee replacement. J Bone Joint Surg Br 73:709-714, 1991.
8. Jenny JY, Boeri C: Computer-assisted implantation of a total knee arthroplasty: A case-controlled study in comparison to classical instrumentation. Rev Chir Orthop Reparatrice Appar Mot 87:645-652, 2001.
9. Krackow KA, Bayer-Thering M, Phillips MJ, Mihalko M: A new technique for determining proper mechanical axis alignment during total knee arthroplasty: Progress toward computer assisted TKA. Orthopedics 22:698-702, 1999.
10. Krackow KA, Phillips MJ, Bayers-Thering M, et al: Computer-assisted total knee arthroplasty: Navigation in TKA. Orthopedics 26:1017-1023, 2003.

11. Lotke PA, Ecker ML: Influence of positioning of prosthesis in total knee replacement. J Bone Joint Surg Am 59:77-79, 1977.

12. Maestro A, Harwin SF, Sandoval MG, et al: Influence of intramedullary versus extramedullary alignment on final total knee arthroplasty component position: A radiological analysis. J Arthroplasty 13:552-558, 1998.

13. Mihalko WM, Krackow KA: Extramedullary, intramedullary and CAS tibial alignment techniques for TKA. Presented at the Annual Meeting of the American Academy of Orthopaedic Surgeons, 2004, San Francisco.

14. Mihalko WM, Krackow KA, Boyle J, et al: Intramedullary and computer navigational femoral alignment in TKA. Presented at the Annual Meeting of the American Academy of Orthopaedic Surgeons, 2004, San Francisco.

15. Mont MA, Urquhart MA, Hungerford DS, Krackow KA: Intramedullary goniometer can improve alignment in knee arthroplasty surgery. J Arthroplasty 12:332-336, 1997.

16. Phillips MJ, Krackow KA, Thering MB: Computer-assisted total knee replacement—results of the first 90 cases using the Stryker navigation system. Presented at the conference on Computer-Assisted Orthopaedic Surgery, 2003, Marbella, Spain.

17. Ritter MA, Faris PM, Keating M, et al: Postoperative alignment of total knee replacement. Clin Orthop 299:153-156, 1994.

18. Sharkey PF, Hozack WJ, Rothman RH, et al: Why are total knee arthroplasties failing today? Clin Orthop 404:7-13, 2002.

19. Sparmann M, Wolke B, Czupalla H, et al: Positioning of total knee arthroplasty with and without navigation support. A prospective, randomised study. J Bone Joint Surg Br 85:830-835, 2003.

20. Stulberg SD, Loan P, Sarin V: Computer-assisted navigation in total knee replacement: Results of an initial experience in thirty-five patients. J Bone Joint Surg Am 84:90-98, 2002.

21. Victor J, Urlus M, Bellemans J, Fabry G: Femoral intramedullary instrumentation in total knee arthroplasty: The role of pre-operative x-ray analysis. Knee 1:123-125, 1994.

22. Whiteside L, Arima J: The anteroposterior axis for femoral rotational alignment in valgus total knee arthroplasty. Clin Orthop 321:168-172, 1995.

23. Windsor RE, Scuderi GR, Moran MC, et al: Mechanisms of failure of the femoral and tibial components in total knee arthroplasty. Clin Orthop 248:15-19, 1989.

CHAPTER 97

Imageless Computer Navigation in Total Knee Arthroplasty: The Simpler Wave of the Future

Aaron A. Hofmann • Amit Lahav

The use of computer-based systems during total knee arthroplasty (TKA) has become more readily accepted and used during recent years. Computer-assisted surgery for total knee replacement was first approved for use in the United States in 2001. Since its introduction there has been rapid expansion of this technology, and several different types of navigation systems have been developed by several different manufacturers. Each new version of the software has incorporated increasingly sophisticated analysis modules to allow not only accurate alignment of the limb and component position but also assessment of ligament balance and knee kinematics.[42] There are an increasing number of references in the orthopedic literature to studies reporting on computer-assisted techniques and early outcomes with these techniques.* Each system affords surgeons the opportunity to maximize clinical outcomes by perfecting their surgical technique. Specifically, component alignment during the procedure must be optimized.[17,18,28]

The significance of component and limb alignment has been extensively studied since the earliest days of TKA. Several early references in the knee arthroplasty literature focusing on outcome and experience with TKA underscore the importance of alignment.[2,26,35] Alignment errors in TKA greater than 3 degrees can be associated with poorer outcomes and accelerated failure. Rotation of the femoral and tibial components has a strong influence on patella tracking, and malrotation of components can lead to patellofemoral complications.[7] Hungerford and Krackow proposed that technical perfection of alignment and component position should be the goals for TKA.[17] Insall found that most failures in TKA could be attributed to incorrect ligament balance or incorrect alignment.[18] Moreland's experience in TKA yielded similar findings and led him to state that component alignment was the most important factor influencing postoperative loosening and instability.[28] The real promise with computer navigation may be its potential to help surgeons avoid outliers when using standard instruments (Fig. 97-1). Outliers represent patients who fall outside the accepted values for alignment. Conventional techniques that use extramedullary alignment guides or intramedullary rods for component orientation can result in component malalignment.[11,31] The computer-assisted technique allows for errors to be verified and corrected intraoperatively. Even an experienced surgeon can obtain (Tables 97-1 and 97-2).

Numerous studies already support the use of computer-assisted systems in knee arthroplasty. In 1999, Krackow et al published a technique that used computer assistance to determine proper mechanical axis alignment during TKA.[23] Jenny and Boeri compared a navigation system with a surgeon-controlled operative technique in 60 TKAs.[20] Radiographic evaluation demonstrated improved accuracy of implantation in the computer-assisted group. Bathis et al showed that computer-assisted TKA gave better correction of alignment of the leg and orientation of the components than the conventional technique did.[5] If implant longevity, pain relief, and function are related to the accuracy with which a TKA is performed, mechanical instrumentation does not result in a high incidence of accuracy when each step of the procedure is measured.[40] Computer-assisted TKA allows more reproducible component positioning, avoids outliers in alignment errors, and assists with soft-tissue balancing.

The incidence of fat embolism syndrome from instrumenting the medullary canal during cemented or cementless TKA is not negligible.[27] Kim found that fat embolism was seen in 65 patients (65%) with a bilateral TKA and 46 patients (46%) with a unilateral TKA. Bone marrow cell embolism was detected in 12 patients (12%) with a bilateral TKA and in 4 patients (4%) with a unilateral TKA.[22] Giachino et al performed a study to determine whether a technique of intraoperative anticoagulation would decrease the incidence or severity of venous embolization after tourniquet release during TKA. Transesophageal echocardiography was performed before and after tourniquet release to detect embolic material in the right atrium. Transient opacification of the right atrium was observed in all patients within the first 30 seconds after tourniquet release. Regional limb heparinization was not effective in reducing the intensity of right atrial opacification.[14] Heparinization does not necessarily reduce the occurrence of embolism. With computer-assisted surgery, violation of the medullary canal is avoided, thereby possibly reducing the occurrence of embolic events.

Computer-assisted systems can generally be grouped into three different types: image-based navigation systems, robotic systems, and image-free navigation systems. Image-based systems require preoperative computed tomography (CT) scans, whereas image-free navigation

*See references 1, 4, 6, 10, 11, 15, 20, 21, 23, 24, 29, 30, 32, 36, 38, 41.

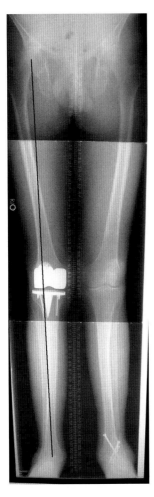

Figure 97–1. Long, standing radiograph of malpositioned total knee arthroplasty components performed with standard instruments.

systems gain all necessary information intraoperatively during a registration process. Computer-integrated instrumentation incorporates highly accurate measurement devices to locate joint centers, track surgical tools, and align prosthetic components. Image-based knee replacement provides a three-dimensional preoperative plan that guides placement of the cutting blocks and prosthetic components. Robot-assisted knee replacement allows one to machine bones accurately without the use of standard cutting blocks. Image-free navigation allows real-time evaluation of deformity and bone cuts and is becoming the standard for computer-assisted knee surgery.

IMAGE-BASED SYSTEMS

In image-based total knee replacement the procedure begins with preoperative planning. To create the preoperative plan, three-dimensional computer models of the patient's femur and tibia are constructed from CT or fluoroscopic data. Once the computer models of the bones have been created, planning software orients the tibial and femoral components and calculates bone resections that align the mechanical axis of the limb and produce the intended implant contact. An intraoperative system determines the position and orientation of the patient's femur and tibia and guides placement of the cutting jigs so that the resections determined in the preoperative plan can be made.[11] Image-based navigation systems include the fluoroscope unit and the CT scanner. Frequent use of the fluoroscope in an operation presents a significant radiation hazard to the surgical staff and patient. A recent technique known as virtual fluoroscopy enhances the fluoroscope's capability for image-guided surgery by optically tracking the position of the C-arm, the surgical instruments, and the patient. Virtuality is achieved by the overlay of surgical instruments onto one or more previously captured fluoroscopic images. A key benefit of virtual fluoroscopy is that it considerably reduces the radiation hazard.[34] CT scan navigation has shown good results in surgeons' hands. Chauhan et al demonstrated that computer-assisted total knee replacement via CT navigation techniques resulted in better alignment of the femoral component and the posterior slope of the tibial component in rotation and flexion and better matching of the femoral and tibial components in rotation in a cadaver model.[8] Perlick et al implanted 100 TKAs with either the computer-assisted technique (50 knees) or the conventional approach (50 knees). Accuracy of implantation was determined on postoperative long-leg coronal and lateral radiographs. A postoperative leg axis between 3 degrees varus and 3 degrees valgus was achieved in 46 patients in the group with computer-assisted implantation and in 36 patients in the control group ($p = .01$). A significant difference was also seen in femoral component alignment in the frontal plane. They concluded that the CT-based navigation system improves the accuracy of TKA, but that higher cost and time-consuming planning will mean that its use is limited to special cases.[33] In image-based knee replacement, analysis of the three-dimensional image data allows the surgeon to determine the size of the implant preoperatively, thereby potentially reducing inventory. Image-based systems also allow comparison of actual placement of the implants relative to the planned placement.

ROBOT-ASSISTED SURGERY

Robot-assisted knee replacement was designed to improve the accuracy and precision of bone resection. Robotic-assisted surgery can aid in drilling the alignment holes for conventional cutting blocks to make the femoral and tibial bone cuts. Robot assistance also provides the capability to machine bone surfaces for alignment or for contact areas for bone ingrowth. The earlier version of these robotic systems, however, used industrial robots, which are not suitable or designed for use in the operating room.[11] Similar to image-guided knee replacement, robot-assisted surgery has the advantage of preoperative imaging, modeling, and planning. The machining capability of a robot may provide a more accurate fit between the prosthesis and bone, thus making the use of cement unnecessary in certain cases.

Table 97–1. Standard Instrumentation—Accuracy of Alignment

AUTHOR	TECHNIQUE	STUDY SIZE	RESULTS

Engh et al[13]	Intramedullary Extramedullary	72 TKAs	Femoral component position
			  IM: 35/40 (87.5%) within ±3 degrees of goal
			  EM: 22/32 (68.8%) within ±3 degrees of goal
			Tibiofemoral alignment
			  IM: 88% correct
			  EM: 73% correct

Dennis et al[12]	Intramedullary Extramedullary	120 TKAs	Tibial component position
			  IM: 72% within ±2 degrees of goal
			  EM: 88% within ±2 degrees of goal

Teter et al[43]	Intramedullary Extramedullary	352 TKAs	Tibial component position
			  IM: 94% within ±4 degrees of goal
			  EM: 92% within ±4 degrees of goal

Teter et al[44]	Intramedullary	201 TKAs	Femoral component position IM: 91.5% within ±4 degrees of goal
Lam et al[25]	Intramedullary	362 TKAs	Femoral component position IM: 92% within ±3 degrees of goal
Jeffcote et al[19]	Extramedullary	350 TKAs	Tibial component position IM: 96.3% within ±2 degrees of goal

Authors' study	CAS Intramedullary Extramedullary	100 TKAs	Femoral component position
			  CAS: 98% within ±3 degrees of goal
			  IM: 90% within ±3 degrees of goal
			Tibial component position
			  CAS: 100% within ±3 degrees of goal
			  EM: 92% within ±3 degrees of goal

Composite table of published results for standard instrumentation. Results of the current study are included for the purpose of comparison.
CAS, computer-assisted system.

IMAGE-FREE NAVIGATION SYSTEMS

Image-free navigation systems use mechanical instruments that are enhanced by their integration with accurate measuring equipment. Reference frames or trackers are used to locate the limb in space (Fig. 97–2). These trackers or frames can be attached to bones and to surgical instruments to track the positions and orientations of each surgical tool relative to the bones. The computer workstation displays the position of the cutting blocks relative to the desired position. Once the jig is oriented properly, it is secured in position and the bone cuts are made with a standard saw.[11]

A radiographic comparison between image-based and image-free navigation systems was conducted by Bathis et al. One hundred thirty patients underwent TKA with a CT-based or a CT-free module of the BrainLAB Vector-Vision Navigation System (Westchester, IL). Postoperative leg alignment and component orientation were determined on long-leg coronal and lateral radiographs. Sixty of 65 patients in the CT-based group and 63 of 65 patients in

Table 97–2. Comparative Studies—Computer-Assisted Technique versus Standard Instrumentation

AUTHOR	SYSTEM	TECHNIQUE	STUDY SIZE	RESULTS

Jenny et al[20]	Orthopilot	CAS Standard	30 TKAs 30 TKAs	Tibiofemoral alignment
				  CAS: 25/30 within ±3 degrees of goal
				  Standard: 21/30 within ±3 degrees of goal

Sparmann et al[37]	Stryker	CAS Standard	240 TKAs	Tibiofemoral alignment CAS > Standard

Hart et al[15]	Orthopilot	CAS Standard	60 TKAs 60 TKAs	Tibiofemoral alignment
				  CAS: 53/60 within ±2 degrees of goal
				  Standard: 42/60 within ±2 degrees of goal

Bathis et al[4]	BrainLab	CAS Standard	50 TKAs 50 TKAs	Tibiofemoral alignment
				  CAS: 48/50 within ±3 degrees of goal
				  Standard: 38/50 within ±3 degrees of goal

Authors' study	Orthosoft	CAS Standard	50 TKAs 50 TKAs	Tibiofemoral alignment
				  CAS: 45/50 within ±3 degrees of goal
				  Standard: 43/50 within ±3 degrees of goal

Composite table of published results for studies comparing a computer-assisted technique with a standard instrumentation technique. Results of the current study are included for the purpose of comparison.
CAS, computer-assisted system.

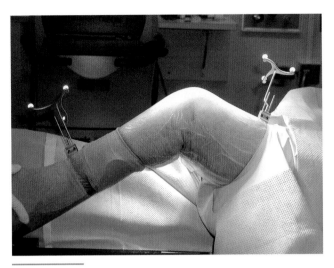

Figure 97–2. **Trackers are placed on the femur and tibia to allow the computer to assess the limb in space.**

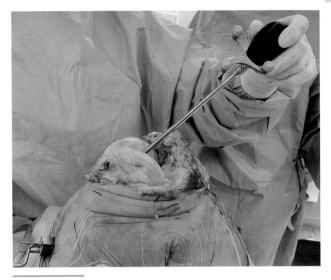

Figure 97–4. A pointer with an attached tracker is used to enter data of the bony landmarks into the computer.

the CT-free group had a postoperative leg axis between 3 degrees varus/valgus. No significant differences were found for varus/valgus orientation of the femoral and tibial components.[3]

The authors compared alignment between 50 TKAs performed with an imageless computer navigation system, Navitrack System-Optical Total Knee Replacement CT-Less device (Orthosoft, Montreal) or Medtronic Trio system (Louisville, CO) (Fig. 97–3), and 50 TKAs performed with standard instrumentation. The purpose of the study was to compare postoperative component alignment between two groups of 50 TKAs, all performed by a single surgeon. The same surgeon used a posterior-referencing TKA system (Natural Knee, Zimmer, Warsaw, IN) in all cases. Long, standing radiographs were collected at 6 weeks' follow-up and measured for component orienta-

tion. When the navigation system was used, 98% (49/50) of all femoral components and 100% (50/50) of all tibial components were placed within ±3 degrees of the radiographic goal position. In the standard instrumentation group, accuracy was decreased to 90% (45/50) and 92% (46/50) within ±3 degrees, respectively. There was a significant difference in standard deviations observed for the navigated cases and the conventional cases when femoral ($p = 0.016$) and tibial ($p = 0.013$) component position was considered. Average tourniquet time was 68 minutes in the navigated group and 57 minutes in the conventional group. Chauhan et al also showed that computer-assisted surgery took longer with a mean increase of 13 minutes ($p = 0.0001$).[9]

This imageless navigation system is straightforward and simple with only a few additional steps needed for tracker placement and validation of the bone cuts. The Navitrack System-Optical Total Knee Replacement CT-Less device consists of a computer workstation, an optical tracking system, surgical instruments, and tracking devices. Tracking devices are affixed to a universal positioning block (UPB) and the pointing instrument, which allows these instruments to be tracked and displayed in real time on a monitor (Figs. 97–4 and 97–5; see also Fig. 97–3). The surgical technique is very straightforward. Intraoperatively, tracking devices are attached to the femur and to the tibia, which allows them to also be displayed in real time on the monitor (Fig. 97–6). The lower extremity is held in extension during placement of the femoral trackers. Two fully threaded $\frac{1}{8}$-inch Steinmann pins are placed in unicortical fashion so that they slightly engage the second cortex of the femur. The inset screws in the tracker are tightened to secure the tracker to the pins. A similar technique is used to place two pins distally on the anteromedial aspect of the tibia for placement of the tibial tracker.

The hip is then taken through a range of motion to establish the center of rotation of the femoral head. Fourteen points are documented during this motion analysis to compute the location of the center of the femoral head.

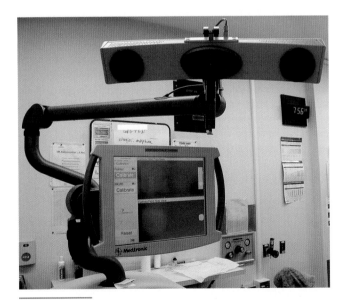

Figure 97–3. An imageless computer navigation system showing the computer screen and infrared camera.

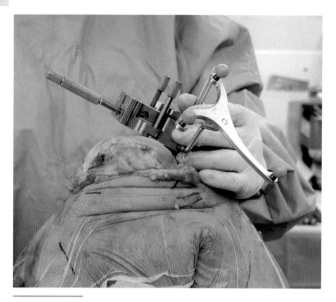

Figure 97–5. Placement of the universal positioning block on the distal end of the femur.

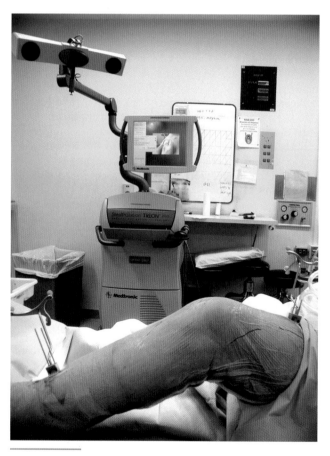

Figure 97–6. Tracking devices are attached to the femur and tibia, which are displayed in real time on a monitor.

The knee is exposed via a standard medial parapatellar, midvastus, or subvastus approach, depending on the surgeon's preference. The pointer instrument is then used to digitize and reference five bony landmarks on the distal end of the femur (see Fig. 97–4) and seven on the proxi-

mal end of the tibia. The landmarks on the femoral side include the intercondylar notch, the medial and lateral epicondyles, and two on the trochlear groove. The UPB with the claws attached is placed on the distal femur to reference the two posterior condyles because the Natural Knee II (Zimmer, Warsaw, IN) system is a posterior-referencing system. The pointer instrument is then used on the tibial side to reference seven landmarks, which include the center of the tibia, the medial third of the tibial tubercle, the posterior cruciate ligament, the most medial and lateral points on the plateau, and the medial and lateral malleoli. Once these points are entered, the intraoperative deformity can be determined and evaluated. The varus-valgus deformity as well as flexion-extension deformity can be saved on the system. At this point the surgeon can also make an evaluation of how correctable the deformity is in real time with numerical values appearing on the computer module. This capability gives the surgeon valuable information for planning soft-tissue–balancing strategies.

Femoral preparation is then initiated. The polyaxial screw to hold the UPB is placed in the distal femur with no entry into the femoral canal. The UPB is positioned on the screw with the posterior condyle claw attached. The surgeon then dials in rotation, flexion/extension, and varus-valgus orientation by manipulating the position of the UPB (see Fig. 97–5). The rotational preference is the posterior condyles, with the posterior claw used for varus cases and the anteroposterior axis for valgus knees. The goal of flexion is 5.0 degrees to account for the anterior bow of the femur. The UPB is dialed down medially or laterally to set a neutral varus-valgus block position with the intact condyle used as a pivot point. A standard distal femoral cutting block is then applied to the UPB, holes for subsequent cutting blocks are drilled, pins are placed to stabilize the block, and the femoral lugholes are drilled through the UPB. The size of the femur is also determined with the pointer. After the distal femoral resection, the UPB is placed flush against the distal cut for validation. The remainder of the femoral preparation is performed in standard fashion with cutting blocks positioned via the drilled lugholes.

Attention is then directed to the tibia. After exposure of the tibia, the pointer instrument can be used to identify four bony landmarks on the tibial plateau, including the most posterior points on the plateau medially and laterally for determination of proper tibial rotation and the least involved portions on the plateau medially and laterally to allow for determination of the natural varus or valgus present at the tibial plateau. An attachment device called a figure-7 tibial guide is impacted into the proximal tibial plateau at the remnant of the anterior cruciate ligament insertion site, and the UPB is set on the device. The rotation, slope, and varus/valgus orientation are established by positioning the UPB. Once these values are adjusted to the desired positions, the depth of resection is set and drill holes are made through the UPB to allow pin placement. The standard tibial cutting guide is then placed over the pins, and the proximal tibia resection is performed.

Trial components can then be placed and the navigation system can evaluate flexion and extension of the knee, as

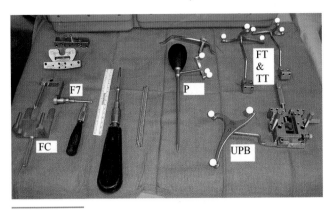

Figure 97-7. The additional instruments needed for the Natural Knee II (Zimmer, Warsaw, IN) computer-assisted total knee arthroplasty: femoral (FT) and tibial trackers (TT), universal positioning block (UPB), pointer (P), figure-7 tibial guide (F7), and posterior femoral claw (FC).

well as the overall alignment axis. The surgeon can evaluate the soft-tissue balancing that has been achieved by manual varus/valgus stress testing. The range of motion of the knee and overall hip-knee-ankle alignment can be documented by the system at the time of trial reduction and again at final component placement. When a cemented technique is used, fine-tuning can be performed during cement setup. This allows for further adjustment of varus-valgus alignment, as well as flexion-extension relationships. All this information can be saved on the system as data points to determine how effectively the deformity was corrected. The threaded pins used for the trackers are removed from the femur and the tibia at the time of wound closure.

There are some features of this imageless computer navigation system that the current authors believe to be advantageous over other computer-assisted systems. The system is truly imageless, and therefore there is no need for preoperative CT imaging or intraoperative fluoroscopy to allow navigation. Another advantage of the system is the fact that it incorporates standard cutting blocks and cutting guides from a preexisting total knee design (Natural Knee II) with a proven clinical track record.[16] The current set has only a few additional instruments (Fig. 97-7). In addition, violation of the intramedullary canal is avoided with this instrumentation. Navigation may lead to improved component survivorship in the long term and a reduction in the complications associated with embolic phenomena that occur with intramedullary instruments.

It is important to realize that computer navigation systems are not all the same and that they cannot be relied on independently. Like all techniques, they can certainly have imperfections. Stulberg et al reported significant concerns about the registration accuracy of the software for the OrthoPilot system.[41] It was thought that the biggest variable leading to inaccuracy was the surgical technique. Their experience indicated that it required approximately 10 procedures to develop a reliable registration technique. The software, however, is constantly being upgraded to provide easier operation of the system and thus facilitate the procedures necessary for data input and understanding. In addition, standard instrumentation can be used to validate computer information before the actual bone cuts. There has also been some concern about bone fractures as a result of tracker placement in the femur or tibia. The authors have not seen this complication in their patient population with unicortical placement of threaded pins.

CONCLUSION

The cost associated with use of any of the systems just described is not minimal at this time. New equipment, including robots, modules, trackers, and computers, along with expenditure for CT scans and fluoroscopy, increase the cost of the operative procedure. With time, however, prices will become more competitive between the manufacturing companies, and more compact computer systems will become available.

The success of total knee replacement depends on several factors, including patient selection, prosthesis design and choice, soft-tissue balancing, and alignment of the limb. Proper rotational and translational alignment of the femoral and tibial components, as well as the limb, is an important factor that can influence the outcome of knee replacement. A reduction in wear and component loosening and an increase in functional performance will be the result.

We predict that computer-assisted surgical techniques will be considered part of the standard of care for primary TKA in the future. Computer-integrated instruments that combine standard cutting guides with highly accurate measurement equipment are a natural extension of current techniques and offer several potential advantages. The improved accuracy has the potential to provide a very real advantage over more traditional techniques. Use of a navigation system provides improved alignment accuracy and can help avoid femoral malrotation and errors in axial alignment.[39] Long-term studies are required to confirm that this improvement in technique will lead to decreased rates of component revision and improved outcomes. Computer navigation would improve component position while minimizing outliers and make a good surgeon even better.

References

1. Amiot LP, Poulin F: Computed tomography–based navigation for hip, knee, and spine surgery. Clin Orthop 421:77-86, 2004.
2. Bargren JH, Blaha JD, Freeman MA: Alignment in total knee arthroplasty. Correlated biomechanical and clinical observations. Clin Orthop 173:178-183, 1983.
3. Bathis H, Perlick L, Tingart M, et al: Radiological results of image-based and non–image-based computer-assisted total knee arthroplasty. Int Orthop 28(2):87-90, 2004.
4. Bathis H, Perlick L, Tingart M, et al: CT-free computer-assisted total knee arthroplasty versus the conventional technique: Radiographic results of 100 cases. Orthopedics 27:476-480, 2004.
5. Bathis H, Perlick L, Tingart M, et al: Alignment in total knee arthroplasty. A comparison of computer-assisted surgery with the conventional technique. J Bone Joint Surg Br 86:682-687, 2004.
6. Berend ME, Ritter MA, Meding JB, et al: Tibial component failure mechanisms in total knee replacement. Clin Orthop 428:26-34, 2004.

7. Berger RA, Rubash HE, Seel MJ, et al: Determining the rotational alignment of the femoral component in total knee arthroplasty using the epicondylar axis. Clin Orthop 286:40-47, 1993.
8. Chauhan SK, Clark GW, Lloyd S, et al: Computer-assisted total knee replacement. A controlled cadaver study using a multi-parameter quantitative CT assessment of alignment (the Perth CT Protocol). J Bone Joint Surg Br 86:818-823, 2004.
9. Chauhan SK, Scott RG, Breidahl W, et al: Computer-assisted knee arthroplasty versus a conventional jig-based technique. A randomised, prospective trial. J Bone Joint Surg Br 86:372-377, 2004.
10. Clemens U, Miehlke RK: Experience using the latest OrthoPilot TKA software: A comparative study. Surg Technol Int 11:265-273, 2003.
11. Delp SL, Stulberg SD, Davies B, et al: Computer assisted knee replacement. Clin Orthop 354:49-56, 1998.
12. Dennis DA, Channer M, Susman MH, et al: Intramedullary versus extramedullary tibial alignment systems in total knee arthroplasty. J Arthroplasty 8:43-47, 1993.
13. Engh GA, Petersen TL: Comparative experience with intramedullary and extramedullary alignment in total knee arthroplasty. J Arthroplasty 5:1-8, 1990.
14. Giachino AA, Rody K, Turek MA, et al: Systemic fat and thrombus embolization in patients undergoing total knee arthroplasty with regional heparinization. J Arthroplasty 16:288-292, 2001.
15. Hart R, Janecek M, Chaker A, et al: Total knee arthroplasty implanted with and without kinematic navigation. Int Orthop 27:366-369, 2003.
16. Hofmann AA, Evanich JD, Ferguson RP, et al: Ten- to 14-year clinical followup of the cementless Natural Knee system. Clin Orthop 388:85-94, 2001.
17. Hungerford DS, Krackow KA: Total joint arthroplasty of the knee. Clin Orthop 192:23-33, 1985.
18. Insall JN, Binazzi R, Soudry M, et al: Total knee arthroplasty. Clin Orthop 192:13-22, 1985.
19. Jeffcote B, Shakespeare D: Varus/valgus alignment of the tibial component in total knee arthroplasty. Knee 10:243-247, 2003.
20. Jenny JY, Boeri C: Computer-assisted implantation of total knee prostheses: A case-control comparative study with classical instrumentation. Comput Aided Surg 6:217-220, 2001.
21. Jenny JY, Boeri C: Unicompartmental knee prosthesis implantation with a non–image-based navigation system: Rationale, technique, case-control comparative study with a conventional instrumented implantation. Knee Surg Sports Traumatol Arthrosc 11:40-45, 2003.
22. Kim YH: Incidence of fat embolism syndrome after cemented or cementless bilateral simultaneous and unilateral total knee arthroplasty. J Arthroplasty 16:730-739, 2001.
23. Krackow KA, Bayers-Thering M, Phillips MJ, et al: A new technique for determining proper mechanical axis alignment during total knee arthroplasty: Progress toward computer-assisted TKA. Orthopedics 22:698-702, 1999.
24. Krackow KA, Phillips MJ, Bayers-Thering M, et al: Computer-assisted total knee arthroplasty: Navigation in TKA. Orthopedics 26:1017-1023, 2003.
25. Lam LO, Shakespeare D: Varus/valgus alignment of the femoral component in total knee arthroplasty. Knee 10:237-241, 2003.
26. Lotke PA, Ecker ML: Influence of positioning of prosthesis in total knee replacement. J Bone Joint Surg Am 59:77-79, 1977.
27. Monto RR, Garcia J, Callaghan JJ: Fatal fat embolism following total condylar knee arthroplasty. J Arthroplasty 5:291-299, 1990.
28. Moreland JR: Mechanisms of failure in total knee arthroplasty. Clin Orthop 226:49-64, 1988.
29. Nishihara S, Sugano N, Ikai M, et al: Accuracy evaluation of a shape-based registration method for a computer navigation system for total knee arthroplasty. J Knee Surg 16:98-105, 2003.
30. Nizard R: Computer assisted surgery for total knee arthroplasty. Acta Orthop Belg 68:215-230, 2002.
31. Novotny J, Gonzalez MH, Amirouche FM, et al: Geometric analysis of potential error in using femoral intramedullary guides in total knee arthroplasty. J Arthroplasty 16:641-647, 2001.
32. Perlick L, Bathis H, Perlick C, et al: Revision total knee arthroplasty: A comparison of postoperative leg alignment after computer-assisted implantation versus the conventional technique. Knee Surg Sports Traumatol Arthrosc 13:167-173, 2004.
33. Perlick L, Bathis H, Tingart M, et al: Navigation in total-knee arthroplasty: CT-based implantation compared with the conventional technique. Acta Orthop Scand 75:464-470, 2004.
34. Phillips R, Peter V, Faure GE, et al: A virtual fluoroscopy system and its use for image guidance in unicompartmental knee surgery. Stud Health Technol Inform 85:341-347, 2002.
35. Ritter MA, Faris PM, Keating EM, et al: Postoperative alignment of total knee replacement. Its effect on survival. Clin Orthop 299:153-156, 1994.
36. Saragaglia D, Picard F, Chaussard C, et al: [Computer-assisted knee arthroplasty: Comparison with a conventional procedure. Results of 50 cases in a prospective randomized study.] Rev Chir Orthop Reparatrice Appar Mot 87:18-28, 2001.
37. Sparmann M, Wolke B, Czupalla H, et al: Positioning of total knee arthroplasty with and without navigation support. A prospective, randomised study. J Bone Joint Surg Br 85:830-835, 2003.
38. Stern SH, Insall JN: Posterior stabilized prosthesis. Results after follow-up of nine to twelve years. J Bone Joint Surg Am 74:980-986, 1992.
39. Stockl B, Nogler M, Rosiek R, et al: Navigation improves accuracy of rotational alignment in total knee arthroplasty. Clin Orthop 426:180-186, 2004.
40. Stulberg SD: How accurate is current TKR instrumentation? Clin Orthop 416:177-184, 2003.
41. Stulberg SD, Loan P, Sarin V: Computer-assisted navigation in total knee replacement: Results of an initial experience in thirty-five patients. J Bone Joint Surg Am 84(Suppl 2):90-98, 2002.
42. Swank ML: Computer-assisted surgery in total knee arthroplasty: Recent advances. Surg Technol Int 12:209-213, 2004.
43. Teter KE, Bregman D, Colwell CW: Accuracy on intramedullary versus extramedullary tibial alignment cutting systems in total knee arthroplasty. Clin Orthop 321:106-110, 1995.
44. Teter KE, Bregman D, Colwell CW: The efficacy of intramedullary femoral alignment in total knee replacement. Clin Orthop 321:117-121, 1995.

Electromagnetic Computer-Assisted Navigation in Total Knee Replacement

David R. Lionberger

The first uses of navigation involved imagery that linked a localizer that measured the geometry of the infrared reflective surfaces and light-emitting diodes or tracking grids applied to a fixed point of the skeleton.[10] Image-guided medical and surgical procedures utilize patient images obtained before or during a medical procedure to guide a physician performing the procedure. Recent advances in imaging technology, especially in imaging technologies that produce highly detailed, two-, three-, and four-dimensional images, such as computed tomography (CT), magnetic resonance imaging (MRI), fluoroscopic imaging (such as with a C-arm device), positron emission tomography, and ultrasound imaging, have increased the interest in image-guided medical procedures. By means of triangulation from a camera array, these reflective devices could calculate minute position changes. However, these were constrained by the necessity of a direct, unobstructed line of sight. If the signal were disrupted by any type of nontransparent object, the signal would change or be blocked, thereby implicating a potential change of position. Because of the sensitivity to signal disruption, it was necessary to build into the navigation system a signal to detect disruption that ensures that false position values are not being conveyed, even though the anatomic specimen may still be in the same position.

Typical image-guided navigation systems generally require dynamic reference frames (DRFs) to track the position of the patient as movement occurs during the procedure. The DRF is affixed to the patient in a generally fixed or rigid fashion. It may also be used as a fiducial marker and may, therefore, be attached to the patient during the acquisition of preoperative images. This enables the image space to be aligned with patient space during the navigated procedure. Trackers are designed to reflect infrared signals from the camera receiver assembly. The visibility for transmission of signals encountered is limited to a 180-degree arc or azimuth. This mandates the trackers to be placed in the optimal location to maintain visibility through a full range of motion for the surgical procedure. Because of the physics of signal resolution and accuracy, the wider the separation of reflector markers of the tracker array, the more accurate the system will be. This mandates a minimal acceptable downsizing of the tracker, which often is obtrusive to surgical exposure as well as easily being caught on instruments in the field of exposure. This necessitates placing the tracker in a remote area by one or more pins to ensure secure fixation.

However, this may result in soft tissue tethering or injury when movement of the extremity is performed. Placing of these trackers also sometimes creates sterility challenges associated with placement.

Various instruments may be used during operative procedures that are desired to be tracked. Even if images are acquired, either intraoperatively or preoperatively, the instrument is generally illustrated and superimposed on the captured image data to identify the position of the instrument relative to the patient space. Therefore, the instrument may include detectable portions such as electromagnetic coils or optical detection points (e.g., light-emitting diodes or reflectors) that may be detected by a suitable navigation system.

Size considerations generally make it difficult to position the tracking sensors near the working end of the jigs. Because of this, the tracking sensors are generally positioned within the handle of the instrument. Therefore, complex calculations and a degree of error may exist to determine the exact position of a distal end of the instrument relative to the position of the detectable sensors. Also the instruments may flex unexpectedly so that the known dimensions are no longer true dimensions of the instrument. Therefore, it may be desirable to provide sensors substantially near the distal tip or end of an instrument positioned within a patient.

Because of problems including fixation, signal acquisition, soft tissue trauma, and operative field disruption from line-of-sight mandates, thought was given to a non–line-of-sight signal that would penetrate soft tissue yet not be affected by the normal examination parameters of the operating room. Because satellite navigation or global positioning systems rely on fairly large sensors with the transmitter and receiver, a tissue-penetrating electromagnetic system with extremely small sensors for localization was considered. The first uses of this technology were for neurosurgical and ear, nose, and throat applications for cranial surgery in infants in whom pin penetration in the soft cranium, 360-degree coordinate measurements, and very accurate three-axis navigation are necessary.

Proving its success in this arena, cardiovascular surgery used the power of ferromagnetic catheter tips forced by electromagnetic field alternation to guide ferrous-tipped catheters into tortuous vessels that were not navigable by traditional intracatheterization techniques. These were tracked by fluoroscopy but had the distinction of reversing the role of an electromagnetic system to steer them rather than track them into extremely tight, convoluted vessels.[1,14]

Electromagnetic tracking techniques have been adopted by the specialties of neurosurgery and ear, nose, and throat disease to provide guidance for many surgical procedures. Despite these applications in the neurosurgical market, integration into orthopedic procedures has been very limited and on a trial basis only. Orthopedic applications have been relegated to a correlative secondary aid for navigation rather than as a primary guidance system.[5-7,13,16,17]

Much of the lack of confidence in electromagnetic technology within the orthopedic market arises from the stability of the signal, metallic interference, and speed of computer computation of positional changes. However, with the advent of redundant transmission magnetic generators referred to as localizers and DRFs constructed with multiple magnetic coils, much of the instability and signal inaccuracy is removed and precision is vastly improved to the same level of accuracy as the industry standard of ± 2 mm and ± 2 degrees of angulation. Achieving this level of accuracy allows electromagnetic tracking to have equivalent status as traditional line of sight infrared navigation systems while maintaining localization through soft tissues.

Safety of magnetism exposure is an age-old debate that has not been completely elucidated even now.[12] As its uses have transcended application to bone and tissue ingrowth, cartilage generation, or pain relief, there are still no published studies implicating detrimental effects. Disruption of the field may thwart proper activation or engagement of the cardiac monitoring and pacemaker capabilities. Difficulties within the confines of cardiac defibrillation and pulsing are being addressed by pacemaker-tolerant circuiting built into many pacemakers.

PHYSICS BEHIND ELECTROMAGNETIC NAVIGATION

By creating a low-intensity magnetic field, sensors are able to read the strength received from the electromagnetic field and produce a microvoltage. The field is produced by a transmitter sometimes referred to as a localizer, which runs off either alternating or direct current. Usually these localizers are a combination of three or more generator coils producing the magnetic strength in intermittent fashions so as to constantly produce an oscillating or varied field, which imparts a stronger sensitivity for the receiver reception. The magnetic field is generally around one gauss (0.0001 Tesla). A receiver placed in a particular position away from a magnetic field will transmit varied electric current depending on its position in relationship to the field strength. However, the electric current produced is based on the change in magnetic field as well as its intensity, hence the rationale behind a pulse or oscillating field. The coil direction in relation to the field produces the maximum strength, whereas a 90-degree polarization negates the electric current produced.

Faraday's law is a relationship derived from *Maxwell's equations*, which are shown below. This relationship states that the magnitude of the electromotive force induced in

a circuit is proportional to the rate of change of the magnetic flux that cuts across the circuit:

Integral Form

$$\oint \vec{E} \cdot d\vec{s} = -\frac{d\Phi_B}{dt}$$

Differential Form

$$\nabla \times E = -\frac{\partial B}{\partial t}$$

Faraday's law is a summary of the ways a voltage may be generated by a change in the magnetic environment. Any change in the magnetic flux, no matter how it is produced, will cause a voltage to be induced into the coil (Fig. 98–1). These changes could be produced by[3]:

- A change in the magnitude of the magnetic field within the coil
- A change in the area of the coil, or the portion of that area that happens to lie within the magnetic field (expand the coil or slide it out of the field)
- A change in the angle between the direction of the magnetic field and the area of the coil

$$\text{Voltage Generated} = -N\frac{\Delta(BA)}{\Delta t}$$

$$\text{Electromotive Force} = -N\frac{\Delta\Phi}{\Delta t}$$

where N = number of turns, ϕ = BA = magnetic force, B = external magnetic field, and A = area of coil.

If the magnetic field is spatially constant across a loop with N turns, the induced electromotive force in the coil of N connected loops can be expressed as N times the electromotive force produced in one loop.

By knowing the field strength, computer calculations can determine the direction of the field strength. The system can then locate and orient the position of the receiver by the electric current it receives from one or more coils. A coil may measure not only field strength but also the direction of the magnetic field such that the XYZ position can be determined. Therefore, pitch and yaw can

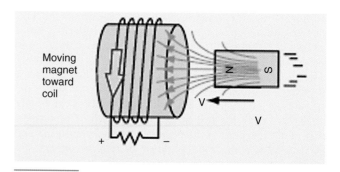

Figure 98–1. The soft iron inside the coil creates a magnetic field when the current is flowing. On the right is the receiver, or DRF, which creates the maximum current when the coil orientation is parallel in the field. Below are resultant formulas describing the energy of both.

be ascertained, which is better known as 5 degrees of freedom; however, the 6th degree, better known as roll, cannot be determined without two or more receiver coils to obtain this final degree of orientation. This is why many vendors are moving to multiple coil receivers in their trackers because rotation has great importance in total knee replacement and other orthopedic surgery.

Transmitter coils or field strength generators are merely solenoids, which are powered through the use of alternating or direct current. There are inherent advantages of both types of technology as there are also disadvantages. For example, in the alternating current system using three-coil technology, the computation is significantly reduced in terms of mathematically determining the position of the instruments. However, the magnet necessary to power the system may be somewhat obtrusive in an operative field if the user desires to create a very large field. Multiple coils can reduce the size of the transmitter but increase the computation power needed to compute for sufficient localization speed.

The transmitter coil array is controlled or driven by the coil array controller, which drives each coil in the transmitter coil array in a time division multiplex or a frequency division multiplex manner. In this regard, each coil may be driven separately at a distinct time or all of the coils may be driven simultaneously with each being driven by a different frequency. On driving the coils in the transmitter coil array with the coil array controller, electromagnetic fields are generated within the patient in the area where the surgical procedure is being performed, which is again sometimes referred to as patient space. This space is a finite area dependent on flux strength and outside interference. The electromagnetic fields generated in the patient space induce currents in sensors positioned in the instrument, such as the paddle probe or pointer. These induced signals from the instrument are delivered to the navigation probe interface through the isolation circuit and subsequently forwarded to the coil array controller. The navigation probe interface also includes amplifiers, filters, and buffers required to directly interface with the sensors in the instrument. Alternatively, the instrument may employ a wireless communications channel as opposed to being coupled directly to the navigation probe interface. Once a signal is activated, a pulse field is oscillated at a set frequency that is sampled by the computer and averaged generally on a per-second update basis, which is then transmitted to the monitor.

The DRF of the electromagnetic tracking system is also coupled to the navigation probe interface to forward the information to the coil array controller. The DRF, which is designed to be fixed to the patient adjacent to the region being navigated, can then detect any movement of the patient as relative motion between the transmitter coil array and the DRF. This relative motion is forwarded to the coil array controller, which updates registration correlation and maintains accurate navigation, further discussed herein. The DRF can be configured as a pair of orthogonally oriented coils, each having the same center, or may be configured in any other non-coaxial or coaxial coil configuration.

Alternating current technology also uses audiofrequency wave energy to transmit to the receiver coil. The receiver coil works much the same way as a transformer because it consists of loops of wire, which create a small electric current. Because of this oscillation system, a time sequence for frequency multiplexed transmission can create a more consistent and sustaining magnetic field that is less susceptible to outside interferences such as metal or environmental factors of other electromagnetic sources. It also is more likely to detect outside interferences capable of disrupting accuracy.

Direct current technology uses coils powered by a direct current source. These coils are cycled sequentially, which are subsequently read by the receiver coil. However, the magnetic fields do not couple energy into loops of wire and, therefore, they require a "hall effect" sensor or flux gate technology. This flux gate technology refers to a larger and more expensive sensor or receiver, which sometimes interferes with navigation issues at a surgical setting.

Originally, some thought that direct current systems would offer the advantage of less interference from metal and other conductive distortions. However, in practice, the effect is a creation of fields from remote metal sources, which actually distort the navigation more than in a pulsed alternating current system. Because of these issues, more emphasis is being placed on alternating current technology than on the more simplified direct current systems.

Industry standards currently achieve a ±2 mm localization accuracy and a ±2 degrees of error in angulatory accuracy.[15] Another term that is commonly utilized to define accuracy is root mean square (RMS) error. This is the normalization of absolute deviation in values obtained by a measure. Currently, an RMS error of ±4 mm of the center of the femoral head for kinematic localization is acceptable to introduce no more than 1 degree of error to knee axis calculations, which is well within the realm of human hand-held jigs. In actuality, many systems are much more accurate than the industry standard; however, to aid in simplicity at the time of surgery, decimal point accuracy is rounded up or down to make navigation more user friendly by eliminating screen clutter. The systems currently available are in some cases dummied down to provide a more simplified navigation for surgeons while improving accuracy logarithmically in terms of the traditional non-navigated instruments.

Part of the exceptional accuracy of the systems stems from the aforementioned transmitter field generation system. Additional precision detection of outside remote signal errors or interference can be gained by smart instruments, which have defined read only memory (ROM) values. By the computer recognizing a particular distinctive discrete sensor, which has its own ROM chip, the device, when plugged in, is able to be individually calibrated both anatomically (femur or tibia) as well as to the highest level of accuracy to the system without user interaction being required. Although single-coil navigation is possible, incorporation of a second or possibly third coil makes the accuracy and precision of the system even more defined. Despite these accuracies, it is important to realize that the bench-tested accuracy of any system is only as good as the environment from which it is utilized. Soft tissue shifts, environmental factors of metal or magnetic distortion, and surgical tactile accuracy all play large roles in the intraoperative accuracy of any system.

SOURCES OF DISTORTION

Inherent with any magnetic system is the interference from other objects in the environment. These can be classified into two general areas of conductive and ferrous distortions.

Conductive distortion is created by a transmission source creating a current in a conductive metal, which results in a "parasitic" field. Examples of materials that create these types of distortions are most steels as well as aluminum or any other highly conductive material. Because titanium is only partially conductive, it remains relatively immune to affecting the field of a nearby coil generation. Even carbon fiber containing Kevlar and other synthetic fibers can create some small conductivity and, therefore, are subject to some small distortion if placed directly in the transmission field (Fig. 98–2).

Ferrous interference is the most frequently referred to and better understood concept, especially given our understanding with MRI interferences. Any object that a magnet is attracted to can be considered ferrous. The stronger the attraction, the more ferrous the metal. Therefore, steels such as the 400 series and 17-4 stainless are highly ferrous. Because aluminum and titanium are not as ferrous, they tend not to "bend" the magnetic field and, therefore, create less distortion. The effects of ferrous metals are seen in both the alternating and direct current systems; however, alternating current systems are less affected by remote ferrous interference.

With knowledge of metal and magnetic interference, a greater understanding of the environment for successful electromagnetic navigation has been ascertained in recent time. A number of axioms have evolved, including:

- Maximizing proximity of the transmitter to the operative field
- Instrumentation selection to minimize ferrous disruption
- Minimization of metal directly between the transmitter and receiver coils, no matter what the metal type
- The larger the metal mass, the greater the distortion
- Encouragement of an electromagnetic friendly environment such as fluoroscopy operative tables and minimization of heavy metals in the immediate vicinity, such as Mayo stands and rails on operative beds

With the recent advancements in sensitivity and distortion, many of these nuisances (e.g., interference sources) have been eliminated. Nonetheless, the more disruption the environment can eliminate, the better the usability of the system.

With the advent of fluoroscopy in the operating room to supplement and confirm three-dimensional anatomic accuracy of tracking, such as in pelvic, spinal, and cranial anatomy, many systems have adopted technology to make possible the use of C-arms and fluoroscopy in proximity to the electromagnetic navigation system. This has inherent interference potential yet is invaluable in subspecialties of spinal and trauma procedures where tracking and three-dimensional small distant relationships become enhanced. Fluoroscopy-guided navigation systems continue to be pursued in the industry; therefore, the compatibility of the system for C-arm is paramount.

ERROR AND ACCURACY

There are a number of accuracy measurements computer-assisted navigation systems can be judged from. The most basic is sensitivity and precision by federal guidelines mandating limits of ±2 degrees of translation accuracy. Before issuing 510K approval, most systems are rounded to the nearest degree and millimeter.

The measures are also subject to other errors such as edge of distortion where interference occurs the closer an object gets to the transmitter receiver field. Drift can also occur as fluctuations in the voltage, temperature, or circuitry relationships change. Or it may be long term in the form of delayed value changes or precision greater than 10 minutes. Voltage stabilization programs embedded in the software elimination field fluctuate with current systems.

Acquisition speed, or the time required to capture, read, and calculate a receiver, varies with different systems. Case in point: stability of the localizer is paramount to prevent the computer from getting fluctuation values from the receivers. Additionally, processing speeds of computers linked to software modifications influence acquisition speed. Sampling may be instantaneous; however, some systems use a mean or average to acquire position values before the program allows the screen to display the numerical readings. In order to enhance usability, the software has a preset value spread before "clipping" the signal, thereby establishing an off-signal or no-signal status. This may be an alert, a color change, or merely a blank screen.

METALLIC DISTORTION ERROR

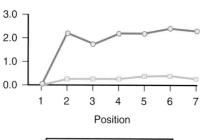

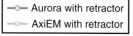

	AxiEM	Aurora
Mean	0.71	1.30
Standard deviation	0.34	0.96
99% Confidence Int.	1.74	4.17
Max	1.59	4.31

Figure 98–2. Distortion from metallic interference is different depending on DC vs. AC transmitter field production.

USE AND TECHNIQUE

Time requirements for this system are no different than others but currently require the surgeon after adoption (usually 15 to 20 cases) to spend about 10 more minutes for registration and data collection over traditional, non-navigated cases. However, by eliminating some of the jig reparation and dismantling, some time-saving steps, such as elimination of preliminary cuts, are possible.

As with many computer-assisted navigation systems, added personnel may be required to enter the data or shift on the various screen options. Many programs feature floor, mouse, or touch-screen capability; however, even this requires the surgeon to temporarily take his or her attention away from the field to the screen. Voice activation commands are also being investigated in commands of various computer functions and consequently are applicable for electromagnetic work as well. Additionally, many programs offer user-specific choices to adapt different procedural sequences to be customized to the surgeon rather than being proprietarily specific.

If one is familiar with the typical infrared tracking system, graduating to an electromagnetic system will prove to be not only easy but also gratifying. Because of the small size of the trackers, a continuous, unobstructed feedback, and downsizing of instrumentation, electromagnetic systems provide an easier platform, which is virtually invisible in the operative field (Fig. 98–3).

Just like infrared systems, the electromagnetic system requires affixing two DRFs to the area around the knee. After soft tissue clearing, the femoral tracker is placed beneath the VMO at the midsagittal line about 4 cm from the joint line to avoid disruption from the femoral component or cutting guides. With the knee in extension, a retractor may be used to move a portion of the soft tissue or expand the incision for positioning of the DRF on a particular portion of the femur; once the portion is removed, the soft tissue is replaced over the DRF (Fig. 98–4).

The tibial tracker is placed on the medial tibial flare low enough to avoid disruption by cutting guide impingement, yet out from the canal so as not to impinge the stem of the tibial tray or its corresponding preparatory instruments. It, too, should be midsagittal with fixation screws pointing posteriorly so as to minimize stem contact (Fig. 98–5).

The DRF is positioned relative to a portion of the anatomy, with single cortical screws, such as a soft tissue

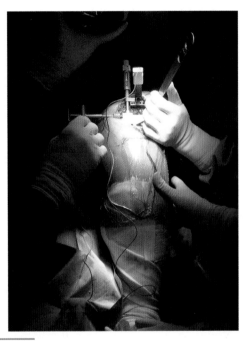

Figure 98–4. Typical subvastus and tibial plateau placement of DRFs on a minimally invasive surgical incision.

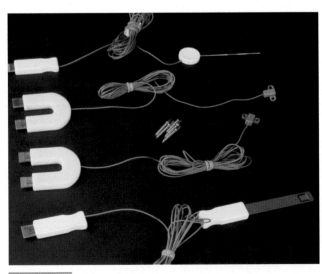

Figure 98–3. Transmitter coils or DRF in order from top to bottom are stylus, femoral and tibial trackers, and paddle probe.

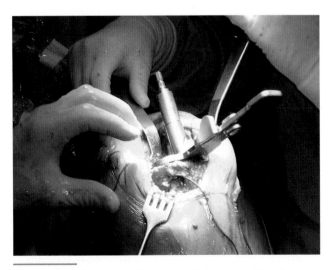

Figure 98–5. The tibial DRF should be placed in the area beneath the medial tibia with the fixation screws pointing away from stem preparation instruments to prevent impingement.

portion for added stability. In addition, the DRF includes antirotation fixators and flexible wings, providing better conformity to the varied contours of the bone. Once the DRF is positioned at the selected location, the incision may be moved back to its initial position, near where the procedure is to be performed. This allows for a transdermal or subdermal placement of the low-profile DRF.

Thus the primary incision, which can be minimally invasive if desired, may be used to both position the DRF and perform a selected procedure. The subdermal placement assists in performing minimally or less invasive procedures.

The features of the DRF do not obstruct the movement of the soft tissue to which the DRF is attached or the soft tissue relative to which the DRF is moving. Thus, the DRF may be positioned and used to determine a movement of a bony portion, a soft tissue portion, and the like, where the DRF is moving and touching the soft tissue portions without interrupting the movement of the various selected portions. Furthermore, the DRF may be substantially wired or wireless to allow for various configurations and purposes. Localizer position is crucial in the electromagnetic setting. Optimal distance from the DRF is 15 cm, but transmission can occur as distant as 500 cm. In practice, a signal can be best transmitted in an unobstructed field with no metal between the localizer and DRF from 5 to 25 cm. However, even in this range, "clipping" may occur if metallic interference is introduced.

Once these are affixed, the landmarks are inputted, including acquiring the hip center through repeated circumduction of the hip. The digitized landmarks are inputted off of a pointer (Fig. 98–6), which are simply:

Medial posterior condyle	Medial tibial plateau
Lateral posterior condyle	Lateral tibial plateau
Medial distal condyle	Tibial eminence
Lateral distal condyle	Tibial tendon insertion
Anterior notch	Medial malleolus
Whiteside's line	Lateral malleolus

In a surgical navigation system, it may be desirable to ensure that the cutting block is positioned at a selected position or orientation. The paddle probe is positioned relative to the cutting block. Once the paddle probe has been fit in the cutting block, the tracking sensor is used to determine a location and orientation of the guide slot.

The best reception for this is to rotate the DRF to the side of the block to minimize metal interferences. This also ensures that the cutting slot or guide surface is positioned relative to the femoral condyles and functional axis (Whiteside's line) in a selected position so as to predict and ensure proper orientation, translation, and rotation. Once positioned for 0 degrees of rotation relative to Whiteside's line or 3 degrees of external relative to functional axis, the right adjustment to prevent notching can be done. Mediolateral centering is a non-navigated function.

The paddle probe allows for a hands-free or single-hand operation of the cutting block. The position of the cutting block can be determined with the instrument by positioning the instrument and using the navigation system.

Most navigation systems have capabilities for kinematic range of motion collection before any cuts are made. This

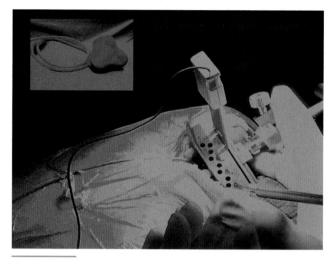

Figure 98–6. Typical operative setup with field generator or triangular localizer inset.

not only provides confidence establishing the playing field of presurgical knee deformity and ranges but also assists in future soft tissue releases and corrected resection requirements necessary to regain the best postoperative function of the knee. As the sequence of resections proceeds, the program is customized to follow an intuitive path of steps to ready the surgeon for navigating each step, such as reserving posterior femoral condyle acquisition until after the tibia is resected so as to optimize visualization (Fig. 98–7).

Then, smart cutting jigs or paddle probes that fit in saw capture guides allow for non-intramedullary preparation of the distal femur or proximal tibia (Fig. 98–8).

Because prediction of size for optimal femoral sizing without violation of the anterior cortex or notching is possible, the system ensures proper restoration of the joint line, adequate extension, and flexion gap distances for proper joint ligament isometry. Referencing posteriorly or anteriorly when exposure allows during the sequences of articular resections makes acquisition more accurate (Fig. 98–9).

Freshening up unsatisfactory cuts to perfect alignment is easily done because the surgeon can maintain an interactive, constant feedback of instruments without losing reception of navigational signals when the surgeon or assistants is in the way of the receiver (Fig. 98–10).

Gap distance measurements available in several systems allow the surgeon actual numerical values of condyle to tray distance in a variety of extension and flexion angles so as to easily make prudent judgments of joint laxity in all positions. Because incisions for minimal interventional surgery restrict visualization, it behooves surgeons to establish better measures and documentation of joint laxity in any position. This can be helped by having the surgeon brace the localizer against the knee at a preset "sweet spot" for best reception. Then, when the assistant moves the knee to determine kinematic measures, the localizer tracks physically with the knee. Once cementing is complete, final verification can be recorded and the DRFs are removed. Because they are inboard to the incision, no special care is used in the closure over that of any

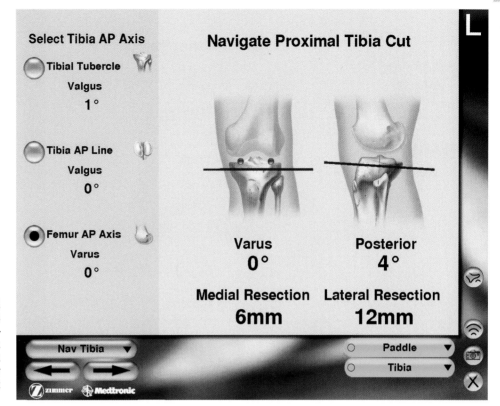

Figure 98–7. Distal femoral resection screen with angles and level of resection in millimeters. Note the activation of the "notch" warning when the resection level falls below the anterior femoral shaft waypoint.

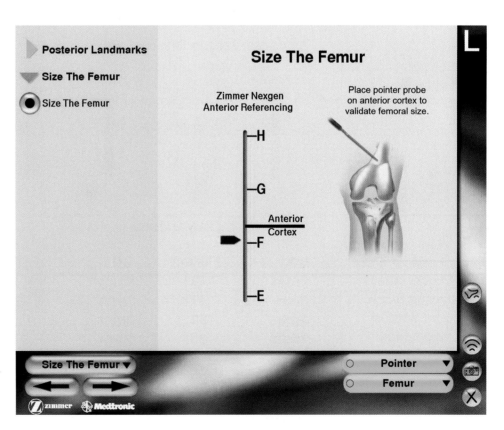

Figure 98–8. Femoral prediction "best size" based on computer-assisted measurements.

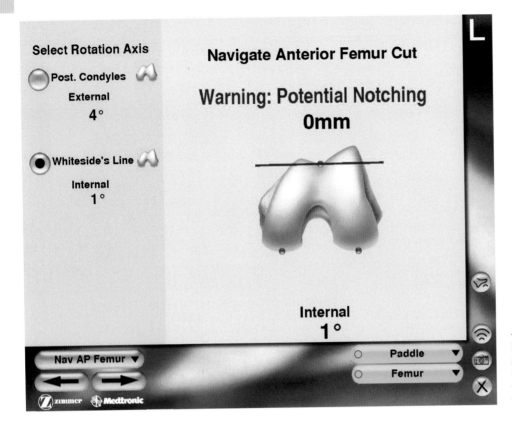

Figure 98–9. Tibial resection screen provides pictorial updates as well as numerical values of angles and resection levels.

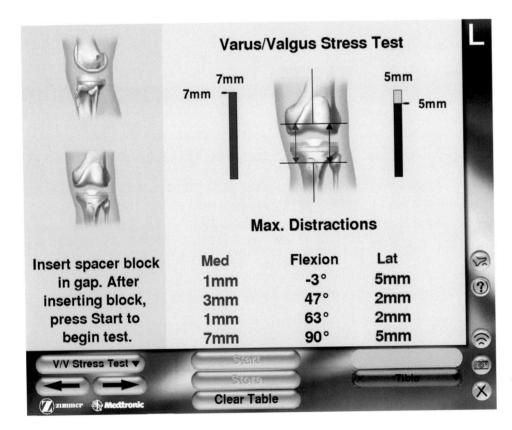

Figure 98–10. Gap distance measurement.

other total knee replacement. Data entered and onscreen shots are then archived to a compact disc from the computer and made available on a disc for PowerPoint, patient, and/or research use. It is prudent to obtain measures with plastic trials before cementing in the event that the large metal mass of some implants does not disrupt the electromagnetic signal after cement application.

ADVANTAGES OF ELECTROMAGNETIC NAVIGATION

One of the most frustrating problems with traditional infrared trackers is the bone and soft tissue trauma they create by attachment using large, ridged pins. Because of the large lever arm on the reflective trackers, ridged bicortical fixation is mandatory to ensure there is no movement of the tracker array. Muscle damage may occur around the anchor pins. These have been reported to induce scar tissue around pin sites, resulting in soft tissue damage, leading to arthrofibrosis or poor postoperative performance. Use of less obtrusive, downsized trackers may minimize this complication.

Additionally, large, bicortical, and multiple hole violations of bone have been implicated in fractures postoperatively, leading users to look for smaller fixation options away from rigid tracker framers. Downsizing of trackers to single cortical mounts on the metaphyseal region, a more load-tolerant area of bone, lessens fracture risks significantly.

The single most enjoyable aspect of electromagnetic tracking over the traditional infrared approach is the disappearance of the assistant or surgeon signal interference from the signal or camera array. Those familiar with infrared computer-assisted navigation can attest to the frustration and difficulties in reception of signals, only to be made worse by an untimely signal interruption at the precise moment the surgeon can least afford it. Electromagnetic tracking simplifies this with the ability to see through the assistant, surgeon, and patient. With electromagnetic friendly instruments and retractors there is less disruption to the signal, which lessens the constraint on the working environment.

Because line of sight is no longer an issue, congestion around a small exposure from personnel allows mobile trackers such as paddle probes to provide real-time verification of the accuracy of a cut. Subsequent revision cuts are made intelligently rather than by cumbersome jigs or trial and error-prone re-cuts.

The most important provision electromagnetic tracking provides is the ability of navigating during minimally invasive surgery. Whether or not one is an advocate of smaller incisions, the invasive, destructive nature of four or more bicortical pins takes away much of what a minimally invasive surgical total joint can provide. When even a small incision allows for placement of the trackers without extending the incision, exceptional guidance can be achieved without interference or alternation of exposure. If one believes precision is as important as minimization of tissue trauma, the use of electromagnetic tracking provides just that.

In summary, as with most navigation systems, the electromagnetic computer-assisted navigation system outcomes would include the following:

1. Reduced outliers are available for acceptable angulation and alignment for implants.
2. Documentation of presurgical and postsurgical kinematics is given as a permanent record or retrievable digital file.
3. Analytical cataloguing and recall for research purposes is made possible.
4. Refinement of first cut to a more perfect cut is likely, owing to a more precise starting point and instantaneous real-time feedback during the cut.
5. Revision of cut inaccuracy is effortlessly done without cumbersome re-cut jigs or their invasive fixation anchors.
6. Avoidance of the femoral canal violation inducing intraoperative pulmonary complication of fat embolisms and lessening of complications associated with inaccuracy of bowing creating flexed femoral components are possible.
7. Predictive measures of many systems on the market make it possible in many instances to provide an intraoperative template of a best-fit scenario. The surgeon can thus rely on more accurate measures instead of less accurate x-ray magnification–corrected plastic template guides.
8. Gap distance measurements are finally obtainable with many new navigation systems, not only in extension but also in a variety of flexion angles, making it possible to check and refine flexion-extension gaps so as to optimize range without giving up stability. These measurements are obtained dynamically and represent a far better solution to balancing isometry and joint line restoration, especially with the downsizing of incisions.
9. Rotational mating of the prosthesis to the anatomic axis of motion is another offshoot of navigation, which can aid in ensuring proper femoral tibial mating as well as in lessening the likelihood of collateral ligament discordance. As more dynamic data through all ranges are available, less collateral mismatch and rotatory incongruities are likely to be created.
10. Given inherent disagreement on the correct positions of the epicondylar axis from limited exposure to the epicondyles in the knee exposures during minimally invasive surgery, reliance on other guidance landmarks is mandatory. Most systems give a choice to the surgeon of Whiteside's line, functional axis, or posterior condyle referencing priority.

Prosthetic-specific, and inventory reduction for, instrumentation by simplification or elimination can not only improve our inventory but also ease the burden on staff and personnel. Tray size reduction, improved instrument turnover, and cost saving or cost shifting from the hospital, surgeon, or patient should eventually be realized.

Through all of the glitz and glamour of bringing a computer to the operating room, we as surgeons have a duty to avoid implying to our patients that the computer automatically makes us better surgeons than those not using the technology. Only decades of review will truly tell the result of what this era of computer technology did to improve our understanding of knee mechanics and whether that translates into more durable and functional knees.

CONS OF ELECTROMAGNETIC NAVIGATION

Just as the line of sight interferes with traditional infrared navigation, electromagnetic navigation can also be influenced by outside sources. One of the most important disruptions comes from ferromagnetic interference. This type of interruption results in the machine's default to be activated and the readings are turned off momentarily. This is absolutely imperative to have engaged in the program lest a surgeon relies on an aging reading that does not represent a current, accurate reception value.

Other signal disrupters are some metals, which may interfere with reception strength. Examples are aluminum, copper, and stainless steels. Yet some metals have a surprisingly low interference constant, such as the 300-series stainless steels (303, 316L) and all of the titanium alloys.

As long as these more disruptive metals are removed from the immediate field of the generator/receiver environment, there does not appear to be a big problem in maintaining adequate signal strength. For example, despite the massive content of aluminum and steel in the operating table, adequate reception of the signal can be maintained, especially with the knee in its typical surgical position in flexion, which places it normally 30 cm away or more from these interfering metals. This metallic interference has been fine-tuned with the use of electromagnetic-friendly instruments, unlike previous trials in electromagnetic tracking in which unstable signals were often encountered.

Edge of distortion interference is another form of potential error unique to electromagnetic navigation. As disruptive fields encroach on the navigation field, cancellation or signal instability can result from ferromagnetic electrical or other magnetic influences. This has been dealt with by computers that detect aberrant signal-to-noise ratios. The computer can detect this "clipping" of the detected strength versus what it should be at the distance to the field when disruption occurs. At this point, the computer either compensates or creates an off-signal status and the system defaults to "no readings." Infrared systems do not experience the same disruption in signal line of sight but may still experience partial fiduciary blockage.

Magnetic signals created by the localizer are also sensitive to movement, just as are their receivers. Therefore, ridged or steady dampening movement during acquisition or measurements improves speed of data registry. If there is any movement in the localizer, the response time on the DRF is lengthened. It is important to stabilize rapid motion, which may be achieved by placing the localizer on a firm platform or support.

The size of the localizer is generally about the size of two softballs. This can be awkward at first, but after a short learning curve the surgical team works around it as if it was not there. If it interferes with standard surgical techniques, it can be moved away. Distance of the localizer from the DRF is somewhat important. Safety of magnetism exposure is an age-old debate that has not been completely elucidated even now.[12] As its uses have transcended application to bone and tissue ingrowth, cartilage generation, or pain relief, there are still no published studies implicating detrimental effects. Disruption of the field may thwart proper activation or engagement of the cardiac monitoring and pacemaker capabilities. Difficulties within the confines of cardiac defibrillation and pulsing are being addressed by pacemaker-tolerant circuiting presently built into many pacemakers.

FUTURE USES OF ELECTROMAGNETIC NAVIGATION

The brightest aspect of electromagnetic technology is its seemingly innocuous, nonobtrusive presence in the operative field. As incisions shrink, so will the patience of surgeons to be saddled with cumbersome technology that either lengthens their day or makes their job more difficult. By short-circuiting steps in knee replacements by smart jigs, smart drills, and prosthetic-specific knowledge-based programs, knee replacement in this coming decade will be much easier. It should be less time-consuming as refinements are made in the software to intuitively lead the surgeon. Through refining the precision to a more consistent product, accuracy, which has never been an issue in computer-assisted surgery, is complemented and assured.[11]

"Smart prostheses" that are bar-coded for identification as well as on-board tracking capability will someday be the norm. To provide the same service while reducing hospital, physician, and implant costs, emerging technology to refine, expedite, and assist the surgeons of tomorrow must continue to be developed. If computerization can accomplish in the private health care sector the same efficiency it has in the business fields, all of us will benefit (Fig. 98–11).

Virtual reality and augmented reality will continue to be developed in the years to come. By using data-gathering gloves and head or eyeglass displays, more flexible tracking and navigating can be achieved. Military applications continue to prove the importance of this in pushing existing capabilities to even more difficult and hard-to-reach goals, such as skeletal deformity as well as revision and trauma surgery, where preservation of remaining soft issue vascular supply is crucial to the success of the operation. The analogy of linking heads-up displays on the windshields of aircraft to heads-down displays on the eyeglasses of pilots in tandem with global positional system guidance (in this case electromagnetic computer-assisted navigational system technology) are examples of the plethora of technology currently available that have yet to be combined. Nonetheless, when all of these aids are given to the average surgeon, it is likely to expand operative effi-

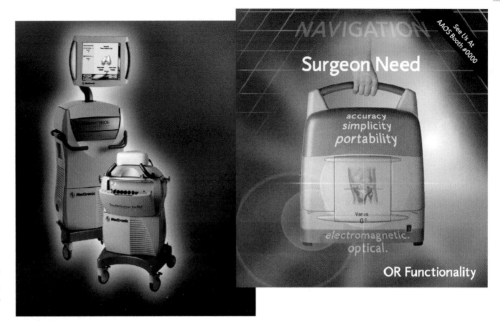

Figure 98–11. Then and now technology reflecting some trends seen in today's downsizing of computers.

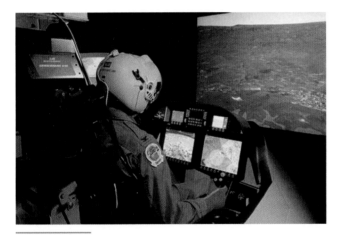

Figure 98–12. Pilot benefiting from today's computer advances.

ciency and accuracy to new horizons for the surgeon while making it far easier on patients in recovery and abbreviating the procedures performed (Fig. 98–12).

References

1. Faddis M, Blume W, Finney J, et al: Novel, magnetically guided catheter for endocardial mapping and radiofrequency catheter ablation. Circulation 106:2980-2985, 2002.
2. Fried MP, Kleefield J, Gopal H, et al: Image-guided endoscopic surgery: Results of accuracy and performance in a multicenter clinical study using an electromagnetic tracking system. Laryngoscope 107:594-601, 1997.
3. Halliday D, Resnick R, Walker J: Fundamentals of Physics, 5th ed. New York, Wiley & Sons, 1997, part III, p 754.
4. International Commission on Non-Ionizing Radiation Protection: Guidelines for limiting exposure to time-varying electric, magnetic and electromagnetic fields (up to 300 GHz). Health Physics 74:494-522, 1998.
5. Koele W, Stammberger H, Lackner A, Reittner P: Image guided surgery of paranasal sinuses and anterior skull base—5 years experience with the Instra Trak-System. Rhinology 40:1-9, 2002.
6. Kottkamp H, Hindricks G, Breithardt G, Borggrefe M: Three-dimensional electromagnetic catheter technology: Electroanatomical mapping of the right atrium and ablation of ectopic atrial tachycardia. J Cardiovasc Electrophysiol 8:1332-1337, 1997.
7. Kottkamp H, Hugl B, Krauss B, et al: Electromagnetic versus fluoroscopic mapping of the inferior isthmus for ablation of typical atrial flutter. Circulation 102:2082-2086, 2000.
8. Manwaring KH, Manwaring ML, Moss SD: Magnetic field guided endoscopic dissection through a burr hole may avoid more invasive craniotomies: A preliminary report. Acta Neurochir Suppl 61:34-39, 1994.
9. Otori N, Haruna S, Yoshiyuki M, Moriyama H: [Endoscopic endonasal surgery with image-guidance.] Nippon Jibiinkoka Gakkai Kaiho 103:1-6, 2000. Japanese.
10. Reinhardt H, Meyer H, Amrein E: A computer assisted device for the intraoperative CT-controlled localization of brain tumors. Eur Surg Res 20:51-58, 1988.
11. Reittner P, Tillich M, Luxenberger W, et al: Multislice CT-image-guided endoscopic sinus surgery using an electromagnetic tracking system. Eur Radiol 12:592-596, 2002.
12. Repacholi M, Greenebaum B: Interaction of static and extremely low frequency electric and magnetic fields with living systems: Health effects and research needs. Bioelectromagnetics (In press). (Summary report of WHO scientific review meeting on static and ELF held in Bologna, 1997).
13. Schwarz Y, Mehta AC, Ernst A, et al: Electromagnetic navigation during flexible bronchoscopy. Respiration 70:516-522, 2003.
14. Solomon S, Magle CA, Acker DE, Venbrux AC: Experimental non-fluoroscopic placement of inferior vena cava filters: Use of an electromagnetic navigation system with previous CT data. J Vasc Interv Radiol 10:92-95, 1999.
15. Victor J, Hoste D: Image-based computer-assisted total knee arthroplasty leads to lower variability in coronal alignment. Clin Orthop Relat Res 428:131-139, 2004.
16. Wagner A, Schicho K, Birkfellner W, et al: Quantitative analysis of factors affecting intraoperative precision and stability of optoelectronic and electromagnetic tracking systems. Med Phys 29:905-912, 2002.
17. Zaaroor M, Bejerano Y, Weinfeld Z, Ben-Haim S: Novel magnetic technology for intraoperative intracranial frameless navigation: In vivo and in vitro results. Neurosurgery 48:1100-1107; discussion 1107-1108, 2001.

CHAPTER 99

Complications of Total Knee Arthroplasty

Marc F. Brassard • John N. Insall • Giles R. Scuderi • Philip M. Faris

GENERAL COMPLICATIONS

Despite the advanced age of most patients and the frequency of associated medical conditions, such as arteriosclerotic heart disease, hypertension, diabetes, and chronic pulmonary disorders, the general complications of knee arthroplasty are relatively few. As with any substantial surgery, the major complications include cerebrovascular accidents, myocardial infarctions, and pulmonary embolism. In the postoperative period, patients are at risk for urinary retention, infections, and deep vein thrombosis (DVT). Considering that total knee arthroplasty (TKA) is a major surgical procedure, however, it is surprising that the operation can be performed so safely, especially when bilateral simultaneous procedures are done.[30,231,270] Several authors studied this aspect and failed to show increased risk with bilateral procedures. The risk of a catastrophic medical event is low in a patient who is monitored carefully. Careful preoperative evaluation is essential, and the patient must be in the best possible medical health. The type of anesthesia is probably not crucial, although we prefer epidural anesthesia. Intraoperative monitoring includes the use of a Swan-Ganz catheter in selected unilateral and most bilateral cases.

SYSTEMIC COMPLICATIONS

Thromboembolism

The importance of thromboembolic disease after TKA is controversial.* DVT occurs in approximately 50% of unilateral cases and in 75% of bilateral cases when no prophylaxis is used. Although DVT occurs mainly in the calf veins (Fig. 99–1), life-threatening emboli do not arise from this region. In contrast to the situation after total hip arthroplasty (THA), isolated proximal vein thrombosis does not seem to occur after knee surgery despite the possible trauma of a pneumatic tourniquet.

Some authors argue that distal thrombosis can be ignored, provided that the patient convalesces normally and is not confined to bed for a lengthy period. We believe this view is too optimistic, although we concede that the risk of a fatal thromboembolus is small and is lower than after THA. In a prospective review of 527 TKAs in 499

*References 48, 79, 80, 96, 97, 113, 124, 132, 148, 197, 200, 202.

patients, Khaw and colleagues,[167] using no prophylaxis other than antithrombotic stockings and relatively early (48 hours) mobilization, found only one death in 3 months from pulmonary embolism (0.19%). This patient had bilateral TKA and had a myocardial infarction 1 day postoperatively with the subsequent pulmonary embolus occurring 22 days postoperatively. Seven (1.3%) other patients developed symptomatic pulmonary embolism and were treated with anticoagulation without sequelae. This lower incidence of fatal pulmonary embolism is supported in other studies by Stulberg and colleagues (0%),[301] Stringer and associates (0%),[300] Khaw and colleagues (0.2%),[167] and Ansari and coworkers (0.4%).[9] Fatal emboli do occur, however, and 3 patients died as a result of emboli in the first 400 arthroplasties performed at the Hospital for Special Surgery. No specific prophylaxis was used at that time; the cause of death was confirmed by autopsy in all cases. We believe that the incidence of fatal pulmonary emboli is underestimated. A certain proportion of calf clots propagate proximally to form the more dangerous clots in the popliteal and femoral veins. This process takes time, however, and the major risk period for a fatal pulmonary embolism after TKA may be in weeks 3 and 4 after surgery (in contrast to the case after THA, in which a clot in the proximal veins may be found in one-fifth of cases after the first week). Because most TKA patients now are discharged after hospitalization of 2 to 3 days, sudden death at home in a patient having no clinical evidence of vein thrombosis may be attributed to myocardial infarction. It also is unlikely that an autopsy would be obtained.

Calf clots may not in themselves be important, but should be regarded as a harbinger of more proximal clotting. Haas and coworkers[113] studied 1329 patients with 1697 TKAs. Thrombosis was found in 808 patients (61%): 53% had thrombosis of the calf vein, and 8% had thrombosis of the proximal veins. The lung scans of 60 patients (4.5%) were positive, and symptomatic pulmonary emboli occurred in 14 patients (1.1%). All of these patients received aspirin as prophylaxis. Venography was performed between postoperative days 4 and 6. A perfusion lung scan obtained on postoperative day 5 to 7 was compared with a preoperative baseline perfusion lung scan. Thrombosis of the calf vein was treated with warfarin (Coumadin); the dosage was adjusted to maintain a prothrombin time at approximately 1.5 times control. Only patients with symptomatic proximal thrombi or symptomatic pulmonary emboli were fully anticoagulated with intravenous heparin.

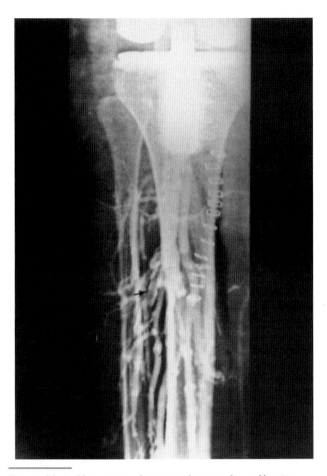

Figure 99–1. Venogram showing clots in the calf veins.

Although the natural history of thromboembolic disease was altered by prophylaxis and treatment, 6.5% of the patients with calf thrombi had a positive lung scan, and 1.6% had symptomatic pulmonary emboli. This finding was compared with the patients who had no venographic evidence of DVT, of whom 1.9% had a positive lung scan, and 0.2% had symptomatic pulmonary emboli. Statistical significance for the difference in lung scan and pulmonary embolus results was $p = 0.001$ and $p = 0.034$. Patients with calf or proximal thrombi were found to have similar rates of positive lung scans and symptomatic pulmonary emboli.

Kakkar and associates[161] used venography and serial fibrinogen imaging to evaluate the progress of calf thrombi in a group of postoperative patients. They found that 23% of calf thrombi propagated to the proximal veins. Doouss[69] performed a similar study and found a 5.6% propagation rate.

DETECTION OF DEEP VEIN THROMBOSIS

Many studies showed that clinical detection of DVT is unreliable. False-positive and false-negative results abound. The current trend in detection of DVT is the use of Doppler ultrasound.[175,342] The sensitivity and specificity of ultrasound are approaching those of the gold standard in detection—contrast venography. The sensitivity of ultrasound is reported to be 89% to 100%, the specificity is 95% to 100%, and the accuracy is 97% to 99%. These numbers apply to thigh clots only, however, between the inguinal ligament and the popliteal vein. Another potential disadvantage of Doppler ultrasound is that the accuracy of the test may vary because it is technician/operator dependent. Della Valle and colleagues[64] found only a 5.7% correlation of a positive duplex ultrasound with symptomatic proven pulmonary embolus. They suggested that a negative ultrasound should not preclude thorough evaluations for pulmonary embolus. Anderson and associates[8] found in patients on prophylactic warfarin that predischarge ultrasound was ineffective in predicting which patients would develop DVT or pulmonary embolism. The distinct advantage of ultrasound over venography is that it is noninvasive and causes minimal discomfort for the patient, allowing for serial examinations after surgery. Another advantage is that it localizes and quantitates the clot, which enables documentation of any changes in size and propagation. Other reliable objective diagnostic methods include iodine-125 fibrinogen scanning, impedance plethysmography, and ascending venography (see Fig. 99–1) for the diagnosis of venous thrombosis and ventilation-perfusion lung scanning and pulmonary angiography for the diagnosis of pulmonary embolism. Iodine-125 fibrinogen scanning provides confusing data after knee surgery, and impedance plethysmography is logistically demanding. Currently, we use Doppler ultrasound on postoperative day 3 and 3 weeks postoperatively. Because we are interested in the natural history of DVT, we obtain a preoperative lung scan and a follow-up scan on postoperative day 3. This protocol may not be necessary as part of the routine screening.

The incidence of DVT after a TKA without prophylaxis is 50% to 84% in the ipsilateral extremity. In the contralateral extremity, it is 3% to 5%.[195] Some confusion arises when discussing DVT based on the location of the thrombus. Most authors agree that thrombi below the popliteal vein are common and probably of little consequence, but they can propagate and become larger thrombi with more serious consequences. Larcom and coworkers[183] determined that proximal DVT occurs in only 5% to 8% of TKA and THA. Many authors[113,137,188,214] agree that isolated proximal venous thrombosis is infrequent after TKA, especially compared with THA.

Newer technology for the detection of DVT is being developed. One new diagnostic modality is magnetic resonance venography.[183] The major advantage of magnetic resonance venography over traditional contrast venography is that it is noninvasive. Its major advantage over venography and Doppler ultrasound is its ability to detect clots in the pelvis, for which both of the other techniques have extremely limited detection capability. Autopsy results from fatal pulmonary embolism show large thrombi that seem to originate in the large veins of the thigh and pelvis immediately before their dislodgment.[183] This finding shows the importance of detecting pelvic DVT. Larcom and coworkers[183] compared magnetic resonance venography with standard contrast venography. They found only a 45% sensitivity of magnetic resonance venography when interpreted by a dedicated magnetic resonance angiographer. This study shows the need for further development of this technique. With improved equipment and more experience in interpretation, however, magnetic resonance venography could become the preferred imaging technique.

PROPHYLAXIS

DVT prophylaxis after TKA is still prudent. With DVT rate 80% after TKA with no prophylaxis, it is mandatory that the patient receive some form of prophylaxis. There is no clear-cut favorite for the one best form of prophylaxis. The most commonly used forms of prophylaxis include aspirin, low-molecular-weight heparin (LMWH), warfarin, heparin, and compression devices. Other methods that have lost popularity include low-molecular-weight dextran, antithrombin III, and elastic stockings. We review the more commonly used agents.

Warfarin has been in use for almost 50 years. Debates are still waged over its advantages and disadvantages. Because warfarin is an oral agent, patient compliance is improved. There is low potential for excessive bleeding if careful control is maintained.[183] This characteristic is also a drawback, however, because monitoring the prothrombin time requires weekly phlebotomy, which many patients find inconvenient and painful. This vigilant monitoring is essential to prevent excessive bleeding complications in the knee and other locations. Another important disadvantage is that the patient cannot take any aspirin or nonsteroidal anti-inflammatory drugs.[195]

Aspirin for the prevention of DVT is another controversial method. Most of the literature published on aspirin is from THA literature. As with warfarin, aspirin is an oral agent, making it is easy to take on discharge from the hospital. Another advantage of aspirin is its low dose and high patient tolerance. Because it is such a small pill, patients have an easier time swallowing it. Also its relatively low cost and over-the-counter availability make aspirin an easier medication to obtain. The major disadvantage of aspirin is gastrointestinal intolerance, ranging from gastrointestinal upset to ulcers. In addition, patients are reluctant to accept this common medication as an effective preventive measure for such a serious complication.[195]

LMWH has gained in popularity. Compared with heparin, LMWH is a smaller and more homogeneous molecule, which accounts for its more favorable binding affinity to activated factors X and II. This mechanism of action results in an antithrombotic effect that is exerted earlier in the clotting cascade and theoretically decreases the risk of concurrent bleeding complications compared with the risk with unfractionated heparin.[13] An advantage of fractionated heparin (LMWH) is that coagulation times do not need to be monitored. Also, side effects (i.e., thrombocytopenia) are decreased compared with heparin, and LMWH half-life is prolonged, which reduces its dosage requirements. Outpatient compliance may be limited because LMWH requires subcutaneous injection. Another limitation may be its restricted use with epidural anesthesia. There have been reports of epidural hematomas forming after the epidural was removed with patients on LMWH. Overall, some authors indicated there is an increase in bleeding complications at the operative wound and at the injection site with the use of LMWH.

Although there is no firm evidence that the rate of fatal pulmonary embolism after TKA is significantly reduced by any form of prophylaxis, our own rate of fatal pulmonary embolism after TKA is 0.6% using intraoperative heparin, postoperative aspirin, antithrombotic stockings, and early mobilization within 24 hours.

New pentasaccharides (fondaparinux), which are selective inhibitors of factor XA, have been evaluated in randomized double-blinded studies. Compared with enoxaparin, fondaparinux reduced the risk of DVT with no difference in morbidity. Current recommendations include beginning fondaparinux with a dose of 2.5 mg daily subcutaneously and continuing for 10 days postoperatively. Postoperative complications, including bleeding and inability to reverse the anticoagulant effect of significant bleeding, may occur.[316] Mechanical compression is one of two types: plantar compression or calf/thigh compression. Plantar compression (foot pumps) (Fig. 99-2) has been gaining in popularity in recent years. The foot pumps work by producing a forceful ejection of blood from the foot into the calf with a pressure of greater than 100 mm Hg (versus traditional calf compression devices providing a pressure of 20 to 30 mm Hg). The pulse wave originates in the plantar venous plexus and flows proximally into the popliteal and femoral veins, which can be shown with venography and Doppler ultrasound.[329] The foot pumps prevent DVT by (1) increasing the venous return; (2) inducing high-flow states, which increase turbulence around venous valves and decrease the formation of thrombi; (3) increasing blood flow and tissue perfusion with the release of endothelium-derived relaxing factor

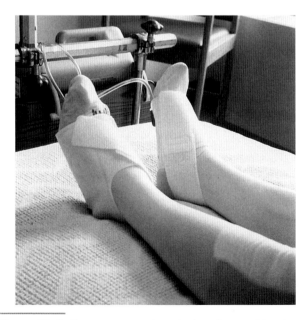

Figure 99-2. Foot compression device. It provides intermittent, pulsatile plantar compression.

and prostacyclin[100]; and (4) enhancing fibrinolysis with use of external pneumatic compression.[7] The advantages of compression devices as a whole include no medications to administer and no monitoring. Additional benefits of foot pumps include decreased postoperative thigh circumference and decreased wound drainage.[329] Disadvantages of external compression devices include patient compliance and the cost of the machines. There has been one report of a peroneal nerve palsy associated with the use of a pneumatic compression device.[250]

The standard external compression devices that compress either the calf or the thigh have advantages similar to the plantar compression devices. Additional advantages of the calf-high sleeves are keeping pressure off the operative site and reducing the prevalence of thrombosis in the calf veins after a TKA.[113] The disadvantage of the thigh-high compression sleeves is that it covers the wound and could compress the operative site.

The question of which mode of DVT prophylaxis should be used has been debated for many years. There have been many conflicting studies, and there is no ideal method for DVT prophylaxis. Warfarin remains one of the most popular methods used today. Most studies show that when warfarin is used alone, it decreases the rate of DVT. Laflamme and coworkers[181] used warfarin in TKA patients and found a DVT incidence of 21% and no pulmonary embolus. They also had a 0.9% incidence of major bleeding and minor bleeding, but no wound problems. Kaempffe and associates[160] compared warfarin and pneumatic compression in THA and TKA patients. In TKA patients, warfarin was more effective than compression (19% versus 32%), but after THA, compression was more effective than warfarin (16% versus 24%). The sample size was small in this study, so the conclusion is limited. Hodge[121] compared warfarin with pneumatic calf compression after TKA; again the sample size was small. In the warfarin patients, he found a DVT incidence of 30% with 6% in the thigh. In the compression group, he found a DVT incidence of 31% with 6% in the thigh. The warfarin group had an increase in expenses of 50% compared with the compression group. Hodge[121] concluded that both forms are safe and effective, but compression devices are more economical.

In a study by Stulberg and colleagues[301] of 517 patients with 638 TKAs, 84% of 49 patients who did not receive prophylaxis experienced ipsilateral DVT. All the patients in this study had postoperative venograms performed for the detection of DVT. The incidence of thrombosis was 57% in the 468 patients who received some form of prophylaxis (aspirin, low-dose heparin, supplemented low-dose aspirin, or warfarin). In 11 patients, there was evidence of thrombosis in the thigh or popliteal veins or both. Of the patients with bilateral TKA, 74% had evidence of thrombosis. No isolated popliteal or femoral clots were encountered.

Other studies compared the other forms of DVT prophylaxis. Haas and associates[113] compared compression devices with aspirin after unilateral and bilateral TKA. In the unilateral group, the incidence of DVT in the compression group was 22% versus 47% in the aspirin group. In the bilateral group, the incidence of DVT in the compression group was 48% versus 68% in the aspirin group.

The authors recommended the use of compression devices in unilateral TKA. Wilson and colleagues[338] compared plantar compression devices with no prophylaxis. In a small sample, they found 0% DVT in the plantar compression group versus 19% in the no prophylaxis group. Westrich and Sculco[329] compared plantar compression and aspirin with aspirin alone. Overall, in unilateral and bilateral TKA, the compression plus aspirin group had a DVT rate of 27% compared with 59% in the aspirin alone group. Significantly, with the proximal thrombi being considered the most likely to embolize, they found no proximal thrombi in the compression group and 14% incidence in the aspirin alone group. Another key point in this study is the patient compliance factor and the amount of time the compression devices were worn. In the group that had DVT, the patients wore the devices an average of 13.4 hr/day. The group that did not experience DVT wore the devices 19.2 hr/day.

Oral anticoagulants, which require no postoperative monitoring, are now in trials and would be a great aid in prophylactic management if they prove efficacious and safe. Many studies have examined the efficacy of LMWH. Colwell and associates[52] compared LMWH with heparin. The incidence of DVT was 24.6% in the LMWH group and 34.2% in the heparin group. Fitzgerald and colleagues[94] compared LMWH with low-dose heparin after TKA. They found that LMWH had a DVT incidence of 25% versus 45% for low-dose heparin. Levine and coworkers[188] compared LMWH with compression stockings. They reported a DVT incidence of 29.8% in the LMWH group and 58.3% in the compression group. In this study, the incidence of bleeding events was similar between the two groups: 2.5% in the LMWH group and 2.4% in the compression group. Leclerc and colleagues[185] compared LMWH with warfarin and found a 36.9% incidence of DVT in the LMWH group compared with 51.7% in the warfarin group. They discovered similar incidence of bleeding events. Spiro and associates[296] examined LMWH and warfarin after TKA. LMWH had a lower incidence of DVT at 25.4% compared with warfarin at 45.4%. Proximal clots also were lower in the LMWH group, 1.7% versus 11.4% in the warfarin group. The investigators found an increased incidence of hemorrhagic complications in the LMWH group, 6.9% compared with 3.4% in the warfarin group.

Currently, no one form of DVT prophylaxis enjoys wide-ranging acceptance because of the side effects, complications, or conflicting data on DVT incidence. The ideal prophylaxis method would be effective immediately postoperatively and last for at least 6 weeks. Currently, this profile of coverage requires two simultaneous methods. Warfarin has been shown to be an effective agent, but it requires several days to become effective. Maynard and colleagues[214] showed that most thromboses form in the intraoperative or immediate postoperative period. Warfarin is not effective in preventing these clots. Maynard and colleagues[214] also showed that all thromboses propagated into or above the popliteal vein despite warfarin therapy initiated at the time of the initial positive venogram. On the basis of this information, the ideal prophylaxis would be effective immediately in the recovery room, such as compression devices. The ideal prophylaxis would remain effective for at least 6 weeks, until the patient resumes normal independent motion, and the native muscles provide the necessary compressive forces.

We are examining a study protocol that evaluates warfarin alone, foot pumps alone, and both methods together. The night of surgery 10 mg of warfarin is given, then no warfarin is given on postoperative day 1. Starting on postoperative day 2, warfarin is given according to the daily prothrombin time. The goal is maintenance of a prothrombin time of 1.3 to 1.5 times the control (2 to 2.5 times the international normalized ratio). The warfarin is continued on discharge home; the patient has weekly monitoring of prothrombin times. We obtain a Doppler ultrasound and lung scan on postoperative day 3 and 3 weeks postoperatively. If the ultrasound at 3 weeks is negative, the warfarin is discontinued. If the ultrasound is positive, the warfarin is continued for 6 weeks. All of the patients wear thigh-high compression stockings from the recovery room to 6 weeks postoperatively.

The most efficacious treatment for preventing DVT and pulmonary embolism is controversial. Although many protocols reduce the incidence of DVT, no single or combined protocol seems to decrease the incidence of fatal pulmonary embolism. Newer pharmaceuticals are being tried, but are, as yet, expensive and not particularly patient-friendly and show no benefit in preventing fatal pulmonary embolism because the incidence of fatal pulmonary embolism after TKA is extremely small (0.4% to 0.8%). Several thousand patients in a prospective, randomized study would be needed to advance one protocol over another.

PROTOCOL FOR PATIENTS WITH DOCUMENTED THROMBOEMBOLIC DISEASE

Positive Venography or Ultrasound

Patients with calf, popliteal, or femoral thrombi are treated with warfarin for 6 weeks. Asymptomatic pulmonary emboli are treated in the same manner. Symptomatic proximal thrombi and symptomatic pulmonary emboli[322] are treated with heparin until the effect of warfarin is established. Based on the discretion of the individual medical consultant, heparin treatment intravenously may be continued for 1 week. Intravenous heparin carries an extreme risk of local bleeding complications and, in our opinion, should be used only in potentially life-threatening situations. This policy sometimes may cause conflict among medical advisors, who often may wish to use heparin in less threatening circumstances. Orthopedic surgeons should plan their own policy and guidelines within their own institution.

Greenfield Filter

When warfarin prophylaxis fails to prevent a pulmonary embolus, when warfarin is contraindicated in a high-risk patient, or when complications develop as a result of anticoagulation, a Greenfield filter should be considered. Vaughn and colleagues[317] reported on its use in 66 patients and found the technique to be safe, easy, and effective.

They inserted the filter preoperatively in 42 patients who were considered at high risk for pulmonary embolus (group I) and postoperatively in 24 patients (group II). The preferred site of insertion was by way of the right internal jugular vein, and a vascular surgeon did the implantations. One patient in group II died of a massive pulmonary embolism 3 days after implantation. At follow-up, none of the remaining patients experienced migration of the filter, and there was no evidence of postphlebitic syndrome or chronic symptomatic edema of the lower extremity.

Fat Embolism Syndrome

The diagnosis of fat embolism can be elusive,[21,35,71,83,228] and we suspect the condition often may pass unrecognized as the cause of transient confusional states after surgery. The syndrome results from the embolization of fat and other debris from the femur or tibia and travels mostly to the lungs. The initial effects in the lungs are mechanical, with an increase in perfusion pressure, engorgement of the vessels in the lungs, and secondary right-sided heart strain. In the presence of hypovolemic shock, the patient may die from acute right-sided heart failure. The delayed effects of fat embolism occur after 48 to 72 hours because of the chemical effects of fat. The pulmonary tissue secretes lipase, which hydrolyzes fat into free fatty acids and glycerol. These free fatty acids increase capillary permeability, cause destruction of alveolar architecture, and damage lung surfactant. The end result of all these changes is hypoxia.[253]

Clinical findings of fat embolism syndrome include tachypnea, dyspnea, profuse tracheobronchial secretions, apprehension, anxiety, delirium, confusion, unconsciousness, and petechial hemorrhage. Laboratory findings are hypoxemia on arterial blood gas and thrombocytopenia less than 150,000 mm^3. Treatment is supportive. Mechanical ventilation may be required in advanced cases. Corticosteroids may be beneficial in diminishing the inflammatory response from the chemical effects of fat emboli.[247]

Monto and colleagues,[228] in a review of the literature, reported 19 cases with 9 deaths, 15 of which were associated with long-stem cemented prostheses, such as the Guepar hinge. Four cases were associated with total condylar arthroplasty. These authors reported one case associated with intramedullary instrumentation. Fahmy and coworkers[83] showed human intramedullary femoral canal pressures of 500 to 1000 mm Hg generated by using standard alignment rod techniques. Venting the canal did not lower the canal pressure significantly. Intramedullary pressures were maintained within normal limits only by overdrilling the femoral canal and gently placing the guide rod. The use of a pneumatic tourniquet does not protect against fat embolism, and with the popularity of intramedullary guidance systems for femoral and tibial components, an increase in the incidence of fat embolism syndrome may be expected. Routinely instrumenting the intramedullary canals of the femur and tibia in bilateral cases should be avoided.

Blood Loss

There is little blood loss during the TKA procedure; most occurs postoperatively through suction drainage.[108,236] Reinfusion drains are useful, but nonetheless one must be prepared for additional blood transfusion, particularly in bilateral cases. Given the current anxiety about receiving blood products, autologous transfusion is the choice of most patients for elective surgery. We recommend obtaining 1 U of blood for each knee arthroplasty to ensure that homologous blood will not be needed. Although retransfusion of the blood may not be strictly necessary, we believe avoidance of postoperative anemia is helpful in promoting more rapid recovery, especially considering the advanced age and myriad medical problems with which arthroplasty patients present. If an adequate preoperative algorithm is used as established at our institution, with adequate treatment of preoperative anemia, the use of autologous blood for primary TKA can be eliminated.

LOCAL COMPLICATIONS

Wound Drainage and Delayed Wound Healing

In a series of 220 total condylar arthroplasties, 49 knees did not have primary wound healing[101] or had some wound drainage. Cultures were taken of 41 knees, of which 35 were negative. The most frequently isolated organism was *Staphylococcus epidermidis*. One case with skin necrosis became secondarily infected (mixed organisms) and eventually developed a deep wound infection. With this exception, early wound drainage was not related to periprosthetic infection.

Altering the skin incision from midline to slightly curved medial parapatella[153,155] and improved techniques in tissue management have increased greatly the incidence of primary wound healing in more recent cases. Continuous passive motion, in routine use since the 1990s, begun immediately postoperatively has not adversely affected wound healing.[320] Johnson[152] recommended that 40 degrees of flexion not be exceeded in the first few days, but we routinely start continuous passive motion in the recovery room at 60 degrees of motion, and we have not seen any increased incidence of wound problems.

Excessive bleeding contributes to postoperative wound drainage and should be controlled. Although Lotke (personal communication, 1999) showed in his own cases that there was no advantage in releasing the tourniquet before wound closure, we recommend that this be done. Frequently, rapid hemorrhage from one of the genicular vessels occurs when the tourniquet is released, and occasionally patients have been returned to the operating room for control of bleeding when the tourniquet was not released (Fig. 99–3). We have found two areas of particular concern: the posterior lateral corner at the level of the tibia, which is supplied by the lateral inferior genicular artery, and the area near the insertion of the posterior cruciate ligament on the tibia. These areas tend to bleed profusely if not properly coagulated. Aneurysm of the medial genicular artery[66,297] secondary to injury during surgery also has been reported. Tourniquet release is recommended after insertion of the components when cement has cured. At the Center for Hip and Knee Surgery, we discontinued the use of continuous passive motion in 1987, do not release the tourniquet before closure, and do not use postoperative drainage systems. To our knowledge, we have had only two patients return to the operating room for hematoma evacuation in more than 10,000 TKAs. Care should be taken to coagulate all bleeding vessels during the course of the procedure, particularly in the areas mentioned previously. All wounds are dressed with a soft compressive dressing, which is changed on postoperative day 2, and motion is begun as active assist with the physical therapist.

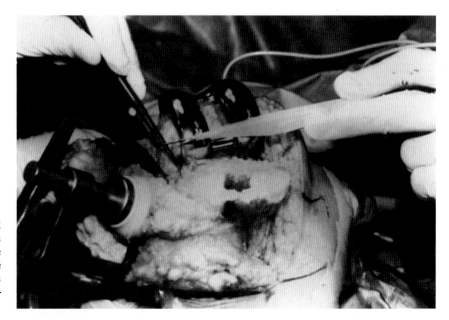

Figure 99–3. Cautery of the lateral genicular artery. Unless this artery is visible, it is advisable to release the tourniquet before closure so that the vessel can be clearly identified. It is the major source of dangerous postoperative bleeding.

Serosanguineous drainage from the incision is common and is a cause for concern only when the drainage is profuse and persistent. If there is no purulence or erythema, initial management should be a compression dressing, immobilization, and observation. Wound healing takes precedence over motion. When there is drainage, antibiotic therapy is controversial because it may mask a deep infection, making it difficult to identify the causative organism. We recommend consulting with an infectious diseases specialist and administering intravenous antibiotics in selected cases. This is a matter of clinical judgment, but we do not consider antibiotics in these circumstances wrong. Prolonged and persistent serosanguineous drainage raises the issue of a capsular defect, which should be surgically repaired. Some authors recommend that if drainage does not stop after 5 days of appropriate treatment, an open débridement should be performed.[264]

Hematoma

A certain amount of bleeding into the knee is normal, and occasionally a profuse amount may exit through the suction drain. In the latter event, we recommend removal of the drain, application of compression dressing, and observation. We also advocate stopping the continuous passive motion and range of motion with therapy. If bleeding continues, as evidenced by tense and painful swelling, the knee must be reopened and the source of the bleeding identified (an argument for intraoperative tourniquet release). Later development of a hematoma is usually secondary to anticoagulant therapy. A period of immobilization and observation is permissible, and many hematomas subside spontaneously. When leakage through the incision occurs, however, it is best to evacuate the hematoma surgically. Another indication to evaluate a hematoma surgically is in the case of impending skin necrosis secondary to excessive soft-tissue extension. The hematoma may be localized to the subcutaneous tissues, but if it is deep there is risk of prosthetic contamination. Probing and squeezing the wound to evacuate a hematoma are not recommended and may lead to retrograde contamination.

Skin Necrosis

In the total condylar knee series, seven patients had skin necrosis or wound separation, three required secondary closure, and two required skin grafts. Skin necrosis (Fig. 99–4) is particularly likely in previously operated knees, especially when midmedial or midlateral incisions are already present and in patients with comorbidities, including rheumatoid arthritis, diabetes mellitus, immunosuppression, malnutrition, peripheral vascular disease, and steroid use.[264] The use of previous incisions involves raising a substantial skin flap, to which making a new incision seems preferable. When there are multiple scars, the most lateral scar should be used; this is done to avoid a large lateral skin flap with multiple scars in it and concern

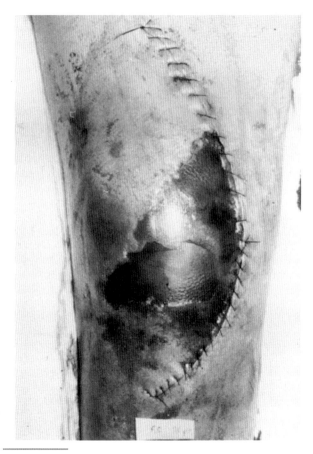

Figure 99–4. Because of its subcutaneous position, skin necrosis is a particular hazard in knee joint replacement. Overaggressive débridement can lead to deep infection. When necrosis occurs, the knee should be immobilized until the eschar separates.

over its viability. Johnson[153] showed a reduction in oxygenation of the skin in the lateral region after skin incisions about the knee through measurement of transcutaneous oxygen. Clarke and associates[46] also have described decreased oxygen tension in the incisional skin margins when using tourniquets. This hypoxia increased with tourniquet tightness. The recommended pressure is 125 mm Hg above the mean blood pressure. Wound problems were recorded at any pressure, however. When the surgeon is faced with ill-placed scars, it may be better to make a "sham" incision 10 to 14 days before the projected arthroplasty or to consider soft-tissue expanders. Postoperative soft-tissue and skin necrosis should be handled early and aggressively. Small areas (<4 cm), especially over the patella or proximal, may be treated by secondary intention healing, split-thickness skin grafts, or local fasciocutaneous flaps. Skin loss over the patellar tendon or tibial tubercle is best treated with muscle flap coverage; usually the medial head of the gastrocnemius rotator flap is adequate. Transverse incisions, such as are made in high tibial osteotomy, can be crossed with impunity. Sometimes part of a previous incision (e.g., incisions used for the fixation of tibial plateau fractures) can be reopened.[61,117,190,206-208,217,237,238,345]

VASCULAR COMPLICATIONS

Arterial complications are rare,[178,255] and the preoperative absence of peripheral pulses has not been regarded as a contraindication to surgery, provided that the capillary circulation was adequate. In a large Mayo Clinic series, Rand[255] found the incidence of arterial insufficiency to be only 0.03% in 9022 TKAs performed between 1971 and 1986. Rush and colleagues[278] reported on arterial complications of TKA in Australia. By means of a questionnaire sent to Fellows of the Australian Orthopaedic Association, a total of 13 cases were reported: 4 with injury to the popliteal artery, 1 with arterial venous fistula involving the lateral genicular artery, and 8 with acute ischemia resulting from superficial femoral or popliteal artery thrombosis. The authors suggested that thrombosis was due to local pressure from the tourniquet and recommended that, in the presence of extensive calcification of the proximal arteries (Fig. 99–5) and poor peripheral pulses, a tourniquet not be used.

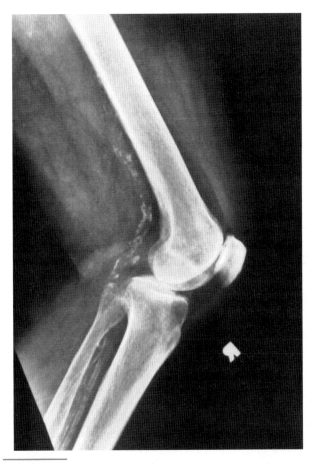

Figure 99–5. Lateral radiograph showing extensive calcification in the femoral, popliteal, posterotibial, posterior tibial, and peroneal arteries. Although this patient had palpable peripheral pulses, knee surgery may result in arterial occlusion by a dislodged clot. Some investigators recommended avoiding a tourniquet. The patient should be watched closely after surgery for evidence of arterial insufficiency.

Absolute vascular contraindications for performing a TKA include the presence of verified vascular claudication with minimal or no activity, active skin ulcerations secondary to arterial insufficiency or venous stasis, and ischemia or frank necrosis in the toes. If there are any questions or doubts, a vascular surgeon should be consulted. Other authors cautioned against the use of a tourniquet after previous bypass surgery. In our own experience, there have been 7 instances of arterial compromise in more than 5000 arthroplasties; 3 resulted in amputation.

When there is concern about the circulation, we recommend a preoperative evaluation by a vascular surgeon. The operation should be scheduled at a time of day when consultant advice is available postoperatively so that prompt investigation with arteriography can be done if the state of the circulation is in doubt. Prompt embolectomy usually restores the circulation. In one of our eventual amputations, embolectomy was delayed beyond the point at which it would have been useful. The other two amputations would not have been prevented by avoidance of a tourniquet. Prolonged observation of postoperative vascular insufficiency is justified only in a setting of extreme vigilance and under the guidance of a vascular surgeon.

NERVE PALSY AND NEUROLOGICAL COMPLICATIONS

Anatomy of the Peroneal Nerve

Although we have encountered two cases of transient paralysis of the popliteal nerve after correction of a severe flexion contracture, most nerve palsies involve the peroneal nerve.[12,60,66,118,119,199,274] This nerve is composed of fibers from the dorsal portion of the L4 and L5 and S1 and S2 nerves. As the nerve courses down from the thigh, it curves laterally behind the head of the fibula to reach the two heads of the peroneus longus. The nerve flattens as it passes between these two heads, separating the bundles and exposing unprotected nutrient vessels. Then the nerve curves around the neck of the fibula and divides into deep and superficial branches.

The deep peroneal nerve continues under the extensor digitorum longus along the anterior aspect of the intraosseous membrane. It sends motor branches to the tibialis anterior, extensor digitorum longus, extensor hallucis longus, and peroneus tertius. The nerve continues distally, ending in the medial and lateral terminal branches, which, among other functions, supply sensation to the first web space of the foot.

The superficial peroneal nerve passes distally between the peronei and extensor digitorum longus. Motor branches are given off to the peroneus longus and peroneus brevis. In the lower one-third of the leg, the nerve branches into the medial and intermediate dorsal cutaneous nerves. These terminal branches complete the sensory innervation of the feet.

Postoperative Clinical Findings

Peroneal nerve palsy is an infrequent but worrisome complication after TKA. The incidence is higher in revision cases than primary TKA.[12] Nerve palsies are seen most commonly after correction of severe flexion and valgus deformities or a combination of the two. Factors that have not been found to be associated with peroneal nerve palsy include age, gender, type of arthritis, and duration of tourniquet. It is most commonly diagnosed within 2 days after TKA.

The prevalence of peroneal nerve palsy has been reported many times in the literature. Mont and associates[225] reviewed the literature and found the cumulative prevalence to be 0.58% (74 of 12,784).[12] Asp and Rand[12] reported an incidence of 0.3% in 8754 TKAs performed at the Mayo Clinic. From January 1974 to December 1980, 2626 TKAs were performed at the Hospital for Special Surgery. During that time, there were 23 peroneal nerve palsies in 22 patients.[274] One patient experienced a peroneal nerve palsy after both TKAs, which were done 5 months apart. The preoperative deformities were varus in 5 knees, neutral alignment in 7 knees, and valgus in 11 knees. In addition, some degree of flexion contracture was found in 14 patients; flexion contracture was severe in 9. Five patients underwent exploration and release of the peroneal nerve, and a nerve palsy developed despite this precaution. These explorations were done in knees with severe flexion contractures (30 degrees and 80 degrees) and in severe valgus deformities (27 degrees, 35 degrees, and 40 degrees).

The time of presentation of the problem varied from discovery in the recovery room to postoperative day 6. Most cases were noted early; eight were found in the recovery room, and another eight were discovered during the first postoperative day. Three were noted on postoperative day 2, two on postoperative day 3, and two on postoperative day 6. The motor fibers of the tibialis anterior and extensor hallucis longus muscles were affected in all cases; a sensory deficit was noticed in 20 cases (87%). The peroneus longus muscle was affected in nine cases (39%). During the early postoperative period, six patients underwent electromyography evaluation; a diffuse motor neuropathy was found in the mild cases, and denervation potentials in muscles supplied by the deep branch of the common peroneal nerve were found in the more severely involved cases.

Treatment and Results

The treatment rendered on discovery of these findings varied according to the discretion of the surgeon involved. The most frequent therapeutic measure was to loosen the Robert Jones dressing and place the knee in a more flexed position. In two cases, this maneuver brought immediate improvement of motor and sensory deficits. The time interval between discovery and the beginning of the return of function ranged from immediately in the two cases mentioned to 6 months. Motor improvement occurred first, with sensory return lagging behind.

In 13 cases, traction secondary to correction of a valgus or flexion deformity or both was the cause of the palsy. In three cases, the palsy was caused by the medial and lateral splints used to hold the knee in full extension with "tight" components and the consequent traction on the nerve by this stretching mechanism. In four cases, the dressing containing the medial and lateral plaster splints was too tight or improperly padded, causing direct pressure on the peroneal nerve. In three cases, no explanation could be determined.

Of the 23 peroneal palsies, 17 were extensive enough to require a footdrop brace. The remaining six cases were mild and did not need any dorsiflexion assist. At follow-up examination, a residual deficit was found in all 18 patients in whom a sensory deficit had been present. Motor power was clinically normal in 6 of the patients (26%); the remaining 17 patients had motor power clinically assessed in the poor to good range. Only two patients, neither of whom had a sensory deficit initially, achieved full clinical recovery, both within 6 months. Four additional patients had complete motor recovery but with a residual sensory deficit.

The following factors contribute to the development of peroneal nerve palsy: (1) stretching of the nerve in valgus and flexion contractures, (2) fascial compression of the nerve and its vascular supply, and (3) direct pressure from the dressing. In rare idiopathic cases, none of the mechanisms listed seem to apply.

Idusuyi and Morrey[142] examined a series of TKA patients seen at the Mayo Clinic from 1979 through 1992. There were 10,321 TKAs performed with 32 postoperative peroneal nerve palsies. The following factors were associated with peroneal nerve palsy: epidural anesthesia for postoperative pain control, previous laminectomy, and preoperative valgus deformity. The relative risk for patients who had previous proximal tibial osteotomy was doubled but not statistically significant. Asp and Rand[12] described a similar Mayo Clinic experience with peroneal nerve palsy. Among 8998 arthroplasties, there were 26 nerve palsies. The circumstances in which the nerve palsies occurred were similar to our own, but recovery was generally better. Complete recovery was more likely when the palsy was initially incomplete. Removal of dressing and flexion of the knee on diagnosis did not always help.

The treatment of chronic peroneal nerve palsy usually consists of an ankle-foot orthosis for a footdrop and passive ankle range of motion to prevent an equinus deformity. Complete recovery of a peroneal palsy is rare. The recovery seen is usually partial, with sensory deficits that may be permanent; residual motor deficits are not usually of clinical significance. Occasional marked weakness, especially of the great toe extensor, may be seen. Asp and Rand[12] studied 26 postoperative peroneal palsies. Palsies were complete in 18 and incomplete in 8. Of the patients, 23 had motor and sensory deficits; 3 had only motor deficits. At 5-year follow-up, recovery was complete for 13 palsies and partial for 12. Complete recovery was more likely in palsies that were incomplete initially. Although most investigators support nonoperative treatment of this complication, others disagree. Krackow and colleagues[176] treated five patients with operative exploration and decompression of the peroneal nerve for a postoperative palsy. The procedure was performed 5 to 45 months after the index TKA. All patients showed improved nerve function. Four of five patients had full peroneal nerve recovery. All patients were able to discontinue their ankle-foot orthosis.

Patients with excessive total deformities apparently are prone to experience peroneal nerve palsies. The large soft-tissue dissections required to balance the more severe deformities may be responsible for increased traction or vascular compromise in this area. The alternative method of bone sacrifice to correct large deformities, although appealing because of the elimination of the need for obtaining soft-tissue balance, does not entirely avoid peroneal nerve palsy. The bone-sacrificing method also leaves a residual leg-length discrepancy that is permanent and may be associated with an extensor lag because of relative lengthening of the quadriceps mechanism. When ligament balance is not attempted, a constrained prosthesis is needed. In younger patients, this may lead to eventual loosening, although, with the constrained condylar prosthesis, this has not happened at the time of writing. In elderly patients at high risk for peroneal nerve palsy, the use of the constrained condylar knee is a suitable alternative. These patients recover much more rapidly than after major release procedures, and because of their age the risk of ultimate loosening is low.

We also have encountered two cases of transient paralysis of the popliteal nerve after correction of severe flexion contractures. In one of these, there was complete recovery, but in the other the recognition of the palsy was delayed because a continued epidural anesthetic interfered with the clinical examination. Although it is sometimes necessary to splint the knee in extension after correction of a severe flexion contracture, evidence of nerve palsy demands immediate removal of the splints and flexion of the knee. If this is done promptly, complete recovery can be expected. In the case of valgus deformities, splinting is not necessary, and the intermittent flexion and relaxation that occurs with immediate continuous passive motion has lessened greatly the occurrence of peroneal nerve palsies. Tight dressings that might press directly on the peroneal nerve also should be avoided.

MECHANICAL COMPLICATIONS

Instability

Instability after knee arthroplasty can be subdivided into three types: extension instability, flexion instability, and genu recurvatum.

EXTENSION INSTABILITY

Instability in extension can be symmetric or asymmetric. Either type is accentuated when there is malposition of the components or overall malalignment of the extremity. Conversely the effects of extension instability are lessened

and sometimes masked altogether when position and alignment are correct.

SYMMETRIC INSTABILITY

Symmetric instability is caused whenever the thickness of the components is less than the extension gap between the bone ends. It can be caused by removal of excessive bone from the distal femur either because of miscalculation or because the collateral ligaments were not tensioned properly.

Over-resection of tibial bone is compensated for by use of a thicker tibial component, which makes up for the extra bone removed. The only adverse consequence is the seating of the prosthesis on more distal and potentially weaker tibial bone. Over-resection of the distal femur has more serious consequences and requires augmentation of the femoral component by blocks attached to the distal femur, which are available in many revision systems. Over-resection is less probable with tensor systems, but also is unlikely to happen when a measured osteotomy (calculated to replace bone with prosthesis) is performed. When it is not due to excessive bone resection, extension instability may be the consequence of abnormal ligament length (i.e., in genu recurvatum and after extensive ligament releases). Although one remedy is to stabilize the knee by using a thicker tibial component, this alters the joint mechanics by moving the joint axis proximally, an action that has secondary effects on ligament tension and stability[211] and patellar function (Fig. 99–6) by creating a low-lying patella. When preoperative and intraoperative assessment of the knee suggests this might happen, the femur should be deliberately under-resected by the initial osteotomy (Fig. 99–7). Later in the procedure, if either spacer blocks or the trial components suggest that further resection is necessary, it can be done by recutting the distal femur. Alternatively, if the osteotomy already has been made, augmentation of the distal femur as described previously can be tried as an alternative to a thicker tibial component.

ASYMMETRIC INSTABILITY

Asymmetric instability is the most frequent variant (Fig. 99–8). Most arthritic knees possess some degree of ligament asymmetry, and if the bone cuts are made without regard to this fundamental anomaly, the arthroplasty is unstable on one side. One of the most common mistakes in technique is to release a tight ligament inadequately because of a natural fear of causing instability. How much instability can be accepted? Here a matter of surgical judgment is involved because, as discussed in Chapter 88, some degree of tightening laterally may be expected, provided that the alignment of the components is satisfactory. As a rule of thumb, we accept only a little medial laxity after correction of valgus (because there is little potential for spontaneous tightening), and we accept lateral laxity after varus correction, provided that the knee cannot be brought back to neutral with the components inserted.

Further medial release should be done if this is possible. We have seen many knees that remained unstable because of insufficient medial release, but few that have been over-released. Laskin and Schob[184] described 4 knees with instability of 68 severe varus deformities requiring medial capsular resection. All of these knees had appeared stable at the time of the operation. One knee had stability improved by inserting a thicker tibial component, and in one a probable neuropathic joint may have contributed to the instability. One knee was revised unsuccessfully by a ligament reconstruction, and the fourth knee required revision to a more constrained prosthesis. In our own practice, we also have seen occasional cases of instability after medial release. The first patient, who underwent

bilateral TKA with varus release, experienced postoperative instability on one side. She responded to 6 weeks of postoperative bracing with an orthosis, and now, 3 years later, the result is highly successful, with no difference in laxity discernible between the two knees. The second patient, who also underwent bilateral TKA with corrective soft-tissue release, had a possible neuropathic joint on one side. The laxity was not noticed in the hospital, but 1 month later it became obvious that the knee was developing a progressive valgus. An orthosis was not successful in this case, perhaps because it was tolerated poorly by the patient. Significant improvement occurred over the next year, however. The patient now has good stability on walking, but notices a medial thrust on stairs. Another iatrogenic cause of asymmetric instability is damage of the medial collateral ligament during surgery (Fig. 99–9). This damage can occur when cutting the proximal tibia or posterior femur. If noticed during surgery, it should be treated by using a constrained condylar prosthesis because operative repair of the ligament is unlikely to be successful.

Apart from such iatrogenic causes, asymmetric instability is rarely due to complete absence of ligaments. This situation might be expected in post-traumatic cases, but even then the torn ligaments normally heal so that the end result is elongation rather than absence. It is often believed that the ligaments in rheumatoid knees are incompetent or sometimes damaged by synovitis, but if so, it must be most unusual. In loose rheumatoid knees, some degree of postoperative stretching can occur so that a tight fit is desirable.

Bone loss accompanying severe instability and deformity is not in itself an indication for a constrained prosthesis. It is a technical mistake to cut back excessively on either the tibia or the femur to produce a flat bone surface. On the tibial side, large asymmetric defects, usually medial, are often found. Resection at the bottom level of the defect removes a large amount of tibial bone; the remaining cancellous bone is weak, and often the cross-sectional area of the tibia is reduced. It is preferable to resect the tibia at the usual level as if no defect existed, then build up the uneven surface on one side with a bone graft. Alternatively an asymmetric tibial component can fill the defect, and several wedge-shaped augments are now available (Fig. 99–10).

Femoral defects are usually lateral. It may be that the indicated level of resection removes bone from the medial femoral condyle, but passes distal to the lateral condyle.

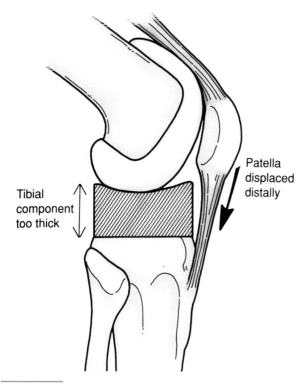

Figure 99–6. If an extra thick tibial component is needed to stabilize the knee, the patella is displaced distally, causing a patella infra. Undersizing of the femoral component in the sagittal plane and anterior malpositioning are possible causes. Excessive distal resection of the femur moving the joint line proximally is another cause.

Tibial component too thick

Patella displaced distally

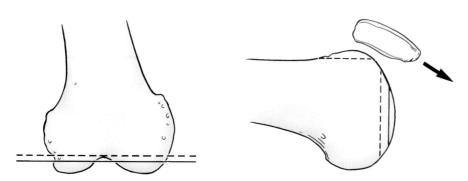

Figure 99–7. In cases with considerable ligamentous laxity, an under-resection of the distal femur may be preferable. The standard femoral resection necessitates a thicker tibial component to take up the slack in the soft tissues and may cause distal migration of the patella. By under-resecting the femur, a desirable patellar position is maintained.

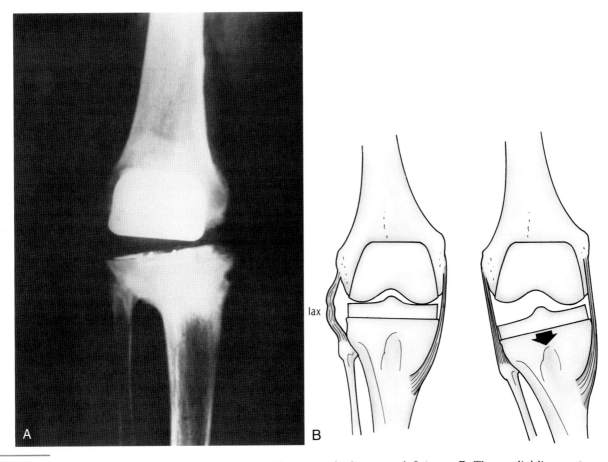

Figure 99–8. **A,** This arthroplasty is unstable, but not because of a ligament deficiency. **B,** The medial ligament was not released; an asymmetric instability remains.

The same solution applies; a distal augment laterally on the femoral component is the preferred solution (Fig. 99–11).

Although stems are a means of gaining extra fixation to the bone, use of a stem should not be confused with constraint in the prosthetic joint itself. Most constrained or hinged prostheses do have long intramedullary stems, however. Particularly in revision operations, constrained prostheses are often used unnecessarily, not because the instability cannot be managed by other means, but because the stabilizing prostheses have a stem.

FLEXION INSTABILITY

The knee is stable in extension but not in flexion. The underlying problem is that the flexion space is relatively too large for the thickness of the tibial component (Fig. 99–12). This situation can arise in numerous ways. First, the femoral component is undersized anteroposteriorly. The remedy is to use a larger femoral component with posterior augments. Second, the knee has a flexion contracture with the trial components. Instead of dealing with the problem by troublesome additional distal femoral resection or posterior capsulotomy, the surgeon may choose to achieve extension by using a thinner tibial component or

by additional tibial resection. Third, lateral release from the distal femur impairs the lateral ligamentous support, which has been the cause of several dislocations of the posterior stabilized knee that we have encountered (Fig. 99–13); it has been reported by Galinat and associates[99] with the posterior stabilized knee and Gebhard and Kilgus[102] with the Kinematic stabilizer. This possibility may not be recognized intraoperatively, but if it is seen, the remedy is either a thicker tibial component or revision to a constrained condylar prosthesis. Fourth, related to that just discussed is the rotational position of the femoral component. After lateral release, lateral laxity should be compensated for by externally rotating the femoral component.[32] A similar type of lateral laxity is created when a transverse tibial osteotomy is done, combined with an anatomic rotational placement of the femoral component (that is referenced from the posterior femoral condyle). Although the normal tibia is described as having a 3-degree medial slope,[163] there is considerable natural variation, with an angle of 6.5 degrees recorded in one normal male volunteer.[230] A knee with this anatomy cut in the manner just described would have a discrepancy of ligament tensions in flexion. We believe the epicondylar axis is the best landmark for determining femoral component rotation. The anteroposterior axis of the femur, tibial shaft, and ligament tension also are methods of confirming rotational position of the femoral component.

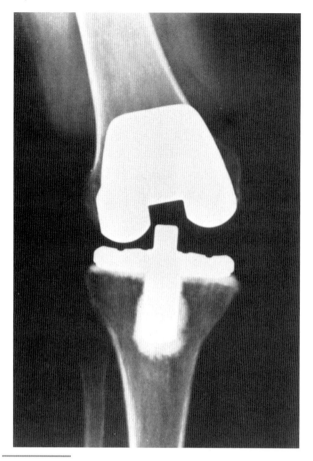

Figure 99–9. Radiograph showing the instability that results from a transected medial collateral ligament. This is not the result of an overzealous medial release.

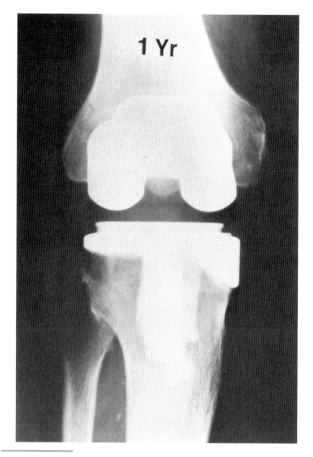

Figure 99–10. A large medial tibial bone deficiency has been compensated by the use of a medial wedge tibial component. The articular surface of the prosthesis is standard total condylar and is not constrained.

Flexion instability is manifest according to the design of the prosthesis. Posterior stabilized designs (see Fig. 99–13) may have episodes of posterior dislocation; when reduced, the knee functions normally again. Often the dislocation is caused by certain activities, such as crossing one leg over the other to put on a shoe or a sock. It is most likely to happen in patients who had a valgus deformity and in patients who rapidly regained flexion probably because the speed of rehabilitation interfered with healing of the lateral structures. Early dislocations should be managed by a period of bracing, avoiding activities known to cause dislocation. Otherwise, recurrent dislocation is treated by inserting a thicker polyethylene tibial component or revision to a constrained condylar prosthesis.

When the prosthesis is a cruciate-retaining model, the remedy may be exchange of the tibial component for a thicker one, but if this is not judged successful intraoperatively, revision of the components to a posterior stabilized or a constrained condylar design should be considered. Manifestation of this instability depends on the constraint in the original tibial component. One study[244] examined 25 patients with flexion instability with a cruciate-retaining device. Of the knee replacements, 22 were revised to posterior stabilized implants, and 3 underwent tibial polyethylene liner exchange only. Nineteen of the 22 patients who had a revision to a posterior stabilized

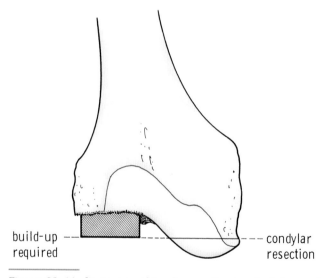

build-up required — — — — — — — — — — condylar resection

Figure 99–11. In some valgus knees, the level of femoral resection may pass distal to the lateral femoral condyle. Lateral augmentation of the femoral component is required.

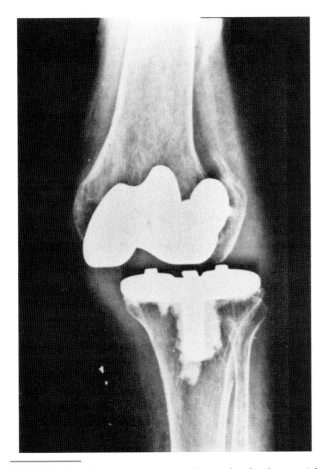

Figure 99–12. Anteroposterior radiograph of a knee with flexion instability. With the knee in flexion, a posterolateral dislocation is observed. This dislocation is caused by inequality between the flexion and extension gaps, and the posterior cruciate ligament is not sufficient to provide stability, particularly when the prosthesis is unconstrained.

implant were improved markedly after the revision surgery. Only one of three patients who had a polyethylene exchange improved. The Knee Society knee scores improved from 45 to 90 points, and function scores improved from 42 to 75 points. We recommend that revision surgery in these cases focus on balancing the flexion and extension spaces and conversion to a posterior stabilized design. Similar results were reported by Waslewski and colleagues[327]; in this study, six of six patients who underwent conversion to a posterior stabilized design improved.

GENU RECURVATUM

The condition of genu recurvatum occurs almost exclusively in patients with rheumatoid arthritis and with muscle paralysis. Recurvatum and anterior subluxation of the tibia have been reported after polycentric arthroplasty in rheumatoid arthritis. Although it is generally true that a knee that does not hyperextend at the conclusion of surgery does not develop recurvatum later, an exception is in patients who lack muscle control. Patients with long-standing weakness from poliomyelitis may experience osteoarthritis and often have recurvatum. An arthroplasty should not be undertaken unless there is good power in the quadriceps muscle, but sometimes a functioning quadriceps is present in an otherwise almost flail extremity. These knees should be approached with great caution because, in the absence of hamstring and calf musculature, a slowly developing recurvatum is likely with any kind of surface replacement. Probably if these knees are to be replaced at all there is an indication for a constrained prosthesis with an extension stop, but the increased risk of loosening with such a device must be weighed carefully before making a decision. In patients with neuromuscular disorders and some collagen vascular disorders (i.e.,

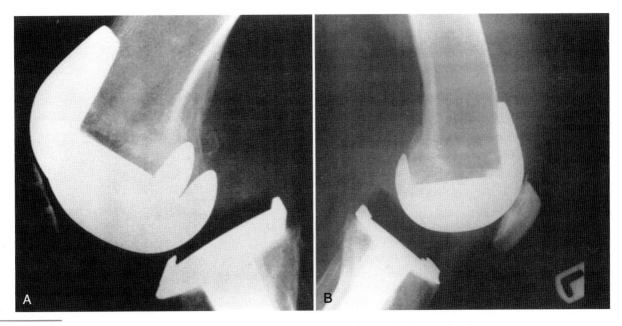

Figure 99–13. **A,** Posterior dislocation of a posterior stabilized prosthesis. **B,** After reduction.

Ehlers-Danlos syndrome), we under-resect the distal femur by 1 to 2 mm. This under-resection may leave patients with a slight flexion contracture, but eventually they return to full extension. Krackow and Weiss[177] described a technique in which the origins of the collateral ligaments are transferred proximally and posteriorly, whereby the cam action of the prosthesis prevents recurvatum.

Inadequate Motion

The range of motion obtained after arthroplasty depends on several factors, including body habitus, patient motivation, adequacy of physical therapy, and prosthetic design. Probably the most important determinant is the range of motion that existed before the arthroplasty. A knee that is extremely stiff to begin with is difficult to mobilize satisfactorily because of quadriceps contracture and capsular fibrosis. Even if an adequate range of motion is achieved in the operating room, this may not be realized postoperatively. For this reason, very stiff or ankylosed knees[2,25,123,241] should be approached with caution and with the expectation that 45 to 60 degrees of flexion is the likely end result. Arthrodesed knees, in which more extensive damage to the extensor mechanism might be expected, and in which the ligaments were probably divided, should not be considered for arthroplasty at all. Two studies have had conflicting results for TKA in ankylosed or arthrodesed knees. Montgomery and colleagues[227] examined 71 patients with 82 TKAs; all had preoperative arc of motion of 50 degrees or less. The average preoperative knee score was 38, average preoperative arc of motion was 36 degrees, average flexion contracture was 22 degrees, and average maximum flexion was 58 degrees. McAuley and associates[215] made similar observations with a mean net gain of range of motion of 44 degress, more than half of which was in reducing flexion contracture. Complication rates were high at 41% with a revision rate of 18.5%. Postoperatively the average knee score was 80, average postoperative arc of motion was 93 degrees, and average maximum flexion was 94 degrees. Postoperatively, no knee had a flexion contracture greater than 10 degrees. McAuley and associates[215] concluded that TKA in ankylosed knees can lead to significant improvement in range of motion and pain.

In contrast to Montgomery's findings,[227] Naranja and coworkers[239] studied 37 knees that were either surgically fused or ankylosed and had a TKA performed. The results included an average 7 degrees lack of extension and 62 degrees of flexion. The total complication rate was 57%. A satisfactory outcome (no pain and an unlimited ambulation distance) was obtained in only 10 patients (27%). The investigators concluded that the lack of consistent adequate motion and the complication rate may suggest that the surgeon reconsider the risks and benefits of this difficult procedure. A linked design is more successful in improving motion than a surface replacement because the ligaments and capsule are not required for stability and can be excised. The difficulty in exposing a very stiff knee has been alluded to, and a quadriceps snip or tibia tubercle osteotomy is recommended. A partial quadricepsplasty can be achieved if only the vastus medialis and rectus femoris components of the quadriceps are resutured, leaving the vastus intermedius and vastus lateralis completely or partially unattached. Extensive soft-tissue releases in all four quadrants are required.

Knee stiffness or decreased range of motion after a TKA is disturbing to the patient and the surgeon. The stiff knee can be painful and lead to decreased use and disability. Reoperation on a stiff knee is no guarantee of success because the success depends on the cause of stiffness. If the stiffness is caused by component malposition, revision of components can be successful. If stiffness is caused by excessive scarring or patella baja, reoperation is limited in its results.[72] Nicholls and Dorr[241] found revision was successful in relieving pain in 12 of 13 knees. Maloney,[205] Christensen and colleagues,[45] and Whiteside and Ohl[334] verified moderate improvement in flexion, function, and pain control with surgical débridement or revision TKA or both. There was no significant improvement in range of motion except in knees that had incorrect component position. Range of motion was not improved in knees that had stiffness from scarring, such as the "stiffening" type of rheumatoid arthritis or in knees that had patella baja. Little or no benefit can be expected from isolated polyethylene exchanges to a thinner polyethylene even when combined with extensive débridement and ligament release.

Our policy is to manipulate knees postoperatively if motion is not regained rapidly, and usually this is done during postoperative weeks 6 to 12 when flexion is not 75 degrees or more by this time. Full muscular relaxation is needed because if tone remains in the quadriceps muscle, the increased resistance may damage the extensor mechanism or possibly cause a fracture adjoining the prosthesis. Epidural anesthesia is convenient, but does not always give the required degree of relaxation; spinal and general anesthesia are better in this respect. The purpose of the manipulation is to overcome intra-articular adhesions, and this can be done with less force when quadriceps resistance is eliminated. We have manipulated approximately 400 knees in this manner. Only two complications have been recorded: One was a supracondylar femoral fracture in a knee that was ankylosed before the arthroplasty, and the other was a patellar ligament avulsion, also occurring in a previously stiff knee. Both of these complications appeared early in our experience, when the value of muscle-relaxing agents was not appreciated, and might have been avoided had the quadriceps been paralyzed.

Some of our patients may not have needed a manipulation and might have regained motion if left alone to continue physical therapy. Fox and Poss[95] studied 343 TKAs performed in a 12-month period, of which 81 (23%) were manipulated, the indication being the failure to achieve 90 degrees of comfortable, active flexion by the end of postoperative week 2. Manipulation did not increase the ultimate flexion of the knee compared with the larger group of knees that were not manipulated at all. Fox and Poss[95] did not address the crucial question of whether the knees chosen for manipulation would have done just as well without. Some patients do not regain flexion of the knee easily after arthroplasty, and in some patients restriction of motion may be permanent. We have seen examples of this in patients who were not manipulated either because a second anesthetic was prevented by a medical problem or because the surgeon involved did not consider manipulation desirable. A selective manipulation is done for the following reasons: (1) It improves the immediate course by allowing more normal function and by making the continued physical therapy easier and less painful, and (2) it prevents permanent restriction of motion in certain patients who are not easily identified until it is too late for manipulation to be effective.

Other intra-articular causes of loss of flexion are an oversized or malrotated femoral component (which may require component revision) and adhesive capsulitis. The latter is likely to follow a hematoma or other wound-healing problem that results in a long delay in physical therapy. Even so, most patients gradually regain motion, given sufficient time. When a lateral retinacular release has not been done, tightening of the lateral capsule makes flexion difficult; in particularly resistant cases, a lateral retinacular release followed by a manipulation sometimes successfully regains motion. In addition, a tight posterior cruciate ligament in a cruciate-retaining knee design can be a cause of loss of flexion and usually is associated with posterior knee pain at the endpoint of flexion. Arthroscopic posterior cruciate ligament resection can be beneficial.

Sympathetic dystrophy is an extreme example of adhesive capsulitis in which the whole joint is chronically swollen, and the capsule is greatly increased in thickness. Usually the other signs associated with a sympathetic dystrophy are present, and the patients invariably complain of excessive pain. The diagnosis of sympathetic dystrophy should be considered especially if the pain is out of proportion to examination findings.

A persistent flexion contracture is usually the result of incorrect bone cuts at surgery or failure to strip and divide the posterior capsule. The latter maneuver is necessary when there is a severe (>30 degrees) preoperative flexion contracture and in practice is mostly limited to rheumatoid knees. Rarely does this degree of contracture develop in gonarthrosis. With this exception, a postoperative flexion contracture is due to removal of an inadequate amount of bone from the distal femur, and normally this should be noticed when inserting the appropriate spacer in extension. If the components already have been fitted, it is tempting to overcome the flexion contracture by excising more bone from the upper tibia; to recut the distal femur requires more reshaping and is a more complicated and troublesome process. If the flexion contracture is relieved by removing extra tibial bone, however, the flexion gap also is enlarged; the result is a posterior sag with posterior cruciate ligament–retaining prosthesis or possible dislocation with cruciate-sacrificing or posterior stabilized devices.[99,102] The distal femur should be recut; only then would the correct flexion balance be retained.

Knee prostheses in current use allow potential motion of 120 degrees or more, whether they are cruciate retaining or cruciate substituting. Clinical studies show an average motion of 110 degrees for the cruciate-retaining Kinematic design[343] and 115 degrees for the posterior stabilized cruciate-substituting design.[145] For various reasons (most importantly, the preoperative range of motion), many knees do not achieve the motion intended by the prosthetic designers, and knee arthroplasty for the purpose of increasing motion alone is generally disappointing. In knees that do not obtain or regain the expected range of motion, component malposition or malrotation, particularly internal rotation of the femoral component, should be considered. Femoral malrotation can be determined with precision by a CT scan, which identifies the femoral epicondyles (Fig. 99–14).

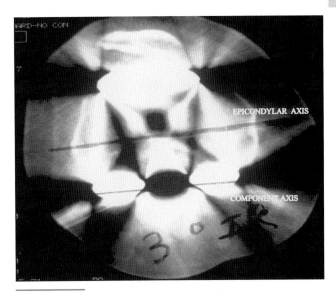

Figure 99–14. CT scan demonstrating 3 degrees of internal rotation of the femoral component compared with reference line through the epicondylar axis.

Loosening

Component loosening, usually of the tibial component, was the most frequent cause of failure with hinged prosthesis and early surface replacements. The results of hinges often appear deceptively good when the follow-up time is short because loosening is a time-related phenomenon and usually heralded by the development of a complete radiolucency at the bone-cement interface (Fig. 99–15). In contrast, with the surface replacements, most component loosening occurs within the first 2 years and is technique related, although the incidence of loosening increases slowly thereafter (Fig. 99–16). A 2-year follow-up examination of a surface replacement model serves as some indication of the security of fixation, whereas similar data for a constrained prosthesis may be misleading. Deburge,[63] using the Guepar prosthesis, reported a 2% loosening rate before 2 years; at 5 years, 15 of the prostheses had aseptic loosening. More sophisticated constrained designs also seem to share this characteristic, albeit to a lesser degree. Kaufer and Matthews,[165] using the spherocentric prosthesis, reported a 7.7% loosening rate after an average follow-up of 34 months. In addition, 10 of the femoral components and 14 of the tibial compo-

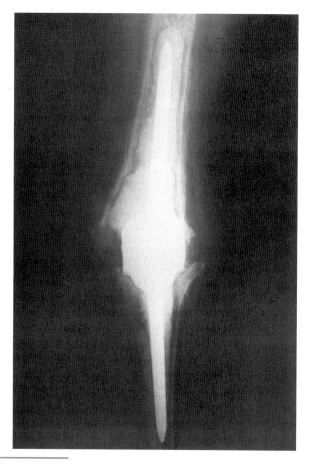

Figure 99–15. With hinge designs, loosening is time related.

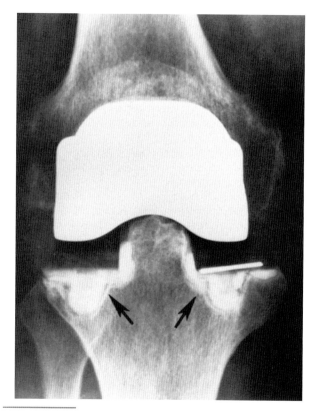

Figure 99–16. Complete radiolucent lines are seen frequently around two-piece polyethylene tibial components (*arrows*).

nents showed a progressive radiolucency, indicating further incipient loosening.

There is reason to believe that the high failure rate caused by tibial component loosening (Fig. 99–17) represents a design problem that is now on the way to solution (Fig. 99–18). High rates of loosening have been reported with polycentric, geometric, and early Freeman-Swanson designs. In addition to loosening, plastic deformation and cold flow were reported with the original UCI prosthesis, indicating that the rigidity of polyethylene can be compromised by excessively thin components and generous cruciate cutouts. Modifications to the tibial components have been made in subsequent designs. The total condylar prosthesis has a one-piece tibial component and a central fixation peg, and no component loosening was seen in 220 knees monitored 3 to 5 years. Reports from the Brigham and Women's Hospital in Boston on the posterior cruciate ligament–retaining, but otherwise similar, Kinematic prosthesis[343] also showed aseptic loosening to be negligible.

We reported the 10- to 12-year follow-up of the same total condylar prosthesis.[319] All had a one-piece polyethylene tibia with a 3.5-cm central peg, and all were cemented. We observed three tibial loosenings and one femoral loosening. All of the tibial component loosenings were positioned in varus (Fig. 99–19). This confirmed our belief that the mechanism of loosening of the tibial component was one of progressive sinkage and migration into

the medial tibia, producing an overall varus position. Hsu and Walker[130] showed experimentally that the ideal position for the Kinematic prosthesis is 7 degrees of femorotibial valgus with the tibia positioned at 90 degrees to the long axis of the tibia. In this situation, the component is loaded with a 51% to 49% distribution between medial and lateral plateaus, at least in a static position.[156] These authors conceded that adduction and abduction motions occurring during the gait cycle would produce different loading patterns in the patient. It seems self-evident that malalignment and malposition should be related to mechanical loosening and perhaps are the main cause of it (Fig. 99–20). There is some evidence for this. Lotke and Ecker[196] showed correlation between malalignment and radiolucent lines. Hvid and Nielsen[141] confirmed these findings. Dorr and Boiardo[70] stated that "prosthetic alignment is the most important factor influencing postoperative loosening and instability." Hsu and and colleagues[129,131] were unable to show an association between varus positioning and component loosening, however, and Smith and colleagues,[294] using a cemented total condylar prosthesis, could find no relationship between either radiolucent lines or loosening and component position. Cornell and associates,[57] also using the total condylar prosthesis, did find a correlation, however, between radiolucency (although not loosening) and varus positioning. Tew and Waugh[310] found the association between positioning and loosening inconclusive. There are possible explanations for these discrepancies. Loosen-

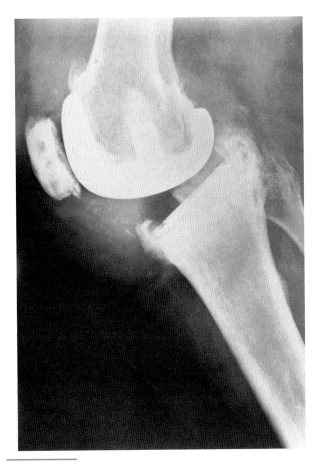

Figure 99–17. Flat tibial components, although one piece, are inadequately supported by the cancellous bone of the upper tibia and are susceptible to sinkage usually in anterior or medial directions.

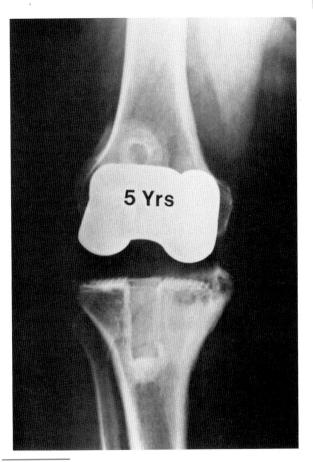

Figure 99–19. The importance of axial alignment. This total condylar knee prosthesis was positioned at surgery in slight varus, which gradually increased over a 5-year period. Collapse of the medial bone support with distortion of the polyethylene can be seen.

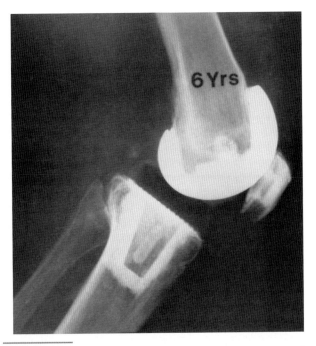

Figure 99–18. The addition of a central fixation peg to the tibial component virtually eliminates tibial component loosening.

ing rates for modern prostheses are low, and not all prostheses positioned in varus loosen. The identification and interpretation of radiolucent lines are confusing to the point that their analysis is probably meaningless (Fig. 99–21), unless the radiolucency is complete and progressive, a circumstance usually accompanied by clinical symptoms (Fig. 99–22). Our own belief is that a lack of statistical correlation between position and loosening is not established, but this is not a reason for carelessness about component positioning. When tibial components fail, they do so into varus, seldom into valgus, and the characteristic bone loss is medial, not lateral. These anecdotal observations, coupled with biomechanical analysis, strongly suggest that positioning remains crucial.

The use of metal-backed tibial components has reduced further the incidence of tibial loosening, presumably by distributing stress more evenly. The earliest version of the posterior stabilized knee had an all-polyethylene tibial component, and at 9- to 12-year follow-up, a 3% tibial loosening rate was recorded.[298] More recently, a minimum 10-year study[49] of the same prosthesis with a metal-backed tibial component showed no tibial loosenings and no complete radiolucent lines. Partial radiolucent lines were seen in 50% of the all-polyethylene components compared with 10% of the metal-backed components. Faris and associ-

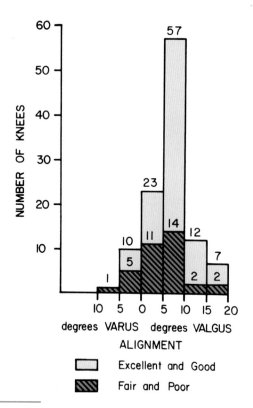

Figure 99–20. Bar graph showing the relationship between postoperative alignment and the clinical rating. The best results were obtained in knees aligned between 5 and 15 degrees of valgus. The relationship between alignment and the clinical result is by no means absolute, however. (From Insall J, Hood RW, Vanni M: The correction of knee alignment in 225 consecutive total condylar knee replacements. Clin Orthop 160:94, 1981.)

ates[85] described an unacceptably high failure rate of 30% at 10 years in all-polyethylene tibial components with coronal flat-on-flat design. All components failed beneath the medial tibial plateau bony collapse and medial tibial subsidence. It was thought that all-polyethylene tibial component success rates are highly design specific and should be used with more conforming designs.

The mechanism of loosening is also of interest. Miller[221] believed that the process was initiated by micromotion between component and bone, postulating that micromotion could be reduced or eliminated by improving the interlock between cement and cancellous bone. This argument, similar to others in joint arthroplasty, may apply more to hip prostheses than to knee prostheses. Another possible mechanism of loosening is that the components sink or subside into the bone. Seitz and coworkers,[291] using CT, showed a loss of bone density for several months after knee arthroplasty, coupled with a tendency for the implant to migrate in a mediolateral direction. Periprosthetic osteolysis is another cause of component loosening. The tibia is the more common site, but there have been documented cases in the literature involving femoral and tibial components. Osteolysis is discussed in more detail in the next section.

Ryd and colleagues[279-282,313] extensively studied fixation of knee prostheses in vivo using roentgenographic stere-

ogrammetric analysis. This technique was developed in Lund by Selvik in 1974 and applied to various orthopedic problems, such as spinal fusion stability, healing of tibial osteotomy, and skeletal growth patterns. It also has been used for assessing hip joint prosthetic loosening. In the knee, three or more tantalum balls of 0.8-mm diameter are implanted into the tibial metaphysis, using a special instrument with needle and piston. Markers also are introduced about 3 mm into the polyethylene tibial component from underneath, using holes made with a dentist's drill. The postoperative reference examination, using a biplanar radiographic technique (Fig. 99–23), is administered to the supine patient before the operated leg has become weightbearing. The follow-up examination is carried out with the patient standing on the operated leg only. Rotations about the transverse and sagittal axes were the only movements determined. The initial study was performed on Marmor unicondylar replacements, all of which were clinically successful. The study showed that none of the prostheses were rigidly fixed to the skeleton, and a degree of micromotion and migration occurred. There was some pattern to migration. Of the six patients studied, five showed posterior and downward migration, and four showed medial tilting away from the central axis of the knee.

Subsequent studies have been performed with cemented and uncemented prostheses, with similar results. Migration was greatest in the first year, after which it tended to stabilize; the direction tended to be medial, posterior, and downward. The mode of fixation was important, and migration was greater for uncemented prostheses. The magnitude was about 1 mm for a cemented total condylar prosthesis and 2.6 mm for an uncemented PCA prosthesis. In another study, the same authors examined 26 patients randomized to cemented or cementless TKA.[313] Using a similar study design, they found the migration between the two groups to be similar. At 1 year, the cemented tibial migration was 1 ± 0.2 mm compared with 1.4 ± 0.22 mm for the cementless TKA. Ryd and Linder[281] published a description of the bone-cement interface in three well-functioning unicondylar replacements that initially had been shown to migrate by roentgenographic stereogrammetric analysis. The three prostheses were removed for reasons other than fixation. The tibial components were solidly fixed to the bone. The three interfaces had a similar distribution of fibrous tissue and fibrocartilage. The peripheral 5 to 10 mm consisted of fibrous tissue, whereas the remainder of the supporting tissue was fibrocartilage. This layer of cartilage always rested on bone sometimes with a seam of osteoid "sandwiched" between the bone and the cartilage. The bone underneath the cartilage was vital. There was a total absence of any cellular reaction in the fibrocartilage.

Ryd's[279-282,313] studies showed that there is no such thing as rigid fixation between prosthesis and bone, and that the normal situation allows some degree of micromotion. Prostheses move or migrate a certain amount early on, then, in most cases, stabilize into a state of equilibrium, which is compatible with satisfactory long-term function. The normal interface between cement and bone consists of fibrocartilage and fibrous tissue with little cellular reaction. This interface probably corresponds with thin, stable

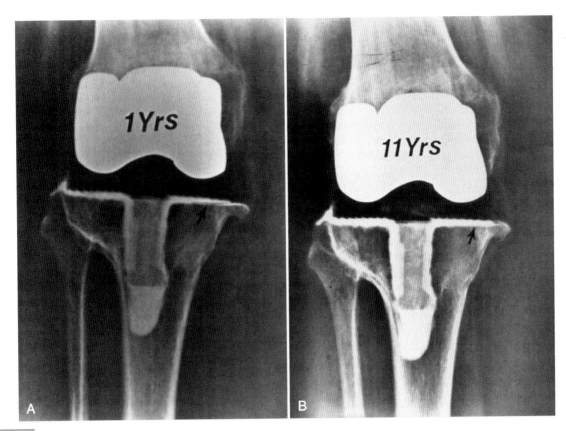

Figure 99–21. **A,** Small partial radiolucency beneath the medial tibial plateau. **B,** Ten years later, the radiolucency is barely perceptible (probably because of a slight difference in projection).

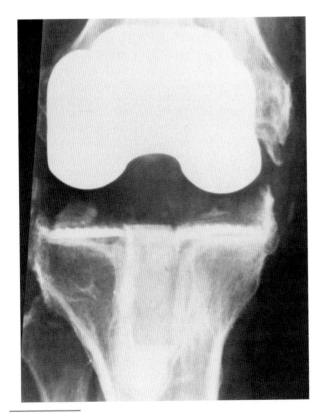

Figure 99–22. With the total condylar prosthesis, a complete radiolucency is attributed to low-grade infection until proved otherwise.

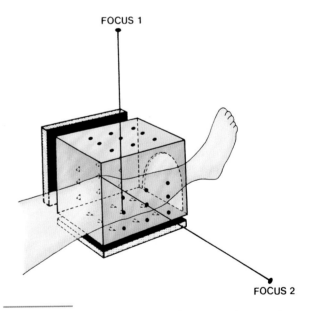

Figure 99–23. Biplanar radiographic setup for roentgenographic stereogrammetric analysis of the knee joint. (From Ryd L, Boegard T, Egund N, et al: Migration of the tibial component in successful unicompartmental knee arthroplasty: A clinical, radiographic, and roentgenstereophotogrammetric study. Acta Orthop Scand 54:408, 1983.)

radiolucencies that can be identified in long-term studies of well-functioning knee arthroplasties. Hvid[139,140] concluded that bone strength may be crucial from the point of view of fatigue. From this information, it can be argued that excessive penetration of cement into the cancellous bone of the knee may be undesirable. It is unlikely that bone trabeculae enclosed within a massive amount of cement remain viable; although the initial mechanical interlock may be improved, the long-term effect may be to transfer the interface to a more distal area of the tibia and into an area in which the strength of the bone is weaker. If one believes this argument, cement penetration should be minimal—2 to 3 mm is ideal.[324] The theoretical argument coincides with clinical observations. Long-term studies of prostheses, using "old-fashioned" cement techniques that gave little bone penetration, have shown extremely good survival. For about 2 years, roughly encompassing 1984 and 1985, we sought greater cement penetration, using low-viscosity cement[221]; however, after realizing that our earlier patients continued to function well, we returned to the earlier cement techniques. Most of our metal-backed tibial components have been fixed, using a thin layer of cement with little attempt to penetrate the cancellous bone.

For bone ingrowth prostheses, close bony apposition, rigid initial fixation,[26,65,302,303,321] and avoidance of early weightbearing to minimize fixation stresses that could prejudice bone ingrowth have been recommended. Bone ingrowth usually does not attach extensively to tibial components, and such bone that does attach to the prosthesis is limited to small areas, usually around fixation lugs.[55] Tibial fixation is mainly by fibrous tissue,[54] although this does seem compatible with good clinical function. Possibly the use of compression screws into the upper tibia would improve the amount of bone ingrowth.[335] The addition of an uncemented central stem has been shown to reduce tilting and sinkage of a proximally cemented tibia, and roentgenographic stereogrammetric analysis has shown the least amount of migration with this type of design.[5,6] Evolution of prosthetic design is perhaps toward a central stem with screws in uncemented prostheses to protect against initial rotational stresses. Cemented and uncemented prostheses migrate, then reach a stage of equilibrium, after which a certain degree of "normal" micromotion occurs without further sinkage or gross movement. The interface in both types of fixation is predominantly of fibrous tissue. Whiteside and Ohl[334] observed the development of bone hypertrophy underneath a stemmed, uncemented tibial component during the first year. Anterolateral sinking was noted in 6 of the first 46 patients, but was not seen again in the series after a design change was made to fix the stem in the bone of the upper tibia more rigidly. Sinkage in these patients was estimated from routine radiographs. Hypertrophy of the bone of the distal femur also was observed around the uncemented femoral components, more posteriorly than anteriorly, and when bone hypertrophy was present, it did not regress.

Alignment is more crucial in cementless knees because cement fixation is not present to help protect against excessive point loading, which may occur with malalignment. With cement fixation, load is distributed more evenly across the tibia, even when malalignment is present. Without cement fixation, this even distribution of load is not present, and a point-load situation is created, which causes necrosis of bone under the overloaded tibial component. Also, without the protective effect of cement fixation, failure of fixation at the opposite condyle occurs from excessive tension at the interface.[72]

Loosening of femoral components is uncommon whether cemented or uncemented. When it does occur, however, it follows a particular pattern in which the bone resorbs posteriorly, allowing the femur to migrate anteriorly and rotate into flexion (Fig. 99–24). King and Scott[169] described a series of 15 loose, cemented duopatellar femoral prostheses. The incidence of femoral loosening is not stated, but in one series at the Hospital for Special Surgery there were 6 femoral loosenings in 430 cemented arthroplasties (1.4%) over a 15-year follow-up period. The mechanism of loosening was similar to that described by King and Scott,[169] who believed that lack of posterior femoral support as a result of either osteoporotic bone or poor technique was the cause. In this region, cancellous bone hypertrophy was reported by Whiteside and Pafford,[335] and this region of the femur is most likely to be highly stressed.

Loosening of the patellar component is associated most often with patellar fractures or with dissociation of polyethylene and metal-back components. Loosening of cemented all-polyethylene patellae in other circumstances is infrequent. The incidence of patella component loosening is about 1%, but has been reported to be 3%.[343] Loosening of the patella was more common with the small central lug, but more recently, the tripod configuration of three small peripheral lugs has become popular. Mason and coworkers[212] reported no loose patella components among 577 tripod configuration patellae at an average of 3 years.

Firestone and associates[93] found loosening rates of 0.6% to 11.1% in several cementless patella component designs. Factors associated with loosening include insertion of the prosthesis with cement into worn or sclerotic bone, malpositioning of the patellar component, subluxation, fracture or avascular necrosis of the patella, osteoporosis, asymmetric resection, loosening of other prosthetic components, and lack of osseous growth into the porous coating.[28,260] Reduction in the rate of loosening of the patella component requires improved bone preparation and cementing techniques, proper patella resection, avoidance of asymmetric or excessive bone removal, and central patella tracking.[13]

Osteolysis

Osteolysis after a TKA is a relatively recently observed phenomenon (Fig. 99–25). Although it is well documented in THA literature in response to particulate debris, it has shown a rapid increase more recently in TKA literature. The cause of osteolysis in the knee is the same as the hip—inflammatory response to particulate debris. The first reported series of osteolysis as a complication was in 1992[248]; the authors reported a 16% incidence in 174

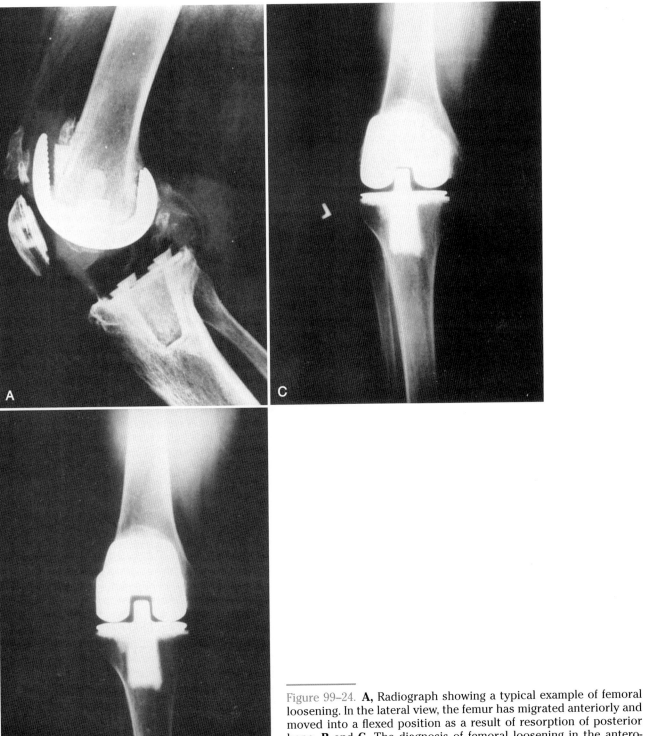

Figure 99–24. **A,** Radiograph showing a typical example of femoral loosening. In the lateral view, the femur has migrated anteriorly and moved into a flexed position as a result of resorption of posterior bone. **B** and **C,** The diagnosis of femoral loosening in the antero-posterior view is not always easy to make. The femur tends to migrate proximally so that there is the appearance of bone over-growth medially or laterally. In this case, the diagnosis of loosening was made because a change in position into varus was noted and was confirmed by overlapping the radiographs.

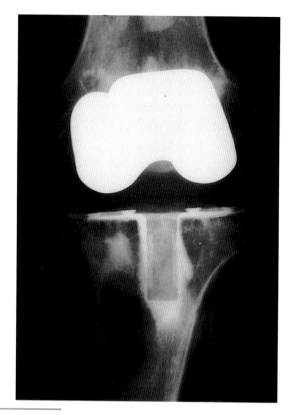

Figure 99–25. Radiograph showing an example of osteolysis involving a prosthesis.

consecutive cementless TKAs, using tibial fixation with bone screws. Since then, there have been reports of osteolysis after cemented and cementless TKA.[78,81,248,271,330]

The presentation of a patient with osteolysis varies. Most patients with well-fixed components are asymptomatic. Other patients present with symptoms of boggy synovitis.[248] Mild or moderate diffuse pain may occur with activity, especially in patients in whom the tibial component is unstable.[248] The radiographic criteria for diagnosis of osteolysis as proposed by Peters and colleagues[248] are a lytic osseous defect that extends beyond the limits of that potentially caused by loosening of the implant alone, absence of cancellous bone trabeculae, and geographic demarcation by a shell of bone.

TKA produces greater wear of the polyethylene surface than THA. Engh and coworkers[78] described four factors that could explain this phenomenon. First is the size of the particles produced, which is related to the type of wear (i.e., delamination and abrasion in TKA); this releases large fragments of polyethylene, rarely seen in THA. Large particles produced in the TKA are relatively bioinert. Second, the synovial cavity of the knee is the most extensive of any synovial joint in the body and has greater capacity to engulf and digest wear debris (i.e., greater resistance to osteolysis). Third, the fixation interface with polymethyl methacrylate is a better seal to potential debris than polymethyl methacrylate in a THA. Fourth, the shear and tensile stresses on polymethyl methacrylate may be less at the knee than at the hip. The modulus of elasticity of polymethyl methacrylate is relatively close to that of the

cancellous bone of the upper tibia and the tibial component. The decreased amount of stress and fatigue means decreased fracture of the cement mantle, which leads to decreased access for debris to bone-cement interface.

When osteolysis appears in the knee after a TKA, it usually appears on the tibial side. This occurrence is probably a multifactorial event. Peters and associates[248] offered three possible factors for this occurrence. First, gravity and weightbearing through the medial side of the knee tend to localize the particulate polyethylene on the tibial side. Second, on the femoral side, if the osteolytic process is initiated along the implant-bone interface, the flanges of the femoral implant tend to obscure a radiographic diagnosis. Last, the addition of screws to the tibial implant provides avenues for the migration of debris into metaphyseal bone.

The incidence of osteolysis around a knee replacement is difficult to assess for many reasons. The first difficulty is obtaining an accurate radiographic assessment at the interface. If there is tibial osteolysis below the tray, and the x-ray angle is from slightly above the joint, this lysis may be missed on x-ray film. Engh and colleagues[78] indicated that femoral lesions are not well recognized as quickly secondary to being hidden by the femoral component on anteroposterior radiograph. Another reason for the difficulty in assessing the incidence of osteolysis is the length of follow-up. Ezzet and coworkers[81] reported a strong correlation between length of follow-up and the prevalence of osteolysis. Before 24 months, no cases of osteolysis were identified; between 24 and 60 months, the incidence was 15%; and at follow-up greater than 60 months, the incidence was 39%.

The reported incidence of osteolysis after a TKA is wide-ranging. Whiteside[330] reported a 0% incidence using the Ortholoc II (Dow Corning Wright, Arlington, TN) components, in which the tibial component is completely covered with porous coating. On the other end of the spectrum, Ezzet and coworkers[81] reported an incidence of 30% in which the tibial component was fixed with cement and screws, and the femoral component was cemented. The actual incidence probably lies between these two reported rates.

Factors that advance osteolysis include tibia components that use screws in cemented and cementless designs. The screw acts as a conduit for debris into the cancellous bone. Ezzet and coworkers[81] recommended that screws not be used at all. Another factor is the design of the components and its coating. Whiteside[330] compared two types of cementless components, Ortholoc II and Ortholoc modular, to study osteolysis rates. The only difference between the two components is that Ortholoc II is completely porous coated, whereas the Ortholoc modular is only partially porous coated with smooth metal bridges connecting the four screw holes. They found a 0% rate of osteolysis with the Ortholoc II component and a 20% rate with the Ortholoc modular. Ezzet and coworkers[81] concluded that the smooth metal tracks conduct debris from the joint cavity to the area surrounding the stem. Whiteside attributed the low osteolysis rate of the Ortholoc II to the full porous coating. They believed there is a gasket effect that prevents polyethylene debris from traveling down the stem. Also, there is protection of the implant-bone interface by the fibrous tissue mantle that permeates the porous coating, preventing polyethylene debris from penetrating. Ezzet and coworkers[81] indicated that a press-fit femoral component may contribute to an increased incidence of osteolysis. Whiteside[330] did not believe that large amounts of polyethylene debris are needed to cause osteolysis as long as free access is available to the medullary canal of the tibia. When the debris enters the medullary canal of the bone, there is no mechanism to remove it from the vicinity, and the macrophage buildup and subsequent osteolysis can become clinically significant. The etiology of the particulate debris, which contributes the most to osteolysis, is controversial. Small particles are generated from tibial post impingement in P.S. knees, from backside wear in all modular designs, and from backside wear in mobile-bearing knees. It is apparent, however, that osteolysis is extremely rare in monoblock tibial designs, especially with net shape molded components.*

Histological analysis of synovial tissue and osteolytic tissue has been performed. The synovial tissue of knees associated with osteolysis shows subsynovial infiltrates consisting of histiocyte and giant cells.[248] Polyethylene and metal particulate debris has been found in specimens. The size and type of material are important. Polyethylene particles less than 3 μm are usually engulfed by giant cells. Polyethylene particles greater than 3 μm are found in the cytoplasm of histiocytes and occasionally within giant cells. Larger particles of metal (>5 μm) usually elicit little cellular response.[248] Histological examinations of osteolytic tissue revealed a hypercellular membrane consisting of sheets of histiocytes and occasional giant cells. There is no necrosis and little associated vascularity.

The treatment of osteolysis around a TKA is controversial. If the implant is stable, and the patient is asymptomatic, one can observe the patient with serial x-ray films on a yearly basis. If the patient is symptomatic or the prosthesis is obviously loose, there are several different options. For patients who are symptomatic, and the prosthesis is not loose, but excessive polyethylene wear is seen, one can remove the defects with a curet, pack with morcellized bone graft, and replace the polyethylene. Engh and colleagues[78] either changed out the polyethylene or performed removal of screws, curettage, and polyethylene exchange. In this series, they reported good results with no tibial defects progressing and no development of new lesions. If the components are grossly loose, revision of components is in order. Because the defects are always larger in situ than they appear on x-ray film, a full armamentarium of revision instruments should be ready. In most of these situations, allograft and the full complement of modular augments should be available. In Engh's series,[78] in which the components were revised and structural allograft was used, four of five patients had excellent fixation interfaces at 2 years. There were no lucencies and no graft resorption. One rheumatoid arthritis patient had 1- to 2-mm radiolucency beneath the tibial plateau without change in component alignment. The patient was pain-free at 6 years. Robinson and coworkers[271] reported on 17 revisions they performed for osteolysis. The original method of component fixation was a mixture of hybrid fixation and cemented and cementless implants. The average time interval from the index surgery to radiographic evidence of osteolysis was 56 months. The prostheses used in the treatment of these 17 revisions were posterior stabilized implants in 65% of cases and a constrained implant in 30%. Osteolytic defects were reconstructed with cement only in 47%, allograft in 30%, and metallic wedges in 35%. No follow-up or outcome data were available from this series.

Fractures

Three types of fractures occur around the prosthesis: (1) intraoperative, (2) stress or fatigue related, and (3) postoperative.

INTRAOPERATIVE FRACTURES

Intraoperative fractures can occur on either the tibial plateau or the femoral condyles. They are most likely to occur when bone is brittle, and when the prosthesis is driven hard onto the bone. Tibial fractures can occur with central stem models when the stem hole is undersized; these are seldom of consequence and require no special treatment. Femoral condyle fractures may occur when the bone is soft, as in rheumatoid arthritis, and the component is driven into the bone more than intended, resulting in a malposition. In posterior stabilizing designs with a central box, insertion of the femoral condyles may split the femur vertically (Fig. 99–26) when the bone cuts for the box are not exactly parallel. If the fracture is stable, no fixation is required, although screws may be needed (see Fig. 99–26). The addition of a stem to the femoral component also may be considered.

Intraoperative fractures are usually nondisplaced with minimal or no comminution. These fractures seldom require any special postoperative management except perhaps a crutch assist for a longer time. Motion does not need to be delayed.

Intraoperative patella fractures are seen most commonly in the revision setting, with removal of the stable component. There are generally two types: horizontal and vertical. Horizontal fractures are more difficult to deal with, mainly secondary to concern over the integrity of the extensor mechanism. Usually a tension band technique is required to stabilize the patella and allow for some early motion. If the tension band is successful, the patella component is not replaced. If the fragments cannot be repaired satisfactorily, other options include patellectomy or, in rare circumstances, an extensor mechanism allograft.

Intraoperative femoral fracture usually involves splitting or fracturing one of the condyles. Another observed fracture is perforation or fracture of the anterior cortex with the alignment rod. The condyles are usually handled with cancellous screws across the condyles or, in situations with greater comminution, a long-stemmed femoral

*References 4, 20, 75, 132, 134, 136, 179, 180, 189, 203, 220, 222, 240, 243, 252, 262, 305, 325, 326, 328.

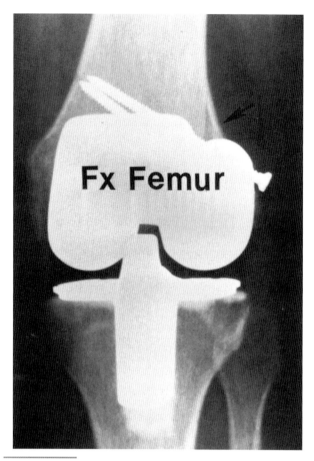

Figure 99–26. An intraoperative fracture of the lateral femoral condyle occurred in this case. After fixation with two screws, the aftercare was uneventful, and weightbearing as usual was permitted.

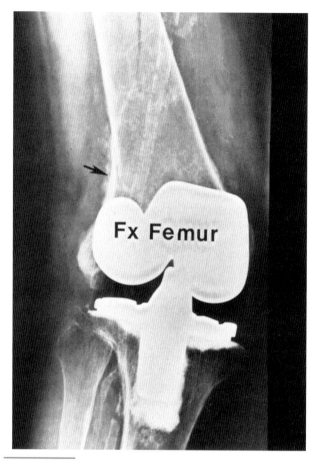

Figure 99–27. In this rheumatoid patient, a lateral soft-tissue release was done to correct a severe valgus deformity. Two months after the operation, pain and a recurrent valgus deformity developed. A stress fracture of the lateral femoral condyle was observed that healed in a position of deformity. The femoral component in this case is apparently not loose, and the knee is painless.

component. The breach of the anterior cortex also is treated with a long-stemmed femoral component.

Intraoperative tibia fractures are usually of the vertical variety. They are caused by impingement of the stem or impaction during surgery. These fractures usually heal well with little intervention. They are best treated with partial weightbearing and full range of motion in the early postoperative period.

STRESS OR FATIGUE FRACTURES

Stress fractures[259] adjoining the components usually occur in the patella (see later discussion) but also occur in the femur (Fig. 99–27) and tibia. These have been seen after a stripping of the lateral femoral condyle for the correction of fixed valgus deformity apparently caused by avascularity of the bone. Stress fracture of the tibia with medial sinkage and displacement of the tibial component also has been seen in a rheumatoid arthritis patient. Stress fractures involving femoral and tibial components usually require revision with the addition of appropriate augments and stems.

Stress fractures of the hip[92] may occur in patients who were unable to walk before surgery. These fractures have

occurred in two of our patients; we also have seen fractures of the pubic rami. These complications might be avoided by prolonged use of crutches or a walker, but in patients at risk it may not be practical.

POSTOPERATIVE FRACTURES

Postoperative periprosthetic fractures are more difficult to treat than intraoperative fractures. Patella and femoral fractures are more common than tibia fractures. The overall incidence is reported to be 0.3% to 2%.[44] Causes of these fractures include trauma, anterior notching of femoral cortex, osteoporosis, prolonged steroid use, preexisting neurological condition, stress shielding caused by rigid implants, pharmacological causes, hormonal influences, rheumatoid arthritis, and arthrofibrosis.[13,42,44] The goal of treatment is to restore the prefracture functional status by achieving fracture union and maintaining proper limb alignment and range of motion with preservation of prosthetic component if stable.

Preoperative assessment and planning are paramount in this situation. In particular, emphasis on the physical examination, evaluating active range of motion, stability of components, presence of extensor lag, palpation for obvious defect in the extensor mechanism, and quadriceps strength, is crucial. Radiographs with a minimum of anteroposterior, lateral, and Merchant views should be obtained. Assessment of the fracture for size and displacement is also essential, as is assessment of the components for obvious signs of loosening. Finally, the patient should be scrutinized for any type of osseous defects, whether from comminution or osteolysis. If surgery is contemplated, a medical consultation is advised secondary to the older age and multiple medical problems of these patients.

Many classification systems have been proposed for these types of fractures. We use a system whereby type I is a nondisplaced fracture with stable components. Type IIA is a displaced fracture with no comminution and stable components. Type IIB is a displaced fracture with comminution and stable components. Type III is either a nondisplaced or displaced fracture with loose components. In general, type I fractures are treated nonoperatively, type II fractures usually require some type of manipulation or fixation or both with retention of components, and type III fractures require revision arthroplasty.

Postoperative patella fractures are often asymptomatic. Occasionally, patients report a sudden onset of pain with knee flexion or difficulty climbing stairs. The causes of patella fractures have been attributed to certain design features of the femoral implant or to patella maltracking, both causing excessive concentrations of patella stress. The integrity of the bone and its capacity for repair of microtrauma also may be compromised by devascularization of the patella during lateral release, resection of the fat pad, or aggressive stripping of soft tissue around the patella.[120,166] Tria and colleagues[314] found an increased rate of patella fracture associated with lateral release in which the lateral superior genicular artery was not preserved. Patellar fractures after TKA can occur with and without patellar resurfacing, although they are more common when a patellar implant has been used.[29,89,110,127,159,266,268,340] Treatment depends on three factors: integrity of extensor mechanism, displacement of the fracture, and prosthetic fixation. A nondisplaced fracture or minimally displaced fracture (<3 mm) may be treated in a knee immobilizer or cylinder cast for 3 to 4 weeks (Fig. 99–28). Surgery is reserved for displaced fractures, disruption of extensor mechanism, and prosthetic loosening. The main goal of treatment is fracture healing, even if that means removing a well-fixed component or not replacing a loose one. Tension band wiring technique can be used with excision of any loose or comminuted pieces of bone that cannot be incorporated properly into the repair. Patellectomy is a last resort.

Postoperative femoral fractures can be difficult to treat. Most fractures that result from a fall or other injury occur in the lower femur adjoining the prosthesis and may be comminuted and displaced.[1,36,56,59,90,120,218,273,293] Fractures seem more likely to occur in this region if the femur was breached at operation by notching of the anterior femoral cortex (Fig. 99–29). Ritter and coworkers[267] do not believe

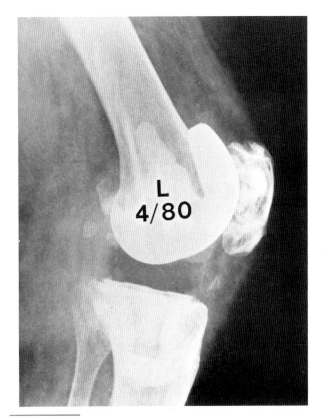

Figure 99–28. A healed fracture of the lower pole of the patella. This patient has an excellent result and no quadriceps weakness.

that femoral notching predisposes to fracture, but others consider it to be a contributing factor. Notching was more likely before a complete range of femoral sizes became available. Size mismatch creates the need to fit a relatively small prosthesis onto a larger bone (Fig. 99–30). Techniques that size the femoral component from the posterior femoral condyles also may predispose the femur to notching because the adjustment cut in between sizes is made anteriorly. Techniques that reference the anterior femoral cortex should decrease this risk; however, when external rotation of the femoral component is performed, notching of the lateral trochlear area can occur.

Supracondylar fractures are often comminuted with displacement of the femoral component posteriorly and laterally (Fig. 99–31). Operative fixation is complicated by the presence of the femoral component, which interferes with fixation of the distal fragment. Periprosthetic fractures have a higher rate of nonunion than other supracondylar femoral fractures in the elderly. This finding has been attributed to premorbid alterations in vascularity at the fracture site as a result of previous surgery, the presence of a metal implant and intramedullary polymethyl methacrylate, or long-term oral corticosteroid administration.

A type I fracture that is nondisplaced with the component well fixed is best treated nonoperatively. The treatment is with a brace or cast brace, allowing for range of motion. In some situations, a long-leg cast may be applied for 3 weeks followed by a brace until healed. Traction

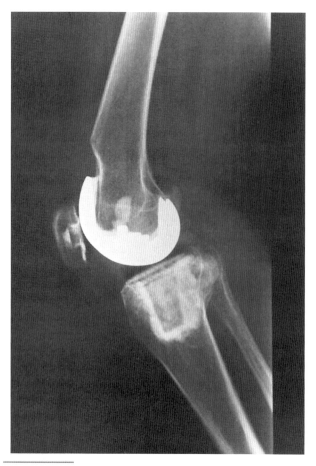

Figure 99–29. Lateral radiograph showing a notch in the femur caused by miscutting the anterior surface. Notching of the femur predisposes to supracondylar fracture.

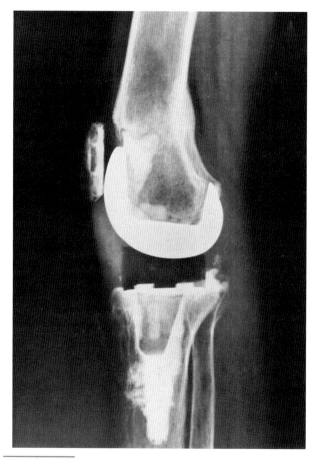

Figure 99–30. The saw has violated the anterior cortex of the femur. The weakened bone makes it susceptible to fracture.

(Fig. 99–32) with a tibial or os calcis pin has lost most of its popularity because of concerns with DVT, pulmonary embolus, pressure sores, and pulmonary infections in this elderly population. The key to nonoperative treatment is close monitoring to ensure there is no displacement of the fracture or alignment changes in the extremity. Operative intervention is necessary in patients with displacement of fracture, in patients with malalignment, in patients who are not able to tolerate the brace, and in patients who have difficulty with the restricted weightbearing. Surgical options include retrograde nail, blade plate (Fig. 99–33), condylar buttress plate, condylar screw, Rush rods, and Zickel supracondylar rods. All have inherent advantages and disadvantages. The intramedullary devices, such as the retrograde nail, Rush rod, and Zickel rod, do not disrupt the fracture site. Retrograde nails cannot be used if the patient has a posterior stabilized femoral component with closed housing or a long-stemmed component. The buttress plate, blade plate, and condylar screw have the disadvantage of requiring a long lateral scar and disruption of the fracture site.

A type II fracture with displacement but stable components usually requires operative intervention. In the appropriate situation, a trial of closed reduction with subsequent bracing or casting may be attempted. This treatment is seldom successful and requires a surgical pro-

cedure. There are many devices to choose from, but there are some important factors to consider when choosing this device, including type of implant; comminution, displacement, and angulation of the fracture; bone quality; and extremity alignment. The selection of devices is similar to devices used for the type I fracture. The buttress plate may be difficult to use in this elderly population secondary to poor bone quality and comminution. If the retrograde nail is to be used, the intercondylar space needs to be ascertained. This is done by knowledge of the prosthesis or measurement on a notch or sunrise radiograph. A minimum of 12 mm is needed.

A type III fracture with loosening of the component usually is treated with a revision. This revision can be accomplished in one of two ways. First, the fracture may be treated first and allowed to heal, and then a revision performed. Alternatively, one may elect to perform the revision as part of the fracture stabilization. We prefer to perform the revision as part of the fracture stabilization, the underlying rationale being early mobilization of the patient. Most patients are elderly with multiple medical problems, and early mobilization decreases the incidence of medical complications and muscle atrophy. If the fracture is treated first, it could take 4 to 6 months to heal. After the revision, it could be another 4 to 6 months for the patient to be independent again. If the revision and

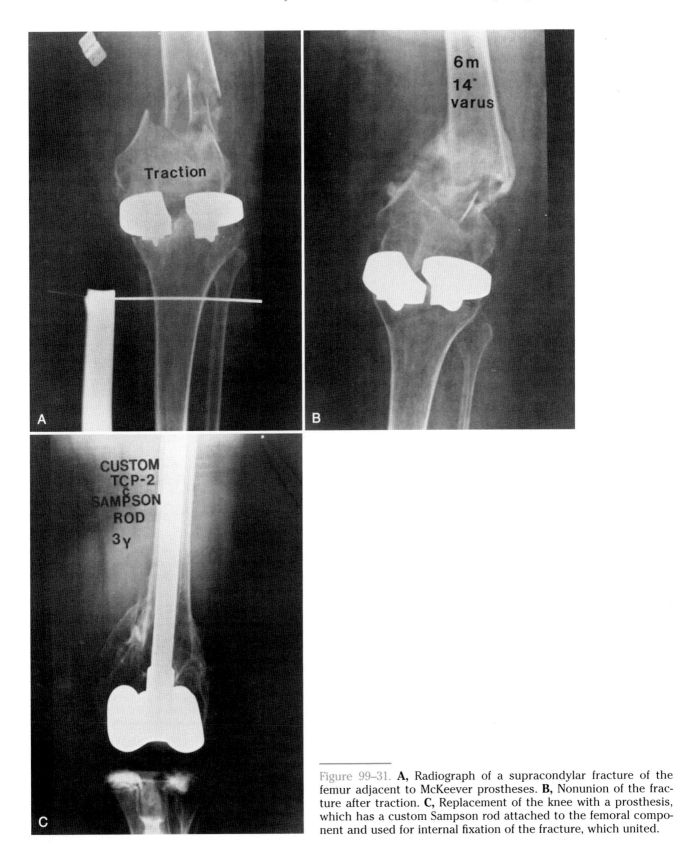

Figure 99–31. **A,** Radiograph of a supracondylar fracture of the femur adjacent to McKeever prostheses. **B,** Nonunion of the fracture after traction. **C,** Replacement of the knee with a prosthesis, which has a custom Sampson rod attached to the femoral component and used for internal fixation of the fracture, which united.

stabilization are performed simultaneously, the total recovery time is usually 4 to 6 months. There are two main advantages to delaying a revision procedure and treating the fracture first: (1) Revision of a knee that has an anatomically healed supracondylar fracture is far easier

than revision of one that has an unstable condylar fragment; (2) a standard revision implant can be used rather than a tumor replacement, a custom-made implant, or a large structural allograft. During the revision, a long-stemmed femoral component should be used. If the

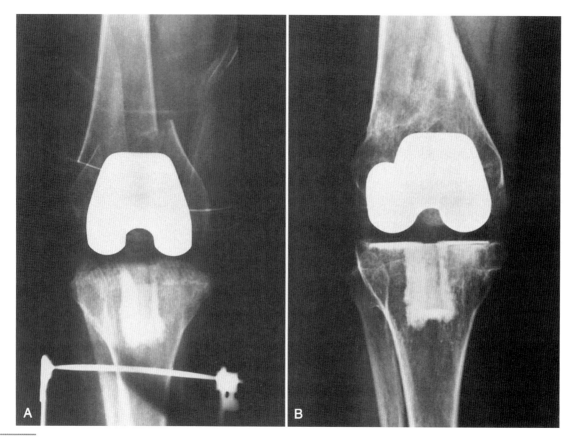

Figure 99–32. **A,** Supracondylar fracture of the femur treated by traction. **B,** Result after the fracture healed. Good alignment and good function were preserved. (From Sisto DJ, Lachiewicz PR, Insall JN: Treatment of supracondylar fractures following prosthetic arthroplasty of the knee. Clin Orthop 196:265, 1985.)

condyles are too comminuted, or there is a large amount of bone loss, one must be prepared with alternatives to replace the deficiencies. Options include allograft,[40] implants made to replace distal femur, allograft-implant composites, and tumor prosthesis. For these cases, it may be necessary to cement the femoral stem extension.

Postoperative periprosthetic tibial fractures are rarer than femoral or patella fractures. The largest published series to date is by Felix and associates,[87] with 83 fractures occurring in the postoperative period. Before that series, the largest series was 15 fractures reported by Rand.[255] The classification system proposed by Felix and associates[87] is the most commonly used system. There are four types, subclassified as A (prosthesis radiographically well fixed), B (loose), and C (intraoperative). Type I fracture involves the tibial plateau, type II fracture is adjacent to the prosthetic stem, type III fracture is distal to the stem, and type IV fracture involves the tibial tubercle.

Treatment of a type IA fracture is nonoperative with a brace or cast, along with protected weightbearing. Type IB, which is more common, is best treated with revision of components and treatment of the depression with bone graft or metal wedges. Type IIA and IIIA fractures, if nondisplaced, can be treated with brace or cast, along with protected weightbearing. If displaced, an attempt at closed reduction and casting is made. If unsuccessful, open reduction and internal fixation is performed. Type IIB and IIIB fractures require revision arthroplasty with long-stemmed components. Nondisplaced type IV fractures are treated in extension with cast or knee immobilizer. Displaced type IV fractures are treated with open reduction and internal fixation.[87]

RESULTS

The results of intraoperative fracture treatment are sparse for many reasons. First, it is rare. Second, it is largely unreported. Lombardi and coworkers[194] reported on 41 intercondylar distal femoral fractures; 6 were identified intraoperatively and treated with a long-stemmed femoral component, screw fixation, or both. All six went on to heal without modification of postoperative regimen. The other 35 fractures were incidental findings on postoperative radiographs. All healed with the standard physical therapy protocol. Felix and associates[87] reported on 19 intraoperative tibia fractures. Eleven were type IC fractures. Nine were fixed intraoperatively, and two were found postoperatively and treated with either a cast or activity modification. Nine of 11 (81%) had no pain or mild occasional pain. One patient had pain with weightbearing and was unable to walk five blocks. The last patient underwent revision for component loosening. Seven were type IIC fractures. Four were seen intraoperatively. Two required no treatment, and two required bone grafting. Three frac-

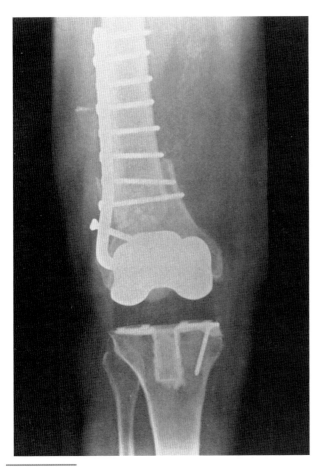

Figure 99–33. Fixation of a supracondylar fracture with a blade plate and screws. A low-grade infection subsequently developed requiring removal of the hardware and the knee implant.

tures were seen on postoperative radiographs; all were treated with a brace or weightbearing restrictions. Six of seven patients had no knee pain at mean follow-up of 50 months. One patient had a type IIIC fracture that was treated with casting and non-weightbearing for 7 weeks. The patient had multiple medical problems and died 8 months after surgery.

More results are available for treatment of postoperative patella fractures. For type I fractures that are nondisplaced or minimally displaced and treated nonoperatively, the results were universally good.[29,104,127,311] The results of operative treatment of displaced patellar fractures, especially with an extensor lag, have been poor.[29,104,127,311] A representative study of treatment of patella fractures was done at the Hospital for Special Surgery.[311] Of 18 patella fractures occurring after a TKA, 4 were treated operatively, and 14 were treated nonoperatively. The results of the four treated operatively were rated good in three and fair in one. Of the 14 nonoperatively treated knees, results were rated excellent in 10 and good in 4. None of this group had demonstrable quadriceps weakness or an extension lag.

The results of nonoperative treatment for nondisplaced femoral fractures are good.[42,218,229] The outcome of treatment of displaced femoral fractures is a little more variable because of the varied treatment options. One study

that examined the use of Rush rods in 22 fractures found that all healed in 3 to 4 months. Two of the fractures healed in 15 degrees of valgus because of technical error. The patients recovered an average of 108 degrees of knee flexion.[269] The results of treatment with plates and screws are, for the most part, encouraging. Healy and colleagues[116] found that 18 of 20 fractures healed after treatment with blade plate, a condylar screw, or a buttress plate. Bone graft was used in 15 of the patients. The postoperative Knee Society scores were equivalent to the prefracture scores. Culp and associates[59] reported that 17 of 20 fractures healed after treatment with a compression plate. There have been reports of poor results with treatment with plates and screws.[56,90,242] Most of the failures and poor outcomes using plates and screws may be attributed to angulation of the fracture (malunion), migration of the condylar screw or plate, nonunion, poor knee motion, and infection.[76] The clinical results of the use of retrograde intramedullary rods is encouraging, but the numbers in most studies are small.[147,216,235,272] Complications of this method of treatment include migration of the rod into the knee joint, femoral shortening, nonunion, loss of motion, and infection.

For type III fractures of the femur that include loosening of the component, requiring use of a revision component, the results are good. Cordeiro and coworkers[56] reported on five fractures treated with a revision stem; all five healed with good results. Kraay and colleagues[174] used a combination long-stemmed prosthesis and allograft in seven patients, all of whom had a satisfactory outcome. McLaren and associates[216] treated 25 knees, most of which received a long-stemmed revision; 24 had a satisfactory outcome.

Chen and colleagues[42] reviewed overall clinical results of management of femoral fractures after TKA. The review incorporated 195 fractures in 12 published studies. Satisfactory results were achieved in 83 of the patients with nondisplaced fractures that were treated without surgery. In the patients with displaced fractures, 64 had satisfactory results with and without surgery. There was no statistically significant difference in satisfactory outcomes between nonoperative and operative treatments (67% versus 61%).

There are few reports of treatment results of postoperative tibia fractures after TKA. Rand and Coventry[259] reported on 15 type IB fractures with loose prostheses. All were treated with revision surgery, and all did well. All the knees with tibia fractures had axial malalignment with increased varus compared with the control group. Lotke and Ecker[196] reported on five fractures of the medial tibial plateau; four of the five tibial components were aligned in varus. Cordeiro and coworkers[56] reported on one tibial fracture that occurred below the prosthesis with loose components (type IIIB) that was treated by a long-stemmed revision. This fracture went on to heal without incident.

Component Breakage

Breakage of components is rare[38,111,232] and usually restricted to hinges and linked designs.[234] Breakage is manifest by instability, pain, and deformity, but does not call for immediate revision. One of our patients had a fracture of the femoral stem associated with an episode of transient pain 3 years after the arthroplasty. Although some instability was present, this patient functioned at a high level with little or no pain for another 5 years before revision became necessary for an increasing varus deformity.

Mechanical failure in surface replacement is rare. We have encountered three fractured femoral components in the early version of the unicondylar and duocondylar prostheses. In these, the femoral runner was made of considerably thinner metal than that used on subsequent designs, and it is not expected that similar fatigue failure will be seen in current models. Fracture of unicondylar metal components also has been reported.[38] Whiteside and coworkers[331] examined fracture of femoral components in cementless TKA. They compared 6172 Ortholoc II femoral components with double-bead layers with 16,230 Ortholoc II femoral components with single-bead layers for fracture of components. They found 32 fractured femoral components in all, 31 of which were in the double-bead layers. The overall minimum rate of failure for the double-bead layers was 0.42, whereas for the single-bead layer it was 0.006. They found that all the failures occurred at the junction between one of the level surfaces and the distal surface of the implant.

Fracture of the metallic tibial tray has been reported on isolated occasions.[111,289] Subsequently, in these designs, the metal tray was strengthened, particularly in the region of the posterior cruciate cutout. We have not seen a metal tray fracture in a cruciate-substituting design.

Polyethylene fractures are generally wear-related as with late catastrophic failure of the tibial inserts of modular components. Catastrophic fractures of the tibial post in posterior stabilized and constrained designs have been reported, however. These failures seem to occur predominately in designs that do not provide adequate anterior clearances and allow anterior post impingement in hyperextension. They also may occur as a result of overflexion of the femoral component or inadequate posterior slope of the tibial component. If impingement occurs, fracture or significant polyethylene wear or both may follow.[37,213,292]

Component Wear

Retrieval analysis of removed total joint implants consistently has revealed polyethylene particles in the synovium.[33,106,107,224] In addition, acrylic debris and occasionally metallic particles have been seen. Inspection of the removed components often reveals embedded cement particles in the polyethylene component with scratching, pitting, and burnishing of the articular surface. Distortion of the polyethylene and gross deformation of the component as a result of cold flow (Fig. 99–34) also may occur and is particularly likely when the tibial polyethylene component is thin. Some earlier designs possessed a component that was deliberately made thin to minimize bone removal and often had a cruciate cutout. This combination led, in some instances, to gross distortion and deformation, which contributed to loosening of the component. (The early UCI design was prone to this type of failure.) It is now considered that, unless the component is reinforced with a metal tray, a minimum thickness of 8 mm is desirable.

Metal femoral components may be observed to have scratches in the highly polished articular surface in more than half of the retrieved specimens. It is believed that some of the debris is generated from free cement particles that have become entrapped between the articular surfaces. Careful surgical technique can lessen cement entrapment; however, even in the absence of evidence of cement or body wear, polyethylene failure at the articular surface may be observed. This failure is manifested by pitting, scratching, burnishing, and abrasion of the surface. The amount of surface failure is highly correlated with the level of patient activity, body weight, and length of implantation and seems to be of a greater degree than noted in retrieval analysis of total hip implants.[125]

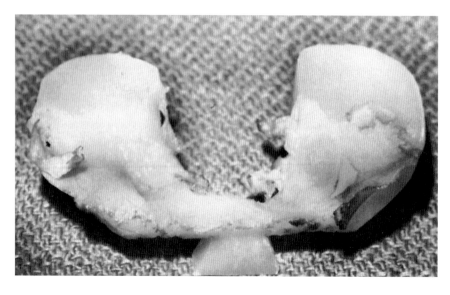

Figure 99–34. Retrieved geometric tibial component showing severe wear.

The type of motion occurring in the articulation is also important. Sliding as opposed to rolling movements causes much greater wear, especially of the delamination type. The kinematic conditions in the joint seem to be of paramount importance.[22] Uncomforming flat surfaces, together with lax ligaments, predispose to various sliding motions.

The durability of a spherically convex polyethylene patellar implant may be questioned in that this shape theoretically causes more wear. Retrieval analysis at the Hospital for Special Surgery of 20 patellar buttons[126] did not indicate that the rate of wear is greater than that of the tibial plateau. There is, however, some deformation of the polyethylene, usually with elongation in the long axis and some flattening of the convex shape where it articulates with the femoral component. Figgie[91] examined all-polyethylene dome patellar components and found a positive correlation between the amount of polyethylene damage and the range of motion achieved postoperatively.

Metal backing of patellar components has not improved the wear performance characteristics, but rather has led to the increase in wear-related complications.[14,15,194,275,304] Up to ten times serum levels of titanium, aluminum, and vanadium can be measured in patients with metal-on-metal contact after metal-backed patellar failure.[307] These extreme levels of debris have been associated with extensive osteolysis and periarticular soft-tissue cysts and masses.[41]

Hsu and Walker[130] more recently studied wear patterns in patellar components. They found that wear occurred regardless of the design shape, although wear was most rapid in dome patellae with metal inlays. A dome patella is only in line contact with the femur until approximately 70 degrees of flexion, after which the patella contacts peripherally with the condylar runners. Contouring the shape of the patella (central convexity and peripheral concavity) greatly improved the wear characteristics, which was better still when the component was metal backed. Even with optimal shape and metal backing, however, wear-through was ultimately predicted because of design constraints on the thickness of the polyethylene (approximately 3 mm). They concluded that currently onset patellar replacements with metal backing should not be used. Inlaying the patellar component allows a thicker layer of plastic, which may be an improvement from the wear point of view, but does not allow polyethylene resurfacing at the margins of the patella, the regions that are subject to the greatest contact pressures when the knee is flexed. There has been a general return to cemented all-polyethylene patellar components, although agreement on this point is not uniform.[53]

Tibial polyethylene wear has emerged as a major clinical problem,[50,78,105,157,168,193] particularly with designs having flat tibial surfaces and thin polyethylene.[43] Isolated cases of wear-through initially were reported for the porous-coated anatomic prosthesis[74] and the variable axis prosthesis. In the described cases, the medial polyethylene wore through to the metal base plate (Fig. 99–35). The original thickness of the components was about 5 mm. These cases were treated by replacing the polyethylene insert with a thicker one. Posterior wear-through to metal has been seen on the Robert Brigham unicondylar design

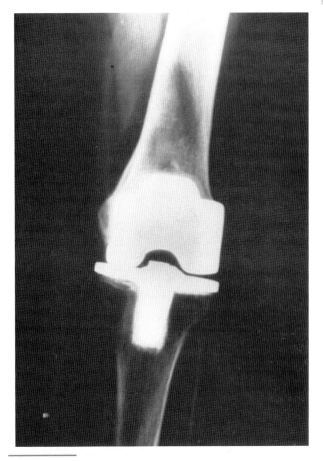

Figure 99–35. Radiograph of a Kinematic prosthesis 5 years postoperatively showing wear-through of the medial tibia.

on 6-mm components[172,173] and on the posterior polyethylene of Kinematic components, in which it was judged that excessive femoral rollback had occurred.

Wear damage to polyethylene is influenced by clinical and design factors.[265] Studies performed on tibial components of a single design showed significant correlation between the amount of polyethylene damage to the articulating surface and patient weight and the length of implantation of the component.[344] Greater wear damage also has been found in patients who achieved better ambulatory status postoperatively.

It seems likely that thinner components also would wear through more commonly, particularly in younger, more active people. The minimum thickness of polyethylene is thought to be about 8 mm at this time. Increasing conformity between the components (Fig. 99–36) improves the wear characteristics, which, on current evidence, is a greater priority than reducing fixation stresses. Even relatively constrained articular shapes have negligible loosening,[290] and it is encouraging that the long-term study of the total condylar prosthesis did not reveal measurable polyethylene wear in any case.[319]

With the increased modularity afforded by metal tibial trays, a new problem has arisen—undersurface or backside wear.[246] This problem is caused by micromotion between the polyethylene insert and the tray (usually made of titanium), causing particulate polyethylene debris to accumulate. In uncemented trays, the debris can filter down the screw holes, initiating osteolysis. Studies documented that, under physiological loading, modular designs have motion between the tray and the polyethylene insert regardless of the locking mechanism.[245] Wasielewski and colleagues[326] examined 67 polyethylene tibial inserts from cementless TKA retrieved at autopsy or revision surgery. The mean implantation time was 62.8 months. Polyethylene cold flow and abrasive wear on the monoarticulating insert surface (undersurface) were assigned a wear severity score (grade 0 to 4). The investigators found that severe grade 4 wear of the tibial insert undersurface was associated with tibial metaphyseal osteolysis or osteolysis around fixation screws. Time in situ was statistically related to grade 4 undersurface wear and tibial metaphyseal osteolysis.

Meniscal-bearing designs, such as the Oxford and LCS (low contact stress), are theoretically the least liable to wear, but the possibility of dislocation of the bearings offsets the advantage to some extent.[16] Although backside wear seems decreased in these designs, it does occur and

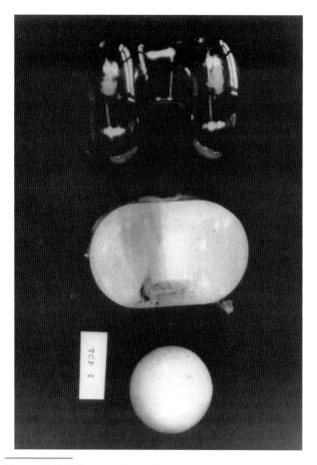

Figure 99–36. Retrieved total condylar prosthesis removed because of infection, after having been implanted for 7 years in an active patient. The appearance of the tibial component shows some burnishing and a few small pits. The patellar component shows slight flattening in one area. There is no other evidence of cold flow, delamination, or cracking of the polyethylene.

has been reported as a cause of bearing dislocation and catastrophic polyethylene failure.[133,135]

Lessons learned from the polished undersurface of the mobile bearing designs may be applied to fixed platform designs. Retrieval analysis of mobile bearing designs has not shown excessive wear of the back insert surface or tibial metaphyseal osteolysis.[31] With studies showing that micromotion occurs between the insert and the tray regardless of locking mechanism, the next step is to polish the trays and analyze wear pattern and debris generation.

Landy and Walker[182] examined 90 retrieved knee prostheses with implant times of up to 10 years. Polyethylene wear was much greater than seen in wear studies of acetabular components in total hip prostheses. Abrasion, burnishing, and deformation were seen in approximately 90 of the components. Cement particles embedded in the surface were found in about half. Delamination, the most severe form of polyethylene degradation, was found in 37 prostheses. Eight flat unicondylar components, which had the longest mean implant times (7.8 years), showed the most severe delamination. Twelve dished unicondylar components (6.3-year implant time) showed less delamination. Six one-piece tibial components, with a mean wear time of 4.3 years, showed much less delamination, almost entirely restricted to the central margin. There was considerable variation in the range of molecular weights between manufacturers and even between different components from the same manufacturer: the wear score for compression-molded components was higher than for other components.

Other factors that also have led to higher wear and failure rates of tibial polyethylene are shelf life (with resultant increased oxidation) of greater than 1.5 years and sterilization via gamma irradiation in air and increased shelf life of the polyethylene surface, leading to a subsurface oxidation line through which subsurface delamination may occur.[51] Landy and Walker[182] concluded that ultra-high-molecular-weight polyethylene is a questionable material for total knee components. Currently a suitable alternative is unavailable, however. The widespread adoption of metal-backed tibial components reduces deformation (Fig. 99–37), but the extra thickness of the metal is obtained either at the expense of greater tibial resection or thinner polyethylene. Apel and colleagues[10] found that thicker (>10 mm) all-polyethylene components behaved similarly to metal-backed components. For this reason and economic ones, we believe there may be some interest in returning to all-polyethylene components or monoblock metal-back tibial augments; however, based on high failure rates of flat-on-flat, all-polyethylene components, all-polyethylene components are extremely design sensitive. They should be used only after long-term clinical data accumulation.[186]

EXTENSOR MECHANISM AND PATELLAR-FEMORAL COMPLICATIONS

Numerous complications involving the extensor mechanism can occur concomitant with TKA.[201]

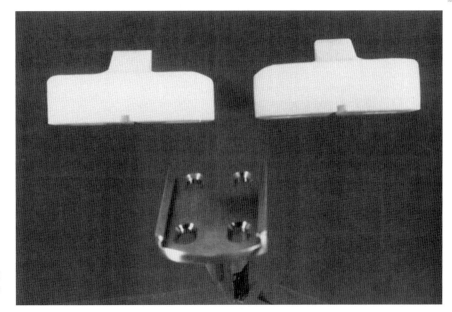

Figure 99–37. Metal tray support of the polyethylene prevents deformation.

Tibial Tubercle Avulsion

Avulsion of the tibial tubercle (Fig. 99–38) is an intraoperative complication that should be avoided rather than treated. Exposure can be difficult in knees that are tight or stiff. With the patella dislocated laterally, considerable traction is exerted on insertion of the patellar ligament. Avulsion of the tubercle during intraoperative maneuvers can happen easily, and if the periosteum tears across, an adequate reconstruction is difficult. Three preventive measures are possible.

First, one can make the vertical capsular incision onto the tibia 1 cm medial to the tibial tubercle so that a cuff of periosteum is reflected in continuity with the ligamentum patellae. If the insertion begins to peel away from the tibial tubercle, the periosteal cuff is taken with the patellar ligament, preserving distal soft-tissue integrity. Second, one can convert the exposure to a quadriceps snip by cutting obliquely at a 45-degree angle across the quadriceps tendon from its apex into the vastus lateralis until the quadriceps tendon and the patella can be turned distally and laterally. The quadriceps snip modification has been described earlier. Third, one can osteotomize the tibial tubercle.[334]

An additional step intraoperatively to avoid tibia tubercle avulsion is to place a towel clip or Steinmann pin into the tibia tubercle. This provides an extra point of fixation/stabilization. If a Steinmann pin or large Kirschner wire is used, it should be smooth rather than threaded to prevent damage to the tendon. During the procedure, it is wise occasionally to assess the amount of tension on the patellar tendon and tubercle. An assistant unwittingly can be placing tension on this area with a retractor.

Avulsion can occur as a result of a manipulation or a fall. It also has been reported as occurring spontaneously during postoperative physical therapy, but probably this is more in the nature of a spontaneous detachment of an insertion already weakened by the operative exposure. A

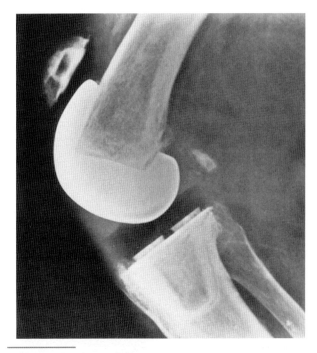

Figure 99–38. The patellar ligament has been avulsed from the tibial tubercle, and the patella is high riding. There is a 40-degree extension lag.

manipulative avulsion is avoidable, provided that the quadriceps muscle is paralyzed by a muscle relaxant before the manipulation is performed.

We know of no satisfactory method of repairing an avulsed tibial tubercle when it is established. Avulsion is most likely when the tibial bone is osteoporotic, and this factor complicates the repair. Open repair by suture, screw, or staple can be done, but often rerupture occurs even after 6 to 8 weeks of immobilization. If the avulsion fracture is nondisplaced, and the component is well fixed, a period of immobilization in extension is the best option. If the component is well fixed, but the fracture is displaced, open reduction and internal fixation with screw fixation should be attempted. If the fracture is displaced or nondisplaced, but the component is loose, a revision of the tibia component plus open reduction and internal fixation of the fracture is the best treatment.

Patellar Ligament or Quadriceps Tendon Rupture

Rupture of the patellar ligament[261] or quadriceps tendon also can occur. The incidence has been reported to range from 0.17% (14 of 8288)[261] to 2.5% (7 of 281).[196] There is an increased incidence in patients who have had a lateral release, secondary to devascularization, previous knee surgery, excision of fat pad, too deep a patellar osteotomy, closed manipulation of the knee, or osteotomy of the tibial tubercle for realignment of the extensor mechanism. The tissues are often of poor quality, making repair difficult. Many treatment options are available, including fixation with wires, staples, screws, or sutures; immobilization; ligament augmentation; and reconstruction with an allograft. None of these techniques have yielded consistently good results. Rand and coworkers[261] cited persistent rupture after treatment in 11 of 18 knees. Cadambi and Engh[34] reported some success in treating this problem. They reported the successful clinical results in seven knees treated with autologous semitendinous tendon graft. This repair was followed by 6 weeks of immobilization in a cast. Only three of seven patients achieved more than 90 degrees of flexion. Emerson and colleagues[73] reported their results using an allograft for a late reconstruction of a rupture of the patellar ligament. In their follow-up, only 3 of 10 allografts failed. With mostly dismal reports on treatment of this problem, prevention is the best treatment.

Patellar Complications

SUBLUXATION AND DISLOCATION

Various technical and design factors may contribute to subluxation and dislocation of the patella (Fig. 99–39).[18,27,109,170,193,219,254]

Depth of the Femoral Trochlea
The design of the femoral sulcus is a compromise. A shallow sulcus predisposes the patella to instability, but an overly deep sulcus offers excessive constraint to the patella, which may lead to patellar component loosening and patellar fracture.

Position of the Femoral Component
Placement of the femoral component in internal rotation increases the lateral soft-tissue tension as the knee is flexed.[263] As discussed elsewhere, some degree of external rotation is preferred (Fig. 99–40). We use the epicondylar axis to set the femoral rotation.

Malrotation of the Tibial Component
Internal rotation of the tibial component gives an external placement of the tibial tubercle, increasing the quadriceps angle and contributing to patellar instability. Malrotation of the tibial component is often the result of inadequate exposure. Sufficient dissection around the tibia to displace the tibial surface anteriorly gives the best visualization of the various landmarks for tibial component placement (Fig. 99–41).

Overall Valgus Alignment
Excessive valgus position increases the quadriceps angle. Reports suggested that often patellar instability occurs in knees that were originally valgus.

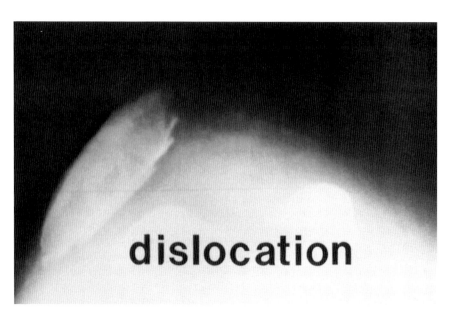

Figure 99–39. Gross rotary malposition of the tibial component leads to patellar dislocation.

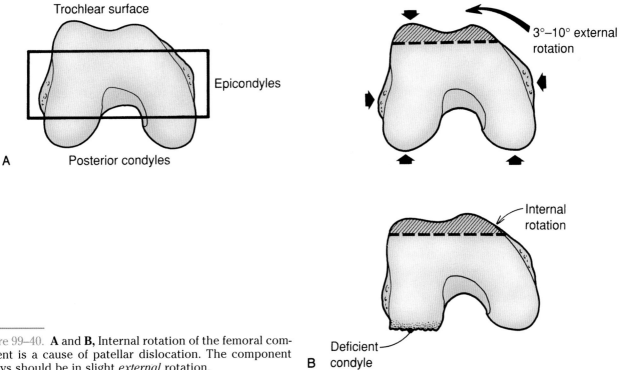

Figure 99–40. **A** and **B,** Internal rotation of the femoral component is a cause of patellar dislocation. The component always should be in slight *external* rotation.

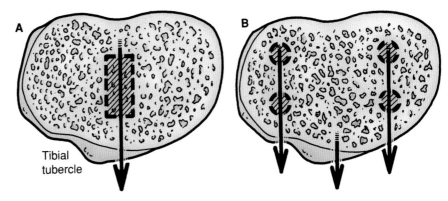

Figure 99–41. **A** and **B,** Alignment of the tibial component is projected at a point slightly medial to the tibial tubercle. Alignment of a symmetric component with the posterior margin of the tibial plateau usually results in some internal rotation of the tibial component. One should err on the side of external rotation.

Tight Lateral Retinaculum

A tight lateral retinaculum can contribute to patellar dislocation.

Patellar tracking problems after TKA have been reported to occur with an incidence of 29%.[150] Subluxation is more common than dislocation.[29] Patients usually complain of anterior knee pain or gross subluxation or dislocation. The treatment of this complication depends on its cause. A patient with mild subluxation and a weak vastus medialis would benefit from intense physical therapy. The components could be malpositioned or malaligned, which could be determined preoperatively with a CT scan (see Fig. 99–14). If this is the cause, a revision would be appropriate. In most of the cases, the treatment is a lateral retinaculum release, sometimes in conjunction with a proximal realignment. We do not recommend a tibial tubercle transposition because of its high complication rate.

Results of surgical treatment for patella instability are good for combined lateral release and proximal realignment procedures. Grace and Rand[109] studied 25 knees with symptomatic lateral patellar instability after TKA. The knees were treated by one of three methods: proximal realignment, combined proximal and distal realignment, or component revision. At 50-month follow-up, 20 knees had normal patellar tracking, and 5 had recurrent instability. Two of nine patients who had a combined realignment had patellar tendon rupture. The authors recommended proximal realignment alone in the absence of component malposition. If the component is malpositioned, component revision should be performed.

Merkow and colleagues[219] reported the experience at the Hospital for Special Surgery. Between 1974 and 1982, 12 dislocations occurred in 11 patients. Trauma was the cause of dislocation in three knees, incorrect tracking of the patella in six, and malrotation of the tibial component in three. Many of the knees were in valgus preoperatively. Dislocations occurred in four different prosthetic designs, suggesting that, in this series, design was not a factor. Unrestrained tibial rotation has been described as predisposing to patellar dislocation by others. Whiteside and associates[332] maintained that the degree of tibial rotation is determined by the ligaments, provided that the ligaments are correctly tensioned during surgery. They believed that rotational constraint in the prosthesis is unnecessary and may predispose to loosening. We believe, however, that knees with initial external rotation deformities of the tibia are managed more easily by a design with rotational constraint, and this feature is useful in managing a patellar dislocation that already has occurred. Altering the rotational position of the tibial component in a design with some constraint is the equivalent to transferring the tibial tubercle.

In Merkow's series,[219] the patellar dislocation was managed by proximal realignment in 10 cases, lateral release in 1 case, and proximal realignment and revision of the tibial component into a more desirable externally rotated position in 1 case. None of the dislocations recurred, and in none was transposition of the tibial tubercle required. We agree with Rand and Bryan[257] that tibial tubercle transposition is inadvisable after TKA because the bone quality is often poor, and the proportion of complications is high. Wolff and coworkers[341] and Whiteside and Ohl[334] claimed that tibial tubercle transposition is effective with good technique. They recommended taking a relatively large fragment of the tibial tubercle so that secure fixation with screws is attainable.

SOFT-TISSUE IMPINGEMENT

In 1982, we described a case in which a fibrous nodule was excised from the suprapatellar region of the quadriceps tendon. This nodule gave rise to what has become known as the *patellar clunk syndrome* (Fig. 99–42).[16,128,312,318] It is associated most commonly with use of a posterior stabilized prosthesis.

The clinical manifestation is postoperative grating and catching on active extension of the knee, signs that usually appear 6 to 12 months after TKA. The radiographs appear entirely normal, and no evidence of patellar subluxation is found. The cause is soft-tissue impingement between the peripatellar synovium and the femoral component. Most often this impingement involves a portion of the suprapatellar synovium, which becomes irritated, inflamed, and swollen. Occasionally a sizable mass can result, which catches within the anterior lip of the intercondylar recess of the femoral component. Because specific implant designs with a short femoral flange have been implicated, it is preferable to select an implant with a long deep femoral sulcus and a smooth transition into the intercondylar recess. These designs have reduced greatly the incidence of patellar crepitus and virtually eliminated the patellar clunk syndrome.

Soft-tissue impingement and patellar clunk syndrome can be cured by the removal of the excess tissue and the "patellar meniscus" that forms around the patellar prosthetic margins. Initially, this removal was done by arthrotomy, but more recently it has been done by arthroscopy.[318] The advantages of using arthroscopy over open arthro-

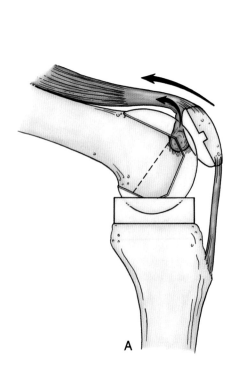

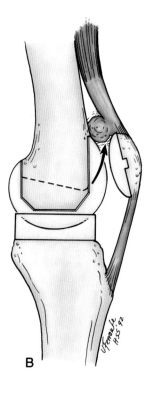

Figure 99–42. **A** and **B,** The patellar clunk syndrome. The cause of this peculiar symptom is a suprapatellar mass of synovium and fibrous tissue that forms a nodule, which is caught between the patella and the femoral component. This nodule typically forms at between 60 and 45 degrees of flexion and can result in locking of the knee in this position. As the knee is brought into terminal extension, the patella can be seen to pop, and the nodule releases from its entrapped position. The symptom can be cured by arthroscopic removal of the fibrous nodule.

A

B

tomy are simplicity, decreased recurrence, decreased risk of infection, and quicker postoperative rehabilitation. Indications for open arthrotomy and excision of nodule are failure of arthroscopic débridement; malpositioned patella component, which can be a cause requiring revision of the component along with excision of nodule; and patella clunk with a loose prosthetic component. With a sharp decline in the incidence of patella clunk secondary to prosthetic design modifications, there are only a few reports of treatment outcomes. Diduch and associates[68] had a success rate of 82% (14 of 17 knees) with a follow-up of 19.9 months after arthroscopic treatment of patella clunk.

UNEXPLAINED PAIN

A certain proportion of patients continue to complain of pain for which there is no apparent explanation. Sometimes the arthroplasty is objectively functioning well and has a good range of motion. The pain may be present continuously or mainly at rest. One of our patients was able to walk considerable distances and climb stairs normally without difficulty. He complained of severe pain when sitting, and because his occupation involved frequent flying, this was a considerable problem for him. Complaints of pain may be associated with lack of motion or flexion contracture, although the components appeared to be well seated and well positioned. We estimate the incidence of these cases to be approximately 1 in 300 arthroplasties. The cause is usually difficult to show. There is an overlap with reflex sympathetic dystrophy,[164] particularly in patients who have restricted motion. It may seem, in retrospect, that the preoperative symptoms were worse than the pathological condition of the knee. Some kind of material allergy has been suspected but never proved, although in one of our patients with a loose metal-on-metal hinge prosthesis we were able to show a skin allergy to cobalt chloride. Low-grade infection is always a possibility.

In the management of these patients, infection must be excluded as much as possible. Aspiration should be attempted, and if sufficient fluid is obtained, cultures can be quite reliable; 90% of our infected knees have been diagnosed by culture of the aspirate. Bone scintigraphy[122,162,251] also may be useful, although technetium-99m scanning after TKA gives highly variable results,[285] in that asymptomatic knees may continue to have abnormal scans indefinitely. Indium scanning[256] was found to be 85% reliable in 18 infected knees. In a group of 20 knees with aseptic loosening, however, the scan results were not given.

When reflex sympathetic dystrophy is suspected, sympathetic block should be tried. If the response is good, a lumbar sympathectomy should be considered. Nicholls and Dorr[241] reported success in surgical revision of stiff and painful knees with improvement of motion and pain. This has not been our experience, and in most cases the results have been disappointing.

A 1996 study[226] examined the role of exploratory surgery in unexplained pain in TKA. Twenty-seven patients underwent exploration of their TKA secondary to severe debilitating pain of an unknown origin. They were divided into two groups: patients with range of motion less than 80 degrees and patients with range of motion greater than 80 degrees. At final follow-up, there were 11 excellent and good results (41%) and 16 fair or poor results (59%). Of the 15 patients with decreased range of motion, 9 (60%) had good or excellent results. The range of motion arc improved from a preoperative 43-degree average to an 81-degree average. For the pain-only group, there were only two excellent or good results (17%). If a problem was identified at surgery, only 3 of 12 knees (25%) had successful outcomes. This study highlights the frustration of performing surgery on patients for unexplained pain. Even when the authors identified a problem at the time of surgery and corrected it, they only had a 25% success rate.

If the workup of a painful TKA is negative, one must consider obtaining fluoroscopically assisted radiographs. In this way, near-perfect perpendicular radiographs can be obtained to evaluate any radiolucencies, especially under the tibial tray. In one study[86] that examined painful TKA without explanation, the authors used fluoroscopic evaluation to study the knees. The authors had 20 patients referred to them for pain and disability after TKA with normal-appearing radiographs. All 20 patients had fluoroscopic radiographs obtained. In 14 of the 20 patients, the diagnosis of aseptic loosening was made with the new radiographs. Each of the patients thought to have a loose component at fluoroscopy did have a loose component at revision. Each patient improved after revision with an increase in the Hospital for Special Surgery score of 26 points.

Great caution is recommended when deciding to revise a knee without good explanation of the pain, and in most cases the condition of the patient either is unimproved or is worse after revision, unless a convincing intraoperative cause is found. Sometimes overgrown soft tissues or an interposed meniscal fragment is found. Because these conditions can be managed without arthrotomy, an arthroscopic examination is recommended before revision is attempted.

INFECTION

Infection is one of the most serious complications.[3,11,17,23,24,39,47,58,62,84,98,103,112,115] Infection usually is classified as acute (<3 months) or chronic (>3 months). The treatment of acute infections is debatable. If the organism is of low virulence, one may attempt an open irrigation and débridement with exchange of polyethylene. This procedure is followed by 6 weeks of intravenous antibiotics and close observation.[17,233,287,308] The most appropriate treatment for a chronic infection is removal of components, débridement, and placement of a cement spacer followed by 6 weeks of intravenous antibiotics. At 6 weeks, the new components may be reimplanted if intraoperative Gram stain and frozen sections are negative.[17,23,47,233,308,336,337,339] The importance of the prevention and management of infection warrants a full-chapter discussion. The treatment options for infection are as follows:

1. Antibiotic suppression
2. Débridement with prosthesis in situ
3. Removal of prosthesis
   a. One-stage reimplantation
   b. Two-stage reimplantation
   c. Pseudarthrosis
   d. "Beef-burger" operation[158]
   e. Arthrodesis[82,88,114,151,154,171,192,209,315,323]

References

1. Aaron RK, Scott R: Supracondylar fracture of the femur after total knee arthroplasty. Clin Orthop 219:136, 1987.
2. Aglietti P, Windsor RE, Buzzi R, et al: Arthroplasty for the stiff or ankylosed knee. J Arthroplasty 4:1, 1989.
3. Ainscow DAP, Denham RA: The risk of haematogenous infection in total joint replacements. J Bone Joint Surg Br 66:589, 1984.
4. Akisue T, Yamaguchi M, Bauer TW, et al: Backside polyethylene deformation in total knee arthroplasty. J Arthroplasty 18:784, 2003.
5. Albrektsson BEJ, Herberts P: ICLH knee arthroplasty: A consecutive study of 108 knees with uncemented tibial component fixation. J Arthroplasty 3:145, 1988.
6. Albrektsson BEJ, Ryd L, Carlsson LV, et al: The effect of a stem on the tibial component of knee arthroplasty: A roentgen stereophotogrammetric study of uncemented tibial components in the Freeman-Samuelson knee arthroplasty. J Bone Joint Surg Br 72:252, 1990.
7. Allenby F, Boardman L, Pflug JJ, et al: Effects of interval pneumatic intermittent compression on fibrinolysis in man. Lancet 2:1412, 1973.
8. Anderson DR, Gross M, Robinson KS, et al: Ultrasonographic screening for deep vein thrombosis following arthroplasty fails to reduce posthospital thromboembolic complications—the postarthroplasty screening study. Chest J 114:119S, 1998.
9. Ansari S, Warwick D, Ackroyd CE, et al: Incidence of fatal pulmonary embolism after 1,390 knee arthroplasties without routine prophylactic anticoagulation, except in high-risk cases. J Arthroplasty 12:599, 1997.
10. Apel DM, Tozzi JM, Dorr LD: Clinical comparison of all-polyethylene and metal-backed tibial components in total knee arthroplasty. Clin Orthop 273:243, 1991.
11. Artz TD, Macys J, Salvati EA, et al: Hematogenous infection of total hip replacements: A report of four cases. J Bone Joint Surg Am 57:1024, 1975.
12. Asp JPL, Rand JA: Peroneal nerve palsy after total knee arthroplasty. Clin Orthop 261:233, 1990.
13. Ayers DC, Dennis DA, Johanson NA, et al: Common complications of total knee arthroplasty. J Bone Joint Surg Am 79:278, 1997.
14. Bayley JC, Scott RD: Further observations on metal-backed patellar component failure. Clin Orthop 236:82, 1988.
15. Bayley JC, Scott RD, Ewald FC, et al: Failure of the metal-backed patellar component after total knee replacement. J Bone Joint Surg Am 70:668, 1988.
16. Beight JL, Yao B, Hozack WJ, et al: The patellar clunk syndrome after posterior stabilized total knee arthroplasty. Clin Orthop 299:139, 1994.
17. Bengtson S, Knutson K, Lindgren L: Treatment of infected knee arthroplasty. Clin Orthop 245:173, 1989.
18. Berger RA, Crossett LS, Jacobs JJ, et al: Malrotation causing patellofemoral complications after total knee arthroplasty. Clin Orthop 356:144, 1998.
19. Bert JM: Dislocation/subluxation of meniscal bearing elements after New Jersey low-contact stress total knee arthroplasty. Clin Orthop 254:211, 1990.
20. Berzins A, Jacobs JJ, Berger R, et al: Surface damage in machined ram-extruded and net-shape molded retrieved polyethylene tibial inserts of total knee replacements. J Bone Joint Surg Am 84:1534, 2002.
21. Bisla RS, Inglis AE, Lewis RJ: Fat embolism following bilateral total knee replacement with the Guepar prosthesis: A case report. Clin Orthop 115:195, 1976.
22. Blunn GW, Walker PS, Joshi A, et al: The dominance of cyclic sliding in producing wear in total knee replacements. Clin Orthop 273:253, 1991.
23. Booth RE Jr, Lotke PA: The results of spacer block technique in revision of infected total knee arthroplasty. Clin Orthop 248:57, 1989.
24. Borden LS, Gearen PF: Infected total knee arthroplasty: A protocol for management. J Arthroplasty 2:27, 1987.
25. Bradley GW, Freeman MAR, Albrektsson BEJ: Total prosthetic replacement of ankylosed knees. J Arthroplasty 2:179, 1987.
26. Branson PJ, Steege JW, Wixson RL, et al: Rigidity of initial fixation with uncemented tibial knee implants. J Arthroplasty 4:21, 1989.
27. Briard J-L, Hungerford DS: Patellofemoral instability in total knee arthroplasty. J Arthroplasty 4:587, 1989.
28. Brick GW, Scott RD: Blood supply to the patella: Significance in total knee arthroplasty. J Arthroplasty 4:575, 1989.
29. Brick GW, Scott RD: The patellofemoral component of total knee arthroplasty. Clin Orthop 231:163, 1988.
30. Brotherton SL, Roberson JR, De Andrade JR, et al: Staged versus simultaneous bilateral total knee replacement. J Arthroplasty 1:221, 1986.
31. Buechel FF: Cementless meniscal bearing knee arthroplasty: 7-12 year outcome analysis. Orthopedics 17:833, 1994.
32. Buechel FF: A sequential three-step lateral release for correcting fixed valgus knee deformities during total knee arthroplasty. Clin Orthop 260:170, 1990.
33. Bullough PG, Insall JN, Ranawat CS, et al: Wear and tissue reaction in failed knee arthroplasty. J Bone Joint Surg Br 58:366, 1976.
34. Cadambi A, Engh GA: Use of a semitendinosus tendon autogenous graft for rupture of the patellar ligament after total knee arthroplasty: A report of seven cases. J Bone Joint Surg Am 74:974, 1992.
35. Caillouette JT, Anzel SH: Fat embolism syndrome following the intramedullary alignment guide in total knee arthroplasty. Clin Orthop 251:198, 1990.
36. Cain PR, Rubash HE, Wissinger HA, et al: Periprosthetic femoral fractures following total knee arthroplasty. Clin Orthop 208:205, 1986.
37. Callaghan JJ, O'Rourke MR, Goetz DD, et al: Tibial post impingement in posterior-stabilized total knee arthroplasty. Clin Orthop 404:83, 2002.
38. Cameron HU, Welsh RP: Fracture of the femoral component in unicompartmental total knee arthroplasty. J Arthroplasty 5:315, 1990.
39. Carlsson AS, Josefsson G, Lindberg L: Revision with gentamicin-impregnated cement for deep infections in total hip arthroplasties. J Bone Joint Surg Am 60:1059, 1978.
40. Chandler HP, Tigges RG: The role of allografts in the treatment of periprosthetic femoral fractures. J Bone Joint Surg Am 79:1422, 1997.
41. Chang FY, Tseng KF, Chen WM, et al: Metal-backed patellar component failure in total knee arthroplasty presenting as a giant calf mass. J Arthroplasty 18:227, 2003.
42. Chen F, Mont MA, Bachner RS: Management of ipsilateral supracondylar femur fractures following total knee arthroplasty. J Arthroplasty 9:521, 1994.
43. Chillag KJ, Barth E: An analysis of polyethylene thickness in modular total knee components. Clin Orthop 273:261, 1991.
44. Chmell MJ, Moran MC, Scott RD: Periarticular fractures after total knee arthroplasty: Principles of management. J Am Acad Orthop Surg 4:109, 1996.
45. Christensen CP, Crawford JJ, Olin MD, et al: Revision of the stiff total knee arthroplasty. J Arthroplasty 17:409, 2002.
46. Clarke MT, Longstaff L, Edwards D, et al: Tourniquet-induced wound hypoxia after total knee replacement. J Bone Joint Surg Br 83:40, 2001.
47. Cohen JC, Hozack WJ, Cuckler JM, et al: Two-stage reimplantation of septic total knee arthroplasty. J Arthroplasty 3:369, 1988.
48. Cohen SH, Ehrlich GE, Kauffman MS, et al: Thrombophlebitis following knee surgery. J Bone Joint Surg Am 55:106, 1973.
49. Colizza WA, Insall JN, Scuderi GR: The posterior stabilized total knee prosthesis: Assessment of polyethylene damage and osteoly-

sis after a ten-year minimum follow-up. J Bone Joint Surg Am 77:1713, 1995.

50. Collier JP, Mayor MB, McNamara JL, et al: Analysis of the failure of 122 polyethylene inserts from uncemented tibial knee components. Clin Orthop 273:232, 1991.

51. Collier MB, Engh CA Jr, Engh GA: Shelf age of the polyethylene tibial component and outcome of unicondylar knee arthroplasty. J Bone Joint Surg Am 86:763, 2004.

52. Colwell CW, Spiro TE, Trowbridge AA, et al, for the Enoxaparin Clinical Trial Group: Efficacy and safety of enoxaparin versus unfractionated heparin for prevention of deep venous thrombosis after elective knee arthroplasty. Clin Orthop 321:19, 1995.

53. Convery FR, Minteer-Convery M, Malcom LL: The spherocentric knee: A re-evaluation and modification. J Bone Joint Surg Am 62:320, 1980.

54. Cook SD, Barrack RL, Thomas KA, et al: Quantitative histologic analysis of tissue growth into porous total knee components. J Arthroplasty 4:533, 1989.

55. Cook SD, Thomas KA, Haddad RJ Jr: Histologic analysis of retrieved human porous-coated total joint components. Clin Orthop 234:90, 1988.

56. Cordeiro EN, Costa RC, Carazzato JG, et al: Periprosthetic fractures in patients with total knee arthroplasties. Clin Orthop 252:182, 1990.

57. Cornell CN, Ranawat CS, Burstein AH: A clinical and radiographic analysis of loosening of total knee arthroplasty components using a bilateral model. J Arthroplasty 1:157, 1986.

58. Cruess RL, Bickel WS, Von Kessler KLC: Infections in total hips secondary to a primary source elsewhere. Clin Orthop 106:99, 1975.

59. Culp RW, Schmidt RG, Hanks G, et al: Supracondylar fracture of the femur following prosthetic knee arthroplasty. Clin Orthop 22:212, 1987.

60. Curley P, Eyres K, Brezinova V, et al: Common peroneal nerve dysfunction after high tibial osteotomy. J Bone Joint Surg Br 72:405, 1990.

61. Cushner FD, Scott WN: Problems after knee arthroplasty—wound complications following total knee arthroplasty. Orthop Blue J 24:905, 2001.

62. D'Ambrosia RD, Shoji H, Heater R: Secondarily infected total joint replacements by hematogenous spread. J Bone Joint Surg Am 58:450, 1976.

63. Deburge A: Guepar hinge prosthesis: Complications and results with two years follow-up. Clin Orthop 120:47, 1976.

64. Della Valle CJ, Steiger DJ, DiCesare PE: Duplex ultrasonography in patients suspected of postoperative pulmonary embolism following total joint arthroplasty. Am J Orthop 386, 2003.

65. Dempsey AJ, Finlay JB, Bourne RB, et al: Stability and anchorage considerations for cementless tibial components. J Arthroplasty 4:223, 1989.

66. Dennis DA, Neumann RD, Toma P, et al: Arteriovenous fistula with false aneurysm of the inferior medial geniculate artery: A complication of total knee arthroplasty. Clin Orthop 222: 255, 1987.

67. Denny-Brown D, Doherty MM: Effects of transient stretching of peripheral nerve. Arch Neurol Psychiatry 54:116, 1945.

68. Diduch DR, Scuderi GR, Scott WN, et al: The efficacy of arthroscopy following total knee replacement. Arthroscopy 13:166, 1997.

69. Doouss TW: The clinical significance of venous thrombosis of the calf. Br J Surg 63:377, 1976.

70. Dorr LD, Boiardo RA: Technical considerations in total knee arthroplasty. Clin Orthop 205:5, 1986.

71. Dorr LD, Merkel C, Mellman MF, et al: Fat emboli in bilateral total knee arthroplasty: Predictive factors for neurologic manifestations. Clin Orthop 248:112, 1989.

72. Dorr LD, Serocki JH: Mechanism of failure of total knee arthroplasty. In Scott WN (ed): The Knee. St. Louis, CV Mosby, 1994, p 1239.

73. Emerson RH Jr, Head WC, Malinin TI: Reconstruction of patellar tendon rupture after total knee arthroplasty with an extensor mechanism allograft. Clin Orthop 260:154, 1990.

74. Engh GA: Failure of the polyethylene bearing surface of a total knee replacement within four years: A case report. J Bone Joint Surg Am 70:1093, 1988.

75. Engh GA, Ammeen DJ: Epidemiology of osteolysis: backside implant wear. AAOS Inst Course Lect 53:243, 2004.

76. Engh GA, Ammeen DJ: Periprosthetic fractures adjacent to total knee implants. J Bone Joint Surg Am 79:1100, 1997.

77. Engh GA, Dwyer KA, Hanes CK: Polyethylene wear of metal-backed tibial components in total and unicompartmental knee prostheses. J Bone Joint Surg Br 74:9, 1992.

78. Engh GA, Parks NL, Ammeen DJ: Tibial osteolysis in cementless total knee arthroplasty. Clin Orthop 309:33, 1994.

79. Evarts CM: Thromboembolism. In Rockwood CA Jr, Green DP (eds): Fractures. Volume 1: Complications. Philadelphia, JB Lippincott, 1975, p 174.

80. Evarts CM: Prevention of venous thromboembolism. Clin Orthop 222:98, 1987.

81. Ezzet KA, Garcia R, Barrack RL: Effect of component fixation method on osteolysis in total knee arthroplasty. Clin Orthop 321: 86, 1995.

82. Fahmy NRM, Barnes KL, Noble J: A technique for difficult arthrodesis of the knee. J Bone Joint Surg Br 66:367, 1984.

83. Fahmy NRM, Chandler HP, Danylchuk K, et al: Blood-gas and circulatory changes during total knee replacement: Role of the intramedullary alignment rod. J Bone Joint Surg Am 72:19, 1990.

84. Falahee MH, Matthews LS, Kaufer H: Resection arthroplasty as a salvage procedure for a knee with infection after a total arthroplasty. J Bone Joint Surg Am 69:1013, 1987.

85. Faris PM, Ritter MA, Keating EM, et al: The AGC all-polyethylene tibial component: A ten-year clinical evaluation. J Bone Joint Surg Am 85:489, 2003.

86. Fehring TK, McAvoy G: Fluoroscopic evaluation of the painful total knee arthroplasty. Clin Orthop 331:226, 1996.

87. Felix NA, Stuart MJ, Hanssen AD: Periprosthetic fractures of the tibia associated with total knee arthroplasty. Clin Orthop 345:113, 1997.

88. Figgie HE III, Brody GA, Inglis AE, et al: Knee arthrodesis following total knee arthroplasty in rheumatoid arthritis. Clin Orthop 224:237, 1987.

89. Figgie HE III, Goldberg VM, Figgie MP, et al: The effect of alignment of the implant on fractures of the patella after condylar total knee arthroplasty. J Bone Joint Surg Am 71:1031, 1989.

90. Figgie MP, Goldberg VM, Figgie HE III, et al: The results of treatment of supracondylar fracture above total knee arthroplasty. J Arthroplasty 5:267, 1990.

91. Figgie MP: Performance of dome shaped patellar components in total knee arthroplasty. Trans Orthop Res Soc 14:531, 1989.

92. Fipp G: Stress fractures of the femoral neck following total knee arthroplasty. J Arthroplasty 3:347, 1988.

93. Firestone TP, Teeny SM, Krackow KA, et al: The clinical and roentgenographic results of cementless porous coated patellar fixation. Clin Orthop 273:184, 1991.

94. Fitzgerald RH, Spiro TE, Trowbridge AA, et al: A randomized and prospective comparison of enoxaparin and warfarin in the prevention of thromboembolic disease following total knee arthroplasty. Orthop Trans 19:335, 1995.

95. Fox JL, Poss R: The role of manipulation following total knee replacement. J Bone Joint Surg Am 63:357, 1981.

96. Francis CW, Pellegrini VD Jr, Stulberg BN, et al: Prevention of venous thrombosis after total knee arthroplasty: Comparison of antithrombin III and low-dose heparin with dextran. J Bone Joint Surg Am 72:976, 1990.

97. Francis CW, Ricotta JJ, Evarts CM, et al: Long-term clinical observations and venous functional abnormalities after asymptomatic venous thrombosis following total hip or knee arthroplasty. Clin Orthop 232:271, 1988.

98. Freeman MAR, Sudlow RA, Casewell MW, et al: The management of infected total knee replacements. J Bone Joint Surg Br 67:764, 1985.

99. Galinat BJ, Vernace JV, Booth RE Jr, et al: Dislocation of the posterior stabilized total knee arthroplasty: A report of two cases. J Arthroplasty 3:363, 1988.

100. Gardner AM, Fox RH: The venous footpump: Influence on tissue perfusion and prevention of venous thrombosis. Ann Rheum Dis 51:1173, 1992.

101. Garner RW, Mowat AC, Hazleman BL: Wound healing after operations on patients with rheumatoid arthritis. J Bone Joint Surg Br 55:134, 1973.

102. Gebhard JS, Kilgus DJ: Dislocation of a posterior stabilized total knee prosthesis: A report of two cases. Clin Orthop 254:225, 1990.

103. Glynn MK, Sheehan JM: The significance of asymptomatic bacteriuria in patients undergoing hip/knee arthroplasty. Clin Orthop 185:151, 1984.

104. Goldberg VM, Figgie HE III, Inglis AE, et al: Patellar fracture type and prognosis in condylar total knee arthroplasty. Clin Orthop 236:115, 1988.

105. Goodfellow J: Knee prostheses: One step forward, two steps back (Editorial). J Bone Joint Surg Br 74:1, 1992.

106. Goodman SB, Fornasier VL, Kei J: The effects of bulk versus particulate polymethylmethacrylate on bone. Clin Orthop 232:255, 1988.

107. Goodman SB, Fornasier VL, Kei J: The effects of bulk versus particulate ultra-high-molecular-weight polyethylene on bone. J Arthroplasty 4:541, 1988.

108. Goodnough LT, Shafron D, Marcus RE: Utilization and effectiveness of autologous blood donation for arthroplastic surgery. J Arthroplasty 5(Suppl):S89, 1990.

109. Grace JN, Rand JA: Patellar instability after total knee arthroplasty. Clin Orthop 237:184, 1988.

110. Grace JN, Sim FH: Fracture of the patella after total knee arthroplasty. Clin Orthop 230:168, 1988.

111. Gradisar IA Jr, Hoffmann ML, Askew MJ: Fracture of a fenestrated metal backing of a tibial knee component: A case report. J Arthroplasty 4:27, 1989.

112. Grogan TJ, Dorey F, Rollins J, et al: Deep sepsis following total knee arthroplasty: Ten-year experience at the University of California at Los Angeles Medical Center. J Bone Joint Surg Am 68:226, 1986.

113. Haas SB, Insall JN, Scuderi GR, et al: Pneumatic sequential-compression boots compared with aspirin prophylaxis of deep-vein thrombosis after total knee arthroplasty. J Bone Joint Surg Am 72:27, 1990.

114. Hagemann WF, Woods GW, Tullos HS: Arthrodesis in failed total knee replacement. J Bone Joint Surg Am 60:790, 1978.

115. Hall AJ: Late infection about a total knee prosthesis. J Bone Joint Surg Br 56:144, 1974.

116. Healy WL, Siliski JM, Incavo SJ: Operative treatment of distal femoral fractures proximal to total knee replacements. J Bone Joint Surg Am 75:27, 1993.

117. Hemphill ES, Ebert FR, Muench: The medial gastrocnemius muscle flap in the treatment of wound complications following total knee arthroplasty. Orthopedics 15:477, 1992.

118. Highet WB, Holmes W: Traction injuries to the lateral popliteal nerve and traction injuries to peripheral nerves after suture. Br J Surg 30:212, 1943.

119. Highet WB, Sanders FK: The effects of stretching nerves after suture. Br J Surg 30:355, 1943.

120. Hirsh DM, Bhalla S, Roffman M: Supracondylar fracture of the femur following total knee replacement: Report of four cases. J Bone Joint Surg Am 63:162, 1981.

121. Hodge WA: Prevention of deep vein thrombosis after total knee arthroplasty. Clin Orthop 271:101, 1991.

122. Hofmann AA, Wyatt RWB, Daniels AU, et al: Bone scans after total knee arthroplasty in asymptomatic patients: Cemented versus cementless. Clin Orthop 251:183, 1990.

123. Holden DL, Jackson DW: Considerations in total knee arthroplasty following previous knee fusion. Clin Orthop 227:223, 1988.

124. Hood RW, Flawn LB, Insall JN: The use of pulsatile compression stockings in total knee replacement for prevention of venous thrombosis: A prospective study. Trans Orthop Res Soc 7:297, 1982.

125. Hood RW, Wright TM, Burstein AH, et al: Retrieval analysis of 70 total condylar knee prostheses. Orthop Trans 5:319, 1981.

126. Hood RW, Wright TM, Burstein AH, et al: Retrieval analysis of twenty polyethylene patellar buttons. Orthop Trans 5:291, 1981.

127. Hozack WJ, Goll SR, Lotke PA, et al: The treatment of patellar fractures after total knee arthroplasty. Clin Orthop 236:123, 1988.

128. Hozack WJ, Rothman RH, Booth RE Jr, et al: The patellar clunk syndrome: A complication of posterior stabilized total knee arthroplasty. Clin Orthop 241:203, 1989.

129. Hsu H-P, Garg A, Walker PS, et al: Effect of knee component alignment on tibial load distribution with clinical correlation. Clin Orthop 248:135, 1989.

130. Hsu H-P, Walker PS: Wear and deformation of patellar components in total knee arthroplasty. Clin Orthop 246:260, 1989.

131. Hsu RWW, Himeno S, Coventry MB, et al: Normal axial alignment of the lower extremity and load-bearing distribution at the knee. Clin Orthop 255:215, 1990.

132. Huang CH, Ho FY, Ma HM, et al: Particle size and morphology of UHMWPE wear debris in failed total knee arthroplasties—a comparison between mobile bearing and fixed bearing knees. J Orthop Res 20:1038, 2002.

133. Huang CH, Liau JJ, Lung CY, et al: The incidence of revision of the metal component of total knee arthroplasties in different tibial-insert designs. Knee 9:331, 2002.

134. Huang CH, Ma HM, Lee YM, et al: Long-term results of low contact stress mobile-bearing total knee replacements. Clin Orthop 416: 265, 2003.

135. Huang CH, Ma HM, Liau JJ, et al: Late dislocation of rotating plat-form in New Jersey low-contact stress knee prosthesis. Clin Orthop 405:189, 2002.

136. Huang CH, Ma HM, Liau JJ, et al: Osteolysis in failed total knee arthroplasty: A comparison of mobile-bearing and foxed-bearing knees. J Bone Joint Surg Am 12:2224, 2002.

137. Hull RD, Raskob GE: Prophylaxis of venous thromboembolic disease following hip and knee surgery. J Bone Joint Surg Am 68:146, 1986.

138. Hunter GA, Dandy D: Diagnosis and natural history of the infected total hip replacement. In The Hip Society: The Hip. Proceedings of the Fifth Open Scientific Meeting of The Hip Society. St. Louis, CV Mosby, 1977.

139. Hvid I: Mechanical strength of trabecular bone. Thesis, University of Aarhus, Denmark, 1988.

140. Hvid I: Trabecular bone strength at the knee. Clin Orthop 227:210, 1988.

141. Hvid I, Nielsen S: Total condylar knee arthroplasty: Prosthetic component positioning and radiolucent lines. Acta Orthop Scand 55:160, 1984.

142. Idusuyi OB, Morrey BF: Peroneal nerve palsy after total knee arthroplasty. J Bone Joint Surg Am 78:177, 1996.

143. Infection in rheumatoid disease (Editorial). BMJ 2:549, 1972.

144. Insall JN: Infection in total knee arthroplasty. Instr Course Lect 31:42, 1982.

145. Insall JN, Lachiewicz PF, Burstein AH: The posterior stabilized condylar prosthesis: A modification of the total condylar design: Two to four year clinical experience. J Bone Joint Surg Am 64:1317, 1982.

146. Insall JN, Thompson FM, Brause DB, et al: Two-stage reimplantation for the salvage of infected total knee arthroplasty. Orthop Trans 6:369, 1982.

147. Jabczenski FF, Crawford M: Retrograde intramedullary nailing of supracondylar femur fracture above total knee arthroplasty: A preliminary report of four cases. J Arthroplasty 10:95, 1995.

148. Jennings JJ, Harris WH, Sarmiento A: A clinical evaluation of aspirin prophylaxis of thromboembolic disease after total hip arthroplasty. J Bone Joint Surg Am 58:926, 1976.

149. Jerry GJ Jr, Rand JA, Ilstrup D: Old sepsis prior to total knee arthroplasty. Clin Orthop 236:135, 1988.

150. Johanson NA: Extensor mechanism failure: Treatment of patella fracture, dislocation, and ligament rupture. In Lotke PA (ed): Master Techniques in Orthopedic Surgery, Knee Arthroplasty. New York, Raven Press, 1995, p 219.

151. Johnson DP: Antibiotic prophylaxis with cefuroxime in arthroplasty of the knee. J Bone Joint Surg Br 69:787, 1987.

152. Johnson DP: The effect of continuous passive motion on wound-healing and joint mobility after knee arthroplasty. J Bone Joint Surg Am 72:421, 1990.

153. Johnson DP: Midline or parapatellar incision for knee arthroplasty: A comparative study of wound viability. J Bone Joint Surg Br 70:656, 1988.

154. Johnson DP, Donell ST: Antibiotic prophylaxis during bilateral knee arthroplasty: Brief report. J Bone Joint Surg Br 70:666, 1988.

155. Johnson DP, Houghton TA, Radford P: Anterior midline or medial parapatellar incision for arthroplasty of the knee: A comparative study. J Bone Joint Surg Br 68:812, 1986.

156. Johnson F, Leitl S, Waugh W: The distribution of load across the knee. J Bone Joint Surg Br 62:346, 1980.

157. Jones SMG, Pinder IM, Moran CG, et al: Polyethylene wear in uncemented knee replacements. J Bone Joint Surg Br 74:18, 1992.

158. Jones WA, Wroblewski BM: Salvage of failed total knee arthroplasty: The "beefburger" procedure. J Bone Joint Surg Br 68:812, 1986.

159. Josefchak RG, Finlay JB, Bourne RB, et al: Cancellous bone support for patellar resurfacing. Clin Orthop 220:192, 1987.

160. Kaempffe FA, Lifeso RM, Meinking C: Intermittent pneumatic compression versus Coumadin: Prevention of deep vein thrombosis in lower extremity total joint arthroplasty. Clin Orthop 269:89, 1991.

161. Kakkar VV, Howe CT, Flanc C, et al: Natural history of postoperative deep-vein thrombosis. Lancet 2:230, 1969.

162. Kantor SG, Schneider R, Insall JN, et al: Radionuclide imaging of asymptomatic versus symptomatic total knee arthroplasties. Clin Orthop 260:118, 1990.

163. Kapandji IA: The Physiology of the Joints. Volume II: The Lower Limb. London, Churchill Livingstone, 1970, p 120.

164. Katz MM, Hungerford DS, Krackow KA, et al: Reflex sympathetic dystrophy as a cause of poor results after total knee arthroplasty. J Arthroplasty 1:117, 1986.

165. Kaufer H, Matthews LS: Spherocentric arthroplasty of the knee. J Bone Joint Surg Am 63:545, 1981.

166. Kayler DE, Lyttle D: Surgical interruption of patellar blood supply by total knee arthroplasty. Clin Orthop 229:221, 1988.

167. Khaw FM, Moran CG, Pinder IM, et al: The incidence of fatal pumonary embolism after knee replacement with no prophylactic anticoagulation. J Bone Joint Surg Br 75:940, 1993.

168. Kilgus DJ, Moreland JR, Finerman GAM, et al: Catastrophic wear of tibial polyethylene inserts. Clin Orthop 273:223, 1991.

169. King TV, Scott RD: Femoral component loosening in total knee arthroplasty. Clin Orthop 194:285, 1985.

170. Kirk P, Rorabeck CH, Bourne RB, et al: Management of recurrent dislocation of the patella following total knee arthroplasty. J Arthroplasty 7:229, 1992.

171. Knutson K, Hovelius L, Lindstrand A, et al: Arthrodesis after failed knee arthroplasty: A nationwide multicenter investigation of 91 cases. Clin Orthop 191:202, 1984.

172. Kozinn SC, Marx C, Scott RD: Unicompartmental knee arthroplasty: A 4.5-6-year follow-up study with a metal-backed tibial component. J Arthroplasty 4:1, 1989.

173. Kozinn SC, Scott R: Unicondylar knee arthroplasty. J Bone Joint Surg Am 71:145, 1989.

174. Kraay MJ, Goldberg VM, Figgie MP, et al: Distal femoral replacement with allograft/prosthetic reconstruction for treatment of supracondylar fractures in patients with total knee arthroplasty. J Arthroplasty 7:7, 1992.

175. Kraay MJ, Goldberg VM, Herbener TE: Vascular ultrasonography for deep venous thrombosis after total knee arthroplasty. Clin Orthop 286:18, 1993.

176. Krackow KA, Maar DC, Mont MA, et al: Surgical decompression for peroneal nerve palsy after total knee arthroplasty. Clin Orthop 292:223, 1993.

177. Krackow KA, Weiss A-PC: Recurvatum deformity complicating performance of total knee arthroplasty: A brief note. J Bone Joint Surg Am 72:268, 1990.

178. Kumar SN, Chapman JA, Rawlins I: Vascular injuries in total knee arthroplasty. J Arthroplasty 13:211, 1998.

179. Kuster MS, Stachowiak GW: Factors affecting polyethylene wear in total knee arthroplasty. Orthop Blue J 25:S235, 2002.

180. Lachiewicz PF, Soileau ES: The rates of osteolysis and loosening associated with a modular posterior stabilized knee replacement. J Bone Joint Surg Am 86:525, 2004.

181. Laflamme GH, Laflamme GE, Beaumont P: Effectiveness and safety of low dose warfarin prophylaxis in cemented total knee prosthesis. J Bone Joint Surg Br 73:112, 1991.

182. Landy MM, Walker PS: Wear of ultra-high molecular-weight polyethylene components of 90 retrieved knee prostheses. J Arthroplasty 3(Suppl):S73, 1988.

183. Larcom PG, Lotke PA, Steinberg ME: Magnetic resonance venography versus contrast venography to diagnose thrombosis after joint surgery. Clin Orthop 331:209, 1996.

184. Laskin RS, Schob CJ: Medial capsular recession for severe varus deformities. J Arthroplasty 2:313, 1987.

185. Leclerc JR, Geerts WN, Desjardins L: Prevention of venous thromboembolism after knee arthroplasty: A randomized double blind trial comparing a low molecular weight heparin fragment (enoxaparin) to warfarin. Blood 246:84, 1994.

186. Lee JG, Keating EM, Ritter MA, et al: Review of the all-polyethylene tibial component in total knee arthroplasty: A minimum seven-year follow-up period. Clin Orthop 260:87, 1990.

187. Lettin AWF, Neil MJ, Citron ND, et al: Excision arthroplasty for infected constrained total knee replacements. J Bone Joint Surg Br 72:220, 1990.

188. Levine MN, Gent M, Hirsh J, et al: Ardeparin (low molecular weight heparin) versus graduated compression stockings for the prevention of venous thromboembolism: A randomized trial in patients undergoing knee surgery. Arch Intern Med 156:851, 1996.

189. Li S, Scuderi G, Furman BD, et al: Assessment of backside wear from the analysis of 55 retrieved tibial inserts. Clin Orthop 404:75, 2002.

190. Lian G, Cracchiolo A III, Lesavoy M: Treatment of major wound necrosis following total knee arthroplasty. J Arthroplasty S24, 1989.

191. Lidwell OM: Clean air at operation and subsequent sepsis in the joint. Clin Orthop 211:91, 1986.

192. Lidwell OM, Elson RA, Lowbury EJL, et al: Ultraclean air and antibiotics for prevention of postoperative infection: A multicenter study of 8,052 joint replacement operations. Acta Orthop Scand 58:4, 1987.

193. Lombardi AV, Engh GA, Volz RG, et al: Fracture/dissociation of the polyethylene in metal-backed patellar components in total knee arthroplasty. J Bone Joint Surg Am 70:675, 1988.

194. Lombardi AV, Mallory TH, Waterman RA, et al: Intercondylar distal femoral fracture. J Arthroplasty 10:643, 1995.

195. Lotke PA: Thrombophlebitis in knee arthroplasty. In Scott WN (ed): The Knee. St. Louis, CV Mosby, 1994, p 1217.

196. Lotke PA, Ecker ML: Influence of positioning of prosthesis in total knee replacement. J Bone Joint Surg Am 59:77, 1977.

197. Lotke PA, Ecker ML, Alavi A, et al: Indications for the treatment of deep venous thrombosis following total knee replacement. J Bone Joint Surg Am 66:202, 1984.

198. Lotke PA, Steinberg ME, Ecker ML: Significance of deep venous thrombosis in the lower extremity after total joint arthroplasty. Clin Orthop 299:25, 1994.

199. Lundborg G, Rydevik B: Effects of stretching the tibial nerve of the rabbit: A preliminary study of the intraneural circulation and barrier function of the perineurium. J Bone Joint Surg Br 55:390, 1973.

200. Lynch AF, Bourne RB, Rorabeck CH, et al: Deep-vein thrombosis and continuous passive motion after total knee arthroplasty. J Bone Joint Surg Am 70:11, 1988.

201. Lynch AF, Rorabeck CH, Bourne RB: Extensor mechanism complications following total knee arthroplasty. J Arthroplasty 2:135, 1987.

202. Lynch JA, Baker PL, Polly RE, et al: Mechanical measures in the prophylaxis of postoperative thromboembolism in total knee arthroplasty. Clin Orthop 260:24, 1990.

203. Mabrey JD, Keshmiri AA, Engh GA, et al: Standardized analysis of UHMWPE wear particles from failed total joint arthroplasties. J Biomed Mater Res 63:475, 2002.

204. Maderazo EG, Judson S, Pasternak H: Late infections of total joint prostheses: A review and recommendations for prevention. Clin Orthop 229:131, 1988.

205. Maloney WJ: The stiff total knee arthroplasty. J Arthroplasty 17:71, 2002.

206. Manifold SG, Cushner FD, Craig-Scott S, et al: Long-term results of total knee arthroplasty after the use of soft tissue expanders. Clin Orthop 380:133, 2000.

207. Marin LA, Salido JA, Lopez A, et al: Preoperative nutritional evaluation as a prognostic tool for wound healing. Acta Orthop Scand 73:2, 2002.

208. Markovich GD, Dorr LD, Klein NE: Muscle flaps in total knee arthroplasty. Clin Orthop 321:122, 1995.

209. Marks KE, Nelson CL, Lautenschlager EP: Antibiotic-impregnated acrylic bone cement. J Bone Joint Surg Am 58:358, 1976.

210. Marsh PK, Cotler JM: Management of an anaerobic infection in a prosthetic knee with long-term antibiotic alone: A case report. Clin Orthop 155:133, 1981.

211. Martin JW, Whiteside LA: The influence of joint line position on knee stability after condylar knee arthroplasty. Clin Orthop 259:146, 1990.

212. Mason MD, Brick GW, Scott RD, et al: Three pegged all polyethylene patellae: Two to six year results. Orthop Trans 17:991, 1994.

213. Mauerhan DR: Fracture of the polyethlyene tibial post in a posterior cruciate-substituting total knee arthroplasty mimicking patellar clunk syndrome. J Arthroplasty 18:942, 2003.

214. Maynard MJ, Sculco TP, Ghelman B: Progression and regression of deep vein thrombosis after total knee arthroplasty. Clin Orthop 273:125, 1991.

215. McAuley JP, Harrer MF, Ammeen D, et al: Outcome of knee arthroplasty in patients with poor preoperative range of motion. Clin Orthop 404:203, 2002.

216. McLaren AC, Dupont JA, Schroeber DC: Open reduction internal fixation of supracondylar fractures above total knee arthroplasties using the intramedullary supracondylar rod. Clin Orthop 302:194, 1994.

217. Menderes A, Demirdover C, Yilmaz M, et al: Reconstruction of soft tissue defects following total knee arthroplasty. Knee 9:215, 2002.

218. Merkel KD, Johnson EW Jr: Supracondylar fracture of the femur after total knee arthroplasty. J Bone Joint Surg Am 68:29, 1986.

219. Merkow RL, Soudry M, Insall JN: Patellar dislocation following total knee replacement. J Bone Joint Surg Am 67:1321, 1985.

220. Mikulak SA, Mahoney OM, Dela Rosa MA, et al: Loosening and osteolysis with the press-fit condylar posterior-cruciate-substituting total knee replacement. J Bone Joint Surg Am 83:398, 2001.

221. Miller J: Improved fixation in total hip arthroplasty using L.V.C. surgical technique. Brochure. Warsaw, IN, Zimmer, 1980.

222. Minoda Y, Kobayashi A, Iwaki H, et al: Polyethylene wear particles in synovial fluid after total knee arthroplasty. Clin Orthop 410:165, 2003.

223. Mintz L, Tsao AK, McCrae CR, et al: The arthroscopic evaluation and characteristics of severe polyethylene wear in total knee arthroplasty. Clin Orthop 273:215, 1991.

224. Mirra JM, Marder RA, Amstutz HC: The pathology of failed total joint arthroplasty. 170:175, 1982.

225. Mont MA, Dellon AL, Chen F, et al: The operative treatment of peroneal nerve palsy. J Bone Joint Surg Am 78:863, 1996.

226. Mont MA, Serna FK, Krackow KA, et al: Exploration of radiographically normal total knee replacements for unexplained pain. Clin Orthop 331:216, 1996.

227. Montgomery WH, Insall JN, Haas SB, et al: Primary total knee arthroplasty in stiff and ankylosed knees. Am J Knee Surg 11:20, 1998.

228. Monto RR, Garcia J, Callaghan JJ: Fatal fat embolism following total condylar knee arthroplasty. J Arthroplasty 5:291, 1990.

229. Moran MC, Brick, Sledge CB, et al: Supracondylar femoral fracture following total knee arthroplasty. Clin Orthop 324:196, 1996.

230. Moreland JR, Hanker GJ: Lower extremity axial alignment of normal males. In Dorr LD (ed): The Knee. Baltimore, University Park Press, 1985, p 55.

231. Morrey BF, Adams RA, Ilstrup DM, et al: Complications and mortality associated with bilateral or unilateral total knee arthroplasty. J Bone Joint Surg Am 69:484, 1987.

232. Morrey BF, Chao EYS: Fracture of the porous-coated metal tray of a biologically fixed knee prosthesis: Report of a case. Clin Orthop 228:182, 1988.

233. Morrey BF, Westholm F, Schoifet S, et al: Long-term results of various treatment options for infected total knee arthroplasty. Clin Orthop 248:120, 1989.

234. Murray DG, Wilde AH, Werner F, et al: Herbert total knee prosthesis: Combined laboratory and clinical assessment. J Bone Joint Surg Am 59:1026, 1977.

235. Murrell GA, Nunley JA: Interlocked supracondylar intramedullary nails for supracondylar fractures after total knee arthroplasty: A new treatment method. J Arthroplasty 10:37, 1995.

236. Mylod AG Jr, France MP, Muser DE, et al: Perioperative blood loss associated with total knee arthroplasty: A comparison of procedures performed with and without cementing. J Bone Joint Surg Am 72:1010, 1990.

237. Nahabedian MY, Mont MA, Orlando JC, et al: Operative management and outcome of complex wounds following total knee arthroplasty. Plast Reconstr Surg 104:1688, 1999.

238. Nahabedian MY, Orlando JC, Delanois RE, et al: Salvage procedures for complex soft tissue defects of the knee. Clin Orthop 356:119, 1998.

239. Naranja RJ, Lotke PA, Pagnano MW, et al: Total knee arthroplasty in a previously ankylosed or arthrodesed knee. Clin Orthop 331:234, 1996.

240. Naudie DDR, Rorabeck CH: Sources of osteolysis around total knee arthroplasty: Wear of the bearing surface. AAOS Inst Course Lect 53:251, 2004.

241. Nicholls DW, Dorr LD: Revision surgery for stiff total knee arthroplasty. J Arthroplasty 5:73, 1990.

242. Nielsen BF, Petersen VS, Vanmarken JE: Fracture of the femur after knee arthroplasty. Acta Orthop Scand 59:155, 1989.

243. O'Rourke MR, Callaghan JJ, Goetz DD, et al: Osteolysis associated with a cemented modular posterior-cruciate-substituting total knee design. J Bone Joint Surg Am 84:1362, 2002.

244. Pagnano MW, Hanssen AD, Lewallen DG, et al: Flexion instability after primary posterior cruciate retaining total knee arthroplasty. Clin Orthop 356:39, 1998.

245. Parks NI, Engh GA, Dwyer KA, et al: Micromotion of modular tibial components in total knee arthroplasty. Orthop Trans 18:611, 1994.

246. Parks NI, Engh GA, Topoleski T, et al: Modular tibial insert micromotion: A concern with contemporary knee implants. Clin Orthop 356:10, 1998.

247. Peltier LF: Fat embolism. Clin Orthop 232:263, 1988.

248. Peters PC, Engh GA, Dwyer KA, et al: Osteolysis after total knee arthroplasty without cement. J Bone Joint Surg Am 74:864, 1992.

249. Petty W, Bryan RS, Coventry M: Infection following total knee arthroplasty. J Bone Joint Surg Br 57:394, 1975.

250. Pittman GR: Peroneal nerve palsy following sequential pneumatic compression. JAMA 261:2201, 1989.

251. Pring DJ, Henderson RG, Rivett AG, et al: Autologous granulocyte scanning of painful prosthetic joints. J Bone Joint Surg Br 68:647, 1986.

252. Puloski SKT, McCalden RW, Macdonald SJ, et al: Tibial post wear in posterior stabilized total knee arthroplasty. J Bone Joint Surg Am 83:390, 2001.

253. Rand JA: Neurovascular complications of total knee arthroplasty. In Rand JA (ed): Total Knee Arthroplasty. New York, Raven Press, 1993, p 417.

254. Rand JA: The patellofemoral joint in total knee arthroplasty. J Bone Joint Surg Am 76:612, 1994.

255. Rand JA: Vascular complications of total knee arthroplasty: Report of three cases. J Arthroplasty 2:89, 1987.

256. Rand JA, Brown ML: The value of indium 111 leukocyte scanning in the evaluation of painful or infected total knee arthroplasties. Clin Orthop 259:179, 1990.

257. Rand JA, Bryan RS: Results of revision total knee arthroplasties using condylar prostheses: A review of fifty knees. J Bone Joint Surg Am 70:738, 1988.

258. Rand JA, Bryan RS, Morrey BF, et al: Management of infected total knee arthroplasty. Clin Orthop 205:75, 1986.

259. Rand JA, Coventry MB: Stress fractures after total knee arthroplasty. J Bone Joint Surg Am 62:226, 1980.

260. Rand JA, Gustilo RB: Technique of patellar resurfacing in total knee arthroplasty. Tech Orthop 3:57, 1988.

261. Rand JA, Morrey BF, Bryan RS: Patellar tendon rupture after total knee arthroplasty. Clin Orthop 244:233, 1989.

262. Rao AR, Engh GA, Collier MB, et al: Tibial interface wear in retrieved total knee components and correlations with modular insert motion. J Bone Joint Surg Am 84:1849, 2002.

263. Rhoads DD, Noble PC, Reuben JD, et al: The effect of femoral component position on patellar tracking after total knee arthroplasty. Clin Orthop 260:43, 1990.

264. Ries MD: Skin necrosis after total knee arthroplasty. J Arthroplasty 17:74, 2002.

265. Rimnac CM, Wright TM: Retrieval analysis of knee replacements. In Scott WN (ed): The Knee. St. Louis, CV Mosby, 1994, p 1251.

266. Ritter MA, Campbell ED: Postoperative patellar complications with or without lateral release during total knee arthroplasty. Clin Orthop 219:163, 1987.

267. Ritter MA, Faris PM, Keating EM: Anterior femoral notching and ipsilateral supracondylar femur fracture in total knee arthroplasty. J Arthroplasty 3:185, 1988.

268. Ritter MA, Keating EM, Faris PM: Clinical roentgenographic and scintigraphic results after interruption of the superior lateral genicular artery during total knee arthroplasty. Clin Orthop 248:145, 1989.

269. Ritter MA, Keating EM, Faris PM, et al: Rush rod fixation of supracondylar fractures above total knee arthroplasties. J Arthroplasty 10:213, 1995.

270. Ritter MA, Meding JB: Bilateral simultaneous total knee arthroplasty. J Arthroplasty 2:185, 1987.

271. Robinson EJ, Mulliken BD, Bourne RB, et al: Catastrophic osteolysis in total knee replacement. Clin Orthop 321:98, 1995.

272. Rolston LR, Christ DJ, Halpern A, et al: Treatment of supracondylar fractures of the femur proximal to a total knee arthroplasty: A report of four cases. J Bone Joint Surg Am 77:924, 1995.

273. Roscoe MW, Goodman SB, Schatzker J: Supracondylar fracture of the femur after Guepar total knee arthroplasty: A new treatment method. Clin Orthop 241:221, 1989.

274. Rose HA, Hood RW, Otis JC, et al: Peroneal-nerve palsy following total knee arthroplasty: A review of the Hospital for Special Surgery experience. J Bone Joint Surg Am 64:347, 1982.

275. Rosenberg AG, Andriacchi TP, Barden R, et al: Patellar component failure in cementless total knee arthroplasty. Clin Orthop 236:106, 1988.

276. Rosenberg AG, Haas B, Barden R, et al: Salvage of infected total knee arthroplasty. Clin Orthop 226:29, 1988.

277. Rubin R, Salvati EA: Infected total hip replacement after dental procedures. Oral Surg 41:18, 1976.

278. Rush JH, Vidovich JD, Johnson MA: Arterial complications of total knee replacement: The Australian experience. J Bone Joint Surg Br 69:400, 1987.

279. Ryd L, Albrektsson BEJ, Herberts P, et al: Micromotion of noncemented Freeman-Samuelson knee prostheses in gonarthrosis: A roentgenstereophotogrammetric analysis of eight successful cases. Clin Orthop 229:205, 1988.

280. Ryd L, Boegard T, Egund N, et al: Migration of the tibial component in successful unicompartmental knee arthroplasty: A clinical, radiographic and roentgenstereophotogrammetric study. Acta Orthop Scand 54:408, 1983.

281. Ryd L, Linder L: On the correlation between micromotion and histology of the bone-cement interface: Report of three cases of knee arthroplasty followed by roentgenstereophotogrammetric analysis. J Arthroplasty 4:303, 1989.

282. Ryd L, Lindstrand A, Stenstrom A, et al: Porous coated anatomic tricompartmental tibial components: The relationship between prosthetic position and micromotion. Clin Orthop 251:189, 1990.

283. Salvati EA, Brause BD, Chekofsky KM, et al: Reimplantation in infected total joint arthroplasty. Orthop Trans 5:449, 1981.

284. Salvati EA, Insall JN: The management of sepsis in total knee replacement. In Savastano AA (ed): Total Knee Replacement. New York, Appleton & Lange, 1980, p 49.

285. Schneider R, Soudry M: Radiographic and scintigraphic evaluation of total knee arthroplasty. Clin Orthop 205:108, 1986.

286. Schoifet SD, Morrey BF: Persistent infection after successful arthrodesis for infected total knee arthroplasty: A report of two cases. J Arthroplasty 5:277, 1990.

287. Schoifet SD, Morrey BF: Treatment of infection after total knee arthroplasty by debridement with retention of the components. J Bone Joint Surg Am 72:1383, 1990.

288. Schurman DJ, Johnson BL Jr, Amstutz HC: Knee joint infections with Staphylococcus aureus and Micrococcus species: Influence of antibiotics, metal debris, bacteremia, blood, and steroids, in a rabbit model. J Bone Joint Surg Am 57:40, 1975.

289. Scott RD, Ewald FC, Walker PS: Fracture of the metallic tibial tray following total knee replacement: Report of two cases. J Bone Joint Surg Am 66:780, 1984.

290. Scuderi GR, Insall JN, Windsor RE, et al: Survivorship of cemented knee replacements. J Bone Joint Surg Br 71:798, 1989.

291. Seitz P, Ruegsegger P, Gschwend N, et al: Changes in local bone density after knee arthroplasty: The use of quantitative computed tomography. J Bone Joint Surg Br 69:407, 1987.

292. Silva M, Kabbash CA, Tiberi JV III, et al: Surface damage on open box posterior-stabilized polyethylene tibial inserts. Clin Orthop 416:135, 2003.

293. Sisto DJ, Lachiewicz PF, Insall JN: Treatment of supracondylar fractures following prosthetic arthroplasty of the knee. Clin Orthop 196:265, 1985.

294. Smith JL Jr, Tullos HS, Davidson JP: Alignment of total knee arthroplasty. J Arthroplasty 4:55, 1989.

295. Spicer DDM, Curry JI, Pomeroy DL, et al: Range of motion after arthroplasty for the stiff osteoarthritic knee. J South Orthop Assoc 11:227, 2002.

296. Spiro TE, Fitzgerald RH, Trowbridge AA, et al: Enoxaparin: A low molecular weight heparin and warfarin for the prevention of venous thromboembolic disease after elective knee replacement surgery. Blood 246:84, 1994.

297. Stanley D, Cumberland DC, Elson RA: Embolization for aneurysm after knee replacement: Brief report. J Bone Joint Surg Br 71:138, 1989.

298. Stern S, Insall JN: Posterior stabilized prosthesis: Results after follow-up on nine to twelve years. J Bone Joint Surg Am 74:980, 1992.

299. Stinchfield FE, Bigliani LU, Neu HC, et al: Late hematogenous infection of total joint replacement. J Bone Joint Surg Am 62:1345, 1980.

300. Stringer MD, Steadman CA, Hedges AR, et al: Deep vein thrombosis after elective knee surgery: An incidence study in 312 patients. J Bone Joint Surg Br 71:492, 1989.

301. Stulberg BN, Insall JN, Williams GW, et al: Deep-vein thrombosis following total knee replacement: An analysis of six hundred and thirty-eight arthroplasties. J Bone Joint Surg Am 66:194, 1984.

302. Stulberg BN, Watson JT, Stulberg SD, et al: A new model to assess tibial fixation in knee arthroplasty: I. Histologic and roentgenographic results. Clin Orthop 263:288, 1991.

303. Stulberg BN, Watson JT, Stulberg SD, et al: A new model to assess tibial fixation: II. Concurrent histologic and biomechanical observations. Clin Orthop 263:303, 1991.

304. Stulberg SD, Stulberg BN, Hamati Y, et al: Failure mechanisms of metal-backed patellar components. Clin Orthop 236:88, 1988.

305. Surface MF, Berzins A, Urban RM, et al: Backsurface wear and deformation in polyethylene tibial inserts retrieved postmortem. Clin Orthop 404:14, 2002.

306. Sutherland CJ, Schurman JR: Complications associated with warfarin prophylaxis in total knee arthroplasty. Clin Orthop 219:158, 1987.

307. Takai S, Yoshino N, Kusaka Y, et al: Dissemination of metals from a failed patellar component made of titanium-base alloy. J Arthroplasty 18:831, 2003.

308. Teeny SM, Dorr L, Murata G, et al: Treatment of infected total knee arthroplasty: Irrigation and debridement versus two-stage reimplantation. J Arthroplasty 5:35, 1990.

309. Teng HP, Lu YC, Hsu CJ, et al: Arthroscopy following total knee arthroplasty. Orthop Blue J 25:422, 2002.

310. Tew M, Waugh W: Tibiofemoral alignment and the results of knee replacement. J Bone Joint Surg Br 67:551, 1985.

311. Thompson FM, Hood RW, Insall JN: Patellar fractures in total knee arthroplasty. Orthop Trans 5:490, 1981.

312. Thorpe CD, Bocell JR, Tullos HS: Intra-articular fibrous bands: Patellar complications after total knee replacement. J Bone Joint Surg Am 72:811, 1990.

313. Toksvig-Larsen S, Ryd L, Lindstrand A: Early inducible displacement of tibial components in total knee prosthesis inserted with and without cement. J Bone Joint Surg Am 80:83, 1998.

314. Tria AJ, Harwood DA, Alicea JA, et al: Patellar fractures in posterior stabilized knee arthroplasties. Clin Orthop 299:131, 1994.

315. Trippel SB: Antibiotic-impregnated cement in total joint arthroplasty. J Bone Joint Surg Am 68:1297, 1986.

316. Turpie AG, Eriksson BI, Bauer KA, et al: New pentasaccharides for the prophylaxis of venous thromboembolism, clinical studies. Chest J 124:371S, 2003.

317. Vaughn BK, Knezevich S, Lombardi AV Jr, et al: Use of the Greenfield filter to prevent fatal pulmonary embolism associated with total hip and knee arthroplasty. J Bone Joint Surg Am 71:1542, 1989.

318. Vernace JV, Rothman RH, Booth RE Jr, et al: Arthroscopic management of the patellar clunk syndrome following posterior stabilized total knee arthroplasty. J Arthroplasty 4:179, 1989.

319. Vince KG, Insall JN, Kelly MA: The total condylar prosthesis: 10- to 12-year results of a cemented knee replacement. J Bone Joint Surg Br 71:793, 1989.

320. Vince KG, Kelly MA, Beck J, et al: Continuous passive motion after total knee arthroplasty. J Arthroplasty 2:281, 1987.

321. Volz RG, Nisbet JK, Lee RW, et al: The mechanical stability of various noncemented tibial components. Clin Orthop 226:38, 1988.

322. Vresilovic EJ, Hozack WJ, Booth RE, et al: Incidence of pulmonary embolism after total knee arthroplasty with low dose Coumadin prophylaxis. Clin Orthop 286:27, 1993.

323. Wade PJF, Denham RA: Arthrodesis of the knee after failed knee replacement. J Bone Joint Surg Br 66:362, 1984.

324. Walker PS, Soudry M, Ewald FC, et al: Control of cement penetration in total knee arthroplasty. Clin Orthop 185:155, 1984.

325. Wasielewski RC: The causes of insert backside wear in total knee arthroplasty. Clin Orthop 404:232, 2002.

326. Wasielewski RC, Parks N, Williams I, et al: Tibial insert undersurface as a contributing source of polyethylene wear debris. Clin Orthop 345:53, 1997.

327. Waslewski GL, Marson BM, Benjamin JB: Early, incapacitating instability of posterior cruciate ligament-retaining total knee arthroplasty. J Arthroplasty 13:763, 1998.

328. Weber AB, Worland RL, Keenan J, et al: A study of polyethylene and modularity issues in >1,000 posterior cruciate-retaining knees at 5 to 11 years. J Arthroplasty 17:987, 2002.

329. Westrich GH, Sculco TP: Prophylaxis against deep venous thrombosis after total knee arthroplasty. J Bone Joint Surg Am 78:826, 1996.

330. Whiteside LA: Effect of porous coating configuration on tibial osteolysis after total knee arthroplasty. Clin Orthop 321:92, 1995.

331. Whiteside LA, Fosco DR, Brooks JG: Fracture of the femoral components in cementless total knee arthroplasty. Clin Orthop 286:71, 1993.

332. Whiteside LA, Kasselt MR, Haynes DW: Varus-valgus and rotational stability in rotationally unconstrained total knee arthroplasty. Clin Orthop 219:147, 1987.

333. Whiteside LA, Mihalko WM: Surgical procedure for flexion contracture and recurvatum in total knee arthroplasty. Clin Orthop 404:189, 2002.

334. Whiteside LA, Ohl MD: Tibial tubercle osteotomy for exposure of the difficult total knee arthroplasty. Clin Orthop 260:6, 1990.

335. Whiteside LA, Pafford J: Load transfer characteristics of a noncemented total knee arthroplasty. Clin Orthop 239:168, 1989.

336. Wilde AH, Ruth JT: Two-stage reimplantation in infected total knee arthroplasty. Clin Orthop 236:23, 1988.

337. Wilson MG, Kelley K, Thornhill TS: Infection as a complication of total knee-replacement arthroplasty: Risk factors and treatment in sixty-seven cases. J Bone Joint Surg Am 72:878, 1990.

338. Wilson NV, Das SK, Kakkar, et al: Thrombo-embolic prophylaxis in total knee replacement: Evaluation of the A-V impulse system. J Bone Joint Surg Br 74:50, 1992.

339. Windsor RE, Insall JN, Urs WK, et al: Two-stage reimplantation for the salvage of total knee arthroplasty complicated by infection: Further follow-up and refinement of indications. J Bone Joint Surg Am 72:272, 1990.

340. Windsor RE, Scuderi GR, Insall JN: Patellar fractures in total knee arthroplasty. J Arthroplasty 4:63, 1989.

341. Wolff AM, Hungerford DS, Krackow KA, et al: Osteotomy of the tibial tubercle during total knee replacement: A report of twenty-six cases. J Bone Joint Surg Am 71:848, 1989.

342. Woolson ST, Pottorff G: Venous ultrasonography in the detection of proximal vein thrombosis after total knee arthroplasty. Clin Orthop 273:131, 1991.

343. Wright J, Ewald FC, Walker PS, et al: Total knee arthroplasty with the Kinematic prosthesis: Results after five to nine years: A follow-up note. J Bone Joint Surg Am 72:1003, 1990.

344. Wright TM, Hood RW, Burstein AH: Analysis of material failures. Orthop Clin North Am 13:33, 1982.

345. Younger ASE, Duncan CP, Masri BA: Surgical exposures in revision total knee arthroplasty. J Am Acad Orthop Surg 6:55, 1998.

CHAPTER 100

Revision of Aseptic Failed Total Knee Arthroplasty

Marc F. Brassard • John N. Insall • Giles R. Scuderi

INDICATIONS FOR REVISION

Causes of mechanical failure of total knee arthroplasty (TKA) are femoral and tibial loosening, osteolysis, instability, subluxation, and dislocation; polyethylene wear; patellar loosening; and lack of motion and malposition of the components.[21,35] The cause of failure of the arthroplasty must be evident because exploration without due reason is not helpful, and the original error, if it is that, must be corrected. One study examined the outcome of exploration of 27 knees for severe pain of unknown origin after TKA. At final follow-up, there were only 41% good and excellent results. Even if the problem was identified at time of surgery, only 25% had successful outcomes.[20] Most mechanical failures are related to problems in either design or technique, and probably a new type of revision prosthesis will be required.

PREOPERATIVE ASSESSMENT

As a general principle, revision surgery should be performed as soon as failure is diagnosed. Once components are loose and have shifted in position, failure is inevitable, and procrastination only results in progressive bone destruction and the creation of larger defects. Likewise, if polyethylene wear-through of tibial or patellar components with exposure of the metal backing (Fig. 100–1) is diagnosed, delay will produce a more massive metallic synovitis. Similarly, polyethylene wear with osteolysis, which at times can be massive, is an indication for early revision. Ligament instability is seldom improved by conservative means. A more satisfactory revision operation is achieved by early intervention.

Preoperatively, all cases must be reviewed carefully, and thought must be given to the type of prosthesis that will be required for the revision. Any special components that may be needed must be ordered. The need for bone graft must also be anticipated. Aspiration is advisable whenever joint fluid is present, and the aspirate should be examined for cells, organisms, and metallic and polyethylene debris, as well as sent for aerobic, anaerobic, and fungal cultures. When infection is seriously considered, fluid should be sent for analysis of protein and glucose levels, and preoperative antibiotics should be avoided. In the preoperative period, reflex sympathetic dystrophy should be ruled out. This diagnosis should especially be considered in situations in which there are no obvious signs of failure of the components and pain is out of proportion to the results of the examination.

An important principle in revision knee surgery concerns identification of the exact failure mode of the preceding arthroplasty. If the mode of failure is not clearly understood, the revision is not likely to succeed. Intraoperative surprises should be very infrequent.

Preoperative planning is essential for successful revision. The size of the original components should be estimated and confirmed whenever possible. If the patient had the previous arthroplasty performed by another surgeon, the operative report should be obtained to ascertain the correct sizes and other pertinent information. Templates for the selected revision components can be helpful. The amount of bone loss to be expected after the components are removed is assessed as well. New revision components of the correct size should preferably be modular to allow intraoperative attachment of augments, wedges, and stems. In our view, the revision proceeds more smoothly when the cruciate ligaments are excised, and both posterior-stabilized and constrained polyethylene inserts are available. Ligament stability and integrity of the extensor mechanism are assessed. The position of previous incisions is noted, and if skin viability is in question, a plastic surgery consultation should be obtained.

SURGICAL TECHNIQUE

Exposure

In the exposure of a revision case, the previous incision should be used whenever possible. Recently, the use of soft-tissue expanders preoperatively in the revision setting has been successful.[10] If the knee is stiff, a quadriceps snip may be anticipated and should be performed early in the procedure to avoid damage to the tibial tubercle. A medial subperiosteal exposure that allows the tibia to be externally rotated and anteriorly subluxated is performed as part of the exposure and may be incorporated into a medial release, if indicated. When eversion of the patella is difficult, the patella may at first be subluxated laterally without eversion while the femoral and tibial components are removed. When a quadriceps snip does not allow adequate exposure, osteotomy of the tibial tubercle should be considered. If tibial tubercle osteotomy is to be performed, a long osteotomy as described by Whiteside and Ohl is the

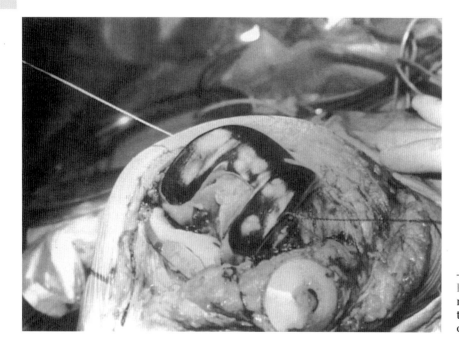

Figure 100–1. Photograph of a kinematic prosthesis showing central wear-through of a metal-backed patellar component.

best option.[32] It is best to leave the lateral soft-tissue attachments to the osteotomized bone and hinge the osteotomy open.

Fixed angular deformities are commonly encountered and should be addressed during the exposure. A fixed varus deformity is corrected by subperiosteal release of the deep and superficial portions of the medial collateral ligament and the pes anserine insertion along the proximal medial aspect of the tibia. The distal insertion of the superficial medial collateral ligament is elevated subperiosteally in an incremental fashion with a periosteal elevator or osteotome. Finally, the semimembranosus and posterior capsule are released to allow full exposure of the proximal end of the tibia. A fixed valgus deformity is unusual in the revision setting; however, if one is present, the most appropriate solution is to make small, multiple horizontal incisions in the lateral structures (posterior capsule, lateral collateral ligament, and iliotibial band) in a "pie-crusting" manner.[5] The small incisions, approximately 1 to 2 cm in length, are made both at the level of the joint and proximally. It is helpful to have some tension on the lateral structure during this procedure, which is accomplished either by placement of laminar spreaders between the femur and tibia or by manual distraction of the leg by an assistant. Severe fixed valgus deformities may require complete release of the lateral supporting structures from the femoral condyle. For patients with a rigid deformity and arthrofibrosis, it may be necessary to perform a femoral peel. Because this procedure involves complete release of the medial and lateral supporting structures, it will be necessary to revise the knee to a constrained design.

Débridement

Débridement of the suprapatellar and parapatellar regions should be done routinely. Failed knees often produce considerable debris of polyethylene, polymethylmethacrylate, and bone fragments that can become incorporated into the synovium. Many times in the presence of a polyethylene or metal synovitis, the synovium is hypertrophic and a complete synovectomy should be performed. The synovectomy also facilitates exposure of the joint.

Removal of Components

When operative inspection reveals granulation tissue, necrotic tissue, or other evidence of infection, the components should be removed, thorough débridement performed, and frozen section tissue examined. Evidence of acute inflammation is a reason for aborting the procedure until microbacterial cultures are available. Closing the wound over an antibiotic-impregnated polymethylmethacrylate spacer (Fig. 100–2) makes subsequent reentry of the knee easier in the event that cultures prove negative.

Revision operations are increasingly being performed for reasons other than loosening. Removal of well-fixed components can be a difficult task, particularly if they are porous coated. Special instruments can facilitate removal, and we have found a large sliding hammer (Fig. 100–3) with various gripping devices invaluable for extraction. We have been using a microsagittal saw blade that is placed directly under and moved parallel to the component to avoid cutting into the bone (Fig. 100–4). Loosening of a well-fixed component can also be achieved by passing flexible osteotomes around the periphery of the components. This action will break down the adhesion between the cement and the component, with the bone left mostly intact. If this technique is done appropriately, the cement is left behind, still attached to the bone. The cement is then removed by cracking it with a small osteotome in a mosaic pattern. The osteotome should be used lightly on the cement to just crack it and prevent any

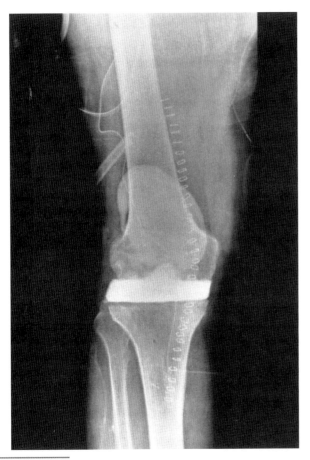

Figure 100–2. Radiograph showing antibiotic-impregnated cement spacers used after removal of an infected implant. The use of spacers contributes to patient comfort and makes reimplantation technically easier.

gouging or iatrogenic bone loss. A diamond-tipped drill may sometimes be required to remove a well-fixed component piecemeal.[34] Shedding of beads can be expected when removing porous-coated implants. When the components are not loose, they must be removed with minimal loss of bone.

Working around the femoral component with a microsagittal saw should free the surfaces up to the fixation pegs or stems. Afterward, thin flexible osteotomes are used to further disrupt the cement-component interface. When the interface is completely severed, an extraction device may be used. This device locks onto the component, and with the slap-hammer attachment, the component is carefully distracted from the bone.

An all-polyethylene tibial component can be separated from the tibial surface with a microsagittal saw to give better access for removal of pegs or stems. For metal-backed components, the microsagittal saw blade can be passed just under the tray in a manner similar to that used for the femur. The key to using the saw blade is to remain parallel to the surface and avoid digging into bone. Once the bond is broken between the cement and the component, stacked osteotomes may be used to gently lift the tray and central stem from the tibia. Again, with the remaining cement, an osteotome is used to crack the

cement gently in a mosaic pattern. Some models allow removal of the polyethylene tibial component to give access to the intramedullary stems. Removal of a cemented porous-coated prosthesis can be a very difficult task, especially with stems designed for bone ingrowth. It may be necessary to disassemble the components to gain access to the stems (Fig. 100–5). In the present situation, with many of the tibial components being modular, it is usually helpful to remove the polyethylene as early as possible. This method will greatly enhance exposure of the tibia and femur.

Polyethylene patellar components can be cut across with an oscillating saw. Removal of metal-backed components, especially cementless components, may be more difficult, and it might be necessary to use a high-speed diamond-edged saw.

With the components out, the bone surfaces are thoroughly cleaned of cement, debris, and granulation tissue. If a small area of cement is difficult to remove from bone, a small oscillating saw blade may also be used. With the saw blade the surgeon has more control over removing the cement and "freshening up" the bone ends. Use of an osteotome, rongeur, or curet to remove this small area of cement may cause further bone loss. In a revision setting in which infection has been ruled out, it is better to leave any remaining well-fixed cement in the canal than to risk excessive bone loss or perforation of the canal when trying to remove it. The soft tissues in the posterior compartment of the knee should also be débrided.

Reconstruction

After removal of the components and thorough débridement is the time to rebuild the knee. The basic principle of revision arthroplasty involves creating a kinematically stable arthroplasty that is well fixed and well aligned. This goal involves management of the residual bone and soft tissue. The key to revision surgery is to create equal flexion and extension gaps; however, when not readily achieved, adjustments need to be made. Adjustments on the femoral side can affect the knee in either flexion or extension, whereas any adjustments on the tibial side will affect both.

When performing revisions, we prefer to use a three-step method: (1) re-creating the flat tibial surface; (2) re-creating the femur and rebuilding the flexion space; and (3) rebuilding the extension space. The tibia is addressed first since it influences both the flexion and extension spaces and establishes a platform onto which the subsequent arthroplasty is built. Familiarity with these steps will aid the surgeon in performing the revision arthroplasty.

RE-CREATE THE TIBIA

After removal of the tibial component, a flat tibial surface perpendicular to the mechanical axis must be created. Minimal bone should be resected to achieve this goal. If there is bone loss, a modular augmentation wedge or

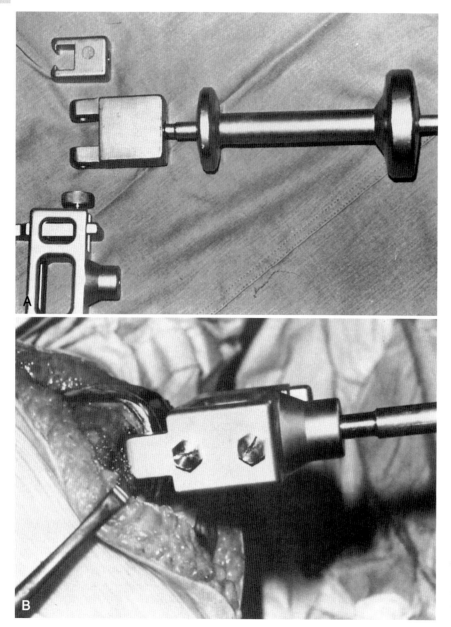

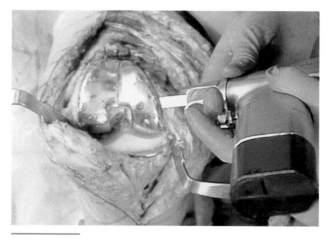

Figure 100–4. Photograph showing the use of a microsagittal saw blade around the femoral component.

Figure 100–3. A sliding hammer with special attachments is very helpful for removing prosthetic components, especially those with stems.

block or even a structural allograft may be needed (Fig. 100–6A). In knees with severe tibial bone loss, we have found it helpful to implant a modular tibial cone to reestablish the proximal end of the tibia (Fig. 100–6B).

RE-CREATE THE FEMUR

Size the Femur
Choosing the correct size of components is an essential step. It is helpful to preoperatively procure the operative notes from the previous procedure. Another useful preoperative step is to template the opposite side to obtain a relative idea of the size. Look at the size of the femoral component that is being removed and determine whether it is appropriate. The remaining bone should be templated

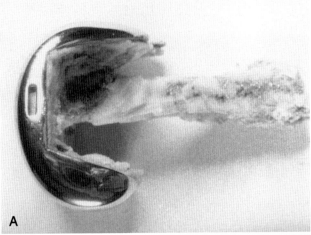

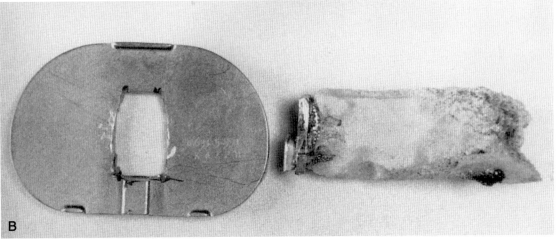

Figure 100–5. Photograph showing porous cemented components that were removed because of infection. This task was very difficult and resulted in some bone loss on the posterior surface of both the femur and tibia. The tibial component could not be extracted until the central peg had been cut from the base plate with a diamond-tipped saw.

in the anteroposterior plane. There is usually posterior bone loss, so templating intraoperatively runs the risk of undersizing the femoral component (Fig. 100–7). The epicondylar width of the femur can also be helpful in selecting the appropriate femoral size.

The danger in selecting an excessively small femoral component is that it will compromise flexion stability. It is better to select a larger femoral component and augment the posterior condyles to restore the anteroposterior dimension. Bone loss is usually most significant in the posterior femoral condyle area, but anterior femoral bone loss can occur and influence sizing, especially sizing of the femoral component in the sagittal position (Fig. 100–8).

Femoral Component Rotation

Correct rotation of the femoral component is vital to knee kinematics and patella tracking. The best way to determine rotation is to identify the medial and lateral epicondyles and establish the epicondylar axis. Rotational adjustments should be made to the residual distal femur,

with shaving of bone from the anterolateral and posteromedial aspect of the femur usually being required if the previous component was rotated internally. To ensure correct femoral component rotation, the posterolateral condyle generally has to be augmented. If a posterior-stabilized or similar prosthesis is used, the intercondylar notch is prepared 90 degrees to the epicondylar axis (Fig. 100–9).

Distal Femur Position

The key to this step is restoring the distance from the joint line, distally and posteriorly. The epicondyles are a useful landmark to determine the joint line, which on average is 25 mm from the lateral epicondyle and 30 mm from the medial epicondyle. Because the tibial cut is established at 90 degrees to the tibial mechanical axis, the joint line of a prosthetic knee of average size is 30 mm from both epicondyles.

After determining the appropriate joint line, the femoral component can be set provisionally to reestablish the distal joint line. Provisional distal augmentation can be

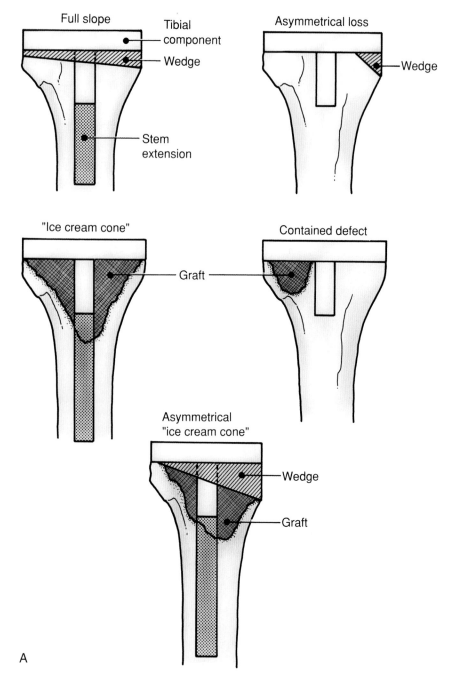

Figure 100–6. **A,** Reconstruction of tibial defects. Symmetric tibial deficiency can be compensated by thicker tibial polyethylene. Stem extension is usually advisable.

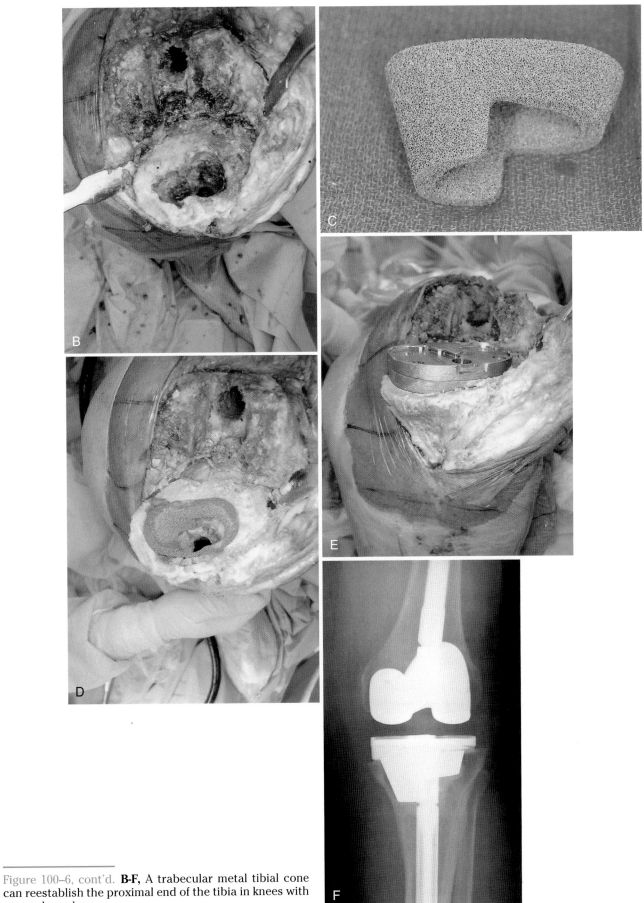

Figure 100–6, cont'd. **B-F,** A trabecular metal tibial cone can reestablish the proximal end of the tibia in knees with severe bone loss.

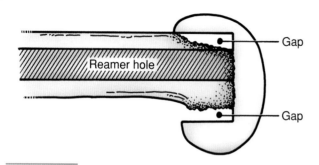

Figure 100–7. The revision femoral component must be sized from measurements of the opposite knee or estimated from the removed components. Typically, there will be gaps anteriorly and posteriorly.

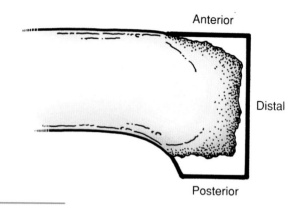

Figure 100–8. Typical bone loss after removal of a femoral component. Distal, anterior, and posterior bone deficiencies are illustrated.

used at this time (Fig. 100–10), especially if there is asymmetric femoral bone loss. The distance from the epicondyles to the posterior joint line is similar to that of the distal joint line and is helpful in confirming the correct femoral component size.

Because this step is provisional, no bone should be resected to fit the augments until the final position and size of the femoral component are determined. Additional adjustments to the position and size of the femoral component may be needed as the flexion and extension gaps are balanced.

REBUILD THE FLEXION SPACE

Balance the Flexion Space
This step requires choosing the correct tibial polyethylene articulation. With the provisional femoral component in place, the thickest tibial polyethylene surface that fills

the flexion space is inserted on the provisional tibial tray (Fig. 100–11).

REBUILD THE EXTENSION SPACE

To assess the extension space, retain the polyethylene used to create the flexion space and bring the knee into full extension. If the gaps are equal and stable, the polyethylene is the correctly sized articulation, and the femoral augments are finalized. Minor adjustments to tibial polyethylene thickness can be made to balance the gaps. If an imbalance is present after minor adjustments are made, refer to the following nine decision points:
1. If the knee is too tight in both flexion and extension, reducing the thickness of the tibial component may be sufficient to balance the knee.

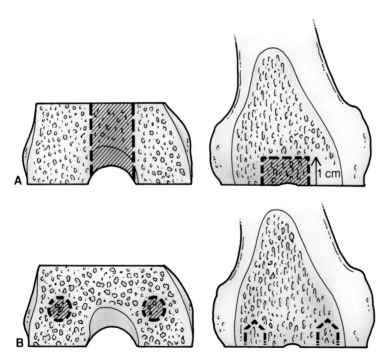

Figure 100–9. Femoral fixation can be enhanced by a central box (**A**), usually found with posterior-stabilized designs, or (**B**) by medial and lateral fixation lugs.

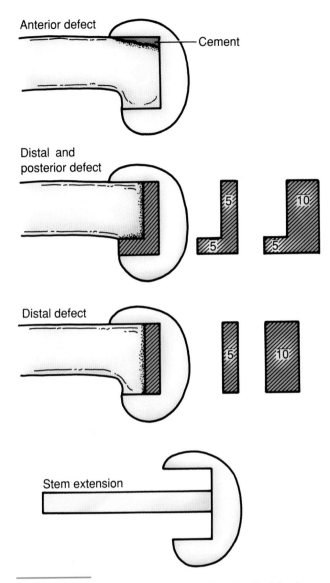

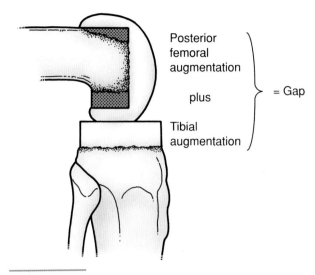

Figure 100–11. During reconstruction, the flexion gap is restored by a combination of posterior femoral and tibial augmentation.

Figure 100–10. Augmentation of the distal end of the femur. The revision femoral component should have a stem extension; usually, both distal and posterior augments are required, although the amount of augmentation at each site may differ. Thus, 5 mm may be sufficient posteriorly, although distal augmentation of 10 mm could be required. This can be judged by considering the spacers needed in flexion and extension and the amount of distal augmentation necessary to restore the joint line.

2. If the knee is tight in flexion but acceptable in extension, there are two options:
   a. Check the sagittal position of the femoral component. If it is positioned too posteriorly, consider using an offset femoral stem extension. This will move the femoral component more anteriorly, but be careful to not overstuff the patellofemoral joint, which will adversely affect motion and patellofemoral tracking.
   b. Downsize the femoral component.
3. If the knee is tight in flexion and loose in extension, consider the following three options:

   a. Check the sagittal position of the femoral component as in point 2, and consider using a thicker tibial component.
   b. Downsize the femoral component, and use a thicker tibial component.
   c. If the femoral component is the correct size, increase the distal femoral augmentation until the extension gap is equal to the flexion gap. A thinner tibial component may be required to balance the knee. Be careful to not move the joint line too far distally because this will adversely affect patellar tracking.
4. If the knee is acceptable in flexion but tight in extension, there are two options:
   a. Either reduce the distal femoral augmentation or resect more distal femoral bone. This will move the femoral component more proximally and increase the extension space.
   b. If a preoperative flexion contracture is present, release the posterior capsule, preferably from the femur.
5. If both the flexion and extension gaps are equal, no further adjustments are necessary.
6. If the knee is acceptable in flexion and loose in extension, the solution is to augment the distal end of the femur so that the extension gap requires the same amount of tibial polyethylene as the flexion gap.
7. The most common problem is that the flexion space is larger than the extension space. If the knee is loose in flexion and tight in extension, the solution is to go through a series of checks and adjustments.
   a. Check the sagittal position of the femoral component. If it is positioned too anteriorly, consider using an offset femoral stem extension. This will move the femoral component more posteriorly and reduce the flexion space.

b. Check the distal position of the femoral component. Consider reducing the distal augmentation or resecting more distal femoral bone.

c. Check the femoral component size. If the size appears to be too small, consider choosing the next larger size, but be careful to not oversize the femur.

d. If the previous maneuvers fail to balance the gaps, there may be a need for a constrained condylar knee (CCK) articulation.

e. Depending on the experience of the surgeon, collateral ligament advancement and reconstruction may be considered.

8. If the knee is loose in flexion and acceptable in extension, moving the femoral component proximally and using a thicker tibial component may solve the problem. If this does not balance the knee, the options in point 7 should be considered.

9. If the knee is symmetrically loose in flexion and extension, a thicker tibial component will solve the problem.

Management of Bone Loss

Bone loss is common in the revision setting. Even unicompartmental replacements (Figs. 100–12 and 100–13) leave substantial asymmetric bony deficiencies.[24] The best way to be prepared for intraoperative surprises is to be well prepared preoperatively. At the time of revision, the surgeon should make sure that all the materials for reconstruction are available, including wedges, blocks, allografts, and special components.

Bone defects can be classified as contained, uncontained, or a combination (Figs. 100–14 and 100–15). A contained defect has an intact cortical rim; an uncontained defect has segmental bone loss with no remaining cortex. Treatment of bone defects depends on two factors: (1) whether the defect is contained or uncontained and (2) the size of the defect. A small (<5 mm) contained defect can be treated with cement or morselized bone graft. The cement can be reinforced with screws and produce good long-term results.[26] Large contained cavitary defects can be treated with autogenous or allograft bone. Small (<5 mm) uncontained defects can also be repaired with cement alone or cement and screws. Intermediate (5 to 10 mm) uncontained defects can be managed with modular wedges.[25] Large (>10 mm) uncontained defects are best managed with modular augments or structural allografts.[4,9,19,27,33]

A useful classification system is the Anderson Orthopaedic Research Institute (AORI) classification.[6] This scheme allows separate classification of the femur and tibia. Type 1 defects have healthy cancellous bone with an undamaged metaphyseal segment, and there is no evidence of component subsidence or osteolysis. Type 2 defects have evidence of bone loss with shortening of the metaphyseal flare and mild to moderate evidence of component subsidence and osteolysis. Type 3 defects have a

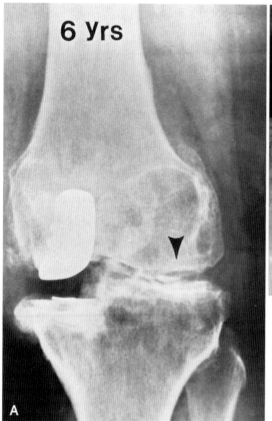

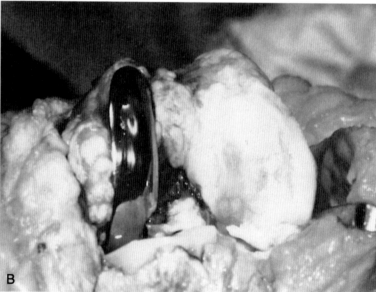

Figure 100–12. The most common reason for failure of unicondylar replacement is progressive arthritis of the unreplaced compartments of the knee. Free or embedded particles of acrylic cement are frequently found.

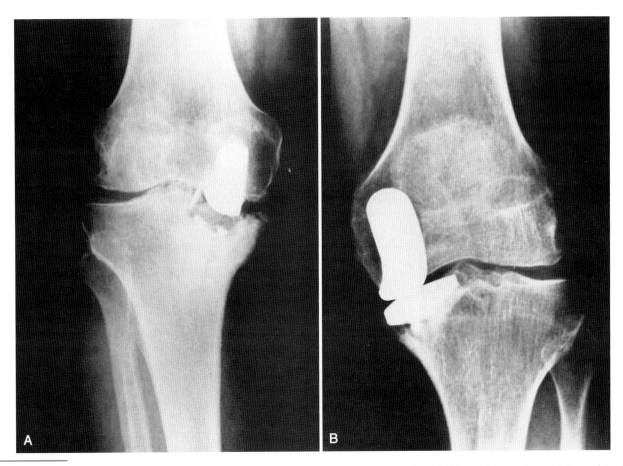

Figure 100–13. **A,** Failed unicompartmental arthroplasty showing the amount of medial bone loss to be anticipated in the tibia. This is an old design. **B,** Radiograph of a more modern type of unicondylar arthroplasty that has also failed because of tibial loosening. A similar degree of medial tibial bone loss can be anticipated.

deficient metaphyseal segment at or above the level of the epicondyles on the femur and at or below the level of the tibial tubercle. In addition, there is considerable component subsidence and osteolysis with a type 3 defect. This scheme is also divided into A for one condyle and B for bicondylar or total plateau involvement. Figure 100–16 presents an algorithmic approach to the management of these types of bone defects.[18]

The use of allograft in managing bone defects has many advantages: restoration of bone stock, biocompatibility, potential for ligamentous reattachment, versatility, and cost-effectiveness. Its disadvantages include donor availability, late resorption, nonunion, fracture, and risk of disease transmission. An absolute contraindication to allograft is a chronic infection. Relative contraindications include immunosuppression, metabolic bone disorders, neuropathic arthropathy, and an inadequate extensor mechanism. The use of bone grafts in anatomically matching sites (e.g., proximal tibia allograft for metaphyseal tibial bone loss) allows for accurate orientation of trabeculae along the lines of force. This may lessen the likelihood of early mechanical failure.[28]

In revisions, severe and extensive bone loss can involve a large portion of the distal femoral metaphysis, possibly including one or both condyles, along with the collateral ligaments. Epicondylar flaring sometimes occurs when a grossly loose femoral component subsides; along with significant femoral bone loss, the distal end of the femur appears to be trumpet shaped. In these situations, reconstruction is complex and requires knowledge of ligament reconstruction and bone-grafting techniques. Surgical options include a tumor-type prosthesis, which may be a constrained or hinged design, or reconstruction with a structural allograft.

Structural allografting of the distal end of the femur depends on the extent of bone loss and the location of the lesion. If the loss is isolated to one entire condyle, it may be possible to reestablish the distal femur with a femoral head allograft. In this case, the femoral head is contoured and matched to the distal femur. Engh et al[7] described a technique whereby the distal femoral defect is prepared with a reamer and the femoral head is prepared with a reverse-shaped reamer. This allows the allograft to mate to the defect. The graft is then secured provisionally to the host, and the construct is prepared to accept the implant. In these cases it is necessary to use a canal-filling stem to secure the implant in place. More extreme cases, with loss of both condyles, including the metaphysis, require either two femoral heads or a distal femoral allograft. Fixation of two femoral heads is similar to the method described earlier but can at times be cumbersome. In this situation, it may be easier to rebuild the metaphyseal bone loss with

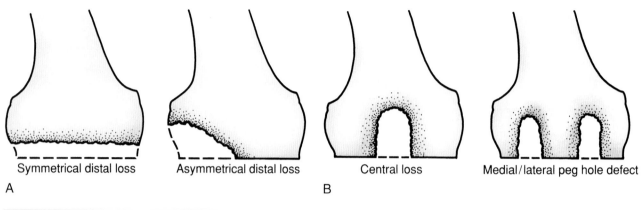

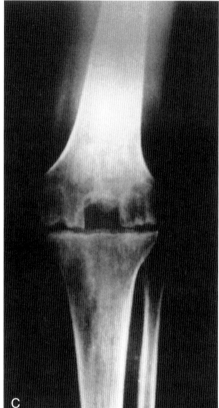

Figure 100–14. **A,** In the coronal plane, distal femoral bone loss may be symmetric or asymmetric. **B,** There may also be contained defects created by central or peripheral fixation lugs. **C,** Radiograph showing defects left after removal of the prosthesis, with a central box on the femur and a central stem on the tibia. Note the good preservation of medial and lateral bone.

a distal femoral allograft that can be fitted onto the residual bone. A distal femoral allograft can also be fitted into the trumpet-shaped or "ice cream cone" defect of the femur that is seen with epicondylar flaring (Fig. 100–17). This apparent widening of the distal end of the femur occurs when the component is grossly loose; along with osteolysis, it results in subsidence of the component. The amount of metaphyseal bone loss can be extensive.

Preparation of the allograft is a two-stage process. While one surgeon prepares the allograft to accept the femoral component, the other surgeon prepares the residual femur. If present, the epicondyles along with the collateral ligaments should be preserved for later attachment. Most likely a constrained implant will be necessary. When positioning the allograft, care must be taken to achieve the correct length and rotation. There are several ways to fix the allograft to the residual bone. One technique is to secure the composite with a canal-filling stem and

supplement the fixation with a plate. Another method requires cementing the stem extension in the femoral diaphysis and securing the construct with cerclage wires. Whereas this technique controls rotation, final fixation is achieved with a press-fit canal-filling stem. In using either method, a step cut can be made in the host femur and allograft to improve rotational stability. When the construct is secure, the epicondyles and collateral ligaments can be reattached to the allograft.

Structural allograft for proximal tibial metaphyseal bone loss is also an appealing option. The type of allograft depends on the size and location of the bone loss. A trumpet-like proximal tibia, which is a contained defect, may easily accommodate one or two femoral heads. An asymmetric uncontained defect may accommodate a femoral head as described before for femoral bone loss. Larger defects, with loss of both the medial and lateral tibial plateaus, can be reconstructed with a proximal tibial

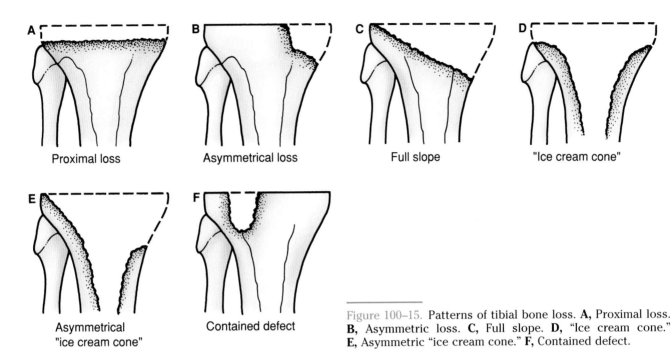

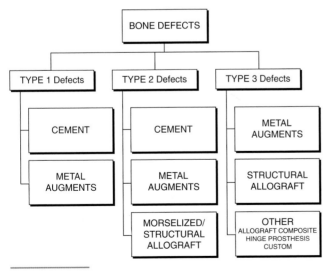

Figure 100–15. Patterns of tibial bone loss. **A,** Proximal loss. **B,** Asymmetric loss. **C,** Full slope. **D,** "Ice cream cone." **E,** Asymmetric "ice cream cone." **F,** Contained defect.

allograft. Rotational stability and fixation are achieved by the techniques described earlier, with a step cut and press-fit canal-filling stem being the best option. If bone loss is so extensive that the tibial tubercle is involved, it will be necessary to have available a proximal tibia with the extensor mechanism still attached. Loss of the collateral ligament attachments necessitates implantation of a constrained knee.

The introduction of trabecular metal tibial cones (see Fig. 100–6B to F) has made it easier to manage type 3 and conical bone defects of the proximal end of the tibia. After preparation of the defect, the porous trabecular metal augment is impacted into place and, with the anticipated

bone ingrowth, becomes incorporated into the proximal tibia. This modular tibial augment reestablishes the proximal tibial surface and provides structural support for the tibial component.

MANAGEMENT OF THE PATELLA

When the components are inserted for a final check, patellar tracking is assessed by means of lateral patellar release and balancing when necessary. If the augments have been chosen correctly, the patellar position will be in the "neutral zone." If not in the neutral zone, altering the distribution of the augments between the femur and tibia should be considered (Fig. 100–18); remember that some pre-revision knees already have patellar infra, which if

Figure 100–16. Algorithm for the management of bone defects. (Redrawn from Lucey SD, Scuderi GR, Kelly MA, Insall JN: A practical approach to dealing with bone loss in revision total knee arthroplasty. Orthopedics 23:1036, 2000).

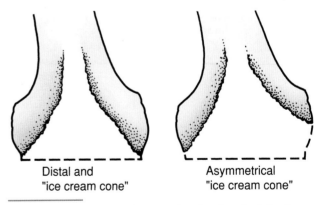

Figure 100–17. Cone defects in the distal end of the femur are usually caused by removal of cemented stemmed components. This very extensive bone loss may be symmetric or asymmetric; bone grafting is often required in addition to augmentation.

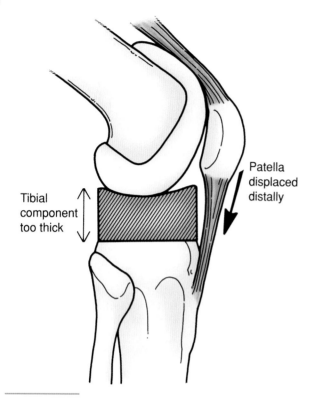

Figure 100–18. If an extra-thick tibial component is needed to stabilize the knee, the patella is displaced distally, thereby causing patella infra. Undersizing of the femoral component in the sagittal plane and anterior malpositioning are possible causes. Excessive distal resection of the femur in which the joint line is moved proximally is another cause.

caused by actual shortening of the patellar ligament must be accepted. In extreme situations, the patellar ligament may be so shortened that the patella actually articulates with the tibial polyethylene. Patellar lengthening and tibial tubercle advancement have been described; however, we believe that there is too much risk of disruption or late failure of the patellar ligament to take this route. We prefer to reduce the size of the patellar bone and omit the patellar prosthesis.

The decision to use a prosthetic patellar component depends not only on the patellar position but also on the amount of remaining bone stock. In most cases it is possible to reshape the patella and cement in a three-peg component. However, the patellar prosthesis can be omitted when the bone stock is insufficient (less than 12 mm) or of very poor quality; the remaining patellar bone is then trimmed so that a reasonable fit in the femoral sulcus is obtained, commonly referred to as a "patelloplasty." At this point the tourniquet is released, and major bleeding points are secured before reapplying the Esmarch bandage and reinflating the tourniquet.

Alternative techniques for the management of deficient patella bone include the bone-grafting technique described by Hanssen[13] and trabecular metal augmentation. If there is a shell of residual patella bone, a trabecular metal patella augment can be sutured in place and a polyethylene patella component cemented onto it (Fig. 100–19).

Final Preparation

The bone surfaces are cleaned with pulsatile lavage. Note that in most revision cases, even with considerable bone loss, the margins of the defect will consist of sclerotic bone or irregular contours. This bone is the strongest available and should not be removed or drilled, and no attempt should be made to obtain a cancellous surface. Even when this is possible, the quality of the bone may be poor and inadequate for providing proper prosthetic support.

The final components are assembled (Fig. 100–20), the selected modular augments and wedges are fixed with screws or cement according to the designer's intention, and the intramedullary stems are attached. It is recommended that these stems be 1 mm larger than the stems used for the trial reduction to get the firmest possible fit.

Use of Stem Extensions

In revision arthroplasty, femoral and tibial bone quality is usually compromised to a variable degree. For this reason, it is preferable to use stem extensions to enhance fixation, especially if a constrained implant is used. There is some debate about whether the femoral and tibial stem extensions should be cemented. This is dependent on the design of the stem extension. Short stem extensions (25 to 30 mm) and long narrow-diameter stem extensions should be cemented. The longer modular stem extensions, which can be canal filling and diaphyseal engaging, can be used in a tight press-fit manner. Offset stems are also helpful because they can better align the implant on the metaphysis (Fig. 100–21) It has been the authors' preference to cement the core prosthesis and insert the stem extensions in a tight press-fit manner. The integrity of the residual bone and the dimensions of the intramedullary canal determine the length and diameter of the stem extensions.

Cementing

Although cementless reconstruction has its advocates,[22,31] cement has many attractions, and its use ensures that the new prosthesis will fit perfectly on bone surfaces, which are inherently irregular. Any bone resection that would otherwise be needed is avoided. Provided that cement is prevented from entering the intramedullary canals, later removal of the prosthesis (e.g., in the event of infection) is not difficult. The objective of cement use is to level the bone ends and provide even loading beneath the prosthesis. Fixation itself is achieved by the component shape and the intramedullary stems (Fig. 100–22).

Two batches of cement are usually required for each component; they should contain an antibiotic powder. If gentamicin-impregnated cement is not available, 1 g of tobramycin powder is used for each bag of cement. The cement is used in the doughy stage and applied to the undersurface of the core femoral component. Because intramedullary cement is to be avoided, care is taken to

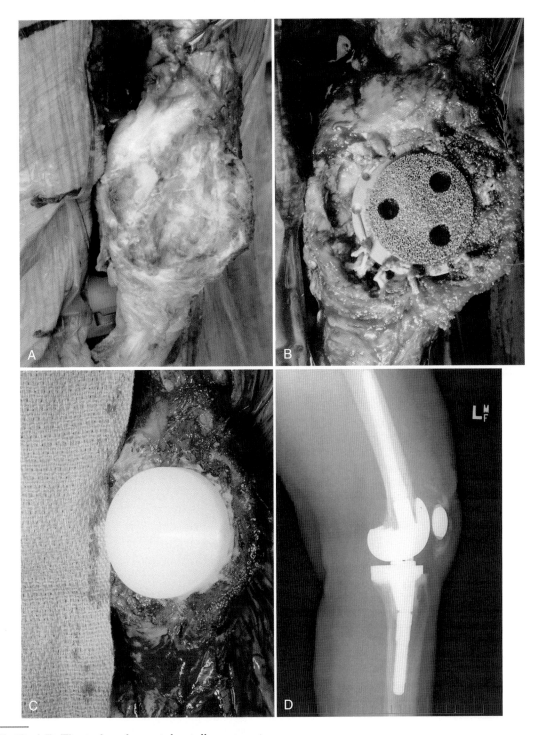

Figure 100–19. **A-D,** The trabecular metal patella augment.

not allow cement to be pushed around the stem. The prosthesis is inserted and gradually impacted into the bone until it is firmly seated on the bony surface. The cement should be doughy because if in a liquid phase, the cement will "leak" from under the prosthesis.

The patellar component, when used, can be cemented with the femur and held with a clamp until cured.

The cement for tibial fixation is then mixed. Once again, it is applied to the underside of the core prosthesis in a doughy condition, and the prosthesis is inserted and

gently impacted into the bone. When morselized graft has been used, insertion of the components must be done gently so that the graft is not displaced into the intramedullary canal (Fig. 100–23).

Aftercare

Aftercare for revision surgery does not differ from that indicated for primary cases, unless there has been exten-

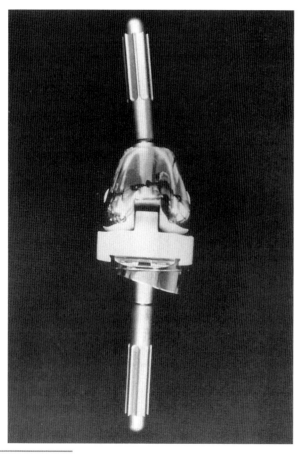

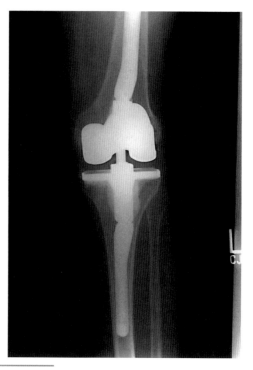

Figure 100–21. Offset stem extensions in revision arthroplasty

Figure 100–20. Modular IB II posterior-stabilized prosthesis with stems and a full wedge augment to the tibia assembled in the operating room for implantation into a knee with a failed implant. There are also augments on the distal end of the femur (not seen). Although this implant has a posterior-stabilized articulation, by changing the polyethylene insert, it could be converted into a constrained condylar knee (CCK). The CCK metal components are compatible with both posterior-stabilized and CCK tibial inserts.

sive bone grafting, which would require some protection in weightbearing. Even with the use of a "quadriceps snip" or a tibial tubercle osteotomy, we still progress with range-of-motion and strengthening exercises. If there is any question regarding fixation of the tibial tubercle osteotomy, motion and quadriceps exercises are limited for 6 to 8 weeks or until the osteotomy is healed.

RESULTS OF REVISION SURGERY

It is difficult to present meaningful results of revision surgery because even more than for primary arthroplasty, techniques are continually evolving. Consequently, the long-term results of revision surgery involve cases in which techniques were used that are not applicable today. Customized components, metal augments, wedges, stems, and allograft techniques are still being refined.

Bertin and colleagues[1] were the first to report revision results with the use of noncemented stems (on the ICLH

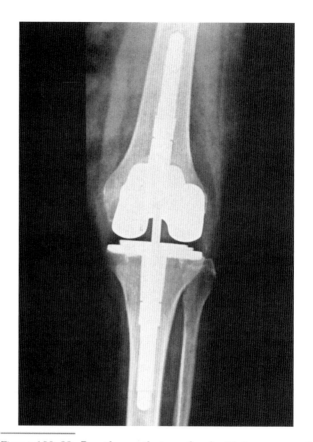

Figure 100–22. Prostheses that are fixed with bone cement as a grouting material at the interface with uncemented stem extensions have been shown by roentgen stereophotogrammetric analysis to have minimal micromotion. It is not necessary for the stems to contact the cortices.

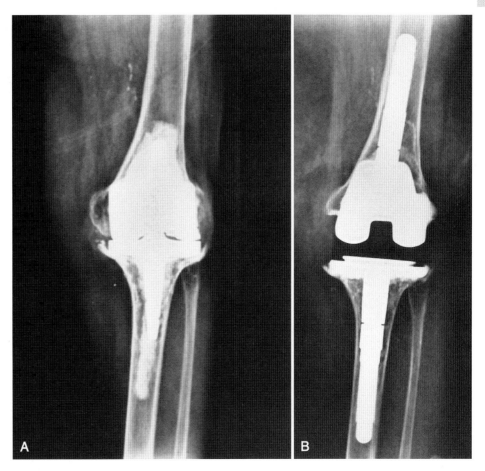

Figure 100–23. **A,** Radiograph showing a loose spherocentric prosthesis. From the distribution of the cement, extensive bone loss was anticipated. **B,** Radiograph taken after revision using constrained condylar knee metal implants with a posterior-stabilized polyethylene insert. The contained defects have been packed with cancellous bone graft. Cement was used to level the bone ends, and the stems were uncemented.

prosthesis); these results were, if anything, better than those with primary arthroplasty. This experience led Freeman (personal communication) to use similar stems for all of his replacements.

The results obtained at the Hospital for Special Surgery with customized prostheses (Fig. 100–24) and the use of augments, wedges, and stems were examined.[29] The infection rate was 5%, and mechanical loosening occurred in 3%, all in cemented and short-stem components. None of the long-stem, noncemented components loosened. Of the noncemented stems, 96% showed a sclerotic halo around the stem and, in most cases, cortical reaction at the distal tip of the stem. Problems of sizing and fit occurred with the custom prosthesis because it was difficult to estimate from preoperative radiographs the exact shape and location of bone defects and, in some cases, the optimal stem size; there were many component misfits, which led to the newer concept of modular design.

The results, though as durable as those of primary arthroplasty, were not equal in quality. In 1982 Insall and Dethmers[15] recorded 89% good and excellent results in a series of cemented revisions. However, the period of follow-up was relatively short, and the incidence of radiolucent lines around the components was high. There were fewer excellent and more good results than in a primary arthroplasty series. Goldberg and colleagues[11] reported the results of 65 consecutive revision TKAs performed for mechanical failure. The types of implants used included total condylar, posterior stabilized, total condy-

lar III, and a kinematic rotating-hinge prosthesis. In this series, 46% of the knees was considered excellent or good and 42% were poor or failures. The infection rate was 4.5%, and multiple revisions did poorly. Jacobs et al[16] reviewed 24 patients with 28 failed TKAs replaced with porous-coated anatomic components. Good and excellent results were achieved in 68%, and there were three failures. Patients who underwent revision operations for severe pain or who had no clearly definable problem were not improved. Friedman and coworkers[8] presented the results of 137 revision total knees at the Brigham and Women's Hospital in Boston. Function instability, motion, and pain all improved after revision, but improvements were significantly less than those seen after primary total knee replacement. A third of the patients still walked with crutches, a walker, or not at all. Loosening was the most common reason for failure. The clinical success rate was 63% for a single revision, and the failure rate at 5 years was 5.8%.

The use of allograft to manage bony defects has had some encouraging results for small and large defects. Whiteside[30] used morselized allograft for localized areas of bone defects in 56 cementless revisions. All 56 knees demonstrated increase density in the grafted zone. For larger defects, Wilde et al[33] reported their results on 12 knees. Five of the knees had contained defects and seven had an uncontained defect; all were treated with structural allograft. Radiographs demonstrated complete incorporation of the graft in 11 of the 12 knees at an average of 23

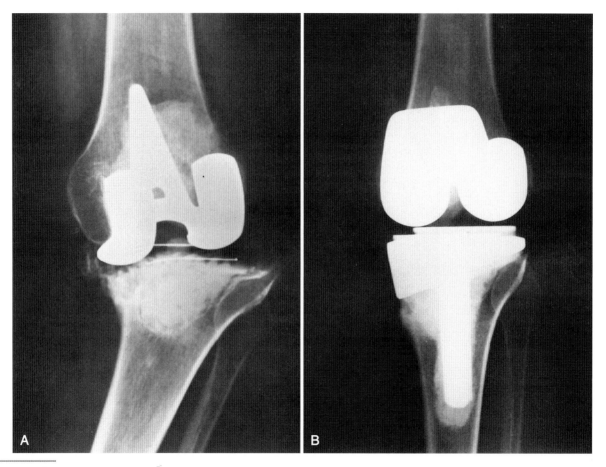

Figure 100–24. For revision of this prosthesis with severe collapse of the medial aspect of the tibia, a custom-made prosthesis with a full wedge was used. The articular surfaces of the revision prosthesis are standard posterior-stabilized condylar design.

months after surgery. Single-photon emission computed tomography scans showed uniform activity in the area of the graft in four of the five knees that were studied. Laskin[17] reported poor results with the use of autogenous bone graft for large bony defects. He examined 26 patients with severe tibial bone loss and secondary varus-valgus instability of greater than 20 degrees treated with TKA and autogenous bone graft. He found that four grafts demonstrated fragmentation and dissolution within the first year with implant subsidence. Needle biopsy in nine other knees 1 year postoperatively revealed osteocytes in the lacunae in only four grafts. In four other knees, complete radiolucency was seen between the graft and the tibial host bone. The overall success rate at 5 years was only 67%.

Other studies of allograft use in mostly uncontained defects have demonstrated good results. Harris and colleagues[14] reported on 14 cases with a 43-month follow-up. Seven of the eight cases (87.5%) that involved the distal end of the femur achieved good or excellent results. Tsahakis et al[28] reported even better results. In their study of 13 large uncontained femoral defects at a mean follow-up of 2.1 years, all 13 demonstrated host-allograft union. In this study all six proximal tibial allografts also healed. Mow and Wiedel[23] likewise reported good results with

uncemented component fixation. They used 15 allografts, including 10 for the proximal end of the tibia. There was 1 failure (at 3 years) as a result of allograft failure. During revision of the failure, they found that the graft had incorporated, but the component lost support with subsequent implant fracture. They concluded that all 15 allografts had healed to host bone.

The use of metal augments in the form of wedges or blocks has produced overall good results in revision knee surgery. Brooks et al[3] compared five different techniques in the treatment of wedge-shaped proximal tibial defects. They concluded that a metal wedge was an acceptable alternative to a custom-made component for reconstruction of tibial bone stock defects. Brand and colleagues[2] reported good results with the use of a metal wedge for proximal tibial defects. In their series, 22 knees (20 patients) were monitored for an average of 37 months. No failures and no loosening of tibial components were reported. However, there was a 27% incidence of nonprogressive radiolucent lines. None of these patients required revision surgery, and all but one patient was pain-free.

The results of our own experience with CCK components and uncemented stems have been examined.[12] There were 68 revision operations, and follow-up ranged from 2 to 10 years. Excellent and good results were obtained in

56 knees, with 11 poor results. Further revision was performed on six knees, all because of infection. A posterior-stabilized tibial insert was used in 49 knees, 43 (88%) of which achieved excellent and good results, with 4 further revisions. The CCK tibial insert was needed to give greater stability in 18 knees, and there were 13 (72%) knees rated excellent and good, with 2 further revisions. The overall infection rate was high (9%), which confirms the wisdom of avoiding intramedullary cement. Survivorship analysis of this group of patients was calculated to be 80% at 10 years, a figure less satisfactory than a similar analysis performed on the total condylar and posterior-stabilized prostheses (90% and 94%, respectively). Thus, even with so-called modern techniques, the results of revision surgery are understandably less satisfactory than those of primary arthroplasty. The point made by Jacobs and coworkers[16] about the poor results of revision surgery performed for pain, without clear definition of the reason, is well taken and cannot be overemphasized. Our own experience confirms this, although we understand how difficult it is to manage a patient with a painful arthroplasty. The temptation to "give it a go" is sometimes irresistible, but the result will be failure.

CUSTOM COMPONENTS

Since the introduction of modularity, custom components have a limited role in revision knee arthroplasty. A custom prosthesis can be considered if one of the following conditions prevails:
1. The bone is so oversized or undersized that standard components will not fit.
2. Stems are needed to enhance fixation, but bone shapes preclude the use of standard devices (for example, when there is a fracture malunion adjacent to the prosthesis [Fig. 100–25] or an offset stem is needed because of peculiarities in intramedullary alignment [Fig. 100–26]; shorter modular stem extensions and offset stems also provide a solution to this problem [Fig. 100–27]).
3. The size or location of the bone loss cannot be accommodated by standard augments.

Otherwise, custom components should be avoided for the following reasons:
1. No instruments have been designed for implanting custom components.

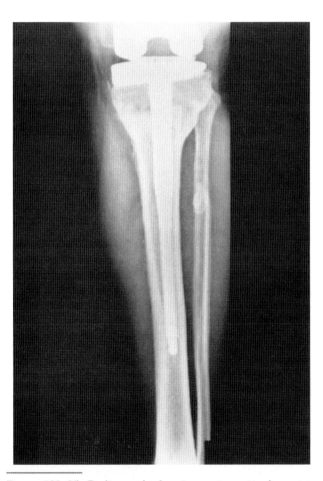

Figure 100–25. Radiograph showing a stem attachment to a tibial component for nonunion of an upper tibial osteotomy. This method has proved very successful and predictable in achieving healing of the fracture.

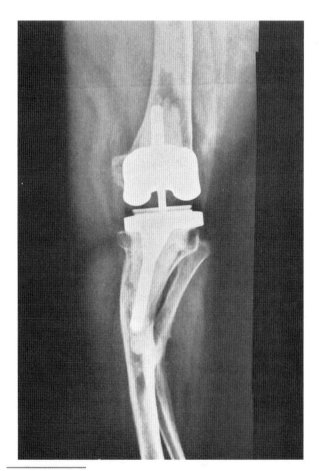

Figure 100–26. This bizarre prosthesis is a posterior-stabilized design used for the revision of a hinged prosthesis. An angulated tibial stem was used because of bone deformity of the upper part of the tibia.

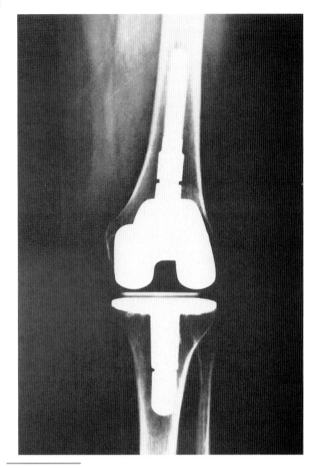

Figure 100–27. Radiograph of a "stubby" stem extension on the tibial component. The stubby stem impinges against the lateral cortex of the tibia. If a longer stem extension had been used, the tibial component would have tilted into valgus. Alternatively, the whole component could be medialized, but this would cause medial overhang of the prosthesis. In this case, an offset stem is required.

2. The use of a custom component does not provide for sizing options intraoperatively.

Generally, the high degree of modularity available with today's knee systems has obviated what little need there is for custom components.

SUMMARY

Revision knee surgery is not straightforward and is not always technically easy. Instruments are not as useful as they are for primary arthroplasty, although the use of stems is helpful in obtaining alignment. Above all, the surgeon should develop a good understanding of the principles of revision knee arthroplasty and perform the appropriate preoperative preparations.

References

1. Bertin KC, Freeman MAR, Samuelson KM, et al: Stemmed revision arthroplasty for aseptic loosening of total knee replacement. J Bone Joint Surg Br 67:242, 1985.

2. Brand MG, Daley RJ, Ewald FC, et al: Tibial tray augmentation with modular metal wedges for tibial bone stock deficiency. Clin Orthop 248:71, 1989.
3. Brooks PJ, Walker PS, Scott RD: Tibial component fixation in deficient tibial bone stock. Clin Orthop 184:302, 1984.
4. Chen F, Krackow KA: Management of tibial defects in total knee arthroplasty. Clin Orthop 305:249, 1994.
5. Clarke HD, Scuderi GR: Correction of valgus deformity in total knee arthroplasty with the pie crust technique of lateral soft tissue releases. J Knee Surg 17:157, 2004.
6. Engh GA: Bone defect classification. In Engh GA, Rorabeck CH (eds): Revision Knee Arthroplasty. Baltimore, Williams & Wilkins, 1997, pp 63-120.
7. Engh GA, Herzwurm PJ, Parks NL: Treatment of major defects of bone with bulk allografts and stemmed components during total knee arthroplasty. J Bone Joint Surg Am 79:1030, 1997.
8. Friedman RJ, Hirst P, Poss R, et al: Results of revision total knee arthroplasty performed for aseptic loosening. Clin Orthop 255:235, 1990.
9. Ghazavi MT, Stockley I, Yee G, et al: Reconstruction of massive bone defects with allograft in revision total knee arthroplasty. J Bone Joint Surg Am 79:17, 1997.
10. Gold DA, Scott WN, Scott SA: Soft tissue expanders prior to total knee replacement in the multioperated knee: A new method to prevent catastrophic skin problems. J Arthroplasty 11:512, 1996.
11. Goldberg VM, Figgie MP, Figgie HE III, et al: The results of revision total knee arthroplasty. Clin Orthop 226:86, 1988.
12. Haas SB, Insall JN, Montgomery W, et al: Revision total knee arthroplasty with use of modular components with stems inserted without cement. J Bone Joint Surg Am 77:1700, 1995.
13. Hanssen AD: Bone grafting for severe patellar bone loss during revision knee arthroplasty. J Bone Joint Surg Am 83:171, 2001.
14. Harris AI, Poddar S, Gitelis S, et al: Arthroplasty with a composite of an allograft and a prosthesis for knees with severe deficiency of bone. J Bone Joint Surg Am 77:373, 1995.
15. Insall JN, Dethmers DA: Revision of total knee arthroplasty. Clin Orthop 170:123, 1982.
16. Jacobs MA, Hungerford DS, Krackow KA, et al: Revision total knee arthroplasty for aseptic failure. Clin Orthop 226:78, 1988.
17. Laskin RS: Total knee arthroplasty in the presence of large bony defects of the tibia and marked knee instability. Clin Orthop 248:66, 1989.
18. Lucey SD, Scuderi GR, Kelly MA, Insall JN: A practical approach to dealing with bone loss in revision total knee arthroplasty. Orthopedics 23:1036, 2000.
19. Mnaymneh W, Emerson RH, Borja F, et al: Massive allografts in salvage revisions of failed total knee arthroplasties. Clin Orthop 260:144, 1990.
20. Mont MA, Serna FK, Krackow KA, et al: Exploration of radiographically normal total knee replacements for unexplained pain. Clin Orthop 331:216, 1996.
21. Moreland JR: Mechanisms of failure in total knee arthroplasty. Clin Orthop 226:49, 1988.
22. Mow CS, Wiedel JD: Noncemented revision total knee arthroplasty. Clin Orthop 309:110, 1994.
23. Mow CS, Wiedel JD: Structural allografting in revision total knee arthroplasty. J Arthroplasty 11:235, 1996.
24. Padgett DE, Stern SH, Insall JN: Revision total knee arthroplasty for failed unicompartmental replacement. J Bone Joint Surg Am 73:186, 1991.
25. Pagnano MW, Trousdale RT, Rand JA: Tibial wedge augmentation for bone deficiency in total knee arthroplasty. Clin Orthop 321:151, 1995.
26. Ritter MA, Keating M, Faris PM: Screw and cement fixation of large defects in total knee arthroplasty. J Arthroplasty 8:63, 1993.
27. Stockley I, McAuley JP, Gross AE: Allograft reconstruction in total knee arthroplasty. J Bone Joint Surg Br 74:393, 1992.
28. Tsahakis PJ, Beaver WB, Brick GW: Technique and results of allograft reconstruction in revision total knee arthroplasty. Clin Orthop 303:86, 1994.
29. Urs WK, Binazzi R, Insall JN, et al: Custom total knee arthroplasty. Orthop Trans 12:711, 1988.
30. Whiteside LA: Cementless reconstruction of massive tibial bone loss in revision total knee arthroplasty. Clin Orthop 248:80, 1989.

31. Whiteside LA: Cementless revision total knee arthroplasty. Clin Orthop 286:160, 1993.
32. Whiteside LA, Ohl MD: Tibial tubercle osteotomy for exposure of the difficult total knee arthroplasty. Clin Orthop 260:6, 1990.
33. Wilde AH, Schickendantz MS, Stulberg BN, et al: The incorporation of tibial allografts in total knee arthroplasty. J Bone Joint Surg Am 72:815, 1990.
34. Windsor RE, Scuderi GR, Insall JN: Revision of well-fixed cemented, porous total knee arthroplasty: Report of six cases. J Arthroplasty 3:87, 1988.
35. Windsor RE, Scuderi GR, Moran MC, et al: Mechanisms of failure of the femoral and tibial components in total knee arthroplasty. Clin Orthop 248:15, 1989.

CHAPTER 101

The Infected Total Knee Replacement

R. Michael Meneghini • Arlen D. Hanssen

Deep infection remains one of the most devastating and challenging complications of total knee replacement (TKR). The complexity and duration of treatment often impart significant physical, emotional, and financial costs to both the patient and treating physicians.[53,103] Patients often require multiple operations and months of recovery and rehabilitation before establishing final function, which in many cases never returns to preoperative levels. Fortunately, treatment of periprosthetic knee infection has become more standardized and predictable with improved clinical outcomes over the past several decades.

The overall scope of prevention, diagnostic, and treatment principles for an infected TKR is complex and variable. Prevention of prosthetic joint infection relies on augmentation of the host's response, optimization the wound environment, and reduction of bacterial contamination in the preoperative, intraoperative, and postoperative period.[48] Definitive diagnosis is often difficult and requires a heightened sense of suspicion. Treatment strategies should focus on establishing a rapid and accurate diagnosis combined with the use of clear and effective treatment algorithms to optimize long-term patient outcomes.

RISK FACTORS AND PREVENTION

Incidence rates of infection after TKR have fallen over the past few decades as a result of improvements in prevention efforts and surgical techniques. The most notable improvement in the reduction of postoperative deep infection occurred with the routine use of perioperative prophylactic antibiotics.[54] Currently, the risk for postoperative infection after TKR is approximately 0.4% to 2%.[16,49,90] Risk factors include patient or host variables, the surgical technique, and a variety of aspects regarding the surgical environment and postoperative management of the knee replacement patient.

Host factors related to a patient's increased susceptibility to infection should be addressed before the procedure. A comprehensive list of host risk factors is presented in Table 101-1. Patients with systemic immunocompromise are clearly at higher risk of infection after total knee arthroplasty (TKA). Patients with rheumatoid arthritis or diabetes mellitus are at increased risk for the development of deep postoperative infection.[12,24,36,79,88,90] Liver or kidney transplantation is an additional risk factor associated with infection in TKA.[108] Human immunodeficiency virus seropositivity[89] and malignancy[12] have also been shown to be independent risk factors for the development of infection after TKA.

The treating surgeon must be aware of the increased risk in these immunosuppressed patient populations and take the necessary measures to minimize the potential for infection and optimize patient outcomes after TKA. Measures such as optimizing the medical treatment of a patient's diabetes mellitus or withholding many of the rheumatoid medications are examples of how the surgeon can optimize such patients' condition in the perioperative period.

Obesity has also been associated with an increased incidence of infection.[90,124] This association may in part be due to the difficulty that obesity imparts on the surgical technique inasmuch as others have not been able to demonstrate an association of obesity with deep infection.[40] Nevertheless, wound-healing issues and the potential increased risk for infection in this patient population must be appreciated before surgery. Previous knee surgery is another risk factor for the development of periprosthetic infection after TKA,[122] and increased rates of infection have also been demonstrated for revision knee procedures.[12,49,90] This increased rate of infection in the revision setting may, in part, represent an expression of occult infection that goes unrecognized in the preoperative period and is manifested after the revision surgery. Patients with previous infection, such as septic arthritis or adjacent osteomyelitis, are at increased risk for subsequent infection.[59,67] In these patients, an acceptably low rate of deep prosthetic infection can be achieved with careful preoperative and intraoperative evaluation combined with the routine use of antibiotic-loaded bone cement (ALBC).[67]

Antibiotic prophylaxis is the single-most effective method of reducing infection in TKA.[54] Cefazolin, a first-generation cephalosporin, meets the majority of these criteria sufficiently and is therefore a prudent choice.[48,101] For patients with a true type I hypersensitivity reaction to penicillin, vancomycin and clindamycin are excellent alternatives.[48] Because of the emergent resistance of organisms to vancomycin, this antimicrobial should not be used for routine prophylaxis unless deemed appropriate by the infection susceptibility patterns of that specific institution.[105] If vancomycin is chosen for prophylaxis, a maximum of two doses is recommended.[105]

The optimal time to administer prophylactic antibiotics is just before the skin incision.[25] Peak serum and bone concentrations of antibiotic in TKA typically occur within 20 minutes of systemic administration, and therefore administration of prophylactic antibiotic 30 to 60 minutes before incision represents the optimal time of delivery.[68] Although the optimal duration of postoperative prophylactic antibiotics has not been conclusively determined, it

Table 101–1. Host Risk Factors Associated with Infection in Total Knee Arthroplasty

Immunocompromise	Debilitation
Rheumatoid arthritis	Advanced age
Steroid therapy	Alcoholism
Diabetes mellitus	Renal failure
Poor nutrition	Liver cirrhosis
Human immunodeficiency virus	Prolonged preoperative hospitalization
Kidney or liver transplantation	
Hypokalemia	Hypothyroidism
Tobacco use	Previous surgery
Obesity	Psoriasis
Concurrent infection	Previous infection
Urinary tract	Infected total knee arthroplasty
Skin	Native joint septic arthritis
Soft tissue	Osteomyelitis

Table 101–2. Appropriate Indications for Prophylactic Low-Dose Antibiotic-Loaded Cement in Total Knee Replacement

PREVIOUS INFECTION	REVISION TOTAL KNEE ARTHROPLASTY
Immunosuppression	Systemic illness
Rheumatoid arthritis	Malignancy
Diabetes mellitus	Renal failure
Immunosuppressive medication	Liver cirrhosis

has been established that a relatively short duration of prophylaxis postoperatively is as effective as longer periods.[76] In 2004, a consensus advisory statement recommended that the first antimicrobial dose begin within 60 minutes before the incision and that prophylactic antibiotics be discontinued within 24 hours after surgery.[20] Although this consensus statement seems appropriate for routine primary TKR, the particular medical and surgical circumstances of each patient must be considered and administration of prophylaxis individualized on a case-by-case basis.

Curtailing risk factors associated with the surgical environment is critical for prevention of infection after TKR. Minimization of operating room personnel[97] and use of methods to reduce wound contamination such as iodophor drapes,[99] clean air,[13,90,98] and wearing of proper surgical attire[31] are all important prevention variables. Another pertinent risk factor for infection is increased duration of the surgical procedure. In a review of 6489 TKRs, the infection rate was significantly higher after procedures with an operative time longer than 2.5 hours.[90]

Intraoperative adjustments to the surgical procedure that are individualized for high-risk patients in an effort to reduce postoperative infection include the use of ALBC for fixation of the prosthesis. Low-dose (less than 2 g antibiotic powder per 40 g of cement) ALBC provides the necessary mechanical characteristics of cement for adequate implant fixation.[4,62] Routine prophylactic use of ALBC in all patients undergoing aseptic primary TKR is not currently supported by the available clinical literature.[45] There have been few prospective, randomized studies investigating the use of prophylactic low-dose ALBC in primary joint arthroplasty.[23,61,78] In a recent prospective, randomized trial comparing 340 primary TKRs with and without the use of prophylactic cefuroxime-impregnated cement, a statistically significant decrease in the infection rate was demonstrated in the group that received antibiotic-impregnated cement.[23] However, on

further evaluation of the study cohort, all infections occurred in patients with diabetes mellitus. It is critical to note that if those with diabetes mellitus were removed from the overall group of study patients, there would be no statistically significant difference in infection rates between groups.

Therefore, with the currently available literature, low-dose prophylactic ALBC can be recommended only for revision TKA and primary TKA in patients at high risk for periprosthetic infection, such as those with systemic immunosuppression or a previous history of infection (Table 101–2). Further investigation, including prospective, long-term outcome studies and cost-benefit analyses, is necessary to fully elucidate whether the benefit of routine use of low-dose prophylactic ALBC outweighs the potential disadvantages, including an increase in antibiotic resistance and potential increase in allergic reactions.

Hematogenous infection of TKA may occur in the early postoperative period or for many years after the arthroplasty. However, there appears to be a time-dependent wound susceptibility that is a fundamental consideration in antibiotic prophylaxis strategies to prevent bacteremia after TKR. The incidence rates of deep periprosthetic infection at the Mayo Clinic from 1969 to 1991 were analyzed.[47] The highest incidence rates for all microorganisms occurred in the first 3 months and gradually decreased to establish a stable incidence rate between 18 and 24 months after the index arthroplasty.[47] As the TKA wound and surrounding tissues heal and the inflammatory reaction subsides over the ensuing 18 to 24 months, the susceptibility of the wound and the subsequent rate of infection decrease to a steady state. In general, invasive procedures that potentially cause bacteremia should simply be avoided in the first 3 to 6 months after TKR.

Antimicrobial prophylaxis for patients with a TKR who undergo an invasive surgical procedure that is a potential source of bacteremia is a source of considerable controversy. The rate of bacteremia after invasive procedures has been reported, and the frequency appears to be highest with oral procedures, followed by genitourinary manipulation, and lowest in association with gastrointestinal procedures.[34] In a retrospective review of 3490 patients who received a TKR, 62 late infections were documented, 7 of which were strongly linked to a dental procedure.[116] The authors reported that these patients had systemic risk

Table 101–3. Patients at Potential Increased Risk of Experiencing Hematogenous Total Joint Infection

PATIENT TYPE	CONDITION PLACING PATIENT AT RISK
All patients for the first 2 years after joint replacement arthroplasty	N/A

Immunocompromised or immunosuppressed patients	Inflammatory arthropathies
	  Rheumatoid arthritis
	  Systemic lupus erythematosus
	Drug-induced immunosuppression
	Radiation-induced immunosuppression

Patients with comorbid conditions (other conditions not listed may apply to this category)	Previous prosthetic joint infections Poor nutrition Hemophilia Human immunodeficiency virus infection Insulin-dependent (type 1) diabetes Malignancy

factors for infection, such as rheumatoid arthritis or diabetes mellitus, and underwent dental procedures longer than 75 minutes in duration.

In 1997, the American Academy of Orthopaedic Surgeons (AAOS) and the American Dental Association (ADA) convened an authoritative panel of orthopedic surgeons, dentists, and infectious disease specialists to investigate the available literature and arrive at a consensus regarding antibiotic prophylaxis before dental procedures. An advisory statement was released that established the first 2 years after arthroplasty as a specific risk factor for all patients.[2] Therefore, when undergoing a high-risk dental procedure, all patients should receive antibiotic prophylaxis in the first 2 years. After that period, only patients considered to be at high risk are given prophylaxis for the remainder of their lifetime. In the subsequent 2003 advisory statement, the AAOS and ADA made some modifications to the classification of patients at potential risk (Table 101–3), but no changes in the recommended antibiotic regimens (Table 101–4).[2]

MICROBIOLOGY

An appreciation and understanding of the microbiology are essential to the management of an infected TKR. Optimal treatment outcomes are achieved by accurately identifying the involved organism and enacting medical and surgical treatment strategies that are directed accordingly. Several reports have documented the distribution of

the most frequent organisms involved in periprosthetic infection.[49,90,117] In all three series, the predominant organisms isolated were gram positive, with *Staphylococcus aureus*, coagulase-negative *Staphylococcus*, and *Streptococcus* species predominating. In a recent report of 116 infected TKRs, the most prevalent organism involved was *S. aureus* (35%), followed by coagulase-negative *Staphylococcus* (15%), *Streptococcus* species (6%), *Escherichia coli* (4%), and methicillin-resistant *S. aureus* (4%).[90] Furthermore, in 9% of patients the infections were polymicrobial, and there was no identifiable organism in 19%.[90] The distribution and pattern of specific organisms will vary among institutions and should be monitored closely for trends and antibiotic resistance as part of a comprehensive infection control program.

Resistance of bacteria to specific antibiotics continues to increase as a result of microbial genetic responses to antibiotics. Particular organisms prone to infecting TKRs have developed particularly troubling patterns of resistance. Methicillin-resistant *S. aureus* and methicillin-resistant coagulase-negative *Staphylococcus* have emerged as common nosocomial pathogens that often require complex antibiotic regimens and subsequently have inferior treatment outcomes.[63] In a study of 35 infected TKRs, those infected with methicillin-sensitive organisms had a treatment success rate of 89% versus only 18% in those with methicillin-resistant infections.[63] Vancomycin is typically the antibiotic of choice in these methicillin-resistant infections; however, vancomycin-resistant *Enterococcus* species have also emerged and represent an uncommon, but devastating periprosthetic pathogen.[96]

Table 101–4. Recommended Antibiotic Prophylaxis Regimens

PATIENT TYPE	SUGGESTED DRUG	REGIMEN
Not allergic to penicillin	Cephalexin, cephradine, or amoxicillin	2 g orally 1 hour before dental procedure
Not allergic to penicillin Not able to take oral medications	Cefazolin or ampicillin	Cefazolin, 1 g, or ampicillin, 2 g, IM or IV 1 hour before dental procedure
Allergic to penicillin	Clindamycin	600 mg orally 1 hour before dental procedure
Allergic to penicillin Not able to take oral medications	Clindamycin	600 mg IV 1 hour before dental procedure

No second doses are recommended for any of the above dosing regimens.

Periprosthetic fungal infections are rare, with *Candida* being the predominant species.[92] A review of 10 cases of candidal periprosthetic joint infection documented successful treatment without relapse in 8 of 10 patients with appropriate antifungal therapy and a two-stage reimplantation.[92] Prosthetic joint infection caused by *Mycobacterium tuberculosis* is also rare. In a review of seven cases, tuberculous prosthetic joint infection most often represented reactivation of previous tuberculous septic arthritis.[11] To decrease the risk of reactivation of quiescent tuberculous infection, consideration should be given to preoperative or perioperative antituberculous prophylaxis.[11]

In the presence of prosthetic implants, most bacteria elaborate a mucopolysaccharide biofilm. This biofilm is a barrier that protects the organism from surfactants, opsonic antibodies, phagocytes, and antibiotic agents, thereby increasing the organism's virulence.[5] These protective biofilms can create an environment for persistent infection despite appropriate antimicrobial therapy, especially when combined with inadequate surgical débridement. Identification and diagnosis of biofilm organisms via traditional culture methods have lacked optimal sensitivity and specificity.[112] Therefore, the development of culture-independent, molecular-based methods such as polymerase chain reaction detection aims to improve our diagnostic ability and subsequent treatment of biofilm organisms. Various antibiofilm strategies directed at disruption of adherent bacteria are the focus of intense research to improve the detection of biofilm organisms and eradicate them.[112] Currently, rifampin is an antibiotic with good biofilm and tissue penetration and has been shown to improve treatment success when used in conjunction with other specific synergistic antimicrobial agents.[126]

DIAGNOSIS

The fundamentals of diagnosis include a high index of suspicion combined with a thorough history, physical examination, plain radiographs, arthrocentesis, and hematological studies. Radionuclide studies and evaluation of surgical tissue specimens are occasionally necessary to establish the diagnosis. The timing of the clinical infection is a critical factor in identification and implementation of the correct treatment strategy (Table 101–5).

Various clinical features have been characterized and classified as a useful guide to select the most appropriate treatment option for an infected TKR.[104] As such, rapid and expedient diagnosis is essential to prevent a delay in diagnosis, which could result in the diagnosis of a late or chronic infection that could have been identified and treated as an early infection.

Pain is the most common initial symptom in a patient with an infected knee TKR and typically occurs at rest. Persistent postoperative pain or progressive pain that fails to abate after surgery is a worrisome sign that may indicate deep infection. Persistent wound drainage is strongly suggestive of infection and should probably be treated by arthrotomy, débridement, and irrigation within the first several weeks after surgery.[118] Cultures of serous wound drainage are difficult to interpret and potentially misleading and are therefore discouraged. Empiric antibiotic use for persistent wound drainage should be avoided because it only suppresses the clinical symptoms of infection, potentially delays diagnosis, and eliminates the possibility of treatment of the infection without removal of the prosthesis.[19,80,102,110]

The diagnosis of early postoperative infection is typically confirmed by joint arthrocentesis because the erythrocyte sedimentation rate (ESR) and C-reactive protein (CRP) levels are nonspecific in the early postoperative period. Although CRP levels typically rise to higher values after TKA than after hip arthroplasty, CRP levels after both TKA and hip arthroplasty peak on postoperative day 2 and decrease to preoperative baseline levels as early as 1 week, but generally 14 to 21 days postoperatively.[15,66,119] In the early postoperative period, assertive management of delayed wound healing or marginal skin necrosis by débridement of necrotic skin and primary wound closure is preferable to empiric antibiotic treatment, prolonged observation, and the eventual development of deep infection.[70]

An acute hematogenous infection is typically manifested as a sudden onset of pain or stiffness in a previously well functioning arthroplasty.[9] Specific risk factors for hematogenous infection should be identified, such as a remote source of infection or a recent invasive procedure causing significant bacteremia.[73] The severity of symptoms in this setting, including pain, effusion, and restricted range of knee motion, facilitates rapid diagnosis. Although the ESR and CRP are typically elevated in these patients, the cornerstone of diagnosis is arthrocentesis with evaluation by Gram stain, quantitative leukocyte count, and

---

Table 101–5. Classification of Deep Periprosthetic Infection

	TYPE 1	TYPE 2	TYPE 3	TYPE 4
Timing	Positive intraoperative culture	Early postoperative infection	Acute hematogenous infection	Late (chronic) infection
Definition	Two or more positive cultures at surgery	Infection occurs within the 1st month after surgery	Hematogenous seeding of previously well functioning arthroplasty	Chronic indolent clinical course; infection present for more than 1 month
Treatment	Appropriate antibiotics	Attempt at débridement with prosthesis salvage	Attempt at débridement with prosthesis salvage or prosthesis removal	Prosthesis removal

culture for aerobic and anaerobic bacteria. Administration of empiric antibiotics for an unexplained painful TKR, without an attempt at definitive diagnosis, is unfortunately quite common, and this approach only complicates subsequent efforts to diagnose deep infection.

In the vast majority of patients, an infected TKA is diagnosed in the subacute or chronic setting. Historical factors such as persistent pain since the arthroplasty, prolonged postoperative wound drainage (Fig. 101–1), antibiotic treatment for difficulties with primary wound healing, and knee stiffness despite extensive rehabilitation efforts may be indicative of deep infection. Comparison of sequential plain radiographs may reveal progressive radiolucencies (Fig. 101–2), focal osteopenia or osteolysis of subchondral bone, and periosteal new bone formation.[83] Additional studies should include a peripheral white blood cell count, CRP, ESR, and aspiration of the affected TKR.

Arthrocentesis is considered an essential element of the workup and evaluation for a suspected deep periprosthetic infection.[8,33,69,111] A synovial fluid leukocyte differential of greater than 65% neutrophils (or a leukocyte count >1.7 × 10³/μL) is a sensitive and specific test for the diagnosis of deep periprosthetic infection in patients without underlying inflammatory disease.[111] Patients should not have been taking antibiotics several weeks before aspiration because this oversight frequently accounts for the inability to isolate organisms. In a series of 69 knees, preoperative aspiration had a sensitivity of 55%, specificity of 96%, and accuracy of 84%.[8] It is important to note that in

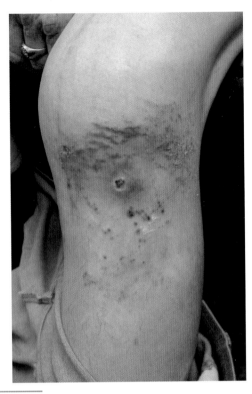

Figure 101–1. Photograph of a chronic sinus tract over the anterolateral aspect of the knee joint in a patient with a chronically infected total knee replacement.

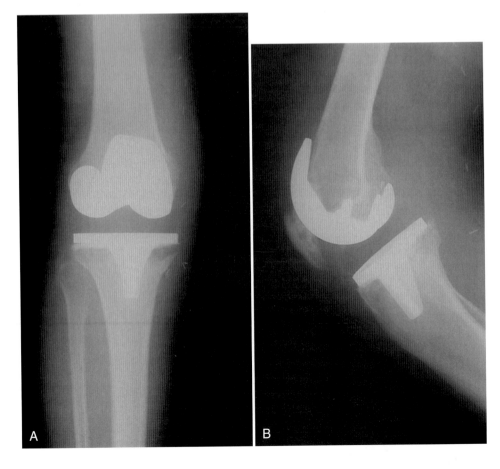

Figure 101–2. Anteroposterior (**A**) and lateral (**B**) radiographs of a patient with a chronically infected total knee arthroplasty. Radiolucencies at the bone-cement interface, which are typically late findings in periprosthetic infection, can be seen inferior to the tibial component on both views.

12 of the infected knees, antibiotics were being taken at the time of aspiration and 7 (58%) of these knee cultures had no growth. After antibiotic therapy was discontinued, four knees were reaspirated and all had a positive culture. The overall sensitivity improved to 75%, the specificity to 96%, and the accuracy to 90%,[8] and these authors recommend routine aspiration before any revision knee arthroplasty. Isolation of microorganisms from the aspirate also helps direct the initial choice of antibiotic after removal of the infected prosthesis.

The use of radioisotope scans to facilitate diagnosis of a chronically infected knee prosthesis is occasionally helpful.[100] A screening technetium 99 study may be useful when the study demonstrates the absence of significant tracer uptake because this finding rules out the possibility of deep infection. Indium 111 leukocyte scanning alone appears to be more accurate (78%) than technetium 99 diphosphonate bone scanning alone (74%); however, the combination of indium 111 leukocyte scanning and technetium 99 sulfur colloid marrow scintigraphy improves the accuracy to 88% to 95%.[100] The use of molecular genetic diagnostic methods with joint aspirates, such as the polymerase chain reaction technique, is potentially promising but remains an experimental modality for diagnosis of an infected joint arthroplasty.[74]

Despite all reasonable efforts to diagnose infection preoperatively, intraoperative evaluation of surgical tissue specimens may be necessary to confirm the diagnosis in difficult cases. Gram stain is notoriously unreliable, with a high percentage of false-negative results and extremely low sensitivity.[6,29] Intraoperative frozen section testing to detect infection has been widely used, but with variable published results.[28,38,71,84,86] This variability is probably due to differences in technique, sampling errors during retrieval of tissue, pathologist experience, and the definition used to declare the presence of infection. The positive predictive value of frozen sections is significantly better ($p < 0.05$) when the index is increased from 5 to 10 polymorphonuclear leukocytes per high-power field.[71] Analysis of intraoperative frozen sections is a reasonable and reliable method when an accomplished and experienced pathologist evaluates appropriate tissue samples.

Though difficult to assess quantitatively, the surgeon's intraoperative evaluation is also very helpful. If there is any reason to suspect deep infection during the course of revision surgery, one should obtain multiple tissue specimens for culture and sensitivity testing and then await the final results. In this setting, a careful review of the history, ESR, and CRP, combined with the results of culture and final interpretation by the pathologist, will often allow a determination of whether infection is present. Our current definition of prosthetic infection includes a combination of clinical signs and symptoms, histological analysis of tissue, and results of culture. A diagnosis of definite infection is made if evaluation of the knee establishes at least one of the following criteria: (1) two or more cultures of material obtained by aspiration or deep tissue specimens obtained at surgery yield the same organism, (2) histopathological evaluation of intra-articular tissue reveals changes of acute inflammation, (3) gross purulence is observed at the time of surgery, or (4) an actively discharging sinus tract is present.[50]

TREATMENT

Once the diagnosis has been established, variables that must be considered before initiating treatment include (1) determination of whether the infection is superficial or deep, (2) the duration of time elapsed between the arthroplasty and diagnosis of infection, (3) identification of host factors that may adversely affect treatment of the infection, (4) appraisal of the soft-tissue envelope surrounding the knee and specifically the integrity of the extensor mechanism, (5) determination of whether the implant is loose or well fixed, (6) consideration of the pathogen or pathogens responsible for the infection, (7) the physician's ability to provide the proper level of care required, and (8) careful assessment of the patient's expectations and functional requirements.

Treatment goals for an infected TKA include eradication of infection, alleviation of pain, and maintenance of a functional extremity. The six basic treatment options include (1) antibiotic suppression, (2) open débridement, (3) reimplantation of another prosthesis (4) arthrodesis, (5) resection arthroplasty, and (6) amputation. With the exception of chronic antibiotic suppression, which does not eliminate infection, the cornerstone treatment options include thorough surgical débridement combined with the appropriate use of antibiotics and optimization of the host response. When confronted with an infected TKR, the treating physician should start by considering the question of whether the prosthesis can be retained or whether removal is required to treat the infection.

Treatment Methods Whereby the Prosthesis Is Retained

ANTIBIOTIC SUPPRESSION

Antibiotic treatment alone will not eliminate deep periprosthetic infection but can be used as suppressive treatment when the following criteria are met: (1) prosthesis removal is not feasible (usually because of a medical condition that precludes an operative procedure), (2) the microorganism has low virulence, (3) the microorganism is susceptible to an oral antibiotic, (4) the antibiotic can be tolerated without serious toxicity, and (5) the prosthesis is not loose.[113] The presence of other joint arthroplasties or a cardiac valvular prosthesis is a relatively strong contraindication to chronic antibiotic suppression as a treatment choice.

In a multicenter study, antibiotic suppression was successful in only 40 of 225 knees (18%).[10] Combining several series reveals that antibiotic suppression was successful in 62 (24%) of 261 knees.[49] Use of a combined regimen of rifampin with a quinolone has been reported to be more successful than treatment with a single antibiotic.[32] Despite the fact that most patients fail to meet all these selection criteria, antibiotic suppression is commonly practiced and unfortunately prolongs the presence of infection and often complicates subsequent treatment attempts. Long-term antibiotic suppression should be rarely initiated and only considered when all treatment criteria are met.

DÉBRIDEMENT WITH PROSTHESIS RETENTION

Open débridement may be indicated for the occasional acute infection in the early postoperative period (type 2) or for acute hematogenous infection (type 3) of a securely fixed and functional prosthesis. Suggested criteria for implementation of this treatment technique include (1) a less than 2-week duration of symptoms of infection, (2) susceptible gram-positive organisms, (3) absence of prolonged postoperative drainage or a draining sinus tract, and (4) no prosthetic loosening or radiographic evidence of infection.[19] A relative contraindication to débridement and attempted salvage of the prosthesis is the presence other joint replacements or a cardiac valve prosthesis.

The results of débridement are difficult to determine because of differences in microbiology and subsequent antibiotic management, variability in the time to treatment, quality of the soft-tissue envelope, extent and completeness of débridement, the status of implant fixation, and the criteria for success in each report. A multicenter study reported a success rate of only 19.5% with open débridement of 154 knees.[10] In a recent literature review, a success rate of 32.6% was reported in 530 infected TKRs treated by open débridement and component retention.[106] Factors identified with failure of open débridement included postoperative drainage longer than 2 weeks in duration, existence of a sinus tract at débridement, hinged prostheses, and immunocompromised hosts.[106]

The importance of the timing of the débridement in relation to the onset of symptoms or the period elapsed since insertion of the prosthesis cannot be overemphasized.[19,81,102,104,109] In a study of 24 infected TKRs treated by open débridement and retention of the component, successful treatment was demonstrated in 100% of the early postoperative infection group (type 2) and 71% of the acute hematogenous group with less than a 30-day duration of symptoms.[81] These authors emphasized strict selection criteria, with patients appropriate for retention of the component demonstrating evidence of infection for less than 30 days.[81] It is quite clear that débridement with prosthesis retention should not be attempted in patients with chronic infections.[18,60,104]

As just detailed, expeditious treatment as soon as possible after the diagnosis of infection has been established is the paramount concern, particularly for *S. aureus*, because delay beyond 48 hours after the onset of symptoms results in a significant decrease in the success rate.[19] The specific organism and its virulence are significant predictors of success after open débridement. It is well documented that *S. aureus* prosthetic joint infection is associated with the lowest success rate after débridement.[27,102,122] In contrast, in a report of 19 cases of infection with penicillin-susceptible streptococcal species in which surgical débridement was performed in all patients within 10 days of symptom onset, treatment success was documented in 89.5% of cases.[80] In a recent report, only 1 (8%) of 13 patients infected with *S. aureus* was successfully treated as compared with 10 (56%) of 18 infected with either *Staphylococcus epidermidis* or a streptococcal species.[27]

Although arthroscopy has been recommended as a method of débridement for an infected TKA, the ability to perform satisfactory débridement of proliferative synovitis and the scarring associated with deep periprosthetic infection is usually limited. Furthermore, modular implants cannot be adequately débrided between the metal tibial tray and polyethylene tibial insert. In a series of 16 infected TKAs treated by arthroscopic débridement, there were four type 2 and 12 type 4 infections.[115] All patients were treated within the first 7 days after the onset of symptoms. Only 6 (38%) of the knees were successfully treated, whereas the remaining 10 knee required prosthesis removal. These results were significantly worse than the 71% success rate obtained with open débridement performed by these authors.[81] They therefore recommend open débridement in preference to arthroscopic débridement for an infected TKA, except for selected circumstances such as medically unstable or anticoagulated patients.

Treatment Methods Whereby the Prosthesis Is Removed

RESECTION ARTHROPLASTY

Definitive resection arthroplasty involves removal of the implant with no intention of subsequent knee reconstruction. The ideal candidate for definitive resection arthroplasty is a patient with polyarticular rheumatoid arthritis and limited ambulatory demands who wishes to be able to sit more readily than feasible with a knee arthrodesis. Patients with less disability are likely to be less satisfied with resection arthroplasty.[37] The primary disadvantage of resection arthroplasty is the frequent occurrence of knee instability associated with pain during transfer or ambulation. In a report of 28 knees in 26 patients who were treated by resection arthroplasty as a salvage procedure for infected TKAs, 89% were free of infection at an average of 5 years after their resection arthroplasty.[37] Functional results were suboptimal: 15 patients were independent walkers but all used walking aids, only 5 had sufficient knee stability for walking without external support, 8 required a knee-ankle-foot orthosis, and 2 used a splint.[37] In 15 knees (15 patients) with infected constrained TKAs treated by resection arthroplasty, infection was eradicated in all knees evaluated at 4-year follow-up.[65]

The three basic fundamentals of the operative technique include (1) initial débridement and removal of all infected tissue and foreign material, (2) temporary fixation with pins or sutures to maintain alignment and apposition of the tibia and femur, and (3) cast immobilization, with weightbearing permitted, for at least 6 months. Although resection arthroplasty usually achieves satisfactory resolution of infection, most patients experience some pain, knee instability, and limited ambulatory capacity. Definitive resection arthroplasty is rarely performed unless the patient has severe polyarticular involvement and limited ambulatory demands.

ARTHRODESIS

Formerly, arthrodesis was considered the gold standard treatment option for an infected TKR because of its excellent potential for resolving infection, alleviating pain, and providing stable knee function. These advantages are offset by the elimination of knee motion, which often makes sitting and other activities cumbersome. Currently, the functional limitations of an arthrodesis seem to be poorly tolerated and unacceptable to most patients. In a report of 30 patients who either experienced spontaneous ankylosis or underwent conversion of TKA to formal arthrodesis, 17 had attempted suicide preoperatively because of unhappiness regarding the affected extremity.[64] Before the procedure, a detailed discussion should be carried out with the patient regarding the physical limitations and functional restrictions imposed by knee arthrodesis.

Indications for arthrodesis after failed TKA include (1) individuals with high functional demands, (2) single-joint disease, (3) young age, (4) disruption of the extensor mechanism, (5) poor soft-tissue envelope requiring extensive reconstruction, (6) systemic immunocompromise, and (7) microorganisms that require highly toxic antibiotic therapy or are resistant to conventional antibiotics.[49] Relative contraindications include (1) bilateral knee disease, (2) ipsilateral ankle or hip disease, (3) severe segmental bone loss, and (4) contralateral extremity amputation.

The fixation techniques most commonly used for knee arthrodesis include external fixation and internal fixation with an intramedullary nail or dual-plate fixation. The type of previous knee implant, the extent of bone deficiency, and the arthrodesis technique affect the success of knee arthrodesis after TKA.[22,30,49] In general, intramedullary nailing appears to be a more reliable technique for achieving union than external fixation techniques, with union achieved in 67% to 100%.[49] The primary disadvantage of intramedullary fixation as compared with external fixation is that if infection recurs, extension of infection along the intramedullary nail can result in extensive osteomyelitis of the femoral and tibial shafts. The primary advantage of external fixation as opposed to intramedullary nailing is that external fixation can be applied at the time of prosthesis removal whereas intramedullary nailing requires a delay between implant removal and nail insertion.

Inherent complications of arthrodesis after TKA include nonunion, recurrent infection, and ipsilateral limb fracture, with the most frequent being nonunion. Causes of nonunion include bone deficiency, persistent infection, poor bone apposition, malalignment, and inadequate immobilization.[49] Specific complications associated with the external fixation technique include neurovascular injury during pin insertion, pin site infection, and fractures through pin sites, with complications reported in 20% to 65% of patients.[94] Complications associated with intramedullary nailing for arthrodesis have been reported in 40% to 56% of cases and include nail breakage and nail migration.[94]

AMPUTATION

Patients with an infected TKR commonly express the fear of eventual amputation. It is rarely indicated except for life-threatening systemic sepsis or persistent local infection associated with massive bone loss. Amputation is estimated to occur in less than 5% of patients treated for an infected TKA.[49] The most common factors leading to amputation include multiple revision attempts for chronic infection, severe bone loss, and intractable pain.[58] Consideration of arthrodesis earlier in the treatment process, when adequate bone stock still remains, rather than repeated attempts at revision surgery in the presence of chronic infection helps reduce the incidence of amputation after failed TKA.

The amputation should be at a level that maximizes function yet facilitates the eradication of infection. Many patients have a cavernous bone defect of the distal end of the femur, and local transposition of the gastrocnemius muscles during the amputation procedure can be extremely helpful for dead space management, as well as optimizing the soft-tissue envelope of the amputation stump. After amputation, many elderly patients remain limited ambulators or are nonambulatory because of the increased energy expenditure required for walking. Of 23 patients treated by above-knee amputation for a failed TKA, only 7 could ambulate regularly, 20 of the 23 used a wheelchair part of the day, and 12 (52%) were confined to the wheelchair.[93]

REIMPLANTATION

Reimplantation, or reinsertion of another prosthesis, has become the primary accepted method of treatment for selected patients with an infected TKR. Generally accepted contraindications for insertion of another prosthesis include (1) persistent or recalcitrant infection, (2) medical conditions that prevent multiple reconstructive procedures, (3) disruption of the extensor mechanism, and (4) a poor soft-tissue envelope about the knee joint.[49]

The optimal duration and route of antibiotic delivery for treatment of an infected knee arthroplasty have not been clearly determined. A 6-week course of intravenous antibiotic administration before reimplantation has provided excellent success rates and is the most commonly accepted clinical standard.[42,57,123] Most 6-week intravenous regimen studies did not routinely use adjunctive methods such as antibiotic-impregnated cement spacers or antibiotic-impregnated cement for fixation of the prosthesis.[57,123] Furthermore, no published trials have directly compared different durations of antibiotic treatment of an infected TKR.

Excellent success with a shorter duration of 3 or 4 weeks of intravenous antibiotics combined with ALBC has been reported.[18,121] In a retrospective analysis of 89 infected TKRs, there were no differences between patients treated with antibiotic-impregnated cement spacers and those treated with 4 weeks or 6 weeks of intravenous antibiotics.[50] Ultimately, the duration of antibiotic therapy should probably be individualized for each patient according to the virulence of the microorganism, comorbid conditions, and whether antibiotic-impregnated spacers or beads are also being used to deliver adjunctive antibiotics.

Immediate Exchange

Reimplantation can be performed as a direct exchange technique or by delayed reinsertion of the new prosthesis (two-stage approach) after antibiotic therapy. Success with direct exchange appears to be dependent on the presence of gram-positive infection, use of ALBC for fixation of the new prosthesis, and prolonged use of antibiotics after the revision surgery.[106] It would appear that the use of ALBC is particularly important because direct exchange procedures performed without the use of antibiotic-loaded cement were successful in only 11 (58%) of 19 knees.[49] When multiple series are combined, the success rate for a one-stage exchange technique using ALBC is 74% (131 of 176 knees).[49]

In an extensive literature review of direct exchange arthroplasty with the use of ABLC, successful control of infection was documented in 33 (89.2%) of 37 infected knees.[106] These authors suggest that factors associated with successful direct exchange include (1) infection by gram-positive organisms, (2) absence of sinus formation, (3) use of ALBC for the new prosthesis, and (4) a prolonged 12-week course of antibiotic therapy.[106] It is important to note that the reports analyzed by these authors primarily involved patients who were treated in the 1980s and that in the current era of drug-resistant organisms and severe bone loss, direct exchange techniques are indicated only in a highly selected group of patients by arthroplasty surgeons familiar with the treatment of periprosthetic infections.

Delayed Two-Stage Reimplantation

Delayed reimplantation after the administration of intravenous antibiotics appears to offer better overall success rates than direct exchange techniques do, and delayed reconstruction is the most commonly accepted approach in North America for treatment of an infected knee arthroplasty.[49] The exact time delay before reimplantation has not been established. Initially, a poor success rate (57%) was reported in 14 patients who underwent insertion of a new prosthesis within several weeks after removal of the infected knee prosthesis.[95] In contrast, the two-stage reimplantation protocol proposed by Insall et al has been a highly effective method of treatment.[57] This protocol includes soft-tissue débridement, removal of the infected prosthesis and cement followed by 6 weeks of intravenous antibiotics, and subsequent reimplantation. The success of this protocol was confirmed in a follow-up report of 64 infected TKRs.[42] These early reports established the commonly accepted time delay of 6 weeks before reimplantation; however, it is important to note that ALBC in the form of spacers or as prosthetic fixation was not used.

Many subsequent studies have used ALBC spacers in the interval between removal of the infected prosthesis and eventual reimplantation, and many also used antibiotic-loaded cement for fixation of the prosthesis at

reimplantation.[49] Use of the adjunctive antibiotic delivery provided by ALBC has gradually led to decreased antibiotic duration and shorter time delays before reimplantation.[49] Although some investigators have shortened this time frame to several weeks, large prospective trials are necessary to settle this issue.

The use of antibiotic-impregnated cement for prosthesis fixation has been reported to exert a beneficial effect at the time of reimplantation.[46] Of 89 infected TKRs treated by reimplantation, ALBC for prosthesis fixation was a significant treatment variable inasmuch as reinfection developed in 7 (28%) of the 25 knees without the use of ALBC versus only 3 (4.7%) of 64 knees in which ALBC was used to fix the prosthesis. This difference was statistically significant irrespective of the duration of intravenous antibiotics ($p = 0.0025$).[46]

On review of the literature regarding treatment of periprosthetic infection, it appears that the overall success rate is greater with the use of delayed reimplantation in a two-stage reconstruction. Early reimplantation in less than 3 weeks without antibiotic-loaded cement provided success in only 11 (58%) of 19 knees, whereas direct exchange techniques with antibiotic-loaded cement for prosthesis fixation were successful in 131 (74%) of 176 knees.[49] In the reports detailing delayed reimplantation, implant fixation without ALBC was successful in 65 (88%) of 74 knees, whereas the use of ALBC resulted in success in 254 (92%) of 277 knees.[49] This would suggest that in general, the best chance for cure is with ALBC used with a two-stage reconstruction and an appropriate time interval between resection and TKA reimplantation.

Antibiotic Cement Spacers

During the time after resection of an infected TKA, before the eventual reimplantation of another prosthesis, local antibiotic therapy is delivered via static or articulating spacer blocks. Most reports have used antibiotic ratios of only 1 g of antibiotic per 40-g batch of bone cement in ALBC.[49,50,122] Currently, most investigators use higher dosage ratios such as 4 to 6 g of antibiotic per 40-g batch of bone cement.[43,51,91] Low-dose ALBC (<2 g antibiotic/ 40 g cement) should be used for prophylaxis in reimplantation, for primary TKAs in high-risk patients, or for fixation of the prosthesis at reimplantation.[45] Higher-dose antibiotic-loaded cement should be reserved for the treatment of active infection and used as spacers because more than 4.5 g of antibiotic powder substantially diminishes the mechanical strength of bone cement and should not be used for prosthesis fixation.[45,51,107]

Antibiotic elution is highly dependent on the porosity of the bone cement, and mixing high doses of powdered antibiotics creates considerable cement porosity, thereby facilitating increased antibiotic elution for at least 4 weeks.[51] Combining two antibiotics in bone cement will improve the elution of both antibiotics, and the two most commonly used antibiotics in clinical practice are vancomycin and tobramycin.[49] The use of at least 3.6 g of tobramycin and 1 g of vancomycin per package of bone cement is recommended to obtain effective elution levels.[75,91] The local levels of antibiotic elution typically far exceed the levels observed in serum during parenteral antibiotic administration.[51] Up to 12 g of antibiotic per 40-g batch of bone cement may be used without prohibiting cement polymerization.[1] The systemic safety of high-dose ALBC for an infected TKR has been established.[107]

The primary functions of block spacers are delivery of local antimicrobial agents and maintenance of collateral ligament length.[17] Potential disadvantages of block spacers include the presence of a foreign body and bone loss incurred while awaiting reimplantation.[21] Essentially, the different types of block spacers include a simple tibiofemoral block, a molded arthrodesis block, articulating mobile spacers, and medullary dowels. The simple tibiofemoral block was the original spacer block; it was preformed and then inserted into the tibiofemoral space after the cement had polymerized. These blocks were shaped as either simple "hockey pucks" or "L-shaped" spacers inserted into the tibiofemoral space. Additional antibiotic beads or thin disks were often placed in the suprapatellar pouch or lateral gutters. Difficulties with this type of block spacer included an inability to match the surfaces of the block with the irregular surfaces of the distal femur and proximal tibia, subluxation of the bony surfaces off the spacer surface, instances of extensor mechanism necrosis, wound breakdown, and progressive bone loss.[21]

The molded arthrodesis block method avoids some of the difficulties encountered with preformed spacer blocks.[51] With this spacer technique the cement is placed within the knee in a doughy state and polymerized within the knee so that it can conform to the irregular contour of the femur and tibia (Fig. 101–3). This macrointerdigitation of the cement into bone defects and the intercondylar notch and extension into the medullary canals and suprapatellar pouch create stability of the knee joint. This stability is helpful for patient comfort and prevents the problems of spacer migration and progressive bone erosion. Removal of these spacers requires fragmentation of the spacer into several large pieces with an osteotome at the time of reimplantation.

The mobile articulating spacer technique allows the patient to place the knee though a range of motion during the period after prosthesis removal before insertion of the new prosthesis.[43,56] These spacers, originally facsimiles of antibiotic-impregnated cement shaped into femoral and tibial components, allowed knee motion through articulation of the acrylic cement surfaces.[43] Eventually, a system of molds was developed to incorporate small metal runners and polyethylene tibial trays so that the cement surfaces were not articulating against each other.[43] One alternative has been to sterilize the prosthesis just removed and then incorporates the femoral component and tibial tray into the antibiotic-loaded spacer.[56]

The theoretic advantages of mobile articulating spacers include the potential for improved functional outcomes and better range of motion, yet conclusive results in this regard have not been realized.[35,39] In a series of 55 patients, 25 with solid spacers and 30 with mobile articulating spacers, there was no difference between the two groups with respect to knee scores or final range of motion.[39] In a recent report of two-stage reimplantation in which 26 septic TKAs treated with static antibiotic spacers were

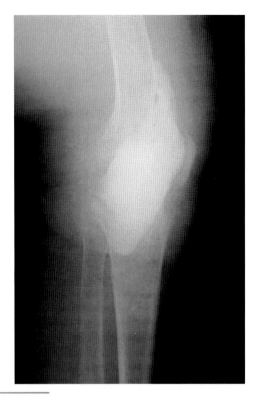

Figure 101–3. Lateral radiograph of a static antibiotic cement spacer molded to conform to the femoral and tibial osseous surfaces with extension into the suprapatellar pouch to prevent scarring and adhesion of the extensor mechanism to the anterior aspect of the femur.

compared with a group of 22 septic TKAs treated with mobile articulating spacers, no difference was found in reinfection rates between the groups at 36 months.[35] The mobile articulating spacer group demonstrated significantly better average range of motion (107.8 degrees) than the static spacer group (93.7 degrees) did at final follow-up.[35] However, these data may be misleading because the study was not a comparative study of concurrent cohorts inasmuch as the static spacer block group was a historical comparison group with different adjunctive treatment methods. Furthermore, articulating spacers appear to simplify the surgical exposure at reimplantation.

Regardless of whether a static or mobile articulating antibiotic-loaded spacer is used, strong consideration should be given to insertion of antibiotic-impregnated cement into the canals (see Fig. 101–6).[51] The infectious process extends into the medullary canals of the femur or tibia in roughly a third of infected knee replacements without stems.[77] Insertion of antibiotic-impregnated medullary dowels is preferable to insertion of ALBC beads because these beads are often extremely difficult to remove at reimplantation. A tapered cement dowel fashioned from the nozzle of a cement gun provides an excellent size and shape to be inserted into and subsequently removed from the medullary canal.[51]

To date, there have been no significant differences between knee scores, functional scores, or range-of-motion arc when the knees are analyzed according to length of delay, type of knee prosthesis used at reimplantation, or the use of a block cement spacer versus a mobile articulating spacer.[50] The final functional result appears to be more dependent on the patient's overall medical and musculoskeletal functional status.[117] Despite the lack of evidence for improved functional outcomes with the use of spacers, the advantages of mechanical stability for the patient and the reduced difficulty of surgical exposure at reimplantation have led to common acceptance and use of these ALBC spacers. Block spacers should be supplemented by external immobilization, such as a brace or cast, while the patient awaits reimplantation. Patients with mobile articulating spacers are encouraged to perform range-of-motion exercises and are allowed up to 50% partial weightbearing.[43] Patients with bilateral infected TKRs are excellent candidates for the use of articulating mobile ALBC spacers.[125]

Period between Resection and Reimplantation

Patients undergoing two-stage reimplantation are typically anemic, with 88% requiring allogeneic blood transfusions, particularly since the two surgeries are temporally close.[87] The presence of infection precludes traditional alternatives such as reinfusion or autologous blood donation; thus, novel blood management practices are required in this patient population. A prospective study of 39 consecutive two-stage reimplantations was conducted to determine whether the use of recombinant human erythropoietin could lower allogeneic transfusion requirements.[26] When compared with a group of 81 patients not receiving recombinant human erythropoietin, the requirement for transfusion was significantly lowered ($p < 0.001$). In patients receiving recombinant human erythropoietin, 52% avoided transfusion for the entire period encompassing both stages of reimplantation.[26]

One of the most important issues for both the patient and surgeon is determination of when it is safe and appropriate to proceed with reimplantation. In just 4 or 6 weeks, the ESR is not expected to normalize; however, the trend should suggest that the values obtained just before reimplantation have improved.[49] CRP levels typically normalize by the 21st day after surgery, and levels that remain elevated may suggest the presence of persistent infection.[15,49,119] Open biopsy or aspiration for culture and sensitivity has been suggested before proceeding with reimplantation.[82] However, a recent study reported 8 false-negative aspirations out of 32 resection TKAs with the use of antibiotic spacers and 6 weeks of intravenous antibiotic treatment before reimplantation.[72] The authors reported that preoperative aspiration before reimplantation has a sensitivity of 0%, a positive predictive value of 0%, and an accuracy of 71% and cannot be recommended for routine use.

It is preferable to base intraoperative decision making on the appearance of the knee joint supplemented by analysis of frozen sections. However, is important to recognize that this method requires considerable experience on the part of the surgeon and pathologist and that the presence of spacers or beads may alter the appearance of the tissues at reimplantation.[28] Analysis of frozen sections at reimplantation to determine the presence of infection has a sensitivity of 25%, specificity of 98%, positive predictive value of 50%, negative predictive value of 9%, and accuracy of 94%.[28] If there is concern about the presence of persistent infection, it is prudent to perform another débridement, insert new ALBC spacers, and await culture and sensitivity testing.

Results of Reimplantation

The midterm to long-term results of reimplantation are beginning to emerge in the literature.[42,44] In two studies of delayed reimplantation protocols with a mean of 7 years' follow-up, both reported that 9% of the knees required component removal for infection and 6% were revised because of aseptic loosening. A recent report of 46 infected TKRs at an average follow-up of 5 years documented a 93.5% success rate with no difference in failure rates between TKRs infected with methicillin-sensitive and methicillin-resistant organisms.[114] These results suggest that the high likelihood of success after two-stage reimplantation for an infected TKA is well maintained through long-term follow-up and that two-stage reimplantation is an acceptable treatment option for infections with resistant and virulent organisms, with only a modest rate of reinfection.

Staged Reimplantation Surgical Technique

Thorough and complete débridement is of paramount concern to ensure treatment success in staged reimplantation of an infected TKR. Careful placement of the skin incision is critical, and when multiple previous incisions are present, use of the most lateral, longitudinal midline incision is recommended. Excision of heavily scarred tissue back to healthy tissue is advised, as well as excision of all sinus tracts. Subcutaneous tissue flap elevation during the approach should be minimized. A formal arthrotomy (Fig. 101–4) is preferred though a medial parapatellar incision, and subperiosteal release of the deep medial collateral ligament allows external rotation of the tibia, which is necessary for adequate exposure. Removal of the tibial polyethylene is then recommended at this point because such removal decreases tension on the joint and releases tension on the extensor mechanism.

Eversion of the patella can be extremely difficult and dangerous during the exposure of an infected TKR and is generally considered unnecessary. Adequate external rotation of the tibia allows lateral translation and subluxation of the extensor mechanism, minimizes the need for lateral retinacular release, and avoids undue tension on the patellar tendon insertion. If additional exposure is necessary, a quadriceps snip may be performed. Formal V-Y turndown and tibial tubercle osteotomy are avoided if possible because of the potential for extensor mechanism necrosis in this setting.

The femoral, tibial, and patellar components are carefully removed to preserve as much viable bone stock as possible. Particular attention is paid to meticulous removal of all cement particles and debris, as well as débridement of any osteolytic defects and nonviable bone. The tibial and femoral intramedullary canals are thor-

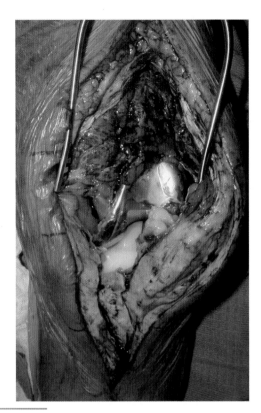

Figure 101–4. Medial parapatellar arthrotomy in a patient undergoing resection of an infected total knee arthroplasty. Gross purulent material and prominent synovial proliferation are present throughout the knee.

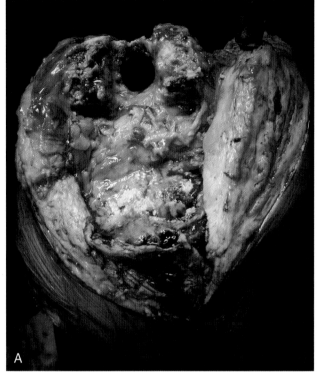

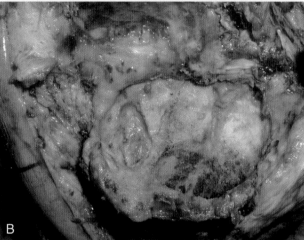

Figure 101–5. **A,** Intraoperative photograph of an infected total knee arthroplasty after initial resection of the prosthetic components. Grossly purulent material is lining the synovium and bone surfaces. **B,** Proximal aspect of the tibia after thorough débridement of purulent debris and necrotic bone. A clean viable bony surface is left for future implantation of a tibial component.

oughly débrided when implants with stems are removed; however, it is not uncommon for the infectious process to extend into the medullary canals, even in the absence of medullary stems. The final step in the débridement process is synovectomy and scar excision in the suprapatellar pouch, medial and lateral gutters, and posterior capsular region. It is helpful to perform this step at the end of the resection and débridement because cement and particulate debris may fall into these areas during removal of the prosthetic components. These fragments are easily identified and removed along with the synovium and scar tissue during the synovectomy. It is critical to perform meticulous and thorough débridement and synovial excision (Fig. 101–5) to viable bone and soft tissue. It is also essential to obtain access and thoroughly débride the posterior aspect of the knee because this is a frequent location for missed cement particles and foreign material. Three to five tissue samples are routinely sent for culture and sensitivity testing.

The knee joint is copiously irrigated and preparation made for placement of the ALBC spacer. The antibiotic-impregnated cement is mixed and placed into the tibiofemoral space in the final stages of polymerization to prevent solid interdigitation into bone and then gently molded to the contour of the distal femur and proximal tibia. Intramedullary antibiotic-loaded cement dowels, when used, are inserted before insertion of the tibiofemoral spacer (Fig. 101–6). The cement from the tibiofemoral spacer is extended into the suprapatellar

space to effectively maintain the length of the extensor mechanism by minimizing scarring and contracture against the anterior aspect of the femur (Fig. 101–7). The wound is closed meticulously over drains. The importance of perfect epidermal apposition to facilitate primary wound healing cannot be overemphasized.

The surgical approach at reimplantation is typically more difficult than at implant removal. As previously mentioned, extensive subperiosteal release of the deep medial collateral ligament from the tibia facilitates anterolateral

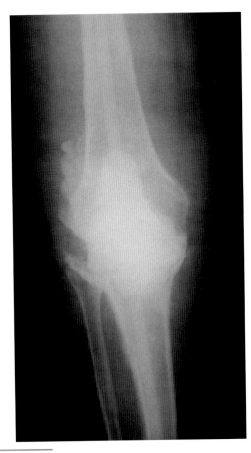

Figure 101–6. Anteroposterior radiograph of a static spacer with medullary antibiotic-loaded bone cement dowels extending into the femoral and tibial canals.

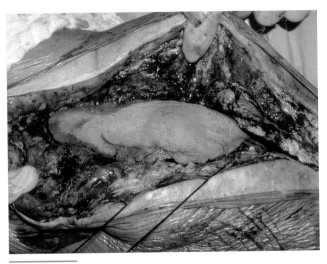

Figure 101–7. Intraoperative photograph of a static molded antibiotic-loaded cement spacer inserted after resection of an infected total knee arthroplasty. Notice the extension into the suprapatellar region to prevent adhesion of the extensor mechanism to the anterior aspect of the femur.

subluxation of the tibia and lateral translation of the patella and extensor mechanism. If removal of the spacer is difficult, the cement spacer is extracted in pieces with an osteotome. Forcible removal of block spacers can result in a periprosthetic fracture of the femur or tibia. Thorough débridement of any residual nonviable synovium and scar tissue is performed, as well as débridement of any necrotic bone. Attention is then turned to implant insertion.

Great care should be taken to place both the femoral and tibial components in the correct rotation. Use of the transepicondylar axis is helpful to prevent inadvertent placement of the femoral component into relative internal rotation. Reimplantation knee arthroplasty is often associated with ligamentous and osseous defects that require implant systems with a more constrained design to achieve stability.[14] Stemmed prosthetic components are typically used in this setting to augment prosthesis fixation against the stress transferred to the associated interfaces from the increased constraint. Although the use of uncemented implants has been recommended for reimplantation, the benefit of antibiotic-loaded cement for prosthesis fixation should be strongly considered in the setting of previous periprosthetic infection (Fig. 101–8).[50,120] Unless one chooses to use an uncemented implant, bone graft is rarely required for the reimplantation arthroplasty. Avoidance of bone graft is accomplished

by using other alternatives such as modular wedges or filling of bone defects with ALBC.

Occasionally after insertion of the new prosthesis it is difficult to close the soft-tissue envelope. Leaving the patellar shell unresurfaced facilitates capsular closure in this setting. Simultaneous use of a gastrocnemius rotational flap during the reimplantation procedure to achieve wound closure has also been reported.[77] Another alternative in patients with multiple skin incisions or a tightly scarred soft-tissue envelope is gradual soft-tissue expansion before reimplantation.[41,85] This procedure has allowed successful wound closure and avoids the use of soft-tissue muscle transposition.

Reinfection after Reimplantation

Reinfection is more likely when treating an infected revision TKA than an infected primary TKA.[55] These patients have more bone loss and compromise of the soft-tissue envelope. Although reimplantation has become a commonly accepted treatment modality for an infected knee prosthesis, the poor outcome of patients who become reinfected after reimplantation can be devastating. In 24 knees treated for reinfection after reimplantation, the final outcome included 10 knees with a successful knee arthrodesis, 5 with infected prostheses maintained by suppressive oral antibiotics, 4 above-knee amputations, 3 persistent pseudarthroses, 1 resection arthroplasty, and 1 uninfected total knee prosthesis.[52] A poor prognosis was associated with the use of a hinged knee design inasmuch as three of the four amputations were performed for failed hinged knee prostheses. A successful arthrodesis at the initial attempt with an external fixation device was more likely for prostheses without stems (75%) than for cemented stemmed prostheses (40%). Long intramedullary arthrodesis was successful in all three attempts. A third attempt at reimplantation was successful in only one (33%) of three attempts.[52]

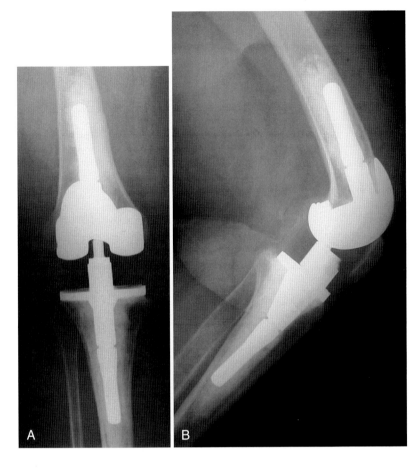

Figure 101–8. Anteroposterior (**A**) and lateral (**B**) radiographs of a reimplantation total knee arthroplasty with a semiconstrained prosthetic design. The femoral and tibial stems were cemented with low-dose antibiotic-loaded bone cement containing gentamicin and vancomycin.

A report of 12 patients who acquired another infection in the reimplanted knee differs with these findings.[7] Three knees were treated by arthrodesis, whereas nine knees underwent another salvage attempt with implant removal, débridement, 6 weeks of parenteral antibiotics, and reimplantation. At an average follow-up of 31 months, the average Knee Society score was 79, the average functional score was 73, and no recurrent infection occurred.[7] Despite these differing viewpoints, the difficulties encountered in obtaining a healed wound, achieving a successful knee arthrodesis, and successfully eradicating infection with nonprosthetic salvage procedures after a failed reimplantation are considerable. The morbidity and increased likelihood of amputation associated with reinfection must be carefully considered and presented to the patient before proceeding with an additional attempt at reimplantation.

References

1. Adams K, Couch L, Cierny G, et al: In vitro and in vivo evaluation of antibiotic diffusion from antibiotic-impregnated polymethylmethacrylate beads. Clin Orthop 278:244-252, 1992.
2. Advisory statement. Antibiotic prophylaxis for dental patients with total joint replacements. American Dental Association; American Academy of Orthopaedic Surgeons. J Am Dent Assoc 128:1004-1008, 1997.
3. Antibiotic prophylaxis for dental patients with total joint replacements. J Am Dent Assoc 134:895-899, 2003.
4. Arciola CR, Campoccia D, Montanaro L: Effects on antibiotic resistance of Staphylococcus epidermidis following adhesion to polymethylmethacrylate and to silicone surfaces. Biomaterials 23:1495-1502, 2002.
5. Arizono T, Oga M, Sugioka Y: Increased resistance of bacteria after adherence to polymethyl methacrylate. An in vitro study. Acta Orthop Scand 63:661-664, 1992.
6. Atkins BL, Athanasou N, Deeks JJ, et al: Prospective evaluation of criteria for microbiological diagnosis of prosthetic-joint infection at revision arthroplasty. The OSIRIS Collaborative Study Group. J Clin Microbiol 36:2932-2939, 1998.
7. Backe HA Jr, Wolff DA, Windsor RE: Total knee replacement infection after 2-stage reimplantation: Results of subsequent 2-stage reimplantation. Clin Orthop 331:125-131, 1996.
8. Barrack RL, Jennings RW, Wolfe MW, Bertot AJ: The Coventry Award. The value of preoperative aspiration before total knee revision. Clin Orthop 345:8-16, 1997.
9. Bengtson S, Blomgren G, Knutson K, et al: Hematogenous infection after knee arthroplasty. Acta Orthop Scand 58:529-534, 1987.
10. Bengtson S, Knutson K: The infected knee arthroplasty. A 6-year follow-up of 357 cases. Acta Orthop Scand 62:301-311, 1991.
11. Berbari EF, Hanssen AD, Duffy MC, et al: Prosthetic joint infection due to Mycobacterium tuberculosis: A case series and review of the literature. Am J Orthop 27:219-227, 1998.
12. Berbari EF, Hanssen AD, Duffy MC, et al: Risk factors for prosthetic joint infection: Case-control study. Clin Infect Dis 27:1247-1254, 1998.
13. Berg M, Bergman BR, Hoborn J: Ultraviolet radiation compared to an ultra-clean air enclosure. Comparison of air bacteria counts in operating rooms. J Bone Joint Surg Br 73:811-815, 1991.
14. Berman AT, O'Brien JT, Israelite C: Use of the rotating hinge for salvage of the infected total knee arthroplasty. Orthopedics 19:73-76, 1996.
15. Bilgen O, Atici T, Durak K, et al: C-reactive protein values and erythrocyte sedimentation rates after total hip and total knee arthroplasty. J Int Med Res 29:7-12, 2001.
16. Blom AW, Brown J, Taylor AH, et al: Infection after total knee arthroplasty. J Bone Joint Surg Br 86:688-691, 2004.

17. Booth RE Jr, Lotke PA: The results of spacer block technique in revision of infected total knee arthroplasty. Clin Orthop 248:57-60, 1989.

18. Borden LS, Gearen PF: Infected total knee arthroplasty. A protocol for management. J Arthroplasty 2:27-36, 1987.

19. Brandt CM, Sistrunk WW, Duffy MC, et al: Staphylococcus aureus prosthetic joint infection treated with débridement and prosthesis retention. Clin Infect Dis 24:914-919, 1997.

20. Bratzler DW, Houck PM: Antimicrobial prophylaxis for surgery: An advisory statement from the National Surgical Infection Prevention Project. Clin Infect Dis 38:1706-1715, 2004.

21. Calton TF, Fehring TK, Griffin WL: Bone loss associated with the use of spacer blocks in infected total knee arthroplasty. Clin Orthop 345:148-154, 1997.

22. Chang CH, Jiang CC: Evaluation of critical postoperative situations in orthopedic patients. J Formos Med Assoc 96:990-995, 1997.

23. Chiu FY, Chen CM, Lin CF, Lo WH: Cefuroxime-impregnated cement in primary total knee arthroplasty: A prospective, randomized study of three hundred and forty knees. J Bone Joint Surg Am 84:759-762, 2002.

24. Chiu FY, Lin CF, Chen CM, et al: Cefuroxime-impregnated cement at primary total knee arthroplasty in diabetes mellitus. A prospective, randomised study. J Bone Joint Surg Br 83:691-695, 2001.

25. Classen DC, Evans RS, Pestotnik SL, et al: The timing of prophylactic administration of antibiotics and the risk of surgical-wound infection. N Engl J Med 326:281-286, 1992.

26. Cushner FD, Locker JR, Hanssen AD, et al: Use of recombinant human erythropoietin in two-stage total knee arthroplasty for infection. Clin Orthop 392:116-123, 2001.

27. Deirmengian C, Greenbaum J, Lotke PA, et al: Limited success with open débridement and retention of components in the treatment of acute Staphylococcus aureus infections after total knee arthroplasty. J Arthroplasty 18(7 Suppl 1):22-26, 2003.

28. Della Valle CJ, Bogner E, Desai P, et al: Analysis of frozen sections of intraoperative specimens obtained at the time of reoperation after hip or knee resection arthroplasty for the treatment of infection. J Bone Joint Surg Am 81:684-689, 1999.

29. Della Valle CJ, Scher DM, Kim YH, et al: The role of intraoperative Gram stain in revision total joint arthroplasty. J Arthroplasty 14:500-504, 1999.

30. Dellinger EP, Gross PA, Barrett TL, et al: Quality standard for antimicrobial prophylaxis in surgical procedures. Infectious Diseases Society of America. Clin Infect Dis 18:422-427, 1994.

31. Der Tavitian J, Ong SM, Taub NA, Taylor GJ: Body-exhaust suit versus occlusive clothing. A randomised, prospective trial using air and wound bacterial counts. J Bone Joint Surg Br 85:490-494, 2003.

32. Drancourt M, Stein A, Argenson JN, et al: Oral treatment of Staphylococcus spp. infected orthopaedic implants with fusidic acid or ofloxacin in combination with rifampicin. J Antimicrob Chemother 39:235-240, 1997.

33. Duff GP, Lachiewicz PF, Kelley SS: Aspiration of the knee joint before revision arthroplasty. Clin Orthop 331:132-139, 1996.

34. Durack DT: Prevention of infective endocarditis. N Engl J Med 332:38-44, 1995.

35. Emerson RH Jr, Muncie M, Tarbox TR, Higgins LL: Comparison of a static with a mobile spacer in total knee infection. Clin Orthop 404:132-138, 2002.

36. England SP, Stern SH, Insall JN, Windsor RE: Total knee arthroplasty in diabetes mellitus. Clin Orthop 260:130-134, 1990.

37. Falahee MH, Matthews LS, Kaufer H: Resection arthroplasty as a salvage procedure for a knee with infection after a total arthroplasty. J Bone Joint Surg Am 69:1013-1021, 1987.

38. Fehring TK, McAlister JA Jr: Frozen histologic section as a guide to sepsis in revision joint arthroplasty. Clin Orthop 304:229-237, 1994.

39. Fehring TK, Odum S, Calton TF, Mason JB: Articulating versus static spacers in revision total knee arthroplasty for sepsis. The Ranawat Award. Clin Orthop 380:9-16, 2000.

40. Foran JR, Mont MA, Etienne G, et al: The outcome of total knee arthroplasty in obese patients. J Bone Joint Surg Am 86:1609-1615, 2004.

41. Gold DA, Scott SC, Scott WN: Soft tissue expansion prior to arthroplasty in the multiply-operated knee. A new method of preventing catastrophic skin problems. J Arthroplasty 11:512-521, 1996.

42. Goldman RT, Scuderi GR, Insall JN: 2-stage reimplantation for infected total knee replacement. Clin Orthop 331:118-124, 1996.

43. Haddad FS, Masri BA, Campbell D, et al: The PROSTALAC functional spacer in two-stage revision for infected knee replacements. Prosthesis of antibiotic-loaded acrylic cement. J Bone Joint Surg Br 82:807-812, 2000.

44. Haleem AA, Berry DJ, Hanssen AD: Mid-term to long-term followup of two-stage reimplantation for infected total knee arthroplasty. Clin Orthop 428:35-39, 2004.

45. Hanssen AD: Prophylactic use of antibiotic bone cement: An emerging standard—in opposition. J Arthroplasty 19(4 Suppl 1):73-77, 2004.

46. Hanssen AD, Osmon DR: Prevention of deep wound infection after total hip arthroplasty: The role of prophylactic antibiotics and clean air technology. Semin Arthroplasty 5:114-121, 1994.

47. Hanssen AD, Osmon DR: The use of prophylactic antimicrobial agents during and after hip arthroplasty. Clin Orthop 369:124-138, 1999.

48. Hanssen AD, Osmon DR, Nelson CL: Prevention of deep periprosthetic joint infection. Instr Course Lect 46:555-567, 1997.

49. Hanssen AD, Rand JA: Evaluation and treatment of infection at the site of a total hip or knee arthroplasty. Instr Course Lect 48:111-122, 1999.

50. Hanssen AD, Rand JA, Osmon DR: Treatment of the infected total knee arthroplasty with insertion of another prosthesis. The effect of antibiotic-impregnated bone cement. Clin Orthop 309:44-55, 1994.

51. Hanssen AD, Spangehl MJ: Practical applications of antibiotic-loaded bone cement for treatment of infected joint replacements. Clin Orthop 427:79-85, 2004.

52. Hanssen AD, Trousdale RT, Osmon DR: Patient outcome with reinfection following reimplantation for the infected total knee arthroplasty. Clin Orthop 321:55-67, 1995.

53. Hebert CK, Williams RE, Levy RS, Barrack RL: Cost of treating an infected total knee replacement. Clin Orthop 331:140-145, 1996.

54. Hill C, Flamant R, Mazas F, Evrard J: Prophylactic cefazolin versus placebo in total hip replacement. Report of a multicentre double-blind randomised trial. Lancet 1:795-796, 1981.

55. Hirakawa K, Stulberg BN, Wilde AH, et al: Results of 2-stage reimplantation for infected total knee arthroplasty. J Arthroplasty 13:22-28, 1998.

56. Hofmann AA, Kane KR, Tkach TK, et al: Treatment of infected total knee arthroplasty using an articulating spacer. Clin Orthop 321:45-54, 1995.

57. Insall JN, Thompson FM, Brause BD: Two-stage reimplantation for the salvage of infected total knee arthroplasty. J Bone Joint Surg Am 65:1087-1098, 1983.

58. Isiklar ZU, Landon GC, Tullos HS: Amputation after failed total knee arthroplasty. Clin Orthop 299:173-178, 1994.

59. Jerry GJ Jr, Rand JA, Ilstrup D: Old sepsis prior to total knee arthroplasty. Clin Orthop 236:135-140, 1988.

60. Johnson DP, Bannister GC: The outcome of infected arthroplasty of the knee. J Bone Joint Surg Br 68:289-291, 1986.

61. Josefsson G, Kolmert L: Prophylaxis with systematic antibiotics versus gentamicin bone cement in total hip arthroplasty. A ten-year survey of 1,688 hips. Clin Orthop 292:210-214, 1993.

62. Joseph TN, Chen AL, Di Cesare PE: Use of antibiotic-impregnated cement in total joint arthroplasty. J Am Acad Orthop Surg 11:38-47, 2003.

63. Kilgus DJ, Howe DJ, Strang A: Results of periprosthetic hip and knee infections caused by resistant bacteria. Clin Orthop 404:116-124, 2002.

64. Kim YH, Kim JS, Cho SH: Total knee arthroplasty after spontaneous osseous ankylosis and takedown of formal knee fusion. J Arthroplasty 15:453-460, 2000.

65. Kramhoft M, Bodtker S, Carlsen A: Outcome of infected total knee arthroplasty. J Arthroplasty 9:617-621, 1994.

66. Laiho K, Maenpaa H, Kautiainen H, et al: Rise in serum C reactive protein after hip and knee arthroplasties in patients with rheumatoid arthritis. Ann Rheum Dis 60:275-277, 2001.

67. Lee GC, Pagnano MW, Hanssen AD: Total knee arthroplasty after prior bone or joint sepsis about the knee. Clin Orthop 404:226-231, 2002.

68. Leigh DA, Griggs J, Tighe CM, et al: Pharmacokinetic study of ceftazidime in bone and serum of patients undergoing hip and knee arthroplasty. J Antimicrob Chemother 16:637-642, 1985.

69. Levitsky KA, Hozack WJ, Balderston RA, et al: Evaluation of the painful prosthetic joint. Relative value of bone scan, sedimentation rate, and joint aspiration. J Arthroplasty 6:237-244, 1991.

70. Lian G, Cracchiolo A 3rd, Lesavoy M: Treatment of major wound necrosis following total knee arthroplasty. J Arthroplasty 4(Suppl):S23-S32, 1989.

71. Lonner JH, Desai P, Dicesare PE, et al: The reliability of analysis of intraoperative frozen sections for identifying active infection during revision hip or knee arthroplasty. J Bone Joint Surg Am 78:1553-1558, 1996.

72. Lonner JH, Siliski JM, Della Valle C, et al: Role of knee aspiration after resection of the infected total knee arthroplasty. Am J Orthop 30:305-309, 2001.

73. Maniloff G, Greenwald R, Laskin R, Singer C: Delayed postbacteremic prosthetic joint infection. Clin Orthop 223:194-197, 1987.

74. Mariani BD, Martin DS, Levine MJ, et al: The Coventry Award. Polymerase chain reaction detection of bacterial infection in total knee arthroplasty. Clin Orthop 331:11-22, 1996.

75. Masri BA, Duncan CP, Beauchamp CP: Long-term elution of antibiotics from bone-cement: An in vivo study using the prosthesis of antibiotic-loaded acrylic cement (PROSTALAC) system. J Arthroplasty 13:331-338, 1998.

76. Mauerhan DR, Nelson CL, Smith DL, et al: Prophylaxis against infection in total joint arthroplasty. One day of cefuroxime compared with three days of cefazolin. J Bone Joint Surg Am 76:39-45, 1994.

77. McPherson EJ, Patzakis MJ, Gross JE, et al: Infected total knee arthroplasty. Two-stage reimplantation with a gastrocnemius rotational flap. Clin Orthop 341:73-81, 1997.

78. McQueen MM, Hughes SP, May P, Verity L: Cefuroxime in total joint arthroplasty. Intravenous or in bone cement. J Arthroplasty 5:169-172, 1990.

79. Meding JB, Reddleman K, Keating ME, et al: Total knee replacement in patients with diabetes mellitus. Clin Orthop 416:208-216, 2003.

80. Meehan AM, Osmon DR, Duffy MC, et al: Outcome of penicillin-susceptible streptococcal prosthetic joint infection treated with débridement and retention of the prosthesis. Clin Infect Dis 36:845-849, 2003.

81. Mont MA, Waldman B, Banerjee C, et al: Multiple irrigation, débridement, and retention of components in infected total knee arthroplasty. J Arthroplasty 12:426-433, 1997.

82. Mont MA, Waldman BJ, Hungerford DS: Evaluation of preoperative cultures before second-stage reimplantation of a total knee prosthesis complicated by infection. A comparison-group study. J Bone Joint Surg Am 82:1552-1557, 2000.

83. Morrey BF, Westholm F, Schoifet S, et al: Long-term results of various treatment options for infected total knee arthroplasty. Clin Orthop 248:120-128, 1989.

84. Musso AD, Mohanty K, Spencer-Jones R: Role of frozen section histology in diagnosis of infection during revision arthroplasty. Postgrad Med J 79:590-593, 2003.

85. Namba RS, Diao E: Tissue expansion for staged reimplantation of infected total knee arthroplasty. J Arthroplasty 12:471-474, 1997.

86. Pace TB, Jeray KJ, Latham JT Jr: Synovial tissue examination by frozen section as an indicator of infection in hip and knee arthroplasty in community hospitals. J Arthroplasty 12:64-69, 1997.

87. Pagnano M, Cushner FD, Hansen A, et al: Blood management in two-stage revision knee arthroplasty for deep prosthetic infection. Clin Orthop 367:238-242, 1999.

88. Papagelopoulos PJ, Idusuyi OB, Wallrichs SL, Morrey BF: Long term outcome and survivorship analysis of primary total knee arthroplasty in patients with diabetes mellitus. Clin Orthop 330:124-132, 1996.

89. Parvizi J, Sullivan TA, Pagnano MW, et al: Total joint arthroplasty in human immunodeficiency virus–positive patients: An alarming rate of early failure. J Arthroplasty 18:259-264, 2003.

90. Peersman G, Laskin R, Davis J, Peterson M: Infection in total knee replacement: A retrospective review of 6489 total knee replacements. Clin Orthop 392:15-23, 2001.

91. Penner MJ, Masri BA, Duncan CP: Elution characteristics of vancomycin and tobramycin combined in acrylic bone-cement. J Arthroplasty 11:939-944, 1996.

92. Phelan DM, Osmon DR, Keating MR, Hanssen AD: Delayed reimplantation arthroplasty for candidal prosthetic joint infection: A report of 4 cases and review of the literature. Clin Infect Dis 34:930-938, 2002.

93. Pring DJ, Marks L, Angel JC: Mobility after amputation for failed knee replacement. J Bone Joint Surg Br 70:770-771, 1988.

94. Rand JA: Evaluation and management of infected total knee arthroplasty. Semin Arthroplasty 5:178-182, 1994.

95. Rand JA, Bryan RS: Reimplantation for the salvage of an infected total knee arthroplasty. J Bone Joint Surg Am 65:1081-1086, 1983.

96. Ries MD: Vancomycin-resistant *Enterococcus* infected total knee arthroplasty. J Arthroplasty 16:802-805, 2001.

97. Ritter MA: Intraoperative controls for bacterial contamination during total knee replacement. Orthop Clin North Am 20:49-53, 1989.

98. Ritter MA: Operating room environment. Clin Orthop 369:103-109, 1999.

99. Ritter MA, Campbell ED: Retrospective evaluation of an iodophor-incorporated antimicrobial plastic adhesive wound drape. Clin Orthop 228:307-308, 1988.

100. Scher DM, Pak K, Lonner JH, et al: The predictive value of indium-111 leukocyte scans in the diagnosis of infected total hip, knee, or resection arthroplasties. J Arthroplasty 15:295-300, 2000.

101. Scher KS: Studies on the duration of antibiotic administration for surgical prophylaxis. Am Surg 63:59-62, 1997.

102. Schoifet SD, Morrey BF: Treatment of infection after total knee arthroplasty by débridement with retention of the components. J Bone Joint Surg Am 72:1383-1390, 1990.

103. Sculco TP: The economic impact of infected joint arthroplasty. Orthopedics 18:871-873, 1995.

104. Segawa H, Tsukayama DT, Kyle RF, et al: Infection after total knee arthroplasty. A retrospective study of the treatment of eighty-one infections. J Bone Joint Surg Am 81:1434-1445, 1999.

105. Shlaes DM, Gerding DN, John JF Jr, et al: Society for Healthcare Epidemiology of America and Infectious Diseases Society of America Joint Committee on the Prevention of Antimicrobial Resistance: Guidelines for the prevention of antimicrobial resistance in hospitals. Infect Control Hosp Epidemiol 18:275-291, 1997.

106. Silva M, Tharani R, Schmalzried TP: Results of direct exchange or débridement of the infected total knee arthroplasty. Clin Orthop 404:125-131, 2002.

107. Springer BD, Lee GC, Osmon D, et al: Systemic safety of high-dose antibiotic-loaded cement spacers after resection of an infected total knee arthroplasty. Clin Orthop 427:47-51, 2004.

108. Tannenbaum DA, Matthews LS, Grady-Benson JC: Infection around joint replacements in patients who have a renal or liver transplantation. J Bone Joint Surg Am 79:36-43, 1997.

109. Tattevin P, Cremieux AC, Pottier P, et al: Prosthetic joint infection: When can prosthesis salvage be considered? Clin Infect Dis 29:292-295, 1999.

110. Teeny SM, Dorr L, Murata G, Conaty P: Treatment of infected total knee arthroplasty. Irrigation and débridement versus two-stage reimplantation. J Arthroplasty 5:35-39, 1990.

111. Trampuz A, Hanssen AD, Osmon DR, et al: Synovial fluid leukocyte count and differential for the diagnosis of prosthetic knee infection. Am J Med 117:556-562, 2004.

112. Trampuz A, Osmon DR, Hanssen AD, et al: Molecular and antibiofilm approaches to prosthetic joint infection. Clin Orthop 414:69-88, 2003.

113. Tsukayama DT, Wicklund B, Gustilo RB: Suppressive antibiotic therapy in chronic prosthetic joint infections. Orthopedics 14:841-844, 1991.

114. Volin SJ, Hinrichs SH, Garvin KL: Two-stage reimplantation of total joint infections: A comparison of resistant and non-resistant organisms. Clin Orthop 427:94-100, 2004.

115. Waldman BJ, Hostin E, Mont MA, Hungerford DS: Infected total knee arthroplasty treated by arthroscopic irrigation and débridement. J Arthroplasty 15:430-436, 2000.

116. Waldman BJ, Mont MA, Hungerford DS: Total knee arthroplasty infections associated with dental procedures. Clin Orthop 343:164-172, 1997.

117. Wasielewski RC, Barden RM, Rosenberg AG: Results of different surgical procedures on total knee arthroplasty infections. J Arthroplasty 11:931-938, 1996.

118. Weiss AP, Krackow KA: Persistent wound drainage after primary total knee arthroplasty. J Arthroplasty 8:285-289, 1993.

119. White J, Kelly M, Dunsmuir R: C-reactive protein level after total hip and total knee replacement. J Bone Joint Surg Br 80:909-911, 1998.

120. Whiteside LA: Treatment of infected total knee arthroplasty. Clin Orthop 299:169-172, 1994.

121. Wilde AH, Ruth JT: Two-stage reimplantation in infected total knee arthroplasty. Clin Orthop 236:23-35, 1988.

122. Wilson MG, Kelley K, Thornhill TS: Infection as a complication of total knee-replacement arthroplasty. Risk factors and treatment in sixty-seven cases. J Bone Joint Surg Am 72:878-883, 1990.

123. Windsor RE, Insall JN, Urs WK, et al: Two-stage reimplantation for the salvage of total knee arthroplasty complicated by infection. Further follow-up and refinement of indications. J Bone Joint Surg Am 72:272-278, 1990.

124. Winiarsky R, Barth P, Lotke P: Total knee arthroplasty in morbidly obese patients. J Bone Joint Surg Am 80:1770-1774, 1998.

125. Wolff LH 3rd, Parvizi J, Trousdale RT, et al: Results of treatment of infection in both knees after bilateral total knee arthroplasty. J Bone Joint Surg Am 85:1952-1925, 2003.

126. Zimmerli W, Widmer AF, Blatter M, et al: Role of rifampin for treatment of orthopedic implant-related staphylococcal infections: A randomized controlled trial. Foreign-Body Infection (FBI) Study Group. JAMA 279:1537-1541, 1998.

CHAPTER 102

Management of Bone Defects

Mark W. Pagnano

Management of bone loss in total knee arthroplasty (TKA) is directed by the extent and location of the bone defects. In primary TKA, the most frequently encountered form of bone loss is a posteromedial tibial plateau defect associated with marked varus angular deformity of the limb (Fig. 102–1). On the femoral side, marked bone loss is rare in the setting of primary TKA. An exception would be a severe valgus limb in which the lateral femoral condyle may have a combination of both distal and posterior bone loss (Fig. 102–2). In revision TKA, marked bone loss is encountered often, and the degree of loss typically exceeds that predicted by preoperative radiographs. Osteolytic defects secondary to wear debris and iatrogenic bone loss caused by the removal of components are major causes of large bony defects (Fig. 102–3). During revision TKA, bone loss from the distal and posterior aspects of the femur must often be addressed (Fig. 102–4). Multiple options can be selected to reconstruct these bone defects, including cement, autograft bone, allograft bone, modular solid-metal wedges and blocks, and porous or trabecular metal augments that can replace bone.

The purpose of this chapter is to review the indications, limitations, detailed surgical techniques, and published clinical results for each of these methods of filling bone defects in TKA. An appropriate understanding of the benefits and limitations of each technique allows the surgeon to deal efficiently and effectively with bone deficiency in TKA. Techniques to address bony defects must not compromise the basic principles of total knee replacement, which include correct limb alignment, correct implant position, balance of the flexion and extension spaces, central tracking of the patella, and adequate range of motion. A bony defect elegantly reconstructed with bone graft, metal wedges, and stems is still doomed to fail if the surgeon does not obtain appropriate limb alignment, component position, and component fixation.

ASSESSMENT OF BONE LOSS

Bone defects in primary TKA are assessed best after making the standard bone cuts. Many defects that initially appear to require some type of augmentation are nearly eliminated by standard bony resection. Often this is true with moderate-sized posteromedial defects of the tibia in a varus knee. Resection of an additional 1 to 2 mm of tibial bone can eliminate some defects entirely, and such additional resection is appropriate if the initial resection was only 8 or 9 mm. Numerous biomechanical studies

have demonstrated that trabecular bone strength in the proximal end of the tibia decreases with greater distance from the joint surface.[24,25,46] These studies have led many to caution against making more than a minimal proximal tibial resection. No study to date, however, has shown a clinically important relationship between tibial component survival and the depth of tibial resection.

Assessment of bone deficiency during revision TKA is best done after removing the components and débriding the osteolytic regions thoroughly (Fig. 102–5). A number of classification schemes can be used to grade the extent of bone loss.[12-14] Most of these schemes distinguish between contained or cavitary defects (those with an intact peripheral cortex) and noncontained or segmental defects (those without a peripheral rim of bone). Although contained defects can often be filled adequately with morselized bone, segmental defects usually require structural graft, solid-metal augments, custom components, or trabecular metal augmentation.[26]

BONE CEMENT

Indications. Small bone defects up to 5 mm in depth, preferably contained defects, can be filled with cement in older patients.

Limitations. The relatively poor biomechanical properties of cement preclude its use in larger or segmental defects, particularly in younger patients.

Bone cement is a useful means to fill small areas of bone deficiency. It is inexpensive, readily fills defects, and does not require any major alteration in the performance of TKA. Cement has, however, relatively poor biomechanical properties. The modulus of elasticity of cement is lower than that of cortical bone, and cement performs poorly when subjected to shear stress. Brooks et al demonstrated that when subjected to axial loads, a simulated peripheral tibial defect filled with cement performs poorly in vitro.[6] Chen and Krackow have shown that it is biomechanically advantageous to convert defects to a step configuration when cement is used[9] (Fig. 102–6). Converting a wedge-shaped defect to a step construct minimizes shear force on the cement. Those authors' laboratory data showed that a 20-degree wedge-shaped defect in the tibia can be converted to a step-shaped construct and filled with cement. In that setting, cement filling of the defect was as strong as a metal augmentation wedge. For larger defects, however, a metal wedge or a solid-metal

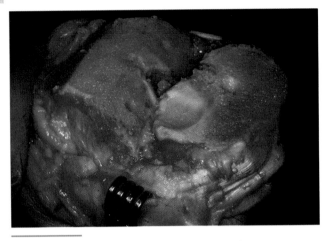

Figure 102–1. The most common bone defect in primary TKA is a posteromedial defect in a varus knee.

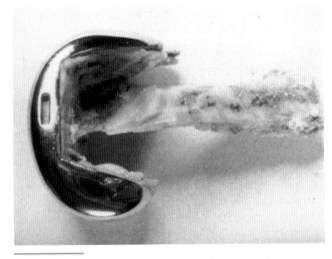

Figure 102–3. Care must be taken when removing components during revision TKA or substantial bone may be lost inadvertently. All exposed prosthetic interfaces must be dissected free before the use of extraction devices.

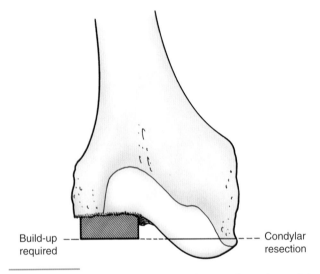

Build-up required — — — — — — — — — — Condylar resection

Figure 102–2. A valgus knee may have a lateral condyle that is deficient both distally and posteriorly. Often, only a minimal amount of distal femoral bone is removed from the lateral condyle in a valgus knee. In some rare cases the level of resection may pass distal to the lateral condyle and require augmentation.

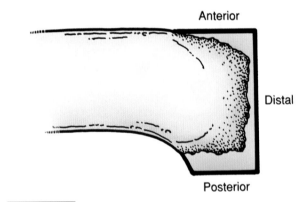

Anterior

Distal

Posterior

Figure 102–4. Distal and posterior femoral bone stock must frequently be augmented at the time of revision TKA.

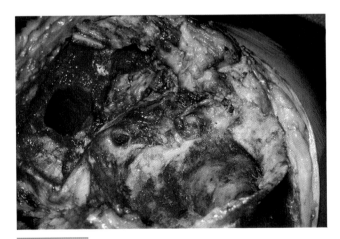

Figure 102–5. After carefully removing the components, the knee should be débrided thoroughly to remove any fibrous tissue associated with areas of osteolysis. At that point, the true extent of bone loss may be assessed accurately.

augmentation block was recommended. Other authors have suggested that cement reinforced with bone screws can be used to fill larger defects.[16,40,41] In vitro biomechanical data suggest that screw reinforcement may result in a slight improvement over bone cement alone when filling defects.

Cement, however, does not restore bone stock, and that may be important in younger patients who face the possibility of future revision. A young patient undergoing primary total knee replacement is probably served better by filling bony defects with autogenous bone rather than cement. In the primary TKA setting, bone is readily available, it will incorporate reliably, and it will

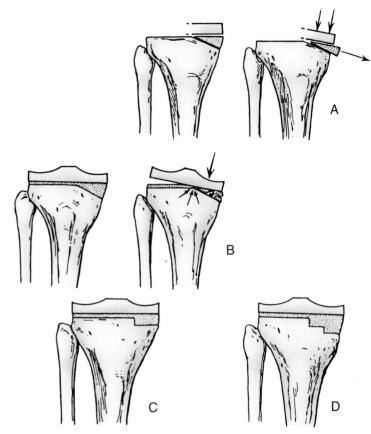

Figure 102–6. It is biomechanically advantageous to convert wedge-shaped bone defects to step-shaped defects when cement is used to fill the defect. **A,** Shear force may weaken the support of the overlying tibial component. **B,** Cement at the periphery of a wedge defect may be exposed to excessive stress. **C** and **D,** A step or terraced configuration will reduce the force and lower the stress on the cement. (From Chen F, Krackow K: Management of tibial defects in total knee arthroplasty. Clin Orthop 305:249-257, 1994.)

restore bone stock should the arthroplasty subsequently fail.

Clinical Results

At early and midterm follow-up the results of cement and cement reinforced with screws to fill tibial defects in TKA have been satisfactory. Ritter et al reported on 47 patients with a minimum of 3 years' and an average of 6.1 years' follow-up after TKA with cement and screw filling of tibial defects.[40,41] The defects were defined as large with a depth of 9 ± 5 mm. Although nonprogressive radiolucent lines were common (27% of cases), there were no signs of cement failure nor any loose prostheses. The authors stated that cement and screw filling of tibial defects has proved to be clinically satisfactory. They have further suggested that the presence of radiolucent lines adjacent to the cement-filled areas may be technique related. After adopting a technique to remove sclerotic bone, expose the underlying cancellous bone, and allow cement interdigitation, Ritter et al found no early radiolucencies. Eleven knees were prepared in that manner, and at 2 years no radiolucencies had developed in that group. Freeman reported good results with the use of cement reinforced with screws for tibial defects.[16] At early follow-up (mean of 32 months), many radiolucent lines were present but none were progressive.

Another technique for using cement augments was reported by Scott et al, who placed prepolymerized cement spacers on the femoral side instead of the more typical metal augments. The short-term follow-up of 10 cases was encouraging, and the authors highlighted the cost savings of these prepolymerized cement augments over metal augments.[43]

Surgical Technique

The tibia is prepared for a standard tibial tray in the typical fashion. The defect is assessed after the initial bone resection. The sclerotic base of the defect is débrided with a high speed bur, and multiple small holes are drilled to encourage cement interdigitation.. If the defect is wedge shaped, it is converted to a step-shaped or terraced defect in an effort to minimize the shear force on the cement construct. The bone is then thoroughly irrigated by pulsatile lavage and dried. For larger defects the cement can be reinforced with screws. Self-tapping cancellous bone screws are placed in the defect and advanced until the head of the screw will be below the level of the prosthesis. Because most tibial baseplates are titanium, titanium screws are favored to limit galvanic corrosion caused by dissimilar metals. The trial component is placed and the screw depth is fine-tuned so that the screw heads do not directly contact the baseplate. The cement is mixed and introduced into the tibia when in a doughy state. Gentle pressurization of the cement into the base of the defect by finger packing is appropriate. Doughy cement is placed over the screw heads and on the underside of the baseplate to ensure that the prosthesis does not directly contact the screws. The tibial component is then inserted, excess cement is removed from the edge of the defect, and the cement is allowed to cure. Stem extensions on the tibial component are not required when small bone defects are filled with cement but should be used in the presence of larger defects or when the bone is markedly osteopenic.

AUTOGENOUS BONE GRAFT

Indications. Autogenous bone grafts are appropriate for defects that are greater than 5 mm in depth or involve more than 50% of a tibial hemiplateau, particularly in younger patients.

Limitations. The availability of autogenous bone is limited.

Autogenous bone is an excellent material to fill defects at the time of TKA. It is readily incorporated, heals reliably, and appears to be durable when used to fill bony defects. Bone can be readily contoured to fit and fill segmental defects, or it can be morselized to fill contained defects. In primary TKA, adequate autogenous bone is often available from the distal femoral resection or the intercondylar resection. In revision TKA, autogenous bone is typically in short supply because of the marked bone loss and the limited need for resection of more bone. An exception would be the trapezoidal bone removed from the intercondylar region when converting from a cruciate-retaining primary knee to a posterior-stabilized revision implant. That autogenous bone can be used to fill small defects in the revision setting.

Clinical Results

Scuderi et al reported good results in 26 TKAs in which autogenous grafting was used.[44] Ninety-six percent good and excellent results were obtained, and the grafts were all seen to be incorporated by 1 year postoperatively. A nonprogressive radiolucency developed in two knees, which in one case was the result of graft collapse. Altcheck et al and Aglietti et al have had similar good results at comparable periods of follow-up.[1,2] Dorr et al reported on 24 knees treated with autogenous graft to fill tibial defects.[12] All patients were monitored for a minimum of 3 years. Bone incorporation was seen in 22 of 24. One graft failed because of collapse, and that failure was linked to postoperative varus limb alignment.

Laskin has reported less satisfactory results with autogenous grafting of tibial defects.[28] Four knees in that series demonstrated graft collapse within 1 year postoperatively. Nine knees underwent biopsy more than 1 year after surgery, and less than half the grafts were found to be living. Of interest is the choice of posterior femoral bone as the autogenous graft material in that series. The author has speculated that the large proportion of cortical and subchondral bone in those graft specimens may have contributed to the poor rate of incorporation and high rate of

failure. The overall success rate in that series was 67% at relatively early follow-up.

To date, there are no studies that report the results for autogenous grafting of femoral bony defects.

Surgical Technique

Sculco has popularized the use of autogenous bone from the distal femoral resection[45] (Fig. 102–7). In that technique the standard tibial resection is carried out. The sclerotic base of the tibial defect is then cut away to expose the underlying cancellous bone. Curettage is performed on any underlying cystic regions in the tibia, and the defects are filled with morselized cancellous autograft. To ensure that graft fixation is not compromised by the keel or stem of the tibial component, the tibia is prepared for the trial component. Next, the flat surfaces of the defect and the bone from the distal femoral resection are opposed and held in place with pins. Typically, the bone from the distal medial aspect of the femur is more substantial and thus a better graft source than bone from the lateral side. The graft is appropriately shaped and then rigidly fixed with screws. The graft-host junction should be free of any gaps. Small defects can be packed with morselized cancellous graft. The graft-host junction is then protected against cement intrusion by caulking the interface. The caulking can be done with Gelfoam or with a small amount of cement itself if the femoral component is cemented separately. The tibial component is then cemented over the graft in standard fashion. For femoral defects a similar technique can be used. The sclerotic bone on the deficient side is removed to expose the underlying cancellous bone. Bone from the opposite condyle is then fixed in place and trimmed appropriately. The femoral component can subsequently be cemented into place.

Windsor et al have suggested an alternative technique for autogenous grafting that involves a so-called self-locking dowel technique.[56] The proximal tibial resection is carried out and the tibia is prepared for the trial tibial component. The defect is then converted to a trapezoidal shape, and the sclerotic base of the defect is removed with a high-speed bur. A matching trapezoid graft is made from the autogenous bone and impacted into place. The press-fit of the graft is temporarily supplemented with K-wire fixation. The tibia is then cemented in standard fashion.

ALLOGRAFT BONE

Indications. Large contained or segmental defects in which autogenous bone is not available or is insufficient to fill the defect are indications for the use of allograft bone.

Limitations.
Union of allograft to host bone is required for long-term success. Large grafts may fail late because they lack the ability to remodel in response to stress.

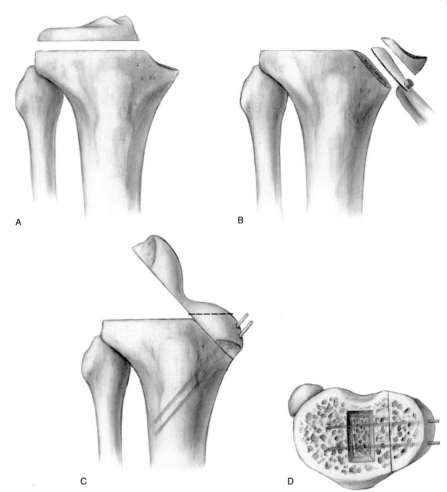

Figure 102–7. Proximal tibial resection (**A**) is carried out and then the sclerotic base of the defect is removed (**B**) with an oscillating saw. The distal femoral graft (**C**) is fixed rigidly in place with bone screws. The construct as viewed from above (**D**), with the graft trimmed and prepared for the tibial component. The tibia is then cemented in place (**E**). (From Sculco TP: Bone grafting. In Lotke PA [ed]: Master Techniques in Orthopedic Surgery, Knee Arthroplasty. New York, Raven Press, 1995.)

Allograft bone is widely used in both revision TKA and revision total hip arthroplasty. The use of morselized cancellous allograft to fill contained defects appears to be both a reliable and durable method. Impacted morselized allograft has been well studied in the hip and has been used successfully to fill large cavitary defects in both the femur and acetabulum.[20,21,33] From a biological standpoint, morselized cancellous allograft lacks osteogenic properties but does possess osteoconductive properties and seems to incorporate much like a cancellous autograft, though at a slower rate. A well-vascularized recipient bed seems to facilitate incorporation of morselized allograft. There is, however, a paucity of scientific data on the use of such techniques in revision TKA.[50]

Large structural allografts are most often used to fill segmental defects at the time of revision total knee replacement.[19,23,27,30,47,49,55] Some reports of large structural allografts, however, have also detailed their use in filling extensive metaphyseal cavitary defects.[47] Allograft bone offers the chance to restore bone stock but requires that the graft unite to the underlying host bone.[17] It is widely available, and the type of bone used can be tailored to the clinical situation, for example, the femoral head, proximal tibia, and distal femur. Allograft bone can potentially provide greater intraoperative flexibility at a lower cost than a custom implant. Disease transmission is a disadvantage with the use of allograft bone,[8] but the risk is low and has been estimated at 1 in a million when strict donor selection criteria and thorough screening methods are used.[7]

Complications with large structural allografts are not uncommon. The long-term success of a structural allograft requires union between the graft and host. Typically, union occurs through a process of external callus formation and then revascularization, followed by creeping substitution and remodeling.[17] If this process occurs too slowly, nonunion may ensue. If the process occurs too rapidly, allograft integrity can be compromised and fracture or collapse may follow. Once the allograft has solidly united to the host bone, it has very limited ability to remodel and it essentially acts like an inert implant. Over long periods that inability to remodel can lead to stress fracture and failure of the allograft construct. For that reason, structural allografts in TKA should be protected by an intramedullary stem that completely bypasses the graft.

Clinical Results

Several groups of authors have reported the results of morselized allograft in revision TKA.[29,42,50,54] Samuelson used morselized allograft to fill large tibial defects in 22 knees. Uncemented tibial components with intramedullary stems were used in all cases. At a minimum of 2 years' follow-up, a third of the implants had migrated but were thought to have reached a stable position. None of the implants were considered clinical failures. Whiteside reported on 56 knees with either contained or segmental tibial defects that were filled with morselized allograft. The tibial components were all of an uncemented design with an extended intramedullary stem. Fixation was further augmented with screws placed through the tibial baseplate. At a minimum 2-year follow-up, nine knees had moderate or severe pain, one tibial component had migrated, three knees were unstable, three patellar dislocations had occurred, and one patellar tendon had ruptured. All grafts showed radiographic evidence of remodeling. Ullmark and Hovelius reported on three patients treated with an impaction allografting technique similar to that described in the hip literature. At 18- to 28-month follow-up, all the patients were doing well clinically. Radiographs revealed incorporation of the allograft bone in two of the three patients.

Clatworthy et al[10] reported a mean 8-year follow-up of 52 revision TKAs with structural allograft for uncontained defects. Thirteen of the TKAs failed, 4 because of infection, 2 with allograft nonunion, 5 because of marked graft resorption, 1 because of tibial loosening, and 1 as a result of continued marked pain. The 10-year survival rate of the allograft was estimated at 72%.

Mow and Weidel used structural allografting in 15 TKAs in which large segmental, cavitary, or combined deficiencies were present.[31] Both femoral and tibial defects were addressed. The allograft-host junction was bypassed with an intramedullary stem in all cases. Follow-up averaged 47 months. Hospital for Special Surgery knee scores improved from 47 before revision to 86 at follow-up. One case failed because of tibial component loosening, and one failed because of progressive lysis. There were no cases of infection. Mnaymneh et al reported the results of 14 structural allografts used to fill large distal femoral or proximal tibial defects.[30] Graft-host union occurred in 12 of these cases. Complications were common in this group, which had been monitored for a mean of 3.3 years. Nonunion occurred in two cases, tibial loosening in two cases, dislocation in one case, and deep prosthetic infection in one case. Tsahakis et al used 48 bulk allografts in 30 revision TKAs.[49] Excellent or good results were reported in 90% of these cases at a mean follow-up of 3.2 years. The authors cemented the prostheses and used intramedullary stems to bypass the allograft in each case. Union was reliably obtained. Complications did occur in three cases and included component failure, loosening, and ligamentous instability. Harris et al used structural allografts in 14 revision TKAs with segmental defects.[23] Six whole tibial allografts, three medial tibial condyles, five whole femurs, and five medial femoral condyles were used. Intramedullary stems were used to bypass the allograft in 11 of the cases. At a mean follow-up of 43 months, 13 of the allografts had united and 11 of the 14 knees were considered clinical successes. Ghazavi et al reported the use of structural allografts in 30 knee revisions.[19] These allografts were used to fill uncontained defects at least 3 cm in depth. A structural allograft was used on the femoral side alone in 16 cases, the tibial side alone in 10 cases, and both the femoral and tibial sides in 4 cases. All allografts were bypassed with an intramedullary stem. There were three deep infections, two cases of tibial loosening, one graft fracture, one graft nonunion, one patellar tendon tear, and one case of wound necrosis. Twenty-three of the 30 knees (77%) were judged to be clinically successful. Wilde et al reported the results of bulk allografts in 12 knees of 10 patients.[55] Allografts were used to fill a segmental defect in seven knees and a contained defect in five knees. Intramedullary stems were used in all cases, and supplemental fixation with a plate or screws was used for each case with a segmental defect. Nonunion occurred in one case. At a mean follow-up of 32 months, radiolucent lines beneath the tibial components were common but were not progressive. Two knees required revision for deep prosthetic infection.

Surgical Technique

MORSELIZED ALLOGRAFT

For contained defects, morselized cancellous or corticocancellous allograft can be efficiently used to restore bone stock. The host bone should be thoroughly débrided of any residual fibrous tissue to create a favorable environment for graft incorporation. For larger metaphyseal defects, the tibial or femoral canal should first be prepared to accept an appropriately sized intramedullary stem. The trial stem should be left in place, and the morselized cancellous allograft can be tightly packed around the stem. For large defects, several femoral heads may be needed. Preparation of the bone is facilitated by the use of a bone mill. To allow efficient packing, the bone should be processed through the bone mill several times to obtain suitably morselized bone. Alternatively, prepackaged morselized corticocancellous allograft can be obtained from several commercial sources. Once the defect has been tightly packed, the trial stem can be removed and the prosthesis and stem cemented in standard fashion.

STRUCTURAL ALLOGRAFT

The host bone is débrided back to healthy bleeding bone to facilitate graft incorporation. When possible, the distal femoral and proximal tibial resections are freshened by removing 1 to 2 mm of bone. Such resection leaves a flat surface on which to seat the prosthesis and maximizes host bone contact with the implant while minimizing further bone sacrifice. The structural allograft is then contoured to fill the defect. In some cases the host and allograft bone can be fashioned into corresponding trapezoidal shapes to maximize fit and intrinsic stability. When a femoral head allograft has been chosen, the host bone may be prepared with an appropriately sized acetabular reamer (Fig. 102–8). Host cortical bone should not be sac-

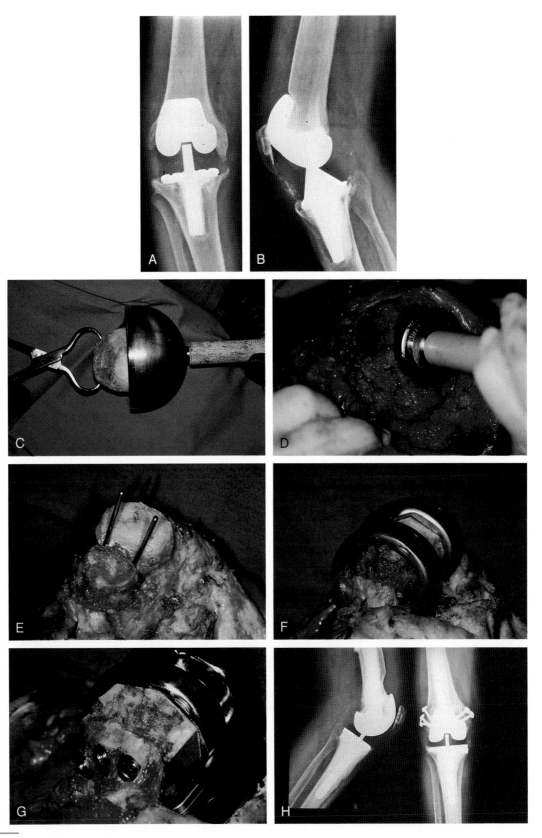

Figure 102–8. **A** and **B**, Anteroposterior and lateral views of a loose TKA with marked femoral and tibial bone loss. **C**, Femoral head allografts are prepared by using female resurfacing reamers. **D**, The host femur is prepared with corresponding small acetabular reamers to allow intimate contact with the allograft femoral heads. **E**, Temporary graft fixation with Steinmann pins. **F**, The distal end of the femur is prepared for the femoral component. **G**, Final graft fixation with cancellous bone screws and cementation of the femoral component with a long intramedullary stem. **H**, Postoperative anteroposterior and lateral views of the construct.

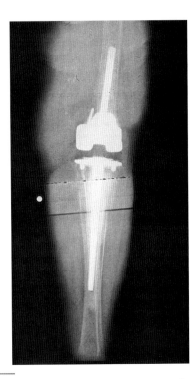

Figure 102–9. A bone-within-bone construct has been used on the tibial side. The proximal tibial allograft was prepared for the tibial prosthesis and then invaginated within the remaining host tibia.

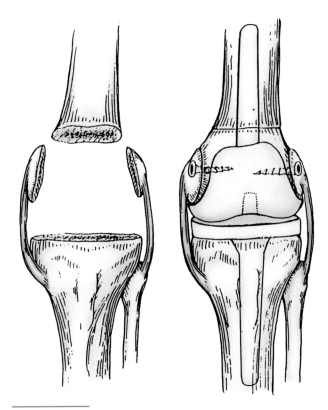

Figure 102–10. When a whole distal femoral allograft is needed, care should be taken to preserve the host bone at the epicondyles. The collateral ligaments can then be secured to the allograft with screws. (From Dennis DA: Structural allografting in revision total knee arthroplasty. In Insall JN, Scott WN, Scuderi GR [eds]: Current Concepts in Primary and Revision Total Knee Arthroplasty. Philadelphia, Lippincott-Raven, 1996.)

rificed. Kirschner wires are used to supplement the mechanical fit between the graft and host bone. Final shaping of the condylar surface of the allograft can be done with the standard knee cutting guides. If the intrinsic mechanical fit of the graft to host is poor, supplemental fixation with cancellous bone screws is appropriate. In cases in which an entire distal femur or proximal tibia are required, the graft-host junction can be step-cut to enhance intrinsic stability. Strut allografts and cables can be used to enhance stability at the host-allograft junction. Alternatively, a so-called bone-within-bone approach has been described for the proximal end of the tibia. In these cases the proximal tibia allograft was invaginated into the remaining host tibia (Fig. 102–9). In all cases, an intramedullary stem is used to bypass the graft and obtain fixation in the diaphyseal region. The prosthesis and stem should be cemented to the condylar surface and to the allograft because bone ingrowth from an avascular allograft to a porous-coated component is unlikely. The intramedullary stem itself may be inserted in a press-fit fashion with diaphyseal cortical contact, or it may be cemented in place. Collateral ligament reattachment can be problematic if allograft reconstruction of the entire distal femur or proximal tibia has been performed. In such cases, it is most appropriate to preserve the host ligament with a portion of bone attached. The ligament and attached host bone can then be fixed to the allograft with a bone screw (Fig. 102–10). Reattachment of the ligament and host bone to allograft bone appears to be the most reliable and durable way to restore appropriate collateral ligament function. Although soft-tissue reattachment to allograft can occur, obtaining appropriate ligament tension has proved problematic. In cases requiring collateral ligament reattachment, it may be prudent to choose a prosthesis designed to provide some inherent medial-lateral constraint, such as a constrained condylar knee. Postoperative management of a patient with a large allograft typically includes protected weightbearing for an extended period, particularly if the prosthesis is largely supported by allograft bone. In such cases full weightbearing should be delayed until there is radiographic evidence of allograft incorporation.

METAL WEDGES AND AUGMENTS

Indications. Modular metal wedges and augments are particularly useful for moderately sized bone defects, particularly in older patients and in revision knee surgery.

Limitations. Metal wedges and augments do not restore bone stock, which may be important in younger patients.

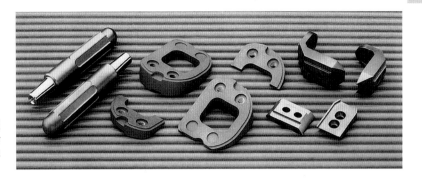

Figure 102–11. Modular metal wedges and blocks come in a variety of sizes and allow intraoperative fabrication of a nearly custom implant.

Modular metal wedges and block augments allow the intraoperative fabrication of a nearly custom implant (Fig. 98–11). By selectively filling distal femoral, posterior femoral, and proximal tibial defects, the surgeon can maximize prosthetic contact with host bone. Metal wedges and blocks are not subject to the problems with incorporation, revascularization, or collapse that can occur with bone graft.[17] Laboratory data have demonstrated that modular wedges perform almost as well as custom implants in transmitting load across tibial defects.[6, 15] Modular implants are less expensive than custom implants and allow more intraoperative flexibility. Templating for a custom implant, particularly estimating the extent of bone loss, is fraught with difficulty. Inappropriate templating can result in the distressing intraoperative situation in which an expensive custom implant does not fit the patient.

Restoration of the joint line, balance of the flexion and extension gaps, and proper femoral rotational alignment can all be facilitated with the use of modular femoral wedges. Distal femoral wedges can compensate for distal femoral bone loss and thus allow the prosthetic joint line to be accurately restored. Reproducing the joint line both improves collateral ligament kinematic function and limits patellar impingement on the tibial component. To obtain equal flexion and extension spaces, it is often necessary to choose a femoral component with an anteroposterior dimension that is greater than that of the remaining host bone. Modular augmentation of the posterior aspect of the femur can fill the gap between the prosthesis and bone and allow the use of an appropriately sized femoral component. Femoral component rotation should be set parallel to a line that connects the medial and lateral epicondyles. Often, selectively augmenting the distal lateral part of the femur slightly more than the distal medial portion aids in positioning the femoral component parallel to the transepicondylar axis. Care must be taken to avoid internal rotation of the femoral component relative to the transepicondylar axis because patellofemoral kinematics will be adversely affected.

On the tibial side, in vitro data have been collected to compare the use of metal wedges versus blocks in association with press-fit stems.[15] In that study, augmentation blocks performed slightly better than metal wedges, but the difference was small. The authors concluded that in clinical practice, the augment that best fills the bone defect should be chosen.

Clinical Results

Early and midterm results with the use of modular metal augments have been favorable.[5,15,34,36,37,52] Long-term results are not available. The durability of the interface between the modular augments and the prosthesis has been questioned, but major problems have not emerged. One clinical retrieval of a cemented metal wedge showed that after 6 years in vivo the interface had maintained 77% of its sheer strength as compared with a freshly cemented wedge[38] (Fig. 102–12). A study by Pagnano et al addressed modular tibial augments in primary TKA and reviewed 25 knees in 21 patients.[34] At a mean follow-up of 4.8 years, excellent and good results were achieved in 96% of patients. Although radiolucent lines were seen beneath the tibial component in 13 knees, none of those lucencies were progressive (Fig. 102–13).

Several studies have addressed the use of modular metal augments in revision TKA. Haas et al reviewed 76 revision knees with modular augments supplemented with press-

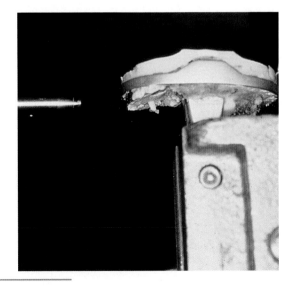

Figure 102–12. One cemented modular tibial wedge was retrieved after 6 years in vivo. The cement-wedge interface maintained 77% of its sheer strength when compared with a freshly cemented wedge.

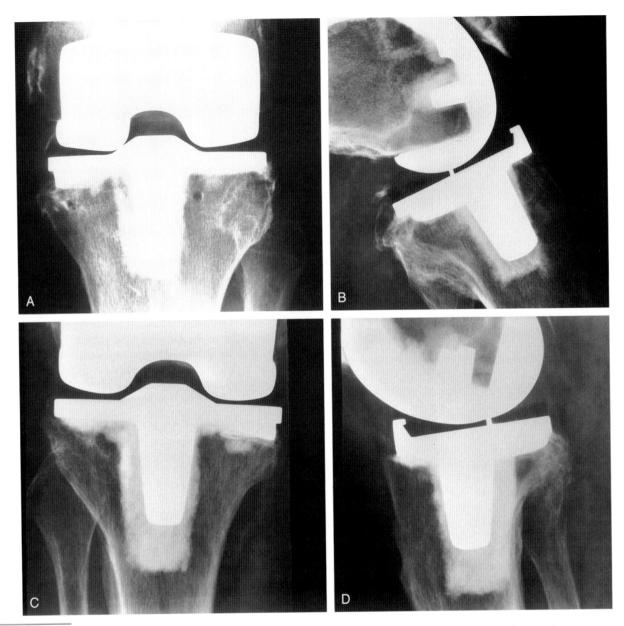

Figure 102–13. Anteroposterior (**A**) and lateral (**B**) views of a cemented modular metal wedge at 5 years demonstrates no radiolucency. Anteroposterior (**C**) and lateral (**D**) views of a cemented modular wedge at 9 years with a nonprogressive radiolucent line beneath the wedge. That line was present in the early postoperative radiographs and showed no progression over a 9-year period.

fit intramedullary stems.[22] The intramedullary rods in that series were sized to obtain a so-called clinical press-fit, but they were not reamed to achieve intimate cortical contact in the diaphysis. At a mean follow-up of 3 years, excellent or good results were found in 84%. Survivorship of the implants was 83% at 8 years. These authors believed that modular augmentation with press-fit rods was a reliable and durable procedure. Vince and Long reviewed 44 revisions with modular augmentations and press-fit intramedullary rods.[51] In 31 cases a posterior-stabilized implant was used, and in 13 a constrained condylar implant was used. At follow-up of 2 to 6 years, 3 of the 13 constrained condylar knees had loosened, in contrast

to none of the 31 posterior-stabilized knees. The authors initially suggested that press-fit rods may be inappropriate when coupled with a constrained condylar implant. Subsequent analysis has suggested that the mechanism of failure in these cases may have been related to suboptimal component alignment in part dictated by the intramedullary stem position. When press-fit stems dictate inappropriate component position, the surgeon must switch to either an offset stem or a smaller cemented stem to avoid component malposition (Fig. 102–14). Rand has studied 41 revision knees in which modular augmentation was used.[39] Modular augments were used for the distal end of the femur alone in 2 knees, the posterior aspect of the

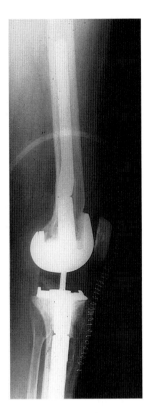

Figure 102–14. Offset intramedullary stems are useful on both the femoral and tibial sides. Here an offset femoral stem brings the femoral component more posterior and allows it to sit flush with the anterior cortex of the distal end of the femur.

femur alone in 16, and both the distal and posterior aspect of the femur in 12 knees. Tibial augments were used medially in 6 knees, both medially and laterally in 4 knees, and as a custom augmentation in 3 knees. Intramedullary stems were used in all cases and included press-fit stems in 17 femurs and 16 tibias and cemented stems in 14 femurs and 13 tibias. At a mean of 3 years' follow-up, excellent and good results were found in 98% of the 41 revisions. There were no cases of loosening. Takahashi and Gustilo used the same implant system and reported satisfactory results in 39 cases at a mean of 20 months' follow-up.[48] Patel et al reported 92% survivorship at 11 years for 102 revision TKAs treated with metal augments for type 2 bone defects.[36]

Surgical Technique

Tibial defects can be addressed with either metal wedges or metal blocks, depending on the extent and location of the bony defect. Large metal wedges that extend from one tibial condyle to the other are also available. Most modular total knee systems have instrumentation that is designed to prepare the host tibia to accept a metal wedge or block. An intramedullary cutting guide can be useful because it

will reproduce the component position that will be dictated by a press-fit intramedullary stem. Care must be taken to ensure that the tibial component is positioned perpendicular to the long axis of the tibia. If a press-fit stem will result in excessive varus or valgus positioning of the tibial component, either a smaller-diameter cemented stem or an offset tibial stem must be used. The surgeon must understand the design limits of the modular knee system that has been chosen. In particular, one should realize that some intramedullary stems are not designed to be inserted with cement. Once proper axial alignment has been verified, the proximal end of the tibia can be cut. In the revision situation this is done as a freshening cut with removal of 1 to 2 mm of bone from the more prominent side to provide a flat surface for the tibial baseplate. The tibial bone loss is surveyed, and an appropriately sized wedge or block is selected. A cutting guide for the block or wedge can then be assembled and a matching bone resection carried out. Care must be taken to set the rotation of the tibial component before resection for the wedge or block. That step ensures that the real component with its modular metal wedge will sit flush with the resection and be appropriately aligned and rotated relative to the femoral component. The trial tibial component with the wedge or block and intramedullary stem is assembled and inserted. If any questions about limb alignment or component position arise, an intraoperative radiograph is obtained. The real components should be assembled and then inspected by the surgeon before cementing. Care must be taken to ensure that the appropriately sized component and stem have been assembled and that the augment positions are correct. If an offset stem has been selected, it must be verified that it is offset in the proper direction. The real prosthesis can then be cemented into place.

Femoral augmentation blocks are used to restore the joint line, fill the flexion space, and ensure that femoral rotational alignment is parallel to the transepicondylar axis. An intramedullary cutting guide is assembled, and the distal femoral cut should be freshened to provided a flat surface on which the revision prosthesis is assembled. Many revision systems will have rod-and-sleeve guides that allow the cuts to be made relative to the position dictated by a press-fit intramedullary rod. The first task is to choose the appropriate femoral component. Preoperative templating of the opposite knee can be useful in determining the proper femoral component size. In many failed TKAs there is marked loss of posterior femoral bone, and one must avoid the temptation to downsize the femoral component to match the existing bone stock. A smaller femoral component may inadequately fill the flexion gap and could result in flexion instability. Once the proper-size component has been selected, the joint line must be reestablished. The most appropriate means in the revision setting is to identify the epicondyles and then measure distally from them. Typically, the joint line is 2.5 cm distal to the medial epicondyle. Distal augmentation blocks are then added to the femoral prosthesis to restore the joint line position. Femoral component rotation should be established by drawing a line across the distal end of the femur that connects the medial and lateral epicondyles.

The intercondylar box cutting guide should then be rotated parallel to that line. When distal femoral augmentation is being used, the box cutting guide should be moved distally a corresponding amount. This maneuver will preserve host bone in the intercondylar region. Finally, posterior femoral wedges are used to fill the gap between the posterior femoral runners and the posterior aspect of the femur. Care is taken to avoid overstuffing the posterior medial side because overstuffing would tend to cause compensatory internal rotation of the femoral component. The real component is then assembled and carefully inspected by the surgeon before cementing.

TRABECULAR METAL AUGMENTS

A recent addition to the revision TKA surgeon's armamentarium has been the introduction of porous metal augmentation cones and wedges. So-called trabecular metal augments, wedges, and cones can address large cavitary or combined cavitary and segmental defects by replacement of bone with this structural material. Trabecular metal is 80% porous and allows an excellent initial press-fit into remaining host bone that promotes bone ingrowth into the material for long-term biological fixation. Trabecular metal can be shaped intraoperatively to fit defects. Unlike structural allograft, however, trabecular metal will of course not resorb over time. The early clinical results at Mayo Clinic with trabecular metal augments for combined cavitary and segmental defects have been encouraging (Fig. 102–15).

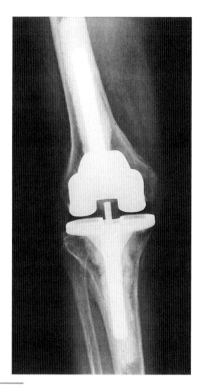

Figure 102–16. **Fully cemented femoral and tibial stems** after revision TKA.

STEMS

Most revision TKAs are cemented, at least at the condylar surface. Controversy still exists regarding cemented or press-fit fixation of intramedullary stems. A common approach is to apply cement to the condylar surface and around the proximal portion of the stem-prosthesis housing, but to press-fit the stem itself.[22] Care is taken with this approach to avoid placing cement at the junction between the stem and baseplate because such cement can markedly interfere with component removal should revision be needed. Good results have been reported with the technique of cemented revision with press-fit intramedullary stems. Other authors have had good results with fully cemented stems (Fig. 102–16). Murray et al used cemented long stems in 40 revision TKAs and found no cases of loosening at an average of 5 years' follow-up.[32] Whaley et al reported the continued follow-up of that same group of patients and found a 96% survival rate at 11 years with the Kinematic Stabilizer revision implant with fully cemented stems.[53] Rand has suggested that the choice of a cemented or press-fit intramedullary stem should be based on bone quality and the effect of the rod on implant alignment.[39] A press-fit stem is preferred in most situations because it facilitates subsequent revision. However, a press-fit stem may not be appropriate in the face of markedly osteopenic bone or marked metaphyseal deformity or in cases in which the press-fit stem would result in limb malalignment or component malposition.[4] Parsley et al[35] evaluated the effect of various tibial stems on mechanical alignment and found that canal-

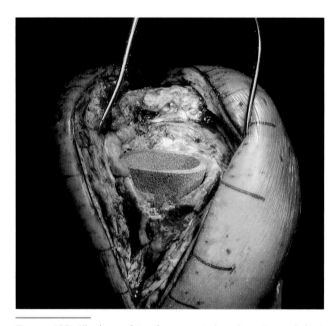

Figure 102–15. A combined segmental and cavitary defect on the tibial side is filled well with a trabecular metal cone. This construct can be fashioned quickly and customized intraoperatively and offers the opportunity for biological fixation in host bone without the risk of resorption that occurs with large structural allografts.

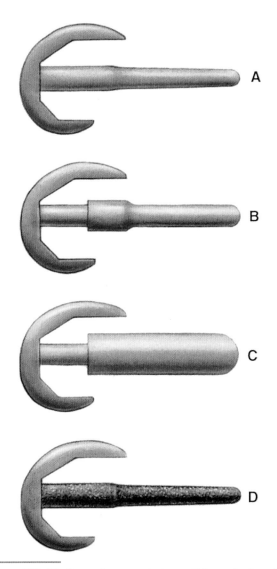

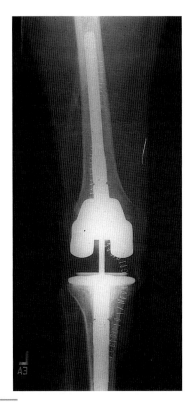

Figure 102–18. **Press-fit stems are often fluted. These stems should not be inserted with cement because the sharp flutes create an unfavorable cement-prosthesis interface.**

Figure 102–17. Smooth tapered stems (**A**) are designed for insertion with bone cement. Stems with complex geometries (**B** and **C**) or with porous coating (**D**) should not be inserted with cement around the stem itself. (From Garino JP, Lotke PA: Fixation techniques in revision total knee surgery. In Lotke PA, Garino JP [eds]: Revision Total Knee Arthroplasty. Philadelphia, Lippincott-Raven, 1999.)

SUMMARY

filling cementless stems helped ensure good tibial alignment. Typically, one should not cement an intramedullary stem that has been designed for insertion in a press-fit fashion (Fig. 102–17). Most rods designed for insertion with cement have gentle rounded surfaces to minimize stress on the cement-prosthesis interface. In contrast, most press-fit stems are fluted. These flutes cause high stress at the bone-cement interface, which could lead to cement mantle fracture (Fig. 102–18). Finally, Barrack et al[3] have drawn attention to the problem of pain at the end of the stem after revision TKA. These authors found end-of-stem pain on the femoral and tibial sides in 11% to 14% of patients both with cemented and with uncemented stems.

Successful reconstruction of a knee with marked bone deficiency requires careful preoperative planning to ensure that the appropriate prosthetic components and allograft bone are available. Small defects localized to one condyle can be successfully addressed with autograft or allograft bone or with a modular metal wedge or block. Alternatively, small defects can be contoured into a step configuration and filled with bone cement. Larger tibial defects can be reconstituted with large modular wedges or blocks and a thicker polyethylene insert (Fig. 102–19). Structural allograft reconstruction of the tibia is typically required when the degree of bone loss results in a flexion-extension gap that exceeds 40 mm. At that point, the thickest modular augments and thickest polyethylene inserts of most modular revision knee systems will fail to fill the gaps adequately. On the femoral side, 12-mm augmentation blocks are commonly available, but defects of greater size will require structural grafts. Any reconstruction that requires extensive bone grafting or modular augmentation is best protected by use of an intramedullary stem that bypasses the defect. The choice of press-fit or cemented intramedullary stem fixation is dictated by the quality of the metaphyseal bone, the extent of bone loss, and the effect of the rod on implant and limb alignment.

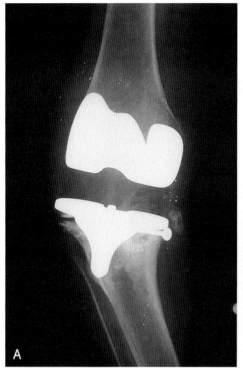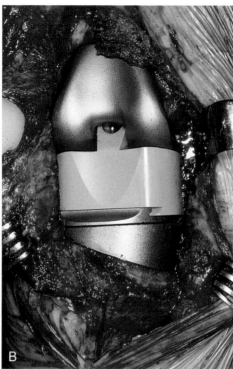

Figure 102–19. **A,** Marked medial tibial bone loss is seen on the preoperative radiograph. **B,** That defect is filled adequately with a full metal wedge and a thick tibial insert.

References

1. Aglietti P, Buzzi R, Scrobe F: Autologous bone grafting for medial defects in total knee arthroplasty. J Arthroplasty 6:287-294, 1991.
2. Altchek D, Sculco TP, Rawlins B: Autogenous bone grafting for severe angular deformity in total knee arthroplasty. J Arthroplasty 4:151-155, 1989.
3. Barrack RL, Rorabeck C, Burt M, Sawhney J: Pain at the end of the stem after revision total knee arthroplasty. Clin Orthop 367:216-225, 1999.
4. Bourne RB, Finlay JB: The influence of tibial component intramedullary stems and implant-cortex contact on the strain distribution of the proximal tibia following total knee arthroplasty. Clin Orthop 208:95-99, 1986.
5. Brand MG, Daley RJ, Ewald FC, et al: Tibial tray augmentation with modular metal wedges for tibial bone stock deficiency. Clin Orthop 248:71-79, 1989.
6. Brooks P, Walker P, Scott R: Tibial component fixation in deficient tibial bone stock. Clin Orthop 184:302-308, 1984.
7. Buck BE, Malinin TI, Brown MD: Bone transplantation and human immunodeficiency virus. An estimate of acquired immunodeficiency virus syndrome (AIDS). Clin Orthop 240:129-136, 1989.
8. Campbell DG, Li P, Stephenson AJ, et al: Sterilization of HIV by gamma irradiation: A bone allograft model. Int Orthop 18:172-176, 1994.
9. Chen F, Krackow K: Management of tibial defects in total knee arthroplasty. Clin Orthop 305:249-257, 1994.
10. Clatworthy MG, Balance J, Brick GW, et al: The use of structural allograft for uncontained defects in revision knee arthroplasty: A minimum five-year review. J Bone Joint Surg Am 83:404-411, 2001.
11. Dennis DA: Structural allografting in revision total knee arthroplasty. In Insall JN, Scott WN, Scuderi GR (eds): Current Concepts in Primary and Revision Total Knee Arthroplasty. Philadelphia, Lippincott-Raven, 1996.
12. Dorr LD, Ranawat CS, Sculco TA, et al: Bone graft for tibial defects in total knee arthroplasty. Clin Orthop 205:153-165, 1986.
13. Elia E, Lotke PA: Results of revision total knee arthroplasty associated with significant bone loss. Clin Orthop 271:114-121, 1991.
14. Engh G, Parks NL: The classification and treatment options for bone defects in revision knee surgery [abstract]. Presented at the Annual Meeting of the American Academy of Orthopedic Surgeons, February 24-28, 1994.
15. Fehring T, Peindl R, Humble R, et al: Modular tibial augmentation in total knee arthroplasty. Clin Orthop 327:207-217, 1996.
16. Freeman MAR, Bradley GW, Revell PA: Observations upon the interface between bone and polymethylmethacrylate cement. J Bone Joint Surg Br 64:489-493, 1982.
17. Garbuz DS, Masri BA, Czitrom AA: Biology of allografting. Orthop Clin North Am 29:199-204, 1998.
18. Garino JP, Lotke PA: Fixation techniques in revision total knee surgery. In Lotke PA, Garino JP (eds): Revision Total Knee Arthroplasty. Philadelphia, Lippincott-Raven, 1999.
19. Ghazavi MT, Stockley I, Yee G, et al: Reconstruction of massive bone defects with allograft in revision total knee arthroplasty. J Bone Joint Surg Am 79:17-25, 1997.
20. Gie GA, Linder L, Ling RSM, et al: Impacted cancellous allografts and cement for revision total hip arthroplasty. J Bone Joint Surg Br 75:14-21, 1993.
21. Gie GA, Linder L, Ling RS, et al: Contained morselized allograft in revision total hip arthroplasty: Surgical technique. Orthop Clin North Am 24:717-725, 1993.
22. Haas S, Insall J, Montgomery W, et al: Revision total knee arthroplasty with use of modular components with stems inserted without cement. J Bone Joint Surg Am 77:1700-1707, 1995.
23. Harris AL, Poddar S, Gitelis S, et al: Arthroplasty with a composite of an allograft and a prosthesis for knees with severe deficiency of bone. J Bone Joint Surg Am 77:373-386, 1995.
24. Harada Y, Wevers HW, Cooke TDV: Distribution of bone strength in the proximal tibia. J Arthroplasty 3:167-175, 1988.
25. Hvid I: Trabecular bone strength at the knee. Clin Orthop 227:210-221, 1988.
26. Insall JN: Revision of aseptic failed total knee arthroplasty. In Insall JN (ed): Surgery of the Knee, 2nd ed. New York, Churchill-Livingstone, 1993.
27. Kraay MJ, Goldberg VM, Figgie MP, Figgie HE III: Distal femoral replacement with allograft/prosthetic reconstruction for treatment of supracondylar fractures in patients with total knee arthroplasty. J Arthroplasty 7:7-16, 1992.
28. Laskin RS: Total knee arthroplasty in the presence of large bony defects of the tibia and marked knee instability. Clin Orthop 248:66-70, 1989.

29. Lonner JH, Lotke PA, Kim J, Nelson C: Impaction grafting and wire mesh for uncontained defects in revision total knee arthroplasty. Clin Orthop 404:145-151, 2002.

30. Mnaymneh W, Emerson RH, Borja F, et al: Massive allografts in salvage revision of failed total knee arthroplasty. Clin Orthop 260:144, 1990.

31. Mow CS, Weidel JD: Structural allografting in revision total knee arthroplasty. J Arthroplasty 11:235-241, 1996.

32. Murray PB, Rand JA, Hanssen, AD: Cemented long stem revision total knee arthroplasty. Clin Orthop 309:116-123, 1994.

33. Nelissen RG, Bauer TW, Weidenhielm LR, et al: Revision hip arthroplasty with the use of cement and impaction grafting. Histological analysis of four cases. J Bone Joint Surg Am 77:412-422, 1995.

34. Pagnano MW, Trousdale RT, Rand JA: Tibial wedge augmentation for bone deficiency in total knee arthroplasty—a followup study. Clin Orthop 321:151-155, 1995.

35. Parsley BS, Sugano N, Bertolusso R, Conditt MA: Mechanical alignment of tibial stems in revision total knee arthroplasty. J Arthroplasty 18(7 Suppl 1):33-36, 2003.

36. Patel JV, Masonis JL, Guerin J, et al: The fate of augments to treat type-2 bone defects in revision knee arthroplasty. J Bone Joint Surg Br 86:195-199, 2004.

37. Rand JA: Bone deficiency in total knee arthroplasty: Use of metal wedge augmentation. Clin Orthop 271:63-71, 1991.

38. Rand J: Augmentation of a total knee arthroplasty with a modular metal wedge. J Bone Joint Surg Am 77:266-268, 1995.

39. Rand J: Modularity in total knee arthroplasty. Acta Orthop Belg 62:180-185, 1996.

40. Ritter MA: Screw and cement fixation of large defects in total knee arthroplasty. J Arthroplasty 1:125-129, 1986.

41. Ritter MA, Keating EM, Faris PM: Screw and cement fixation of large defects in total knee arthroplasty. A sequel. J Arthroplasty 8:63-64, 1993.

42. Samuelson KM: Bone grafting and noncemented revision arthroplasty of the knee. Clin Orthop 226:93-101, 1988.

43. Scott G, Patel M, Braden M: Use of prepolymerized cement spacers to augment the femoral component in revision total knee arthroplasty: A clinical outcome and laboratory experiment. J Arthroplasty 18:769-774, 2003.

44. Scuderi GR, Insall JH, Haas SB, et al: Inlay autogenic bone grafting of tibial defects in primary total knee arthroplasty. Clin Orthop 248:93-97, 1989.

45. Sculco TP: Bone grafting. In Lotke PA (ed): Master Techniques in Orthopedic Surgery, Knee Arthroplasty. New York, Raven Press, 1995.

46. Sneppen D, Christensen P, Larsen H, Vang PS: Mechanical testing of trabecular bone in total knee replacement. Development of an osteopenetrometer. Int Orthop 5:251-256, 1981.

47. Stockley I, McAuley JP, Gross AE: Allograft reconstruction in total knee arthroplasty. J Bone Joint Surg Br 74:393-397, 1992.

48. Takahashi Y, Gustilo R: Nonconstrained implants in revision total knee arthroplasty. Clin Orthop 309:156-162, 1994.

49. Tsahakis PJ, Beaver WB, Brick GW: Technique and results of allograft reconstruction in revision total knee arthroplasty. Clin Orthop 303:86-94, 1994.

50. Ullmark G, Hovelius L: Impacted morsellized allograft and cement for revision total knee arthroplasty: A preliminary report of 3 cases. Acta Orthop Scand 67:10-12, 1996.

51. Vince KG, Long W: Revision knee arthroplasty: The limits of press fit medullary fixation. Clin Orthop 317:172-177, 1995.

52. Werle JR, Goodman SB, Imrie SN: Revision total knee arthroplasty using large distal femoral augments for severe metaphyseal bone deficiency: A preliminary study. Orthopedics 25:325-327, 2002.

53. Whaley AL, Trousdale RT, Rand JA, Hanssen AD: Cemented long-stem revision total knee arthroplasty. J Arthroplasty 18:592-599, 2003.

54. Whiteside LA: Cementless revision total knee arthroplasty. Clin Orthop 286:160-167, 1993.

55. Wilde AW, Schickendantz MS, Stulberg BN, et al: The incorporation of tibial allografts in total knee arthroplasty. J Bone Joint Surg Am 72:815-824, 1990.

56. Windsor RE, Insall JN, Sculco TP: Bone grafting of tibial defects in primary and revision total knee arthroplasty. Clin Orthop 205:132-137, 1986.

Extensor Mechanism Disruption after Total Knee Arthroplasty

Kelly G. Vince • Cass Nakasone

Disruption of the extensor mechanism after total knee arthroplasty (TKA) is devastating to the patient and surgeon. This complication rivals deep infection as the worst outcome of a knee replacement because of the serious functional impairment and the profound difficulty of restoring knee function. Sharkey and colleagues in Philadelphia reported the reasons for revision surgery in over 200 cases. Significant extensor lag from rupture, patella baja, or patellectomy accounted for 6.6% of revisions, the majority of which occurred within 2 years of the primary arthroplasty.[39] The anatomic location of the rupture (quadriceps tendon, patellar bone, or patellar tendon) has implications for prevention, prognosis, and treatment (Fig. 103–1). Quadriceps tendon rupture can sometimes be prevented by the orientation of the arthrotomy. Transverse patellar fractures require surgery only if there is an extensor lag or the patellar component has loosened. Disruption of the patellar tendon or its attachment to either the patella or the tibial tubercle is the most resistant to reconstruction and requires elaborate surgery. In general, repairs that succeed in the absence of an arthroplasty are not appropriate after a knee prosthesis has been implanted. Sadly, extensor mechanism rupture is often associated with sepsis or global knee instability, further limiting the chance for restoration of function. Arthrodesis or amputation may result.

Extensor mechanism complications, including maltracking, patellar component wear and loosening, patellar fracture, and extensor rupture, have been reviewed.[38,47,51,53,63,67] A few publications, including this one, focus exclusively on problems that functionally separate the quadriceps muscle from the tibial tubercle.[18,60,61]

INCIDENCE AND PREVENTION OF QUADRICEPS TENDON RUPTURE

Prevention is supremely important because disruption of the extensor mechanism renders an otherwise successful knee arthroplasty virtually useless. Corrective surgery is difficult and fraught with complications. The results are at best compromised, and at worst the entire limb may be in jeopardy.

The quadriceps tendon is probably the least likely site of extensor disruption. Sinha, Crossett, and Rubash,[60,61] in a excellent review of extensor mechanism disruption after TKA, cite a 1.1% (3 of 281) incidence of quadriceps tendon rupture after TKA, quoting Lynch et al.[46] This number (from 1987) should be considered high by current standards. In a recent, comprehensive study of the problem, Dobbs and colleagues from the Mayo Clinic identified 24 primary TKA patients with either a partial or complete quadriceps tendon rupture among their patients.[17] During the same time interval (1976 to 2002), 23,800 primary, condylar-type knee replacements were performed, for an incidence of 0.1%. Because of the difficulties with such a large database, this incidence may be underreported. The true risk nationwide probably lies somewhere between 0.1% and 1.0%.

Systemic factors beyond the control of the surgeon may increase the risk for quadriceps tendon rupture. Fernandez-Baillo et al suggested that rheumatoid arthritis might have been a risk factor in the case that they reported.[21] Dobbs and colleagues[17] added diabetes mellitus, chronic renal failure, obesity, and hyperthyroidism as risk factors in their review of the literature on quadriceps tendon rupture with or without knee arthroplasty.[28,46,62,64]

Lynch and colleagues from the University of Western Ontario identified aggressive resection of patellar bone at the time of resurfacing as potentially jeopardizing the attachment of the quadriceps tendon to the patella.[46] Similarly, a lateral patellar retinacular release that extends proximally and then medially across the tendon may predispose to rupture. An insidious cause of quadriceps tendon rupture may be the location and orientation of the arthrotomy. If the very common medial parapatellar approach strays transversely across the quadriceps tendon (especially if it does so close to the proximal part of the patella), many, if not all the longitudinal fibers of the tendon will be transected with little soft tissue for repair. Such an arthrotomy will be held together only by sutures until the surgery heals (Fig. 103–2).

An arthrotomy that transects the quadriceps tendon medially to laterally has been described as the "wandering resident approach" (because of its inadvertent origins) for a difficult exposure.[29] It seems best, with this approach, to cross the tendon proximally and thus maintain a long section for "side-to-side" closure. In this respect, the "wandering resident" approach resembles the "quadriceps snip"[3,24] (which also originated inadvertently, but has not been associated with an increased risk for quadriceps tendon rupture). Ideally, none of the structures that resist the huge tensile force (quadriceps tendon, patella, patellar tendon and its attachments to the patella and the tibia) on the extensor mechanism in normal knee function should be violated by the surgical approach or patellar preparation.

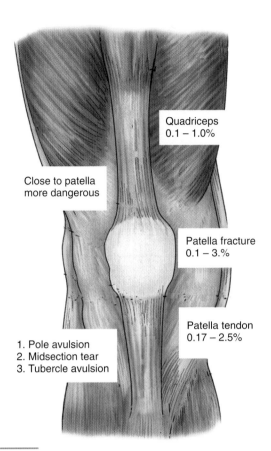

Figure 103–1. The incidence of extensor mechanism rupture after total knee arthroplasty is difficult to quantify. Quadriceps tendon rupture may be easier to treat unless the rupture is transverse and close to the superior pole of the patella. Not all patellar fractures result in rupture of the extensor mechanism—but it may be the most common cause of extensor lag. Inferior rupture may result from avulsion of the patellar tendon from the patella, a midsubstance tear, or avulsion from the tibial tubercle. Such ruptures are invariably problematic.

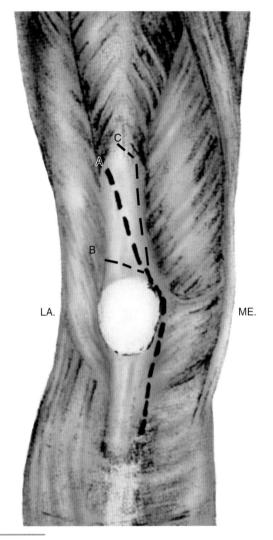

Figure 103–2. Line A depicts the "wandering resident" arthrotomy, recommended for difficult exposure. Line C is the standard "quadriceps snip" exposure, which is easily and safely created from a standard medial approach when necessary. Line B is to be avoided. The more horizontal the arthrotomy and the closer to the patella, the more likely a chronic extensor mechanism rupture that cannot easily be repaired. (Reprinted from Hendel D, Weisbort M, Garti A: "Wandering resident" surgical exposure for 1- or 2-stage revision arthroplasty in stiff aseptic and septic knee arthroplasty. J Arthroplasty 19:757, 2004.)

TREATMENT OF QUADRICEPS TENDON RUPTURE

Few treated cases of quadriceps tendon rupture after knee arthroplasty have been reported. A technique described by C. Scuderi in 1958 for the treatment of quadriceps tendon rupture in the absence of knee arthroplasty[57] was applied successfully by Fernandez-Baillo to a knee replacement patient. This repair was reinforced with Dacron tape and the knee immobilized in a cast for 6 weeks.[21] Sinha and colleagues alluded to "attempted primary repair and Achilles tendon reconstruction"[60] for ruptured quadriceps tendons with mixed results. Extensor mechanism allografts, originally described for rupture of the patellar tendon, may also be used to repair the quadriceps tendon (Fig. 103–3).[11,18,48]

Dobbs, Hanssen, and colleagues[17] reported good results with conservative treatment in patients with "partial"

quadriceps tendon tears. By contrast, 7 of 11 patients with complete tears who underwent surgical reconstruction experienced poor outcomes and a high complication rate. The technique in 10 was adapted from Scuderi's 1958 surgery,[57] "with or without" drill holes in the patella. Two patients had the reconstruction reinforced with Marlex mesh (C.R. Bard, Murray Hill, NJ), which these surgeons recommend and illustrate in their manuscript. Complications in the surgically reconstructed cases were legion: four with rerupture, one with recurvatum and instability, and two with deep periprosthetic infection necessitating resection arthroplasty that ended in amputation for one patient. Motion was maintained in the successful cases,

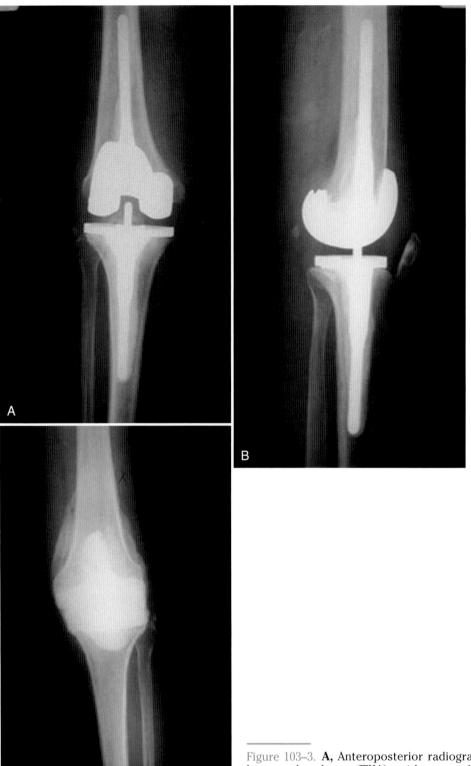

Figure 103–3. **A,** Anteroposterior radiograph of an infected revision total knee arthroplasty (TKA) with a nonlinked constrained prosthesis. **B,** Lateral radiograph of a failed, infected revision TKA with extreme patella baja/infra secondary to quadriceps tendon rupture. **C,** Nonarticulating antibiotic-impregnated cement spacer block.

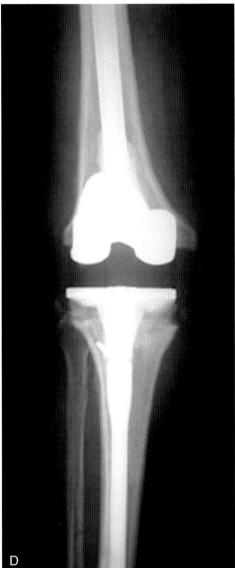

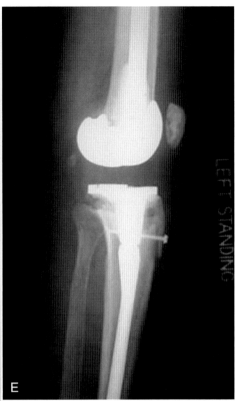

Figure 103–3, cont'd. **D,** Anteroposterior radiograph of a second revision/reimplantation TKA with uncemented stem extensions, a non-constrained prosthesis, and a proximal tibial allograft with an extensor mechanism attached. **E,** Lateral radiograph of the reimplantation with a combined proximal tibial and extensor mechanism allograft. A single screw has been added to the tubercle to resist avulsion.

with 0 to 10 degrees of extensor lag and flexion ranging from 60 to 125 degrees. In one of their patients, a revision knee arthroplasty was performed concurrent with the extensor reconstruction. The role of concurrent revision arthroplasty to address potential causes of extensor rupture has not been evaluated in the literature.

INCIDENCE AND PREVENTION OF TRANSVERSE PATELLAR FRACTURES

Patellar fractures may or may not interrupt the extensor mechanism. Those that do not are usually longitudinal (vertical), can be treated without surgery unless a patellar component has worn or loosened, and may result from rotational positioning problems of the tibial and femoral components.[47,63,67] Accordingly, not all patellar fractures are pertinent to our discussion because we are concerned here only with those that result in significant extensor lag.

Nor is the older literature on patellar fractures pertinent because improvements in implant design and surgical technique have made old theories of etiology and old figures on incidence irrelevant. Sinha et al indicated that the incidence of all patellar fractures after TKA ranges from 0.27%[71] to 5.4%.[32] The incidence with the original Insall-Burstein posterior-stabilized prosthesis is as high as 8.4%, attributable to larger (thicker) patellar components, increased flexion, and a higher level of activity.[33] Most of these fractures were longitudinal without disruption of the extensor. Modifications of femoral component designs, in particular, the trochlear groove, have reduced the incidence of patellar fracture with this and other knee prostheses, thus highlighting the role of implant geometry in patellar fractures.

All studies of patellar fracture conclude that transverse fractures with extensor mechanism disruption (and extensor mechanism lag) are problematic. Goldberg and colleagues segregated patellar fractures after arthroplasty by anatomic site in a 1988 paper. Goldberg types II (fractures involving the implant-cement interface or quadriceps mechanism) and IIIA (inferior pole fracture with patellar ligament rupture) result in extensor discontinuity. These accounted for 6 of 36 (16.7%) and 8 of 36 (22.2%) fractures, respectively, thereby establishing that somewhat less than half of all patellar fractures led to disruption of the extensor in that era.[26]

Hozack and colleagues, also in 1988, focused primarily on whether the patellar fracture was displaced or not, then whether the component was loose, and finally on the integrity of the extensor.[30] Patellar complications may be associated with lateral tracking of the extensor. Vertical fractures, with or without component loosening, seem to result from a patella that wants to dislocate laterally and a patellar button that fits congruently in the femoral trochlear groove, resisting dislocation. Patellar fractures complicating TKA should probably be evaluated by computed tomography (CT) for rotational positioning, and a full revision may be necessary to correct tracking problems.[47]

Keating and colleagues identified 177 patellar fractures in 4583 TKAs (3.9%). They segregated them into 22 vertical fractures with a well-fixed implant and an intact extensor mechanism, 21 with disruption of the extensor mechanism of less than 1 cm, 17 with disruption of the extensor by more than 1 cm, and 114 with a loose component but an intact extensor mechanism. This study identifies 177 of 4583 cases with a significantly "ruptured extensor" (0.37%), thus making the complication unusual.[37] Ortiguera and Berry, from the Mayo Clinic, published another study with a broad scope.[50] They identified 85 (0.68%) fractures after 12,464 TKAs. This figure is fivefold less than Keating's observation. Complete capture of all complications will be more difficult as cohort size and geographic distribution increase. Consistent with other studies, only 12 (0.09%) fractures were associated with extensor mechanism rupture. The low incidence confirms that few surgeons will often encounter this difficult problem in their practice. Both recent studies indicate that the best results, no matter what type of fracture, occurred when conservative management was feasible. When surgery was necessary, the results were generally poor.

Much of the old discussion on risk factors for patellar fracture after TKA was conjectural. The true risk factors for patella fractures that threaten the integrity of the extensor mechanism and how they can be avoided are difficult to define. Postulated risk factors fall into the following categories: (1) patellar maltracking and avascular necrosis (including the effect of lateral patellar retinacular release, fat pad excision, and thermal necrosis from cement), (2) weak or damaged bone and tendon (osteoporosis, revision surgery, excessive bone resection, clamping of tendon, bone cysts), (3) component design (prominent femoral trochlea, thick patellar prosthesis, size and alignment of patellar fixation holes), and (4) large tensile force in the extensor mechanism (male gender, patient size and activity, manipulation under general anesthesia, degree of flexion). Without establishing which factors are the most dangerous, there is general assent that most are deleterious.

RISK FACTORS FOR EXTENSOR MECHANISM DISRUPTION THROUGH THE PATELLA

Extensor mechanism maltracking probably heightens the risk for all patellar complications, including fracture. If internal rotation of the femoral and/or tibial components is at the root of a patellar fracture, most treatment options short of revision arthroplasty are likely to produce poor results. Hozack et al reviewed their patellar fractures in 1988,[30] predating studies that clearly identified the relationship between internally rotated components and patellar complications.[6,10] Revision surgery was not generally done, and the results, consistent with subsequent studies on the surgical treatment of extensor mechanism rupture through the patella, were poor.[37,50] The results may have benefited from concurrent revision arthroplasty.

Whether avascular necrosis or patellar maltracking has a greater impact on the development of patellar fractures is unknown. The relationship between avascular necrosis, more frequent after lateral patellar retinacular release,[58] and maltracking, however, is not often appreciated. If femoral and/or tibial components have been internally rotated, this will lead to maltracking that is apparent at surgery and, consequently, a greater likelihood of lateral patellar retinacular release. Does the release cause avascular necrosis, which in turn increases the risk for fracture?[28,55,56] If so, is it not maltracking that leads to the release and in some cases the rotational position of the femoral and tibial components that leads to the release? Component positioning is certainly the factor most directly under the control of the surgeon.

Other factors postulated, but in no way proven, to increase the risk for fracture via avascular necrosis include compromise of the patellar blood supply by excision of the infrapatellar fat pad[15] and thermal necrosis of bone from the heat of polymethylmethacrylate cement as it polymerizes.[15,27] Hughes and colleagues investigated the effect of surgical dissection on patellar blood flow during surgery with a laser Doppler device. The blood supply decreased to 60.4% of normal after medial arthrotomy and then decreased another 10.4% after resection of the patellar fat pad. Lateral patellar retinacular release brought the vasculature to 43.6%, and ultimately, loss of the superolateral geniculate brought the blood supply to 30.6% of normal.[31] The threshold at which a patella is likely to suffer avascularity and necrosis has not been established.

Kayler and Lyttle concluded that the "prepatellar" or anterior blood supply was very important in a study of cadavers. The intraosseous blood vessels of the patella were compromised by cutting the patella and resecting the fat pad, even when the arthrotomy was performed more than a centimeter away from the patella.[36] Ogata et al studied the effects of surgical dissection on patellar blood flow in monkeys with a hydrogen washout technique. Patellar blood flow decreased to 65% after medial arthrotomy, and complete removal of the fat pad lowered the blood supply to 49% of control. Lateral release and fat pad removal reduced the blood supply to 17% of control.[49]

The fat pad contributes to the blood supply of the patella. However, the link has not yet been established between patellar fracture and removal of the infrapatellar fat pad. Many surgeons routinely remove this structure without an apparent increase in the incidence of patellar fractures, let alone disruption of the extensor mechanism. The complete story may invoke all effects, with maltracking increasing force on the patella and also leading to lateral patellar retinacular release. The worst patellar fractures in one study correlated with higher degrees of malalignment, in an era before CT had been applied to arthroplasties.[22] A study of the rotational position of components by CT in knees with patellar fractures would be illuminating.

Thermal necrosis of bone may result from polymerization of polymethylmethacrylate bone cement, but to a depth that is unlikely to result in structural impairment and fracture. In fact, when this effect is avoided completely with uncemented patellar implants, the incidence of patellar fracture appears to be higher.[28,55] Indeed, even the saws that are used to cut the patella have been associated with high temperature in the bone.[43]

Bone may be weakened not only by avascular necrosis but also as a result of "over-resection" for patellar resurfacing, osteoporosis, osteoarthritic cysts, and previous fracture. The implications for fracture of weakened bone cannot be refuted. In general, surgeons have been encouraged to resect an amount of bone equal in thickness to the known thickness of the polyethylene patellar component. A frequent concern is that an inordinately thick resurfaced patella will result in a stiff knee. A biomechanical test measured a 22% increase in anterior patellar strain with a conventional resurfacing prosthesis and a 28% increase with an inset-style patellar prosthesis. Increased strain is likely to increase the risk for fracture. Progressive over-resection of bone was significantly more detrimental with inset designs.[72]

Does this information help in the debate over whether the patella should be left unresurfaced? Controversy persists regarding whether residual pain in an unresurfaced patella is a greater problem than extensor mechanism complications after a prosthesis has been applied. Sinha et al, in their careful review of patellar fractures, found three factors that statistically increased the risk for patella fracture: patellar resurfacing, lateral patellar retinacular release, and revision surgery.[60]

Boyd and colleagues from Harvard compared 396 knees that underwent patellar resurfacing with 495 in which the patellae were left unresurfaced. Complications occurred about a year earlier in the group with resurfacing. There was a higher incidence of patellar tendon rupture (0.75% versus 0.40%) and patellar fracture (0.75% versus zero) after resurfacing. However, chronic peripatellar pain occurred in 0.25% of the resurfaced patellae as compared with 10.3% of the unresurfaced patellae.[9] These results, published in 1993, are likely to have been improved on in the passing decade. Grace and Sim described a significant difference in the incidence of patellar fracture after patellar resurfacing: 9 of 2719 (0.33%) versus 3 of 5530 (0.05%) ($p < 0.05$).[27] If comfort and function are hypothesized to be superior with resurfacing, these studies do not

so much argue against resurfacing of the patella as they do argue in favor of superior surgical technique and advanced implant designs.

The statistical significance of lateral patellar retinacular release has been expounded by Healy et al in 1995,[28] Scott et al in 1982,[56] and Tria et al in 1994.[65] Again, it is difficult to argue against performing lateral release and even more difficult to discern whether this effect originates from avascularity, maltracking, or a combination of the two. In general, with improved designs, greater understanding of the importance of rotational positioning of femoral and tibial components, and improved surgical approaches,[8] the incidence of lateral patellar retinacular release and (one hopes) patellar fracture has decreased.

The final statistically significant feature associated with patella fractures is revision surgery. Multiple surgeries have a deleterious effect by virtue of thinner, weaker, often osteolytic bone; compromised vascularity; and poor flexion. Grace and Sim found patellar fractures in 3 of 495 revision knee arthroplasties (0.61%) and 9 of 7754 primary replacements (0.12%) ($p < 0.05$).[27]

TREATMENT OF PATELLAR FRACTURES

Patellar fractures must be treated differently, depending on whether a knee arthroplasty is in place. Without an arthroplasty, the patella is a normal size and shape. The blood supply is intact, and it is important to reestablish articular congruence to avoid painful arthritic deterioration. Tension band wiring based on the principles of Pauwel is often the favored technique. Accordingly, the fracture fragments are held together by two parallel wires, around which stainless steel suture is wrapped in a "figure of 8" and then tightened. These wires induce a force vector across the anterior aspect of the patella that may even be strong enough to create a gap on the articular side. With knee flexion, the femoral condyle theoretically compresses the gap and forces the fracture fragments together.[66] It should be noted that this mechanism has been difficult to prove in experimental models.[70]

A resurfaced patella, by contrast, cannot be expected, even theoretically, to benefit from tension band wiring. There is barely enough room to admit the parallel pins. The deep surface of the bone, usually forced together by tension banding, no longer exists, and thus the principles are not applicable. Furthermore, if the patella was not avascular at the time of fracture, there is a strong possibility that the surgical approach has compromised the blood supply, so important for fracture healing. Tension band wiring is not recommended for patellar fractures complicating knee arthroplasty (Fig. 103–4).

Despite displacement of the fracture fragments, loosening of the patellar prosthesis, and even an acute extensor lag, it is probably best to temporize before recommending open reduction and internal fixation of a fractured, resurfaced patella. The knee joint can usually be immobilized in extension and re-evaluated within 2 weeks. Many of these patellae are relatively avascular and fragmented. Immediate surgery can only remove a loose component

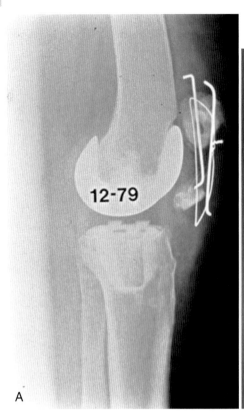
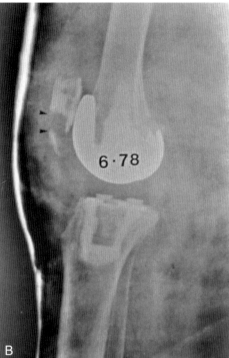

Figure 103–4. **A,** Lateral radiograph (dated December 1979) showing failed tension band wiring of a transverse patellar fracture that had resulted in an extensor mechanism rupture. This type of fixation is no longer recommended for patellar fractures in the presence of knee arthroplasty. **B,** Lateral radiograph (dated June 1978) of a total knee arthroplasty immobilized in plaster after an inferior pole fracture of the patella resulting in extensor mechanism lag. This is a good first step and will succeed in many cases. (Courtesy of John Insall.)

and perhaps cerclage the residual bone fragments. With time, the fracture fragments may coalesce into a mass that is large enough to hold a new patellar prosthesis (Fig. 103–5). After 4 to 6 weeks, a persistent lag or a loose component will necessitate surgery. Some of these patients eliminate their extensor lag, in which case surgery can be limited to removal or revision of a loose button. CT scanning may help determine whether the rotational positioning of the tibial and femoral components could be improved by concurrent revision arthroplasty.

Keating and colleagues observed that four of nine patients with patellar fractures and loose components suffered infection complicating simple removal of the components. Both patients in whom open reduction plus internal fixation was performed ended with nonunion of the fragments. The authors recommended nonoperative treatment and acknowledged the advantage of patellectomy with repair of the residual tendon.[37]

Ortiguera and Berry described 12 of 85 fractures complicating knee arthroplasty that also had disruption of the extensor mechanism. One patient treated by prolonged immobilization without surgery achieved a pain-free state with a 5-degree lag. Of six who underwent open reduction and internal fixation, only one achieved bone union. Five had partial patellectomy and tendon advancement to bone, with three requiring additional surgery. Six of the 12 suffered complications, 5 underwent reoperations, and 7 had pain, patellar instability, or extensor weakness.[50] Both these publications illustrated failed tension band wiring.[37,50] The "basket plate," a new fixation device for inferior pole avulsion fractures of the patella (in the absence of knee replacement), has been described.[35] Though as yet untried in the presence of a knee replace-

ment, it is likely to fail for many of the same reasons as tension band wiring: limited bone stock and avascularity. In short, although cerclage fixation is often recommended for patellar fractures with an extensor lag, there are no good data to substantiate this recommendation, other than the abysmal results with tension band wiring. Delayed surgery may be best.

PATELLAR TENDON RUPTURE AND AVULSION

Patellar tendon rupture or avulsion is uncommon and profoundly debilitating. It is reported in 0.17%[54] to 2.5%[1] of patients with total knee replacements. Because of its rarity, large studies have not been conducted and the ideal treatment is uncertain. Conventional wisdom recommended arthrodesis in these cases, but the resulting disability is severe. More functionally appealing reconstructions have been described, including a case of a chronic, neglected patellar tendon rupture in the presence of severe osteoarthritis that was treated by patellectomy and TKA with advancement of the tendon.[14] Surgeons have sutured the tendon end into a trough in the tubercle and then supplemented the repair with tension band wiring.[2] Fujikawa et al treated 25 such cases with a Leeds-Keio synthetic ligament repair and obtained good results in the 18 whom they were able to monitor.[23] Other techniques include cast immobilization with or without operative repair and reconstruction with semitendinosus, fascia lata, or hamstring tendon autogenous graft; Dacron 4-mm vascular graft (U.S. Catheter and Instrument, Glen Falls, NY); and

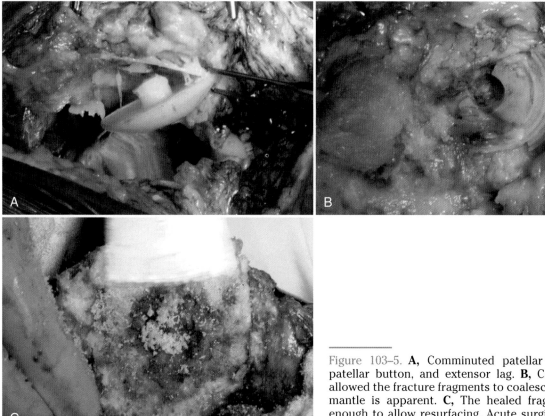

Figure 103–5. **A,** Comminuted patellar fracture, a loose patellar button, and extensor lag. **B,** Cast immobilization allowed the fracture fragments to coalesce. Residual cement mantle is apparent. **C,** The healed fragments were thick enough to allow resurfacing. Acute surgical intervention is unlikely to succeed.

bovine xenograft.[54] Zanotti et al used the bone–patellar tendon–bone complex that is used for anterior cruciate ligament reconstructions with some success.[73] The patella was fused to the proximal end of the tibia in an unusual case of ruptured patellar tendon complicating a knee arthroplasty in the presence of metabolic bone disease.[39]

Reconstruction with an intact unit consisting of an allograft tibial tubercle, patellar tendon, patella, and quadriceps tendon was reported by Emerson et al in 1990.[19] Several studies of this and other techniques have been published in small numbers of patients.[1,16,19,20,45,48,52] These pioneering efforts have established several important principles of the extensor mechanism allograft technique.

TREATMENT WITH AN EXTENSOR MECHANISM ALLOGRAFT

The largest series of extensor mechanism allografts involved 36 patients and was published by Nazarian and Booth in 1999.[48] Other studies of the surgical reconstruction of ruptured patellar tendons are smaller, with 7 to 20 patients whose average age ranged from 64 to 74 years.[1,5,16,19,20,45,48] The average follow-up ranged from 23 to 43 months after the initial reconstruction.[1,16,19,20,45,48] The indications for surgical reconstruction were rupture of the extensor mechanism between the tibial tubercle and the inferior pole of the patella in the majority (33% to 86%).[1,19,20,45,48] Previous patellectomy was the second most common indication for reconstruction and accounted for

15% to 44% of cases.[1,19,20,48] Quadriceps tendon rupture was the third indication for extensor mechanism allografting (15% to 31%),[1,19,48] followed by patella fractures (10% to 14%).[1,48] Extensor mechanism allografts have been used to treat debilitating extensor lag after TKA as a result of previous patellectomy.[42]

In general, extensor mechanism allograft reconstruction is considered a salvage procedure. It does not achieve the results of primary arthroplasty or revision surgery that is uncomplicated by extensor rupture. The average postoperative Knee Society scores range between 52 and 88 points[1,19,20,45,48] and the average maximum postoperative knee flexion from 98 to 108 degrees.[1,19,20,45,48] Thirty percent to 100% of patients had an extension lag ranging from 4.3 to 59.0 degrees after reconstruction.[1,19,20,45,48] The proportion of reconstructions requiring revision or additional surgery ranged between 15% and 86%.[1,19,20,45,48] Failure rates (defined as repeat surgery or an extensor lag exceeding 30 degrees) were as high as 100%.[1,19,20,45,48] Nonetheless, when the reconstruction works, it gives the best possible functional results for a devastating complication.

TECHNICAL CONSIDERATIONS— RESURFACING OF ALLOGRAFT PATELLA

Resurfacing an allograft patella is controversial, but usually considered unnecessary. In their original patients, Emerson et al resurfaced all allograft patellae.[19,20] By 1990,

31% were resurfaced with an all-polyethylene component and 69% with metal-backed buttons.[19] In their 1994 report, 60% of their patellae were resurfaced with an all-polyethylene component and only 40% with metal-backed implants.[20] Complications related to the patellar components developed in 2 (13.3%) of their original 15 patients. One patient had catastrophic wear of a metal-backed component. It was revised to an all-polyethylene component that sustained a nondisplaced patellar fracture. In the second patient, loosening of a cemented all-polyethylene component resulted in "mechanical" problems. They were the first to question the need to resurface the insensate allograft patella and to warn of complications.[1,19,20] Whether an unresurfaced patella is stronger or more durable than a resurfaced allograft has not been resolved.

TECHNICAL CONSIDERATIONS—FREEZE-DRIED VERSUS FRESH FROZEN ALLOGRAFT

In 1994, Emerson et al reported one patellar tendon rupture, patella fracture, wear-through of a metal-backed patellar component, and loosening of a cemented all-polyethylene component in allograft reconstructions. All occurred with freeze-dried, irradiated allografts.[20] Their series consisted of nine freeze-dried allografts and six fresh frozen allografts. Although they did not condemn freeze-dried allografts, they questioned their strength.[20] Subsequent series have implanted only fresh frozen allografts.[1,19,48]

Fresh frozen allografts have suffered complications. Leopold et al reported a 14.0% incidence of patellar tendon rupture in their fresh frozen allografts.[45] Nazarian and Booth reported a 6% incidence and Burnett et al a 29% incidence of patellar tendon rupture in their series using only fresh frozen allografts.[1,48] Nazarian and Booth reported that 17% failed at the quadriceps tendon anastomosis, whereas Burnett et al experienced an 8% incidence of the same.[11,48] In analyzing their failed reconstructions, Leopold et al reported that 29% of allografts exhibited attenuation of the quadriceps tendon and 14% demonstrated attenuation of the patellar tendon.[45]

TECHNICAL CONSIDERATIONS—GRAFT TENSION

When Emerson et al first described this technique in 1990, they recommended tensioning the graft such that 60 degrees of knee flexion could be obtained with the assistance of gravity alone while the patient remained anesthetized on the operating table.[19] They reported an overall failure rate of 44% with this technique. Thirty-three percent had a residual extensor lag averaging 28.3 degrees. In 1999, Leopold et al reported that 100% of their patients exhibited a residual extensor lag averaging 59.0 degrees.[45] In analyzing their failed reconstructions, they noted attenuation of the quadriceps and patellar tendon in 29.0% and 14%, respectively.[44] They suggested that allograft attenua-

tion may be an important cause of progressive postoperative extensor lag and recommended that the grafts be placed under more tension than originally described. Nazarian and Booth supported greater intraoperative graft tensioning in their report of 36 extensor mechanism reconstructions earlier that same year.[48] They sutured the allograft under maximal tension with the knee in full extension. Furthermore, the patients were cast immobilized in extension for 6 weeks. Nazarian and Booth reported an overall failure rate of 22%, with 42.0% exhibiting a residual extensor lag averaging 13.0 degrees.

In 2004 (from the same unit as Leopold), Burnett et al retrospectively compared their seven original patients[11] (Emerson technique[19]) with 13 patients treated by extensor mechanism reconstruction as described by Nazarian and Booth.[48] All in the first group failed, with average extensor lags of 59.0 degrees and average knee scores of 52. In contrast, all of the second group were successes, with an average extensor lag of 4.3 degrees and an average knee score of 88. They concluded that placing the graft under tight tension with the knee in full extension dramatically improved the results. Although some surgeons have hypothesized that the grafts themselves stretch, there is probably considerable elongation from a quadriceps muscle that has been chronically retracted, scarred, and shortened in the thigh.

ALTERNATIVE TECHNIQUE—ACHILLES TENDON ALLOGRAFT

The first report of extensor mechanism reconstruction with an Achilles tendon allograft appeared in 1998 by Wascher and colleagues.[69] In 2002, Crossett et al published a small series of extensor mechanism reconstructions with an allograft Achilles tendon and an attached calcaneal bone block.[16] The study included nine patients (average age, 70 years) with an average follow-up of 28 months. We may reasonably compare these results with those described by Nazarian and Booth, representing the best results and the largest extant series. Nazarian and Booth studied 36 patients with an average age of 71 years and average follow-up of 43 months.[48] Patellar tendon rupture accounted for 100% and 55% of the extensor mechanism disruptions in Crossett and colleagues' and Nazarian and Booth's studies, respectively. Postoperative mean knee scores were comparable at 81 (Crossett et al) and 75 (Nazarian and Booth) points. Seventy percent and 60% of patients achieved full active extension in the Achilles tendon group and the extensor mechanism group, respectively. Crossett et al[16] reported that 30% had a residual extensor lag with an average magnitude of 3.0 degrees, whereas Nazarian and Booth[48] reported that 40% of their patients had a residual lag averaging 13.0 degrees. Both groups reported that 22% of patients required revision of the extensor mechanism reconstruction.[16,48] Barrack and colleagues described very good results after eight Achilles tendon allograft and six extensor mechanism allograft reconstructions.[5] Although it is difficult to make firm conclusions with the data available, reconstruction of extensor mechanism failures as a result of complex disruption with an Achilles tendon allograft appears to be a reasonable surgical option.

ALTERNATIVE TECHNIQUE— SEMITENDINOSUS AUTOGENOUS RECONSTRUCTION

In 1992 Cadambi and Engh reported their experience reconstructing patellar ligament disruption after TKA with an autogenous semitendinosus graft.[13] No case included rupture proximal to the inferior pole of the patella. They reported seven cases at an average of 30 months after surgery. The average age of their patients at the time of reconstruction was 78 years. Their average postoperative knee score was 73 points (Nazarian and Booth: 75 points), and the average postoperative knee flexion was 80 degrees (Nazarian and Booth: 98 degrees). Seventy percent of their patients continued to have a residual extension lag averaging 4.4 degrees (Nazarian and Booth: 40% and 13.0 degrees). Fifty percent had a flexion contracture averaging 5.4 degrees. None required repeat surgery or were considered failures. No patient had an extensor lag greater than 10 degrees.

ALTERNATIVE TECHNIQUE— GASTROCNEMIUS FLAP

Gastrocnemius flaps that include a portion of the Achilles tendon have been rotated into place and used to reconstruct the patellar tendon.[12,34] Jauregito and colleagues from the University of Chicago described seven patients whose ruptured extensor mechanisms were reconstructed in this way. Six were available for assessment 26 to 41 months after reconstruction. All patients who had required a walker preoperatively ambulated with or without a cane, and wheelchair patients progressed to use of a walker. Two of them had previously undergone patellectomy.[34] This procedure may be one that is particularly useful for patients in need of a gastrocnemius flap for soft-tissue coverage. However, restoration of the patellar fulcrum is an appealing part of the extensor mechanism allograft.

Seven years later, Busfield and colleagues from the University of California in San Francisco reported a similar experience for a ruptured extensor mechanism in seven patients with a TKA (plus an additional two with no arthroplasty but a ruptured extensor and previous septic arthritis).[12] In four patients an Achilles tendon allograft had already failed, and in two the arthroplasty had been infected. Some patients were infected with human immunodeficiency virus or had hemophilia or diabetes. One died after surgery, and another, with reflex sympathetic dystrophy, elected to have an above-knee amputation. A third, originally with an arthroplasty as conversion of an arthrodesis, suffered late wound problems requiring a free flap. The technique is promising and was reserved in this series for the most severely disabled and medically compromised individuals. Bickels et al, in resecting tumors about the knee, reported a variety of techniques for reconnecting the patellar tendon to the tibia if tumor margins required that it be removed when a limb salvage arthroplasty was implanted. They believed that reattachment of the patellar tendon to the prosthesis plus reinforcement with an autologous bone graft and a gastrocnemius flap was reliable.[7] There are no reports of the gastrocnemius flap as a first choice in the treatment of a ruptured extensor mechanism complicating a standard knee replacement.[70] This technique might assist healing and enhance the long-term results, particularly of the proximal anastomosis.

ALTERNATIVE TECHNIQUE—COMBINED PROXIMAL TIBIAL ALLOGRAFT AND EXTENSOR MECHANISM ALLOGRAFT

Special situations arise when significant proximal tibial bone loss from osteolysis or gross deficiencies of the soft-tissue envelope accompany rupture of the extensor mechanism. Each of these situations has led to innovation. Large proximal tibial defects and extensor mechanism rupture may be treated with an allograft that includes the proximal tibial bone, as well as the tendons and the patella.[71] This technique was illustrated in Figure 103–3.

SPECIAL CIRCUMSTANCE— INTRAOPERATIVE DISRUPTION

Bipartite patellae may be problematic for patellar resurfacing, but it should definitely be distinguished from fibrous union of old fractures. In both situations, the patellae can be left unresurfaced. Internal fixation in this region is probably inadvisable, unless the fracture fragments have separated in surgery (Fig. 103–6). Gelinas and Ries encountered a vertical patellar fracture in a revision patella weakened by osteolysis and opted for cerclage and implantation of a cemented prosthetic button.[25] Alternatively, this configuration can be left with the so-called gull wing osteotomy and be bone-grafted.[68] Transverse fractures are rarely encountered intraoperatively and would be more likely during difficult revision arthroplasties. No data exist, but cerclage wiring and perhaps a patellectomy with repair of the tendon might be advisable. New patellar implants made of porous, elemental tantalum in conjunction with cerclage wiring may provide a useful option. Immediate allografting would also be reasonable.

SURGICAL TECHNIQUE—EXTENSOR MECHANISM ALLOGRAFT

Of all the reconstructions described, the extensor mechanism allograft has been used most frequently and is the most universally applicable. Fresh frozen graft material is favored because of superior mechanical strength. In many cases, rupture of the extensor will be accompanied by

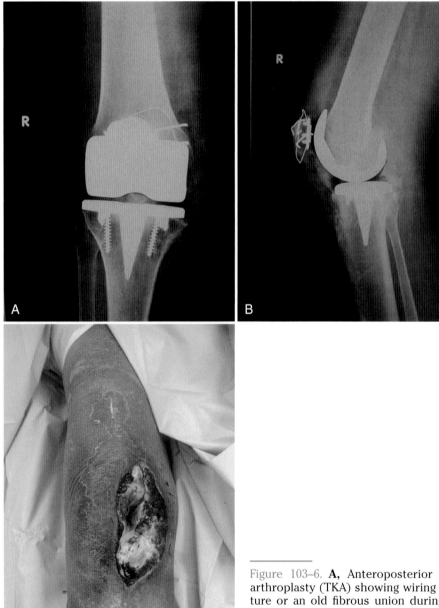

Figure 103–6. **A,** Anteroposterior radiograph of a primary total knee arthroplasty (TKA) showing wiring of either an acute, intraoperative fracture or an old fibrous union during primary TKA. **B,** Lateral radiograph showing cerclage fixation and an inferior third transverse fracture. **C,** The fixation wires eroded through the skin and led to infection with profound soft-tissue loss.

other problems in the arthroplasty that may have contributed to the extensor problems or that resulted from chronic extensor lag. Accordingly, concurrent revision arthroplasty is often advantageous. Preoperative CT scanning may be instructive.

The skin incision should follow an existing scar. When the patellar tendon or its attachment to the patella has been completely disrupted, the arthrotomy is best made directly over the center of the tubercle. This allows the residual soft tissue to be split, elevated medially and laterally, and then closed over top of the tubercle graft. In some situations it is desirable to preserve what may be left of the patient's own extensor, as in an allograft for a previous patellectomy. In this case, if the graft fails, a subsequent reconstruction may be feasible with the patient's own tissue, albeit without a patella.

Revision arthroplasty should be completed before the allograft is installed. The mode of tibial allograft tubercle fixation will have to be selected before completing the revision to maintain the option of passing wires around the tibial stem extension. The allograft tubercle bone will usually have to be reduced in size so that it fits into a trough on the host bone. If too wide, the medial and lateral cortices of the host tibia will be destroyed. The surgeon holds the allograft as the assistant holds the bone saw firmly and without moving on the operating table. In this respect the saw has become a "table saw." Saw blades with finer teeth will work most efficiently—large teeth break the graft or make it difficult to hold.

An oblique cut on the proximal surface of the graft (the anterior cortex is shorter than the deeper surface) will enable it to wedge into the trough under a cortical bridge.

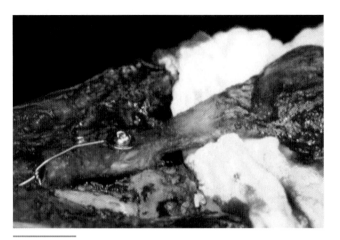

Figure 103–7. The allograft tubercle can be attached to the host with wires, screws, or a combination of both as shown here. Tight fit of the graft into a trough on the tubercle is probably the most important aspect of this junction.

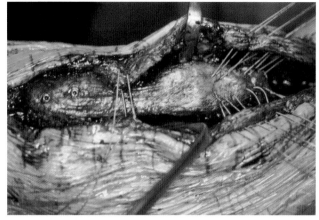

Figure 103–8. The array of sutures on the *right* of the figure illustrates the importance of placing and clamping all sutures before tying and to approximate the tension in the graft at this point. To the *left* we see that the arthrotomy will cover the graft completely.

Once the dimensions of the allograft tubercle have been set, its shape can be marked on the host. A transverse piece of host tibial bone should be preserved distal to the tibial prosthesis to enhance fixation. The location of the tubercle will also determine the height of the patella relative to the femoral component and should be selected carefully. The trough should be slightly smaller than the graft—a mallet will be required for impaction. The graft may be retained with wires around the tibial stem or through drill holes. Lag screws, usually the "small fragment" type, have also been used with advantage. A combination of one screw proximally and a fine-gauge stainless steel wire wound around it, crossed into a figure "8," and then passed distally through a transverse hole in the host tibia, will substitute for two screws. These screws can, however, erode through the skin and should probably be countersunk (Fig. 103–7).

There is no general agreement on the technique for the proximal anastomosis, except that the extensor mechanism should be very tight once the graft has been installed. Frequently, once the quadriceps tendon has been connected, the knee will spontaneously bend only a few degrees. The two layers of the quadriceps in the midline may be separated to "sandwich" the allograft tendon between them. In general, the entire graft patellar tendon, the patella, and the quadriceps tendon will all be installed inside the knee joint and covered by the capsule and extensor mechanism.

Heavy nonresorbable suture is passed down from the outside of the knee, through the top of the host quadriceps tendon at a relatively proximal location. Then the needle comes down to the superficial graft tendon and is passed through and out of the deep surface. If the host quadriceps tendon has been split, the suture is carried through the deep level and then back up through each level. This suture is clamped but not tied because to do so makes it very difficult to place other similar sutures (Fig. 103–8). At least four of them will be positioned. They establish preliminary fixation, position of the graft relative to the host, and extensor mechanism tension. The host

patella, if present, may be thinned and sutured to the allograft patella through drill holes. This helps bring the host quadriceps down to a more anatomic level and provides a bone-to-bone junction that may strengthen the proximal junction. Krakow-style sutures can be placed along the edge of the graft and up into the host for longitudinal strength.[40,41] If one is placed medially and one laterally, the ends can be tied to each other. The arthrotomy is closed over the top of the graft, usually with absorbable No. 1 suture. The patella is not resurfaced.

The knee is placed in a bulky, padded cotton dressing (Jones dressing), often with plaster reinforcement. The dressing is removed after several days, when most surgeons would apply a long-leg cast. Our preference is a hinged knee brace that can be removed for hygiene and that has drop locks for ambulation and dial locks for gentle, passive motion up to a predetermined limit, usually about 30 degrees after the first 2 weeks. This brace is useful for 3 months as the limits of the dial lock are increased. Active extension is prohibited for about 12 weeks, and either crutches or a walker is necessary.

Previous infection makes a difficult situation much worse. There is good reason to recommend arthrodesis for an infected arthroplasty without an extensor mechanism. Nonetheless, in some circumstances a two-stage reimplantation may be planned with an extensor allograft at the time of reimplantation. It is this situation where the medial gastrocnemius muscle flap may prove to be advantageous, although no data are as yet available. Extensor allografts may be repeated successfully. Septic failure, especially in the presence of extensive bone loss, may best be treated with an above-knee amputation. Sadly, by the time that the patient agrees to fusion, there is usually too little bone to accomplish this goal. Most of these patients are older and ill and have had numerous disappointing operations. An above-knee prosthesis has the advantage of flexion, which facilitates riding in a car, bus, train, or airliner. This highlights the serious implications of a ruptured extensor mechanism, perhaps the most feared complication in knee arthroplasty surgery.

CONCLUSIONS

Personal experience combined with the successes, failures, hypotheses, opinions, and data in the literature leads to some (subjective) conclusions. The question "Why has the extensor mechanism ruptured?" should always be addressed. Tracking problems are common in many extensor mechanism complications, and a CT scan can be very instructive to the surgeon and help with the decision regarding whether an allograft should be performed alone or with a revision.

The problem in treating all disruptions of the extensor, regardless of anatomic location, is solid reconnection of the quadriceps muscle to the tibial tubercle. Simple repair does not seem to work for any disruption, although the quadriceps tendon is the most likely to succeed, especially if tissue layers are overlapped. Augmentation of some kind is almost always preferred.

The extensor allograft, though intended for distal rupture, can reinforce a chronic quadriceps rupture and replace a chronically fractured patella in the presence of avascular necrosis and a debilitating extensor lag. The weak link will not be the osseous union of the tubercle, but the junction between the host and allograft quadriceps tendons.

Knees with a concurrent infection and ruptured extensor may do very well with a two-stage reimplantation protocol and an extensor allograft. Many require tissue transfer procedures for coverage of the joint. A knee that has failed one two-stage reimplantation protocol with a graft should probably not have a second reimplant with an extensor graft. Despite the heavy sense of loss by the patient and failure by the surgeon, an above-knee amputation may be best. Removal of the problem arthroplasty with the limb often provides the patient and family with comfort that has been missing and the necessary escape from the hospital.

References

1. Abrahamowicz M, Du Berger R, Krewski D, et al: Bias due to aggregation of individual covariates in the Cox regression model. Am J Epidemiol 160:696-706, 2004.
2. Abril JC, Alvarez L, Vallejo JC: Patellar tendon avulsion after total knee arthroplasty. A new technique. J Arthroplasty 10:275-279, 1995.
3. Barrack RI: Specialized surgical exposure for revision total knee: Quadriceps snip and patellar turndown. Instr Course Lect 48:149-152, 1999.
4. Barrack RL, Lyons T: Proximal tibia—extensor mechanism composite allograft for revision TKA with chronic patellar tendon rupture. Acta Orthop Scand 71:419-421, 2000.
5. Barrack RL, Stanley T, Allen Butler R: Treating extensor mechanism disruption after total knee arthroplasty. Clin Orthop 416:98-104, 2003.
6. Berger RA, Crossett LS, Jacobs JJ, Rubash HE: Malrotation causing patellofemoral complications after total knee arthroplasty. Clin Orthop 356:144-153, 1998.
7. Bickels J, Wittig JC, Kollender Y, et al: Reconstruction of the extensor mechanism after proximal tibia endoprosthetic replacement. J Arthroplasty 16:856-862, 2001.
8. Bindelglass DF, Vince KG: Patellar tilt and subluxation following subvastus and parapatellar approach in total knee arthroplasty. Implication for surgical technique. J Arthroplasty 11:507-511, 1996.
9. Boyd AD Jr, Ewald FC, Thomas WH, et al: Long-term complications after total knee arthroplasty with or without resurfacing of the patella. J Bone Joint Surg Am 75:674-681, 1993.
10. Briard JL, Hungerford DS: Patellofemoral instability in total knee arthroplasty. J Arthroplasty 4(Suppl):S87-S97, 1989.
11. Burnett RS, Berger RA, Paprowsky WG, et al: Extensor mechanism allograft reconstruction after total knee arthroplasty. A comparison of two techniques. J Bone Joint Surg Am 86:2694-2699, 2004.
12. Busfield BT, Huffman GR, Nahai F, et al: Extended medial gastrocnemius rotational flap for treatment of chronic knee extensor mechanism deficiency in patients with and without total knee arthroplasty. Clin Orthop 428:190-197, 2004.
13. Cadambi A, Engh GA: Use of a semitendinosus tendon autogenous graft for rupture of the patellar ligament after total knee arthroplasty. A report of seven cases. J Bone Joint Surg Am 74:974-979, 1992.
14. Chen CF, Chen WM, Lee KS, et al: Advanced osteoarthritic knee with neglected patellar tendon rupture treated with total patellectomy and total knee arthroplasty. J Arthroplasty 19:793-796, 2004.
15. Clayton ML, Thirupathi R: Patellar complications after total condylar arthroplasty. Clin Orthop 170:152-155, 1982.
16. Crossett LS, Sinha RK, Sechriest VF, Rubash HE: Reconstruction of a ruptured patellar tendon with Achilles tendon allograft following total knee arthroplasty. J Bone Joint Surg Am 84:1354-1361, 2002.
17. Dobbs RE, Hanssen AD, Lewallen DG, Pagnano MW: Quadriceps tendon rupture after total knee arthroplasty. Prevalence, complications, and outcomes. J Bone Joint Surg Am 87:37-45, 2005.
18. Emerson RH: Extensor mechanism rupture. In Fu F, Harner CD, Vince K (eds): Knee Surgery. Philadelphia, Williams & Wilkins, 1994, pp 1483-1489.
19. Emerson RH Jr, Head WC, Malinin TI: Reconstruction of patellar tendon rupture after total knee arthroplasty with an extensor mechanism allograft. Clin Orthop 260:154-161, 1990.
20. Emerson RH Jr, Head WC, Malinin TI: Extensor mechanism reconstruction with an allograft after total knee arthroplasty. Clin Orthop 303:79-85, 1994.
21. Fernandez-Baillo N, Garay EG, Ordonez JM: Rupture of the quadriceps tendon after total knee arthroplasty. A case report. J Arthroplasty 8:331-333, 1993.
22. Figgie HE 3rd, Goldberg VM, Giggie MP, et al: The effect of alignment of the implant on fractures of the patella after condylar total knee arthroplasty. J Bone Joint Surg Am 71:1031-1039, 1989.
23. Fujikawa K, Ohtani T, Matsumoto H, Seedhom BB: Reconstruction of the extensor apparatus of the knee with the Leeds-Keio ligament. J Bone Joint Surg Br 76:200-203, 1994.
24. Garvin KL, Scuderi G, Insall JN: Evolution of the quadriceps snip. Clin Orthop 321:131-137, 1995.
25. Gelinas JJ, Ries MD: Treatment of an intraoperative patellar fracture during revision total knee arthroplasty. J Arthroplasty 17:1066-1069, 2002.
26. Goldberg VM, Figgie HE 3rd, Inglis AE, et al: Patellar fracture type and prognosis in condylar total knee arthroplasty. Clin Orthop 236:115-122, 1988.
27. Grace JN, Sim FH: Fracture of the patella after total knee arthroplasty. Clin Orthop 230:168-175, 1988.
28. Healy WL, Wasilewski SA, Takei R, Oberlander M: Patellofemoral complications following total knee arthroplasty. Correlation with implant design and patient risk factors. J Arthroplasty 10:197-201, 1995.
29. Hendel D, Weisbort M, Garti A: "Wandering resident" surgical exposure for 1- or 2-stage revision arthroplasty in stiff aseptic and septic knee arthroplasty. J Arthroplasty 19:757-759, 2004.
30. Hozack WJ, Goll SR, Lotke PA, et al: The treatment of patellar fractures after total knee arthroplasty. Clin Orthop 236:123-127, 1988.
31. Hughes SS, Cammarata A, Steinmann SP, Pellegrini VD Jr: Effect of standard total knee arthroplasty surgical dissection on human patellar blood flow in vivo: An investigation using laser Doppler flowmetry. J South Orthop Assoc 7:198-204, 1998.
32. Insall JN, Hood RW, Flawn LB, Sullivan DJ: The total condylar knee prosthesis in gonarthrosis. A five to nine-year follow-up of the first one hundred consecutive replacements. J Bone Joint Surg Am 65:619-628, 1983.
33. Insall JN, Lachiewicz PF, Burstein AH: The posterior stabilized condylar prosthesis: A modification of the total condylar design. Two to four-year clinical experience. J Bone Joint Surg Am 64:1317-1323, 1982.

34. Jaureguito JW, Dubois CM, Smith SR, et al: Medial gastrocnemius transposition flap for the treatment of disruption of the extensor mechanism after total knee arthroplasty. J Bone Joint Surg Am 79:866-873, 1997.

35. Kastelec M, Veselko M: Inferior patellar pole avulsion fractures: Osteosynthesis compared with pole resection. J Bone Joint Surg Am 86:696-701, 2004.

36. Kayler DE, Lyttle D: Surgical interruption of patellar blood supply by total knee arthroplasty. Clin Orthop 229:221-227, 1988.

37. Keating EM, Haas G, Meding JB: Patella fracture after post total knee replacements. Clin Orthop 416:93-97, 2003.

38. Kelly MA: Extensor mechanism complications in total knee arthroplasty. Instr Course Lect 53:193-199, 2004.

39. Kempenaar JW, Cameron JC: Patellotibial fusion for patellar tendon rupture after total knee arthroplasty. J Arthroplasty 14:115-117, 1999.

40. Krackow KA, Thomas SC, Jones LC: A new stitch for ligament-tendon fixation. Brief note. J Bone Joint Surg Am 68:764-766, 1986.

41. Krackow KA, Thomas SC, Jones LC: Ligament-tendon fixation: Analysis of a new stitch and comparison with standard techniques. Orthopedics 11:909-917, 1988.

42. Kulkarni S, Sawant M, Ireland J: Allograft reconstruction of the extensor mechanism for progressive extensor lag after total knee arthroplasty and previous patellectomy: A 3-year follow-up. J Arthroplasty 14:892-894, 1999.

43. Larsen ST, Ryd L: Temperature elevation during knee arthroplasty. Acta Orthop Scand 60:439-442, 1989.

44. Leopold SS, Berger RA, Patterson L, et al: Serum titanium level for diagnosis of a failed, metal-backed patellar component. J Arthroplasty 15:938-943, 2000.

45. Leopold SS, Greidanus N, Paprosky WG, et al: High rate of failure of allograft reconstruction of the extensor mechanism after total knee arthroplasty. J Bone Joint Surg Am 81:1574-1579, 1999.

46. Lynch AF, Rorabeck CH, Bourne RB: Extensor mechanism complications following total knee arthroplasty. J Arthroplasty 2:135-140, 1987.

47. Malo M, Vince KG: The unstable patella after total knee arthroplasty: Etiology, prevention, and management. J Am Acad Orthop Surg 11:364-371, 2003.

48. Nazarian DG, Booth RE Jr: Extensor mechanism allografts in total knee arthroplasty. Clin Orthop 367:123-129, 1999.

49. Ogata K, Shively RA, Shoenecker PL, Chang SL: Effects of standard surgical procedures on the patellar blood flow in monkeys. Clin Orthop 215:254-259, 1987.

50. Ortiguera CJ, Berry DJ: Patellar fracture after total knee arthroplasty. J Bone Joint Surg Am 84:532-540, 2002.

51. Parker DA, Dunbar MJ, Rorabeck CH: Extensor mechanism failure associated with total knee arthroplasty: Prevention and management. J Am Acad Orthop Surg 11:238-247, 2003.

52. Prada SA, Griffin FM, Nelson CL, Garvin KL: Allograft reconstruction for extensor mechanism rupture after total knee arthroplasty: 4.8-year follow-up. Orthopedics 26:1205-1208, 2003.

53. Rand JA: Extensor mechanism complications following total knee arthroplasty. J Knee Surg 16:224-228, 2003.

54. Rand JA, Morrey BF, Bryan RS: Patellar tendon rupture after total knee arthroplasty. Clin Orthop 244:233-238, 1989.

55. Rorabeck CH, Angliss RD, Lewis PL: Fractures of the femur, tibia, and patella after total knee arthroplasty: Decision making and principles of management. Instr Course Lect 47:449-458, 1998.

56. Scott RD, Turoff N, Ewald FC: Stress fracture of the patella following duopatellar total knee arthroplasty with patellar resurfacing. Clin Orthop 170:147-151, 1982.

57. Scuderi C: Ruptures of the quadriceps tendon; study of twenty tendon ruptures. Am J Surg 95:626-634, 1958.

58. Scuderi G, Scharf SC, Meltzer LP, Scott WN: The relationship of lateral releases to patella viability in total knee arthroplasty. J Arthroplasty 2:209-214, 1987.

59. Sharkey PF, Hozack WJ, Rothman RH, et al: Insall Award paper. Why are total knee arthroplasties failing today? Clin Orthop 404:7-13, 2002.

60. Sinha R, Crossett LS, Rubash HE: Extensor mechanism rupture. In Insall J, Scott NW (eds): Surgery of the Knee. Philadelphia, Churchill Livingstone, 2001, pp 1863-1873.

61. Sinha R, Rubash HE: Extensor mechanism rupture. In Callaghan J, Rosenberg AG, Rubash HE, Simonian PT (eds): The Adult Knee. Philadelphia, Lippincott, Williams & Wilkins, 2003, pp 1351-1358.

62. Siwek CW, Rao JP: Ruptures of the extensor mechanism of the knee joint. J Bone Joint Surg Am 63:932-937, 1981.

63. Spitzer A, Vince K: Patellar considerations in total knee arthroplasty. In Scuderi GR (ed): The Patella. New York, Springer-Verlag, 1995, pp 309-331.

64. Trepte CT, Kirgis A: [Spontaneous ruptures of the extensor system of the knee following joint replacement in patients with rheumatoid arthritis.] Z Orthop Ihre Grenzgeb 126:519-525, 1988.

65. Tria AJ Jr, Harwood DA, Alicea JA, Cody RP: Patellar fractures in posterior stabilized knee arthroplasties. Clin Orthop 299:131-138, 1994.

66. Tscherne H, KC, and LP: Fractures about the knee. In Fu FH, Harner CD, Vince K (eds): Knee Surgery. Baltimore, Williams & Wilkins, 1994, pp 1027-1058.

67. Vince KG, McPherson EJ: The patella in total knee arthroplasty. Orthop Clin North Am 23:675-686, 1992.

68. Vince K, Roidis N, Blackburn D: Gull-wing sagittal patellar osteotomy in total knee arthroplasty. Tech Knee Surg 1:106-112, 2002.

69. Wascher DC, Summa CD: Reconstruction of chronic rupture of the extensor mechanism after patellectomy. Clin Orthop 357:135-140, 1998.

70. Weber MJ, Janecki CJ, McLeod P, et al: Efficacy of various forms of fixation of transverse fractures of the patella. J Bone Joint Surg Am 62:215-220, 1980.

71. Webster DA, Murray DG: Complications of variable axis total knee arthroplasty. Clin Orthop 193:160-167, 1985.

72. Wulff W, Incavo SJ: The effect of patella preparation for total knee arthroplasty on patellar strain: A comparison of resurfacing versus inset implants. J Arthroplasty 15:778-782, 2000.

73. Zanotti RM, Freiberg AA, Matthews LS: Use of patellar allograft to reconstruct a patellar tendon–deficient knee after total joint arthroplasty. J Arthroplasty 10:271-274, 1995.

CHAPTER 104

Transfusion Avoidance, Blood Loss Management, and Total Knee Arthroplasty

Fred Cushner

Modern surgical techniques have reduced the amount of blood loss during total knee arthroplasty (TKA) procedures, but despite these advances, a significant amount of blood loss still occurs. Acute postoperative anemia and risks of allogeneic transfusion remain of great concern to the patient and surgeon. The practice of strict transfusion triggers has been largely abandoned, although resulting anemia remains a concern. Allogeneic transfusions traditionally have been used to ameliorate the occurrence of anemia, but the incidence of disease transmission, allergic reactions, fluid overload, transfusion reactions, and immunosuppression from allogeneic transfusions is increased.[14,17,28,36,55,86] This chapter discusses the risks of allogeneic transfusion and reviews conservation protocols. Conservation techniques for the preoperative, intraoperative, and postoperative periods are reviewed, and blood management protocols are presented.

RISK OF INFECTION

Historically, 50% of patients undergoing total joint arthroplasty receive an allogeneic blood transfusion. The risks of allogeneic transfusions are well described in the literature.[1,2,4,57,58,75,80] These concerns often are focused on the transmission of viral agents, such as hepatitis and human immunodeficiency virus. Newer concerns also have been raised; West Nile virus transmission has been discussed as a potential infectious agent after allogeneic transfusions.[10]

Allogeneic transfusions often have been implicated in the increased incidence of infections after surgery. Houbiers and colleagues[46] looked at 697 patients undergoing abdominal surgery, and multivariate analysis identified allogeneic transfusions as a significant risk factor for postoperative infection. Kendall and colleagues[56] described immunosuppression secondary to allogeneic transfusions in 34 patients undergoing total hip arthroplasty. This study had the additional goal of trying to determine whether allogeneic transfusions result in postoperative immunosuppression, and these authors concluded that immunosuppression does occur. According to these Kendall and colleagues,[56] the lymphocyte function is impaired, and the immunosuppression may increase the risk of deep prosthesis infection.

The Kendall study[56] documented the occurrence of immunosuppression, and Murphy and associates[64] showed increased risk of postoperative infection in patients receiving total hip arthroplasty. In this study,

higher infection rates were noted in patients who received allogeneic transfusions. The patients also showed a benefit of higher blood parameters. Increased hematocrit and hemoglobin levels during the preoperative period proved of benefit in this series.

Other authors have shown an increased benefit of higher postoperative blood levels. Keating and coworkers[54] assessed patient vigor and defined a concise, patient-based instrument to measure the patient's vigor after joint arthroplasty. Among the objective criteria studied, there was a significant correlation between vigor and hematocrit value: the higher the postoperative blood levels, the higher the vigor scale. The question remains whether increased vigor translated into shorter hospital stay or quicker recovery and progression in the rehabilitation process.

Disease transmission may be the main concern for patients and surgeons, but other factors also are important. There may be other negative consequences of the immunosuppression in addition to the benefits of increased vigor and fewer medical complications. Lotke and colleagues[61] showed decreased medical complications when anemia was not allowed to occur, and autologous blood was immediately transfused. This is another example of the benefit of higher postoperative blood values.

RISK FACTORS FOR TRANSFUSION

One of the best ways to determine which patient requires allogeneic infusion is to evaluate preoperative blood values.[15,27,32] Checking the hemoglobin and hematocrit before scheduling the indicated procedure may reduce allogeneic transfusions. We evaluated transfusion rates in patients undergoing TKA.[23] In this study, we found preoperative hematocrit values were the best predictor for allogeneic needs. Nuttall and colleagues[68] had similar findings and noted the importance of preoperative hemoglobin. The patient received a transfusion, but the important factor in these two studies was the preoperative blood values. Patients who began with higher preoperative hemoglobin concentrations were able to tolerate the 10% hematocrit loss that occurs after joint arthroscopy surgery. Patients who were anemic in the preoperative process would be anemic during the postoperative process and require transfusion.

The relationship between preoperative hemoglobin values and transfusion requirements was seen not only in

TKA, but also in total hip arthroplasty. Nuttall and colleagues[68] evaluated 299 patients who had undergone total hip arthroplasty in an attempt to predict the risk factors for allogeneic transfusions. In this series, they found that in most cases the predonated blood was not transfused, leading to blood wastage and increased cost. Nuttall and colleagues[68] concluded that if the patients who did not need to donate could be eliminated, unnecessary donations would be avoided, and cost savings would occur. The preoperative hemoglobin concentrate is judged to be the most significant indication in preventing allogeneic transfusions. Sculco and Gallina[76] evaluated 1405 patients who underwent total joint arthroplasty. They looked at the hemoglobin concentration measurement before surgery and found that they are inversely related to the frequency of allogeneic transfusions: the lower the preoperative blood values, the higher allogeneic transfusion rates. In a large multicenter study, Bierbaum and coworkers[9] evaluated 9482 patients undergoing major orthopedic surgery. This study not only showed increased transfusions, with patients with hemoglobin values less than 13 g/dL, but also a more complicated postoperative course was noted in patients receiving a transfusion. In this series, transfusions were associated with an increase in infection rate, fluid overload, and a longer hospital stay. These studies suggest that presurgical goals should be maximized by checking hemoglobin levels before surgery.

PREOPERATIVE BLOOD MANAGEMENT

Preoperative Autologous Donations

In the late 1980s, the standard of care for a patient undergoing TKA was the preoperative donation of autologous blood. Although commonplace in the United States, preoperative autologous donation (PAD) is limited in other areas of the world. PAD does have some limitations. Patients who are anemic in the preoperative period are excluded from donating blood. PAD is convenient for the physician, but can be inconvenient for the patient. It is often assumed that after donating blood, the patient returns to the predonation status; this is often not the case. Several studies have shown that PAD may cause further anemia and is not only wasteful, but also may lower the patient's preoperative blood levels.[13,25,81] The patient donates the blood, does not return to baseline, and arrives for the surgery in an anemic state. The patient is more at risk for allogeneic transfusion because of the autologous donation.

Hatzidakis and coworkers[41] performed a retrospective analysis of 489 consecutive patients undergoing total joint arthroplasty. This study was limited because predonation blood values were available only on 149 of the 489 patients. A decrease in hemoglobin concentration from the time of the donation to the time of surgery was reported; the average decrease was 1.22 g/dL. This study questioned the benefit of PAD in patients with predonation hemoglobin concentrations greater than 15 g/dL. In younger patients, a lower threshold was accepted. The authors did not recommend PAD for patients with predonation status greater than 13 g/dL.

Lotke and colleagues[61] evaluated medical complications after TKA. This study initially was done to evaluate the controversy regarding the administration of preoperative autologous blood. The question remained that if the blood is donated, should all of it be given back, or should a strict transfusion criteria apply. The result of the study showed that patients who received an immediate transfusion of their PAD had fewer medical complications compared with patients who did not receive their PAD until their hemoglobin concentration was less than 9 g/dL ($p < 0.002$). An immediate transfusion of PAD was suggested to be particularly important in critically ill elderly patients because of their increased risk of cardiac and nonsurgical complications. This study concluded that the increase in the hemoglobin level, as a result in the immediate return of PAD, improved the outcome in these patients.

Other authors have shown that as a result of a PAD program, the patients have more anemia in the preoperative period.[23,32,68] A 1- to 2-U PAD program does not cause a significant erythropoietic response, and anemia is noted before surgery. Because no erythropoietic response occurs, patients do not return to their baseline level before their donations. Postsurgical transfusion may not always result in the desired hemoglobin concentrations because stored autologous blood may show a decrease in number of red blood cells.

We evaluated our PAD program. Between 1993 and 1995, 2 U of PAD were obtained on average compared with 1 U of PAD obtained in the years between 1995 and 1997. Our studies showed a 3% decrease in hematocrit values for every unit donated before surgery.[25] Although the hematocrits were similar with 1 U achieved in protocols preoperatively, an increase was noted in the 2-U PAD program. When 1 U was donated, a 3% decrease in hematocrit was noted before surgery. When 2 U were donated, a 6% decrease from baseline was noted; 2 U of PAD resulted in more anemia before the surgical procedure. We also reviewed our results of a 1-U PAD program with automatic infusion of the donated blood and found it to be the potential best-case scenario for PAD. All patients were given their PAD immediately after surgery, resulting in 0% wastage. Despite ordering the PAD unit 1 month before surgery, significant anemia was noted. A 1.3 g/dL decrease was noted between predonation and presurgical testing.[69] We refer to this occurrence as "orthopedic induced anemia." As a result of the prescribed PAD donations, the patients were anemic before their planned surgical procedure. As documented by others, the use of PAD results in anemia, and the patients do not return to the predonation hemoglobin and hematocrit values. Although the allogeneic infusion rate was low for this series, we believe this reflects the acceptance of lower hemoglobins in the immediate postoperative period. Had historical transfusion triggers been followed (hemoglobin concentration <10 g/dL), a transfusion rate of 30% would have been found. In addition, 50% of patients were discharged with hemoglobin concentrates less than 9 g/dL. Overall, allogeneic rates were low, but this should not be misconstrued as efficacy of a 1-U PAD program.

The protocols based on work of Lotke and colleagues[61] showed fewer medical complications with the actual infusion of the donated unit. Our institution has abandoned the aforementioned protocol based on the apparent lack of efficacy. This protocol may place patients at risk because the 100% autologous rate exposes them to donation error. Goldman and associates[34] reviewed autologous error rates in Canada and found an error rate of 6/149. Not all of these errors were related to labeling (48%) or component preparation (25%). One patient received the wrong unit of donated blood, which is a common occurrence. According to the College of American Pathologists,[20] 0.9% of the 3852 institutions studied had at least 1 U of PAD given to the wrong patient. Cost is an issue of PAD, for this is not an inexpensive procedure. The costs of a PAD program are related to procurement and the cost connected with giving the blood. There is also a cost of the wastage: Several series have shown that autologous wastage rate is 50% to 75%. Billote and colleagues[12] evaluated PAD in patients who were receiving total hip arthroplasty and found no benefit in PAD for nonanemic patients undergoing primary hip replacement. Each patient donated 2 U of autologous blood, with an additional cost of $758 per patient. Etchason and coworkers[30] studied the cost of the PAD program and concluded that increased protection afforded by autologous blood is limited and may not justify the increased cost. The cost has been raised in the discussion of use of erythropoietin (EPO) (see next section).

Use of Erythropoietins

The importance of proper hemoglobin concentrations was discussed earlier. The surgeon is often limited in his or her ability to maximize the patient's predonation hemoglobin values. Until more recently, we participated in a PAD program. Unhappy with the anemia caused by donations, we have now put our patients on a new protocol. We obtain hemoglobin concentrations at the time of surgical scheduling, and based on the hemoglobin concentrations, we identify the patients who are at risk for a transfusion. A patient with a hemoglobin concentration greater than 10 g/dL and less than 13 g/dL receives 40,000 U of recombinant human EPO at 3 weeks, 2 weeks, and 1 week before surgery. Iron supplementation also is prescribed for patients placed on the EPO injection. Nearly 75% of our patients avoid autologous donations because they have hemoglobin values greater than 13 g/dL; only 25% need to participate in the donation and the EPO injections. We compared 50 patients who received EPO injections with 50 patients participating in the autologous program with automatic reinfusion.[21] The patients receiving EPO had higher blood parameters preoperatively, postoperatively, and on discharge than the patients who participated in the autologous program. Additionally, our overall cost was reduced because the autologous program was used in 25% of the patients with EPO compared with 100% in previous protocols. Treating 25% of patients with EPO injections is significantly less costly than using an autologous donation program for 100% of the patients, especially in light of potential risks with an automatic reinfusion protocol.

Insall-Scott Institute Protocol

We have abandoned the use of autologous blood for unicompartmental TKAs and use a patient-specific approach. We check hemoglobin values before surgery and identify patients at increased risk; approximately 25% of patients receive the EPO injections. The other patients, with a predonation hemoglobin greater than 13 g/dL, are scheduled for surgery without any PAD or recombinant human EPO prescriptions. The patients receive their injections before surgery from our office or from their primary care physician. This approach maximizes the hemoglobin and hematocrit levels not only before surgery, but also during the perioperative period.

INTRAOPERATIVE BLOOD MANAGEMENT

PAD and EPO injections are attempts in the preoperative period to reduce the need for allogeneic transfusions. Several options exist in regards to intraoperative blood management of the TKA patient. The preoperative measures work by attempting to maximize the ability of patients to tolerate the intraoperative blood loss. To avoid transfusions, addressing the amount of intraoperative blood loss also may be beneficial. In this section, hypotensive anesthesia, blood salvage, hemodilution, topical hemostatic agents, and specialized cautery are reviewed.

Acute Normovolemic Hemodilution

Acute normovolemic hemodilution involves simultaneous removal of whole blood from a patient immediately before surgery and replacement with acellular fluids (crystalloid or colloid) to maintain normal blood volume. This technique is recommended when the potential for blood loss may exceed 20% in patients with hemoglobin greater than 10 g/dL. It is a cost and preoperative time commitment for preoperative autologous donations, with the possibility of clerical error or bacterial contamination. Acute normovolemic hemodilution is common, however, in patients with coronary, renal, pulmonary, or significant liver disease. It is often impractical in most total joint programs because of the relatively short duration of the procedure and lesser blood loss.[52]

Combined data from 16 randomized control studies of 615 patients showed that acute normovolemic hemodilution reduced the likelihood of allogeneic transfusions in patients undergoing surgery by 31%. The likelihood of allogeneic transfusion in patients undergoing surgery was reduced in cardiac and miscellaneous procedures, but not in orthopedic surgery. The patients were required to have at least 1000 mL withdrawn, and there had to be no transfusion protocols in place.[65] In contrast, Shulman and Grecula[79] found that acute normovolemic hemodilution reduced allogeneic transfusions from 2.4% to 0.6%. This is a 75% reduction in primary revision hip replacements. Acute normovolemic hemodilution has been found to be as effective as preoperative autologous donation in total hip and total knee replacements.[35] Acute normovolemic hemodilution may not be necessary when blood loss is expected to be less than 1000 mL intraoperative blood salvage.[11]

Intraoperative Blood Salvage

Blood salvage requires a return of the patient's autologous blood loss during surgery. Often the indicated TKA is performed under tourniquet control, and these devices are used during the postoperative period, when most of the blood loss occurs after the tourniquet is placed down. The use of drains is discussed in depth in the section on postoperative blood loss management.

Hypotensive Anesthesia

Hypotensive anesthesia is a technique for reducing intraoperative blood loss by significantly lowering the mean arterial pressure during surgery. Hypotensive anesthesia may reduce intraoperative blood loss, but it depends on the relative decrease in pressure and the type of anesthesia.[5,66,78] The reduction in blood loss does not seem to be related to cardiac output.[77] Hypotensive anesthesia associated with tissue hypoperfusion and complications can occur, including death. Patients with underlying cardiac, cerebral, or peripheral vessel disease are more at risk. The possibility of increased deep vein thrombosis events also has been raised. In the total joint arthroplasty literature, several studies evaluating hypotensive anesthesia have been described. In a study of 30 total hip arthroplasties, spinal anesthetic with mean arterial pressure maintained at 70 mm Hg was compared with hypotensive epidural anesthesia (mean arterial pressure 50 to 60 mm Hg). Intraoperative blood loss was decreased from 900 mL to 400 mL, and total perioperative blood loss was decreased by 45%, significantly lowering the number of transfusion units in the hypotensive group.

A similar study was done in total joint arthroplasty patients.[51] A hypotensive epidural anesthesia protocol was used and compared with a spinal anesthetic. Total perioperative blood loss was decreased by nearly 800 mL in the hypotensive group, resulting in 38% fewer patients requiring transfusion and 75% less blood per transfusion. Inhalational anesthetics and hypotensive anesthesia also have worked to reduce intraoperative blood loss significantly in total hip replacements.[84]

Tissue Hemostasis

A more direct method to reduce intraoperative blood loss is obtained through improved tissue hemostasis within the operative field. Topically or locally active agents, including thrombin, collagen, and fibrin glues, have been reported. These agents are efficacious in reducing postoperative blood loss and perioperative exposure to allogeneic blood transfusions. In several randomized controlled trials, fibrin sealants reduced the rate of exposure to allogeneic red blood cell transfusions by approximately 54%.[16] The use of fibrin tissue adhesive significantly reduced mean postoperative blood loss from 800 mL to 360 mL in a study of 58 patients undergoing joint surgery.[60]

A fibrin tissue adhesive was sprayed on the internal aspects of the operating field before skin closure. In addition to the direct mechanism of action, the fibrin sealants contain various amounts of antifibrinolytics, increasing their efficacy.[60] With any homologous blood protection, there is a small risk of viral transmission from fibrin sealants prepared from pooled human plasma.

The specialized cautery units enhance maintenance of operative hemostasis. One example of such technology is the Tissue-Link device (Tissue-Link, Dover, NH), which reduces hemostasis via collagen shrinking at cooler temperatures over broader fields and with less tissue destruction than standard electrocautery devices. Randomized prospective studies dedicated to the study of this cautery device are in its early stages. Further studies are needed to predict its effect on decreasing transfusion rates and maximizing postoperative blood values. The device costs approximately $500 per use; a cost-benefit analysis needs to be done when more studies are available. It can be speculated that a dryer operative field likely would lead to decreased levels of intraoperative and postoperative blood loss and less exposure to allogeneic blood during a patient's hospital stay.

Pharmacological Strategies

Pharmacological strategies to decrease transfusion requirements in patients undergoing surgery have been studied extensively.[52,72] Few articles on this topic are in the orthopedic literature, however. One such drug class is the antifibrinolytics. Fibrinolysis is stimulated by surgical trauma and further augmented by the use of a tourniquet. Antifibrinolytics act to increase hemostasis within a surgical site, by enhancing the clotting mechanism. The use of antifibrinolytics to minimize perioperative blood transfusion was reviewed.[42] Despite notable heterogeneity in the various trials, aprotinin seems to reduce the need for red blood cell transfusion and the need for reoperation because of bleeding, without serious adverse effects, including thromboembolism events and renal failure. Mostly in cardiac surgery, aprotinin was found to reduce the rate of allogeneic blood transfusions by 30%. Similar trends in efficacy were seen with tranexamic acid and aminocaproic acid, but the data are sparse. Eight trials directly comparing tranexamic acid with aprotinin have been done, and no significant difference has been reported. A trend toward an increased risk of transfusion with tranexamic acid over aprotinin was seen (relative risk increase of 21%).[83]

TRANEXAMIC ACID

Tranexamic acid inhibits fibrinolysis by blocking the lysine-bonding sites of plasminogen to fibrin. Several studies have shown the efficacy of tranexamic acid in reducing postoperative blood loss and transfusion requirements of TKA[6,43,44,47,82,83,85] and total hip arthroplasty[7,29]; blood loss reductions of 25% to 50% have been noted.[6,7,29,43,44,47,82,83,85] Additionally, in direct comparison studies, tranexamic acid has proved more efficacious than decompression in acute normovolemic hemodilution in patients undergoing TKA.[87,88] Some studies found no effect of tranexamic acid in TKAs.[8] Optimal timing of administration is not well defined. Several clinical studies have shown the efficacy of tranexamic acid boluses when given before surgery,[7,47] at deflation of the tourniquet,[6,44,83] and for various times after surgery.[42,88] The timing and duration of additional boluses and continued transfusions have varied in these studies. Generally, dosing is 10 to 20 mg/kg. In our institution, we use 10 mg/kg before surgery and at the time of the tourniquet deflation. Anaphylaxis has been noted to occur if the patient is given numerous doses. Caution should be used if the patient undergoes a procedure involving an infected TKA, where exposure can occur on two occasions within a 6- to 8-week period. By 6 months, the incidence of anaphylaxis decreases, but caution is advised. The surgeon should be familiar with the packaging label before prescribing this drug.

APROTININ

Aprotinin is a naturally occurring proteinase inhibitor, derived from bovine lung. It inhibits plasmin, trypsin, and kallikreins of different origins and has antifibrinolytic properties. Aprotinin also may have effects on the intrinsic coagulation pathway and platelet adhesion. It has been used with success in cardiac, vascular, and major liver surgery. The mechanism of aprotinin in orthopedic surgery has not yet been elucidated fully.[73,74]

The use of aprotinin has been studied in orthopedic surgery, including large operations for malignancy, infection, trauma, revision surgery, and bilateral joint replacement. Most of these studies showed an advantage of aprotinin over placebo. In a prospective study, no difference was noted in a medium dose of aprotinin (2 million KIU, followed by infusion of 0.5 million KIU/hr). Aprotinin did not lower preoperative blood loss or transfusion requirements relative to placebo.[3] Aprotinin in primary joint replacement has had mixed results.[3,74] Medium doses of aprotinin had no significant effect on fibrinolysis variables, reduction of postoperative bleeding, and transfusion requirements in TKA or estimated blood loss, hemoglobin levels, and transfusion requirements in THA. Similarly, a small dose of aprotinin was not effective in reducing blood loss transfusion needs in patients undergoing unilateral primary THA.[49] Other authors have found aprotinin to be successful in reducing blood loss during THA. Janssens and colleagues[48] reduced blood loss by 26% and transfusion units from 3.4 U to 1.8 U, with so-called high-dose protocols.

Although use of antifibrinolytics can reduce intraoperative blood loss, pharmacy and hospital costs are increased. The cost of these drugs is high, and there is theoretical risk of increased deep vein thrombosis complications, although Haas and coworkers[40] found no significant increased risk of deep vein thrombosis with the use of these drugs. Aprotinin is expensive, but also may be a savings in transfusion requirements and hospital cost. More investigation is needed before use of aprotinin; specifically, more TKA studies are needed before its use can be recommended for postoperative blood management.

POSTOPERATIVE MANAGEMENT

Drain Usage

Most blood loss in a TKA procedure occurs in the postoperative period, and techniques have been developed to salvage this shed blood. Numerous types of drains exist and basically differ on whether the cells are washed or unwashed and whether red cells are used for reinfusion. Faris[31] studied the quality of shed blood and its reinfusion and found that the shed blood was well tolerated, although a febrile reaction was noted in 2% of patients receiving the blood. Most of these febrile reactions occurred in patients receiving blood greater than 6 hours drainage time at the time of reinfusion. In this study, efficacy was not established, and the author since has abandoned the use of reinfusion drains.

Other authors have shown different results. Groh and colleagues[38] and Majkowski and associates[62] performed retrospective studies marking the efficacy of postoperative drain usage. In a survey of American Association of Hip and Knee Surgeons members,[21] most respondents were found to use drains in the postoperative period; 62% always used a drain compared with 24% who never used a drain. Occasional use of a drain also was reported. The survey found that 47% of respondents used a reinfusion type of drain, which was removed in approximately 24 to 36 hours.

Jones and associates[50] conducted a postoperative review of 43,000 hip replacements and 33,000 knee replacements performed in the United Kingdom. They evaluated the use of autologous salvage drains in hip and knee patients. The authors concluded that based on these findings, reinfusion drains seemed to be a cost-effective means of reducing the requirement of allogeneic blood in hip and knee arthroplasty. In this series, 21% of the reinfusion drain group compared with 45.7% in the suction drain group required allogeneic transfusions. In another series, Grosvenor and colleagues[39] looked at the efficacy of postoperative blood salvage after hip arthroplasty in patients with and without deposited autologous blood. The results of this study showed that postoperative blood salvage significantly reduced the risk of allogeneic transfusions. The patients who were treated with postoperative blood salvage were approximately 10 times more likely to acquire allogeneic transfusions than patients who had a non-reinfusion drain.

Mont and coworkers[63] recommended a new approach, designing a study to evaluate the efficacy of an intraoperative surgeon decision to use a reinfusion drain. In the TKA group, 84% of the patients in the standard group had reinfusion, similar to the 85% in the reinfusion drain group. The surgeon cannot predict intraoperatively whether a patient would require a reinfusion drain; however, in more than 94% of the cases, by 90 minutes, a decision can be made whether a reinfusion drain was necessary. This study also concluded that a drain can be placed and converted to a reinfusion drain if it was thought this could be efficacious.

Friederichs and coworkers[33] compared the use of a postoperative salvage drain with the practice of autologous donations. This study also included the perioperative blood salvages that are safe and cost-effective, making it possible to discontinue the practice of predonating blood for TKA and TKA in a patient with hematocrit greater than 37%. This is the practice at our institution because PAD has been abandoned for patients with hemoglobin values greater than 13 g/dL.

A decision can be made whether to use washed or unwashed cells. We switched to the OrthoPAT system, in the attempt to improve the quality of blood returned to the patient. Such a system has the benefits of a washed cell device without the additional costs of a cell-saver type system. We believe that a lower volume of better quality packed red blood cells is advantageous, and further studies are currently being done to test the efficacy of this system.

There may be a negative effect to not using a drain with regards to the appearance of the wound. Holt and associates[45] reported that patients who do not receive a drain experience the same degree of blood loss as patients in whom a drain was used. In the absence of a drain, the wound exhibited greater ecchymosis and drainage. This type of finding easily could be attributed erroneously to the anticoagulant, but appear to be related to the failure to use a postoperative drain in these patients. Niskanen and colleagues[67] also showed more wound drainage when a postoperative drain was not used.

Most surgeons use a drain after elective TKA. Although this practice can debated based on current literature, the studies about TKA show a significant decrease in the transfusion rates when postoperative salvage devices are used. Further studies are needed to evaluate the efficacy of these newer washed cell systems.

Special Situations

INFECTED TOTAL KNEE ARTHROPLASTY

Blood loss after revision for infected TKA is documented in the literature. Pagnano and colleagues[70] reviewed transfusion data of 75 infected TKAs and noted an overall transfusion rate of 88%. Only 12% of the patients avoided needing allogeneic transfusion throughout the two-stage reimplantation process. Transfusion after the resection of the affected prosthesis did not prevent subsequent allogeneic transfusions at the time of prosthesis reimplantation.

In a follow-up study, Cushner and associates[24] looked at the use of recombinant human EPO two-stage knee arthroplasty for infection. This was a multicenter prospective study to determine if EPO could be used to lower the transfusion requirements after two-stage arthroplasty for infection. The study enrolled 41 consecutive patients undergoing successful two-stage arthroplasty, who received EPO, 40,000 U subcutaneously, after prosthesis resection and antibiotic spacer placement. Although there was no difference in hemoglobin levels before resection arthroplasty or on postoperative day 3 between the study group or the control group, hemoglobin levels after reimplantation were higher in the patients who received EPO (12.4 g/dL versus 11.3 g/dL in the control group). The average increase in hemoglobin in the interval between stages was higher in the treatment group (3.2 mg/dL versus 1.7 mg/dL). The transfusion rate decreased from 83% of patients in the control group to 34% in the study group, showing the efficacy of this approach. One could make a case to delay the reimplantation until acceptable hemoglobin values can be achieved, to reduce the risks of allogeneic transfusions further. In a patient already compromised by infection, using allogeneic transfusions is beneficial. We are trying to record the use of tranexamic acid to reduce further this allogeneic transfusion rate after infected knee replacements.

REVISION OF TOTAL KNEE ARTHROPLASTY

Revision arthroplasty has been associated with increased blood loss in transfusion rates. Churchill and coworkers[18] reported that 15% of patients who did not participate in a PAD program before a revision TKA received transfusions compared with 80% of patients who underwent TKA who predonated blood. In this study, sample size was small, probably too small to show a significant treatment effect. In contrast, Bierbaum and colleagues[9] reported more than 476 revisions of TKA from a series of 9482 patients having joint arthroplasty. In all, 22% of patients who had revision TKA received an autologous transfusion, and 21% received an allogeneic transfusion. When only patients who did not participate in the PAD program were evaluated, an allogeneic transfusion rate of 30% was reported (meaning 2.4 U). In the PAD group, 11% of the patients required breakthrough allogeneic transfusions, and this rate increased to 18% when only patients who participated in the PAD program were considered. Cases for more than 331 surgeons were included in the study, and no specific treatment approach, transfusion criteria, or postoperative protocol was followed.

At our institution, all patients were treated comparably and received transfusions on the basis of symptoms of anemia and not a transfusion trigger.[22] In this series, 100 patients undergoing TKA revision were evaluated for factors predicting allogeneic transfusions. As noted with primary TKAs, the importance of the preoperative hemoglobin cannot be overstated, especially in a revision candidate. The preoperative hemoglobin levels were the most effective in predicting the need for allogeneic transfusion.

Patients with preoperative hemoglobin values less than 13 g/dL were significantly more likely to have a transfusion. Gender also played a role; the mean preoperative hemoglobin for women was 12.1 g/dL compared with 14.1 g/dL for men. Women had a higher allogeneic transfusion rate of 19.2%. The ability to participate in a PAD program was detrimental to the patient's preoperative hemoglobin status.

BILATERAL TOTAL KNEE ARTHROPLASTY

Most of the available evidence of blood loss in transfusion and management is from unilateral TKA data. The probable benefits are greater when a bilateral TKA is done. Keating and associates[53] reported a 5.42 g/dL decrease in hemoglobin in a patient who underwent bilateral TKA compared with a 3.85 g/dL decrease for in unilateral TKA patients. In the bilateral TKA group, 82% of patients with baseline hemoglobin values of 10 to 13 g/dL received a transfusion compared with 60% of patients with baseline hemoglobin greater than 13 g/dL. In a small study, Goodnough and colleagues[37] also noted increased blood loss with bilateral TKA throughout the length of hospital stay. Drainage was noted postoperatively at 1367 ± 560 mL for the unilateral group compared with 2773 ± 494 mL for the bilateral group. Only one of the nine bilateral patients required allogeneic transfusions.

Conversely, in the prospective comparison of 100 consecutive bilateral TKAs and 100 consecutive unilateral TKAs, Lane and coworkers[59] found 17% of bilateral TKA patients required allogeneic transfusion compared with 1% of the unilateral TKA patients. A total of 1.72 U of postoperative salvage blood was used in the bilateral group. Despite the use of allogeneic transfusions and blood salvage, however, lower postoperative hemoglobin values were noted in the bilateral group (9.5 g/dL) compared with the unilateral group (10.1 g/dL).

Cohen and colleagues[19] also evaluated blood management for bilateral versus unilateral TKA. They reported greater blood loss (692 mL versus 440 mL) and a greater need for allogeneic blood in the bilateral TKA group; 50% of the bilateral TKA patients who donated preoperatively required allogeneic transfusion compared with 8% of the unilateral TKA patients. Bilateral TKA patients also were noted to have lower hematocrit levels before surgery (38.8% versus 41%) and at discharge (30% versus 34%). Bierbaum and coworkers[9] looked at blood management in 9482 patients treated by 330 orthopedic surgeons in the United States. Of this group, 429 of the patients underwent bilateral TKA, and 49% of the patients underwent unilateral TKA. A high allogeneic transfusion rate was noted (28%) in the bilateral TKA group compared with an allogeneic transfusion rate of only 11% in the unilateral group.

We reported a series of 170 bilateral TKAs.[26] The patients in this series participated in the PAD program, which resulted in preoperative anemia before the start of the bilateral TKA procedure. As a result, we have since converted our PAD program. We now require only 2 U of PAD before bilateral TKA. If hemoglobin decreases to less than 13 g/dL because of the donations, EPO supplementation is provided.

CONCLUSION

The surgeon can play a role in not only minimizing the exposure to allogeneic blood, but also maximizing the patient's hemoglobin at the time of discharge. The number one factor preventing allogeneic transfusion is the preoperative hemoglobin and hematocrit. The practice of autologous blood donations should be questioned, and newer protocols, which emphasize a patient-specific approach, seem to be beneficial. Cushner and colleagues[69] reported the effects of orthopedic surgery–induced anemia and questioned the autologous donation process. Another study by Pierson and coworkers[71] showed a patient-specific approach, in which determination can be made based on the patient's preoperative blood status, assessing patients who are most at risk from allogeneic transfusion.

References

1. Alter HJ, Nakatsuji Y, Melpolder J, et al: The incidence of transfusion-associated hepatitis G virus infection and its relation to liver disease. N Engl J Med 336:747, 1997.
2. Alter HJ, Purcell RH, Shih JW, et al: Detection of antibody to hepatitis C virus in prospectively followed transfusion recipients with acute and chronic non-A, non-B hepatitis. N Engl J Med 321:1494, 1989.
3. Amar D, Grant FM, Zhang H, et al: Antifibrinolytic therapy and perioperative blood loss in cancer patients undergoing major orthopaedic surgery. Anesthesiology 8:337, 2003.
4. Ammann AJ, Cowan MJ, Wara DW, et al: Acquired immunodeficiency in an infant: Possible transmission by means of blood products. Lancet 1:956, 1983.
5. An HS, Mikhail WE, Jackson WT, et al: Effects of hypotensive anesthesia, nonsteroidal anti-inflammatory drugs, and polymethylmethacrylate on bleeding in total hip arthroplasty patients. J Arthroplasty 6:245, 1991.
6. Benoni G, Fredin H: Fibrinolytic inhibition with tranexamic acid reduces blood loss and blood transfusion after knee arthroplasty: A prospective, randomized, double-blind study of 86 patients. J Bone Joint Surg Br 78:434, 1996.
7. Benoni G, Fredin H, Knebel R, Nilsson P: Blood conservation with tranexamic acid in total hip arthroplasty: A randomized, double-blind study in 40 primary operations. Acta Orthop Scand 72:442, 2001.
8. Benoni G, Lethagen S, Nilsson P, Fredin H: Tranexamic acid, given at the end of the operation, does not reduce postoperative blood loss in hip arhtroplasty. Acta Orthop Scand 71:250, 2000.
9. Bierbaum BE, Callaghan JJ, Galante JO, et al: Analysis of blood management in patients having total hip or knee arthroplasty. J Bone Joint Surg Am 81:2, 1999.
10. Biggerstaff BJ, Petersen LR: Estimated risk of West Nile virus transmission through blood transfusion during an epidemic in Queens, New York City. Transfusion 42:1019, 2002.
11. Billote DB, Abdoue AG, Wixson RL: Comparison of acute normovolemic hemodilution and preoperative autologous blood donation in clinical practice. J Clin Anesth 12:31, 2000.
12. Billote DB, Glisson SN, Green D, Wixson RL: Efficacy of preoperative autologous blood donation: Analysis of blood loss and transfusion practice in total hip replacement. J Clin Anesth 12:537, 2000.
13. Billote DB, Glisson SN, Green D, Wixson RL: A prospective, randomized study of preoperative autologous donation for hip replacement surgery. J Bone Joint Surg Am 84:1299, 2002.

14. Brunson ME, Alexander JW: Mechanisms of transfusion-induced immunosuppression. Transfusion 30:651, 1990.

15. Canadian Orthopedic Peri-operative Erythropoietin Study Group: Effectiveness of peri-operative recombinant human erythropoietin in elective hip replacement. Lancet 341:1227, 1993.

16. Carless PA, Henry DA, Anthony DM: Fibrin sealant use for minimizing perioperative allogeneic blood transfusion. Cochrane Database of Systematic Reviews 3, 2003.

17. Cascinu S, Fedeli A, Del Ferro E, et al: Recombinant human erythropoietin treatment in cisplatin-associated anemia: A randomized double-blind trial with placebo. J Clin Oncol 12:1058, 1994.

18. Churchill WH, Chapman RH, Rutherford CJ, et al: Blood product utilization in hip and knee arthroplasty: Effect of gender and autologous blood on transfusion practice. Vox Sang 66:182, 1994.

19. Cohen RG, Forrest CJ, Benjamin JB: Safety and efficacy of bilateral total knee arthroplasty. J Arthroplasty 12:497, 1997.

20. Cooper ES, Walker RH, Schmidt PJ, Polesky HF: The 1990 comprehensive blood bank surveys of the College of American Pathologists. Arch Pathol Lab Med 117:125, 1993.

21. Cushner FD, et al: Presented 2003 AAOS Meeting, San Francisco.

22. Cushner FD, Foley I, Kessler D, et al: Blood management in revision total knee arthroplasty. Clin Orthop 404:247, 2002.

23. Cushner FD, Friedman RJ: Blood loss in total knee arthroplasty. Clin Orthop 269:98, 1991.

24. Cushner FD, Locker JR, Hanssen AD, et al: Use of recombinant human erythropoietin in two-stage total knee arthroplasty for infection. Clin Orthop 392:116, 2001.

25. Cushner FD, Scottt WN: Evolution of blood transfusion management for a busy knee practice. Orthopedics 22:s145, 1999.

26. Cushner FD, Scott WN, Scuderi GR, et al: Blood loss and transfusion in bilateral total knee arthroplasty. J Knee Surg 28:102-107, 2005.

27. De Andrade JR, Jove M, Landon G, et al: Baseline hemoglobin as a predictor of risk of transfusion and response to epoetin alfa in orthopedic surgery patients. Am J Orthop 8:533, 1996.

28. Dodd RY: The risk of transfusion-transmitted infection. N Engl J Med 327:419, 1992.

29. Ekback G, Axelsson K, Ryttberg L, et al: Tranexamic acid reduces blood loss in total hip replacement surgery. Anesth Analg 91:1124, 2000.

30. Etchason J, Petz L, Keeler E, et al: The cost effectiveness of pre-operative autologous blood donations. N Engl J Med 332:740, 1995.

31. Faris PM: Unwashed filtered shed blood collected after knee and hip arthroplasty. J Bone Joint Surg Am 73:1169, 1991.

32. Faris PM, Ritter MA, Ables RI, the American Erythropoietin Study Group: The effects of recombinant human erythropoietin on perioperative transfusion requirements in patients having a major orthopaedic operation. J Bone Joint Surg Am 78:62, 1993.

33. Friederichs MG, Mariani EM, Bourne MH: Perioperative blood salvage as an alternative to predonating blood for primary total knee and hip arthroplasty. J Arthroplasty 17:298, 2002.

34. Goldman M, Remy-Prince S, Trepanier A, Decary F: Autologous donation error rates in Canada. Transfusion 37:523, 1997.

35. Goodnough LT, Despotis GJ, Merkel K, Monk TG: A randomized trial comparing acute normovolemic hemodilution and preoperative autologous blood donation in total hip arthroplasty. Transfusion 40:1054, 2000.

36. Goodnough LT, Skikne B, Brugnara C: Erythropoietin, iron, and erythropoiesis. Blood 96:823, 2000.

37. Goodnough LT, Verbrugge D, Marcus RE: The relationship between hematocrit, blood lost, and blood transfused in total knee replacement: Implications for postoperative blood salvage and reinfusion. Am J Knee Surg 8:83, 1995.

38. Groh GI, Buchert PK, Allen WC: A comparison of transfusion requirements after total knee arthroplasty using the Solcotrans Autotransfusion System. J Arthroplasty 3:281, 1990.

39. Grosvenor D, Goyal V, Goodman S: Efficacy of postoperative blood salvage following total hip arthroplasty in patients with and without deposited autologous units. J Bone Joint Surg Am 82:951, 2000.

40. Haas S, Mueller E, Fritsche H: Effect of aprotinin on the incidence of thrombosis and postoperative bleeding. Thromb Haematol 54:99, 1985.

41. Hatzidakis AM, Mendlick RM, McKillip T, et al: Preoperative autologous donation for total joint arthroplasty: An analysis of risk factors for allogeneic transfusion. J Bone Joint Surg Am 82:89, 2000.

42. Henry DA, Moxey AJ, Carless PA, et al: Anti-fibrinolytic use for minimizing perioperative allogeneic blood transfusion. Cochrane Database for Systematic Reviews 3, 2003.

43. Hiipala S, Strid L, Wennerstrand M: Tranexamic acid (Cyklokapron) reduces perioperative blood loss associated with total knee arthroplasty. Br J Anaesth 74:534, 1995.

44. Hiippala ST, Strid LJ, Wennerstrand MI, et al: Tranexamic acid radically decreases blood loss and transfusions associated with total knee arthroplasty. Anesth Analg 84:839, 1997.

45. Holt BT, Parks NL, Engh GA, Lawrence JM: Comparison of closed-suction drainage and no drainage after primary total knee arthroplasty. Orthopedics 20:1121, 1997.

46. Houbiers JG, van de Velde CJ, van de Watering LM, et al: Transfusion of red cells is associated with increased incidence of bacterial infection after colorectal surgery: A prospective study. Transfusion 37:126, 1997.

47. Jansen AJ, Andreica S, Claeys M, et al: Use of tranexamic acid for an effective blood conservation strategy after total knee arthroplasty. Br J Anaesth 83:596, 1999.

48. Janssens M, Joris J, David JL, et al: High dose aprotinin reduces blood loss in patients undergoing total hip replacement surgery. Anesthesiology 80:23, 1994.

49. Jeserschek R, Clar H, Aigner C, et al: Reduction of blood loss using high-dose aprotinin in major orthopaedic surgery: A prospective, double-blind, randomized and placebo-controlled study. J Bone Joint Surg Br 85:174, 2003.

50. Jones HW, Savage L, White C, et al: Postoperative autologous blood salvage drains—are they useful in primary uncemented hip and knee arthroplasty? A prospective study of 186 cases. Acta Orthop Belg 70:466, 2004.

51. Juelsgaard P, Larsen UT, Sorensen JV, et al: Hypotensive epidural anesthesia in total knee replacement without tourniquet: Reduced blood loss and transfusion. Reg Anesth Pain Med 26:105, 2001.

52. Keating EM, Meding JB: Perioperative blood management practices in elective orthopaedic surgery. J Am Acad Orthop Surg 10:393, 2002.

53. Keating EM, Meding JB, Faris PM, et al: Predictors of transfusion risk in elective knee surgery. Clin Orthop 6:50, 1998.

54. Keating EM, Ranawat CS, Cats-Baril W: Assessment of postoperative vigor in patients undergoing elective total joint arthroplasty: A concise patient- and caregiver-based instrument. Orthopedics 22:s119, 1999.

55. Keating EM, Ritter MA: Transfusion options in total joint arthroplasty. J Arthroplasty 17:125, 2002.

56. Kendall SJ, Weir J, Aspinall R, et al: Erythrocyte transfusion causes immunosuppression after total hip replacement. Clin Orthop 381:145, 2000.

57. Kleinman S, Busch MP, Schreiber GB: The incidence/window period model and its use to assess the risk of transfusion-transmitted human immunodeficiency virus and hepatitis C virus infection. Transfus Med Rev 11:155, 1997.

58. Lackritz EM, Satten GA, Aberle-Grasse J, et al: Estimated risk of transmission of the human immunodeficiency virus by screened blood in the United States. N Engl J Med 333:1685, 1995.

59. Lane GJ, Hozack WJ, Shah S, et al: Simultaneous bilateral versus unilateral total knee arthroplasty: Outcomes analysis. Clin Orthop 345:106, 1997.

60. Levy O, Martinowitz U, Oran A, et al: The use of fibrin tissue adhesive to reduce blood loss and the need for blood transfusion after total knee arthroplasty: A prospective, randomized, multicenter study. J Bone Joint Surg Am 81:1580, 1999.

61. Lotke PA, Barth P, Garino JP, Cook EF: Predonated autologous blood transfusions after total knee arthroplasty: Immediate versus delayed administration. J Arthroplasty 14:647, 1999.

62. Majkowski RS, Currie IC, Newman JH: Postoperative collection and reinfusion of autologous blood in total knee arthroplasty. Ann R Coll Surg Engl 73:381, 1991.

63. Mont MA, Low K, LaPorte DM, et al: Reinfusion drains after primary total hip and total knee arthroplasty. J South Orthop Assoc 9:193, 2000.

64. Murphy P, Heal JM, Blumberg N: Infection or suspected infection after hip replacement surgery with autologous or homologous blood transfusions. Transfusion 31:212, 1991.

65. NHS Centre for Reviews and Dissemination: The efficacy of technologies to minimize peri-operative allogeneic transfusion (Struc-

tured Abstract). University of York, York, UK, Database of Abstracts of Review of Effectiveness, 2003.

66. Niemi TT, Pitkanen M, Syrjala M, Rosenberg PH: Comparison of hypotensive epidural anesthesia and spinal anesthesia on blood loss and coagulation during and after total hip arthroplasty. Acta Anesth Scand 44:457, 2000.

67. Niskanen RO, Korkala OL, Haapala J, et al: Drainage is of no use in primary uncomplicated cemented hip and knee arthroplasty for osteoarthritis: A prospective randomized study. J Arthroplasty 15: 567, 2000.

68. Nuttall GA, Santrach PJ, Oliver WC Jr, et al: The predictors of red cell transfusions in total hip arthroplasties. Transfusion 36:144, 1996.

69. Orthopaedic induced anemia: The fallacy of autologous blood donation program. Clin Orthop Rel Res 431:116-123, 2005.

70. Pagnano M, Cushner FD, Hansen A, et al: Blood management in two-stage revision knee arthroplasty for deep prosthetic infection. Clin Orthop 367:238, 1999.

71. Pierson JL, Hannon TJ, Earles DR: A blood-conservation algorithm to reduce blood transfusions after total hip and knee arthroplasty. J Bone Joint Surg Am 86:1512, 2004.

72. Porte RJ, Leebeek FWG: Pharmacological strategies to decrease transfusion requirements in patients undergoing surgery. Drugs 2:2193, 2002.

73. Samama CM, Dietrich W, Horrow J, et al: Structure, pharmacology, and clinical use of antifibrinolytic agents. In: Handbook of Experimental Pharmacology: Fibrinolytics and Antifibrinolytics. New York, Springer, 2000, p 559.

74. Samama CM, Langeron O, Rosencher N, et al: Aprotinin versus placebo in major orthopedic surgery: A randomized, double-blinded, dose-ranging study. Anesth Analg 95:287, 2002.

75. Schreiber GB, Busch MP, Kleinman SH, Korelitz JJ: The risk of transfusion-transmitted viral infections. N Engl J Med 334: 1685, 1996.

76. Sculco TP, Gallina J: Blood management experience: Relationship between autologous blood donation and transfusion in orthopedic surgery. Orthopedics 22:s129, 1999.

77. Sharrock NE, Mineo R, Go G: The effect of cardiac output on intraoperative blood loss during total hip arthroplasty. Reg Anesth 18:24, 1993.

78. Sharrock NE, Mineo R, Urquhart B, Salvati EA: The effect of two levels of hypotension on intraoperative blood loss during total hip arthroplasty performed under lumbar epidural anesthesia. Analg Anesth 76:580, 1993.

79. Shulman G, Grecula MJ, Hadjipavlou AG: Intraoperative autotransfusion in hip arthroplasty. Clin Orthop 369:119, 2002.

80. Stevens CE, Aach RD, Hollinger FB, et al: Hepatitis B virus antibody in blood donors and the occurrence of non-A, non-B hepatitis in transfusion recipients: An analysis of the transfusion-transmitted viruses study. Ann Intern Med 101:733, 1984.

81. Stowell CP, Chandler H, Jove M, et al: An open-label, randomized study to compare the safety and efficacy of peri-operative epoietin alfa with pre-operative autologous blood donation in total joint arthroplasty. Orthopedics 22:s105, 1999.

82. Tanaka N, Sakahashi H, Sato E, et al: Timing of the administration of tranexamic acid for maximum reduction in blood loss in arthroplasty of the knee. J Bone Joint Surg Br 83:702, 2001.

83. Tenholder M, Cushner FD: Intraoperative blood management in joint replacement surgery. Orthopedics 27(6 Suppl):s663, 2004.

84. Thompson GE, Miller RD, Stevens WC, Murray WR: Hypotensive anesthesia for total hip arthroplasty: A study of blood loss and organ function (brain, heart, liver, and kidney). Anesthesiology 48:91, 1978.

85. Veien M, Sorensen JV, Madsen F, Juelsgaard P: Tranexamic acid given intraoperatively reduces blood loss after total knee replacement: a randomized, controlled study. Acta Anesth Scand 46:1206, 2002.

86. Walker R: Transfusion risks. Am J Clin Pathol 88:371, 1987.

87. Zohar E, Fredman B, Ellis M, et al: A comparative study of the postoperative allogeneic blood-sparing effect of tranexamic acid versus acute normovolemic hemodilution after total knee replacement. Anesth Analg 89:1382, 1999.

88. Zohar E, Fredman B, Ellis MH, et al: A comparative study of the postoperative allogeneic blood-sparing effects of tranexamic acid and of desmopressin after total knee replacement. Transfusion 41:1285, 2001.

CHAPTER 105

Prevention of Thrombophlebitis in Total Knee Arthroplasty

Richard J. Friedman

Venous thromboembolism (VTE) is a potentially life-threatening complication for patients undergoing elective knee arthroplasty. Both mechanical and pharmacological means of prophylaxis have been used with varying degrees of success. Warfarin has proved to be effective in total hip replacement, although less so in total knee arthroplasty (TKA), whereas relatively newer classes of agents, such as the low-molecular-weight heparins (LMWHs) and factor X inhibitors, have been approved for thromboprophylaxis in knee surgery patients and are proving to be an acceptable alternative. This chapter reviews the current status of anticoagulant therapy in TKA patients based on the clinical trial data available to date. Recommendations will then be made, as far as possible, on the best course of action for effective anticoagulant prophylaxis in TKA patients.

KNEE SURGERY AND THROMBOTIC RISK

TKA is one of the most commonly performed orthopedic procedures. Statistics show that 381,000 TKA procedures were performed in 2002 in the United States, with the aim of relieving pain and restoring function and mobility.[61]

Deep vein thrombosis (DVT) is the most common post-operative complication of TKA and the most frequent cause of hospital readmission. Patients undergoing major orthopedic surgery on the lower limbs, such as TKA or total hip arthroplasty (THA), are at particularly high risk for DVT when compared with other surgical or medical patients, with the incidence of total DVT after TKA ranging from 41% to 85%.[2] The incidence of thrombi in the proximal veins, which have been shown to give rise to a higher rate of embolization than do thrombi in more distal veins, is thought to range from 5% to 22%.[31] Pulmonary embolism (PE), a potentially fatal complication of DVT that occurs when a fragment of a thrombus breaks off and embolizes in the lungs, is less well documented, but published studies have reported rates of 0% to 10% for total PE and 0% to 1.7% for fatal PE.[11,31] In addition to being a major cause of death, DVT can also be a significant cause of morbidity through recurrent thrombosis or the post-thrombotic syndrome and can result in pain, swelling, and leg ulceration in advanced cases.[65]

The surgical procedure itself carries with it an intrinsic risk for DVT. Injury to the venous endothelium as a result of operative positioning and manipulation, thermal injury from bone cement, anterior tibial subluxation, and flexion of the knee for an extended time may result in foci of vascular damage that represent an increased risk for thrombosis. The trauma of the procedure itself results in sustained activation of tissue factor and other clotting factors, which then localize at sites of vascular injury and in areas of venous stasis. Postoperative reduction in levels of antithrombin III and inhibition of the endogenous fibrinolytic system may allow continued growth of the thrombus. In addition to the risks associated with surgery itself, the risk for DVT can be compounded by the presence of acquired or congenital risk factors such as advanced age, obesity, cancer, and inherited coagulation disorders.[3] Because patients undergoing TKA are frequently of advanced age, have concomitant disease, and may be less mobile for prolonged periods, risk can quickly accumulate.

In addition to the burden of mortality and morbidity associated with DVT and PE, these events also impose substantial demands on health care resources.[13,63,72] One study showed that the total medical cost for orthopedic surgery patients in whom in-hospital VTE developed was approximately $18,000 higher than in those in whom it did not.[64] This finding has been supported by several studies showing that effective thromboprophylaxis in patients undergoing major orthopedic surgery is a cost-effective strategy.[35,37,46,59]

Therefore, from both a clinical and economic perspective there is a strong rationale for effective thromboprophylaxis in patients undergoing major knee surgery. Yet despite the availability of prophylactic measures, modern surgical techniques, and an increased awareness of the problem that has encouraged physicians to mobilize patients early, DVT remains a significant potential complication of knee surgery.

There are many reasons for prophylaxis in TKA patients in addition to preventing death from a fatal PE. Aside from preventing nonfatal PE and primary proximal and distal DVT, both of which can cause the patient significant morbidity in postoperative recovery and increase the cost to the health care system, there are other long-term potential complications from a thromboembolic episode that need to be prevented, including recurrent proximal and distal DVT, chronic pulmonary hypertension, and the post-thrombotic syndrome with chronic venous stasis ulcers.

OPTIONS FOR THROMBOPROPHYLAXIS IN KNEE SURGERY

Methods of thromboprophylaxis for TKA patients include pharmacological interventions, mechanical interventions, and a combination approach using both. The ideal pharmacological prophylactic agent should be efficacious and cost-effective, require little to no monitoring, and have minimal to no side effects or complications.

Pharmacological Thromboprophylaxis

Anticoagulants used for thromboprophylaxis in orthopedic surgery patients act at a variety of sites in the coagulation cascade (Fig. 105–1). Currently available agents include warfarin, LMWHs, and factor Xa inhibitors (fondaparinux), whereas newer agents such as direct thrombin inhibitors are also now emerging.[75] Unfractionated heparin (UFH) has been widely used for treatment and thromboprophylaxis in medical and surgical patients, but its lower efficacy in TKA patients combined with issues of practicality (need for intravenous administration and laboratory monitoring) has caused it to be used less frequently in this patient population.[15,18] A comparison of the old and new anticoagulants is presented in Table 105–1.

WARFARIN

Warfarin (Coumadin) has formed the mainstay of anticoagulant therapy for more than 50 years. In a class of agents known as vitamin K antagonists, warfarin is one of the most widely used drugs for thromboprophylaxis. It acts by inhibiting the cyclic interconversion of vitamin K and its 2,3-epoxide, thus leading to limited carboxylation of the vitamin K–dependent clotting factors II, VII, IX, and X. This action results in inhibition of the extrinsic coagulation pathway (see Fig. 105–1). The anticoagulant effect is delayed for 24 to 36 hours, the time necessary for replacement of normal clotting factors with the decarboxylated form; however, the full anticoagulant effect does not occur until some 72 to 96 hours later when all the vitamin K–dependent factors have been completely replaced.[6] Warfarin has been the standard for hip arthroplasty and remains one of the most widely used and effective methods of thromboprophylaxis in THA. Fewer data are available on its safety and efficacy in TKA patients.

The efficacy of dose-adjusted warfarin in patients undergoing TKA has been assessed in a number of randomized clinical trials, and an analysis of nine of these studies has produced relative risk reductions of approximately 27% in the incidence of pooled DVT when compared with no preventive measures.[30] The incidence of venographically detected asymptomatic DVT has been shown to be relatively high (25% to 50%) after warfarin therapy, and although the majority of such events remain clinically silent, 10% to 20% of calf vein thrombi extend to the proximal leg veins, where thrombosis is associated with a major risk for PE.[50] In contrast to asymptomatic DVT, the incidence of symptomatic VTE is low in patients receiving warfarin. In one study, the incidence of symptomatic VTE in 257 TKA patients who received warfarin for 10 days at doses adjusted to achieve an international normalized ratio (INR) of 1.8 to 2.5 was 0.8%.[67]

Although warfarin offers the convenience of oral administration, its use in clinical practice can be complicated. It has a narrow therapeutic window (Fig. 105–2) and shows considerable interindividual variability in its dose-response relationship.[17] With a narrow therapeutic window, an INR of less than 2.0 will be associated with a low risk of bleeding but reduced efficacy and therefore an

SIMPLIFIED COAGULATION CASCADE: ALL SITES

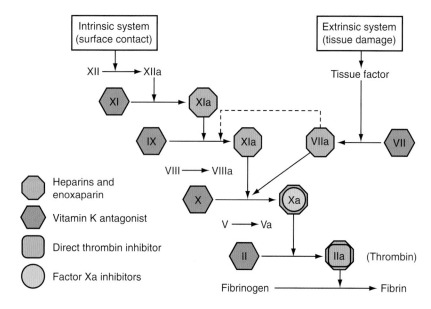

Figure 105–1. Sites of action of anticoagulant drugs used in thromboprophylaxis

Table 105–1. Old and New Anticoagulants: An Overview of Action and Administration

	UFH	WARFARIN	LMWH	FONDAPARINUX	XIMELAGATRAN
Dosing route	IV	**Oral**	SC	SC	**Oral**
Fixed dose	No	No	**Yes**	**Yes**	**Yes**
Inhibits clot-bound thrombin	No	No	No	No	**Yes**
Extended use	No	**Yes**	**Yes**	**Yes**	**Yes**
Risk for HIT	Yes	**No**	Yes	**No**	**No**
Monitoring necessary	Yes	Yes	**No**	**No**	**No**
Rapid onset/offset	**Yes**	No	**Yes**	No	**Yes**
Interactions	**No**	Yes	**No**	**No**	**No**

Green is an advantage; red is a disadvantage.
HIT, heparin-induced thrombocytopenia.

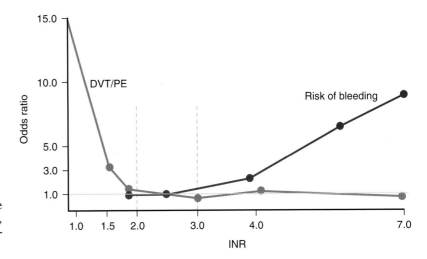

Figure 105–2. The narrow therapeutic range of warfarin. DVT, deep vein thrombosis; INR, international normalized ratio; PE, pulmonary embolism.

increased risk for DVT and PE. If the INR rises above 3.0, the risk for thromboembolic complications is low, but the risk of bleeding, both at the surgical site and remote bleeding, rises exponentially. Furthermore, warfarin is subject to numerous dietary and drug interactions,[82] and the need for regular dose adjustments to achieve and maintain a target INR can lead to additional problems such as nonadherence to medication or communication difficulties between the physician and patient.[6] Therefore, it is very difficult to keep the patient inside that narrow therapeutic window where both efficacy and safety exist.

LOW-MOLECULAR-WEIGHT HEPARINS

LMWHs are derived from UFH by chemical or enzymatic depolymerization and have a mean molecular weight of 4000 to 5000 daltons. Like heparin, LMWHs produce their major anticoagulant effect by activating antithrombin. This interaction increases the inhibitory activity of antithrombin III against procoagulatory serine proteases such as factors IIa (thrombin), IXa, and Xa (see Fig. 105–1). When compared with UFH, LMWHs offer a more favorable pharmacokinetic profile and more predictable dose response, plus a reduced risk of heparin-induced

thrombocytopenia—a potentially serious complication of heparin therapy that can lead to platelet aggregation and risk for venous and arterial thrombosis.[39] Because of the reduced anti–factor IIa activity relative to anti–factor X activity, monitoring of the activated partial prothrombin time is not required, thus allowing subcutaneous administration of a fixed dose without the need for laboratory monitoring. Accordingly, LMWHs are suitable for extended thromboprophylaxis outside the hospital setting[44] because the risk for VTE may persist for several weeks beyond the time of hospital discharge (currently 3 to 4 days postoperatively).[27]

Extensive data have shown that LMWHs are effective and safe in the prevention of VTE after TKA. A study published in 1994 concluded that LMWH was significantly more efficacious than low-dose warfarin in TKA. The incidence of DVT was found to be 26% (6% proximal) in the LMWH group versus 43% (10% proximal) in the warfarin group. Safety was similar between groups, with no increased risk of bleeding.[28] For six randomized studies comparing LMWHs with warfarin, the pooled incidence of DVT was found to be 33% and 48%, respectively, and that of proximal DVT was 7.1% and 10.4%, respectively.[25,36,38,45,47,55]

The superior efficacy of LMWH over warfarin has also been confirmed in a number of meta-analyses. In one

Table 105–2. Risk for Venous Thromboembolic Events (with 95% CI) in a Meta-analysis of 14 Randomized Trials of Thromboprophylaxis in TKA Patients

	TOTAL DVT	PROXIMAL DVT	DISTAL DVT	SYMPTOMATIC PE	FATAL PE	MAJOR BLEEDING	MINOR BLEEDING
LMWH	31.3% (26.8-36.1)	5.9% (4.0-8.5)	24.4% (20.3-29.0)	0.2% (0.06-0.6)	0% (0-0.2)	2.4% (1.8-3.3)	16.4% (10.2-25.4)
UFH	39.3% (24.3-56.7)	5.4% (2.0-11.2)	21.5% (14.0-30.6)	0.4% (0.01-2.3)	0% (0-1.6)	0.9% (0.3-2.3)	18.3% (13.1-24.9)
Warfarin	45.6% (40.2-51.0)	10.2% (8.7-11.9)	24.4% (20.3-29.0)	0.4% (0.1-0.9)	0% (0-0.3)	1.3% (0.2-2.7)	14.3% (7.6-25.3)
Placebo	60.2% (55.7-64.5)			0% (0-10.9)	0% (0-4.2)		

CI, confidence interval; DVT, deep vein thrombosis; LMWH, low-molecular-weight heparin; PE, pulmonary embolism; TKA, total knee arthroplasty; UFH, unfractionated heparin.

analysis of data from 10 randomized trials involving approximately 3000 patients, the relative risk for DVT in patients receiving LMWH was 0.73 versus treatment with warfarin or dose-adjusted UFH, whereas the relative risks for proximal DVT and PE were 0.58 and 0.55, respectively.[41] A further meta-analysis of 14 studies involving a total of 3482 patients found that the total risk for DVT was 31.3% in LMWH-treated patients versus 45.6% in warfarin-treated patients and 60.2% in patients receiving placebo (Table 105–2).[11] LMWH produced significantly greater reductions in total ($p = 0.0001$), distal ($p = 0.0001$), and proximal ($p = 0.0002$) DVT when compared with warfarin, an observation that has clinical relevance in light of the fact that proximal DVT is associated with a much higher risk for PE.

FACTOR Xa INHIBITORS

Anticoagulants that block the propagation of coagulation by direct or indirect inhibition of factor Xa or its respective cofactors are now emerging. Fondaparinux is a synthetic analogue of the pentasaccharide sequence involved in binding UFH or LMWH to antithrombin III, the major endogenous inhibitor of factor Xa and thrombin (see Fig. 105–1). Binding of fondaparinux to antithrombin III leads to increased inactivation of factor Xa and acts as an indirect factor Xa inhibitor. The drug has a predictable dose response, a long plasma half-life of approximately 17 hours, and 100% bioavailability, thus permitting once-daily subcutaneous injection without laboratory monitoring.[75]

The antithrombotic efficacy of fondaparinux has been evaluated in a randomized, double-blind trial involving 1049 patients undergoing elective major knee surgery.[7,73] Thromboprophylaxis was administered for 5 to 9 days, starting 6 hours postoperatively. The incidence of documented VTE on day 11 was 12.5% in patients receiving fondaparinux (2.5 mg) versus 27.8% in those receiving enoxaparin (30 mg), a relative risk reduction of 55.2% ($p < 0.001$). However, major bleeding was significantly more common with fondaparinux than with enoxaparin (2.1% versus 0.2%, respectively; $p = 0.006$).

There are other limitations to the use of fondaparinux in TKA. The drug should not be used in patients who are older than 75 years, weigh less than 50 kg, or have a creatinine clearance less than 30 mL/min because the risk of bleeding is increased significantly. With a long half-life of 17 to 20 hours, the surgeon must wait 2.5 days after the last dose for the drug to clear sufficiently so that bleeding is not increased if one has to reoperate.

In addition to fondaparinux, an oral direct inhibitor of factor Xa is also under development. In a recent study, DPC 906 (razaxaban) was compared with enoxaparin in a phase II dose-ranging study in patients undergoing TKA. In the 656-patient trial, razaxaban administered at 25 mg twice daily was considered to have efficacy and safety similar to that of enoxaparin, 30 mg twice daily.[54]

DIRECT THROMBIN INHIBITORS

In contrast to indirect thrombin inhibitors, which act by catalyzing antithrombin, heparin cofactor II, or both, direct thrombin inhibitors bind to thrombin itself and thus block the interaction of thrombin with its substrate.[74] One such agent is ximelagatran, a prodrug of melagatran, which is a reversible inhibitor of thrombin. Currently in phase III trials, melagatran has a stable and reproducible pharmacokinetic profile plus a wide therapeutic window that dispenses with the need for anticoagulant monitoring.[8,17,26] Oral bioavailability, measured as the plasma concentration of melagatran, is approximately 20%, with most of the remaining 80% being excreted renally. Despite the relatively low bioavailability, the pharmacokinetics is stable and the drug allows fixed dosing with no clinical monitoring.

Direct thrombin inhibitors offer a number of potential advantages over indirect inhibitors. Because they do not bind to plasma proteins, they offer a more predictable anticoagulant effect than indirect inhibitors do, and they also have the advantage of being effective against both circulating and clot-bound thrombin (whereas heparins are ineffective against clot-bound thrombin, which remains biologically active).

However, a big part of the attraction lies in their oral route of administration, which provides added convenience and encourages patient compliance (particularly in the outpatient setting). As we have seen, warfarin provides convenient oral administration but has a delayed onset of action and requires regular laboratory monitoring. As such, the search has continued for an alternative oral agent that is both effective and safe. Ximelagatran may represent such an alternative.

The efficacy of ximelagatran in patients undergoing TKA has been investigated in the randomized, double-blind, phase III trials EXULT A and EXULT B, which involved 2301 and 2303 patients, respectively, who received ximelagatran, 24 or 36 mg twice daily starting on the morning after surgery, or warfarin (target INR of 2.5) starting on the evening of the day of surgery.[17,26] In both studies, ximelagatran, 36 mg, was significantly more efficacious than warfarin (20.3% versus 27.6%, $p = 0.003$ in EXULT A; 22.5% versus 31.9%, $p < 0.001$ in EXULT B). Safety was similar, with no significant differences in major or minor bleeding between the two groups.

ASPIRIN

Aspirin (acetylsalicylic acid) is appealing to the clinician because of its easy administration, minimal bleeding complications, and relative cost-effectiveness. It irreversibly binds and inactivates cyclooxygenase on circulating platelets, which in turn inhibits thromboxane production, a prostacyclin required for platelet aggregation. Aspirin has been shown to be less effective than other prophylactic measures in a number of clinical trials. In one randomized clinical trial comparing enoxaparin and aspirin with venographic endpoints, the overall DVT rate after TKA was 79%, with a proximal rate of 33%.[32] Other studies have shown DVT rates between 47% and 80%, with most of the clots being distal.

BLEEDING ISSUES

All forms of pharmacological thromboprophylaxis must be managed properly to minimize the risk of bleeding. In terms of bleeding risk, meta-analyses comparing LMWHs and warfarin have shown that when compared with warfarin, the use of LMWHs is not associated with an increased risk for bleeding complications (see Table 105–2). The meta-analysis performed by Howard and Aaron[41] found that LMWHs are more effective than warfarin, UFHs, or placebo in preventing DVT after TKA, but importantly, they were also found to be as safe. This result is supported in studies by Leclerc et al[55] and Heit et al,[38] who reported no differences in major or minor bleeding during or after TKA.

As demonstrated in the study of Leclerc et al, patients not receiving any pharmacological prophylaxis still have a bleeding rate of 2% to 3%, and this has been consistent in the literature throughout the years. Bleeding is multifactorial and, as such, will occur in placebo patients. It is important for the surgeon to minimize the risk for additional bleeding when using pharmacological agents by using the drugs at the proper doses and with the appropriate dosing schedule.

Mechanical Thromboprophylaxis

Mechanical methods of thromboprophylaxis include graduated compression stockings (GCSs), intermittent pneumatic compression (IPC) devices, and venous foot pumps (VFPs). They act by increasing the speed of venous blood flow and the volume of blood returned from the extremities to the heart.

IPC devices can play a role in the prevention of DVT, particularly in patients who have contraindications to anticoagulation treatment. IPC devices have been found to be effective in a number of small studies involving TKA patients.[10,34,43,58] However, patients must wear the devices for 17 to 20 hours each day, and this is not practical or realistic when they are getting out of bed and bearing full weight on the first postoperative day and being discharged 3 to 4 days postoperatively.

GCSs have been shown to reduce the risk of DVT by approximately 57% in patients undergoing hip replacement surgery,[2] but conversely, the limited data available in TKA patients suggest that GCSs have little effect on the risk for VTE in this group.[42,56] This may reflect technical issues in TKA, such as the use of a thigh tourniquet, which impairs venous drainage, damages the endothelium, and confines coagulation factors below the tourniquet, thus increasing the risk for thrombosis. In general, GCSs are not considered an adequate means of thromboprophylaxis for TKA patients.[31]

The use of VFPs is based on the large volume of blood contained in the foot and the beneficial effects of the physiological foot pump.[71] Two small trials have found that VFPs are effective in TKA patients,[76,80] whereas others have shown that this approach is less effective than therapy with LMWHs.[9,62] VFPs may have value in the early postoperative stage when used in conjunction with pharmacological thromboprophylaxis, but VFP use as the sole method of thromboprophylaxis is not recommended.[2]

As stated, to be most effective, mechanical forms of prophylaxis should be applied either during or immediately after surgery and worn continuously, at least until the patient is fully ambulatory. Mechanical means of thromboprophylaxis generally require 17 to 21 days of treatment to be effective, yet knee surgery patients are typically discharged 3 days after surgery. This means that the usefulness of mechanical methods can be limited by poor compliance, incorrect use, and the inability to continue thromboprophylaxis after hospital discharge. There is increasing interest in the "stacked modality" approach whereby several types of thromboprophylaxis are used concurrently, such as the combination of IPC or foot pumps with LMWH or warfarin. Results from the Global Orthopaedic Registry (GLORY) suggest that North American surgeons are three times more likely to adopt this approach than surgeons elsewhere are.[21]

THROMBOPROPHYLAXIS IN KNEE ARTHROSCOPY

Although VTE is a recognized complication after TKA, less is known about the risk for thromboembolic events in patients undergoing arthroscopic procedures on the knee, which are among the most commonly performed orthopedic procedures, particularly in younger patients.[31] Arthroscopy has traditionally been considered a low-risk procedure and is widely performed without thromboprophylaxis. However, prospective studies have suggested that, in the absence of thromboprophylaxis, the incidence of DVT in patients undergoing knee arthroscopy can be as high as 18%, with an incidence of proximal DVT of up to 5%.[20,22,23,48,60,70,79,81] In one particular study, DVT occurred in 7.8% of patients undergoing elective knee arthroscopy, and the risk for DVT was increased in patients with a previous history of thrombosis (relative risk, 8.2; $p < 0.005$) or with two or more risk factors for VTE (relative risk, 2.94; $p < 0.05$).[22] Operative arthroscopy appears to be associated with a higher risk than diagnostic arthroscopy, possibly as a result of the more complex operational technique involving a longer surgical procedure and longer tourniquet time.

Two studies have investigated the effect of thromboprophylaxis with LMWH in patients undergoing knee arthroscopy.[60,81] In the first study, the incidence of DVT in patients treated with reviparin for 7 to 10 days was 0.85% versus 4.1% in patients receiving no thromboprophylaxis, a relative risk reduction of 79.3%.[81] In the second study, 130 patients were randomized to receive dalteparin for 4 weeks or no prophylaxis.[60] The incidence of DVT detected by bilateral compression ultrasonography in the two groups was 1.5% and 15.6%, respectively ($p = 0.004$).

THROMBOPROPHYLAXIS IN TRAUMA SURGERY

Lower limb fractures below the femur are common in patients of all ages, and there is an increasing trend toward surgical repair.[31] However, there has been little study of the risk for VTE in patients with such fractures. Data from four prospective studies suggest that in the absence of thromboprophylaxis, venographically documented DVT occurs in 10% to 45% of patients with isolated lower limb injuries, whereas 5% to 8% have proximal DVT.[1,40,49,53] Risk factors for VTE in these patients include advanced age, fractures, and obesity, but it remains to be established whether surgical management is itself a risk factor.[40,53] Fractures proximal to the knee appear to be associated with a higher risk for VTE than more distal fractures do.[1]

The efficacy of LMWHs in the prevention of VTE in patients with isolated lower leg injuries has been evaluated in four randomized clinical trials.[49,51-52] Three of these trials reported a significant reduction in the incidence of DVT in patients receiving LMWH as compared with placebo.[1,49,52]

RISK STRATIFICATION

Although a strong case can be made for the extended use of thromboprophylaxis in many patients undergoing TKA, it is important to recognize that this strategy may not be necessary in all patients and that thromboprophylaxis should be tailored to the risk for VTE in an individual patient. Risk stratification can be difficult, however. The use of signs or symptoms of early DVT is unreliable because physical findings are nonspecific and many VTE events are asymptomatic.[77] Indeed, in many cases, the first sign of VTE may be death from PE.[57] Routine screening of patients for symptomatic DVT is logistically difficult and expensive and is inefficient in identifying patients at risk for clinical VTE.[14]

Multiple risk factors determine the risk for VTE in a given patient.[31] They may be grouped into inherited risk factors, such as congenital thrombophilias, and clinical risk factors, such as age, obesity, previous VTE, and the duration and type of surgery.[12] Many hospitalized patients will have more than one risk factor. In a study in Massachusetts, for example, 80% of hospitalized patients with a first diagnosis of VTE had three or more risk factors for VTE.[4] The presence of multiple risk factors has a cumulative effect leading to a high overall level of risk.[3,68,77]

A number of risk assessment models have been developed to predict the level of risk in a given patient from the number of risk factors present,[66,69] but their use has been limited because of their complexity. Current risk assessment models are simpler and include specific recommendations for thromboprophylaxis in different groups of patients. One such model, developed by Caprini et al,[12] assigns surgical patients a score based on the presence of predefined risk factors within the 24 hours preceding surgery. This score allows the level of risk to be categorized into low, moderate, high, or very high, with specific recommendations for thromboprophylaxis being made in each case (Fig. 105-3). Thus, patients at low risk for VTE (no more than one risk factor) require no specific measures other than early ambulation; patients at moderate or high risk (two to four risk factors) should receive appropriate mechanical or pharmacological thromboprophylaxis, whereas those at highest risk should receive aggressive therapy with combinations of drugs and IPC or GCSs. This risk assessment model provides clinicians with a rational strategy for risk stratification, with accountability and systematic assessment.

DURATION OF THROMBOPROPHYLAXIS

DVT occurs in 41% to 85% of patients undergoing TKA, and there is increasing evidence that a high proportion of these events occur after discharge from the hospital.[31] For example, in a review of data from 24,059 patients undergoing primary TKA, the incidence of symptomatic VTE at 3 months was 2.1%; the median time to diagnosis was 7 days, and in 47% of cases VTE was diagnosed after discharge from hospital.[78] A meta-analysis of six randomized trials comparing extended (4 to 5 weeks) and conventional (7 to 15 days) thromboprophylaxis with LMWH in patients undergoing hip or knee arthroplasty showed that the risk for clinical VTE was reduced by 50% in those receiving extended thromboprophylaxis ($p = 0.009$).[16] However, five of the six studies were based on THA patient populations, and when extrapolating combined THA and TKA data, it should be remembered that, in terms of VTE prevention, TKA differs from THA with respect to the incidence and efficacy of prophylactic measures.[31]

Step 1: Exposing risk factors associated with clinical setting			
Assign 1 factor	Assign 2 factors	Assign 3 factors	Assign 5 factors
☐ Minor surgery	☐ Major surgery* ☐ Immobilizing plaster cast ☐ Medical or surgical patients confined to bed > 72 hours ☐ Central venous access	☐ Myocardial infraction ☐ Congestive heart faliure ☐ Severe sepsis/infection	☐ Elective major lower extremity arthroplasty ☐ Hip, pelvis, or leg fracture ☐ Stroke ☐ Multiple trauma ☐ Acute spinal cord injury

* Operations in which the dissection is important or that last longer than 45 minutes, including laparoscopic procedures,
Baseline risk factor score (if score = 5, go to step 4): _____

Step 2: Predisposing risk factors associated with patient

Assign 1 factor unless otherwise noted

	Molecular	
Clinical setting	Inherited	Acquired
☐ Age 40 to 60 years (1 factor) ☐ Age over 60 years (2 factors) ☐ History of DVT/PE (3 factors) ☐ Pregnancy or postpartum (<1 month) ☐ Malignancy (2 factors) ☐ Varicose veins ☐ Inflammatory bowel disease ☐ Obesity (>20% ideal body weight) ☐ Combined oral contraceptive/ hormonal replacement therapy	☐ Factor V Leiden/activated protein C resistance (3 factors) ☐ Antithrombin III deficiency (3 factors) ☐ Proteins C and S deficiency (3 factors) ☐ Dysfibrinogenemia (3 factors) ☐ Homocysteinemia (3 factors) ☐ 20210A prothrombin mutation (3 factors)	☐ Lupus anticoagulant (3 factors) ☐ Antiphospholipid antibodies (3 factors) ☐ Myeloproliferative disorders (3 factors) ☐ Disorders of plasminogen and plasmin activation (3 factors) ☐ Heparin-induced thrombocytopenia (3 factors) ☐ Hyperviscosity syndromes (3 factors) ☐ Homocysteinemia (3 factors)

Total additional predisposing risk factors score: _____

Step 3: Total risk factors (exposing + predisposing): _____
Step 4: Recommended prophylactic regimens for each risk group

Low risk (1 factor)	Moderate risk (2 factors)	High risk (3–4 factors)	Highest risk (5 or more factors)
No specific measures	LDUFH (every 12 h), LMWH, IPC and GCS†	LDUFH (every 8 h), LMWH, and IPC	LMWH, oral anticoagulants, IPC‡ (+ LDUFH or LMWH), GCS† (+ LDUFH or LMWH)
Early ambulation		GCS† (+ LDUFH or LMWH)	Adjusted-dose heparin

Abbreviations: LDUFH, low-dose unfractionated heparin; IPC, intermittent pneumatic compression; GCS, graduated compression stockings.

† Combining GCS with other prophylactic methods (LDUFH, LMWH, or IPC) may give better protection.

‡ Data show benefit of plantar pneumatic compression in orthopedic total joint arthroplasty and leg trauma and can be used when IPC is not feasible or tolerated.

Figure 105–3. The risk assessment model developed by Caprini et al.[12] (From Caprini JA, Arcelus JI, Reyna JJ: Effective risk stratification of surgical and nonsurgical patients for venous thromboembolic disease. Semin Hematol 38[Suppl 5]:12-19, 2001.)

When compared with THA, there is less evidence to support extended thromboprophylaxis in TKA patients, and therefore strong recommendation has been lacking. In a meta-analysis of studies involving approximately 13,000 patients receiving 7 to 10 days' thromboprophylaxis with LMWHs or warfarin, the 3-month incidence of symptomatic VTE in TKA patients was 2.4%.[24] Similarly, in a study by Comp et al, the total VTE risk seen in 438 TKA patients who received enoxaparin (30 mg every 12 hours for 7 to 10 days followed by 40 mg once daily for 3 weeks) was 17.5% versus 21% in patients who received placebo (Fig. 105–4).[19,27] Previous thromboembolic studies with various agents have demonstrated efficacy when patients have received pharmacologic prophylaxis for 7 to 10 days. However, thromboprophylaxis is often discontinued on discharge from the hospital, and the duration of hospitalization for many major orthopedic surgery procedures has decreased

significantly during the last decade. Data from the U.S. Hip and Knee registry, for example, indicate that the mean duration of hospitalization for TKA patients decreased from 4.5 days to 3.7 days ($p < 0.001$) between 1996 and 2001.[5] Thus, thromboprophylaxis will need to be continued outside the hospital setting if it is to be effective throughout the period of greatest risk. Patients are typically discharged from the hospital on postoperative day 3 or 4, yet risk normally peaks at day 10 and remains until day 28. Therefore, thromboprophylaxis should be continued for a minimum of 7 to 10 days postoperatively, which means that patients should receive out-of-hospital prophylaxis for approximately 1 week after discharge to receive the minimum 7 to 10 days of prophylaxis. Risk stratification can help determine which patients would benefit from extended prophylaxis out to 28 to 35 days. In terms of cost savings, postdischarge thromboprophylaxis has been shown to be cost-effective when compared

CLINICAL VIEWS

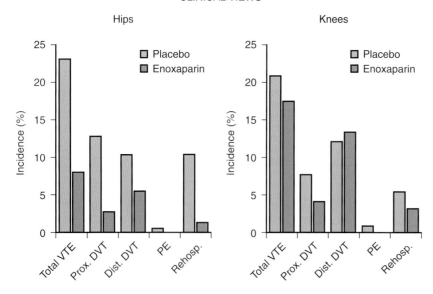

Figure 105–4. Incidence of venous thromboembolic events in total knee arthroplasty patients receiving postdischarge thromboprophylaxis with enoxaparin.[19,27] (From Comp PC, Spiro TE, Friedman RJ, et al: Prolonged enoxaparin therapy to prevent venous thromboembolism after primary hip or knee replacement. J Bone Joint Surg Am 83:336-345, 2001.)

with the cost of treating thromboembolic events or the cost of laboratory monitoring with drugs such as warfarin or UFH, although these data were collected for THA patients.[29]

THE SEVENTH ACCP GUIDELINES FOR KNEE SURGERY PATIENTS

The American College Chest Physicians (ACCP) guidelines are developed with the use of evidence-based medicine.[31] Orthopedic surgeons review the available literature and make graded recommendations for treatment on the basis of the quality of the data. Grade 1 recommendations are made when there is clear evidence of benefit or risk, and grade 2 recommendations are made when the evidence is less clear. The level of evidence is graded A (consistent results from randomized clinical trials), B (inconsistent results from randomized trials or the presence of major methodological weaknesses), or C (observational studies or generalizations from randomized trials in one patient group to another group; a grade C+ recommendation is made if such generalization was considered to be secure or the evidence from observational studies was considered to be overwhelmingly compelling).[33]

For patients undergoing elective TKA, the seventh ACCP guidelines recommend routine thromboprophylaxis with one of the following regimens (grade 1A)[31]:

- Warfarin: administered at doses adjusted to produce a target INR of 2.5 (range, 2.0 to 3.0); treatment should be started the night before or the night of surgery
- LMWH: 30 mg subcutaneously every 12 hours starting 12 to 24 hours after surgery or 2500 U starting 4 to 6 hours after surgery and then increased to 5000 U the following day

- Fondaparinux: 2.5 mg subcutaneously starting 6 to 8 hours after surgery

No specific recommendations for the choice of drug are made because a higher priority is placed on minimizing bleeding complications than on preventing venographically diagnosed thrombosis. Low-dose UFH or aspirin or VFPs are not recommended as a sole thromboprophylactic measure. IPC is best used as an alternative to anticoagulant therapy.

Routine thromboprophylaxis is not recommended in patients undergoing knee arthroscopy (grade 2B). Thromboprophylaxis with LMWH is suggested for patients at higher than usual risk as a result of preexisting risk factors or a prolonged or complicated procedure (grade 2B).

The guidelines recommend that for patients undergoing TKA, thromboprophylaxis with LMWHs, warfarin, or fondaparinux be given for at least 10 days. Out-of-hospital thromboprophylaxis is warranted in this situation because the duration of hospital stay is generally less than 5 days. Patients considered at high risk for VTE, such as those with a history of thromboembolism, cancer, obesity, or advanced age, may benefit from extended thromboprophylaxis for up to 28 to 35 days.

Decisions about the timing of thromboprophylaxis should be based on the relative efficacy and risk of bleeding associated with the drug in question. The guidelines state that for all major orthopedic procedures, "the decision about timing of prophylaxis should be based on the efficacy-to-bleeding tradeoffs." For each of the antithrombotic drugs, the ACCP recommends that clinicians consider the manufacturer's suggested dosing guidelines. In particular, clinicians should take into consideration renal impairment when deciding on doses of LMWHs, fondaparinux, the direct thrombin inhibitors, and other antithrombotic drugs that are cleared by the kidneys, particularly in the elderly and patients at high risk for bleeding.

CONCLUSIONS

TKA is a major orthopedic procedure that carries a significant risk for postoperative VTE. Thromboembolic events are associated with substantial morbidity and mortality and impose heavy demands on health care resources. Effective thromboprophylaxis should therefore be an important feature of the management of patients undergoing TKA.

Thromboprophylaxis with LMWHs, warfarin, or fondaparinux has been shown to be effective in reducing the risk for VTE after TKA, and it seems likely that novel anticoagulants currently under development will also be evaluated in this situation. The availability of evidence-based guidelines for thromboprophylaxis, together with simple and convenient methods of risk stratification in individual patients, offers the opportunity for widespread use of effective thromboprophylaxis in patients undergoing TKA.

References

1. Abelseth G, Buckley RE, Pineo GE, et al: Incidence of deep-vein thrombosis in patients with fractures of the lower extremity distal to the hip. J Orthop Trauma 10:230-235, 1996.
2. Agu O, Hamilton G, Baker D:. Graduated compression stockings in the prevention of venous thromboembolism. Br J Surg 86:992-1004, 1999.
3. Anderson FA Jr, Spencer FA: Risk factors for venous thromboembolism. Circulation 107(Suppl 1):I9-I16, 2003.
4. Anderson FA Jr, Wheeler HB, Goldberg RJ, et al: A population-based perspective of the hospital incidence and case-fatality rates of deep vein thrombosis and pulmonary embolism. The Worcester DVT Study. Arch Intern Med 151:933-938, 1991.
5. Anderson FA Jr, White K: Hip and Knee Registry Investigators. Prolonged prophylaxis in orthopedic surgery: Insights from the United States. Semin Thromb Hemost 28(Suppl 3):43-46, 2002.
6. Ansell J, Hirsh J, Poller L, et al: The pharmacology and management of the vitamin K antagonists: The Seventh ACCP Conference on Antithrombotic and Thrombolytic Therapy. Chest 126(3 Suppl):204S-233S, 2004.
7. Bauer KA, Eriksson BI, Lassen MR, et al: Fondaparinux compared with enoxaparin for the prevention of venous thromboembolism after elective major knee surgery. N Engl J Med 345:1305-1310, 2001.
8. Berkowitz SD, Francis CW, McElhattan J, Colwell CW Jr: Bleeding indicators and wound complications with ximelagatran and warfarin after TKR: Findings from 3 clinical trials [abstract 1771]. Blood 104(11):491S, 2004.
9. Blanchard J, Meuwly JY, Leyvraz PF, et al: Prevention of deep-vein thrombosis after total knee replacement. Randomised comparison between a low-molecular-weight heparin (nadroparin) and mechanical prophylaxis with a foot-pump system. J Bone Joint Surg Br 81:654-659, 1999.
10. Bottner F, Sculco TP: Nonpharmacologic thromboembolic prophylaxis in total knee arthroplasty. Clin Orthop 392:249-256, 2001.
11. Brookenthal KR, Freedman KB, Lotke PA, et al: A meta-analysis of thromboembolic prophylaxis in total knee arthroplasty. J Arthroplasty 16:293-300, 2001.
12. Caprini JA, Arcelus JI, Reyna JJ: Effective risk stratification of surgical and nonsurgical patients for venous thromboembolic disease. Semin Hematol 38(Suppl 5):12-19, 2001.
13. Caprini JA, Botteman MF, Stephens JM, et al: Economic burden of long-term complications of deep vein thrombosis after total hip replacement surgery in the United States. Value Health 6:59-74, 2003.
14. Cipolle MD, Wojcik R, Seislove E, et al: The role of surveillance duplex scanning in preventing venous thromboembolism in trauma patients. J Trauma 52:453-462, 2002.
15. Clagett GP, Anderson FA Jr, Geerts W, et al: Prevention of venous thromboembolism: The Fifth ACCP Conference on Antithrombotic and Thrombolytic Therapy. Chest 114(Suppl):531S-560S, 1998.
16. Cohen AT, Bailey CS, Alikhan R, Cooper DJ: Extended thromboprophylaxis with low molecular weight heparin reduces symptomatic venous thromboembolism following lower limb arthroplasty—a meta-analysis. Thromb Haemost 85:940-941, 2001.
17. Colwell CW, Berkowitz SD, Comp PC, et al: Randomized, double-blind comparison of ximelagatran, an oral direct thrombin inhibitor, and warfarin to prevent venous thromboembolism (VTE) after total knee replacement (TKR): EXULT B [abstract 39]. Blood 102(11), 2003.
18. Colwell CW Jr, Spiro TE, Trowbridge AA, et al: Efficacy and safety of enoxaparin versus unfractionated heparin for prevention of deep venous thrombosis after elective knee arthroplasty. Enoxaparin Clinical Trial Group. Clin Orthop 321:19-27, 1995.
19. Comp PC, Spiro TE, Friedman RJ, et al: Prolonged enoxaparin therapy to prevent venous thromboembolism after primary hip or knee replacement. Enoxaparin Clinical Trial Group. J Bone Joint Surg Am 83:336-345, 2001.
20. Cullison TR, Muldoon MP, Gorman JD, Goff WB: The incidence of deep venous thrombosis in anterior cruciate ligament reconstruction. Arthroscopy 12:657-659, 1996.
21. Cushner F, Friedman R, Anderson F, et al: Concomitant use of mechanical and pharmacological methods of prophylaxis for venous thromboembolism after total hip and knee arthroplasty: Findings from the Global Orthopaedic registry (GLORY) [abstract P1439]. J Thromb Haemost 1(Suppl 1):1439, 2003.
22. Delis KT, Hunt N, Strachan RK, Nicolaides AN: Incidence, natural history and risk factors of deep vein thrombosis in elective knee arthroscopy. Thromb Haemost 86:817-821, 2001.
23. Demers C, Marcoux S, Ginsberg JS, et al: Incidence of venographically proved deep vein thrombosis after knee arthroscopy. Arch Intern Med 158:47-50, 1998.
24. Douketis JD, Eikelbloom JW, Quinlan DJ, et al: Short-duration prophylaxis against venous thromboembolism after total hip or knee replacement. A meta-analysis of prospective studies investigating symptomatic outcomes. Arch Intern Med 162:1465-1471, 2002.
25. Fitzgerald RH Jr, Spiro TE, Trowbridge AA, et al: Enoxaparin Clinical Trial Group. Prevention of venous thromboembolic disease following primary total knee arthroplasty. A randomized, multicenter, open-label, parallel-group comparison of enoxaparin and warfarin. J Bone Joint Surg Am 83:900-906, 2001.
26. Francis CW, Berkowitz SD, Comp PC, et al: EXULT A Study Group. Comparison of ximelagatran with warfarin for the prevention of venous thromboembolism after total knee replacement. N Engl J Med 349:1703-1712, 2003.
27. Friedman RJ: Extended thromboprophylaxis after hip or knee replacement. Orthopedics 26(2 Suppl):S225-S230, 2003.
28. Friedman RJ, Davidson BL, Friedman J, et al: RD heparin compared with warfarin for prevention of venous thromboembolic disease following total hip or knee arthroplasty. J Bone Joint Surg Am 76:1174-1185, 1994.
29. Friedman RJ, Dunsworth GA: Cost analyses of extended prophylaxis with enoxaparin after hip arthroplasty. Clin Orthop 370:171-182, 2000.
30. Geerts WH, Heit JA, Clagett GP, et al: Prevention of venous thromboembolism: The Sixth ACCP Conference on Antithrombotic and Thrombolytic Therapy. Chest 119(Suppl):132S-175S, 2001.
31. Geerts WH, Pineo GF, Heit JA, et al: Prevention of venous thromboembolism: The Seventh ACCP Conference on Antithrombotic and Thrombolytic Therapy. Chest 126(3 Suppl): 338S-400S, 2004.
32. Graor RA, Stewart JH, Lotke PA: RD heparin (ardeparin) vs aspirin to prevent deep venous thrombosis after hip or knee replacement surgery. Chest 102:118S, 1993.
33. Guyatt G, Schünemann HJ, Cook D, et al: Applying the grades of recommendation for antithrombotic and thrombolytic therapy: The Seventh ACCP Conference on Antithrombotic and Thrombolytic Therapy. Chest 126:179S-187S, 2004.
34. Haas SB, Insall JN, Scuderi GR, et al: Pneumatic sequential-compression boots compared with aspirin prophylaxis of deep-vein thrombosis after total knee arthroplasty. J Bone Joint Surg Am 72:27-31, 1990.
35. Haentjens P, De Groote K, Annemans L: Prolonged enoxaparin therapy to prevent venous thromboembolism after primary hip or

knee replacement. A cost-utility analysis. Arch Orthop Trauma Surg 124:507-517, 2004.

36. Hamulyak K, Lensing AW, van der Meer J, et al: Subcutaneous low-molecular-weight heparin or oral anticoagulants for the prevention of deep-vein thrombosis in elective hip and knee replacement? Fraxiparine Oral Anticoagulant Study Group. Thromb Haemost 74:1428-1431, 1995.

37. Hawkins DW, Langley PC, Krueger KP: A pharmacoeconomic assessment of enoxaparin and warfarin as prophylaxis for deep vein thrombosis in patients undergoing knee replacement surgery. Clin Ther 20:182-195, 1998.

38. Heit JA, Berkowitz SD, Bona R, et al: Efficacy and safety of low molecular weight heparin (ardeparin sodium) compared to warfarin for the prevention of venous thromboembolism after total knee replacement surgery: A double-blind, dose-ranging study. Ardeparin Arthroplasty Study Group. Thromb Haemost 77:32-38, 1997.

39. Hirsh J, Raschke R: Heparin and low-molecular-weight heparin: The Seventh ACCP Conference on Antithrombotic and Thrombolytic Therapy. Chest 126(3 Suppl):188S-203S, 2004.

40. Hjelmstedt A, Bergvall U: Incidence of thrombosis in patients with tibial fractures. Acta Chir Scand 134:209-218, 1968.

41. Howard AW, Aaron SD: Low molecular weight heparin decreases proximal and distal deep venous thrombosis following total knee arthroplasty. A meta-analysis of randomized trials. Thromb Haemost 79:902-906, 1998.

42. Hui AC, Heras-Palou C, Dunn I, et al: Graded compression stockings for prevention of deep-vein thrombosis after hip and knee replacement. J Bone Joint Surg Br 78:550-554, 1996.

43. Hull R, Delmore TJ, Hirsh J, et al: Effectiveness of intermittent pulsatile elastic stockings for the prevention of calf and thigh vein thrombosis in patients undergoing elective knee surgery. Thromb Res 16:37-45, 1979.

44. Hull RD, Raskob GE, Pineo GF, et al: Subcutaneous low-molecular-weight heparin compared with continuous intravenous heparin in the treatment of proximal-vein thrombosis. N Engl J Med 326:975-982, 1992.

45. Hull R, Raskob G, Pineo G, et al: A comparison of subcutaneous low-molecular-weight heparin with warfarin sodium for prophylaxis against deep-vein thrombosis after hip or knee implantation. N Engl J Med 329:1370-1376, 1993.

46. Hull RD, Raskob GE, Pineo GF, et al: Subcutaneous low-molecular-weight heparin vs warfarin for prophylaxis of deep vein thrombosis after hip or knee implantation. An economic perspective. Arch Intern Med 157:298-303, 1997.

47. Iobst CA, Friedman RJ: The role of low molecular weight heparin in total knee arthroplasty. Am J Knee Surg 12:55-60, 1999.

48. Jaureguito JW, Greenwald AE, Wilcox JF, et al: The incidence of deep venous thrombosis after arthroscopic knee surgery. Am J Sports Med 27:707-710, 1999.

49. Jorgensen PS, Warming T, Hansen K, et al: Low molecular weight heparin (Innohep) as thromboprophylaxis in outpatients with a plaster cast: A venografic controlled study. Thromb Res 105:477-480, 2002.

50. Kearon C: Natural history of venous thromboembolism. Circulation 107(Suppl 1):I22-I30, 2003.

51. Kock HJ, Schmit-Neuerburg KP, Hanke J, et al: Thromboprophylaxis with low-molecular-weight heparin in outpatients with plaster-cast immobilisation of the leg. Lancet 346:459-461, 1995.

52. Kujath P, Spannagel U, Habscheid W: Incidence and prophylaxis of deep venous thrombosis in outpatients with injury of the lower limb. Haemostasis 23(Suppl 1):20-26, 1993.

53. Lassen MR, Borris LC, Nakov RL: Use of the low-molecular-weight heparin reviparin to prevent deep-vein thrombosis after leg injury requiring immobilization. N Engl J Med 347:726-730, 2002.

54. Lassen MR, Davidson BL, Gallus A, et al: A phase II randomized, double-blind, five-arm, parallel-group, dose-response study of a new oral directly-acting factor Xa inhibitor, razaxaban, for the prevention of deep vein thrombosis in knee replacement surgery—on behalf of the razaxaban investigators [abstract L11]. Blood 102:(11), 2003.

55. Leclerc JR, Geerts WH, Desjardins L, et al: Prevention of venous thromboembolism after knee arthroplasty. A randomized, double-blind trial comparing enoxaparin with warfarin. Ann Intern Med 124:619-626, 1996.

56. Levine MN, Gent M, Hirsh J, et al: Ardeparin (low-molecular-weight heparin) vs graduated compression stockings for the prevention of

venous thromboembolism. A randomized trial in patients undergoing knee surgery. Arch Intern Med 156:851-856, 1996.

57. Lindblad B, Eriksson A, Bergqvist D: Autopsy-verified pulmonary embolism in a surgical department: Analysis of the period from 1951 to 1988. Br J Surg 78:849-852, 1991.

58. McKenna R, Galante J, Bachmann F, et al: Prevention of venous thromboembolism after total knee replacement by high-dose aspirin or intermittent calf and thigh compression. BMJ 280:514-517, 1980.

59. Menzin J, Colditz GA, Regan MM, et al: Cost-effectiveness of enoxaparin vs low-dose warfarin in the prevention of deep-vein thrombosis after total hip replacement surgery. Arch Intern Med 155:757-764, 1995.

60. Michot M, Conen D, Holtz D, et al: Prevention of deep-vein thrombosis in ambulatory arthroscopic knee surgery: A randomized trial of prophylaxis with low–molecular weight heparin. Arthroscopy 18:257-263, 2002.

61. National Center for Health Statistics: Nationwide inpatient surgery 2002. Available from http://www.cdc.gov/nchs/fastats/ insurg.htm (cited 2004 December 15).

62. Norgren L, Toksvig-Larsen S, Magyar G, et al: Prevention of deep vein thrombosis in knee arthroplasty. Preliminary results from a randomized controlled study of low molecular weight heparin vs foot pump compression. Int Angiol 17:93-96, 1998.

63. Ollendorf DA, Vera-Llonch M, Oster G: Cost of venous thromboembolism following major orthopedic surgery in hospitalized patients. Am J Health Syst Pharm 59:1750-1754, 2002.

64. Oster G, Ollendorf DA, Vera-Llonch M, et al: Economic consequences of venous thromboembolism following major orthopedic surgery. Ann Pharmacother 38:377-382, 2004.

65. Prandoni P, Lensing AW, Cogo A, et al: The long-term clinical course of acute deep venous thrombosis. Ann Intern Med 125:1-7, 1996.

66. Prevention of venous thromboembolism. International consensus statement (guidelines according to scientific evidence). Int Angiol 16:3-38, 1997.

67. Robinson KS, Anderson DR, Gross M, et al: Ultrasonographic screening before hospital discharge for deep venous thrombosis after arthroplasty: The post-arthroplasty screening study. A randomized, controlled trial. Ann Intern Med 127:439-445, 1997.

68. Rosendaal FR: Venous thrombosis: A multicausal disease. Lancet 353:1167-1173, 1999.

69. Second Thrombembolic Risk Factors (THRiFT II) Consensus Group: Risk of and prophylaxis for venous thromboembolism in hospital patients. Phlebology 13:87-97, 1998.

70. Stringer MD, Steadman CA, Hedges AR, et al: Deep vein thrombosis after elective knee surgery. An incidence study in 312 patients. J Bone Joint Surg Br 71:492-497, 1989.

71. Styf J: The venous pump of the human foot. Clin Physiol 10:77-84, 1990.

72. Sullivan SD, Kahn SR, Davidson BL, et al: Measuring the outcomes and pharmacoeconomic consequences of venous thromboembolism prophylaxis in major orthopaedic surgery. Pharmacoeconomics 21:477-496, 2003.

73. Turpie AG, Bauer KA, Eriksson BI, Lassen MR: Fondaparinux vs enoxaparin for the prevention of venous thromboembolism in major orthopedic surgery: A meta-analysis of 4 randomized double-blind studies. Arch Intern Med 162:1833-1840, 2002.

74. Weitz JI, Crowther M: Direct thrombin inhibitors. Thromb Res 106:V275-V284, 2002.

75. Weitz JI, Hirsh J, Samama MM: New anticoagulant drugs: The Seventh ACCP Conference on Antithrombotic and Thrombolytic Therapy. Chest 126(3 Suppl):265S-286S, 2004.

76. Westrich GH, Sculco TP: Prophylaxis against deep venous thrombosis after total knee arthroplasty. Pneumatic plantar compression and aspirin compared with aspirin alone. J Bone Joint Surg Am 78:826-834, 1996.

77. Wheeler HB: Diagnosis of deep vein thrombosis. Review of clinical evaluation and impedance plethysmography. Am J Surg 150:7-13, 1985.

78. White RH, Romano PS, Zhou H, et al: Incidence and time course of thromboembolic outcomes following total hip or knee arthroplasty. Arch Intern Med 158:1525-1531, 1998.

79. Williams JS Jr, Hulstyn MJ, Fadale PD, et al: Incidence of deep vein thrombosis after arthroscopic knee surgery: A prospective study. Arthroscopy 11:701-705, 1995.

80. Wilson NV, Das SK, Kakkar VV, et al: Thrombo-embolic prophylaxis in total knee replacement. Evaluation of the A-V impulse system. J Bone Joint Surg Br 74:50-52, 1992.

81. Wirth T, Schneider B, Misselwitz F, et al: Prevention of venous thromboembolism after knee arthroscopy with low-molecular weight heparin (reviparin): Results of a randomized controlled trial. Arthroscopy 17:393-399, 2001.

82. Wittkowsky AK: Drug interactions update: Drugs, herbs, and oral anticoagulation. J Thromb Thrombolysis 12:67-71, 2001.

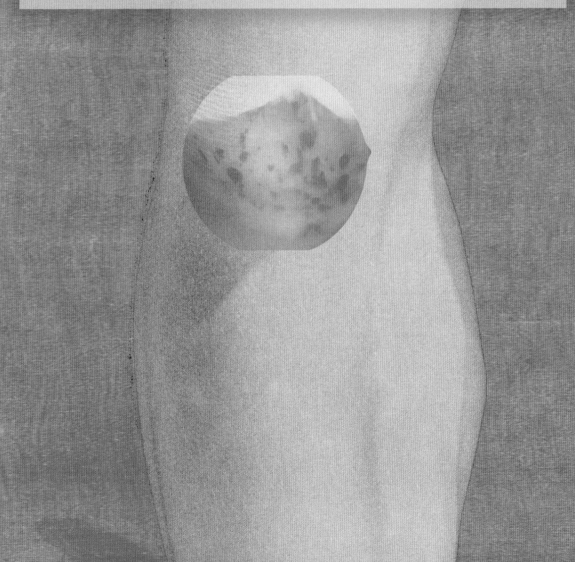

SECTION XII

Tumors about the Knee

CHAPTER 106

Evaluation of Patients with Bone Lesions about the Knee

Ginger E. Holt

Evaluation of a patient with a bone lesion about the knee requires a thorough history and physical examination, imaging studies, and sometimes associated laboratory tests to formulate a differential, make a diagnosis, and provide appropriate treatment. The differential diagnosis will then determine the need for further investigation (e.g., biopsy).

HISTORY

Symptoms

Bone tumors about the knee are brought to clinical attention for a variety of reasons. The more common initial symptoms include pain, a mass, decreased range of motion, or a finding incidental to the these symptoms. Bone lesions may be painful because of primary or secondary reasons. Primary bone pain results from rapid intraosseous and soft-tissue pressure caused by tumor expansion and malignant tumor cell proliferation. Secondary pain results from mechanical instability and is caused by destruction of cortical bone by the tumor. It is exacerbated by weightbearing. The extreme form of mechanical instability gives rise to a pathological fracture.

A soft-tissue mass may arise from direct tumor extension through cortical bone or may be the result of extension through the haversian canal system, as in the case of Ewing's sarcoma. The resulting soft-tissue mass may be the initial symptom noted by the patient or be the result of diminished range of motion secondary to a mechanical block. A characteristic nocturnal pain pattern relieved by aspirin or nonsteroidal anti-inflammatory drugs in association with characteristic findings on plain radiography or computed tomography (CT) is diagnostic of an osteoid osteoma.[7]

As important as initial symptoms are to defining the nature of a bone lesion about the knee, a lack of symptoms can be as important. Discovery of a benign bone tumor may be the result of a radiographic finding that is incidental to the initial symptoms.

Age

Although many bone tumors may have a similar appearance and clinical features, patient age can narrow the differential diagnosis, with certain conditions being more likely to occur in a specific age range (Fig. 106–1).[19] For example, a lytic epiphyseal lesion in a skeletally immature patient is more likely to be a chondroblastoma, whereas a giant cell tumor of bone must be considered in a skeletally mature patient.[20]

Activity Level

Assessing activity level, participation in contact sports, or a recent history of trauma may be helpful in determining a bone lesion's cause. Patients who have had a sudden increase in activity level may be at risk for a stress fracture (proximal end of the tibia). A patient who has sustained direct trauma to the thigh or calf may have an apparent bone tumor that is actually heterotopic ossification.

Past Medical History

The past medical history can be helpful in uncovering significant diagnostic information. A personal history of cancer may lead to several diagnostic possibilities. A lytic bone lesion in a patient with a personal history of cancer is metastatic disease until proved otherwise.[1] A patient with a medical history of metastatic carcinoma treated with radiation therapy may have a postradiation sarcoma, whereas patients who have undergone chemotherapy and/or radiation treatment may have osteonecrosis. A patient who has had a previous lesion treated with radiation therapy may also have postradiation necrosis of the bone.[10] A past medical history of local or systemic infection should lead to evaluation for potential osteomyelitis. Patients with a history of chronic obstructive pulmonary disease, asthma, or conditions commonly treated with steroids should be questioned about their steroid history and consideration made for osteonecrosis.[4]

A family history of benign familial osteochondromatosis should be obtained.[14] Li-Fraumeni syndrome is a well-known example of an inherited predisposition for cancer. Germline mutations of the p53 gene predispose patients to many cancers, including osteosarcoma.[3]

PHYSICAL EXAMINATION

Patients with a bone lesion about the knee require an in-depth physical examination to elucidate potential clues

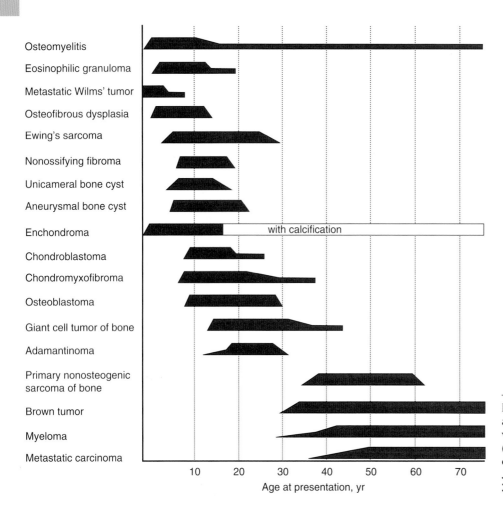

Figure 106–1. Range of patient ages at presentation for the various radiolucent lesions. (From Springfield DS: Radiolucent lesions of the extremities. J Am Acad Orthop Surg 2:306-316, 1994.)

about the diagnosis. Examination of the integumentary system may provide diagnostic details to narrow down a differential. Café au lait spots may be indicative of neurofibromatosis, whereas cutaneous angiomas are associated with Maffucci's syndrome. Previous skin incisions or draining sinuses should be evaluated to determine whether previous trauma or surgery may be the cause of underlying osteomyelitis. A long-standing, draining sinus may be indicative of a Marjolin ulcer and suggest underlying squamous cell carcinoma. Other skin lesions associated with an underlying bone tumor may suggest not only bacterial but also fungal infection such as blastomycosis.

A complete physical examination includes a lymph node survey. An underlying bone lesion with enlarged lymph nodes may be diagnostic of lymphoma. A patient with a suspected metastatic bone lesion should undergo a directed examination of the thyroid, prostate, or breasts because a primary tumor may be found.

IMAGING

Local

Plain radiography remains the most specific noninvasive means to establish a differential diagnosis for primary

bone tumors. Plain radiographs in two perpendicular planes should be the initial imaging study obtained to evaluate an orthogonal bone tumor about the knee. Commonly, the benign or malignant nature of a tumor can be determined on plain radiographic evaluation. To formulate a differential diagnosis, Enneking's four questions should be asked of any bone tumor[5]: (1) location, (2) what the tumor is doing to the bone, (3) what the bone is doing to the tumor, and (4) whether underlying matrix is present. Location of the tumor includes diaphyseal, metaphyseal, or epiphyseal locations or surface tumor.

If the diagnosis is not clear after plain radiographic evaluation, a more specific examination may be warranted. The next test obtained is based on the question being asked.

Computed tomography (CT) is the best tool to evaluate cortical bone, the endosteal skeleton, or erosion and lesion mineralization.[8] Magnetic resonance imaging (MRI) provides information on anatomy, including bone and soft tissue, as well as definitive tumor margins.[21] MRI can give specific information about the matrix of the tumor. An expansile bone lesion that is multiloculated with multiple fluid-fluid levels is suggestive of an aneurismal bone cyst. A lesion that is dark on both T1- and T2-weighted sequences is suggestive of a fibrous lesion such as an extra-abdominal desmoid, whereas a tumor that is bright on both T1- and T2-weighted images is suggestive of a lesion high in water content such as a myxoma.

Systemic Imaging

Systemic staging includes evaluation for multifocal disease, metastatic disease from a primary bone tumor, or the source of metastatic disease causing a secondary bone tumor.

A whole-body technetium 99–labeled methylene diphosphonate (^{99m}Tc-MDP) bone scan is useful in evaluating multifocal skeletal disease.[15] Although such imaging may assist in determining an alternative biopsy site if the underlying diagnosis is unknown, it rarely aids in narrowing the differential diagnosis.

A CT scan of the chest, abdomen, and pelvis will determine the origin of metastatic disease in approximately 85% of cases.[17] These scans serve as systemic staging for primary malignant bone tumors as well.

[^{18}F]2-flouro-2-deoxy-D-glucose positron emission tomography uses the glucose metabolism of tumors to detect tumor activity.[16] This mechanism of systemic staging is most useful for melanoma, adenocarcinoma, and lymphoma.

LABORATORY EVALUATION

Serum and urine tests are for the most part nonspecific and should be ordered selectively. An elevated white blood cell count, erythrocyte sedimentation rate (ESR), and C-reactive protein suggests infection, although the ESR may be elevated in many malignant tumors. Prostate-specific antigen should be tested in males with lytic bone lesions to evaluate for prostate cancer. Serum protein electrophoresis and urine protein electrophoresis are useful in evaluating multiple myeloma. Alkaline phosphatase may be elevated in primary bone tumors (osteosarcoma) and Paget's disease. Serum calcium and parathyroid hormone levels are increased in the brown tumors of hyperparathyroidism. Serum lactate dehydrogenase and alkaline phosphatase have been shown to have prognostic significance inasmuch as patients with elevated levels have shorter survival times than do those with normal values.[13] Calcium levels should be checked in patients with a bone tumor, especially those undergoing surgery, because these patients oftentimes have hypercalcemia. Urine tests include N-telopeptide and urine hydroxyproline. These tests may be helpful in evaluating bone turnover in Paget's disease or osteoporosis.

DIFFERENTIAL DIAGNOSIS

See Table 106–1 and Figure 106–2.

BIOPSY

Biopsy is the final procedure in the assessment of a bone lesion and is a complex, cognitive skill. A biopsy must be well planed and executed to maximize treatment and minimize risk. Poorly planned incisions and soft-tissue contamination can negate limb salvage surgery. Mankin and colleagues[11,12] have determined that patients were adversely affected when biopsy of a skeletal sarcoma was performed by nontrained musculoskeletal oncologists. The recommendation of these studies was that lesions suspected of being malignant be referred before biopsy to a specialist in the care of malignant bone tumors.

Needle versus Open Biopsy

The decision to perform needle versus open biopsy is based on many factors. The comfort of the treating pathologist in making a diagnosis from a limited tissue source such as a needle biopsy specimen versus an open biopsy specimen is a consideration. It may also depend on the availability of operative time in performing a biopsy. The lesion itself may not be amenable to needle biopsy. Liquid

Table 106–1. Differential Diagnosis by Tumor Location

NOT TUMOR	BENIGN	MALIGNANT
Diaphyseal		
Infection	Osteoid osteoma	Osteosarcoma
Stress fracture	Osteoblastoma	Ewing's sarcoma
	Fibrous dysplasia	Lymphoma
	Histiocytosis	Myeloma
Metaphyseal		
Infection	Osteoblastoma	Osteosarcoma
Brown tumor	Aneurysmal bone cyst	Chondrosarcoma
Bone infarct	Unicameral bone cyst	Lymphoma
Paget's disease	Giant cell tumor	Metastatic disease
	Enchondroma	
	Chondromyxoid fibroma	
	Nonossifying fibroma	
Epiphyseal		
Infection	Chondroblastoma (skeletally immature)	Osteosarcoma
Osteochondral defect	Giant cell tumor (skeletally mature)	Clear cell chondrosarcoma

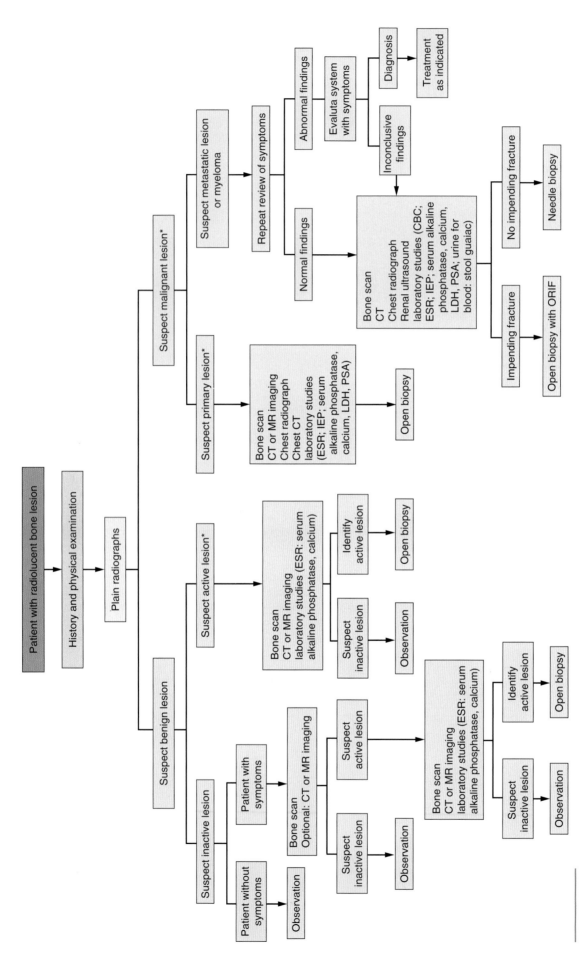

Figure 106–2. Algorithm for the evaluation of a patient with a radiolucent lesion of an extremity. Asterisk indicates a point at which referral is indicated if the evaluating physician is not prepared to treat the patient. CBC, complete blood cell count; LDH, lactate dehydrogenase; ORIF, open reduction and internal fixation; PSA, prostate-specific antigen (From Springfield DS: Radiolucent lesions of the extremities. J Am Acad Orthop Surg 2:306-316, 1994.)

tumors, such as Ewing's sarcoma or myeloma, may have a low yield with needle biopsy and could require open biopsy. Lesions that appear to have a large necrotic center or have a large associated hematoma may be poorly represented on a needle biopsy sample. These lesions should be considered for open biopsy. The ability to obtain an adequate amount of tissue for future treatment, including genetic evaluation, may also be a determining factor regarding whether needle or open biopsy should be performed. The more information the orthopedist can provide to the pathologist, the more accurate the diagnosis.

Biopsy Technique

There are several general issues involved in the technique of open biopsy. An initial consideration is withholding parenteral antibiotics until tissue for culture is obtained. Once intraoperative tissue has been obtained for culture, antibiotics may be administered. In general, a biopsy should include a direct line from the skin to the tumor. Developing flaps should be avoided, and strict hemostasis must be maintained to minimize tumor spread. A biopsy approach that avoids contamination of a neurovascular structure is paramount. The definitive procedure must be considered when performing the biopsy. Some specific techniques regarding anatomic sites may be considered. When performing a biopsy of the distal end of the femur, the biopsy itself should avoid the quadriceps tendon and harvest bone just medial or lateral to it. When returning for definitive resection, this technique spares the quadriceps tendon from resection. Biopsy of the proximal end of the tibia must avoid the patellar tendon. An attempt should be made to bury the hematoma within the anterolateral muscle tissue because biopsy over the subcutaneous aspect of the tibia oftentimes results in continued drainage and infection. Biopsy of the proximal part of the fibula is best performed anteriorly to avoid contamination or potential damage to the peroneal nerve. When performing a biopsy of the popliteal fossa, a short oblique biopsy may be appropriate because the definitive procedure will probably require a "lazy S"–shaped incision.[18]

STAGING OF BONE TUMORS

After a complete history and physical examination, local and systemic evaluation, and diagnosis of the tumor type and grade, a tumor may be staged. Systems exist for both benign and malignant bone tumors. In general, staging allows for predicting the risk for metastatic disease and therefore determining the appropriate treatment.

Benign bone tumors may be staged by the Campanacci system[2] or the Enneking system.[6] The Campanacci system is based on plain radiographs. Latent lesions (stage A) are contained with the bone. Active lesions (stage B) remain within the bone, but have a responsive cortical reaction. Aggressive lesions (stage C) breach the cortex. The Enneking, or Surgical Staging System (SSS), is based on compartmental anatomy. In the Enneking system a benign bone tumor is stage 0.

Malignant bone tumor staging consists of the Enneking system/SSS or the American Joint Commission on Cancer (AJCC) Staging System.[9] In the Enneking system, malignant bone tumors are graded by histology and compartment status.

Histologically, tumors are graded as low or high grade, whereas compartment status is evaluated by confinement of the tumor to a compartment (intracompartmental) or no such confinement (extracompartmental). Histologically, stage I tumors are low-grade lesions and stage II tumors are high-grade lesions. Compartmental status is determined as stage A when the tumor remains with the bony compartment, and stage B represents an extracompartmental tumor. Stage III defines metastatic tumors, whether they are low or high grade. The majority of malignant tumors are high grade and extracompartmental (stage IIB lesions). The Enneking system does not apply to Ewing's sarcoma or rhabdomyosarcoma.

The AJCC Staging System uses the TNM classification scheme. It determines the prognosis based on tumor size (T1, ≤8 cm; T2, >8 cm), grade (G1, G2, low grade; G3, G4, high grade), lymph nodes (+/−), and metastases (+/−). Both systems are outlined in Table 106–2.

Table 102–2. Staging Systems

STAGING SYSTEM	STAGE	STAGE DESCRIPTION	PROGNOSTIC FACTORS
Surgical Staging System (SSS)	IA: low grade, intracompartmental IB: low grade, extracompartmental IIA: high grade, intracompartmental IIB: high grade, extracompartmental III: any metastasis	G1 T1 M0 G1 T2 M0 G2 T1 M0 G2 T2 M0 Any G, any T, M1	G1: low grade G2: high grade T1: intracompartmental T2: extracompartmental M1: any metastases
American Joint Committee on Cancer (AJCC) Staging System	IA: low grade, ≤8 cm IB: low grade, >8 cm IIA: high grade, ≤8 cm IIB: high grade, >8 cm III: skip metastases in primary bone IVA: any size, any grade, lung metastases IVB: any size, any grade, lymph nodes involved	T1; G1,2; N0; M0 T2; G1,2; N0; M0 T1; G3,4; N0; M0 T2; G3,4; N0; M0 T3, any G, N0 M0 Any T, any G, N0 M1a Any T, any G, N, any M	T0: no evidence of primary tumor T1: ≤8 cm in greatest dimension T2: >8 cm in greatest dimension T3: discontinuous tumors in primary bone site G1: well differentiated, low grade G2: moderately differentiated, low grade G3: poorly differentiated, high grade G4: undifferentiated, high grade

SUMMARY

The most critical aspect in evaluating a patient with a bone lesion about the knee is to make a diagnosis. Arriving at this vital juncture requires a thorough history, physical examination, imaging studies, appropriate differential diagnosis, and ultimately, an appropriately executed biopsy. Staging follows the diagnosis of a malignant tumor to aid in prognosis and treatment. Once an accurate diagnosis and staging are complete, treatment can follow.

References

1. Aaron A: Current concepts review: Treatment of metastatic adenocarcinoma of the acetabulum and the extremities. J Bone Joint Surg Am 794:917-932, 1994.
2. Campanacci M, Baldini N, Boriani S, et al: Giant-cell tumor of bone. J Bone Joint Surg Am 69:106-114, 1987.
3. Chompret A: The Li-Fraumeni syndrome. Biochimie 84:75-82, 2002.
4. Cryess RL: Steroid-induced osteonecrosis: A review. Can J Surg 24:567-571, 1981.
5. Enneking WF: Musculoskeletal Tumor Surgery. New York, Churchill Livingstone, 1983, pp 3-60.
6. Enneking WF, Spanier SS, Goodman MA: A system for the surgical staging of musculoskeletal sarcoma, 1980. Clin Orthop Rel Res 153:106-120, 1980.
7. Frassica FJ, Waltrip RL, Spouseller PD, et al: Clinicopathologic features and treatment of osteoid osteoma and osteoblastoma in children and adolescents. Orthop Clin North Am 27:559-574, 1996.
8. Gitelis S, Wilkins R, Conrand EU III: Benign bone tumors. J Bone Joint Surg Am 77:1756-1782, 1995.
9. Greene FL, Page DL, Fleming ID, et al: American Joint Commission on Cancer Staging Manual, ed 6. New York, Springer-Verlag, 2002.
10. Holt GE, Griffin AM, Pintilie M, et al: Fractures following radiotherapy and limb-salvage surgery for lower extremity soft tissue sarcomas. A comparison of high dose versus low dose radiotherapy. J Bone Joint Surg Am 87:315-319, 2005.
11. Mankin HJ, Lange TA, Spanier SS: The hazards of biopsy in patients with malignant primary bone and soft-tissue tumors. J Bone Joint Surg Am 64:1121-1127, 1982.
12. Mankin HJ, Mankin CJ, Simon MA: The hazards of the biopsy, revisited. Members of the Musculoskeletal Tumor Society. J Bone Joint Surg Am 78:656-663, 1996.
13. Meyers PA, Heller G, Healey JH, et al: Osteogenic sarcoma with clinically detectable metastasis at initial presentation. J Clin Oncol 11:449-453, 1993.
14. Ozaki T, Kawai A, Sugihara S, et al: Multiple osteocartilaginous exostosis. A follow-up study. Arch Orthop Trauma Surg 115:255-261, 1996.
15. Peabody TD, Gibbs CP Jr, Simon MA: Evaluation and staging of musculoskeletal neoplasms. J Bone Joint Surg Am 80:1204-1218, 1998.
16. Rougraff BT, Kneisl JS, Simon MA: Skeletal metastases of unknown origin: A prospective study of a diagnosis strategy. J Bone Joint Surg Am 75:1276-1281, 1993.
17. Schulet M, Brecht-Krauss D, Werrer M, et al: Evaluation of neoadjuvant therapy response of osteogenic sarcoma using FDG PET. J Nucl Med 40:1637-1643, 1999.
18. Simon MA, Biermann JS: Biopsy of bone and soft-tissue lesions. J Bone Joint Surg Am 75:616-621, 1993.
19. Springfield DS: Radiolucent lesions of the extremities. J Am Acad Orthop Surg 2:306-316, 1994.
20. Turcotte RE, Kurt AM, Sim FH, et al: Chondroblastoma. Hum Pathol 24:944-949, 1993.
21. Wetzel LH, Levine E, Murphey MD:A comparison of MR imaging and CT in the evaluation of musculoskeletal masses. Radiographics 7:851-874, 1987.

CHAPTER 107

Surgical Treatment of Benign Bone Lesions

R. Lor Randall

Benign bone lesions are relatively common entities. Overall, the knee is the most common location for most of these growths. Evaluation of a patient with a bone lesion about the knee is discussed in Chapter 106. This chapter focuses on the more common benign bone lesions. A brief review of the staging system of benign lesions is presented first.

STAGING FOR BENIGN BONE TUMORS

Stage 1 lesions are considered latent. They generally are asymptomatic, but not always. Although they can progress, they usually resolve. Initially, these lesions should be observed. Stage 2 lesions are considered active. They tend not to resolve spontaneously and are less well demarcated, consistent with stage 1 lesions. Frequently, stage 2 lesions require surgical intervention with aggressive treatment. Recurrence is frequent. Stage 3 lesions are aggressive lesions and exhibit extensive destruction. Treatment often requires wide, en-bloc resection.

SPECIFIC CONDITIONS AND THEIR TREATMENT

Treatment of benign growths of bone is a function of their symptoms. Most benign bone lesions about the knee can be observed if they do not cause the patient any problems. Benign bone lesions rarely cause internal derangement to the knee with the exception of chondroblastomas. This section discusses common types of benign bone tumor seen by practicing orthopedic surgeons specializing in knee surgery.

Benign Bone-Forming Tumors

OSTEOID OSTEOMA

The most common benign osteoid-forming tumor is osteoid osteoma, accounting for 10% of all benign bone tumors. This tumor is more common in males than in females, and the peak incidence is in the second decade of life. The proximal femur is the most favored location, but it can arise in the distal femur, proximal tibia, or less

likely the fibula. Dull aching pain is the most frequent symptom. Osteoid osteoma has been attributed to otherwise unexplainable knee pain.[19,31] If the nidus is close to a joint or actually in the joint (which can occur in approximately 15% of cases),[2] inflammatory synovitis results and suggests the diagnosis of a pyarthrosis or rheumatoid disease.[63] If the bony reaction is focal and intense, the lesion can take on the appearance of an exostosis.[40] Osteoid osteomas can mimic pes anserinus syndrome.[53] Generally, symptoms are relieved with nonsteroidal anti-inflammatory drugs secondary to a high concentration of prostaglandins in the nidus.[12,22,38,46,67] Osteoid osteoma may have a unique pathogenic nerve supply as well, a finding that may be common among bone tumors.[48]

The characteristic radiographic feature of osteoid osteoma is the central lytic nidus, which measures 1 cm in diameter. In the common cortical lesion (Fig. 107–1), there is an extensive reactive sclerosis creating a fusiform bulge on the bone surface. If the nidus is more centrally located in metaphyseal bone, less sclerosis is seen, and the radiographic appearance is less diagnostic. Technetium bone scans are invariably positive. A CT scan is helpful to locate the lesion anatomically in preoperative planning.[3] MRI may miss the nidus, making the establishment of the diagnosis more difficult.[18]

Previously, some investigators believed that the osteoid osteoma was an inflammatory process, such as a Brodie's abscess, which has a similar clinical and radiographic appearance. Currently, it is accepted that osteoid osteoma is a true osteoid-forming neoplasm and is lacking lymphocytes or plasma cells. Histologically the nidus shows aggressive but benign woven bone formation, with large numbers of osteoblasts and osteoclasts in a vascular fibrous stroma. No chondroid areas are seen.

Most cases of osteoid osteoma are stage 1 lesions; they resolve spontaneously and can be treated symptomatically with aspirin or nonsteroidal anti-inflammatory drugs.[5] If the patient fails such treatment, surgical intervention is warranted. If surgery is undertaken, it is important to eradicate the entire symptomatic nidus. Removal of a large amount of the surrounding sclerotic bone should be avoided because it can severely weaken the bone and may result in a pathological fracture. For open techniques, if the lesion is in cortical bone, adequate exposure is required so that the surgeon can visualize the bulging cortex. Intralesional resection via the "bur-down" technique generally is preferred over en-bloc resection. The nidus can be identified visually by the hyperemic pink color in the reactive bone adjacent to it. Simple curettage

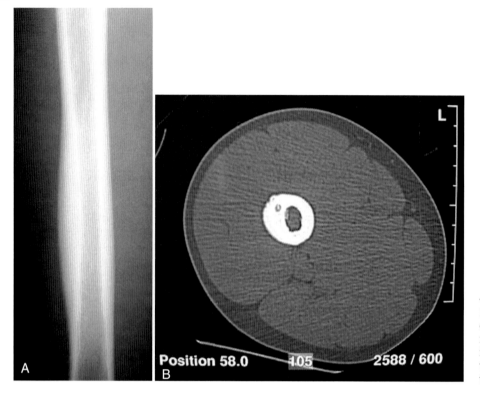

Figure 107–1. Osteoid osteoma of the femur. **A,** Anteroposterior radiograph shows dense bone formation, yet a nidus is difficult to appreciate. **B,** CT scan reveals the nidus readily.

of the nidus followed by high-speed burring to advance the margin another 2 to 3 mm is all that is necessary. If the lesion is not visible on the surface, as in the case of a medullary lesion, radiographic markers should be placed intraoperatively before placing the round cortical window. Alternatively, percutaneous radiofrequency ablation is another, less invasive method of treating osteoid osteoma and is my preferred method of treatment (Fig. 107–2). This technique continues to gain wide acceptance as a preferable management modality.[8,13,14,34,56] Depending on location, CT guidance may or may not be necessary.[42]

OSTEOBLASTOMA

Osteoblastoma is a large osteoid osteoma (Fig. 107–3).[17] Its incidence about the knee is less than osteoid osteoma, and it accounts for 1% of all bone tumors overall. Osteoblastomas arise more commonly in males than in females and occur in the second decade of life, the same age group as osteoid osteomas. Infrequently, these lesions are found in the metaphyses of distal femur (raising suspicion about a possible osteosarcoma). Osteoblastomas lesions are usually stage 1 to 2 lesions. Radiographically, osteoblastoma has a more lytic and destructive appearance than osteoid osteoma. Its nidus, which is greater than 1 or 2 cm, has a less sclerotic reactive bone at the periphery and may take on the appearance of an aneurysmal bone cyst. Histologically the nidus of the osteoblastoma is nearly identical to that of the osteoid osteoma and shows excessive osteoblastic activity and osteoid formation with numerous giant cells in a vascular fibrous stroma. Treatment usually consists of a vigorous curettage of the lesion, which may require a bone graft if instability results.

Radiofrequency ablation also may prove useful in the management of this lesion.

OSTEOFIBROUS DYSPLASIA

Osteofibrous dysplasia is a rare condition that is seen almost exclusively in the tibia of children younger than 10 years old. It is more common in boys than in girls and is frequently asymptomatic. It commonly affects the diaphysis and results in anterior cortical bowing. Osteofibrous dysplasia can occur in the fibula and even more rarely can be seen bilaterally. True involvement of the knee is exceptionally rare.

In osteofibrous dysplasia, the lytic changes seen in the anterior tibial cortex are surrounded by sclerotic margins, creating a soap-bubble appearance similar to the radiographic picture of fibrous dysplasia and adamantinoma. Some studies suggest that osteofibrous dysplasia may be a precursor to adamantinoma.[24,27,35,37,43,50,60,61] Histologically the lytic lesion shows a benign trabecular alphabet-soup pattern in a fibrous stroma. The histological findings are similar to the findings in fibrous dysplasia, although the lesions of fibrous dysplasia lack the prominent surface layer of osteoblasts seen in osteofibrous dysplasia and can be distinguished by a variety of clinical, immunohisto-chemical,[36,58] and molecular markers.[59] These lesions are stage 1 to 2.

Surgical treatment in osteofibrous dysplasia should be reserved for patients in whom the disease is poorly controlled by conservative treatment or patients who have a high possibility of impending fracture and progressing deformity.[49] Early attempts at surgical curettage and grafting may result in a high failure rate because of recurrence.

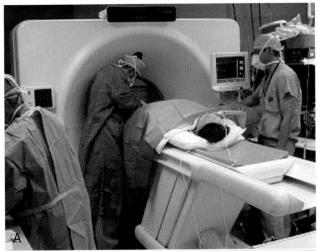

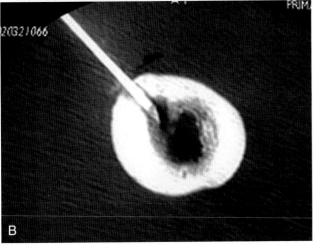

Figure 107–2. **A** and **B,** CT-guided radiofrequency ablation of a femoral osteoid osteoma.

For this reason, it is generally suggested that if intervention is necessary, it be deferred until patients reach adolescence, when there is an improved chance that the disease may arrest after surgery.[65]

Benign Chondroid-Forming Tumors

ENCHONDROMA

Enchondroma refers to a centrally located chondroma of bone. These tumors are relatively common lesions, accounting for greater than 10% of benign bone tumors. Although approximately 50% of cases arise in the small tubular bones of the hands and feet, the distal femur is second only to the proximal humerus for next most common location. It develops in growing bones as a hamartomatous process, but is frequently asymptomatic and may avoid detection until the patient reaches adulthood, at which time the lesion may be discovered in association with a pathological fracture or as an incidental finding on a routine radiographic examination. Radiographs of enchondromas show geographic lysis of

normal trabecular bone with sharp margination and central calcification (Fig. 107–4). Infrequently, there is cortical erosion or dilation of the bone about the knee. When such features are present, one must consider the possibility of a low-grade chondrosarcoma. Enchondromas are stage 1 or 2 lesions.

Multiple enchondromatosis, or Ollier's disease, is a rare nonfamilial dysplasia that is typically seen on one-half of the body and appears similar to fibrous dysplasia. When it is bilateral, one side tends to be more involved than the other. This condition can be quite extensive with significant involvement of metaphyseal areas resulting in bowing and shortening of the long bones (Fig. 107–5). Such dramatic changes are rarely seen in cases of a solitary enchondroma. Varus deformities can be severe and may be managed by a variety of techniques.[11] In patients with Maffucci's syndrome, enchondromatosis is seen in association with multiple soft-tissue hemangiomas.

A large solitary enchondroma in a large bone converts to a low-grade chondrosarcoma in fewer than 5% of cases, and the conversion takes place during adulthood. A secondary chondrosarcoma in enchondromatosis can arise in 20% of cases and may be related to inactivation of particular tumor-suppressor genes.[7]

There is no need to treat an asymptomatic patient with a solitary enchondroma. If the patient has a pathological fracture, it is usually best to allow the fracture to heal and at a later date to perform a simple curettage and bone grafting procedure, which usually results in good function and a low chance of recurrence. Patients with Ollier's disease or Maffucci's disease must be followed carefully because of the increased risk of malignant degeneration.

PERIOSTEAL CHONDROMA

A benign chondroma seen on the surface of a bone is a periosteal chondroma. Patients may have more than one lesion, and the most common location is on the proximal humeral metaphysis. The distal femur is a relatively common site as well, and intra-articular involvement has been reported.[20,23,57] Radiographically, these lesions often have a thin shell of bone and appear to lie on the cortical surface (Fig. 107–6). These lesions are stage 1 to 2. Periosteal chondromas can grow to a sizable mass, but anything larger than 4 cm would suggest a peripheral primary chondrosarcoma. Management of patients with periosteal chondromas generally consists of observing the lesion at intervals to ensure that it does not continue growing as the patient reaches adulthood. In cases in which simple local resection without bone graft is indicated, the procedure is associated with a low recurrence rate.

OSTEOCHONDROMA

Although nonossifying fibroma of bone is the most common benign tumor of bone, solitary osteochondroma is the second most common. Because they are generally more symptomatic than nonossifying fibromas, orthope-

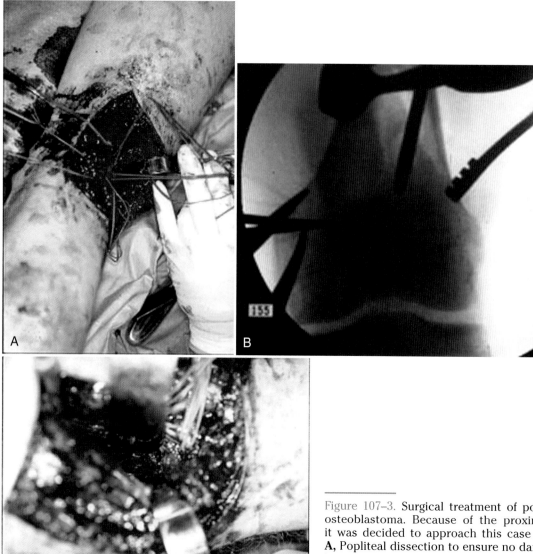

Figure 107–3. Surgical treatment of posterior distal femur osteoblastoma. Because of the proximity of the vessels, it was decided to approach this case in an open manner. **A,** Popliteal dissection to ensure no damage to neurovascular structures. **B,** Intraoperative fluoroscopy to localize the lesion. **C,** The cavity after curettage.

dic surgeons are more likely to see osteochondromas. Similar to enchondroma, osteochondroma is a developmental or hamartomatous process that arises from a defect in the outer edge of the growth plate on the metaphyseal side, resulting in an exostosis that always points away from the joint of origin as the lesion advances from the growth plate during the growing years.

The bony base of an osteochondroma is in direct communication with the medullary canal of the bone from which it arises. These lesions can be either pedunculated, as is commonly seen around the knee (Fig. 107–7), or can be sessile. There must be an associated cartilaginous cap on the bony base to make the diagnosis of osteochondroma. This cap has the histological features of a normal growth plate during the growing years. Osteochondroma growth plate activity subsides, however, at the same time as the activity in the larger plate from which the osteochondroma arose.

A familial form of osteochondroma, multiple hereditary exostoses, is an autosomal dominant disorder that is one-tenth as common as solitary osteochondroma. Three genetic loci have been determined to be involved with multiple hereditary exostoses involving the *EXT* gene. This condition can vary from quite mild to extensive involvement with symmetric limb shortening. The metaphyseal portions of long bones are deformed and widened (Fig. 107–8). The histological findings in multiple exostoses are similar to the findings in solitary osteochondroma.

Conversion of solitary osteochondroma to chondrosarcoma occurs only during adulthood. The overall rate of conversion for all types of solitary lesions is quite rare.[28] In multiple hereditary exostoses, there is a less than 1% chance of malignant conversion to secondary chondrosarcoma in the cartilaginous cap, especially in the larger, more proximal lesions.

Osteochondromas are stage 1 lesions. Symptoms are caused by mechanical effects on surrounding structures. Most children and adults with a solitary osteochondroma are asymptomatic and do not require surgical treatment.

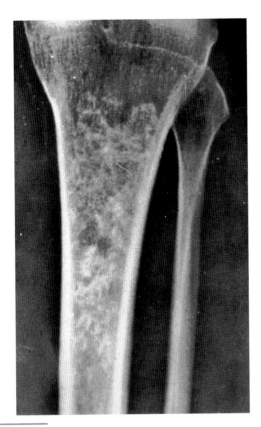

Figure 107–4. Anteroposterior radiograph of the proximal tibia shows loss of the normal bone trabecular pattern with central calcification. There is no endosteal scalloping or dilation.

In some cases, the lesion may be palpable and irritating. Surgical removal is appropriate in these cases to address the symptoms only and not as a prophylaxis for chondrosarcomatous degeneration. Likewise in multiple hereditary exostoses, symptomatic lesions are addressed surgically as needed. Corrective osteotomy occasionally is required because of angulatory deformity about the knee. In adults with a solitary osteochondroma or with multiple exostoses, if a previously quiescent lesion begins to enlarge, it should be removed. The surgical margin should be wide enough to include the entire cartilaginous cap because this is where malignant degeneration can occur.

CHONDROBLASTOMA

The term *chondroblastoma* suggests a benign cartilage-forming tumor, but this epiphyseal lesion of childhood has a histological appearance that is more typical of the benign metaphyseal-epiphyseal giant cell tumor of young adulthood. The chondroblastoma is about one-fifth as common as the giant cell tumor. It differs from other bone tumors in that it almost always is associated with epiphyseal or apophyseal bone. Most cases arise in the second decade of life, and males are affected more often than females. Although the most common location is the outer portion of the proximal humeral epiphysis, other common locations are the distal femoral and proximal tibial epiphyseal areas. Because of its proximity to a joint, chondroblastoma can present with a symptomatic joint effusion.

In cases of chondroblastoma, the radiograph shows a lytic tumor with a sharp sclerotic margin and central stippled or flocculated calcification occurring in the

Figure 107–5. **A,** Full-length lower extremity antero-posterior radiograph shows the windswept deformity secondary to Ollier's disease. **B,** Anteroposterior radiograph of the right knee of the patient in **A.**

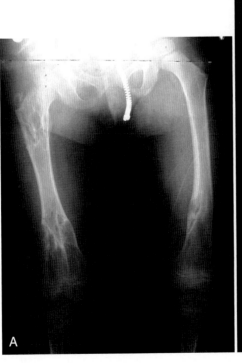

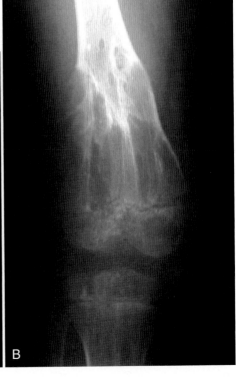

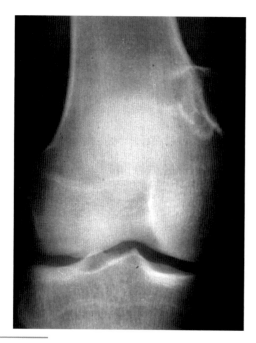

Figure 107–6. Anteroposterior radiograph of the knee shows a periosteal chondroma of the anteromedial distal femur.

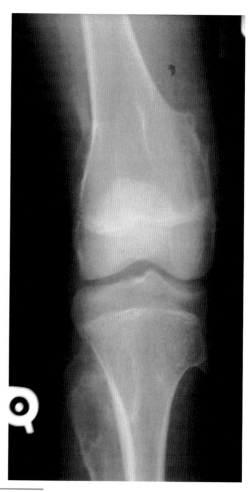

Figure 107–8. Anteroposterior radiograph of the knee shows the typical metaphyseal flaring and numerous osteochondromas seen in multiple hereditary exostoses.

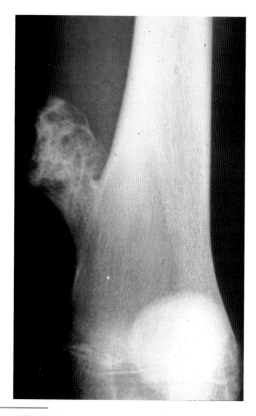

Figure 107–7. Anteroposterior radiograph of the knee shows a typical pedunculated osteochondroma.

chondroid portion of the tumor. As the growth plate closes, the tumor can expand gradually into the metaphyseal area and sometimes becomes quite aneurysmal. Chondroblastoma has the histological appearance of a giant cell tumor, with numerous macrophages seen usually in areas of hemorrhage. The stromal cells of the chondroblastoma are polyhedral, similar to those of a giant cell tumor, but with associated halos that give the chondroblastoma a "chicken wire" appearance. Although chondroid metaplasia in chondroblastoma is not easy to find, it must be present to establish the diagnosis firmly. Most chondroblastomas are stage 2 lesions, but some can be stage 3.[44]

The spontaneous conversion of chondroblastoma to a malignant tumor is extremely rare. As with the case of giant cell tumors, conversion to sarcoma can occur after radiation treatment, however. Although chondroblastoma is considered benign, it has been reported to metastasize to the lung on rare occasions.[51] Nevertheless, it carries an excellent prognosis.[51] Treatment for chondroblastoma consists of aggressive intralesional resection with curettage and reconstruction with bone graft or bone cement (polymethyl methacrylate). Local recurrence with this technique is less than 10%. With recurrent disease, more aggressive marginal or wide resection may be necessary.

Radiofrequency ablation of these lesions is starting to be performed at major centers that see a large number of these lesions.

Benign Fibrous Tumors of Bone

FIBROUS CORTICAL DEFECT

Fibrous cortical defects or cortical desmoids are small hamartomatous fibromas seen almost exclusively in the metaphyseal areas of the lower extremities of growing children. The distal femur is the most common site, followed by the distal tibia and the proximal tibia. They can be multiple, and 25% of normal children have these asymptomatic lesions at 5 years of age. The lesions tend to disappear as the result of bone remodeling before skeletal maturity. If excessive stress is placed across the lesions, they can become symptomatic and can cause findings of increased activity on an isotope bone scan.

In the case of fibrous cortical defects, microscopic studies show benign-appearing fibroblasts with an occasional area of histiocytes, foam cells, and benign giant cells. The radiographic appearance is so characteristic of this entity (Fig. 107–9) that a biopsy is usually not necessary. These are stage 1 lesions and generally can be observed.

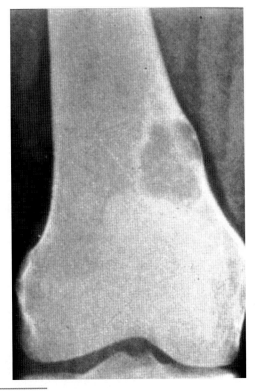

Figure 107–9. Anteroposterior radiograph of the distal femur shows a large fibrous cortical defect, which also could be called a nonossifying fibroma.

NONOSSIFYING FIBROMA

Just as osteoblastoma is considered a larger or more extensive form of osteoid osteoma, nonossifying fibroma is considered a larger form of fibrous cortical defect. It is typically seen in the lower extremity of children. Because of its size, it may not resolve entirely by skeletal maturity and can persist into adult life. If the lesion is quite large, approaching 50% of the diameter of the bone, pathological fracture may ensue. The fracture healing process may facilitate resolution of the lesions. Careful consideration to fracture prophylaxis should be reserved for large lesions. Nonossifying fibromas are stage 1 lesions. Similar to fibrous cortical defects, nonossifying fibroma does not require biopsy because the radiographic appearance is so characteristic. Large lesions placing the bone at risk of pathological fracture may be treated with curettage and bone grafting. With nonossifying fibroma, there may be multiple lesions that take on the appearance of fibrous dysplasia and can be associated with café-au-lait skin defects.

FIBROUS DYSPLASIA

Fibrous dysplasia can present in a variety of ways: monostotic, polyostotic, and with or without associated syndromes. Most cases are diagnosed before age 30, and there is a distinct female predilection. The monostotic presentation is more common than the polyostotic presentation. This condition is a dysplastic anomaly of bone-forming mesenchymal tissue with an inability to produce mature lamellar bone. The bone is arrested in the woven state with a resultant proliferation of spindle cell fibroblasts. In the polyostotic form, it tends to involve one side of the body rather than bilaterally. Nevertheless, it can involve any bone of the body. The most common location is the proximal femur, where it results in the so-called shepherd's crook deformity (Fig. 107–10). Other areas frequently involved include the tibia, pelvis, humerus, radius, and ribs. It is unusual for focal involvement of the knee. If a patient presents with knee pain with a history of fibrous dysplasia, it is important to obtain hip and pelvis radiographs.

In addition to bony involvement, patients can have café-au-lait skin pigmentation. These patches usually have a rough border, in contrast to the smooth border of the patches seen in neurofibromatosis. Patients with fibrous dysplasia may have associated endocrine problems; 5% of patients with the polyostotic form of fibrous dysplasia also exhibit precocious puberty (McCune-Albright syndrome). Other associated endocrine abnormalities include hyperthyroidism, acromegaly, Cushing's disease, and hypophosphatemic osteomalacia. Polyostotic fibrous dysplasia with soft-tissue myxomas is known as Mazabrand's syndrome. Fibrous dysplasia also can involve the skull and jawbones, mimicking ossifying fibroma of the jaw.

In fibrous dyplasia, microscopic findings include an alphabet-soup pattern of metaplastic woven bone scattered through a benign fibrous tissue stroma. This woven stroma lacks osteoblastic rimming. Foam cells, giant cells,

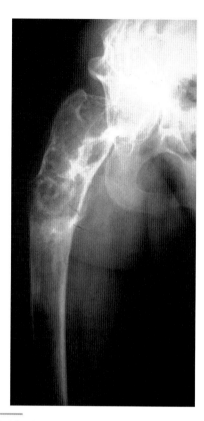

Figure 107–10. Anteroposterior radiograph of the proximal femur shows the typical "shepherd's crook" deformity of the proximal femur. Early hip symptoms may present as knee pain.

and cholesterol deposits can be seen. Large cystic areas and areas of cartilage formation are commonly present.

More recent research has potentially implicated a mutation in the signal-transducing G proteins interrupting cellular communication at the transmembrane cell surface receptor–intracellular signal transduction pathway.[39] The C-fas oncoprotein may be involved as well.[39]

Fibrous dysplasia tends to be active during the growing years, then burns out in adult life. Fewer than 1% of lesions convert to osteosarcoma, fibrosarcoma, or chondrosarcoma.[25] If there is conversion, it almost always occurs during adulthood. Generally, this disease is stage 1 or 2. In pediatric patients with active disease, curettage and grafting should be avoided because of high recurrence rates. The goals in managing pediatric patients are the prevention and treatment of deformity, especially in the lower extremity. Most cases should become quiescent with skeletal maturity. If not, the best surgical management in adults consists of rigid fixation, preferably with an intramedullary implant, with realignment osteotomies as needed.[21] This treatment has a higher success rate in adult patients than in pediatric patients. Medical management with bisphosphonates has been shown to be beneficial in some cases.[10] Irradiation is contraindicated because it may lead to irradiation-induced sarcoma at a later date.[26]

Cystic Lesions of Bone

SIMPLE BONE CYST

Simple bone cyst is a common pseudotumor of bone and is the most frequent cause of pathological fractures in children. Bone cysts typically affect patients between 5 and 15 years old and occur more often in boys than in girls. They are found in the proximal humerus in 50% of cases, but they also can be seen in the proximal tibia (Fig. 107–11) and distal femur. Patients are asymptomatic until a pathological fracture occurs. Fractures seem to arise from the central metaphyseal side of an epiphyseal or apophyseal growth plate. The cystic process continues to grow away from the physis. When it remains in contact with the physis, it is termed *active*. When it separates, it is termed *inactive*. Radiographs typically show a solitary cyst that is centrally located in the metaphyseal area and has marked thinning of the adjacent cortical bone and a pseudoloculated appearance (see Fig. 107–11). The bone cyst is filled with a clear serous fluid, and there is increased pressure during the active phase. The fact that this pressure gradually decreases as the cyst becomes inactive suggests a hydrodynamic mechanism.

The cyst cavity is lined with a fibrinous membrane that contains giant cells, foam cells, and a slight osteoid formation and is similar to the fibrous tissues seen in other fibrous bone lesions, including fibrous dysplasia. The periosteal covering in the area of a cyst is normal, and the pathological fractures heal normally and in most cases do not require surgery. The cyst usually persists after fracture union and requires further treatment. Bone-resorbing factors, such as matrix metalloproteinases, prostaglandins, interleukin-1, interleukin-6, tumor necrosis factor-α, and oxygen free radicals, have been shown in the cyst fluid.[30] Elevated nitrate and nitrite levels also have been noted to be higher in the cyst fluid than in serum.[29]

Historically the standard treatment for a solitary bone cyst was aggressive curettage or resection followed by bone grafting.[52] In patients with active disease, the recurrence rate was 30% to 50%, and repeated grafting was frequently necessary.[15] In patients with inactive disease, particularly patients older than age 15 years, the surgical results were much better, and the recurrence rate was lower. Solitary bone cysts are generally considered stage 1 lesions; occasionally, they may be stage 2. Currently, treatment is a function of location. In weightbearing bones, such as the proximal tibia, lesions should be treated aggressively. Initial management usually involves aspiration/injection with either bone marrow or corticosteroid. The injections are carried out with bone biopsy needles and are repeated three to five times at intervals of 2 to 3 months, depending on the radiographic response. The best results are when the patient is between 5 and 15 years old, at which time the disease is active, and macrophage activity is greatest in the cyst lining. Curettage and bone grafting also may be an effective modality. Indirect, limited curettage through a small bone window employing a flexible nail to break up septations followed by percutaneous bone grafting is beginning to be used at referral centers with promising early results. For realized fractures in

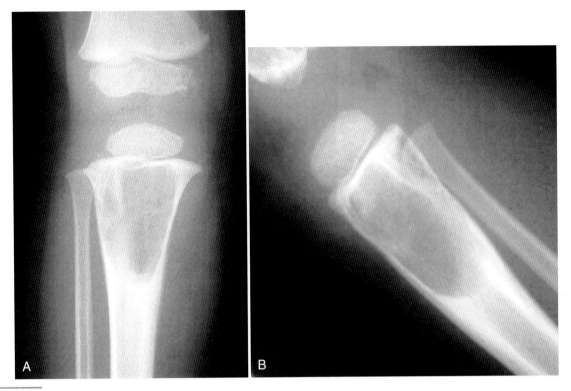

Figure 107–11. Anteroposterior **(A)** and lateral **(B)** radiographs of a child with a simple bone cyst of the proximal tibia. These generally are asymptomatic until a fracture occurs.

preadolescents, flexible nails are an acceptable internal fixation device.[55] Sarcomas can take on the radiographic appearance of a solitary bone cyst. For this reason, if needle aspiration does not reveal cystic fluid, or if it is not possible to inject contrast material and obtain radiographic confirmation of a cystic lesion, referral should be made to a tertiary center.

ANEURYSMAL BONE CYST

Aneurysmal bone cyst is a hemorrhagic lesion that has many characteristics of giant cell tumor, but is only half as frequent. Although giant cell tumor is rare in patients younger than age 20, 75% of the cases of aneurysmal bone cyst occur in patients 10 to 20 years old. Aneurysmal bone cyst and giant cell tumor are more common in females than in males. The distal femur is the most frequently affected site, followed by the proximal tibia, so knee surgeons are likely to see these entities in their practices (Fig. 107–12).

Initially, aneurysmal bone cyst appears on radiographs as an aggressive osteolytic lesion with extensive permeative cortical destruction that gives the impression of a malignant process, such as Ewing's sarcoma or hemorrhagic osteosarcoma. Next, a large aneurysmal bulge occurs outside the bone, with a thin reactive shell of bone forming at the outer edge (Fig. 107–13). Less soap-bubble pseudoseptation is seen in an aneurysmal bone cyst than in a solitary cyst.

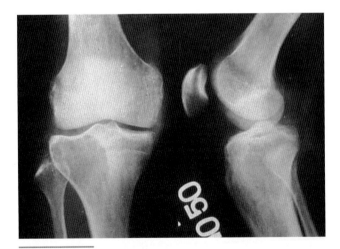

Figure 107–12. Anteroposterior and lateral radiographs of the knee show an eccentric radiolucent mass that turned out to be an aneuysmal bone cyst.

At the time of biopsy, the aneurysmal bone lesion exhibits large hemorrhagic cysts, but bleeding is typically modest. The hemorrhagic cysts are broken up by thick spongy fibrous septa that histologically contain great numbers of large giant cells and have thin osteoid seams. Even if a few mitotic figures are seen, the diagnosis of a benign lesion can remain. A carefully placed biopsy with multiple samples is needed to rule out other well-known skeletal tumors that may show an aneurysmal component,

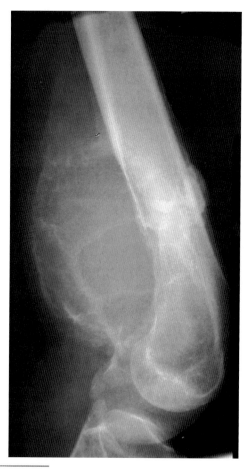

Figure 107–13. Lateral radiograph of the distal femur reveals an aggressive process that was concerning for a telangiectatic osteosarcoma, but was actually an aneurysmal bone cyst.

including giant cell tumor, chondromyxoid fibroma, and malignant hemorrhagic osteosarcoma. Aneurysmal bone cyst may arise secondarily as a morphological variant of some other underlying neoplastic process.[41] Similar to the solitary bone cyst, this cyst may have a hydraulic pressure origin that is secondary to hemorrhage and could be traumatically induced. Abnormal cytogenetic findings have been noted in aneurysmal bone cysts, however, which may suggest a distinct cellular pathogenetic etiology.[4] Aneurysmal bone cyst is a stage 2 or 3 lesion and frequently symptomatic.

If an aneurysmal cyst is left untreated, it may involute spontaneously, during which time it develops a heavy shell of reactive bone at the periphery. This involutional process can be hastened by surgical curettage and bone grafting. Radiation is no longer recommended. Another option for treating extremely large lesions is repeated embolization to reduce the rate of hemorrhagic expansion.[66]

Giant Cell Tumor of Bone

Numerous types of tumors contain giant cells, but are not true benign giant cell tumors. Most of the variants are seen in children and include aneurysmal bone cyst, chondroblastoma, simple bone cyst, osteoid osteoma, and osteoblastoma. Hemorrhagic osteosarcoma is the most malignant of the variants, and it is difficult to distinguish from an aggressive benign giant cell tumor. The brown tumor of hyperparathyroidism is a non-neoplastic variant seen in primary and secondary hyperparathyroidism. Only after all of the variant conditions are excluded can the diagnosis of benign giant cell tumor be made.

Five percent to 10% of all benign bone tumors are true giant cell tumors, occurring most frequently in the third decade of life. They are found more frequently in women than in men. In about half of the cases, the tumor is found about the knee and can arise in the patella.[1] The tumor is usually painful for several months before diagnosis and can cause a pathological fracture. It also can cause a painful effusion because of its juxtaposition to a major joint. Giant cell tumors may present as stage 2 or 3 disease and less frequently as stage 1. On radiograph, the lesion appears lytic in nature and is located in the epiphyseal-metaphyseal end of a long bone (Fig. 107–14). The lesion grows toward the joint surface and frequently comes into contact with articular cartilage, but rarely breaks into the joint.

Similar to chondroblastoma, benign giant cell tumor has a 1% to 5% chance of metastasizing to the lung.[62] Recurrent tumors have a 6% chance. Pulmonary staging is an important component in the initial evaluation and follow-up of giant cell tumor of bone. The prognosis for survival with this complication is favorable, and the tumors may resolve spontaneously. Benign giant cell tumor rarely can convert later to a malignant condition, such as an osteosarcoma or malignant fibrous histiocytoma,[45] and may be related to older radiation therapy techniques[54]; this has come into question with newer radiation therapy modalities.[9,16,47]

Currently, most surgeons elect an aggressive curettage, followed by the use of adjuvant phenol, hydrogen peroxide, or liquid nitrogen and by the subsequent packing of the defect with bone cement or bone graft. With this approach, the recurrence rate is 10% to 25%.[6,64] Treatment of recurrent giant cell tumor about the knee generally consists of another attempt at curettage, margin expansion, and local adjuvant therapy or a resection of the involved area and reconstruction with a large osteoarticular allograft, endoprosthesis, or an excisional arthrodesis. When giant cell tumor infrequently involves an expendable bone, such as the proximal fibula or ilium, it should be primarily resected. En-bloc resection continues to be used for multiple recurrent tumors, intensive soft-tissue involvement, or massively destructive cases. Embolization also may prove palliative or curative in unresectable cases. For advanced, multiply recurrent or aggressive metastatic cases, investigators are developing experimental medical protocols that employ serial embolization and systemic therapy, although this is generally reserved for axial disease.[32,33] Close follow-up for locally recurrent disease and pulmonary involvement is crucial. Chest x-ray every 6 to 12 months for the first 2 to 3 years at least is a reasonable consideration.

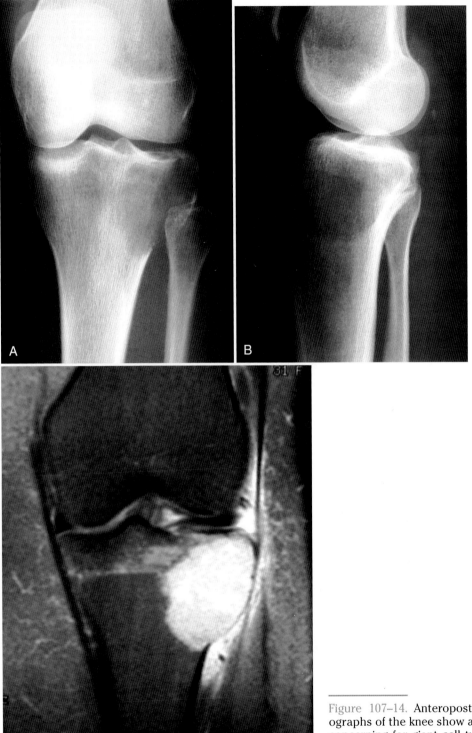

Figure 107–14. Anteroposterior (A) and lateral (B) radiographs of the knee show a lytic lesion of the proximal tibia concerning for giant cell tumor. C, Coronal MRI shows the proximity to the joint.

CONCLUSION

Knee surgeons must be familiar with the basic clinical aspects of benign bone lesions because the knee is a common site for a variety of lesions. Distinguishing benign from malignant conditions is paramount. Consultation with an experienced orthopedic oncologist is always encouraged if there are any questions or concerns about a more aggressive process.

References

1. Agarwal S, Jain UK, Chandra T, et al: Giant-cell tumors of the patella. Orthopedics 25:749, 2002.
2. Allen SD, Saifuddin A: Imaging of intra-articular osteoid osteoma. Clin Radiol 58:845, 2003.
3. Athwal GS, Pichora DR, Ellis RE, Rudan JF: A computer-assisted guidance technique for the localization and excision of osteoid osteoma. Orthopedics 27:195, 2004.
4. Baruffi MR, Neto JB, Barbieri CH, et al: Aneurysmal bone cyst with chromosomal changes involving 7q and 16p. Cancer Genet Cytogenet 129: 177, 2001.
5. Bottner F, Roedl R, Wotler K, et al: Cyclooxygenase-2 inhibitor for pain management in osteoid osteoma. Clin Orthop 393:258, 2001.
6. Boutou-Bredaki S, et al: Prognosis of giant cell tumor of bone: Histopathological analysis of 15 cases and review of the literature. Adv Clin Pathol 5:71, 2001.
7. Bovee JV, van Reggen JF, Cleton-Jansen AM, et al: Malignant progression in multiple enchondromatosis (Ollier's disease): An autopsy-based molecular genetic study. Hum Pathol 31:1299, 2000.
8. Cantwell CP, Obyrne J, Eustace S: Current trends in treatment of osteoid osteoma with an emphasis on radiofrequency ablation. Eur Radiol 14:607, 2004.
9. Chakravarti A, Spiro IJ, Hug EB, et al: Megavoltage radiation therapy for axial and inoperable giant-cell tumor of bone. J Bone Joint Surg Am 81:1566, 1999.
10. Chapurlat RD, Hugueny P, Delmas PD, Meunier PJ: Treatment of fibrous dysplasia of bone with intravenous pamidronate: Long-term effectiveness and evaluation of predictors of response to treatment. Bone 35:235, 2004.
11. Chew DK, Menelaus MB, Richardson MD: Ollier's disease: Varus angulation at the lower femur and its management. J Pediatr Orthop 18:202, 1998.
12. Ciabattoni G, Tamburrelli F, Greco F: Increased prostacyclin biosynthesis in patients with osteoid osteoma. Eicosanoids 4:165, 1991.
13. Cioni R, Armillotta N, Bargellini I, et al: CT-guided radiofrequency ablation of osteoid osteoma: Long-term results. Eur Radiol 14:1203, 2004.
14. Davis KW, Choi JJ, Blankenbaker DG: Radiofrequency ablation in the musculoskeletal system. Semin Roentgenol 39:129, 2004.
15. Dormans JP, Hanna BG, Johnston DR, Khurana JS: Surgical treatment and recurrence rate of aneurysmal bone cysts in children. Clin Orthop 421:205, 2004.
16. Feigenberg SJ, Marcus RB Jr, Zlotecki RA, et al: Radiation therapy for giant cell tumors of bone. Clin Orthop 411:207, 2003.
17. Frassica FJ, Waltrip RL, Sponseller PD, et al: Clinicopathologic features and treatment of osteoid osteoma and osteoblastoma in children and adolescents. Orthop Clin North Am 27:559, 1996.
18. Gaeta M, Minutoli F, Pandolfo I, et al: Magnetic resonance imaging findings of osteoid osteoma of the proximal femur. Eur Radiol 14:1582, 2004.
19. Georgoulis AD, Papageorgiou CD, Moebius UG, et al: The diagnostic dilemma created by osteoid osteoma that presents as knee pain. Arthroscopy 18:32, 2002.
20. Gonzalez-Lois C, Garcia-de-la-Torre P, Santos Briz-Terron A, et al: Intracapsular and para-articular chondroma adjacent to large joints: Report of three cases and review of the literature. Skeletal Radiol 30:672, 2001.
21. Guille JT, Kumar SJ, MacEwen GD: Fibrous dysplasia of the proximal part of the femur: Long-term results of curettage and bone-grafting and mechanical realignment. J Bone Joint Surg Am 80:648, 1998.
22. Hasegawa T, Hirose T, Sakamoto R, et al: Mechanism of pain in osteoid osteomas: An immunohistochemical study. Histopathology 22:487, 1993.
23. Hasegawa Y, Ishimura M, Tamai S, Fujisawa Y: Chondromatosis within a meniscal cyst of the knee. Arthroscopy 11:115, 1995.
24. Hazelbag HM, Wessels JW, Mollevangers P, et al: Cytogenetic analysis of adamantinoma of long bones: Further indications for a common histogenesis with osteofibrous dysplasia. Cancer Genet Cytogenet 97:5, 1997.
25. Huvos AG, Higinbotham NL, Miller TR: Bone sarcomas arising in fibrous dysplasia. J Bone Joint Surg Am 54:1047, 1972.
26. Inoue YZ, Frassica FJ, Sim FH, et al: Clinicopathologic features and treatment of postirradiation sarcoma of bone and soft tissue. J Surg Oncol 75:42, 2000.
27. Kahn LB: Adamantinoma, osteofibrous dysplasia and differentiated adamantinoma. Skeletal Radiol 32:245, 2003.
28. Kivioja A, Ervasti H, Kinnunen J, et al: Chondrosarcoma in a family with multiple hereditary exostoses. J Bone Joint Surg Br 82:261, 2000.
29. Komiya S, Kawabata R, Zenmyo M, et al: Increased concentrations of nitrate and nitrite in the cyst fluid suggesting increased nitric oxide synthesis in solitary bone cysts. J Orthop Res 18:281, 2000.
30. Komiya S, Minamitani K, Sasaguri Y, et al: Simple bone cyst: Treatment by trepanation and studies on bone resorptive factors in cyst fluid with a theory of its pathogenesis. Clin Orthop 287:204, 1993.
31. Kornberg A, Stangl M, Scheele J, Hammer C: Chronic persistent knee pain after repeated diagnostic arthroscopy: Osteoid osteoma, a primarily overlooked diagnosis in a young woman. Arch Orthop Trauma Surg 121:291, 2001.
32. Lackman RD, Khoury LD, Esmail A, Donthineni-Rao R: The treatment of sacral giant-cell tumours by serial arterial embolisation. J Bone Joint Surg Br 84:873, 2002.
33. Lin PP, Guzel VB, Moura MF, et al: Long-term follow-up of patients with giant cell tumor of the sacrum treated with selective arterial embolization. Cancer 95:1317, 2002.
34. Lindner NJ, Ozaki T, Roedl R, et al: Percutaneous radiofrequency ablation in osteoid osteoma. J Bone Joint Surg Br 83:391, 2001.
35. Maki M, Athanasou N: Osteofibrous dysplasia and adamantinoma: Correlation of proto-oncogene product and matrix protein expression. Hum Pathol 35:69, 2004.
36. Maki M, Saitoh K, Horiuchi H, et al: Comparative study of fibrous dysplasia and osteofibrous dysplasia: Histopathological, immuno-histochemical, argyrophilic nucleolar organizer region and DNA ploidy analysis. Pathol Int 51:603, 2001.
37. Maki M, Saitoh K, Kaneko Y, et al: Expression of cytokeratin 1, 5, 14, 19 and transforming growth factors-beta1, beta2, beta3 in osteofibrous dysplasia and adamantinoma: A possible association of transforming growth factor-beta with basal cell phenotype promotion. Pathol Int 50:801, 2000.
38. Makley JT, Dunn MJ: Prostaglandin synthesis by osteoid osteoma. Lancet 2:42, 1982.
39. Marie PJ: Cellular and molecular basis of fibrous dysplasia. Histol Histopathol 16:981, 2001.
40. Marinelli A, Giacomini S, Bianchi G, et al: Osteoid osteoma simulating an osteocartilaginous exostosis. Skeletal Radiol 33:181, 2004.
41. Martinez V, Sissons HA: Aneurysmal bone cyst: A review of 123 cases including primary lesions and those secondary to other bone pathology. Cancer 61:2291, 1988.
42. Mastrokalos DS, Passler HH, Tibesku CO, Wrazidlo W: Computed tomography-guided endoscopic removal of an osteoid osteoma from the femur. Arthroscopy 17:62, 2001.
43. McCaffrey M, Letts M, Carpenter B, et al: Osteofibrous dysplasia: A review of the literature and presentation of an additional 3 cases. Am J Orthop 32:479, 2003.
44. Mirra JM, Ulich TR, Eckardt JJ, Bhuta S: "Aggressive" chondroblastoma: Light and ultramicroscopic findings after en bloc resection. Clin Orthop 178:276, 1983.
45. Mori Y, Tsuchiya H, Karita M, et al: Malignant transformation of a giant cell tumor 25 years after initial treatment. Clin Orthop 381: 185, 2000.
46. Mungo DV, Zhang X, O'Keefe RJ, et al: COX-1 and COX-2 expression in osteoid osteomas. J Orthop Res 20:159, 2002.
47. Nair MK, Jyothirmayi R: Radiation therapy in the treatment of giant cell tumor of bone. Int J Radiat Oncol Biol Phys 43:1065, 1999.
48. O'Connell JX, Nanthakumar SS, Nielsen GP, Rosenberg AE: Osteoid osteoma: The uniquely innervated bone tumor. Mod Pathol 11:175, 1998.
49. Ozaki T, Hamada M, Sugihara S, et al: Treatment outcome of osteofibrous dysplasia. J Pediatr Orthop B 7:199, 1998.
50. Putnam A, Yandow S, Coffin CM: Classic adamantinoma with osteofibrous dysplasia-like foci and secondary aneurysmal bone cyst. Pediatr Dev Pathol 6:173, 2003.
51. Ramappa AJ, Lee FY, Tang P, et al: Chondroblastoma of bone. J Bone Joint Surg Am 82:1140, 2000.
52. Randall RL, Nork SE, James PJ, et al: Aggressive aneurysmal bone cyst of the proximal humerus. Clin Orthop 370:212, 2000.

53. Rochwerger A, Curvale G, Demortiere E, et al: Pes anserinus syndrome and osteoid osteoma. Clin J Sport Med 10:72, 2000.

54. Rock MG, Sim FH, Unni KK, et al: Secondary malignant giant-cell tumor of bone: Clinicopathological assessment of nineteen patients. J Bone Joint Surg Am 68:1073, 1986.

55. Roposch A, Saraph V, Linhart WE: Flexible intramedullary nailing for the treatment of unicameral bone cysts in long bones. J Bone Joint Surg Am 82:1447, 2000.

56. Rosenthal DI, Hornicek FJ, Torriani M, et al: Osteoid osteoma: Percutaneous treatment with radiofrequency energy. Radiology 229:171, 2003.

57. Sakai H, Tamai K, Iwamoto A, Saotome K: Para-articular chondroma and osteochondroma of the infrapatellar fat pad: a report of three cases. Int Orthop 23:114, 1999.

58. Sakamoto A, Oda Y, Iwamoto Y, Tsuneyoshi M: A comparative study of fibrous dysplasia and osteofibrous dysplasia with regard to expressions of c-fos and c-jun products and bone matrix proteins: A clinicopathologic review and immunohistochemical study of c-fos, c-jun, type I collagen, osteonectin, osteopontin, and osteocalcin. Hum Pathol 30:1418, 1999.

59. Sakamoto A, Oda Y, Iwamoto Y, Tsuneyoshi M: A comparative study of fibrous dysplasia and osteofibrous dysplasia with regard to G_{salpha} mutation at the Arg201 codon: Polymerase chain reaction-restriction fragment length polymorphism analysis of paraffin-embedded tissues. J Mol Diagn 2:67, 2000.

60. Sarisozen B, Durak K, Ozturk C: Adamantinoma of the tibia in a nine-year-old child. Acta Orthop Belg 68:412, 2002.

61. Sherman GM, Damron TA, Yang Y: CD99 positive adamantinoma of the ulna with ipsilateral discrete osteofibrous dysplasia. Clin Orthop 408:256, 2003.

62. Szendroi M: Giant-cell tumour of bone. J Bone Joint Surg Br 86:5, 2004.

63. Szendroi M, Kollo K, Antal I, et al: Intraarticular osteoid osteoma: Clinical features, imaging results, and comparison with extraarticular localization. J Rheumatol 31:957, 2004.

64. Turcotte RE, Wunder JS, Isler MH, et al, Canadian Sarcoma Group: Giant cell tumor of long bone: A Canadian Sarcoma Group study. Clin Orthop 397:248, 2002.

65. Wang JW, Shih CH, Chen WJ: Osteofibrous dysplasia (ossifying fibroma of long bones): A report of four cases and review of the literature. Clin Orthop 278:235, 1992.

66. Wathiong J, Brys P, Samson I, Maleux G: Selective arterial embolization in the treatment of an aneurysmal bone cyst of the pelvis. JBR-BTR 86:325, 2003.

67. Wold LE, Pritchard DJ, Bergert J, Wilson DM: Prostaglandin synthesis by osteoid osteoma and osteoblastoma. Mod Pathol 1:129, 1988.

CHAPTER 108

Surgical Management of Malignant Bone Tumors around the Knee

Michael D. Neel

Surgical management of malignant tumors about the knee requires a basic understanding of tumor biology and knowledge of common tumors and their clinical and radiographic behavior. To successfully treat malignant tumors, it is essential that the general principles of sarcoma surgery be understood, including staging of a bone tumor, appropriate biopsy techniques, patient selection for limb salvage surgery versus amputation, and methods of resection and reconstruction. In this chapter, principles of limb salvage surgery, patient selection criteria, and principles of resection and reconstruction will be discussed. The initial workup, including staging and biopsy of a bone tumor, is discussed in another chapter. Reconstructive options that will be reviewed in this chapter include arthrodesis, allograft reconstruction, and rotationplasty. Reconstruction with a megaprosthesis or allograft-prosthetic composite is reviewed in another chapter. Common malignant bone tumors around the knee include osteosarcoma, chondrosarcoma, Ewing's sarcoma, and lymphoma of bone, and these tumors will also be reviewed.

TUMOR BIOLOGY

Primary malignant tumors have the capacity to metastasize to distant sites. They are also locally aggressive, destroy bone, and involve adjacent soft-tissue structures. Malignant tumors are typically subclassified as low, intermediate, or high grade based on the histological grade. Grade is a feature of the amount of cellular activity, cellular pleomorphism, mitotic activity, and tumor necrosis. It is reflective of the tumor's aggressiveness.

Malignant bone tumors spread locally by centrifugal tumor expansion. As the tumor cells divide and the mass grows, normal tissue is compressed. Microscopic "pseudopods" of tumor invade normal surrounding tissue. In an effort to control the tumor, an inflammatory response is established adjacent to the tumor. This reactive zone consists of inflammatory cells, edematous tissue, and neovascularity feeding the advancing tumor. The compressed normal tissue produces a pseudocapsule about the mass. Thus, the surrounding soft tissue around the malignant tumor is slowly invaded by satellites of advancing tumor. To remove the tumor completely, resection must proceed well beyond the reactive zone and into normal adjacent soft tissue or bone to avoid leaving satellites behind.[10] Unfortunately, current imaging modalities such as magnetic resonance imaging (MRI), positron emission tomography, bone scans, and other types of imaging cannot adequately identify microscopic tumor extension. Frequently, the edematous tissue can be well identified, but this really gives no clear information regarding the presence or absence of tumor satellites.

This aggressive local spread of tumor is frequently halted by anatomic barriers such as cortical bone, periosteum, cartilage, synovium, and fascia. These "barriers" are relative and do not offer an absolute stopping point for tumor growth. They can be breached with extension of tumor beyond their confines. However, they do serve to force tumor growth into a longitudinal pattern. Tumors can extend for great distances along bone and soft-tissue planes and acquire a large bulky size before being detected. Tumors that remain within the confined bone or soft-tissue compartment are termed "intracompartmental."[2] Those that extend out of the compartment of origin and involve adjacent structures are termed "extracompartmental." As the tumor spreads, it frequently displaces rather than encases neurovascular structures. Occasionally, these structures can be circumferentially engulfed by tumor but tend to remain patent and functional unless significantly compressed by a large mass. Destruction of bone and the presence of a soft-tissue mass can lead to pain, the most common initial symptom of malignant tumors of bone. The subcutaneous nature of the distal femur and proximal tibia lend to early detection of a soft-tissue mass associated with a bone tumor.

PRINCIPLES OF SURGICAL MANAGEMENT

On completion of appropriate staging and determination of an accurate diagnosis, attention is turned toward treatment. Cure of malignant tumors requires local control of tumor, as well as control of systemic disease. Surgical management of malignant bone tumors is often the foundation for local control. The principles of surgical management are outlined here. Adjuvant treatment of common malignant tumors is found in the section for each of the common bone malignancies.

Surgical Margins

In collecting, analyzing, and reporting surgical data, it is imperative to have a language that is common among surgeons regarding what surgical procedure has been performed. The relationship between the surgical plane of resection of the tumor and the surrounding tissue is what is termed the surgical margin. Enneking[2] established a nomenclature to describe oncological surgical procedures in terms of four surgical margins. The margin can be achieved by either amputation or a limb salvage procedure.

Intralesional margins are achieved if the surgical plane of dissection is through the tumor with gross residual disease left behind. This is typically the case when a biopsy is performed but also occurs with curettage or a debulking procedure. Tumor is obviously left behind and the procedure is not curative of malignant bone tumors. This margin is appropriate only in the palliative setting or for very low-grade lesions amenable to local control with curettage alone.

Marginal margins are achieved when the plane of dissection is the pseudocapsule itself. The main body of the tumor easily peels away from the surrounding pseudocapsule. This leads the surgeon to inadvertently perform a "shell-out" procedure. Failure to recognize that histologically there is a real potential to have satellites of tumor within and beyond the pseudocapsule results in lack of an adequate margin. Several studies have demonstrated the high rate of tumor cells in this reactive zone after a shell-out or gross total resection. Even after adjuvant therapy, local recurrence is high with a marginal margin. For this reason, tumor bed re-excision is often recommended after gross total resection or shell-out procedures are performed. In tumors treated preoperatively with chemotherapy or radiation, a marginal margin can be accepted only adjacent to vital structures such as a neurovascular bundle. In this situation, the preoperative treatment would have (one hopes) sterilized any microscopic satellite lesions in these areas.

Wide margins are the most commonly achieved margins when dealing with bone malignancies. The resection plane is beyond the pseudocapsule and the reactive zone. It results in a cuff of normal tissue surrounding the tumor. The specimen contains the biopsy track (skin and underlying soft tissue), the body of the tumor, the pseudocapsule, the reactive zone, and a cuff of normal tissue. How thick that cuff must be is subject to study and debate. It must be realized that the thickness of the cuff is not as important as the concept that the cuff be wide enough to be beyond any satellite or skip lesions that may be present. A wide margin must be achieved in both bone and soft tissue to adequately treat high-grade malignant lesions (Fig. 108–1).[10]

Radical margins are achieved when the involved bone and soft-tissue component is resected in its entirety. An extracompartmental resection is thus achieved. When managing tumors that are extracompartmental, the entire involved bone and involved adjacent musculature must be excised to be considered a radial resection. Radical margins are not typically necessary for bone sarcomas.

Patient Selection for Limb Salvage versus Amputation

In the modern age of treatment, most patients are candidates for limb-sparing resections. Several factors play a role in determining which patients should or should not undergo a limb salvage procedure. Local anatomic extent, involvement of major neurovascular structures, adjacent soft-tissue attachments, and reconstructive options all play a role in determining the most appropriate procedure. Additionally, response to chemotherapy may render a previously unresectable lesion resectable. Adjuvant therapy can influence the decision for limb salvage or amputation. The decision to attempt limb salvage versus amputation lies with the surgeon's ability to achieve an appropriate oncological margin. If the appropriate oncological margin is able to be obtained, it must be determined whether the reconstruction will provide a stable construct to support the limb. The functional result of a limb-sparing procedure must be as good as or better than an amputation.

Principles of Tumor Resection

Once a patient is considered a candidate for limb salvage, careful preoperative planning of the resection and reconstruction is essential to achieve a successful outcome. Review of the initial and interval imaging studies during the course of treatment allows the surgeon to plan the definitive surgery. Bone resection is determined by initial tumor imaging and typically involves 3- to 5-cm resection of bone to achieve a wide surgical margin. In some instances, this margin may be as close as 1 cm. Subchondral bone provides an excellent barrier to tumor extension. Even when the tumor extends into epiphyseal bone it is rare for it to extend into the joint, which allows tumor resection of the proximal tibia or distal femur in an intra-articular fashion. Tumors that involve the proximal end of the tibia often require removal of the proximal end of the

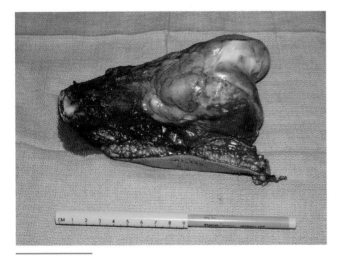

Figure 108–1. Surgical specimen demonstrating wide margins after resection of the distal end of the femur. Note the cuff of normal tissue surrounding the tumor and inclusion of a biopsy tract.

fibula through the proximal tibiofibular joint if the joint is in danger of tumor penetration or in close proximity to tumor. Proximal fibula tumors are usually treated by resection of the fibula alone, but may require removal of the proximal tibiofibular joint in an extra-articular fashion, as well as a small portion of the adjacent tibia. Large tumors or tumors with intra-articular extension require resection in an extra-articular fashion. If tumor has extended into the knee joint or if there is contamination from a previous ill-planned biopsy, the joint must be removed en bloc by resection beyond the capsular attachments at the proximal tibial and distal femoral levels. The patella and extensor mechanisms are resected along with the joint. The resection must include any skip metastases in the bone or soft tissues.

Special consideration is also made for a skeletally immature child who has significant growth remaining. Resection of the distal femoral and proximal tibial physes can result in significant limb length inequality. Special reconstruction options must be considered for these growing children. Amputation, rotationplasty, and an expandable prosthesis are reconstructive options in this group of patients. The resection level may be influenced by the desire to save the physis, but the best oncological margin is always what determines the resection level.

Once the bone margins are determined, consideration is turned to soft-tissue resection. Most tumors of the distal end of the femur are adequately covered by deep layers of soft tissue. Frequently, a sufficient amount of the quadriceps mechanism may be spared to provide an appropriate functional result. Commonly, only a small portion of the vastus medialis obliquus or vastus lateralis is removed with resection of the biopsy track. The remainder of the quadriceps, patella, and patellar tendon can be spared. Typically, the deep soft-tissue margin (serving as coverage over the tumor) is provided by the vastus intermedius. In large bulky tumors, more extensive quadriceps resection may be required. Such resection may have an effect on function and should be considered when deciding on amputation versus limb salvage. The neurovascular bundle may be displaced by the sarcoma but is not usually encased by tumor and can be spared. The cruciate ligaments, collateral insertions, and gastrocnemius insertions are all removed off the distal end of the femur; as a consequence, a constrained design is required if arthroplasty is the method of skeletal reconstruction. The adductors are divided as well. The pes anserinus and hamstring insertions on the tibia and fibula are usually left intact when performing distal femoral resections. Resection of ligamentous insertions always includes a short cuff of tissue to ensure adequate margins. Typically, the resection is performed by first dissecting through soft tissue in a manner that allows the biopsy track to be removed with the specimen, performing the arthrotomy and continuing with the soft-tissue dissection, and then osteotomizing the femur. Often, the posterior soft tissues are more easily approached after the femoral osteotomy has been performed. The specimen is removed and inspected by the surgeon and pathologist for margins. Attention is then turned toward reconstruction.

On the tibial side, tumors frequently involve the tibial tubercle, and therefore division of the patellar tendon is required. It must be reconstructed to provide an adequate extensor mechanism. The pes anserinus and hamstring insertions are divided near the bone with a cuff of normal tissue. On the femoral side the gastrocnemius and adductor insertions are spared. The cruciate and collateral attachments are removed from the proximal end of the tibia as well when resecting a proximal tibial lesion.

PRINCIPLES OF RECONSTRUCTION

When choosing the optimal reconstruction, the surgeon must consider the patient's age and functional demands, as well as the anticipated bone and soft-tissue deficits. Bone loss must be reconstructed with either local grafts, allografts, endoprosthetic replacements, or a combination of these options. Soft-tissue defects, such as the extensor mechanism, can be reconstructed with local advancement flaps or allograft reconstruction. In the case of extensive bone and soft-tissue loss, arthrodesis may be the appropriate reconstructive method. In a young child, rotationplasty affords the ability to resect the tumor and reconstruct the knee in a semiamputated fashion. These techniques will be reviewed. Megaprostheses and allograft-prosthetic composites are the two most commonly used reconstructions and are discussed elsewhere. Osteoarticular allografts may still be considered for reconstruction in young patients to avoid resurfacing of the uninvolved articulation. No single option is good for all patients.

Arthrodesis

Before the availability of endoprosthetic joints, resection followed by arthrodesis was the only viable option for surgical reconstruction after limb salvage procedures. With the advent of successful modular oncology megaprostheses, fewer patients undergo arthrodesis. Arthrodesis is typically accomplished with the use of local grafts from the opposite side of the resected joint or large bulk intercalary allografts. In either case, the fusion is held in place with intramedullary rods and/or plates and screws to provide stability to the construct and promote healing of the graft-host junction. The knee joint is fused in a position that allows easy swing-through of the extremity during the swing phase of normal gait. The desired position is 5 degrees of valgus, 10 to 15 degrees of knee flexion, and slight external rotation. The extremity is typically shortened by 1 cm to maximize gait mechanics.[10] Once healed, the arthrodesis provides a durable, stable reconstruction. Unfortunately, the lack of knee motion is a functional deficit that most patients dislike.

LOCAL AUTOGRAFTS

As reported by Enneking and Shirley, the use of local autografts can produce a durable reconstruction with reliable consolidation.[3] The technique described uses a segment of adjacent bone and fibula to bridge the resection gap. Fixation is maintained with an intramedullary rod. An essential component of preoperative planning is determination of the length of resection. Defects greater than a third the length of the bone require consideration of alternative methods of reconstruction because of an inability to achieve adequate stability. Radiographs in both planes help determine the most appropriate size and length of rod. Most manufacturers can provide off-the-shelf interlocking fusion rods. For patients with small-diameter bones or unusually large femoral bows, a custom device may be required. After appropriate reaming, a guide rod is placed in retrograde fashion through the proximal end of the femur and out the piriformis fossa. A spacer made from polymethylmethacrylate is then placed temporarily in the segmental defect to maintain length while placing the rod. The rod should extend to within 3 to 4 cm of the ankle joint. The rod is then placed in antegrade fashion down the femur, across the defect, and into the tibia.

Local grafts are now harvested. For distal femoral resections, a segment of anterior tibia is harvested. It consists of the anterior half of the bone. The length is 2 cm longer than the resection segment because the graft will be "keyed" into the native bone on either side of the defect. The overall length of the leg will be planned to be 1 cm short. A bridge of bone measuring 3 cm should be left at the proximal end of the tibia to provide structural support for the graft. For proximal tibial resections, the anterior cortex of the femur is harvested in similar fashion. Next the fibula is harvested. Care is taken to protect the peroneal nerve. Sufficient length of fibula is harvested to span the defect. The fibula is then placed in the posterior aspect of the defect and fixed with screws or Steinmann pins. The proximal end of the fibula is beveled to provide additional surface area for healing.

The spacer is now removed and graft placed into the defect. The graft is countersunk into the remaining bone. The segment is measured to ensure that the reconstructed defect is 1 cm shorter than the removed specimen to shorten the extremity by 1 cm overall. The graft is then fixed to the bone proximally and distally. Additional graft is placed around the fusion areas to promote healing and consolidation. Proximal and distal interlocking screws are then applied. Local muscle flaps may be used if needed to provide soft-tissue coverage. Flaps also provide vascular soft tissue to assist in consolidation of fusion. The wound is closed over drains. Toe-touch weightbearing is allowed until the graft consolidates at about 4 to 6 months.

LARGE BULK ALLOGRAFT

With the advent of bone and tissue banking, the use of bulk allograft for arthrodesis has been popularized. Bulk allografts have the advantage of reconstruction of larger defects than possible with local grafts. Fixation can be achieved with intramedullary rods, plates and screws, or a combination of these methods.

Preoperative measurements are used to order the appropriate size of allograft. Typically, a distal femoral graft is used. The length should be several centimeters longer than the anticipated resection length to allow intraoperative flexibility. After resection and inspection, the specimen is measured. The graft is then cut to match the defect minus 1 cm. Preparation for rodding proceeds as detailed earlier, with the allograft reamed 1 to 2 mm larger than the rod selected to ensure ease of rod insertion through the graft. The rod is inserted in antegrade fashion into the femur, allograft, and then the tibia. Short derotational and compression plates may be used at the proximal and distal junctions to provide stability and promote healing of the allograft to the host bone.

Alternatively, the allograft can be secured with plates and screws instead of an intramedullary rod with supplemental plates. Typically, two 4.5 large-fragment dynamic compression plates or locking plates are used. The graft is inserted as previously described. Plates are placed on the anterior and anterolateral positions and span the proximal and distal junctions. A few screws are placed in the graft. Multiple screws have been implicated in allograft fracture. Compression techniques are used to provide stability and promote fusion.

In either method of fixation, additional graft material can be applied at both junctions. A gastrocnemius muscle flap is recommended for soft-tissue coverage. It also provides the junction with a covering of well-vascularized tissue. With either technique, the patient is allowed toe-touch weightbearing until consolidation occurs at about 4 to 6 months.[12]

Rotationplasty

Rotationplasty is another method of reconstruction after resection of tumors about the knee and is commonly used for treatment of a skeletally immature patient. Tumors of the distal femur and proximal tibia can be reconstructed with this technique. Rotationplasty essentially uses the ankle joint as the knee joint. By rotating the foot 180 degrees, the plane of motion in the ankle is in the same plane as the knee joint (Fig. 108–2). After resection of the tumor, the foot and ankle are rotated and brought up to the level of the contralateral knee joint. The residual tibia is then fixed to the femur. Eventually, the extremity is fitted for a special prosthesis in which the foot fits into a special component. The reconstruction essentially functions as a below-knee amputation.[10] Without the restrictions entailed with an endoprosthesis, a patient with a rotationplasty has very few functional limitations. The durability of the reconstruction limits the necessity for future surgery when compared with other reconstructions. In addition, rotationplasty may also be considered for patients with extensive intra-articular involvement or large associated soft-tissue masses. This procedure provides the ability to perform an extra-articular resection of the knee and achieve a wide margin for large, extensive sarcomas.

One of the disadvantages of rotationplasty is the obvious cosmetic appearance of the extremity. However, in most circumstances the rotated foot is contained within the special prosthetic in which it is fitted. With careful patient selection and preoperative counseling, patients

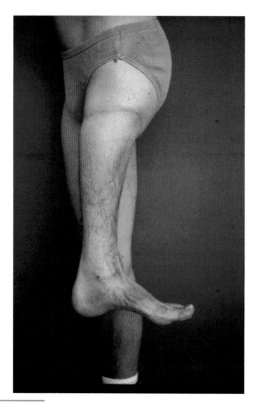

Figure 108–2. Clinical appearance of a patient with a Van Ness rotationplasty. (Courtesy of Dr. Norbert Lindner.)

have not demonstrated any significant increase in psychosocial disturbances when compared with those receiving other types of reconstruction. Rotationplasty is an excellent alternative to amputation in a properly selected patient.[6,10]

As with other reconstructions, extensive preoperative planning is essential to achieve a successful outcome. The level of ankle placement is based on patient age and anticipated future growth of the contralateral extremity. To accommodate for the resection and rotation, a unique circumferential skin incision is made. With some variations, it is essentially a modified rhomboid shape with the long axis oriented along the anterior aspect of the thigh.[4] Circumferential incisions along the thigh and calf are then connected with a posterior lateral incision. The level of the proximal circumferential incision for distal femoral resection is a few centimeters above the bone resection level. The tibial incision is just distal to the level of the tibia tubercle. The neurovascular bundle is exposed and protected as usual for resections about the knee. En bloc resection of the vessels with subsequent reanastomosis may be required for tumor involvement. Osteotomy is performed at the predetermined level. A Steinmann pin is placed proximal to the osteotomy and then a second is placed in the tibia perpendicular to the first to provide a guide to rotation during fixation of the bones. Intra-articular or extra-articular resection is then performed as required, followed by soft-tissue resection in a transverse fashion above and below the tumor with appropriate margins. As per the preoperative planning, the tibia is divided at the proper level. The foot and ankle are then rotated, brought up to the level of the resected femur, and

fixed with plates and screws. The neurovascular bundle is typically coiled to prevent kinking. Wound closure is performed over drains. Postoperatively, the extremity is dressed with a compression dressing to avoid undue swelling. Early weightbearing is allowed with an ischial-bearing prosthesis. Eventually the limb is fitted with a modified prosthesis in which weightbearing is achieved through the foot fitted into a special platform. Function is similar to a below-knee amputation.

COMMON MALIGNANT BONE TUMORS OF THE KNEE

Osteosarcoma

Osteosarcoma is a neoplastic process in which osteoid is produced by malignant cells. A variety of histological subtypes can occur and produce a range of clinical entities. The subtypes have been organized into classic (conventional), parosteal, periosteal, high-grade surface, telangiectatic, low-grade central, and small cell osteogenic sarcoma. Osteosarcoma is further subclassified by whether it arises as a primary de novo lesion or as a secondary lesion. Secondary lesions can arise from Paget's disease, osteogenesis perfecta, and multiple hereditary exostosis or as radiation-induced tumors.[13]

Osteosarcoma is the most common malignant bone tumor of childhood. Classic osteosarcoma has a peak incidence in the second decade with male predominance. Parosteal osteogenic sarcoma has a slightly older mean age of 30 years. Secondary tumors and radiation-induced tumors have a much higher peak age at onset, between 35 and 45 years. The vast majority of osteosarcomas, approximately 80%, appear in the long tubular bones. The knee is a favored site, with approximately 40% to 45% of osteosarcomas arising in the femur and 15% to 20% in the tibia. The tumor is typically metaphyseal. The parosteal variant is most commonly seen in the posterior aspect of the distal end of the femur. Pain is the most common initial complaint across all subtypes. The notable exception is parosteal osteogenic sarcoma, which is typically manifested as a painless mass.

In these young active patients, pain is often attributed to injury, overuse, or "growing pains" commonly seen around the knee. The insidious, constant nature of the pain, which steadily increases in severity and duration, is usually cause for alarm and referral to a clinician. Night pain and pain associated with weightbearing also typically herald the presence of a malignant process. The average duration of symptoms before initial evaluation is about 3 months.[10] Serum alkaline phosphatase will be elevated in approximately 50% of patients.

Conventional osteosarcoma may have a lytic, blastic, or mixed mineralization pattern on plain radiographs. Parosteal lesions will appear as a lobulated ossified mass. Periosteal reaction, Codman's triangle, cortical disruption, and a soft-tissue mass are seen in over 90% of patients and are all features common to high-grade subtypes. MRI is performed to better evaluate the extent of bone and soft-tissue involvement so critical to surgical planning. Moreover, MRI is the most sensitive tool for identifying skip metastases. Prognostic factors that seem to most significantly influence the outcome in patients with osteosarcoma are the extent of disease at initial evaluation and the presence of a high-grade lesion. Tumors that are large in size or located in an anatomic site that precludes appropriate wide margins have a poorer prognosis. Response to induction chemotherapy as measured by tumor necrosis of the resected specimen has been shown to be of prognostic value.[7]

Surgical removal of the primary tumor for local control plus administration of chemotherapy for systemic control is the foundation of modern treatment protocols for osteosarcoma. Radiation is reserved for unresectable lesions or metastatic disease but really has no role outside the palliative setting.[8]

Chondrosarcoma

Chondrosarcoma is the second most common malignant bone tumor. It is characterized as a neoplastic process producing cartilage from malignant cells and is typically classified according to grade, anatomic location, or the presence of primary versus secondary lesions. Common clinical subtypes include conventional chondrosarcoma, secondary chondrosarcoma arising from osteochondroma, mesenchymal chondrosarcoma, dedifferentiated chondrosarcoma, and clear cell chondrosarcoma. It has a 60% male preponderance, with a peak incidence in the third to sixth decade. Treatment is more often determined by the grade of the lesion than by any other classification.[10] Fortunately, the knee is not commonly involved and most chondrosarcomas are low grade. Benign aggressive active lesions can be very similar histologically to low-grade lesions. Before performing any biopsy, consultation should be obtained with an experienced radiologist and pathologist familiar with evaluating this difficult tumor.

Pain is the most common initial symptom and occurs in more than 75% to 95% of patients with chondrosarcoma.[14] By comparison, less than 5% of benign enchondromas produce pain. With the incidental finding of a painless enchondroma, the incidence of chondrosarcoma is less than 1%. Most chondrosarcomas are initially seen after a "protracted" clinical course of several months consistent with the common low-grade nature of the lesion. Simon and Springfield have found that lesions greater than 6 cm are at an increased risk of being a high-grade lesion and deserve careful observation and follow-up.[10]

The radiographic appearance of chondrosarcoma corresponds to the subtype of tumor. Low-grade lesions exhibit features in common with benign aggressive lesions. Matrix calcification is an indication of low- to intermediate-grade lesions. High-grade lesions have a more aggressive radiographic appearance, as expected. In the long bones, chondrosarcoma tends to occur in metadiaphyseal or diaphyseal locations, with epiphyseal lesions usually being consistent with a clear cell subtype. More than 60% are calcified.[10] Endosteal scalloping is frequently seen in all cartilage tumors regardless of grade. It is thought that endosteal scalloping involving greater than 50% of the cortex is consistent with a more aggressive lesion. Periosteal reaction is not a common characteristic except in very active enlarged lesions. Many lesions will have mixed areas of calcification and radiolucency suggestive of a malignant process. There is not usually a crisp border or area containing reactive bone noted radiographically.

Secondary chondrosarcomas, especially those associated with osteochondromas, can be difficult to differentiate from their benign counterparts. Associated soft-tissue masses, large cartilaginous caps greater than 2 cm and adjacent radiolucency, and cortical erosions are indicative of malignant transformation of these lesions. A cartilaginous cap greater than 1 to 2 cm in adults or greater than 2 to 3 cm in children should raise suspicion for possible malignant transformation of an osteochondroma.

Computed tomography is helpful in determining the amount of cortical disruption, periosteal reaction, soft-tissue mass, and matrix calcification present within the lesion. MRI can be used to determine the thickness of the cartilage cap. Cross-sectional imaging is important for determining the extent of local tumor and adjacent soft tissues involved and identifying any aggressive features that will help with the diagnosis. This coupled with the clinical manifestations and plain film findings is essential for determining the aggressiveness of a particular lesion. Review of these critical images with the pathologist is very important when a biopsy is indicated.

Treatment of chondrosarcoma is primarily surgical. Low-grade lesions that are readily resectable with wide margins typically require only surgery. High-grade and dedifferentiated lesions are frequently treated with neoadjuvant chemotherapy protocols because of the high risk for systemic spread. No clear-cut chemotherapy protocol has shown to improve long-term survival in patients with chondrosarcoma. Radiation therapy is used only in the palliative setting. The prognosis for patients with chondrosarcoma is best based on the grade of the lesion.[5]

Ewing's Sarcoma

Ewing's sarcoma is a high-grade malignant tumor of bone and soft tissue that consists of "small round blue" cells. The cells produce scant osteoid matrix scattered throughout sheets of blue cells. These cells fill the trabeculae of the normal surrounding bone. It is the third most common bone tumor and the second most common malignant bone tumor in childhood. The commonly used term "Ewing's sarcoma" is giving way to the more accurate term "primitive neural ectodermal tumor" or "Ewing's sarcoma family of tumors" (ESFT).[8,14] Terc-Carel et al demonstrated that 80% to 90% of ESFT have the distinct t(11;22)(q24;q12) translocation. This cytogenetic abnormality helps in differentiating the lesion from neuroblastoma and other histologically similar lesions.[10,11]

ESFT has a peak age at onset in the second decade of life with a slight male predilection. The tumor most commonly occurs in long tubular bones; there is a 15% incidence of ESFT occurring around the knee.[10,14] Pain and swelling are the most common initial symptoms. A low-grade fever and an elevated sedimentation rate and white blood cell count are not uncommon. The presence of abnormal laboratory studies, a soft-tissue mass, and fever often causes this tumor to be confused with osteomyelitis with an associated soft-tissue abscess. Grossly, the tumor can appear to have an almost liquid-like consistency, which can also cause confusion with chronic osteomyelitis.

On plain radiographs, the lesion appears within the metadiaphyseal or diaphyseal region of bone as a permeative lesion with poorly defined margins and no reactive rim of bone. Areas of radiolucency and radiodensity can be seen within the lesion itself. An associated soft-tissue mass is frequently present. "Onion skinning" (layered, wave-like periosteal reaction) of the bone is a common feature. Determination of soft-tissue size and the extent of bony destruction is best evaluated with MRI and is essential for surgical planning.

Treatment consists of neoadjuvant chemotherapy followed by surgery, radiation therapy, or a combination thereof for local disease control and subsequent additional chemotherapy. The impact of surgery on survival is somewhat controversial. Because of the excellent response to chemotherapy and its radiosensitivity, ESFT has traditionally been treated with these modalities for local and systemic control. Initially, surgery was reserved for "expendable bones," those that were easily resected with wide margins. Now there is a growing trend toward managing these tumors more aggressively with surgery. More recent studies seem to indicate that surgery alone can yield acceptable rates of local control, thereby avoiding the morbidity of radiotherapy.[9]

Lymphoma of Bone

Primary lymphoma of bone is a lymphoproliferative malignancy arising in bone. Lymphoma can be a single, solitary bone lesion or one of multiple bony sites without any evidence of soft-tissue involvement. It can also arise as a bone lesion in association with soft-tissue involvement (lymph nodes, liver, spleen, etc.). Lymphoma can arise primarily in the bone or occur in the bone in a metastatic fashion. Histologically, lymphoma shows a diffuse proliferation of cells with very little matrix. Reticulum stains are positive. Immunohistochemistry and flow cytometry are helpful in diagnosing and differentiating the lesion.[14] The peak age of onset is in the sixth decade with a male preponderance. Lymphoma is rare in patients younger than 20.[14] Lymphoma of bone tends to arise in the pelvis and proximal end of the femur. Around the knee, approximately 8% occur in the distal femur and 4% in the proximal tibia. Within the bone itself it tends to be diffuse within the metadiaphyseal region and involves the entire bone.[14] Patients typically complain of progressive, constant pain and a soft-tissue mass. About 25% of patients will have a pathological fracture, usually with a history of minimal trauma. Occasionally, patients will have only minimal complaints.

Lymphoma of bone is typically manifested as a permeative, destructive process on plain films. Areas of radiolucency are commonly found adjacent to radiodense areas. A moth-eaten permeative appearance is common. Because of their rapid growth and the tendency to "percolate" through the trabeculae, most lesions do not demonstrate any periosteal reaction. There will be little to no reactive bone, and the borders of the tumor are quite indistinct. The cortex may be thickened and give the indication of a more indolent process. A soft-tissue mass, often quite large, is frequently seen.[14] MRI is helpful in determining the local extent of disease and subtle changes in the bone, such localized bone marrow edema.

The mainstay of treatment is chemotherapy and radiation therapy, with surgery limited to resection for extensive bone loss or fracture. Patients with lymphoma of bone have a 40% to 50% survival rate at 5 years.[1]

CONCLUSION

Surgical treatment of malignant tumors about the knee requires careful preoperative planning to achieve appropriate oncological results. Skillful skeletal and soft-tissue reconstruction is essential for functional success. Such treatments should be performed by surgeons with appropriate experience. Rewarding results can often be achieved in these patients.

References

1. Dubey P, Ha CS, Besa PC, Fuller L, et al: Localized primary malignant lymphoma of bone. Int J Radiat Oncol Biol Phys 37:1087, 1997.
2. Enneking WF: Musculoskeletal Tumor Surgery, vol 1. New York, Churchill Livingstone, 1983.
3. Enneking WF, Shirley PD: Resection arthrodesis for malignant and potentially malignant lesions about the knee using intramedullary rod and local bone grafts. J Bone Joint Surg Am 59:223, 1977.
4. Gebhart MJ, McCormack RR Jr, Healy JH, et al: Modification of the skin incision for the Van Ness limb rotationplasty. Clin Orthop 216:179, 1987.
5. Marcove RC, Mike V, Hutter RVP, et al: Chondrosarcoma of the pelvis and upper end of the femur. J Bone Joint Surg Am 54:582, 1980.
6. Merkle KD, Gebhard M, Springfield DS: Rotation plasty as a reconstructive operation after tumor resection. Clin Orthop 270:231, 1991.
7. Picci P, Bacci G, Campanacci M, et al: Histologic evaluation of necrosis in osteosarcoma induced by chemotherapy; regional mapping of viable and nonviable tumor. Cancer 56:15, 1985.
8. Rodriguez-Galindo C, Shah N, McCarville MB, et al: "Outcome after local recurrence of osteosarcoma: The St. Jude Children's Research Hospital Experience (1970-2000). Cancer 100:1928, 2004.
9. Rodriguez-Galindo C, Spunt SL, Pappo AS: Treatment of Ewing's sarcoma family of tumors." Current status and outlook for the future. Med Pediatr Oncol 4:267, 2003.
10. Simon M, Springfield D (eds): Surgery for Bone and Soft Tissue Tumors. Philadelphia, Lippincott Raven, 1998.
11. Turc-Carel C, Phillip I, Berger MP, et al: Chromosome study of Ewing's sarcoma (ES) cell lines. Consistency of a reciprocal translocation t(11;22)(q24;q12). J Cancer Genet Cytogenet 12:1, 1984.
12. Weiner SD, Scarborough M, Vander Griend RA: Resection of arthrodesis of the knee with an intercalary allograft. J Bone Joint Surg Am 78:185, 1996.
13. Wold L, McCleod R, Sim F, Unni K (eds): Atlas of Orthopaedic Pathology. Philadelphia, WB Saunders, 2003.

Suggested Reading

Malawar M, Sugarbaker PH (eds): Musculoskeletal Cancer Surgery, Treatment of Sarcoma and Allied Diseases. Boston, Kleuwer, 2001.

CHAPTER 109

Allograft-Prosthetic Composite Reconstruction of the Knee

C. P. Beauchamp • I. D. Dickey

The goal of surgical management of musculoskeletal tumors about the knee is to obtain wide surgical margins and preserve a functional mobile knee, and in general, quite satisfactory results can be achieved.[31] Reconstruction options to attain a mobile knee include the use of an osteoarticular allograft, an oncology prosthesis, or an allograft-prosthetic composite reconstruction, with the latter two being the most common.[39,40] Each method of reconstruction has its advantages and disadvantages. The choice of a specific option needs to be based on a multitude of factors because one method is not necessarily better than the others.

An osteoarticular allograft has the advantage of providing a biological solution to the problem, and in the absence of complications, the results can be quite good.[1-3] The disadvantages, however, can be considerable. Problems with fixation, nonunion, delayed weightbearing, fracture, graft dissolution, ligamentous instability, degenerative arthritis, extensor weakness, and disease transmission are just some of the complications inherent with this method of reconstruction.[4,11,34,37]

Reconstruction with an endoprosthesis has the advantage of being predictable. These implants are modular, readily available, and easily implanted and deal with bone loss very well.[15,16] Fixation is often immediate, weightbearing can be started early, stability is built in,[28] and disease transmission is eliminated. There are two main concerns, however. First is the issue of soft-tissue attachment, namely, the extensor mechanism and the difficulty of obtaining secure, functional fixation. Current metallic prostheses do not provide an attachment surface that has an environment for stable, functional soft-tissue ingrowth because they are a nonbiological construct with the current metal coatings that are being used. Attempts at ensuring soft-tissue attachment to metal have, to date, not been successful. Efforts to reconstitute the extensor mechanism have included securing the native tendon to transposed gastrocnemius fascia or into the fibula. Incorporation and maintenance of appropriate tension are difficult to achieve and often inconsistent. Thus, quadriceps pull is weak in extension of the knee, as reflected in the persistent degree of extensor lag often found in this patient group. The other major potential disadvantage is the long-term durability of the device itself inasmuch as they are often implanted in a young patient population.[43] This is further compounded by the long lever arms that are present on the points of weakness of these devices as a result of the large defects that they must bridge.[25,26,47]

Allograft-prosthetic reconstruction of the proximal end of the tibia combines the benefits of osteoarticular allografts (soft-tissue extensor reconstruction) with all the advantages of prosthetic replacement such that reconstruction of all or part of the extensor mechanism from the quadriceps tendon to the tibial tubercle is possible by taking advantage of the secure allograft patellar tendon insertion[20] (Fig. 109–1). The combination of bulk allograft and metallic prosthesis provides a biological construct to which tendons and ligaments can not only be attached but also be incorporated with time. Long-term durability remains an issue, but many of the major disadvantages of osteoarticular allografts are diminished or eliminated with the addition of a prosthesis. It must be acknowledged that with the choice of allograft-prosthetic reconstruction, the cost, supplies needed, and surgical time can be greater because the procedure is technically more demanding with longer operating room/anesthesia times and a potentially high complication rate.[19,38,41,45] Allograft-prosthetic reconstruction was first performed and continues to be performed in the belief that these risks are outweighed by the benefit of a more biological reconstruction that leads to a better-functioning limb. Distal femoral allograft-prosthetic composites, on the other hand, offer little if any advantage over endoprosthetic replacement.[9,10,29] In general, whenever a bulk allograft is used, there is potential concern regarding nonunion, dissolution, infection, fracture, disease transmission, and serious wound complications postoperatively.[5,12,35,37,41] In addition, if anything less than a fully constrained device is used, instability can become a problem.

Anecdotal information has long purported the superiority of an allograft-prosthetic composite over an endoprosthesis with regard to extensor mechanism strength and subsequent function, which has been the argument used to justify the use of such composites. It has also been thought that an endoprosthesis is subject to functional impairment secondary to weakness of the extensor mechanism reconstruction. What has never been objectively determined is whether there is a clinically relevant difference between these two reconstructive options with respect to validated outcome scores and biomechanical function as determined by gait analysis.[6,38,45] The few studies published to date have primarily looked at the long-term survival of the reconstruction choice and not at the functional difference between surviving reconstructive options. Most of these studies examine and compare outcome scores only, with no formal analysis of dynamic function.[6,45]

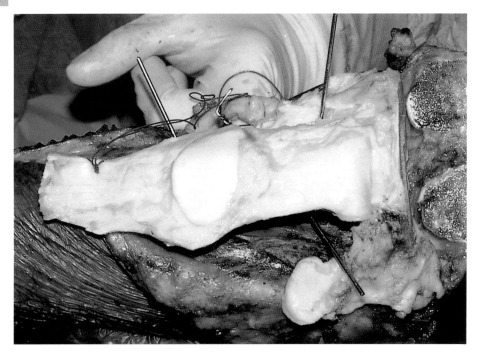

Figure 109–1. The advantage of an allograft-prosthetic composite is the presence of soft-tissue attachments. Here the extensor mechanism can be reconstructed in a variety of ways, depending on the defect. The proximal tibia, proximal femur, proximal humerus, and proximal ulna all require secure soft-tissue attachments.

BASIC PRINCIPLES OF ALLOGRAFT-PROSTHETIC RECONSTRUCTION

Fixation Needs to Span the Graft

One of the major complications of using allografts is graft fracture. This problem is aggravated by graft dissolution. One of the advantages of using a prosthesis with an allograft is that the prosthesis can not only reconstruct the joint surface but also provide graft fixation and maintain the strength of the allograft. That is why it is important to span the entire length of the graft and extend into host bone. Fixation by any means should not stop within the substance of the allograft.[21,22]

Allograft Host Fixation Needs to Be Rigid

Until recently there have been limited options for press-fit fixation. Conventional primary components were fixed to segmental allografts, and allograft-host fixation was accomplished with either a rod or a plate. A locked intramedullary nail cannot provide adequate rigid fixation, and hence the risk of nonunion is increased. Plate fixation provides good rigid fixation but brings with it an increase risk of allograft fracture and fragmentation. In general, avoid the use of plates with allografts. If you must, try to use minimal screw fixation and consider filling the allograft with bone cement to provide increased strength of the allograft. Current-generation prosthetics have a tremendous range of reconstructive capabilities. There are options for stem fixation that include long-stemmed cemented stems, smooth press-fit stems, fluted stems, locked stems, and fully porous-coated stems. Thus far, no studies have compared the various forms of fixation, but

in general, the basic principle is to fix the prosthesis to the allograft with cement and obtain a rigid press fit to the host bone. Fully porous-coated stems are now available around the knee. We have had the best results in the proximal end of the femur with the use of cemented allografts with long porous-coated femoral stems in the host bone.

Avoid Gaps at the Graft-Host Junction

Good contact between the host and the graft is critical to healing. Some authors have championed the need for or desirability of a step cut. We have found it technically very difficult to achieve a satisfactory step cut that is without significant gaps, especially if a line-to-line press-fit stem is used. The ultimate fit of the step cut is determined by the final alignment established by the fit within the host canal. We have found a simple butt joint to be easier to manage. To fine-tune the final fit a small bevel is made before stem insertion on the endosteal side of the allograft on the end that matches the host. When the allograft-prosthetic composite is almost seated, a thin high-speed bur can remove a small amount of bone to allow an exact fit without scoring the implant. A step cut or an oblique osteotomy does increase the surface area of contact, thereby increasing the likelihood of healing, and it provides additional stability. It is ideally used if the implant does not interfere with the final fixation of the graft-host junction (Fig. 109–2).

Cementing into Host Bone Is Okay

We believe that a press-fit stem is ideal, but unfortunately for tumor reconstruction, many patients receive

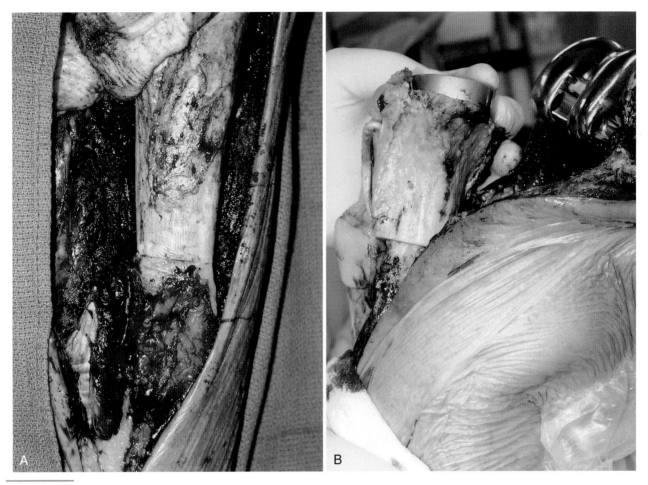

Figure 109–2. **A** and **B**, Appearance of graft-host junctions immediately after the stem was cemented through the allograft into the host bone. The graft-host junction must be a perfect fit and held under compression while the cement hardens.

chemotherapy, which has a detrimental effect on bone ingrowth.[14,23,24] Cementing the composite may be a better choice *if* certain conditions can be met. The major problem with cement in an allograft-prosthetic reconstruction is with the cement technique itself. The usual method described is cementation in two steps, first cementing the prosthesis to the graft and, second, cementing the composite to the host bone. This method results in a poor cement technique in both instances. When cementing the prosthesis to the allograft, it is difficult to contain the cement within the graft without it all running out both ends of the graft. When cementing into the host bone, it is difficult to keep the cement out of the graft-host junction, thus contributing to problems with healing. If cement is chosen as the method of fixation, we cement the stem into the allograft and the host bone at the same time with standard third-generation techniques. Insertion of the stem into the host bone does not have an effect on the graft-host junction relationship, so rigid provisional fixation can be used to hold the graft in place and the prosthesis can be inserted in one step. Thus, it is true that cement should be avoided in host bone, unless it can be used in one step with good pressurization.

Size Does Matter

Infection remains one of the leading causes of failure of allograft-prosthetic composite reconstructions and is a significant concern whenever bulk allografts are used.[35] Wound-healing complications continue to be a major contributing factor to the development of infection. Management of the soft-tissue envelope is the key to avoidance of soft-tissue wound-healing problems. One advantage of using an allograft with a prosthesis is the option of using a slightly smaller graft to allow for a relative increase in the soft-tissue envelope. Accurate sizing of osteoarticular allografts is critical to their success, but the same does not hold true for composite reconstructions. In the revision situation, however, canal diameter does come into play and may be the limiting factor in selection of the graft if a press-fit configuration is chosen. Most allografts are of relatively small diameter with respect to older patients with failed implants, and to fit a press-fit stem of sufficient diameter, you may have to use a large allograft. Fortunately, this does not apply to short distal femoral reconstructions because the metaphyseal region will permit a large-diameter stem.

Soft-Tissue Coverage

With all reconstructions around the knee, good reliable coverage of the implant and allograft is essential. The threshold for the use of local muscle flaps with a skin graft should be very low, and if one must err, it is better to exercise this option than to deal with the consequences of infection.

Anticipate, Anticipate . . .

Anything that can go wrong can and will go wrong. If you do not have the luxury of a large bone bank in your facility, consider the following scenarios. We have encountered all of these problems.

1. Have a plan if your graft becomes contaminated. Dropping the graft on the floor is a disaster. As soon as the graft is brought to the patient, we suture it to the patient with a single safety suture.
2. Are you sure that it will fit? We check all grafts with a repeat in-house radiograph to be sure. Will the prosthesis you have chosen fit both the graft and the host?
3. Grafts can be mislabeled. If we are certain that we will be using a graft, we try to thaw the graft before the procedure is begun. This is not possible if the graft may not be used.
4. Some grafts come without soft-tissue attachments. If soft-tissue attachments are necessary for your reconstruction, be certain that they are there first.

ALLOGRAFT-PROSTHETIC COMPOSITE RECONSTRUCTION OF THE TIBIA—TECHNIQUE

This method of reconstruction has the advantage of allowing for numerous reconstructive options of the extensor mechanism. Any or all of the allograft extensor mechanism can be replaced. We use osteoarticular allografts that are stored with all of the capsular and ligamentous soft tissues attached. The entire extensor mechanism, quadriceps tendon, patella, and patellar ligament are retained with the allograft. Ideally, up to 15 cm of quadriceps tendon can be retrieved with the allograft. The remaining host tissues determine the method of reconstruction. Typically, a constrained rotating-hinge device is selected[28]; however, ligamentous reconstruction with a conventionally constrained implant can be chosen, but this can lead to a risk of ligament failure and subsequent instability. We use a constrained (rotating-hinge) device in almost all cases because otherwise the ligamentous reconstruction required only adds more complexity to an already complex reconstruction.

Choose an allograft of the appropriate length and diameter with the soft tissues attached as described earlier. The graft proximally should be no larger in circumference at the plateau and, in fact, preferably smaller than the resected specimen to facilitate soft-tissue coverage.

Remove capsule and ligaments that will not be used. Use a safety suture through tissue on the allograft and sew it to the patient to protect against dropping the allograft on the floor. The resected tibia is cut at a right angle and a butt joint is used for this method of reconstruction (Fig. 109–3). The allograft is cut at the same distance as the resected specimen. The remaining host tibia is then prepared for the tibial stem by reaming to the appropriate size. The distal portion of the tibial allograft is similarly prepared. The allograft is attached to the host tibia provisionally (Fig. 109–4) by using two specially prepared bone clamps that are fixed to the allograft and host bone with K-wires (see Fig. 109–1). The clamps are simply modified by drilling holes in the jaws of the bone clamp. These holes allow for wires to be driven into the cortex of the allograft and the host bone to secure the clamps to the bone. Such fixation permits compressive force to be applied to the bone clamps. Standard cerclage cables are passed under the jaws of the bone clamps so that with the application of tension, the two clamps are drawn together and provide enough compression at the graft-host junction site that stable temporary fixation is obtained. The K-wires must not penetrate into the intramedullary canal of the allograft or host bone or they will interfere with reaming of the allograft-host composite. The principle is

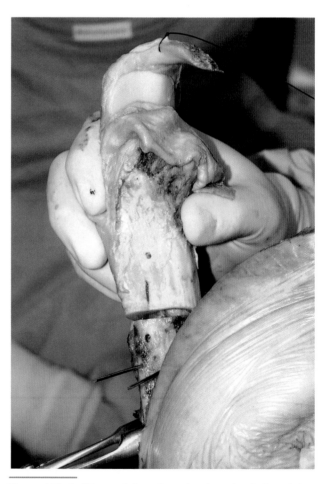

Figure 109–3. **The graft-host junction is a simple butt joint; this allows for accurate total contact and permits compression.**

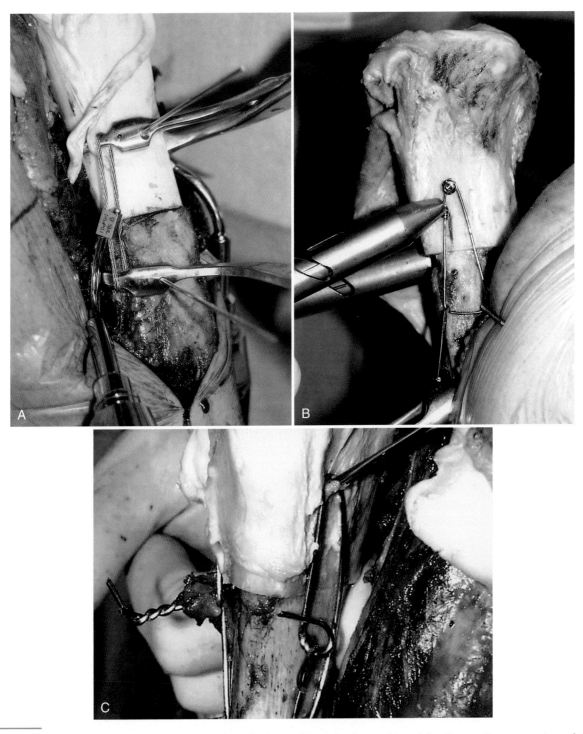

Figure 109–4. **A,** The authors current preferred method to achieve both provisional fixation and compression while the allograft is prepared as though the tibia were completely intact. The K-wires penetrate the bone clamps, and the cables provide compression and fixation; the K-wires do not enter the intramedullary canal of the graft or the host bone so that the canal can be reamed. **B** and **C,** Two alternative methods of achieving provisional fixation with readily available instruments. The K-wires or screws penetrate a single cortex only and do not interfere with the medullary canal.

similar to skull traction. At this point the allograft-host construct is prepared in standard fashion to accept a stemmed tibial tray. Most implants come in stem lengths of 180 mm and longer. After the proximal tibia is cut, use a high-speed bur to remove most of the proximal meta-

physeal bone; the remaining allograft and host bone can be reamed together if necessary. The provisional fixation should be stable enough to allow for gentle reaming. The canal is then plugged and the tibial component cemented its entire length. Cement offers the advantage of allowing immediate weightbearing and predictable fixation with preservation of allograft-host junction compression. It also reduces the risk of nonunion (Fig. 105–5). Allograft union is directly related to the rigidity of fixation. Cementing into the allograft with distal press fitting is an option. The stem is inserted through the allograft and into the host until it engages the host bone distally, and cement is then injected into the prepared metaphyseal bone. The prosthesis is then impacted the last centimeter to engage the cement proximally. The practical issues and possible disadvantages of noncemented distal fixation are worth addressing. Currently, the leading fixed rotating-hinge designs that have the necessary requisite modular stems for the tibial component are of a bone on-growth variety. These assembled implants rely on the hoop stress of the host tibia and the splines (for rotational stability), which are a frequent feature of these designs, for distal fixation and rely heavily on cement for proximal stability. Although this strategy may be reasonable with an intact tibia in the revision setting, relying on the proximal cement mantle in the allograft-prosthetic composite setting where there is a bony discontinuity does not seem prudent given that immediate rigidity is the key to bony union. In addition, the stem is usually highly polished and does not encourage the desired long-term stability via bone on-growth. A long, fully porous-coated ingrowth modular stem is in development by several of the major

implant manufacturers and is available on a custom basis, but this option is very expensive, difficult to obtain, and certainly not available as an on-the-shelf item to provide realistic flexibility in the operating room. Thus, our current preference in achieving reliable host-graft junction union is to cement the whole construct. As other ingrowth stems become available, this implant selection merits re-evaluation.

EXTENSOR MECHANISM REPAIR

The simplest reconstructive situation is when the entire patellar ligament is present. The host ligament is sewn in pants-over-vest fashion[32] to the allograft ligament with the allograft tissue placed deep to the host tissue. More tissue from the allograft can also be used. The allograft patella can be removed, with the periosteum left intact so that a long strip of tissue can be split and passed around the host patella and woven into the quadriceps tendon of the host bone (Fig. 109–6). If necessary, the allograft patella and quadriceps tendon can be incorporated into the remaining host tissue. If the allograft patella is used, it can be either resurfaced or left intact. It has been our preference to resurface it, but we have no data to support that opinion (Fig. 109–7).

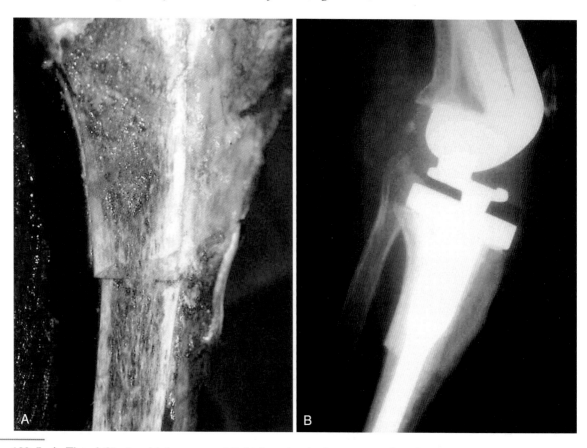

Figure 109–5. **A,** The ability to obtain a cement-tight junction is demonstrated in this patient in whom we were able to preserve his tibial tubercle. This is the appearance of the graft-host junction after the allograft was osteotomized to accept the patient's own tubercle. We replace at least 10 cm of the anterior tibial cortex if we are reconstructing the extensor mechanism through bone. **B,** Typical radiograph of a graft-host junction from a different patient with no extravasation of bone cement.

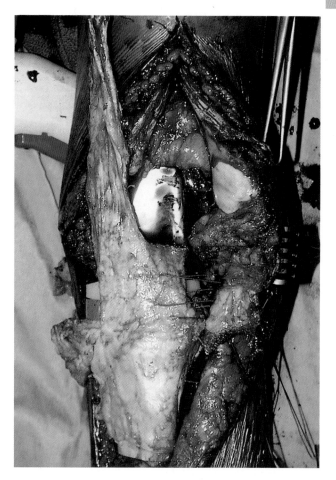

Figure 109–6. Our current method of reconstructing the extensor mechanism when the patient's entire extensor mechanism can be preserved. The patient's own patellar ligament is sewn over top of the allograft patellar tendon. The allograft patella is removed, and the remaining allograft tendon complex is sewn around the medial aspect of the patella and woven into the host quadriceps mechanism.

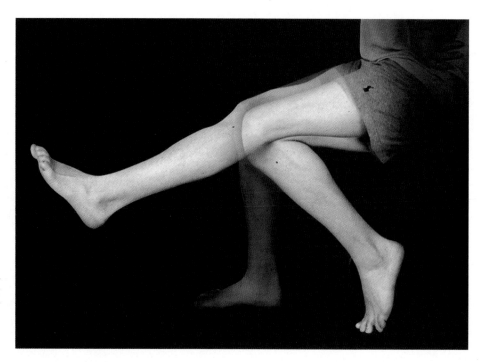

Figure 109–7. Postoperative appearance at 6 months showing a minimal flexion deformity and no extensor lag. Tibial allograft–prosthetic composite for stage IIA osteosarcoma.

ALLOGRAFT-PROSTHETIC COMPOSITE RECONSTRUCTION OF THE DISTAL FEMUR

For reasons outlined earlier we would normally reconstruct distal femoral defects with a prosthesis.[29] Authors have described the usefulness of an allograft-prosthetic composite reconstruction in the situation of a failed endoprosthesis, the allograft being valuable in restoring bone and assisting in issues of fixation caused by loosening, osteolysis, and ectasia of the remaining host bone. The use of a distal femoral allograft may a good choice if fixation options are limited in the host bone because of remaining bone available or preexisting implants.

Select an allograft of the appropriate length and canal diameter that would allow for the fixation method of your choice: press-fit or cement fixation. As in the proximal end of the femur, it is our preference to fix with a press-fit, fully porous-coated stem, with the prosthesis cemented into the allograft. The graft is prepared on the back table in an allograft vise with standard arthroplasty instruments. Ligaments and soft tissues are removed or retained, depending on the level of constraint of the implant that the surgeon chooses. The osteotomy used to remove the tumor is a simple right-angle cut, and the allograft is fitted to the host bone with a butt joint if the entire stem is cemented. A provisional compression system is used as described earlier. This method cannot be used if the stem is press-fitted because the geometry of the stem will determine the fit of the butt joint. In this situation, the stem is first cemented to the allograft on the back table. The portion of the stem that is press-fitted is first coated with a plastic film to prevent cement from coating it (Fig. 109–8). The cement is injected into the graft and pressurized as much as possible, the prosthesis is inserted, and the plastic coating is removed before the cement sets. The resulting composite is then carefully driven into place while making adjustments to the allograft-host interface with a high-speed bur or small saw as the two surfaces are coming together. Supplemental fixation with a plate or onlay struts can provide additional fixation and rotational control. Plates are best avoided because they are associated with an increased risk of graft fracture and resorption. Step cuts provide improved rotational control as well as increased surface area for healing, but the same problem of fit exists as when a press-fit stem is used, and it is the final insertion that determines the orientation of the osteotomy. It is technically challenging to achieve a tight junction. The soft tissues are repaired as determined by the level of constraint selected. A rotating-hinge implant requires no capsular or ligamentous repair.

ALLOGRAFT EXTENSOR MECHANISM TRANSPLANTATION

Absence of the extensor mechanism presents a very difficult problem to manage.[7,13,46] It occurs rarely in oncological situations but is more commonly a problem with primary or, more often, revision knee arthroplasty patients.[8,17,18,27,36] Most common are traumatic ruptures with and without a history of an underlying inflammatory

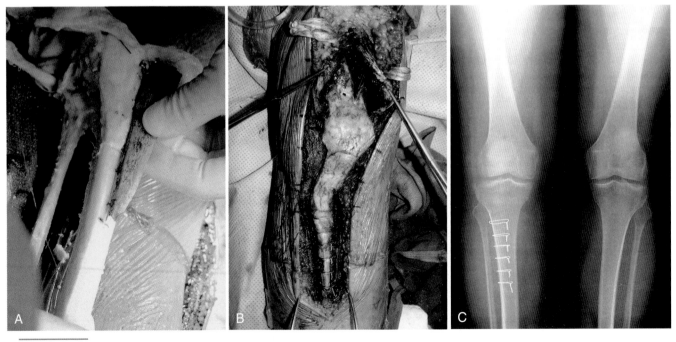

Figure 109–8. **A,** Ten centimeters of bone is replaced with allograft in continuity with the extensor mechanism. **B,** Fixation is achieved with numerous 18-gauge wires without penetrating the allograft bone. The extensor mechanism with unresurfaced patella is woven through the remaining extensor mechanism in a patient with a chronic extensor disruption after a revision total knee replacement. **C,** Postoperative radiograph of the tibial tubercle reconstruction.

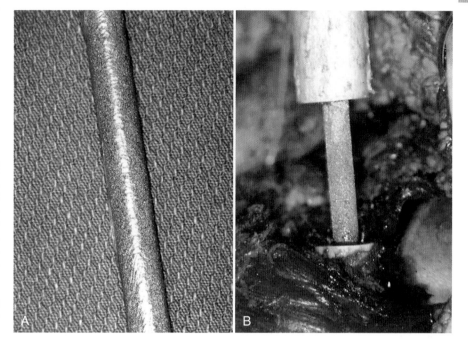

Figure 109–9. Reconstruction of the distal end of the femur with an allograft-prosthetic composite using a press-fit stem. **A,** The stem is cemented into the femoral allograft. To protect the porous-coated stem it is first coated with a thin plastic adhesive, which is removed after cementation. **B,** The stem is then inserted into the host bone. Note the butt joint rather than the technically more challenging step cut.

condition.[30,33,42,44] There are few options available to repair this problem, extensor allograft reconstruction being one. This situation is fortunately rare; consequently, there are few reports on the results of treatment.

In general, attempts to repair this problem with local tissue have been unrewarding.[34] We use a variation of the technique described by Emerson et al.[17,18] If there is a major absence of the extensor mechanism involving the patellar ligament, we replace the quadriceps tendon, patella, patellar ligament, tibial tubercle, and anterior cortex of the tibia with an allograft (Fig. 109–9). Again, as mentioned earlier, the patella is variable with respect to the choice to resurface. Certainly in a patient without a prosthesis we do not resurface it. Approximately 10 cm of anterior tibial cortex is transplanted and fixed with wires. We try to avoid screw fixation in allografts to minimize the risk of resorption. The results reported with this technique have been quite satisfactory, and we have not had any failures to date except in patients who have had a deep infection.

References

1. Aho AJ: Half-joint allograft transplantation in human bone tumours. Int Orthop 9:77-87, 1985.
2. Aho AJ, Ekfors T, Dean PB, et al: Incorporation and clinical results of large allografts of the extremities and pelvis. Clin Orthop 307:200-213, 1994.
3. Alho A, Karaharju EO, Korkala O, et al: Allogeneic grafts for bone tumor. 21 cases of osteoarticular and segmental grafts. Acta Orthop Scand 60:143-153, 1989.
4. Barrack RL, Lyons T: Proximal tibia–extensor mechanism composite allograft for revision TKA with chronic patellar tendon rupture. Acta Orthop Scand 71:419-421, 2000.
5. Berrey BH, Lord CF, Gebhardt MC, Mankin HJ: Fractures of allografts. Frequency, treatment, and end-results. J Bone Joint Surg Am 72:825-833, 1990.
6. Brien EW, Terek RM, Healey JH, Lane JM: Allograft reconstruction after proximal tibial resection for bone tumors. An analysis of function and outcome comparing allograft and prosthetic reconstructions. Clin Orthop 303:116-127, 1994.
7. Burks RT, Edelson RH: Allograft reconstruction of the patellar ligament. A case report. J Bone Joint Surg Am 76:1077-1079, 1994.
8. Cadambi A, Engh GA: Use of a semitendinosus tendon autogenous graft for rupture of the patellar ligament after total knee arthroplasty. A report of seven cases. J Bone Joint Surg Am 74:974-979, 1992.
9. Capanna R, Morris HG, Campanacci D, et al: Modular uncemented prosthetic reconstruction after resection of tumours of the distal femur. J Bone Joint Surg Br 76:178-186, 1994.
10. Choong PF, Sim FH, Pritchard DJ, et al: Megaprostheses after resection of distal femoral tumors. A rotating hinge design in 30 patients followed for 2-7 years. Acta Orthop Scand 67:345-351, 1996.
11. Clohisy DR, Mankin HJ: Osteoarticular allografts for reconstruction after resection of a musculoskeletal tumor in the proximal end of the tibia. J Bone Joint Surg Am 76:549-554, 1994.
12. Conrad EU, Gretch DR, Obermeyer KR, et al: Transmission of the hepatitis-C virus by tissue transplantation. J Bone Joint Surg Am 77:214-224, 1995.
13. Cushing MV, Lundy DW, Keating JG, Ogden JA: Patellar ligament reconstruction using allograft patellar ligament: A case report. Am J Orthop 28:263-266, 1999.
14. Dick HM, Malinin TI, Mnaymneh WA: Massive allograft implantation following radical resection of high-grade tumors requiring adjuvant chemotherapy treatment. Clin Orthop 197:88-95, 1985.
15. Eckardt JJ, Eilber FR, Rosen G, et al: Endoprosthetic replacement for stage IIB osteosarcoma. Clin Orthop 270:202-213, 1991.
16. Eckardt JJ, Matthews JG 2nd, Eilber FR: Endoprosthetic reconstruction after bone tumor resections of the proximal tibia. Orthop Clin North Am 22:149-160, 1991.
17. Emerson RH Jr, Head WC, Malinin TI: Reconstruction of patellar tendon rupture after total knee arthroplasty with an extensor mechanism allograft. Clin Orthop 260:154-161, 1990.
18. Emerson RH Jr, Head WC, Malinin TI: Extensor mechanism reconstruction with an allograft after total knee arthroplasty. Clin Orthop 303:79-85, 1994.
19. Ghazavi MT, Stockley I, Yee G, et al: Reconstruction of massive bone defects with allograft in revision total knee arthroplasty. J Bone Joint Surg Am 79:17-25, 1997.
20. Gitelis S, Piasecki P: Allograft prosthetic composite arthroplasty for osteosarcoma and other aggressive bone tumors. Clin Orthop 270:197-201, 1991.
21. Harris AI, Gitelis S, Sheinkop MB, et al: Allograft prosthetic composite reconstruction for limb salvage and severe deficiency of bone at the knee or hip. Semin Arthroplasty 5:85-94, 1994.

22. Harris AI, Poddar S, Gitelis S, et al: Arthroplasty with a composite of an allograft and a prosthesis for knees with severe deficiency of bone. J Bone Joint Surg Am 77:373-386, 1995.

23. Hejna MJ, Gitelis S: Allograft prosthetic composite replacement for bone tumors. Semin Surg Oncol 13:18-24, 1997.

24. Hornicek FJ Jr, Mnaymneh W, Lackman RD, et al: Limb salvage with osteoarticular allografts after resection of proximal tibia bone tumors. Clin Orthop 352:179-186, 1998.

25. Horowitz SM, Glasser DB, Lane JM, Healey JH: Prosthetic and extremity survivorship after limb salvage for sarcoma. How long do the reconstructions last? Clin Orthop 293:280-286, 1993.

26. Horowitz SM, Lane JM, Otis JC, Healey JH: Prosthetic arthroplasty of the knee after resection of a sarcoma in the proximal end of the tibia. A report of sixteen cases. J Bone Joint Surg Am 73:286-293, 1991.

27. Hungerford DS: Management of extensor mechanism complications in total knee arthroplasty. Orthopedics 17:843-844, 1994.

28. Kawai A, Healey JH, Boland PJ, et al: A rotating-hinge knee replacement for malignant tumors of the femur and tibia. J Arthroplasty 14:187-196, 1999.

29. Kawai A, Muschler GF, Lane JM, et al: Prosthetic knee replacement after resection of a malignant tumor of the distal part of the femur. Medium to long-term results. J Bone Joint Surg Am 80:636-647, 1998.

30. Kelly DW, Carter VS, Jobe FW, Kerlan RK: Patellar and quadriceps tendon ruptures—jumper's knee. Am J Sports Med 12:375-380, 1984.

31. Kneisl JS, Finn HA, Simon MA: Mobile knee reconstructions after resection of malignant tumors of the distal femur. Orthop Clin North Am 22:105-119, 1991.

32. Krackow KA, Thomas SC, Jones LC: A new stitch for ligament-tendon fixation. Brief note. J Bone Joint Surg Am 68:764-766, 1986.

33. Larsen E, Lund PM: Ruptures of the extensor mechanism of the knee joint. Clinical results and patellofemoral articulation. Clin Orthop 213:150-153, 1986.

34. Leopold SS, Greidanus N, Paprosky WG, et al: High rate of failure of allograft reconstruction of the extensor mechanism after total knee arthroplasty. J Bone Joint Surg Am 81:1574-1579, 1999.

35. Lord CF, Gebhardt MC, Tomford WW, Mankin HJ: Infection in bone allografts. Incidence, nature, and treatment. J Bone Joint Surg Am 70:369-376, 1988.

36. Lotke PA: Management of extensor mechanism complications. Orthopedics 21:1046-1047, 1998.

37. Mankin HJ, Gebhardt MC, Jennings LC, et al: Long-term results of allograft replacement in the management of bone tumors. Clin Orthop 324:86-97, 1996.

38. Mascard E, Anract P, Touchene A, et al: [Complications from the hinged GUEPAR prosthesis after resection of knee tumor. 102 cases.] Rev Chir Orthop Reparatrice Appar Mot 84:628-637, 1998.

39. Sim FH, Beauchamp CP, Chao EY: Reconstruction of musculoskeletal defects about the knee for tumor. Clin Orthop 221:188-201, 1987.

40. Simon MA: Limb salvage for osteosarcoma. J Bone Joint Surg Am 70:307-310, 1988.

41. Simonds RJ, Holmberg SD, Hurwitz RL, et al: Transmission of human immunodeficiency virus type 1 from a seronegative organ and tissue donor. N Engl J Med 326:726-732, 1992.

42. Siwek CW, Rao JP: Ruptures of the extensor mechanism of the knee joint. J Bone Joint Surg Am 63:932-937, 1981.

43. Unwin PS, Cannon SR, Grimer RJ, et al: Aseptic loosening in cemented custom-made prosthetic replacements for bone tumours of the lower limb. J Bone Joint Surg Br 78:5-13, 1996.

44. Webb LX, Toby EB: Bilateral rupture of the patella tendon in an otherwise healthy male patient following minor trauma. J Trauma Injury Infect Crit Care 26:1045-1048, 1986.

45. Wunder JS, Leitch K, Griffin AM, et al: Comparison of two methods of reconstruction for primary malignant tumors at the knee: A sequential cohort study. J Surg Oncol 77:89-99, discussion 100, 2001.

46. Zanotti RM, Freiberg AA, Matthews LS: Use of patellar allograft to reconstruct a patellar tendon–deficient knee after total joint arthroplasty. J Arthroplasty 10:271-274, 1995.

47. Zwart HJ, Taminiau AH, Schimmel JW, van Horn JR: Kotz modular femur and tibia replacement. 28 tumor cases followed for 3 (1-8) years. Acta Orthop Scand 65:315-318, 1994.

CHAPTER 110

Megaprostheses for Reconstruction after Tumor Resection about the Knee

Mary I. O'Connor

Resection of the distal femur or proximal tibia for tumor necessitates reconstruction of the skeletal defect to restore limb function. This chapter focuses on the use of megaprostheses for reconstruction after distal femoral or proximal tibial resection for treatment of neoplasm.

RATIONALE FOR THE USE OF MEGAPROSTHESES

Options for reconstruction after distal femoral or proximal tibial resection include the use of a megaprosthesis (implant designed to replace the resected large bone segment) or the combined use of a structural allograft with a revision-type arthroplasty implant (allograft-prosthetic composite). In the past, one perceived advantage of an allograft-prosthetic composite was the potential for bone stock restoration. However, long-term studies show that little of the structural allograft actually becomes remodeled to viable bone[9] and that resorption of the allograft and fracture can occur over time.[2] Allograft-prosthetic composites do provide the potential for effective host tendon healing to allograft tendon, a critical advantage in reconstruction of the extensor mechanism after proximal tibial resection, as discussed in the previous chapter. Although new implant materials (e.g., trabecular metal) show great potential for effective healing of host tissue and tendon to metal prostheses, such implants are currently in the design stage.

After resection of the distal end of the femur for tumor, an allograft-prosthetic composite has no clear advantage over a megaprosthesis. In this setting, collateral and cruciate ligament function is best reconstructed with a constrained arthroplasty articulation. Furthermore, a megaprosthesis is appropriate for patients who will receive chemotherapy or radiation therapy after surgery, modalities that would increase the risk for allograft infection and nonunion.

INDICATIONS

A segmental modular rotating-hinge megaprosthesis knee system is appropriate for distal femoral reconstruction after tumor resection. Segmental modular systems allow for intraoperative determination of the implant size based on the extent of bone resection necessary for appropriate oncological resection. A rotating-hinge design is favored over a fixed hinge, which permits motion in only flexion-extension. A rotating hinge allows motion in flexion-extension, in rotation, and longitudinally along the axis of the extremity by permitting some distraction of an inner bearing component with its outer articulation. When compared with a fixed-hinged design, such features minimize stress transfer to the fixation interface and decrease the risk of aseptic loosening.

After proximal tibial resection, a segmental modular rotating-hinge megaprosthesis knee system is appropriate for patients who require postoperative irradiation or have an extensor mechanism that cannot be reconstructed with an allograft-prosthetic composite (Fig. 110–1). Although chemotherapy can retard bone healing at the allograft-host bone junction, administration of postoperative chemotherapy is not an absolute contraindication to the use of an allograft-prosthetic composite in the proximal tibia.

In skeletally immature patients, expandable implants will compensate for the loss of growth from resection of the involved physis. Noninvasive means of expansion have been developed that simplify the use of these implants. The implants are not yet approved by the Food and Drug Administration.

METHODS OF FIXATION OF MEGAPROSTHESES

Fixation of the intramedullary stems of the femoral and tibial components may be achieved by various methods. Cement fixation is commonly used and has been shown to be effective in long-term studies. Cement fixation should be considered for patients with poor-quality bone and those who will require postoperative radiotherapy. Some surgeons will press-fit stems if a good press-fit is obtained intraoperatively.[14] Preliminary results with use of hydroxyapatite coating on the intramedullary stem component of megaprostheses to achieve stable uncemented fixation are favorable.[5,16]

With either press-fit or cemented stems, implant systems will typically have the option of a porous-coated collar on the intramedullary stem component (Fig. 110–2). This design feature is intended to encourage the formation of extracortical bone bridging, or bone that forms between the host bone and this collared portion of the implant (Fig. 110–3). Bone graft material is placed in

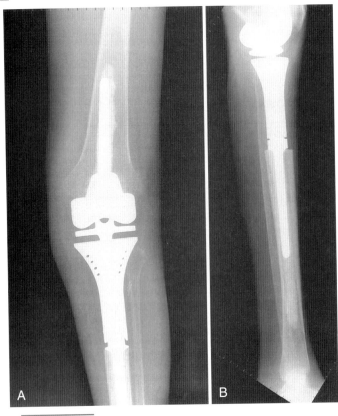

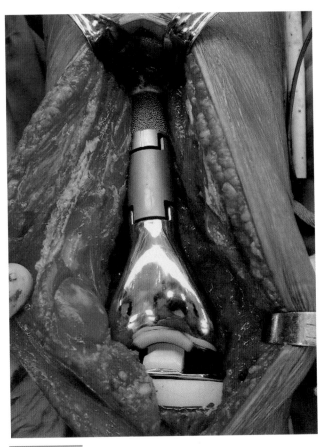

Figure 110–1. Proximal tibial replacement knee arthroplasty after sarcoma resection. **A,** Anteroposterior view. Suture holes in the proximal tibial body to assist with reconstruction of the extension mechanism. **B,** Lateral view.

Figure 110–2. Intraoperative photograph of a modular distal femoral replacement knee arthroplasty. The femoral component is composed of a distal articulating body, an intercalary segment to provide appropriate length, and a proximal intramedullary stem with a porous-coated collar. Bone graft has not yet been applied to the junction of the host bone and the porous-coated collar of the implant. The patella was not resurfaced.

this region before wound closure to promote bone bridging. Ward et al postulated that extracortical bridging between the host bone and implant with either bone or soft tissue may retard osteolysis by preventing implant debris–containing synovial fluid from contacting the bone-implant or bone-cement interface (Fig. 110–4).[25]

The degree of development of extracortical bone bridging has been variable. In the distal end of the femur, extracortical bridging develops more commonly posteriorly[6,13,15] and along the compression side of the femur.[13] Chao et al noted that the total percentage of the length of the porous-coated region that was covered with bone formation in the distal femur and knee was 75% ± 31% in 15 implants with a follow-up of 2 to 21 years.[6] The formation of this extracortical bone bridging stabilized by 2 years after surgery. These authors also found that the prevalence of stem loosening was very low, thus suggesting that extracortical bone bridging improved long-term fixation. Kawai et al noted an association between extracortical bone bridging and higher limb function scores.[14]

Although clinical data suggest that the presence of extracortical bone bridging is helpful in achieving long-term success, the actual bone callus of the extracortical bone bridging may not, however, actually grow into the porous coating of the implant. Lucent lines may be observed between the extracortical bone and the porous surface.[13] Furthermore, histological analysis of five

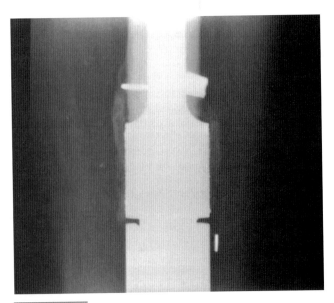

Figure 110–3. Close-up radiograph of the host bone–implant junction illustrating extracortical bone bridging.

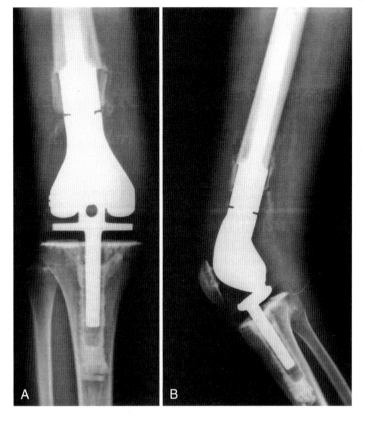

Figure 110–4. Distal femoral replacement knee arthroplasty after sarcoma resection. **A,** Anteroposterior view showing all polyethylene tibial components. The metal inner bearing component allows some longitudinal distraction between the inner bearing and the cemented tibial component. Polyethylene bushings, an axle, and a polyethylene extension bumper compose the remainder of the articular portion. The femoral component, in this case, consists of only the articular body component and the stem. Bone graft has been placed to promote extracortical bone bridging. **B,** Lateral view. The patella has been resurfaced on this patient.

retrieved tumor megaprostheses showed no bone ingrowth into the porous-coated segment of the implant despite radiographs of these implants suggesting bone ingrowth into the porous-coated segment.[20] Rather, transmitted light microscopy showed fibrous tissue between the extracortical bone and the porous coating. Nonetheless, the presence of this extracortical bone/fibrous tissue may increase prosthetic stability. With the application of new implant material that more effectively promotes the ingrowth of bone (e.g., trabecular metal), true bone ingrowth may occur with future implant designs.

A relatively new method of achieving bone ingrowth fixation of a megaprosthesis is compliant prestress fixation. Developed by James O. Johnston, a porous-coated titanium surface with a conical section is mounted transverse to the axis of the femur. Compression of the implant against host bone occurs through Belleville spring washers tightened by a bolt over an intramedullary traction bar. One retrieved specimen showed 70% new bone formation along the bone-metal interface with an average of 42% bone ingrowth into the transverse porous-coated titanium surface.[4] Further experience with this method should be forthcoming.

SURGICAL TECHNIQUE

Distal Femoral Replacement Arthroplasty

Although the degree of bone and soft-tissue resection is dictated by the location of tumor, the extent of quadriceps

removal influences postoperative function. In patients who underwent distal femoral resection for tumor and reconstruction with a distal femoral replacement arthroplasty, resection of the vastus lateralis and vastus intermedius (and preservation of the vastus medialis) resulted in a more physiological gait and more physiological knee-loading pattern than seen in patients with resection of the vastus medialis (and preservation of the vastus lateralis).[1] The importance of these data is in the location of the biopsy: if the surgeon has a choice, the preferred location of the biopsy should be lateral to allow preservation of the vastus medialis.

Primary distal femoral sarcomas should be resected with a wide margin. The entire lower extremity should be included in the sterile field to permit more proximal dissection if needed. A sterile tourniquet should be used. The previous biopsy site is excised en bloc with the specimen. The superficial femoral vessels may be identified in the adductor canal before the femoral osteotomy if there is any concern regarding compromise of the vasculature by tumor. Otherwise, the uninvolved muscles may be mobilized (typically, the rectus femoris and either the vastus lateralis or vastus medialis), with the vastus intermedius left intact around the femur. The medial and lateral intermuscular septum is cut along the long axis of the femur, and a cuff of tissue is left as a tumor margin. The anterior femoral and corresponding anterior tibial cortexes are marked with the knee in full extension to aid in placement of the distal femoral component in proper rotation. The level of the femoral osteotomy is marked, and the vastus intermedius and any additional muscle to be transected at this level are then cut. The underlying vessels are protected during the osteotomy. The marrow at the proximal osteotomy margin is sent for frozen section analysis to confirm a negative margin. The proximal aspect of the resection specimen (distal aspect of the femoral osteotomy level) is then retracted anteriorly, medially, or laterally to facilitate transection of the remaining soft tissues. The middle geniculate branch is identified and ligated. The popliteal vessels are easily identified and protected. The heads of the medial and lateral gastrocnemius muscles are detached, again leaving a cuff of tissue on the specimen. The knee capsule and collateral and cruciate ligaments are transected; this step may be done after the osteotomy to facilitate distal femoral mobilization. Negative margins are confirmed on frozen section analysis. After resection of the distal femur, the proximal end of the tibia is prepared with a perpendicular bone cut as in a standard knee arthroplasty. The proximal tibia is prepared for the stem portion of the tibial component. The femoral canal is prepared for either a cemented, press-fit, or composite fixation application. The patella may or may not be resurfaced, depending on the status of the articular cartilage.[7] Trial components are placed to assess for limb length, soft-tissue tension, and proper patellar tracking. After the final implant is inserted, the prostheses should be completely covered with soft tissue. If inadequate muscle remains, a gastrocnemius muscle flap should be considered. The implant should not be left in a subcutaneous position. A deep drain should be placed and perioperative antibiotics administered. Wound healing takes priority over early knee motion. Typically, most patients gain excellent flexion; active extension is dependent on the quality of the quadriceps remaining.

Proximal Tibial Replacement Arthroplasty

Proximal tibia sarcomas should be resected with a wide margin. A tourniquet may be placed high on the thigh; if there is any concern regarding the potential for more proximal dissection, a sterile tourniquet is appropriate. The biopsy site is included in the en bloc resection. In all possible areas, a margin of deep soft tissue should remain over the resected specimen. The patellar tendon is cut to permit a safe tumor margin while preserving as much length for subsequent repair as possible. The knee capsule, collaterals, and cruciates are cut at the level of the knee joint. The posterior tibial vessels and nerve are protected. Before specimen removal, rotation of the distal femur relative to the remaining tibia should be marked to assist in placement of the implant in proper rotation. The remaining proximal tibia is prepared to receive the intramedullary stem of the implant. The distal femur is resurfaced. The patella may or may not be resurfaced.

The main challenge with proximal tibia resection is reconstruction of the extensor mechanism. With the use of a megaprosthesis, a common reconstructive technique is rotation of the medial head of the gastrocnemius to both cover the implant and provide a repair site for the patellar tendon.[18] The limb is initially protected in extension, and gradual flexion is subsequently permitted. Others have described use of a Trevira tube fixed to the megapros-

thesis by nonabsorbable sutures; the extensor tendon and gastrocnemius flap are then sutured to the Trevira tube. In retrieved specimens from various anatomic locations, histological findings showed fibrous tissue ingrowth into the Trevira tube without a foreign body or inflammatory reaction.[10]

CLINICAL RESULTS

Limited data comparing megaprostheses and allograft-prosthetic composites performed at the same institution are available. Wunder et al reviewed their experience with the use of an irradiated allograft-prosthetic composite or megaprosthesis after resection of the distal femur or proximal tibia for sarcoma. Reconstructive failure occurred in 6 of 11 (55%) allograft-prosthetic composites versus 10 of 64 (16%) megaprostheses. Statistically significant improvement in limb salvage was observed with megaprostheses (95%) as compared with allograft-prosthetic composites (64%). Functional outcomes were also significantly improved in patients with megaprostheses.[27] However, irradiation of the allografts in this series may have contributed to the high rate of allograft fracture (36%) by decreasing the mechanical strength of the grafts. In addition, the smaller number of allograft-prosthetic composites and the relatively higher use of allografts in the proximal tibia may have influenced these results because this location has a known higher rate of complications than the distal femur.

Distal Femur

The results of megaprosthetic replacement of the distal femur are influenced by prosthetic design. Early Stanmore fixed-hinge megaprostheses had a 10-year probability of implant survival of 68% (168 patients).[21] With introduction of the rotating-hinge articulation, stress transmission to the bone-cement interface lessened, and loosening rates decreased.

Using the Kinematic rotating-hinge distal femoral replacement prosthesis, Choong et al reported a 90% implant survival rate at 2 to 7 years in 30 patients, with 20 patients having good to excellent function and flexion of 120 degrees or more.[7] Five- to 10-year results of custom endoprosthetic replacement for tumors of the distal end of the femur showed an 83% implant survival rate at 6 years in 48 patients, 44 with a Kinematic and 4 with a Noiles S-ROM rotating-hinge implant.[23] Slightly better results were reported by Bickels et al with an overall prosthetic survivorship of 93% at 5 years and 88% at 10 years in 110 patients with custom, modular, or expandable distal femoral megaprostheses.[3] Using press-fit stems in a majority of the 25 distal femoral patients, Kawai et al reported a prosthetic survival rate at 5 years of 88% with the Finn rotating-hinge implant.[14]

Failures of distal femoral replacements have been primarily due to aseptic loosening or extensor mechanism dysfunction. Ward et al[23] found greater body weight and poorer range of knee motion to be predictors of failure. In another study from the same institution, failure as a result of aseptic loosening was found to be more likely in men and in patients younger than 26 years at either initial or revision surgery.[26] Choong et al reported nine complication in 7 of their 30 patients, including extensor mechanism problems in 4, post-traumatic periprosthetic femur fracture in 2, post-traumatic aseptic loosening in 1, wound infection in 1, and temporary peroneal nerve palsy in 1. Because of the patellar complications encountered and the lack of functional difference between patients who underwent patellar resurfacing and those who did not, Choong et al recommended only selective patellar resurfacing.[7]

The extent of bone resection appears to influence the survival of distal femoral replacement implants. Cobb et al reported a 94% survival rate of the implant at 10 years with distal resections of less than 40% of the femur versus a 49% survival rate with resection of more than 40%.[8] Kawai et al studied patients who underwent distal femoral resection and reconstruction with a Lane-Burstein semi-constrained-hinge segmental knee prosthesis (Biomet, Warsaw, IN) (82 patients) or a Finn rotating-hinge segmental knee implant (Biomet) (31 patients). Five- and 10-year Kaplan-Meier prosthetic survival rates were 71% and 50%. Univariate analysis showed that patients with more than 40% resection of the distal end of the femur and those with complete resection of the quadriceps had significantly worse prosthetic survival, with aseptic loosening being the primary cause of late failure.[15] Ward et al used supplemental fixation with a cemented interlocking pin through the femoral stem and into the femoral head and neck in patients with extensive bone resection and less than 4 inches of retained diaphysis below the lesser trochanter.[23] Although the degree of bone resection performed is dictated by the extent of tumor, only the amount of bone necessary to provide an adequate margin should be resected to promote implant longevity.

Proximal Tibia

Megaprosthetic replacement of the proximal tibia is not as successful as in the distal femur. Grimer et al reported their experience in 151 patients over a period of 20 years. Nearly two-thirds of these implants were a fixed-hinge design (Stanmore hinged knee, Stanmore, UK). At 10 years the probability of additional surgical procedures was 70% and the risk of amputation was 25%. A very high early infection rate of 36% was reduced to 12% with the use of a medial gastrocnemius rotational flap to provide appropriate deep soft-tissue coverage of the prosthesis.[11]

Others have reported similar poor long-term results, with infection and loosening being the primary causes of failure. Malawer and Chou reported less than a 50% prosthetic survival rate at 4 years in 13 cases.[17] Kawai et al reported a 5-year prosthetic survival rate of 58% in a small series of 7 patients, all with a rotating-hinge implant.[14]

Complications

Complications associated with megaprosthetic reconstruction about the knee include aseptic loosening, infec-

tion, extensor mechanism dysfunction, and mechanical problems involving the implant. Aseptic loosening is the most common cause of failure at long-term follow-up and, as discussed earlier, is related to the extent of bone resection. The rate of infection in more current clinical series ranges from 3% to 8%,[7,14,23] with this improvement over historical results related to improved management of soft tissues, particularly the use of muscles flaps.

Mechanical problems pertaining to hinge design can occur.[22,24] Ward et al studied the association between the length and taper of the center rotational stem and the stability of several different rotating-hinge implants.[23] Their results were that the Howmedica, Techmedica, Intermedics/Sulzer Medica, and Wright Medical Technology/Dow Corning Wright designs required at least 39 mm of distraction before dislocation. The S-ROM rotating-hinge design dislocated with only 26 mm of distraction, and the Biomet knee dislocated at 33 or 44 mm of distraction, depending on the thickness of the polyethylene tray used. The authors concluded that rotating-hinge designs with short, tapered central rotational stems without a mechanical stop to distraction may dislocate in patients in whom bone and soft-tissue resection permits excessive distraction.

Rotatory laxity of the Kinematic rotating-hinge distal femoral prosthesis was studied by Kabo et al and found to be greater than in the nonoperative knee at both 2 and 3 years after surgery, with the peak at 2 years.[12] Residual soft tissues play an important role in preventing excessive in vivo axial rotation. The authors noted that their results implied that maturation of periprosthetic scar strength may vary among individuals and may take 2 years.

Revision of Failed Hinged Megaprostheses

Revision of failed hinged implants is challenging because of loss of bone and functional soft tissues. Revision of a failed fixed-hinge implant to another fixed-hinge implant is not likely to be successful[19,21]; a rotating-hinge device should be considered.

Revision of a failed rotating-hinge megaprosthesis to another rotating-hinge megaprosthesis is often successful. Wirganowicz et al reported second failures in 9 of 48 megaprosthetic revisions (the majority involved the distal femur).[26] Time from the index procedure to the first revision was similar to the time from the first revision to the second revision. In their total series of 64 failed megaprostheses (42 involving the distal femur and 7 the proximal tibia), the 7-year failure rate was 31% for primary reconstructions and 34% for revision procedures. Shin et al reported a 5-year survival probability of revision megaprosthesis about the knee of 72% at 5 years and 38% at 10 years.[19] They concluded that reoperation for failed initial segmental replacement implants is feasible and effective.

SUMMARY

Megaprostheses for reconstruction of skeletal defects about the knee after tumor resection are successful in most patients. The degree of bone and soft-tissue resection is determined by the extent of tumor. As much bone and soft tissue as possible should be spared. A device with a rotating-hinge design is preferred to a fixed hinge. Good muscular soft-tissue coverage of the implant is important to minimize wound-healing problems and infection. Patients should be counseled to avoid activities stressful to their limb. Although the reconstructed knee is not "normal," preservation of the limb in these patients is highly gratifying.

References

1. Benedetti MG, Catani F, Donati D, et al: Muscle performance about the knee joint in patients who had distal femoral replacement after resection of a bone tumor. An objective study with use of gait analysis. J Bone Joint Surg Am 82:1619-1625, 2000.
2. Berrey BH Jr, Lord CF, Gebhardt MC, Mankin HJ: Fractures of allografts. Frequency, treatment, and end-results. J Bone Joint Surg Am 72:825-833, 1990.
3. Bickels J, Wittig JC, Kollender Y, et al: Distal femur resection with endoprosthetic reconstruction: A long-term followup study. Clin Orthop 400:225-235, 2002.
4. Bini SA, Johnston JO, Martin DL: Compliant prestress fixation in tumor prostheses: Interface retrieval data. Orthopedics 23:707-711, discussion 711-702, 2000.
5. Blunn GW, Briggs TW, Cannon SR, et al: Cementless fixation for primary segmental bone tumor endoprostheses. Clin Orthop 372:223-230, 2000.
6. Chao EY, Fuchs B, Rowland CM, et al: Long-term results of segmental prosthesis fixation by extracortical bone-bridging and ingrowth. J Bone Joint Surg Am 86:948-955, 2004.
7. Choong PF, Sim FH, Pritchard DJ, et al: Megaprostheses after resection of distal femoral tumors. A rotating hinge design in 30 patients followed for 2-7 years. Acta Orthop Scand 67:345-351, 1996.
8. Cobb JP, Grimer R, Unwin P, Walker P: Less is more in massive replacements about the knee [abstract]. J Bone Joint Surg Br 76:140, 1994.
9. Enneking WF, Mindell ER: Observations on massive retrieved human allografts. J Bone Joint Surg Am 73:1123-1142, 1991.
10. Gosheger G, Hillmann A, Lindner N, et al: Soft tissue reconstruction of megaprostheses using a trevira tube. Clin Orthop 393:264-271, 2001.
11. Grimer RJ, Patel N, Sneath R: Endoprosthetic replacement of the proximal humerus. Presented at the Eighth International Symposium on Limb Salvage, 1995, Florence, Italy, p 62.
12. Kabo JM, Yang RS, Dorey FJ, Eckardt JJ: In vivo rotational stability of the kinematic rotating hinge knee prosthesis. Clin Orthop 336:166-176, 1997.
13. Kaste SC, Neel MD, Meyer WH, et al: Extracortical bridging callus after limb salvage surgery about the knee. Clin Orthop 363:180-185, 1999.
14. Kawai A, Healey JH, Boland PJ, et al: A rotating-hinge knee replacement for malignant tumors of the femur and tibia. J Arthroplasty 14:187-196, 1999.
15. Kawai A, Lin PP, Boland PJ, et al: Relationship between magnitude of resection, complication, and prosthetic survival after prosthetic knee reconstructions for distal femoral tumors. J Surg Oncol 70:109-115, 1999.
16. Kay RM, Kabo JM, Seeger LL, Eckardt JJ: Hydroxyapatite-coated distal femoral replacements. Preliminary results. Clin Orthop 302:92-100, 1994.
17. Malawer MM, Chou LB: Prosthetic survival and clinical results with use of large-segment replacements in the treatment of high-grade bone sarcomas. J Bone Joint Surg Am 77:1154-1165, 1995.
18. Malawer MM, McHale KA: Limb-sparing surgery for high-grade malignant tumors of the proximal tibia. Surgical technique and a method of extensor mechanism reconstruction. Clin Orthop 239:231-248, 1989.
19. Shin DS, Weber KL, Chao EY, et al: Reoperation for failed prosthetic replacement used for limb salvage. Clin Orthop 358:53-63, 1999.
20. Tanzer M, Turcotte R, Harvey E, Bobyn JD: Extracortical bone bridging in tumor endoprostheses. Radiographic and histologic analysis. J Bone Joint Surg Am 85:2365-2370, 2003.
21. Unwin PS, Cobb JP, Walker PS: Distal femoral arthroplasty using custom-made prostheses. The first 218 cases. J Arthroplasty 8:259-268, 1993.
22. Wang CJ, Wang HE: Early catastrophic failure of rotating hinge total knee prosthesis. J Arthroplasty 15:387-391, 2000.
23. Ward WG, Eckaardt JJ, Johnston-Jones KS, et al: Five to ten year results of custom endoprosthetic replacement for tumors of the distal femur. In Brown KLB (ed): Complications of Limb Salvage: Prevention, Management and Outcome: 6th International Symposium, Montreal, September 8 to 11, 1991. Montreal, Isols, 1991 pp 483-493.
24. Ward WG, Haight D, Ritchie P, et al: Dislocation of rotating hinge total knee prostheses. A biomechanical analysis. J Bone Joint Surg Am 85:448-453, 2003.
25. Ward WG, Johnston KS, Dorey FJ, Eckardt JJ: Extramedullary porous coating to prevent diaphyseal osteolysis and radiolucent lines around proximal tibial replacements. A preliminary report. J Bone Joint Surg Am 75:976-987, 1993.
26. Wirganowicz PZ, Eckardt JJ, Dorey FJ, et al: Etiology and results of tumor endoprosthesis revision surgery in 64 patients. Clin Orthop 358:64-74, 1999.
27. Wunder JS, Leitch K, Griffin AM, et al: Comparison of two methods of reconstruction for primary malignant tumors at the knee: A sequential cohort study. J Surg Oncol 77:89-99, discussion 100, 2001.

CHAPTER 111

Metastatic Disease about the Knee: Evaluation and Surgical Treatment

Timothy A. Damron

According to the latest cancer statistics, at least 1,368,030 new cancer cases are diagnosed annually in the United States.[8] Cancers with a propensity for bone metastases rank among the most commonly diagnosed types of new cancer. Both breast and prostate cancer rank first in the number of new cases for women and men, respectively. Lung cancer ranks second for both men and women, kidney cancer ranks seventh among men, and thyroid cancer ranks eighth among women.[8]

Metastatic disease to bone occurs less commonly about the knee than it does in more proximal femoral sites, but the distal end of the femur is not an uncommon site of metastatic lesions or pathological fractures.[4] Metastatic disease is particularly rare distal to the knee joint, as it is distal to the elbow in the upper extremity. Metastatic disease to the tibia has been estimated to account for only 4% of pathological fractures, although lesions in this location are probably more frequent.[6,9] In part, the less frequent involvement by metastatic disease in these sites presents a challenge to orthopedic management because of the paucity of literature available on which to base guidelines.

In addition, the relatively distal location in the extremity presents its own challenges for both diagnosis and treatment. Both the distal femur and the proximal tibia are composed predominately of cancellous metaphyseal bone, so lesions may become quite large before they are evident radiographically. Supracondylar femur and tibial plateau fractures in the elderly population most commonly affected by metastatic disease frequently occur in osteoporotic bone, thus making fixation difficult even without tumor involvement. The presence of tumor increases the level of difficulty. Currently available fixation devices designed specifically for the distal femur do not allow the surgeon to accomplish the goal of protecting the entire femur, including the intertrochanteric region and femoral neck, from the coexistent or subsequent development of other lesions. Plate and screw devices designed for the proximal end of the tibia carry the same limitation below the knee, whereas intramedullary devices for the proximal tibia may be technically challenging.

Hence, metastatic disease about the knee is a topic of great interest to the orthopedic oncologist and general orthopedic surgeon alike. Comparatively little is known, and much research is needed. This chapter describes the general treatment principles of metastatic disease to bone, evaluation of patients with suspected metastatic disease, prediction of pathological fracture, and surgical management.

TREATMENT PRINCIPLES

Operative management of metastatic lesions to the distal femur or proximal tibia should follow the same principles of treatment as for metastatic lesions to any site. The most important principle is that recovery time from surgery should not outlast the patient's expected survival. Even patients with a 4- to 6-week life expectancy are likely to benefit from improved quality of life if the operative intervention improves their overall function. Although recovery time after intramedullary rodding or plate fixation is relatively short, poor fixation requiring a prolonged period of restricted weightbearing to allow healing does not benefit the patient. Cement supplementation or prosthetic replacements that obviate the need for bone healing and allow full weightbearing immediately decrease the recovery time and benefit the patient. Hard and fast rules regarding minimum life expectancy to warrant operative intervention are less important than an individualized assessment of the patient in conjunction with the medical oncologist and family members. In general, a patient should be expected to survive the hospitalization and a period between 30 and 90 days postoperatively. A moribund, immediately preterminal patient is not considered a good operative candidate.

The corollary to the minimum survival rule is that the operation should result in a stable reconstruction that allows immediate weightbearing and durability for the patient's shortened life span. The improved function and pain relief provided by an immediately stable construct will translate into improved quality of life over the period of limited survival. Although a cemented endoprosthetic reconstruction will usually accomplish this goal, the same ends may often be achieved by internal fixation. In a fracture situation, supplementing internal fixation with bone cement will often allow immediate weightbearing, but fixation durability relies on fracture healing. If the patient survives long enough and the fracture fails to heal, the construct will probably fail. Healing of pathological fractures is slowed both by local disease progression and by radiotherapy, but it is also closely related to the underlying disease process and expected survival. Patients with metastatic lung cancer, for instance, rarely survive longer than 3 to 6 months, so their fractures rarely heal. Some fractures in patients with breast carcinoma metastases will heal, given appropriate treatment, since many will live longer than 6 months. Even the best reported healing rate for pathological fractures, which occurred for multiple myeloma, was only 67%.[3]

The role of methylmethacrylate as an adjunct to treatment of pathological fractures is well established, both for internal fixation devices and for endoprostheses. As a supplement to lower extremity internal fixation devices, bone cement improves pain relief and ambulation over that of internal fixation alone, particularly in metaphyseal regions such as those about the knee. In contrast, when metastatic lesions occur in diaphyseal locations, a number of series have demonstrated the success of intramedullary rodding without adjuvant bone cement. Even in diaphyseal locations, however, cement adds stability to the construct, so its use in addition to intramedullary rodding remains controversial. As the means of fixation for endoprostheses, bone cement obviates the need for healing by bony ingrowth into porous-coated implants, which can be hampered not only by the underlying disease process but also by radiotherapy.

One of the most important, but often neglected axioms for orthopedic treatment of metastatic disease is protection of the entire bone proximal and distal to the lesion (Fig. 111–1). This is especially important when addressing preexisting bone lesions that may progress to weaken the bone or cause fracture, but it is also recommended to prophylactically address new sites that may arise as the disease progresses. With fixation of the distal femur with either a retrograde intramedullary nail or a long-stemmed femoral total knee component, the intertrochanteric region and femoral neck remain unprotected and are frequent sites of metastasis. Failure to consider proximal femoral impending pathological fractures may result in pathological fracture proximal to an internal fixation or prosthetic device. Before operative intervention, radiographs of the entire affected bone should be reviewed.

Finally, radiotherapy should be used postoperatively to protect the entire instrumented region of the bone. When intramedullary reaming is performed, the entire bone should receive irradiation. Failure to irradiate postoperatively leads to a higher rate of implant failure and lower functional benefit overall.[12] Consultation should be obtained with a radiation oncologist either preoperatively or in the early postoperative course for this purpose. When incisions are laterally placed, they can often be avoided by anterior-posterior/posterior-anterior radiation treatment, but incisions within the actual radiation field should usually be allowed to heal completely before initiating radiotherapy.

EVALUATION

Before treatment may be undertaken, the correct diagnosis must be established. The diagnosis of metastatic disease as the cause of a specific new bone lesion in any location should never be assumed unless the patient already has biopsy-proven metastatic disease. The danger lies in incorrectly treating a primary bone sarcoma as a metastatic lesion, with typically disastrous results for the patient and the physician. In the age group beyond 40 years, sarcomas are rare in comparison to metastatic

disease, multiple myeloma, and lymphoma, but they do occur. Furthermore, solitary metastatic lesions from renal cell or thyroid carcinoma may be treated by resection for cure rather than internal fixation, so this scenario should also be given due consideration. Even in a patient with a history of malignancy that has a propensity for bone involvement, the first bone metastasis should usually be proven by biopsy before proceeding with operative intervention. Beyond the consideration of mistreating a sarcoma, some lesions, such as those from metastatic renal carcinoma, myeloma, and thyroid carcinoma, are notorious for being highly vascular. Consideration should be given to preoperative embolization of these vascular lesions.

Primary malignancies with a propensity for bone involvement include breast, prostate, lung, kidney, and thyroid carcinoma, although nearly all primary sites have been reported to involve bone. Most breast and prostate bone metastases occur in patients with an established diagnosis of the corresponding primary, whereas the most common sources for a bone metastasis without an established primary are lung and renal carcinoma.

For patients without an established diagnosis, a comprehensive evaluation should seek any history of previous biopsies or tumor excision, however remote (Table 111–1). Physical examination should also be comprehensive, including assessment of the breast or prostate, abdomen, and thyroid, and may best be performed by an internist or oncologist. Lymphadenopathy should also be sought. Serological examination, including serum and urine protein electrophoresis for multiple myeloma and prostate-specific antigen in males, should be performed along with assay of serum calcium to identify hypercalcemia. Radiographic evaluation, including chest radiographs and mammography, when appropriate, should be done initially, followed by chest computed tomography (CT) and abdominal/pelvic evaluation by CT or ultrasound. This approach will reveal the diagnosis in approximately 85% of patients.[11]

Table 111–1. Key Elements in the Evaluation of a Patient with Metastatic Disease of Unknown Primary

KEY ELEMENT	FEATURES OF METASTATIC DISEASE TO EVALUATE
History	Carcinomas, biopsies, purpose of hysterectomy/TURP
Physical examination	Breast or prostate examination, thyroid, abdominal masses, lymphadenopathy
Laboratory evaluation	CBC, SPEP/UPEP, PSA, LDH, calcium
Radiographic evaluation	Chest radiograph, radiographs of the entire affected bone
Total skeleton technetium 99 bone scan
Computed tomography of chest/abdomen/pelvis

CBC, complete blood count; LDH, lactate dehydrogenase; PSA, prostate-specific antigen; SPEP, serum protein electrophoresis; UPEP, urine protein electrophoresis; TURP, transurethral resection of prostate.

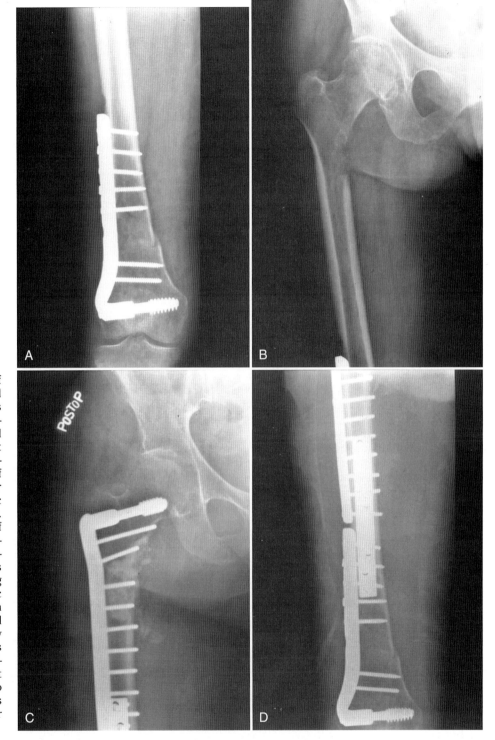

Figure 111–1. Importance of imaging the entire affected long bone and adjacent joints before surgery. **A,** Anteroposterior radiograph of the distal end of the femur in a patient who underwent open reduction and internal fixation of a pathological supracondylar femur fracture with a dynamic condylar screw (DCS) device. The patient complained of groin pain in the early postoperative period. **B,** A subsequent right hip radiographs show a lytic lesion involving the right subtrochanteric femur. **C,** Because of an impending fracture proximal to the already placed screw device, another DCS was placed proximally. **D,** To minimize the stress riser effect at the junction between the two lateral plates, the gap was spanned with a 90:90 anterior femoral plate.

Biopsy, when necessary to establish the diagnosis, should follow the principles outlined in Chapter 106. Submitting intramedullary reaming material as a biopsy specimen during placement of a retrograde nail for a distal femoral lesion is not appropriate when the diagnosis is in doubt. The same can be said for reaming material obtained during placement of a tibial intramedullary nail for a proximal tibial lesion. If the patient is subsequently found to have a sarcoma, the entire knee joint as well as the reamed

portion of the femur or tibia would have to be considered contaminated. A straight, longitudinal, laterally placed extracapsular incision is appropriate for distal femur lesions. However, when the distal femoral cortex is breached medially and there is soft-tissue extension in that direction, a medial biopsy is preferred. The proximal tibia is more commonly biopsied anteromedially. When possible, the defect in the cortex in either the distal femur or proximal tibia should be made through the thin metaphyseal bone to minimize the additional weakening that occurs when the more structurally sound diaphyseal cortex is breached. When biopsy of a small metaphyseal or epiphyseal lesion establishes the diagnosis of metastatic disease, curettage and cementation of the region with or without reinforcement pins followed by postoperative irradiation may suffice as treatment.

Although the surgical treatment principles for multiple myeloma are essentially the same as those for metastatic carcinoma, the diagnosis of multiple myeloma can usually be based on the finding of a monoclonal spike on serum protein electrophoresis or Bence Jones proteins in urine. Hence, biopsy is less frequently needed once the serological diagnosis of multiple myeloma is established.

PREDICTION OF IMPENDING FRACTURE

Prediction of fracture risk from bone lesions is an evolving field, but the classic guidelines suggest that prophylactic fixation should be entertained for any bone lesion that involves greater than 50% of the cortical bone, is greater than 2.5 cm in maximal dimension, is accompanied by a lesser trochanteric fracture, or has failed radiotherapy treatment.[5] However, these guidelines are relatively insensitive and fail to take into account numerous other potentially important variables. Mirels' scale for prediction of pathological fracture is based on four variables[10] (Table 111–2). Each variable is assigned 1 to 3 points based on the relative risk of fracture for the individual lesion, and the total number of points defines the risk for fracture. In his original article, Mirels set the definition of an impending pathological fracture at a total of 9 points, which corresponded in his series to a 33% risk for fracture. Prophylactic fixation was recommended for lesions that meet Mirels' definition of impending fracture. Prospective evaluation of this system has shown its reliability across experience levels, but has also confirmed its low specificity for prediction of fracture.[2]

The distal femur and proximal tibia are uncommon sites of pathological fracture, in large part because of the rarity of occurrence of metastatic disease in these anatomic locations. According to Mirels' scale for prediction of fracture risk in pathological lesions, sites in the lower extremity other than the subtrochanteric region are weighted equally for fracture risk. Hence, both distal femoral and proximal

tibial lesions carry the same risk implications as a diaphyseal femoral lesion. However, unlike devices available for the proximal femur and the femoral diaphysis, apart from antegrade femoral nailing for distal femoral diaphyseal lesions, the devices and techniques used for prophylactic fixation of the distal femur do not allow prophylactic stabilization of the proximal femur, where metastases may subsequently develop.

More recently, the extent of axial cortical involvement has been found to more specifically predict fracture risk in one study.[13] Structural rigidity analysis has been applied by using data from CT, magnetic resonance imaging, and bone densitometry for benign bone lesions, and this technique holds promise for metastatic lesions as well.[7] However, neither of these techniques has been evaluated prospectively, so their use remains confined to research at this time.

ORTHOPEDIC MANAGEMENT

Nonoperative management is appropriate for many bone lesions caused by metastatic disease or multiple myeloma. Some patients require no treatment, but such treatment is restricted to immediately preterminal patients and those whose medical comorbid conditions do not allow operative intervention. Some patients may be observed with only routine radiographic follow-up. Such patients should be restricted to those with small asymptomatic lesions. In general, even small lesions, if symptomatic, should be considered for radiotherapy to achieve pain relief and to prevent progression. When nonoperative treatment is elected, bracing is an option. For distal femoral lesions, a knee-ankle-foot orthosis with drop-lock hinges may provide stability when standing. For proximal tibial lesions, either a similar knee-ankle-foot orthosis or a patellar tendon–bearing orthosis may be elected.

With the preceding exceptions, many patients with pathological fractures or impending pathological fractures around the knee will require operative treatment. The specific procedure is determined by the location and size of the lesion and by the presence or absence of a pathological fracture.

Surgical treatment of metastatic disease of the distal femur includes prophylactic stabilization for impending fractures, open reduction and internal fixation of pathological fractures, and resection with endoprosthetic reconstruction for large lesions or complicated pathological fractures that preclude fixation (Table 111–3) Techniques for prosthetic reconstruction with the use of megaprostheses and allograft-prosthetic composites in the distal femur and proximal tibia are discussed in Chapters 109 and 110.

Prophylactic stabilization of the distal femur may be divided into three areas: distal diaphysis, distal metaphysis, or epiphysis. In actuality, the metastatic lesion may affect more than one of these areas. In these cases, the most distal extent of the lesion often dictates the available options. For the *distal femoral diaphysis*, an antegrade intramedullary reconstruction nail is preferred when the tip of the nail will be two diaphyseal widths distal to the lesion and the distal interlocking screws are in uninvolved

---

Table 111–2. Mirels' Scoring System for Pathological Fracture Risk in Long Bones

VARIABLE	SCORE		
	1	2	3
Site	Upper limb	Lower limb	Peritrochanteric
Pain	Mild	Moderate	Functional
Lesion	Blastic	Mixed	Lytic
Size*	$<1/3$	$1/3-2/3$	$>2/3$

*Proportion of shaft diameter.
From Mirels H: Metastatic disease in long bones. A proposed scoring system for diagnosing impending pathologic fractures. Clin Orthop 249:256-264, 1989.

Table 111–3. Surgical Treatment Options for Distal Femoral Impending and Pathological Fractures

SURGICAL TREATMENT OPTIONS	DISTAL FEMORAL ANATOMIC SITE			
	Distal Diaphysis	*Metaphysis (Supracondylar)*	*Epiphysis (Condylar)*	*Meta-epiphyseal Combination*
Antegrade locked reconstruction with intramedullary rodding	X			
Retrograde locked intramedullary rodding				
Without cement	X	x		
With cement augmentation	x	X		
Plate fixation augmented with bone cement		X	X	
Curettage and cementation with or without pins*		X	X	x
Long-stemmed cemented total knee arthroplasty with augmentations		x	X	x
Resection and distal femoral replacement endoprosthetic reconstruction		x	x	X

*Generally reserved for small lesions or after biopsy for diagnosis alone.
X, viable option; x, limited indications.

bone (Fig. 111–2). This is the only option that will provide adequate prophylactic protection of the proximal femur, including the femoral neck, from a pathological fracture in a proximal bone lesion, should one be present or develop there. Cephalomedullary nails (antegrade femoral reconstruction nails with a tip-of-trochanter insertion site) are an excellent option here.

When the *distal femoral metaphysis* (supracondylar femur) is involved by a lesion that is considered an impending fracture, an antegrade nail is not usually a viable alternative because the lesion extends to the end of the intramedullary canal. The options here include plate fixation supplemented by bone cement, retrograde intramedullary stabilization, and curettage and cementation with or without pins. Options for plate fixation in the supracondylar femur continue to evolve. Traditionally, a dynamic condylar screw has been used when 5 cm or more of distal bone is intact, a blade plate when the distal bone is limited to 3 cm or less, and a condylar buttress plate when the distal bone is even more severely compromised. The recent availability of locking plates provides another option that combines the advantage of multiple potential points of distal fixation previously available only with a condylar buttress plate with the distal rigidity of a blade plate. It is biomechanically superior to a condylar buttress plate in its initial stability and technically easier to apply than a blade plate. Further study is needed to define the precise role of locking condylar plates in the treatment of impending supracondylar femur fractures. In general, metaphyseal bone lesions treated by any means of plate stabilization should be supplemented with the use of bone cement.

Retrograde intramedullary stabilization fails to protect the proximal femur and relies on adequate remaining distal bone to provide secure fixation for the interlocking screws. This technique is contraindicated when there is an impending proximal femoral fracture lesion already present, and care should be taken to allow room for proximal femoral fixation should such a lesion develop later. Supplementation with bone cement may be needed if distal interlocking screw fixation is used. Nuts are available for the distal interlocking screws when bone quality in the region is poor.

Curettage and cementation alone or combined with intramedullary pins has been reserved for small lesions of the distal metaphysis. These techniques are especially appropriate when a small, asymptomatic lesion must be approached for diagnostic purposes only and would otherwise not warrant surgical treatment as a true impending pathological fracture. Aggressive curettage of the lesion should be accomplished to allow the bone cement to interdigitate with intact bone trabecula. Preexisting sites of cortical transgression should be used for intramedullary access, when feasible, to avoid further weakening of the intact bone. Fully threaded Steinmann pins may be inserted into the femoral canal before introduction of the bone cement, similar to the technique used for giant cell tumors of bone. Alternatively, Rush rods or other similar relatively flexible pins have been inserted in retrograde manner through the epicondyles and into the distal femoral diaphysis, followed by distal femoral cementing of the defect.[14] From a biomechanical perspective, these techniques are probably inferior to either intramedullary rodding or plate stabilization. Furthermore, they fail to provide adequate prophylactic stabilization of the remaining femur. Hence, their use should be restricted and done with caution.

Epiphyseal lesions in the distal femur from metastatic disease are rare, and fixation is problematic because there is no bone distally to allow internal fixation. For small lesions requiring access for diagnostic purposes, the curettage and cementing techniques discussed earlier may suffice. For larger, but truly epiphyseal lesions, conventional long-stemmed total knee arthroplasty, supplemented by buildup with cement or metal augments to address the distal defects, may suffice. Although these stems are needed to transfer the stress well beyond the area of deficiency, they are rarely long enough to protect the entire remaining bone. For lesions that involve the epiphysis and supracondylar region, resection and reconstruction with megaprostheses should be considered.

The indications for *distal femoral resection* in the presence of only an impending pathological fracture are twofold. The first indication is when inadequate bone remains to allow secure fixation even when supplemented with bone cement (Fig. 111–3). The second indication is

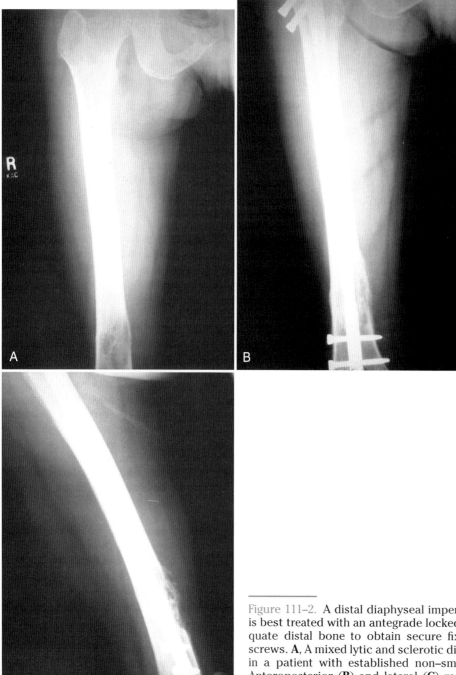

Figure 111–2. A distal diaphyseal impending pathological femoral fracture is best treated with an antegrade locked reconstruction nail if there is adequate distal bone to obtain secure fixation with the distal interlocking screws. **A**, A mixed lytic and sclerotic distal femoral diaphyseal bone lesion in a patient with established non–small cell lung carcinoma is shown. Anteroposterior (**B**) and lateral (**C**) radiographs show the postoperative appearance after antegrade reconstruction nailing. This nail protects the proximal end of the femur and achieves fixation distal to the lesion, but if the lesion had been any further distal, another option might have been needed.

a solitary renal cell or thyroid metastasis, where resection for cure may be of benefit. These techniques are discussed in Chapter 110.

Internal fixation for pathological fractures of the distal femur are similar to those used for impending fractures, but here, the fixation device must provide rigid fixation if it is to achieve the goal of immediate stability. Hence, curettage and cementation alone or supplemented with Steinmann pins or flexible nails is not an acceptable

alternative in this situation. As for impending distal femoral diaphyseal lesions, an antegrade, distally locked intramedullary nail should be used whenever possible. However, many of these lesions are too distal to achieve adequate intramedullary nail length distal to the fracture. In these situations, a retrograde nail may be used, but with careful consideration of the lack of proximal femoral protection provided by this device. In the presence of proximal disease combined with a distal fracture, sometimes a

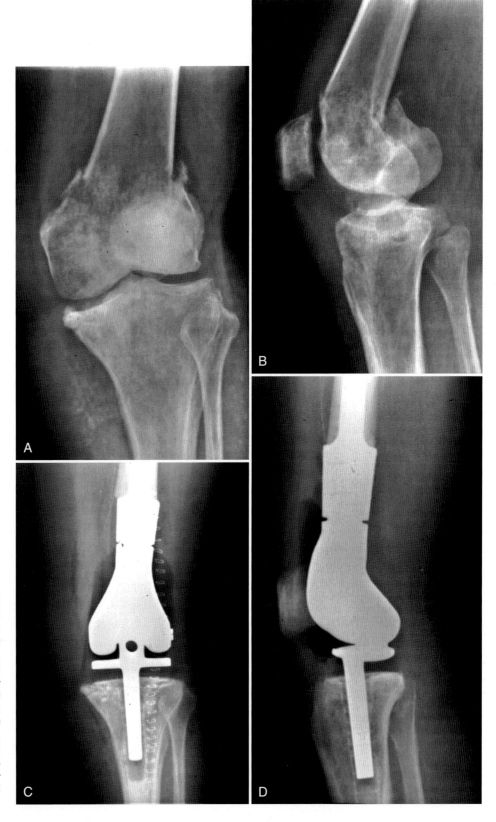

Figure 111–3. Distal femoral replacement should be used for very limited indications, although in some cases there is no better alternative. Anteroposterior (A) and (B) lateral radiographs of a pathological supracondylar fracture of the distal end of the femur. Because of the extensive degree of distal destruction, the patient underwent distal femoral resection with a distal femoral endoprosthetic cemented replacement (C and D).

combination of devices must be used, such as a dynamic hip screw device proximally and a retrograde rod distally or a proximal endoprosthetic reconstruction or cephalomedullary nail combined with a plate and screw device distally. In the situation in which two devices are being used to cover the entire femur, overlap of at least two diameters of the bone should be the goal. The screws in the region overlapping the rod may be angled around the rod, or cerclage cables around or attached to the plate may be used instead. When the lesion is too extensive or too distally placed for even a retrograde intramedullary rod, a plate and screw device is often the best alternative. The options for plate and screw fixation of the distal femur have been discussed earlier in the section on impending distal femoral fractures. The advantage of these techniques, particularly when supplemented by bone cement, is that they have the potential to provide rigid fixation. However, they have the limitation of not protecting the proximal femur, so the remaining bone should be carefully evaluated in advance.

The surgeon must have a lower threshold for *resection after pathological fractures of the distal femur* than for the impending fracture situation when adequate fixation cannot be achieved with the usual techniques. Resection for a solitary thyroid or renal cell metastasis remains an option even in the setting of pathological fracture, although the potential for soft-tissue dissemination increases the likelihood of local recurrence.

Proximal tibial metastatic bone lesions may require operative intervention for the same reasons as the distal femur: prophylactic fixation of impending fractures, internal fixation of fractures, and resection with endoprosthetic reconstruction (Table 107–4). Paralleling the difficulties in the distal femur, epiphyseal and metaphyseal lesions are difficult to address in a fashion that protects the remainder of the bone. The added concern in the proximal tibia is the presence of the extensor mechanism, which must be maintained or reconstructed after resection.

For *proximal tibial epiphyseal lesions*, as for those in the distal femoral epiphysis, curettage and cementing should be restricted to small lesions. Larger epiphyseal lesions that represent impending fractures may be resected and spanned with long-stemmed tibial components on a total knee replacement. Lesions extending into the epiphysis but more extensively involving the metaphysis may be treated either by a combination of curettage, internal fix-

ation with a plate and screws, and cementing or by resection and endoprosthetic reconstruction.

For *proximal tibial metaphyseal impending fractures*, the options include both antegrade locked tibial rodding and plate fixation. If adequate proximal bone remains to provide acceptable proximal interlocking screw fixation through an intramedullary nail, the goal of protecting the entire tibia can be achieved. However, when the extent or proximal location of the tibial metaphyseal lesion precludes adequate fixation with an intramedullary nail, plate fixation is the better internal fixation option (Fig. 111–4). More conventional proximal tibial buttress plates, as well as newer locking plates, are both now available for internal fixation of the proximal tibia. Regardless of the fixation choice, supplementary curettage and cementing are advisable in this location to allow adequate stability for early weightbearing.

When the *impending proximal tibial lesion is located in the proximal diaphysis*, antegrade tibial intramedullary nailing is the technique of choice (Fig. 111–5). The decision to use cement as an adjunct to intramedullary stabilization of long bones is controversial. The more distal and the smaller the lesion, the less likely cement is needed, particularly for stabilization of an impending fracture.

For pathological fractures of the proximal tibia, the options are essentially the same as those already described for impending fractures. However, cementing alone is not a viable alternative. For *fractures of the proximal tibial epiphysis*, resection or curettage of the fractured segment usually requires endoprosthetic replacement. Whether this can be accomplished with long-stemmed standard total knee components and buildup blocks or proximal tibial replacement depends on the extent of the lesion.[1] Fractures through the rare isolated epiphyseal lesion can usually be handled with conventional components, but fractures through lesions extending into the metaphysis often require proximal tibial replacement, which is discussed in Chapter 110.

Fractures of the proximal tibial metaphysis are analogous to supracondylar femoral fractures. Intramedullary stabilization here will rarely provide adequate proximal fixation, so plates and screws, supplemented with bone cement, usually represent the internal fixation of choice. Extensive involvement that precludes adequate internal fixation, however, requires resection and reconstruction. Proximal diaphyseal tibial fractures should be treated by

Table 111–4. Surgical Treatment Options for Proximal Tibial Impending and Pathological Fractures

SURGICAL TREATMENT OPTIONS	PROXIMAL TIBIAL ANATOMIC SITE Meta-epiphyseal Combination	Epiphysis	Metaphysis	Proximal Diaphysis
Resection and proximal tibial replacement with endoprosthetic reconstruction	X	x		
Long-stemmed cemented total knee arthroplasty with augmentations	x	X	x	
Curettage and cementation with or without pins*		X	x	
Plate fixation augmented with bone cement		X	X	x
Locked antegrade tibial intramedullary rodding		x	x	X

*Generally reserved for small lesions or after biopsy for diagnosis alone.
X, viable option; x, limited indications.

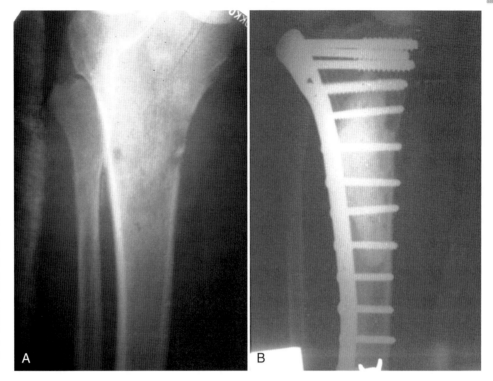

Figure 111–4. This woman with metastatic uterine carcinoma to bone had a painful lytic destructive lesion of the proximal tibial metaphysis with a probable nondisplaced pathological fracture. **A**, Appearance after curettage and cementation with lateral tibial buttress plate stabilization. **B**, Immediate postoperative view.

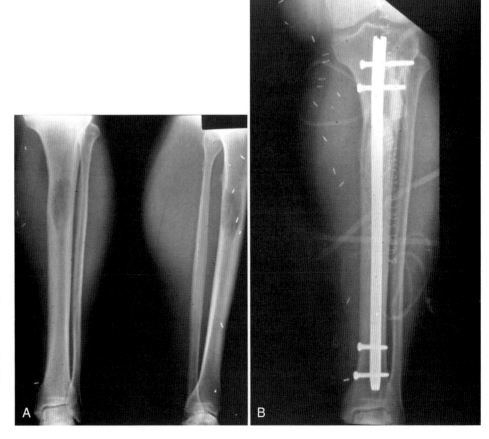

Figure 111–5. **A**, Two-view radiographs of the tibia show a proximal tibial diaphyseal lytic lesion in a patient with multiple bone metastases from a renal primary. **B**, A postoperative radiograph shows an antegrade intramedullary locked rod in place.

intramedullary stabilization when enough proximal tibial bone remains to allow secure fixation of the proximal interlocking screws. If not, plate stabilization with the longest plates possible to protect as much of the bone as possible should be chosen. Consideration should be given to supplementary cementing.

References

1. Beauchamp CP, Sim FH: Lesions of the tibia. In Dim FH (ed): Diagnosis and Management of Metastatic Bone Disease. A Multidisciplinary Approach. New York, Raven Press, 1988, pp 207-212.
2. Damron TA, Morgan H, Prakash D, et al: Critical evaluation of Mirels' rating system for impending pathologic fractures. Clin Orthop 415(Suppl):S201-S207, 2003.
3. Gainor BJ, Buchert P: Fracture healing in metastatic bone disease. Clin Orthop 178:297-302, 1983.
4. Getty PJ, Awan AM, Peabody TD: Metastatic disease of the distal femur. In Heiner JP, Kinsella TJ, Zdeblick TA (eds): Management of Metastatic Disease to the Musculoskeletal System. St Louis, Quality Medical Publishing, 2002, pp 459-468.
5. Haentjens P, Casteleyn PP, Opdecam P: Evaluation of impending fractures and indications for prophylactic fixation of metastases in long bones. Review of the literature. Acta Orthop Belg 59(Suppl 1):6-11, 1993.
6. Heiner JP: Metastatic disease of the tibia, foot, and ankle. In Heiner JP, Kinsella TJ, Zdeblick TA (eds): Management of Metastatic Disease to the Musculoskeletal System. St Louis, Quality Medical Publishing, 2002, pp 469-477.
7. Hong J, Cabe GD, Tedrow JR, et al: Failure of trabecular bone with simulated lytic defects can be predicted non-invasively by structural analysis. J Orthop Res 22:479-486, 2004.
8. Jemal A, Tiwari RC, Murray T, et al: Cancer statistics, 2004. CA Cancer J Clin 54:8-29, 2004.
9. Leeson MC, Makley JT, Carter JR: Metastatic skeletal disease distal to the elbow and knee. Clin Orthop 206:94-99, 1986.
10. Mirels H: Metastatic disease in long bones. A proposed scoring system for diagnosing impending pathologic fractures. Clin Orthop 249:256-264, 1989.
11. Rougraff BT, Kneisl JS, Simon MA: Skeletal metastases of unknown origin. A prospective study of a diagnostic strategy. J Bone Joint Surg Am 75:1276-1281, 1993.
12. Townsend PW, Smalley SR, Cozad SC, et al: Role of postoperative radiation therapy after stabilization of fractures caused by metastatic disease. Int J Radiat Oncol Biol Phys 31:43-49, 1995.
13. Van der Linden YM, Dijkstra PD, Kroon HM, et al: Comparative analysis of risk factors for pathological fracture with femoral metastases. J Bone Joint Surg Br 86:566-573, 2004.
14. Wilkins RM, Sim FH: Lesions of the femur. In Dim FH (ed): Diagnosis and Management of Metastatic Bone Disease. A Multidisciplinary Approach. New York, Raven Press, 1988, pp 199-205.

CHAPTER 112

Soft-Tissue Tumors of the Knee

Kimberly Templeton

Soft tissue tumors about the knee reflect the same benign and malignant histological features as those at other anatomic locations. However, when compared with other locations, the diagnosis of tumor at the knee may be delayed because of difficulty differentiating it from the more common sports injuries or degenerative changes in the knee. These more common diagnoses occur in patients in the same age range at which soft-tissue tumors occur. In addition, patients frequently relate a history of trauma before the diagnosis of tumor.

CLINICAL FEATURES

Patients with tumor may have a painless mass but, especially with intra-articular neoplasms, may also complain of joint pain, locking, or effusion, further complicating the clinical picture. In a retrospective review of patients with benign or malignant bone or soft-tissue tumors about the knee, Muscolo et al[19] found that 3.7% of these patients had previously undergone an invasive diagnostic or therapeutic procedure for a presumptive diagnosis of a sports-related injury, such as meniscal lesions, patellofemoral subluxation, or anterior cruciate ligament rupture. These patients were re-examined, including evaluation by magnetic resonance imaging (MRI), because of lack of improvement after the initial procedure. Over half these patients ultimately underwent a more extensive oncological procedure than would have been offered on the basis of the original studies as a result of soft-tissue contamination during the initial procedure or progression of the tumor because of delay in diagnosis. Lewis and Reilley,[15] in a review of tumors originally misdiagnosed as sports-related injuries, found that half these tumors were soft-tissue neoplasms, with synovial sarcoma being the most frequent diagnosis.

Soft-tissue tumors about the knee may arise from the surrounding soft tissue and have an incidence similar to that of benign and sarcomatous masses seen at other anatomic locations. Benign lesions include lipomas, extra-abdominal desmoids, and peripheral nerve sheath tumors. Malignant lesions include synovial sarcoma, rhabdomyosarcoma, malignant fibrous histiocytoma, lymphoma, and soft-tissue metastases from remote carcinoma. Soft-tissue masses may also originate from within the intra-articular space and include synovial chondromatosis and pigmented villonodular synovitis (PVNS). Cystic lesions, such as Baker's cysts, meniscal cysts, and proximal tibiofibular cysts, may also be manifested as juxta-articular masses. Rarely, non-neoplastic entities such as calcific hemorrhagic bursitis of the infrapatellar or prepatellar bursae[24] or gouty tophus[2] have been described as mimicking soft-tissue masses of the knee.

The clinical features of soft-tissue tumors about the knee vary, depending on whether the mass is intra-articular or in the surrounding soft tissue. Patients with tumors in the adjacent soft tissue typically have a mass that may have been present for months to years. The mass may or may not have been noted to enlarge. These masses are typically painless, unless there is erosion into the underlying bone or involvement of adjacent nerves. Lesions within the joint may produce symptoms such as effusion, locking, or pain. In addition, PVNS may be associated with recurrent hemarthrosis. Cystic lesions, such as Baker's or meniscal cysts, may also cause symptoms referable to the underlying joint pathology. Patients with proximal tibiofibular cysts may have symptoms from compression of the peroneal nerve. Patients may relate an episode of trauma that initially drew attention to the mass.

The age of the patient may also help in the diagnosis, especially with the malignant neoplasms. Rhabdomyosarcoma is typically seen in younger patients, synovial sarcoma is more common in younger adults, and malignant fibrous histiocytoma is seen in older patients.

EVALUATION

Physical examination should be used to evaluate the location, whether superficial or deep, and the approximate size of the mass. Lesions greater than 5 cm in greatest dimension and deep are more likely to be malignant. However, approximately a third of soft-tissue sarcomas arise from subcutaneous tissue. Change in character of the mass with position of the knee should also be evaluated. For example, Baker's cysts typically become less tense with knee flexion and firmer with knee extension. Position relative to the joint should likewise be determined, although meniscal and Baker's cysts may dissect away from the joint and true neoplasms may exist at the joint line. The presence of a knee effusion should also be evaluated. This may be useful in ruling in or out intra-articular pathology, such as PVNS or synovial chondromatosis, as well as degenerative changes potentially associated with juxta-articular cysts. Distal neurological examination may reveal changes resulting from nerve compression, such as with a proximal tibiofibular cyst, or direct nerve involvement by a tumor. However, the latter is unusual. Proximal lymph node examination may reveal involvement by lymphoma.

Radiographic evaluation initially consists of plain films, which will help confirm that the palpable mass is arising from the soft tissue and not the underlying bone or periosteum. In addition, secondary involvement of the bone can be determined. Subchondral cysts, especially if present on both sides of the joint, suggest intra-articular pathology such as PVNS or synovial chondromatosis. Frequently, the masses are seen as only soft-tissue shadows on the films. Some lesions, such as synovial sarcoma, synovial chondromatosis, and mesenchymal chondrosarcoma, may exhibit mineralization within the lesion. Ultrasound can help confirm the cystic nature of lesions such as Baker's cysts.

MRI can further help delineate the location and composition of the lesion and can assist in the evaluation of lesions whose diagnosis cannot be determined from physical examination and other radiographic modalities (Fig. 112–1). MRI can confirm the cystic nature of Baker's and meniscal cysts, as well as identify any associated intra-articular pathology. These cysts are typically homogeneous, with high signal on T2-weighted images. However, there may be some heterogeneity because of hemorrhage or debris. If the image is not characteristic, especially if there is no associated intra-articular pathology, the diagnosis of meniscal or Baker's cysts should be made with caution.[18] MRI may confirm the cartilaginous nature of synovial chondromatosis, which may or may not be mineralized and detected on plain films. Lipomas are easily detected with MRI; they should have the same appearance as subcutaneous tissue, especially on fat-suppressed sequences. Most other soft-tissue masses do not have a characteristic appearance on MRI. Enhancement of the lesion with gadolinium helps confirm the neoplastic nature of the lesion. Heterogeneity, as well as involvement of adjacent tissue, is suggestive, but not diagnostic of malignancy.

When the diagnosis remains in question after MRI or malignancy is suspected, the histology should be confirmed by biopsy. The biopsy may be either needle or open, depending on the clinical situation, comfort of the pathologist in working with the small amount of tissue obtained with a needle biopsy, or the need for tissue for additional studies. Whichever method of biopsy is chosen, the location of the biopsy should be planned so that it is in an area that can be easily excised at the time of definitive surgery if the tumor proves to be malignant. For open biopsies, the incision should be longitudinal, and soft-tissue flaps should not be developed to decrease the degree of surrounding soft-tissue contamination.

DIFFERENTIAL DIAGNOSIS

Cystic Lesions

Cystic lesions adjacent to the knee may reflect involvement of the bursae related to the patella, pes anserinus, iliotibial band, or collateral ligaments.[17] However, symptomatic cysts are more commonly found in the popliteal space (Baker's cyst), at the joint line (meniscal cysts), or within the joint (intra-articular ganglion cysts). The first two are typically associated with intra-articular pathology.

Baker's cysts typically arise in adults between the tendons of the semimembranosus and medial head of the gastrocnemius (Fig. 112–2). The prevalence of Baker's cysts increases with age. These cysts are filled with joint

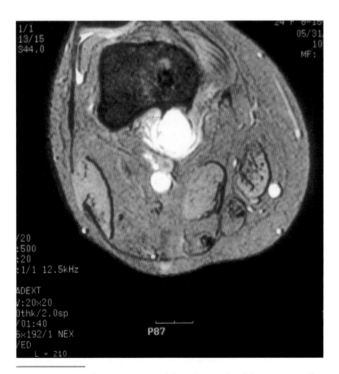

Figure 112–1. Sixteen-year-old with a palpable mass in the popliteal fossa. A T2-weighted axial view shows a lesion arising from the posterior aspect of the femur, consistent with a periosteal chondroma.

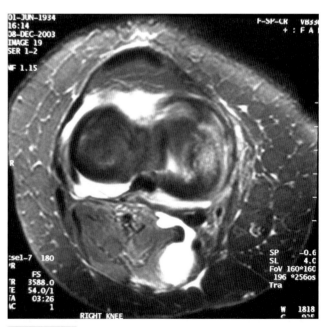

Figure 112–2. T2-weighted axial image of the knee demonstrating a Baker's cyst emanating between the semimembranosus and medial head of the gastrocnemius.

fluid and reflect intra-articular pathology such as meniscal tears or degenerative joint disease. In patients with Baker's cysts, 82% are found on MRI to have an associated meniscal tear, most commonly medial, and 13% to have a tear of the anterior cruciate ligament.[10] Adult patients may complain of aching and a feeling of fullness in the posterior aspect of the knee, as well as symptoms from the associated knee pathology.[4] Rupture of the cysts can cause acute pain and swelling in the posterior aspect of the knee and leg. Treatment of cysts in adults is targeted at the underlying joint pathology. In a follow-up study of patients treated arthroscopically for intra-articular lesions without addressing the popliteal cysts, chondral lesions were the most relevant prognostic factor for persistence of the cyst.[21] If the cyst persists and remains symptomatic, open excision, with suturing or cauterization of the stalk emanating from the joint, may be undertaken.

Unlike adults, popliteal cysts in pediatric patients are not usually associated with intra-articular pathology. Patients typically have a mass in the posterior medial aspect of the knee. In pediatric patients, these cysts are usually asymptomatic. Popliteal cysts in children generally resolve and do not require operative intervention.

Meniscal cysts are located more medial or lateral than a popliteal cyst. They are typically, but not exclusively associated with a meniscal tear. The diagnosis is more straightforward if the lesion is homogeneous on MRI. The lesions may be lobulated and septate.[23] Treatment is aimed at the underlying meniscal pathology.

Intra-articular ganglion cysts are not associated with other intra-articular pathology. They may be found in the infrapatellar fat pad, adjacent to the anterior cruciate ligament, or adjacent to the posterior cruciate ligament, with the latter being the most common in the series by Kim et al.[13] The clinical findings of intra-articular ganglion cysts vary according to the location of the cyst. Lesions in the infrapatellar fat pad may be characterized by a palpable mass. Patients with cysts in the intercondylar notch may have pain, especially in a squatting position.[13] Patients may also have symptoms of knee locking. MRI is typically diagnostic in these cases, with the cysts usually demonstrating homogeneous high signal on T2-weighted images. Symptomatic cysts may be removed via an open procedure or arthroscopically.

In a review of 654 MRI scans of the knee, the prevalence of proximal tibiofibular cysts was found to be 0.76%.[12] Only half of these cysts were symptomatic. When proximal tibiofibular joint cysts are symptomatic, an anterior soft-tissue mass is typically present (Fig. 112–3). With time, these cysts may lead to compromise of peroneal nerve function. Removal of these cysts may require dissection of the cyst from the epineurium[5] but can lead to recovery of at least some degree of nerve function.

Intra-articular Pathology

PVNS is a condition of unknown etiology, with both inflammatory and neoplastic causes suggested. Its propensity for local recurrence, including recurrence in the subcutaneous tissue adjacent to arthroscopy portals,[16] may

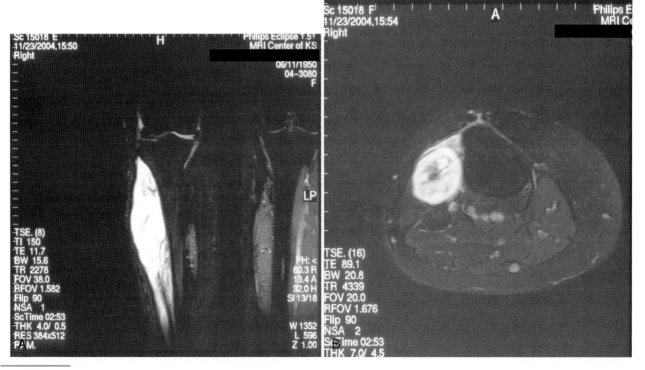

Figure 112–3. **A,** Coronal T2-weighted image showing a cystic structure arising from the proximal tibiofibular joint. The patient had a painful anterior leg mass and footdrop. **B,** Axial T2-weighted image of the proximal part of the leg showing the cyst in the anterior compartment compressing the deep peroneal nerve.

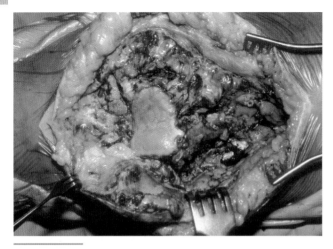

Figure 112–4. Intraoperative appearance of pigmented villonodular synovitis demonstrating extensive involvement of the knee.

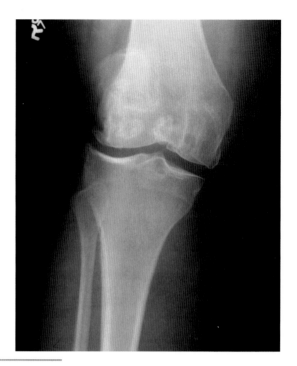

Figure 112–5. Anteroposterior radiograph of the knee in a 45-year-old women with recurrent pigmented villonodular synovitis. Subchondral cysts and marginal osteophytes are seen on the femur and tibia.

point toward a neoplastic origin. It can affect any joint, with involvement of the knee being the most frequent. PVNS may occur in a localized or diffuse form (Fig. 112–4). Patients typically have recurrent knee swelling (hemarthrosis) and pain. Making the diagnosis can be difficult, with an average delay of longer than 4 years.[9] Plain films do not demonstrate any mineralized lesions, which helps distinguish PVNS from synovial chondromatosis. MRI typically demonstrates a knee effusion, as well as multiple intra-articular masses that are low signal on T1- and T2-weighted images because of the presence of hemosiderin.[23] This appearance of hemosiderin is considered diagnostic for PVNS. Erosion into adjacent bone may be seen on both plain films and MRI, although bone involvement is less common in the knee than in other joints such as the hip. Bone involvement is thought to be due to the presence of a narrow joint space (Fig. 112–5).[3] However, Uchibori et al[25] found increased production of matrix metalloproteinases 1 and 9, thus suggesting an additional mechanism for bone and cartilage loss in PVNS. Treatment requires removal of the abnormal tissue, either a discrete mass and subtotal synovectomy in the localized form or total synovectomy in the more diffuse form. Removal may be accomplished through either open or arthroscopic procedures. Arthroscopy is less invasive, with more rapid rehabilitation and decreased risk of joint stiffness, but in some cases it may not provide adequate exposure, especially with diffuse disease. Some patients may require both anterior and posterior approaches, particularly for lesions adjacent or posterior to the posterior cruciate ligament.

PVNS has a propensity for local recurrence, especially in the diffuse form. Zvijac et al[28] reported a 14% local recurrence rate after arthroscopic partial or total synovectomy, all of the recurrences occurring in patients with diffuse disease. Adjuvant therapy, such as external beam radiotherapy or radiosynovectomy, has been suggested for the treatment of diffuse or recurrent PVNS. In a small series, Shabat et al[22] found no complications with the use of yttrium 90 after synovectomy, and all patients achieved excellent results. de Visser et al[8] reported an equal distribution of excellent and fair functional results after radiosynovectomy for recurrent disease. However, in a retrospective study of 40 patients with primary or recurrent diffuse PVNS treated by open synovectomy with or without adjuvant radiotherapy, Kingsley et al[14] reported an 18% local recurrence rate. All recurrences in this series were in patients receiving radiosynovectomy or external beam radiation therapy.

Primary synovial chondromatosis is a condition characterized by the metaplastic formation of cartilaginous nodules in the synovium (Fig 112–6).[7] It is typically monarticular. Symptoms include joint pain, swelling, and occasional mechanical symptoms. Plain radiographs may show nodules with stippled calcification within the joint, along with occasional secondary degenerative changes. However, these nodules are calcified/ossified in only two-thirds of cases. Nodules that are more cellular histologically are less likely to be calcified or ossified. The cartilaginous nature of the lesions can be confirmed by MRI, especially lesions not well visualized on plain films. The lesions demonstrate heterogeneous high signal on T2-weighted images, with areas of signal void reflecting calcification/ossification. Treatment consists of removing the loose bodies and/or partial synovectomy. Davis et al[7] reported a 15% local recurrence rate, which they thought was due to inadequate removal of loose bodies and/or involved synovium. Malignant degeneration to secondary chondrosarcoma is rare. Multiple recurrences or rapid deterioration in symptoms may indicate malignant degeneration.[7]

Other lesions reported in the knee include those composed of fat, both solitary intra-articular lipomas and the

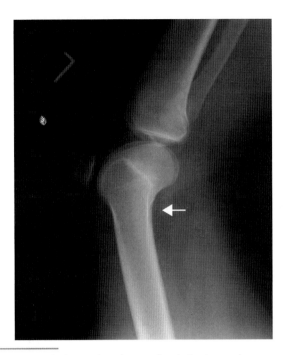

Figure 112–6. Lateral radiograph of the knee demonstrating a mineralized lesion posterior to the knee (arrow), consistent with synovial chondromatosis. At the time of surgery, multiple smaller lesions were found within the joint.

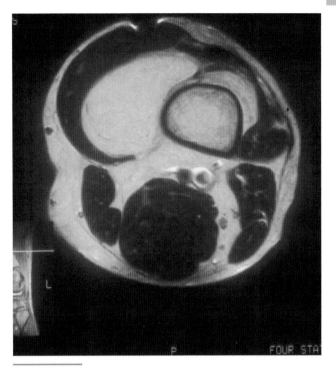

Figure 112–7. T1-weighted axial image of the distal part of the thigh showing a fatty lesion deep to the vastus medialis, consistent with lipoma.

more diffuse lipoma arborescens. Patients with intra-articular lipomas typically complain of a painless soft-tissue mass, mild joint swelling, and pain.[27] Rarely, they may experience acute locking of the knee, especially if the mass is located within the intercondylar notch. These lesions are uncommon and thought to arise from tissue adjacent to the cruciate ligaments. Lipoma arborescens is a more common condition, but of unknown etiology. It is thought to be a reactive process associated with inflammatory, traumatic, or degenerative joint disease. Lipoma arborescens is characterized by replacement of subsynovial tissue by mature fat, which results in villous proliferation of the synovium.[26] This proliferation is most commonly found in the suprapatellar and lateral recesses of the knee. Patients typically have a slow-growing painless mass and intermittent joint effusion. Both these entities are readily diagnosed by their MRI appearance. Lipoma arborescens can be differentiated from PVNS on MRI by its high signal on T1-weighted images as a result of the lipomatous nature of the former lesion.

Benign Soft-Tissue Neoplasms

Benign soft-tissue masses may occur adjacent to the knee in a proportion similar to that in other anatomic locations. Lipomas, hemangiomas, extra-abdominal desmoid tumors, and schwannomas commonly occur in this area. The first two are typically superficial. However, they may arise from deeper structures originating in the thigh, whether intramuscular or intermuscular, with extension to the level of the knee. These masses are usually painless and exhibit gradual, if any increase in size. Approximately one-eighth of extra-abdominal desmoids occur in the thigh or popliteal fossa.[6] These tumors may slowly increase in size and are firm to palpation on initial evaluation. The tumors may result in distal neurological or vascular compromise if they originate in the popliteal fossa. Schwannomas are typically slowly enlarging masses. Despite their location adjacent to nerves, they are usually painless without demonstration of distal neurological compromise. These may arise from large or small nerves.

MRI is useful in the evaluation of these tumors. Lipomas should be homogeneous high signal on T1-weighted images, with occasional demonstration of septations (Fig. 112–7). They should be uniformly low signal on fat-suppressed images. If there are areas of heterogeneity on T1-weighted images or areas of high signal on fat-suppressed images, the diagnosis of lipoma should be questioned. Extra-abdominal desmoids show low signal intensity on both T1- and T2-weighted images. However, this appearance is not diagnostic and requires biopsy for confirmation. MRI may also be suggestive of a schwannoma because the mass is seen to be adjacent to a nerve. There may be cystic areas noted within the schwannoma, especially in larger lesions.

Treatment of benign soft-tissue masses of the knee is identical to treatment in other locations. Other confounding factors, however, are potential involvement of the popliteal structures. If diagnosis of the lesion is confirmed by MRI, such as with a lipoma, and the lesion is asymptomatic and not enlarging, observation is warranted. If the diagnosis is confirmed but the lesion is symptomatic or enlarging, marginal resection is the treat-

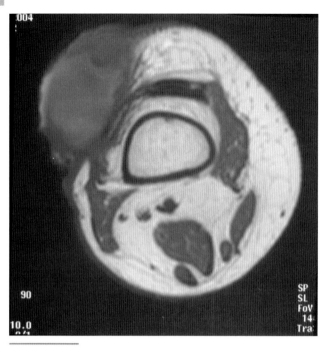

Figure 112–8. T1-weighted axial image of the distal part of the thigh showing a lateral, superficial, heterogeneous lesion. The pathological diagnosis was malignant fibrous histiocytoma.

ment of choice, except in the case of desmoids, for which wide margins should be attempted. If the diagnosis is not certain, biopsy is recommended.

Malignant Soft-Tissue Tumors

Malignant tumors reflect the histological findings described in other locations. These tumors may arise from the adjacent muscle, such as rhabdomyosarcoma in children, synovial sarcoma in adolescents and young adults, and malignant fibrous histiocytoma (Fig. 112–8) or liposarcoma in older adults. Occasionally, lesions may originate in the popliteal fossa, such as malignant peripheral nerve sheath tumors. Malignant lesions rarely arise from within the joint; tumors reported in this location have been synovial chondrosarcoma and synovial sarcoma.[20] The tumors as initially seen as enlarging masses. They are usually pain-free, unless there is involvement of the adjacent neurovascular or bony structures. MRI of these lesions demonstrates heterogeneity, seen best on T2-weighted images. However, this appearance is not diagnostic. Staging studies to evaluate for potential metastatic disease are performed in patients with lesions that are worrisome for sarcoma. Specifically, computed tomography of the chest is performed because soft-tissue sarcomas primarily metastasize via a hematogenous route. Histological diagnosis is obtained after open or needle biopsy.

Options for treatment of soft-tissue sarcoma include amputation and limb salvage. With adequate treatment, both have statistically equivalent rates of overall survival.

If wide resection of the tumor would leave adequate tissue for limb function, limb-sparing resection is preferred. If only a marginal surgical margin can be obtained because of the proximity of neurovascular structures, limb salvage may still be appropriate if adjuvant radiotherapy can be administered. In addition, vascular bypass/reconstruction may be performed if a wide resection necessitates en bloc removal of a segment of blood vessel(s). Preoperative radiation therapy necessitates resection through an irradiated bed, with an increased risk for wound complications. Postoperative radiation therapy requires irradiation of the entire tumor bed exposed at the time of surgery, thereby resulting in a larger volume of irradiated tissue and increased risk for long-term complications such as lymphedema. Chemotherapy is an additional modality to consider. However, the impact of chemotherapy on local recurrence or long-term survival has not been definitively elucidated. It may be considered in patients with large, deep-seated, high-grade tumors.

Additional factors must be considered when contemplating limb salvage for tumors around the knee. The proximity of the neurovascular structures in the popliteal fossa may make wide resection difficult, if not impossible. In addition, irradiation in this area may lead to loss of nerve function, especially the peroneal nerve.[1] There may also be fibrosis of the joint capsule leading to decreased range of motion of the knee. Moreover, the proximity of the physes of the distal femur and proximal tibia may place them at risk of injury. Fletcher et al[11] reported on the development of varus and valgus deformities of the knees in children treated for synovial sarcoma with brachytherapy or external beam radiation.

SUMMARY

Soft-tissue tumors of the knee may present diagnostic challenges because typical symptoms such as pain and swelling may be attributed to more common conditions, such as intra-articular injury or arthritis. Symptoms out of proportion to a reported traumatic episode or that persist longer than anticipated warrant further evaluation. The presence of a palpable soft-tissue mass, either at the joint itself or in adjacent soft tissue, should also lead to further diagnostic evaluation. Frequently, plain films may be diagnostic, such as in the case of synovial chondromatosis. In some instances, other modalities such as MRI may be needed. Treatment of benign and malignant soft-tissue masses is similar to that in other anatomic locations. In the case of malignant tumors, however, limb salvage may be complicated by the proximity of the vessels and nerves in the popliteal fossa, as well as the femoral and tibial physes in children.

References

1. Alektiar KM, McKee AB, Jacobs JM, et al: Outcome of primary soft tissue sarcoma of the knee and elbow. Int J Radiat Oncol Biol Phys 54:163-169, 2002.

2. Bond JR, Sim FH, Sundaram M: Radiologic case study: Gouty tophus involving the distal quadriceps tendon. Orthopedics 27:90-92, 2004.

3. Cheng XG, You YH, Liu W, et al: MRI features of pigmented villonodular synovitis (PVNS). Clinical Rheumatol 23:31-34, 2004.

4. Curl WW: Popliteal cysts: Historical background and current knowledge. J Am Acad Orthop Surg 4:129-133, 1996.

5. Damron TA, Rock MG: Unusual manifestations of proximal tibiofibular joint synovial cysts. Orthopedics 20:225-230, 1997.

6. Damron TA, Sim FH: Soft-tissue tumors about the knee. J Am Acad Orthop Surg 5:141-152, 1997.

7. Davis RI, Hamilton A, Biggart JD: Primary synovial chondromatosis: A clinicopathologic review and assessment of malignant potential. Hum Pathol 29:683-688, 1998.

8. de Visser E, Veth RP, Pruszczynski M, et al: Diffuse and localized pigmented villonodular synovitis: Evaluation and treatment of 38 patients. Arch Orthop Trauma Surg 119:401-404, 1999.

9. Edwards MR, Tibrewal S: Patello-femoral joint pain due to unusual location of localized pigmented villonodular synovitis—a case report. Knee 11:327-329, 2004.

10. Fielding JR, Franklin PD, Kustan J: Popliteal cysts: A reassessment using magnetic resonance imaging. Skeletal Radiol 20:433-435, 1991.

11. Fletcher DT, Warner WC, Neel MD, Merchant TE: Valgus and varus deformity after wide-local excision, brachytherapy and external beam irradiation in two children with lower extremity synovial cell sarcoma: Case report. BMC Cancer 4:57, 2004.

12. Ilahi OA, Younas SA, Labbe MR, Edson SB: Prevalence of ganglion cysts originating from the proximal tibiofibular joint: A magnetic resonance imaging study. Arthroscopy 19:150-153, 2003.

13. Kim MG, Kim BH, Choi JA, et al: Intra-articular ganglion cysts of the knee: Clinical and MR imaging features. Eur Radiol 11:834-840, 2001.

14. Kingsley RC, Barr SJ, Winalski C, et al: Treatment of advanced primary and recurrent diffuse pigmented villonodular synovitis of the knee. J Bone Joint Surg Am 84:2192-2202, 2002.

15. Lewis MM, Reilly JF: Sports tumors. Am J Sports Med 15:362-365, 1987.

16. Lu KH: Subcutaneous pigmented villonodular synovitis caused by portal contamination during knee arthroscopy and open synovectomy. Arthroscopy 20:9-13, 2004.

17. McCarthy CL, McNally EG: The MRI appearance of cystic lesions around the knee. Skeletal Radiol 33:187-209, 2004.

18. Mountney J, Thomas NP: When is a meniscal cyst not a meniscal cyst? Knee 2:133-136, 2004.

19. Muscolo DL, Ayerza MA, Makino A, et al: Tumors about the knee misdiagnosed as athletic injuries. J Bone Joint Surg Am 85:1209-1214, 2003.

20. Namba Y, Kawai A, Naito N, et al: Intraarticular synovial sarcoma confirmed by SYT-SSX fusion transcript. Clin Orthop 395:221-226, 2002.

21. Rupp S, Seil R, Jochum P, Kohn D: Popliteal cysts in adults. Prevalence, associated intraarticular lesions, and results after arthroscopic treatment. Am J Sports Med 30:112-115, 2002.

22. Shabat S, Kollender Y, Merimsky O, et al: The use of surgery and yttrium 90 in the management of extensive and diffuse pigmented villonodular synovitis of large joints. Rheumatology 41:1113-1118, 2002.

23. Stacy GS, Heck RK, Peabody TD, Dixon LB: Neoplastic and tumor-like lesions detected on MR imaging of the knee in patients with suspected internal derangement. AJR Am J Roentgenol 178:595-599, 2002.

24. Stahnke M, Mangham DC, Davies AM: Calcific haemorrhagic bursitis anterior to the knee mimicking a soft tissue sarcoma: Report of two cases. Skeletal Radiol 33:363-366, 2004.

25. Uchibori M, Nishida Y, Tabata I, et al: Expression of matrix metalloproteinases and tissue inhibitors of metalloproteinases in pigmented villonodular synovitis suggests their potential role for joint destruction. J Rheumatol 31:110-119, 2004.

26. Vilanova JC, Barcelo J, Villalon M, et al: MR imaging of lipoma arborescens and the associated lesions. Skeletal Radiol 32:504-509, 2003.

27. Yamaguchi S, Yamamoto T, Matsushima S, et al: Solitary intraarticular lipoma causing sudden locking of the knee: A case report and review of the literature. Am J Sports Med 31:297-299, 2003.

28. Zvijac JE, Lau AC, Hechtman KS, et al: Arthroscopic treatment of pigmented villonodular synovitis of the knee. Arthroscopy 15:613-617, 1999.

Index

Note: Page numbers followed by f, t, and b refer to figures, tables, and boxed material, respectively.